AF335233

Focus on
MACULAR DISEASES

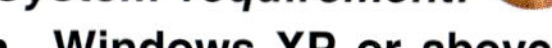

System requirement:
- **Windows XP or above**
- **Power DVD player (Software)**
- **Windows media player version 10.0 or above**
- **Quick time player version 6.5 or above**

Accompanying DVD ROM is playable only in Computer and not in DVD player.

Kindly wait for few seconds for DVD to autorun. If it does not autorun then please follow the steps:
- Click on my computer
- Click the **DVD drive labelled JAYPEE** and after opening the drive, kindly double click the file **Jaypee**

Focus on
MACULAR
DISEASES

Sandeep Saxena MS MAMS

Member, National Academy of Medical Sciences, India
Visiting Professor, UNC-Chapel Hill, Chapel Hill, USA
Fellow, Barnes Retina Institute and Anheuser-Busch Eye Institute, St. Louis, USA
Fellow, New York-Presbyterian Hospital, New York, USA

Professor
Department of Ophthalmology
King George's Medical University
Lucknow, India

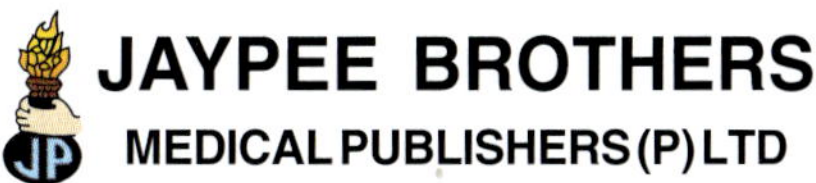

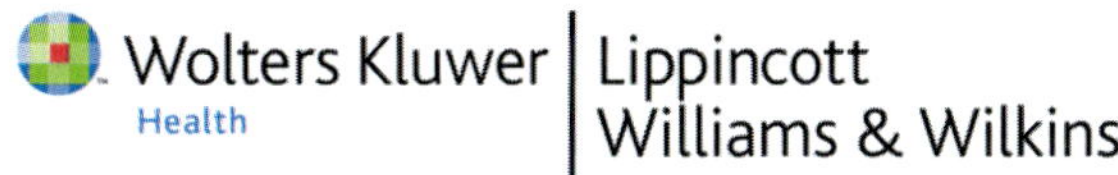

First published in India in 2007 by
Jaypee Brothers Medical Publishers (P) Ltd, New Delhi, India.
EMCA House, 23/23B Ansari Road, Daryaganj, New Delhi 110 002, India
Phones: +91-11-23272143, +91-11-23272703, +91-11-23282021, +91-11-23245672
Fax: +91-11-23276490, +91-11-23245683
e-mail: jaypee@jaypeebrothers.com, Visit our website: www.jaypeebrothers.com

First published in USA by The Lippincott Williams & Wilkins, 530 Walnut Street, Philadelphia, PA
19106, USA. Exclusively worldwide distributor except South East Asia (India, Nepal, Sri Lanka,
Bhutan, Pakistan, Bangladesh).

ISBN 978-0-7817-9129-8

To
My Parents
Dr RC Saxena and Mrs Madhu Saxena

Travis A Meredith MD, Matthew A Thomas MD, Harvey Lincoff MD,
Maurice B Landers III MD, Lawrence A Yannuzzi MD and Stanley Chang MD

for showing me the new horizons in Macula

and my family
Sangeeta, Shreeya and Aishwarya

Contributors

Levent Akduman MD
Assistant Professor
St Louis University Eye Institute
St Louis University
St Louis, USA

Shashank Bidaye MS
Retina Foundation
Ahmedabad, India

Muna Bhende MS
Senior Vitreoretinal Consultant
Sankara Nethralaya
Chennai, India

Jyotirmay Biswas MS
Director, Uveitis Department
Sankara Nethralaya
Chennai, India

Wai-Man Chan FRCP, FRCS
Consultant Ophthalmologist
Hong Kong Hospital
Hong Kong, PRC

Robert F Degenring MD
Vitreoretinal Associate
Department of Ophthalmology
Cologne Hospitals
Cologne, Germany

Satpal Garg MD
Professor
Dr RP Centre for Ophthalmic Sciences
All India Institute of Medical Sciences
New Delhi, India

Amod Gupta MS
Professor and Head
Department of Ophthalmology
Post Graduate Institute of Medical Education and Research
Chandigarh, India

Vishali Gupta MS
Associate Professor
Department of Ophthalmology
Post Graduate Institute of Medical Education and Research
Chandigarh, India

Murali M Gurran MS
Retina Foundation
Ahmedabad, India

Nancy M Holekamp MD
Barnes Retina Institute
Washington University School of Medicine
St Louis, USA

Nazimul Hussain MS
Vitreoretinal Consultant
L.V. Prasad Eye Institute
Hyderabad, India

Michael Jones MD
St Louis University Eye Institute
St Louis University
St Louis, USA

Vinay K. Khanna PhD
Scientist
Industrial Toxicology Research Center
Lucknow, India

Kiran Kumari MPhil
Electrodiagnostic Department
Sankara Nethralaya
Chennai, India

Teresa TY Lau MRCS
Clinical Fellow
Prince of Wales Hospital
Hong Kong, PRC

David TL Liu MRCS
Ophthalmology Specialist
Prince of Wales Hospital
Hong Kong, PRC

Asheesh Mehrotra MD
Childrens Hospital of Wisconsin
Milwaukee, USA

Travis A Meredith MD
Professor and Chairman
Department of Ophthalmology
University of North Carolina at Chapel Hill
Chapel Hill, USA

Carsten H Meyer MD
Assistant Professor
Department of Ophthalmology
Phillips-University
Marburg, Germany

Amit Nagpal DNB
Associate Consultant, Vitreoretinal and Oncology Services
Sankara Nethralaya
Chennai, India

Kamal Nagpal MS
Retina Foundation
Ahmedabad, India

Manish Nagpal MS, DOMS, FRCS
Retina Foundation
Ahmedabad, India

Bijoy K Nair MPhil
Electrodiagnostic Department
Sankara Nethralaya
Chennai, India

Narendra GV MS
Retina Foundation
Ahmedabad, India

Masahito Ohji MD
Professor and Chairman
Shiga University of Medical Science
Seta Tsukinowa-cho
Otsu, Japan

Aditya B. Pant PhD
Scientist
Industrial Toxicology Research Center
Lucknow, India

Priya Ravi BS
Electrodiagnostic Department
Sankara Nethralaya
Chennai, India

Parveen Sen MS
Consultant, Vitreoretinal service
Sankara Nethralaya
Chennai, India

P Mahesh Shanmugam DO, PhD, FRCS
Associate Professor
Department of Ophthalmology and Visual Sciences
The Chinese University of Hong Kong, Hong Kong Eye Hospital
Hong Kong, PRC

Sandeep Saxena MS, MAMS
Professor
Department of Ophthalmology
King George's Medical University
Lucknow, India

Osamu Sawada MD
Assistant Professor
Shiga University of Medical Science
Seta Tsukinowa-cho, Otsu, Japan

Ramandeep Singh MS
Department of Ophthalmology
Post Graduate Institute of Medical Education and Research
Chandigarh, India

Prachi Srivastava PhD
Industrial Toxicology Research Center
Lucknow, India

S Sudharshan DO
Consultant, Uveitis Department
Sankara Nethralaya
Chennai, India

Matthew A Thomas MD
Barnes Retina Institute
Washington University School of Medicine
St Louis, USA

Pradeep Venkatesh MD
Associate Professor
Dr RP Centre for Ophthalmic Sciences
All India Institute of Medical Sciences
New Delhi, India

Arun Bhargava MS
Sankara Nethralaya
Chennai, India

Arindam Chakravarti MS
Sankara Nethralaya
Chennai, India

Foreword

The world grows smaller every day. One of the benefits of this is the improving level of medical knowledge and care available to physicians and patients everywhere.

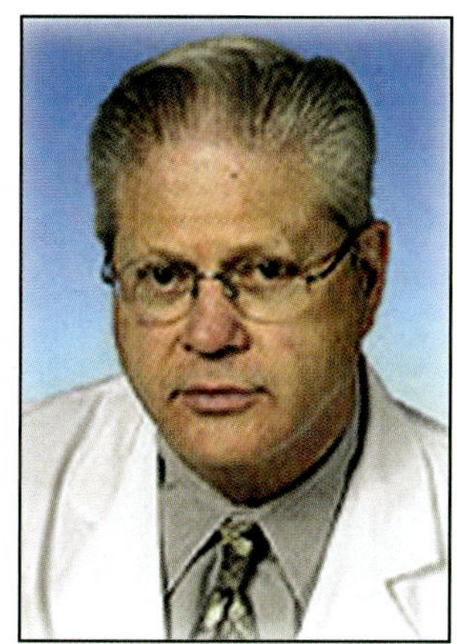

In *Focus on Macular Diseases*, Dr Saxena and a group of colleagues from around the world have produced a timely and highly informative text, further demonstrating how rapidly the information revolution is making available the expertise of the best doctors to patients in all corners of the globe.

The first five chapters of the book deal with contemporary techniques of detailed evaluation of the macula, covering the optical coherence tomography examination, microperimetry, the multifocal electroretinogram, the scanning laser ophthalmoscope and Heidelberg retina angiograph, along with fluorescein angiography and indocyanine green angiography. These chapters are extremely valuable to modern retinologists, particularly the sections on the optical coherence tomography and the multifocal electroretinogram.

The next five chapters deal with the outpatient treatment of macular diseases, and cover laser treatment for diabetic macular edema, laser treatment of other macular diseases, the use of intravitreal triamcinolone in macular diseases, photodynamic therapy treatment, and interestingly, an optimistic chapter detailing the use of transpupillary thermotherapy in cases of age-related macular degeneration with choroidal neovascularization.

Next is an excellent survey chapter on vascular endothelial growth factor, and the currently available anti-vascular endothelial growth factor drugs, and their use in treating age-related macular degeneration.

The final discussion of the medical management of age-related macular degeneration is covered in a well-written chapter on antioxidants and age-related macular degeneration.

A remarkably inclusive and exhaustively referenced chapter on surgery of the macula; written by internationally acclaimed experts, is clearly one of the highlights of the book.

The chapter on surgery for retinal vein occlusion presents an extensive review of radial optic neurotomy for central retinal vein occlusion, and sheathotomy for branch retinal vein occlusion. The authors' summary states that neither of these procedures, on their own, have been clearly proven to offer any therapeutic benefit, and that any benefit they may offer in combination with other procedures, including vitrectomy, intravenous thrombolysis with tissue plasminogen activator, etc. await the results of controlled clinical trials.

An overview of macular involvement in posterior uveitis is succinct, as one might expect in a book of this nature. The discussions of conditions affecting macular function are good.

Macular involvement in intraocular tumors is again an extensively referenced presentation on ocular oncology seen from the point of view from the retinologist examining the macula for an explanation of a patient's decreased central vision.

In summary, this is a timely, well written and exhaustively referenced book, combined with visual references (figures and surgical videos), which will be a welcome addition to the library of retinologists around the world.

Maurice B Landers III MD
Professor
Department of Ophthalmology
University of North Carolina at Chapel Hill
Chapel Hill, USA

Preface

Diagnosis and treatment of macular diseases is a continuously advancing field as new technologies are being introduced at a rapid rate. As new medications, lasers and instruments are introduced, one must learn their intricacies for applying them to the treatment of macular diseases. In turn, the adoption of new technology brings with it the need to learn new skills and develop new treatment algorithms. Advancing capabilities furthermore allows intervention for new indications.

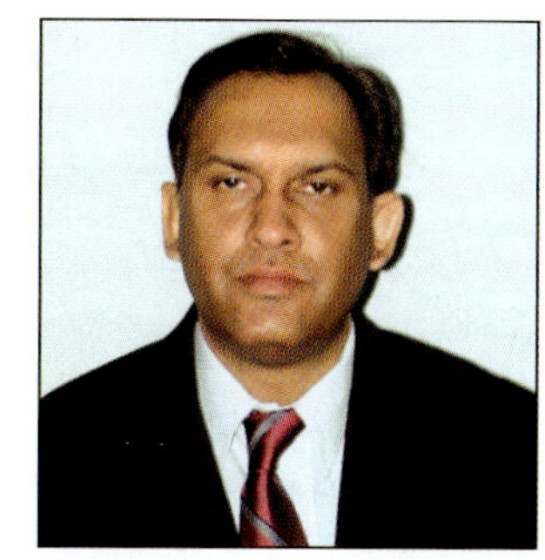

As techniques, indications, and equipment evolve, better outcomes result but may also be accompanied by new sets of complications. Coping up with these changes is vital. New technology and surgical approaches must be adapted to the specific socioeconomic conditions and disease presentations in different parts of the world.

Focus on Macular Diseases provides a comprehensive text combined with integrated visual reference, in the form of black and white and colored figures and surgical videos of treatable macular disorders. This book attempts to update the state-of-the-art diagnostic and treatment modalities in macular diseases in a lucid, authoritative and well-illustrated manner.

The value of this book lies in the quality and expertise of the text chapters and surgical video contributors.

The book is intended for the experienced ophthalmologists, postgraduates as well as those in training. This pragmatic book provides an understanding of the diagnosis and management of treatable macular diseases which are so important in the everyday practice.

Sandeep Saxena

Contents

DVD CONTENTS

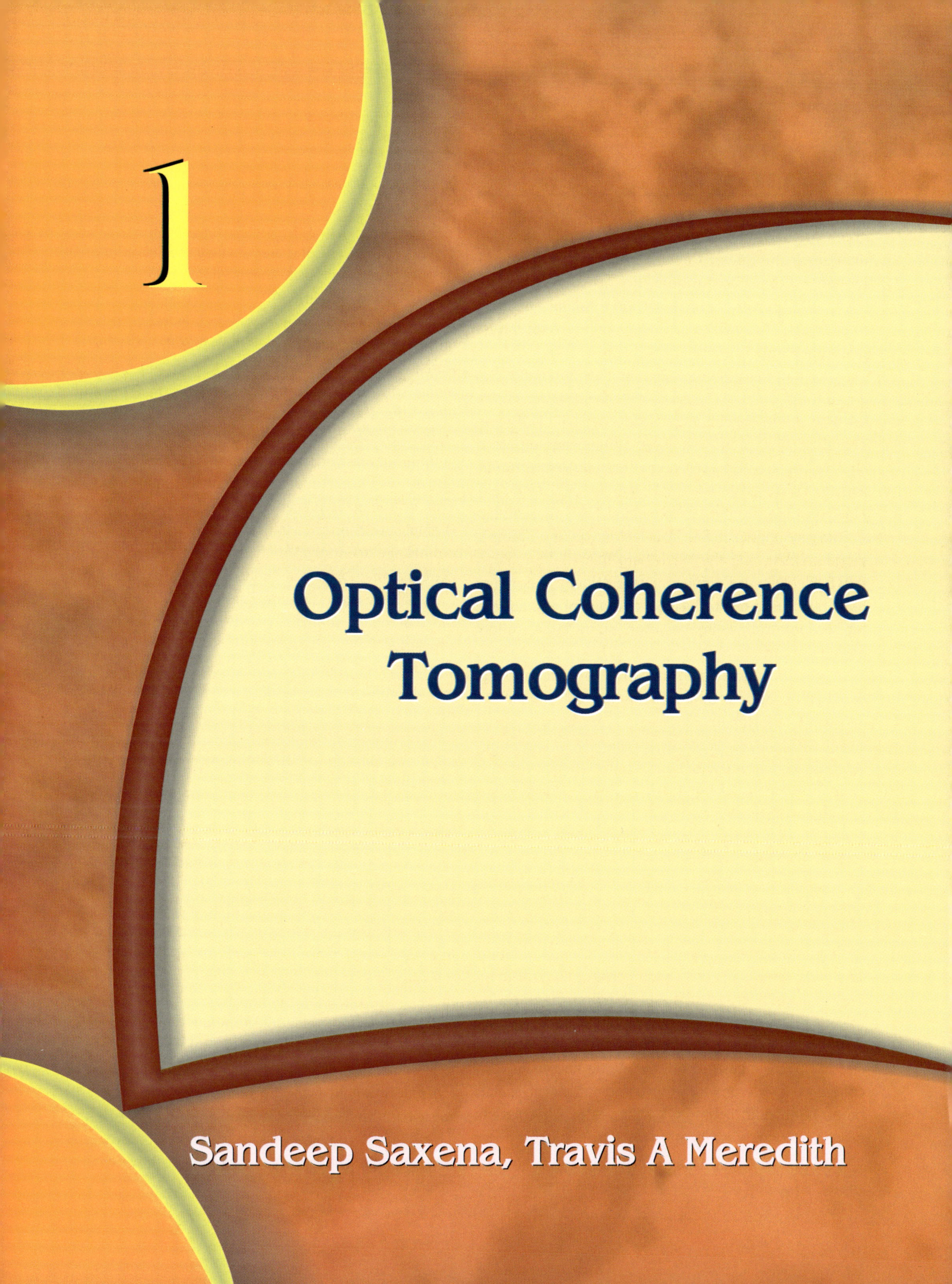

Optical Coherence Tomography

INTRODUCTION

Fundus photography, fluorescein and indocyanine green angiography, are among the frequently used imaging techniques to evaluate macular pathology. However, these techniques do not give detailed information regarding cross-sectional retinal anatomy, and do not provide quantitative retinal thickness measurements.

New emerging medical imaging technologies can improve not only the diagnosis and clinical management but also the understanding of pathogenesis of disease. Therefore, they promise to have a significant impact in clinical practice and research. Imaging instruments, including optical coherence tomography (OCT; Carl Zeiss Meditec Inc., Dublin, California, USA), the Retinal Thickness Analyzer (RTA; Talia Technology Inc., Tampa, Florida, USA), and the Heidelberg Retinal Tomograph (HRT; Heidelberg Engineering, Heidelberg, Germany) have been used to produce cross-sectional and surface topographic retinal images, and quantitative retinal thickness data.

A need has existed in medicine for a technology capable of 'optical biopsy,' imaging at or near the resolution of histopathology without excisional biopsy.[1] Advances in optics, fiberoptics, and laser technology have led to the development of a non-contact, high-resolution optical biomedical imaging technology, called Optical Coherence Tomography (OCT).[2-5] In 1990, OCT was invented at the Massachusetts Institute of Technology in Boston. In 1993, the first *in vivo* human retina images were obtained. In 1995, the first clinical retinal images were obtained.

Optical coherence tomography is a new technique for high-resolution cross sectional visualization of retinal structure.[6] Optical coherence tomography achieves 2- or 3-dimensional cross-sectional imaging of retina by measuring the echo delay and intensity of back-reflected infrared light from internal tissue structures. Using a classic optical measurement technique known as low-coherence interferometry [7-13] in combination with special broad-bandwidth light, OCT achieves high-resolution, cross-sectional visualization of tissue morphologic characteristics at depths significantly greater than the penetration depth offered by conventional bright-field and confocal microscopy.

A- and B-scan ultrasonography require physical contact with the eye and are routinely used in ophthalmic diagnosis, with a typical longitudinal resolution of 150 μm.[14,15] Imaging with OCT is analogous to ultrasound B-scan in that distance information is extracted from the time delays of reflected signals. However, the use of optical rather than acoustic waves in OCT provides a much higher (≤ 10 micron) longitudinal resolution in the retina versus the 100-micron scale for ultrasound. This is due to the fact that that the speed of light is nearly a million times faster than the speed of sound. Use of optical waves also allows a non-contact and noninvasive measurement. This technique is presently being used increasingly to evaluate and manage a variety of retinal diseases. Optical coherence tomography has been used to identify epiretinal membranes and macular holes, to differentiate macular holes from simulating lesions, to identify lamellar macular holes, macular cysts, vitreomacular traction, subretinal fluid, pigment epithelial detachment, and choroidal neovascularization. It can be used to identify and quantify macular edema, and to measure retinal thickness changes in response to therapy.[16] The ability to non-excisionally evaluate tissue can have a significant impact on the diagnosis and management of a wide range of diseases.[17]

BASIC PRINCIPLE

Optical coherence tomography is based on the principle of Michelson interferometry.[7-13] Low-coherence infrared light coupled to a fiberoptic travels to a beam-splitter and is directed through the ocular media to the retina and to a reference mirror, respectively. Light passing through the eye is reflected by structures in different retinal tissue layers. The distance between the beam-splitter and reference mirror is continuously varied. When the distance between the light source and retinal tissue is equal to the distance between the light source and reference mirror, the reflected light from the retinal tissue and reference mirror interacts to produce an interference pattern. The interference pattern is detected and then processed into a signal. The signal is analogous to that obtained by A-scan ultrasonography using light as a source rather than sound. A two-dimensional image is built as the light source is moved across the retina. The image is in the form of a series of stacked and aligned A-scans, which produces a two-dimensional cross-sectional retinal image that resembles that of a histology section. This imaging method thus can be considered a form of *in vivo* histology. Digital processing aligns the A-scans to correct for eye motion. Digital smoothing techniques are used to further improve the signal-to-noise ratio.[18]

IMAGE DISPLAY

Stratus OCT (OCT-3; Carl Zeiss Meditec Inc., Dublin, California, USA) is an advanced imaging device. It can be used in the absence of dilation in many individuals, and usually requires a 3 mm pupil for adequate visualization. The imaging lens is positioned 1 cm from the eye to be examined and adjusted independently until the retina is in focus. An infrared-sensitive charge-coupled device videocamera documents the position of the scanning beam on the retina.

The OCT image can be displayed on a gray scale where more highly reflected light is brighter than less highly reflected light. Alternatively, it can be displayed in color whereby different colors correspond to different degrees of reflectivity. On the currently commercially available OCT scanners, highly reflective structures are shown with bright colors (red and white), whereas those with low reflectivity are represented by darker colors (black and blue). Those with intermediate reflectivity appear green.

IMAGE RESOLUTION

Optical coherence tomographic image resolution depends on several factors. Resolution can be considered in the axial (Z axis) or transverse (X-Y) planes.

Axial resolution depends on the wavelength and bandwidth of the incident light. Shorter wavelength light, in the 800 nm range, is not absorbed as much as longer wavelength light by high water content structures such as the cornea and vitreous. This property allows adequate light penetration to the retina, and excellent axial resolution. Hence, light with a broader spectral bandwidth enhances axial resolution by producing a shorter coherence light beam. Current commercial scanners employ a low coherence super luminescent diode source (820 nm). The presently available model Stratus OCT (OCT-3) has a theoretical axial resolution ≤10 microns.

VOLUMETRIC OPTICAL COHERENCE TOMOGRAPHY

Jaffe and Caprioli[18] have coined the term "volumetric optical coherence tomography (VOCT)" to quantify retinal thickness throughout the macula. To obtain such tomogram using commercially available software on the Stratus OCT, the retinal thickness map (RTM) scan mode and analysis function, or the fast retinal thickness map (FRTM) scan mode and analysis function, is used. With these scan modes, six radial scans are obtained.

In the RTM mode, each of the six individual scans is manually acquired sequentially by the operator, while, in the FRTM mode, each of the sequential scans is obtained automatically by the OCT software. Each of the six scans is oriented radially, 30 degrees from one another, and intersect at the foveal center. Each radial scan (typically obtained at a scan length of approximately 6 mm) produces a cross-sectional image. The OCT software locates the inner retina at the vitreoretinal interface and the outer retina at the retinal pigment epithelial-photoreceptor outer segment interface, based on differences in the image reflectance patterns. The software then places a line on the inner retina and another on the retinal pigment epithelium. A retinal thickness measurement is determined as the distance between these lines at each measurement point along the scan's X-axis. From these scans, a surface map reconstruction is created. The surface map is displayed as a false color image whereby retinal thickness at each point is represented by a different color. Bright colors (for example, red and white) represent thick regions, and dark colors (for example, blue and black) represent thin areas. Intermediate thickness regions are displayed as green and yellow. Because the data point density is greater centrally than peripherally, interpolated thickness measurements of regions further from the fovea are determined from fewer measurements, and may be less accurate, than those in central regions.[18]

Typical RTM or FRTM scan and analysis OCT printout yields a lot of data. These include:

- Cross-sectional images for each of the six radial scans
- Measurement of central foveal thickness (calculated as the mean and standard deviation of the retinal thickness at the intersection of the six radial scans)
- Measurement of retinal thickness in nine separate regions in the macula
- Surface map reconstruction display
- Measurement of retinal volume contained under the area represented by the surface reconstruction.

The central foveal thickness measurement is particularly useful, as it includes the thickness measurement variability among the six radial scans. Typically, this variability is less than 5%. Volumetric scanning is especially useful to quantify changes in retinal thickness. Thickness measurements determined by this technique are reproducible.[19]

STRATUS OCT

Stratus OCT is an interferometer that resolves retinal structures by measuring the echo delay time of light (broad bandwidth near-infrared light beam; 820 nm) that is reflected and backscattered from different microstructural features in the retina. The instrument electronically detects, collects, processes and stores the echo delay patterns from the retina. With each scan pass, the instrument captures from 128 to 768 longitudinal (axial) range samples, i.e. A-scans. Each A-scan consists of 1024 data points over 2 mm of depth. Thus the instrument integrates from 131,072 to 786,432 data points to construct a cross-sectional image (tomogram) of retinal anatomy. It displays the tomograms in realtime using a false color scale that represents the degree of light backscattering from tissues at different depths in the retina. The system stores the scans, which can be selected for later analysis.

The instrument delineates intraretinal, cross-sectional anatomy with axial resolution of ≤10 microns and transverse resolution of 20 microns. Its software package includes 19 scan acquisition protocols and 18 analysis protocols. The videocamera enables to view the patient's fundus and to store video and scan images together. The data management system enables storage of patient histories, for monitoring patients over time. Images and data can be archived on rewritable DVD-RAM discs. The inkjet printer generates color hard copy.

ADVANTAGES OF OPTICAL COHERENCE TOMOGRAPHY

There are several advantages of OCT as a diagnostic imaging technique:
1. It is non-contact unlike ultrasound and noninvasive, unlike fluorescein angiography.
2. Patients, especially children, easily tolerate it.
3. It is extremely helpful in providing quantitative information regarding macular thickness changes over time.
4. It is a valuable teaching tool for the physicians as well as patients.

DISADVANTAGES OF OPTICAL COHERENCE TOMOGRAPHY

Although OCT is an extremely valuable technique, there are limitations and potential pitfalls to its use:
1. Optical coherence tomographic images are degraded in the presence of media opacity, for example dense cataract.
2. Scan quality is dependent on the skill of OCT operator.
3. Optical coherence tomographic scanning may not be possible with uncooperative patients.
4. Measurements of foveal thickness may be inaccurate if the scan is not centered over the fovea.

COMPARISON OF OPTICAL COHERENCE TOMOGRAPHY WITH STANDARD TECHNIQUES

Stereofundus-photographs and fluorescein angiography are the other methods of evaluating macular thickness. Retinal thickening determined by stereofundus photography correlates well with that measured by OCT. Macular hyperfluorescence seen on fluorescein angiography correlates well with increased retinal thickness measured by OCT. However, occasionally, eyes with macular hyperfluorescence do not appear thickened by OCT, and, conversely, some eyes without macular hyperfluorescence look thickened by OCT. Fundus photography, fluorescein angiography, and OCT, together, provide complementary information regarding macular disorders.

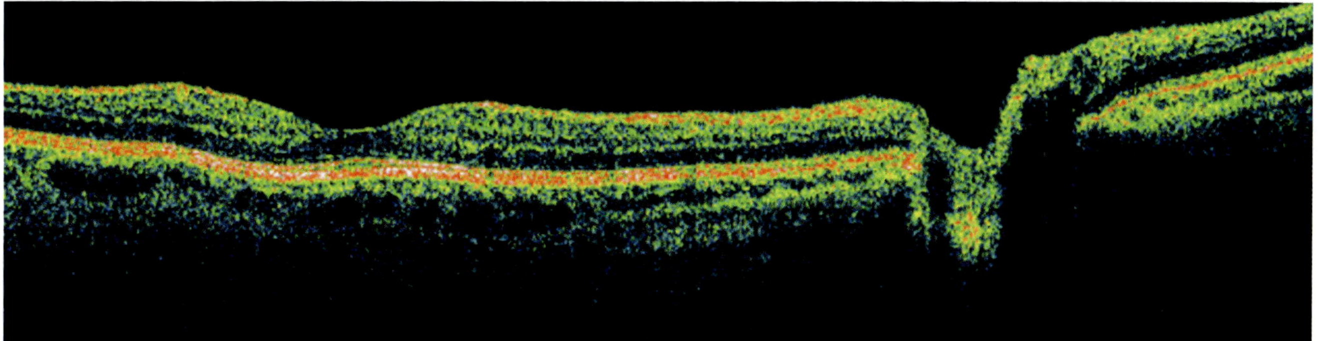

FIGURE 1.1: Collage photograph of a normal OCT scan showing the macula and the optic nerve.

Fundus photography, unlike OCT, does not yield objective quantitative measurements of retinal thickening, and neither fundus photography nor fluorescein angiography gives information about cross-sectional retinal morphology or high-magnification surface topographic images. However, fluorescein angiography can provide information about the origin of macular fluid leakage, and retinal vascular abnormalities, while fundus photography may demonstrate subtle macular lesions not seen by OCT or clinical examination.

COMPARISON OF OPTICAL COHERENCE TOMOGRAPHY WITH COMMERCIALLY AVAILABLE INSTRUMENTS

The HRT and RTA are the other commercially available instruments, in addition to OCT, to measure retinal thickness and to evaluate retinal morphology. All can effectively measure retinal thickness in normal eyes, and in eyes with macular edema. There is a high degree of correlation between retinal thickness determined by OCT and that measured by RTA.[20-23] For patients with very early diabetic retinopathy without clinically significant macular edema, RTA may be more sensitive than OCT to detect macular thickening. However, RTA may produce a larger number of falsely elevated retinal thickness measurements, and produces retinal images less effectively than OCT in eyes with media opacity.[21,22,24] The HRT may be more effective than OCT and RTA to image the outer retina in the presence of retinal hemorrhage and hard exudates.[25] The HRT can also demonstrate surface topology. However, images are acquired relatively slowly.

NORMAL OCT SCAN

On a normal 10 mm horizontal scan passing through the fovea, one can clearly demarcate two major landmarks; namely, the optic disk and fovea (Figure 1.1).

The optic disk is seen towards the right of the tomogram and can be easily identified by its contour. The central depression represents the optic head cup and the stalk continuing behind is the anterior part of optic nerve. The fovea is seen towards the left of the tomogram and can be easily identified by characteristic thinning of the retinal layers. The vitreous anterior to the retina is non-reflective and is seen as a dark space. The interface between the non-reflective vitreous and backscattering retinal layers is the vitreoretinal interface.

Retinal morphology and macular OCT imaging correlate well, with alignment of areas of high and low reflectivity to specific retinal and choroidal elements (Figure 1.2). Resolution of retinal structures by OCT depends on the contrast in relative reflectivity of

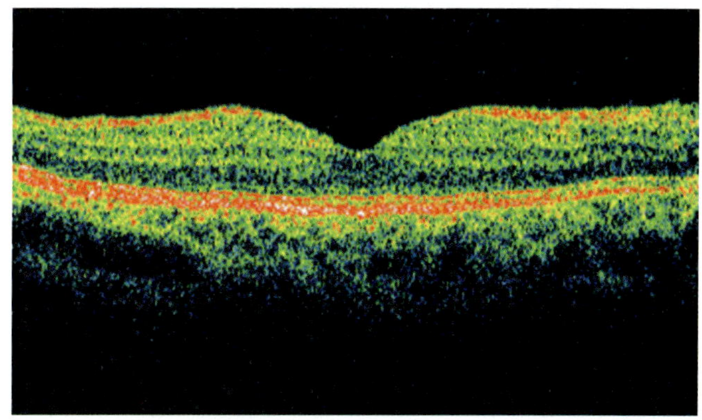

FIGURE 1.2: Normal macula on an OCT scan.

adjacent structures. The nerve fiber layer and ganglion cell layers are reflective, and are seen as bright colors on the false color map. The nuclear layers appear hyporeflective, while interconnecting plexiform layers and axonal layers are relatively hyper-reflective. Typically, the photoreceptor outer segments appear slightly hyporeflective compared with the other retinal layers. The retinal pigment epithelium/choriocapillaris complex is seen as a hyper-reflective band. The retinal blood vessels within the neurosensory retina show backscatter and also cast a shadow behind. The choroid is also highly reflective, although it is frequently not well resolved because of light reflection by the overlying retinal pigment epithelium.

OPTICAL COHERENCE TOMOGRAPHY INTERPRETATION

An OCT image can have two modes of interpretation: objective and subjective. For an accurate interpretation, one needs to combine both these modalities.

The purpose of OCT is to detect abnormalities in the retina, in terms of thickness, morphology, and reflectivity. OCT reading must be done in two stages (Table 1.1):

    I. Qualitative and quantitative analysis.
    II. Deduction and synthesis.

Table 1.1: OCT interpretation

I.   **Qualitative analysis**
Morphological Study
- Morphological variations: overall retinal structural changes, changes in retinal outline, intraretinal structural changes and morphological changes in the posterior layers
- Anomalous structures: Preretinal, epiretinal, intraretinal and subretinal
- Reflectivity study: Hyper-reflectivity, hyporeflectivity, and shadow areas

II. **Quantitative analysis**
- Thickness, volumetry and surface mapping
- Deductive and synthetic study is performed comparing all the analytical data, the results of the clinical examination and all the other available data
- The OCT software offers the protocols for both qualitative as well as quantitative estimation.

QUALITATIVE ANALYSIS

Morphological Study

Deformation of Retina

a. Concavity: In cases of high myopia and posterior staphyloma in myopia, OCT reveals the presence of pronounced concavity, which can become less evident if the scan is processed using the alignment function.

b. Convexity: Convexity is often observed in cup-shaped detachment of the retinal pigment epithelium and subretinal cysts.

Deformation of Retinal Profile

a. Disappearance of the foveal depression: This is a sign of clinically significant macular edema.

b. Epiretinal membrane: It may be separated from the retina, in contact with it, or adhered to it and may cause folds of retinal surface.

c. Macular pseudo-holes and lamellar holes.

d. Macular hole: The OCT helps in identifying and classifying macular holes, as well as determining their diameter and the extent of detachment.

Intraretinal Structural Changes

a. Pseudoholes.

b. Cysts due to cystoid macular edema.

c. Cotton-wool spots consist of superficial hyper-reflective retinal nodules, which are in contact with superficial retinal layers in the nerve fiber layer. They are located at the margins of ischemic lesions of the nerve fibers.

d. Hard exudates occur at the margin of an edematous area and normal retina. They are hyper-reflective in an OCT scan.

Posterior Morphological Changes

a. Retinal pigment epithelial detachments deform the posterior limit of retina on OCT scan, forming a steep angle with the choriocapillaris.

b. Serous retinal detachment of the retina protrude less, and form shallow angles with the retinal pigment epithelium.

c. Drusens produce irregularities and wavy undulations of the pigment epithelium and choriocapillaris.

d. Choroidal neovascular membrane in young or myopic patients are usually visualized as nodular, rounded fusiform structure located in front of the retinal pigment epithelium. This is also true in cases of early neovascular age-related macular degeneration. They may be associated with edema or serous retinal detachment. When choroidal neovascular membranes have had several weeks or months to develop they are much more difficult to detect and may appear as thickening of the retinal pigment epithelium. Occult choroidal neovascular membranes are difficult to identify.

Reflectivity Study

When pathology is present, reflectivity may be increased or decreased, or a shadow zone may be observed on an OCT scan. Vertical structures, such as photoreceptors, are less reflective than horizontal structures, such as nerve fibers.

High Reflectivity
- Pigment accumulation
- Hypertrophy of retinal pigment epithelium
- Nevus
- Scar
- Neovascularization
- Hard exudates
- Nerve fiber (normal)
- Retinal pigment epithelium-choriocapillaris complex (normal)

Medium Reflectivity
- Plexiform layer (normal)

Low Reflectivity
- Retinal edema
- Cystoid edema
- Nuclear layer (normal)
- Photoreceptors (normal)
- Cavities/cysts
- Pigment epithelial detachment
- Serous retinal detachment

Shadow Areas

An area of dense, hyper-reflective tissue produces a screen that may be complete or incomplete, thereby creating a shadow area on OCT scan that conceals the elements lying behind it.

Anterior shadow and screen effects
- Hemorrhage
- Exudates
- Retinal vessel (normal)
- Posterior shadow and screen effects
- Retinal scars
- Pigment epithelial hypertrophy/hyperplasia
- Pigment accumulation
- Choroidal nevi

QUANTITATIVE ANALYSIS

Retinal Thickness/Volume

This analysis protocol obtains two circular maps for each eye that depict thickness and volume of retina. It can be displayed either as retinal thickness or retinal volume. The output display includes all the elements of the retinal thickness/volume analysis, with a slightly different arrangement to accommodate the table. The output display has the same layout for both thickness and volume analysis. The upper map always presents retinal thickness using a color code. The color scale appears to the right. The lower map shows either average retinal thickness (in microns) or average volume (in mm^3) in each area. A key of the map circle diameters appears at right below the color scale. The default diameters are 1, 3 and 6 mm. On the lower right, numeric information for each eye includes: Foveal thickness which represents the calculation of average thickness in microns +/- the standard deviation for the center point, where all the scans intersect; and total macular volume of the retinal map area in mm^3.

Mean foveal thickness refers to the average of retinal thickness values in the central 1000 microns central disk, and central foveal thickness refers to the average of 6 values of retinal thickness at the intersection of the six radial scans.

Retinal Thickness/Volume Tabular

This analysis protocol gives the same information as above. It obtains not only all the output of the Retinal thickness/volume analysis, but also a data table that includes thickness and volume quadrant averages, ratios and differences among the quadrants and between the eyes.

Retinal Thickness/Volume Change

This analysis protocol helps assess changes in retinal thickness or volume between examinations. The default output displays thickness change between examinations.

The output has the same layout for both thickness and volume change analysis. The upper map always presents retinal thickness change using a color code. The color scale appears to the right. The lower map shows the change in either average retinal thickness (in microns) or average volume (in mm^3).

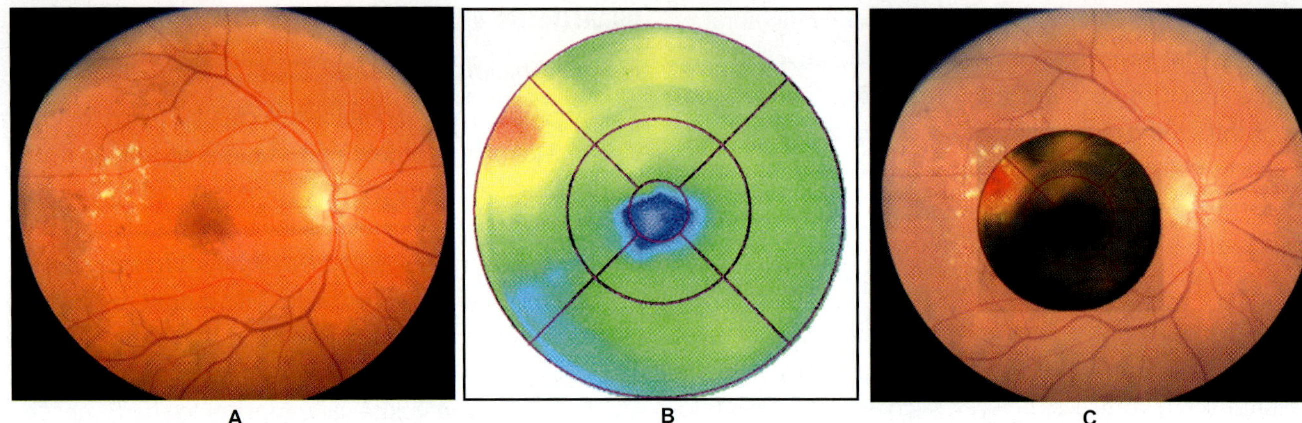

A   B   C

FIGURES 1.3 A to C: Macular map thickness of the OCT scan, depicting macular thickness, can be overlaid on a color fundus photograph to correlate topographically, the macular thickness corresponding to that underlying area.

OPTICAL COHERENCE TOMOGRAPHY-ASSISTED PATIENT EVALUATION

FUNDUS PHOTOGRAPH-OCT OVERLAY

Circular map of the OCT scan, depicting macular thickness, can be overlaid on a color fundus photograph. This helps correlate topographically, the macular thickness corresponding to that underlying area (Figures 1.3A to C).

SIX-UP PHOTOGRAPH DISPLAY

In the office, 6-up display of OCT scan (macular thickness) and color fundus photographs of the last visit and the present visit helps in assessment of the current status of the macula (Figure 1.4). It is a noninvasive, quick and useful method of patient evaluation.

DIABETIC MACULAR EDEMA

The quantitative assessment of macular edema was one of the first uses of OCT. Optical coherence tomography is being widely used to detect and monitor diabetic macular edema, using the scan profile and macular mapping.[26]

SCAN PROFILE

The OCT scan profile allows the evaluation of intraretinal changes of:

a. The shape of the inner boundary of the thickened macula, and

b. The presence of possible subretinal detachment or incomplete vitreomacular separation.

These findings are often missed on clinical examination. The scan profile mode of OCT allows accurate definition of the different characteristics of diabetic macular edema, such as diffuse swelling, cystoid cavities, and hard exudates. [26]

Intraretinal Changes

Diffuse Swelling
Diffuse swelling appears as a thickening of the retina without definite cystic spaces. The outer plexiform layer and outer nuclear layer are often more prone to thickening and hyporeflectivity (Figures 1.5A to G). [27]

Cystoid Cavities
Cystoid cavities are hyporeflective spaces of various sizes, mainly located in the outer retina (Henle fiber and outer plexiform layers), and sometimes in the inner plexiform layer. In advanced stages of diabetic macular edema, one or several large central cysts are responsible for significant thickening of the foveola. These hyporeflective spaces, which, in bidirectional scans look like individual "cysts", appear as if they were interconnected in a three-dimensional representation (Figures 1.6A to F).[28]

Foveolar Detachment
In some cases, diabetic macular edema is combined with a foveolar detachment which is not detected or even suspected on biomicroscopy. In such cases, the macula

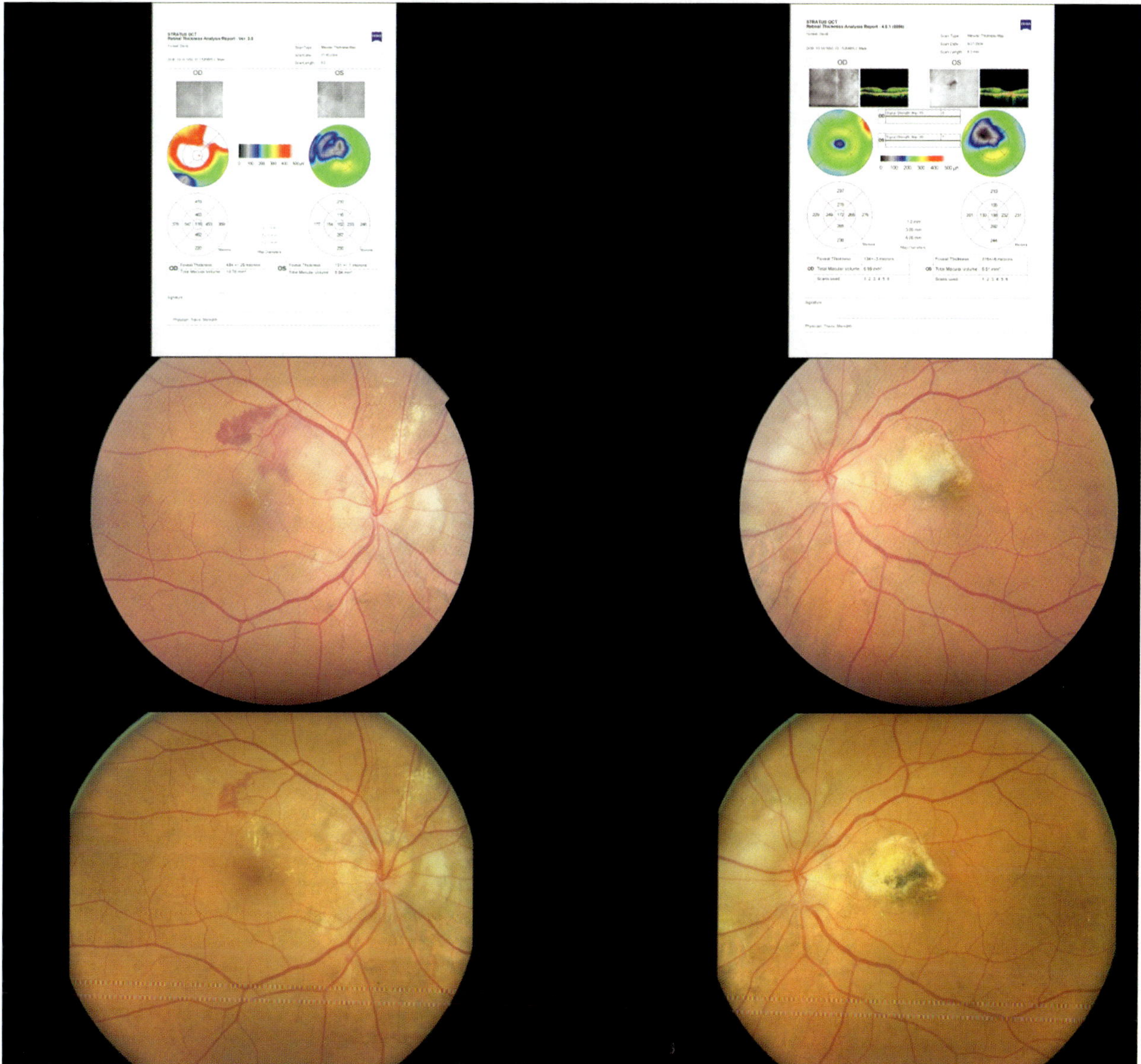

FIGURE 1.4: Six-up display of OCT scan (macular thickness) and color fundus photographs of the last visit and the present visit helps in assessment of the current status of the macula.

usually thickens significantly and contains prominent cystoid cavities (Figures 1.7A to G). Extrafoveal focal edema may also result in the migration of subretinal fluid to the subretinal space, despite the absence of major foveal cystic changes or thickening. In that case the foveal detachment is not usually due to any vitreoretinal traction. [29-31] Foveolar detachment has been observed in 15% of eyes with diabetic macular edema. [30] However, in a series of 78 eyes with macular edema examined by OCT,

the presence of foveal elevation did not correlate with poorer visual acuity, compared to other cases with the same macular thickening. [32]

Hard Exudates

Hard exudates appear as hyper-reflective intraretinal deposits, mostly located in the outer plexiform layer of the retina. They mask the reflectivity of the underlying tissue. [33] They may accumulate in the fovea, resulting in

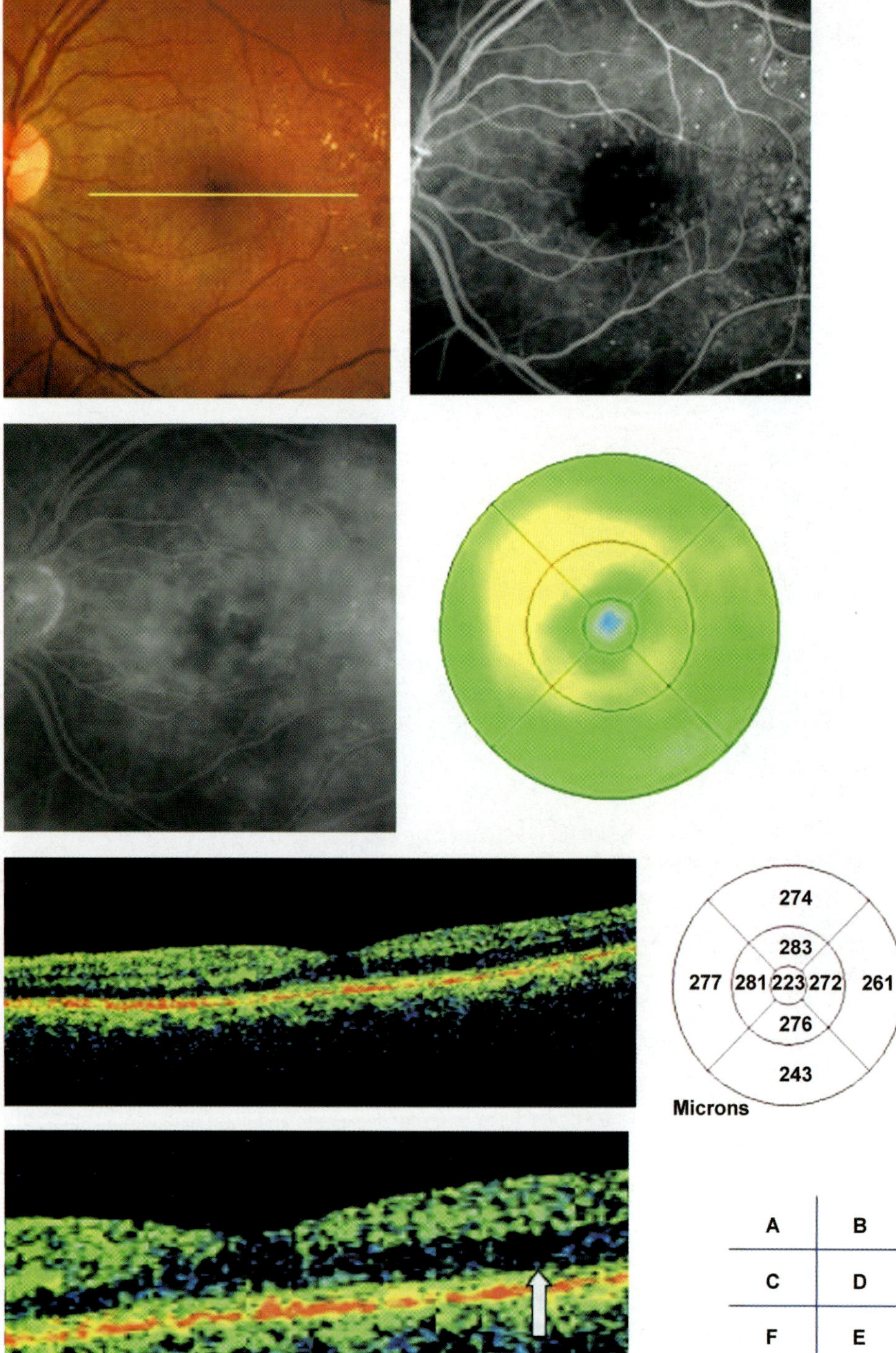

FIGURES 1.5A to G: Non-cystoid diffuse macular edema in moderate non-proliferative diabetic retinopathy. (A) Color fundus photograph showing microaneurysms, punctate hemorrhages and a few scattered hard exudates. (B) Fluorescein Angiography, early phase. Note the numerous microaneurysms and minimal enlargement of the foveal avascular zone. (C) Fluorescein angiography, late phase. Diffuse leakage is visible. (D and E) Retinal thickness map; the color code indicates moderate diffuse macular thickening. Mean thickness values are at the upper limit of normal. (F) Horizontal 6 mm linear scan. The macular profile seems normal, except for the foveal depression, which is shallower than usual, indicating a diffuse swelling of the macula. (G) Detail. Hyporeflective space in the outer nuclear layer (arrow), indicating accumulation of intraretinal fluid. The visual acuity of this eye is 20/20 (Prof Alain Gaudric MD, France).

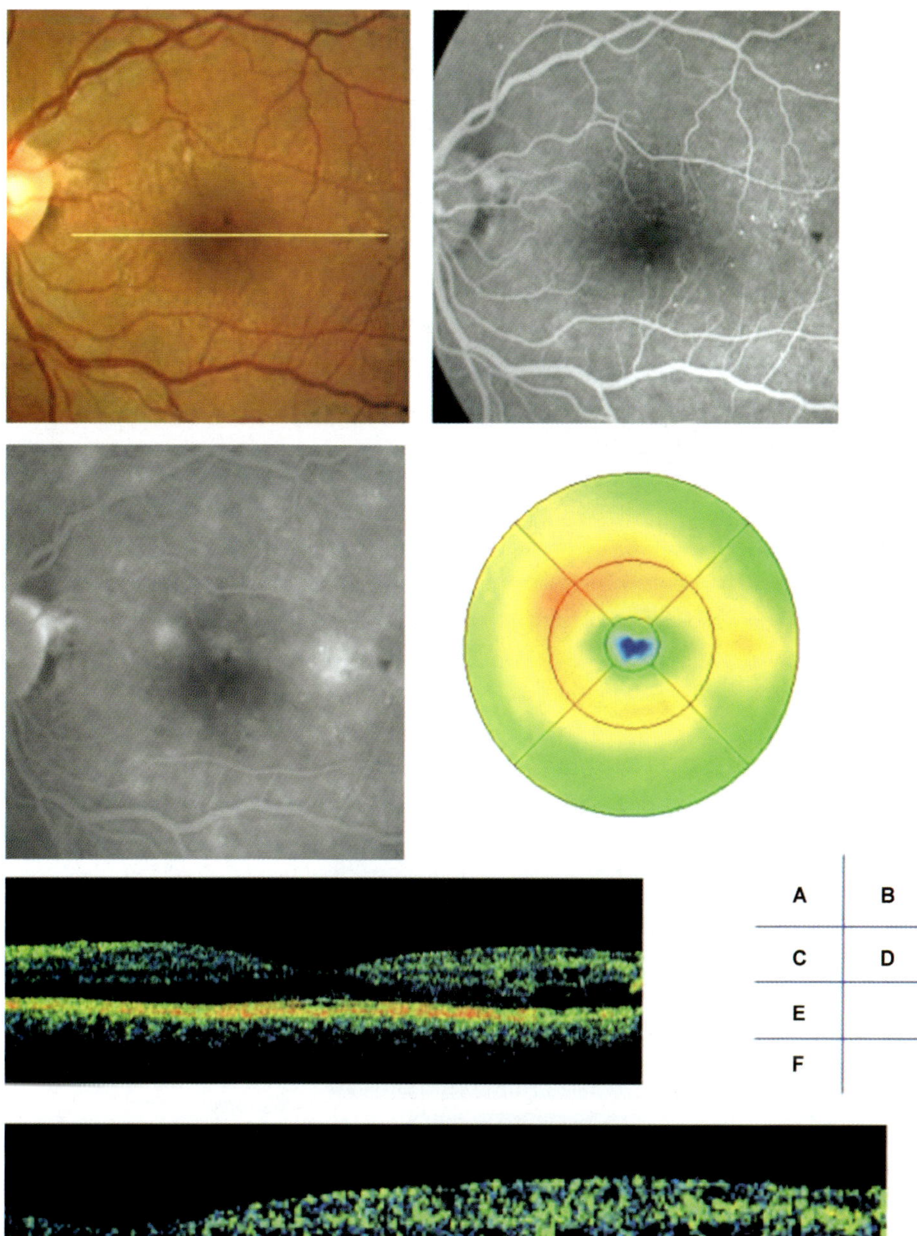

FIGURES 1.6A to F: Non-cystoid macular edema in moderate non-proliferative diabetic retinopathy. (A) Color fundus photograph showing an irregular retinal reflex. Punctate hemorrhages and minimal hard exudates are visible. (B) Fluorescein angiography, early phase showing numerous microaneurysms and a small area of capillary closure, temporal to the macula. (C) Fluorescein angiography, late phase. Note the diffuse leakage in the macular area. (D) Retinal thickness maps; despite diffuse perimacular thickening, the foveal center has remained almost normal (dark blue). (E) Horizontal 6 mm scan. The foveal pit contour is normal. The micro cystic changes temporal to the macula correspond to the area of focal leakage. (F) Detail: note the large cystic spaces in the outer nuclear layer (ONL). Smaller cysts are also present in inner retinal layers. The visual acuity of this eye is 20/32 (Prof Alain Gaudric MD, France).

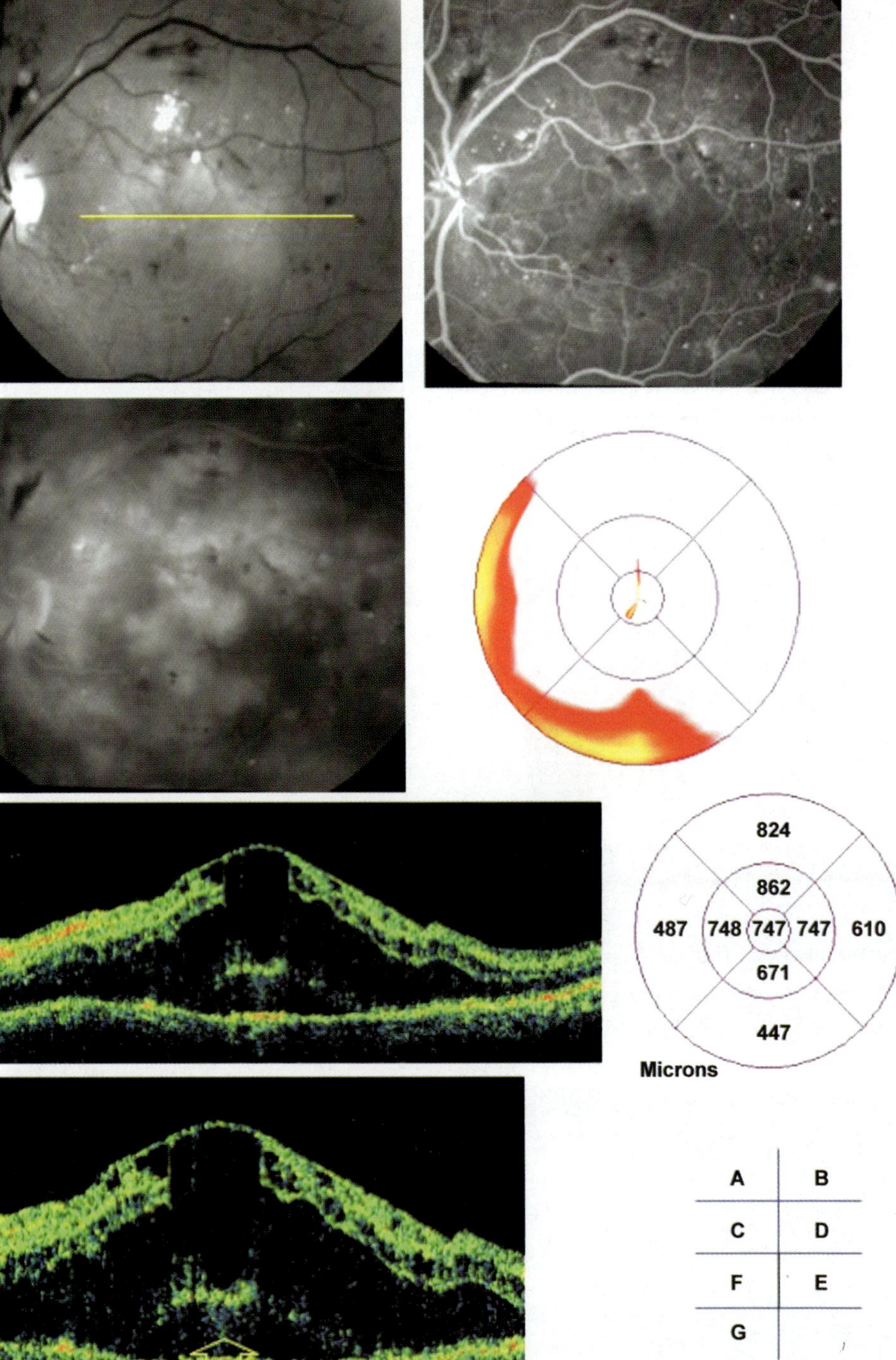

FIGURES 1.7A to G: Severe cystoid macular edema in mild proliferative diabetic retinopathy. (A) Red-free photograph of the posterior pole showing intraretinal hemorrhages and hard exudates. (B) Fluorescein angiography, early phase; note the areas of capillary non-perfusion, intraretinal microvascular anomalies, and early preretinal new vessels. (C) Fluorescein angiography, late phase disclosing the severe cystoid macular edema. (D and E) Retinal thickness maps; color map shows severe macular thickening. Central average thickness has increased to 747 µm. (F) Horizontal 6 mm scan ; a large central foveal cyst surrounded by smaller ones has resulted in significant macular thickening. (G) Detail; note that the intraretinal cystic spaces have mainly developed in the outer retinal layers. A small foveolar detachment is present (large arrow). The visual acuity of this eye is 20/100 (Prof Alain Gaudric MD, France).

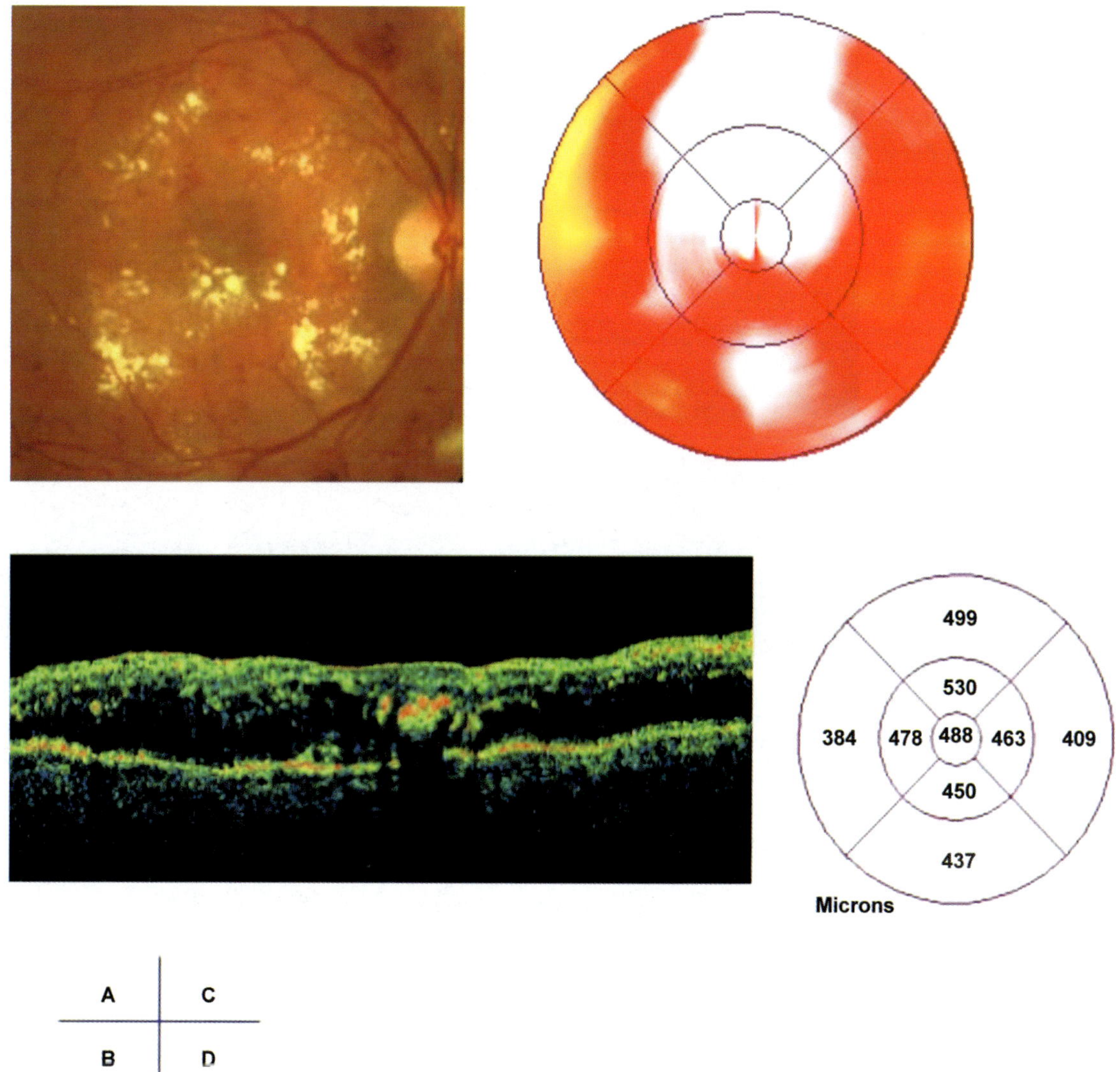

FIGURES 1.8A to D: Severe macular edema with hard exudates in nonproliferative diabetic retinopathy. (A) Color fundus photograph showing several rings of hard lipid exudates, which join in the fovea; (B) Horizontal 6 mm scan showing diffuse swelling and thickening of the macula, and the accumulation of hard exudates in the outer part of the fovea. (C and D) Retinal thickness maps showing that retinal thickening is maximal in the circinate hard exudates. Foveal thickness is 488 µm (Prof Alain Gaudric MD, France).

macular thickening (Figures 1.8A to D). However, in other cases, the foveal thickness is normal or nearly normal although the exudates surrounding the focal edema accumulate in the fovea. Such a situation occurs as the exudates deposit occurs at the limit of the area of fluid reabsorption. In such cases, OCT helps to distinguish between resorption exudates and exudates surrounding an active focus of edema.

Centrofoveal exudates accumulate in the inner foveola at the border of an area of retinal thickening. Visual acuity may be only moderately impaired in such cases (Figures 1.9A to F). Subfoveal plaques of exudates form a subfoveal deposit. They are associated with atrophy of the macular tissue, which explains the poor vision of the eyes affected (Figures 1.10A to C). [26]

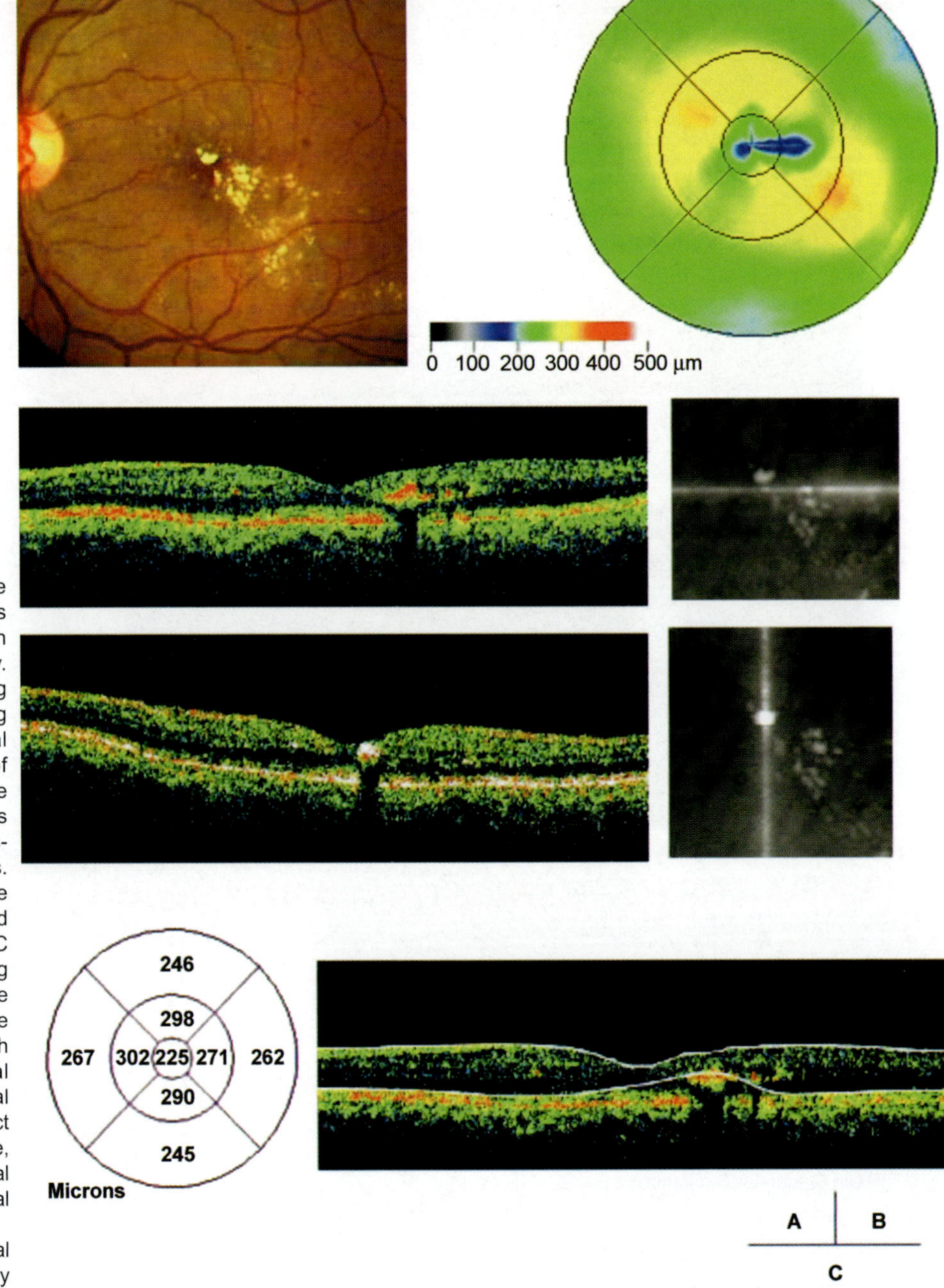

FIGURES 1.9A to F: Apparently severe macular edema. Hard exudates involving the center of the macula in non-proliferative diabetic retinopathy. (A) Color fundus photograph showing temporoinferior hard exudates involving the foveal center. (B and E) Retinal macular map showing two areas of moderate focal retinal thickening: the superonasal and inferotemporal areas of the macula. The latter area corresponds to the circinate hard exudates. The color code tends to show that the thickness of the foveal center and temporal parafoveal zone is normal. (C and D) Horizontal retinal scan showing hard intraretinal exudates on the temporal edge of the macula. The vertical scan passes exactly through hard exudates involving the foveal center. (F) Analysis of the horizontal scan of the mapping shows an artifact due to the presence of a hard exudate, which explains the misleadingly normal appearance of the temporal parafoveal area.

Despite the presence of a central intraretinal hard exudate, and probably because the fovea has in fact moderately thickened, visual acuity is 20/25. The visual prognosis should be good after focal laser photocoagulation (Prof Alain Gaudric MD, France).

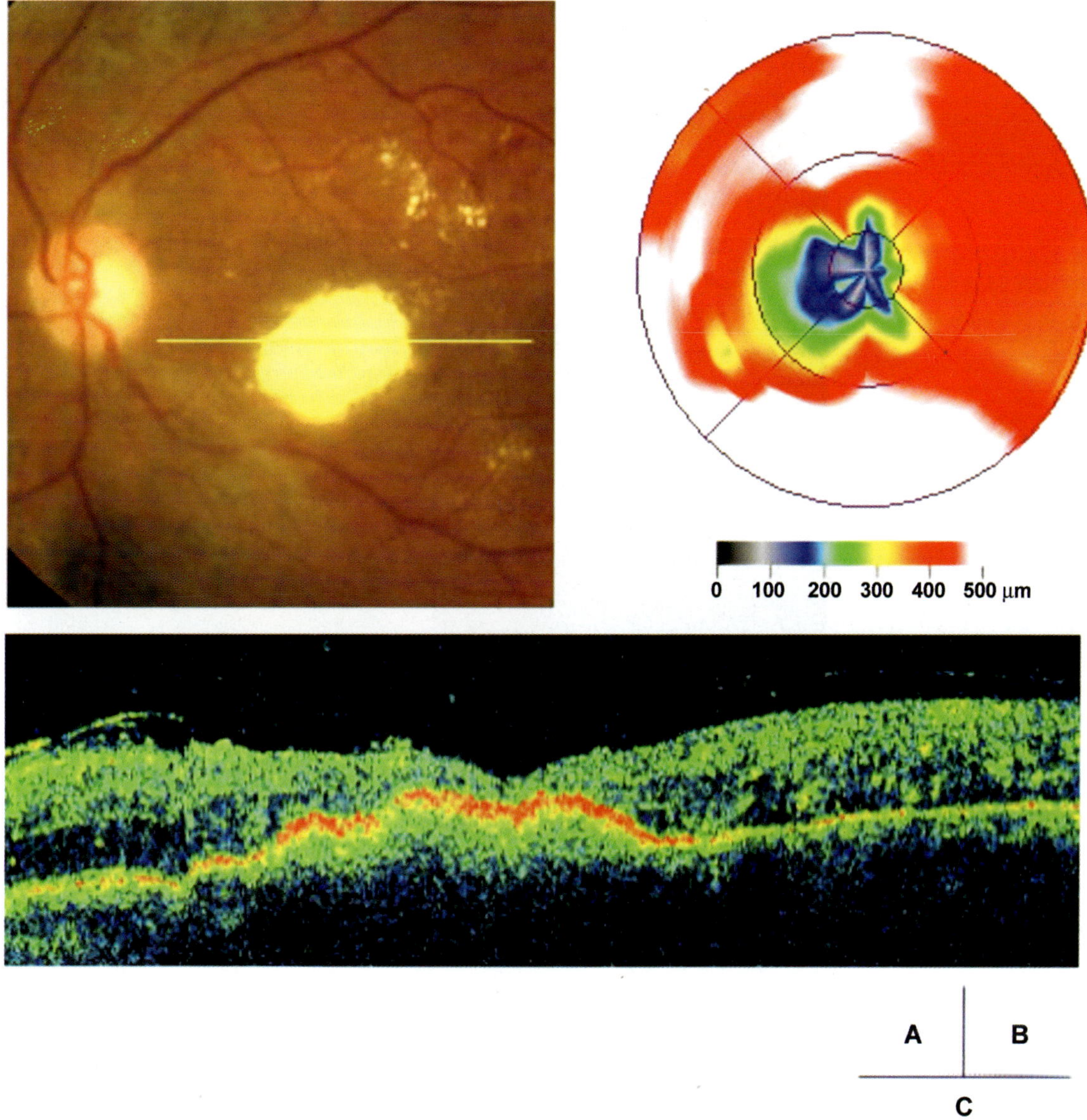

FIGURES 1.10A to C: Severe macular edema with a subfoveal plaque of lipid exudates in non-proliferative diabetic retinopathy. (A) Color photograph showing a compact yellow subfoveal plaque of hard lipid exudates. (B) Retinal macular map showing diffuse retinal thickening, except at the fovea, which seems atrophic, despite an artifactual pattern. (C) Horizontal retinal scans showing the hyper-reflectivity and thickness of subfoveal hard exudates. The underlying retinal tissue is indeed atrophic (Prof Alain Gaudric MD, France).

Inner Retinal Boundary

In OCT scans passing through the macular center, the shape of the inner retinal boundary indicates the severity of central macular edema. The earliest sign of foveolar edema on OCT scans is the flattening of the foveal pit (Figures 1.11A to G).

When macular edema is definitely present, the inner retinal boundary tends to be dome-shaped (Figures 1.12A to F). A dome-shaped profile is more frequently observed when the posterior hyaloid remains attached to the macular center. However, this convex profile may also exist if the posterior hyaloid is detached. In rare cases, the macular center rises steeply and exhibits concave slopes. This is typically the case when a thick, hyper-reflective, taut posterior hyaloid is attached to the top of the elevated macular center, and causes tractional diabetic macular edema. [34-36]

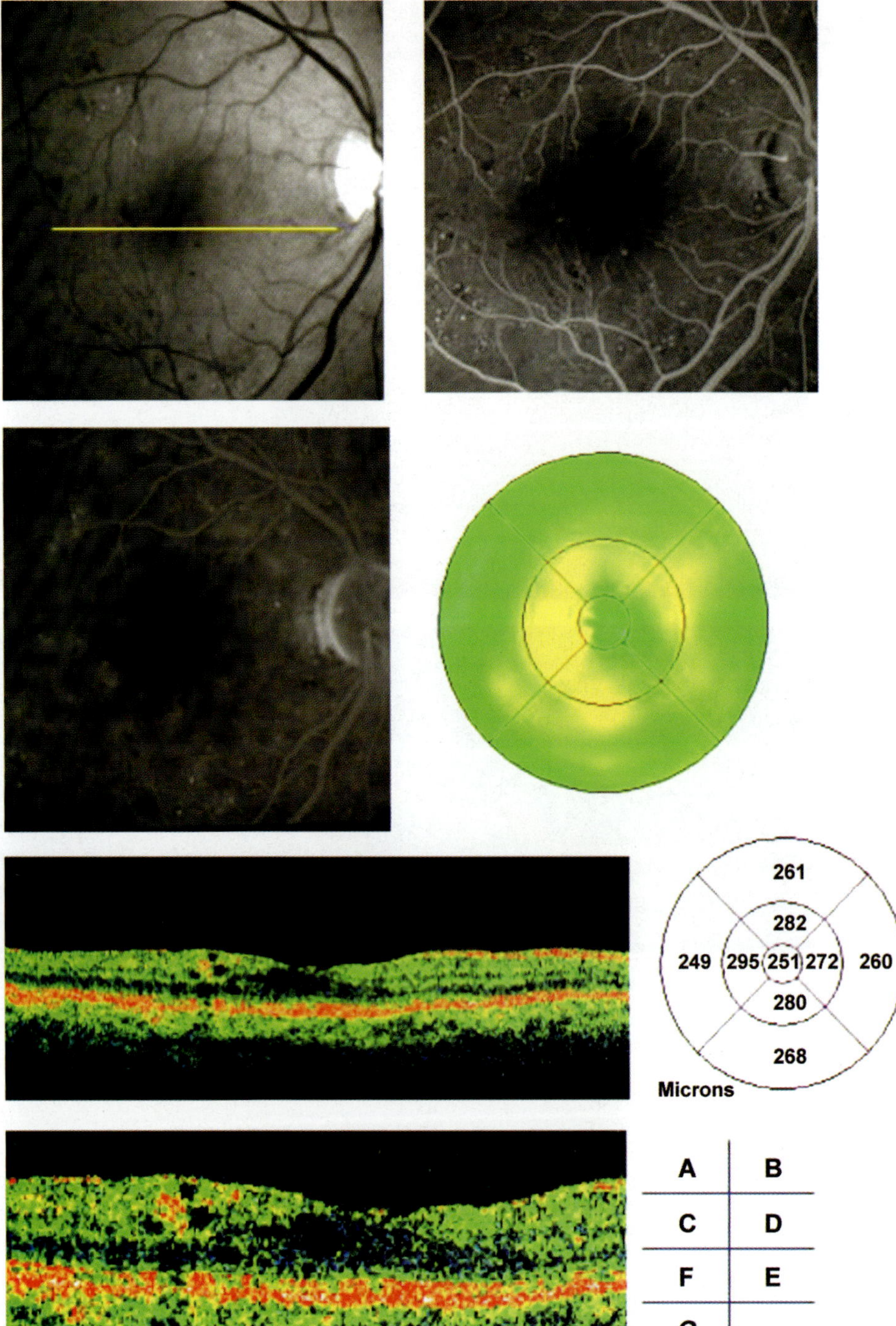

FIGURES 1.11A to G: Early cystoid macular edema in moderate non proliferative diabetic retinopathy. (A) Red-free photograph: showing numerous punctate hemorrhages in the posterior pole. (B) Fluorescein angiography, early phase. Many microaneurysms are visible. (C) Fluorescein angiography, early phase; mild diffuse macular leakage, without a cystoid appearance. (D and E) Retinal thickness maps show diffuse, moderate macular thickening, with flattening of the foveal depression. Mean thickness of the central area is slightly increased (251 μm). (F) Horizontal 6 mm scan disclosing slight moderate thickening of the macula and flattening of the foveal depression. There is a cystoid cavity in the temporal part of the fovea, and numerous micro-cystic changes are visible which were not seen on fluorescein angiography. (G) Detail showing the cystoid spaces. The visual acuity of this eye is 20/25 (Prof Alain Gaudric MD, France).

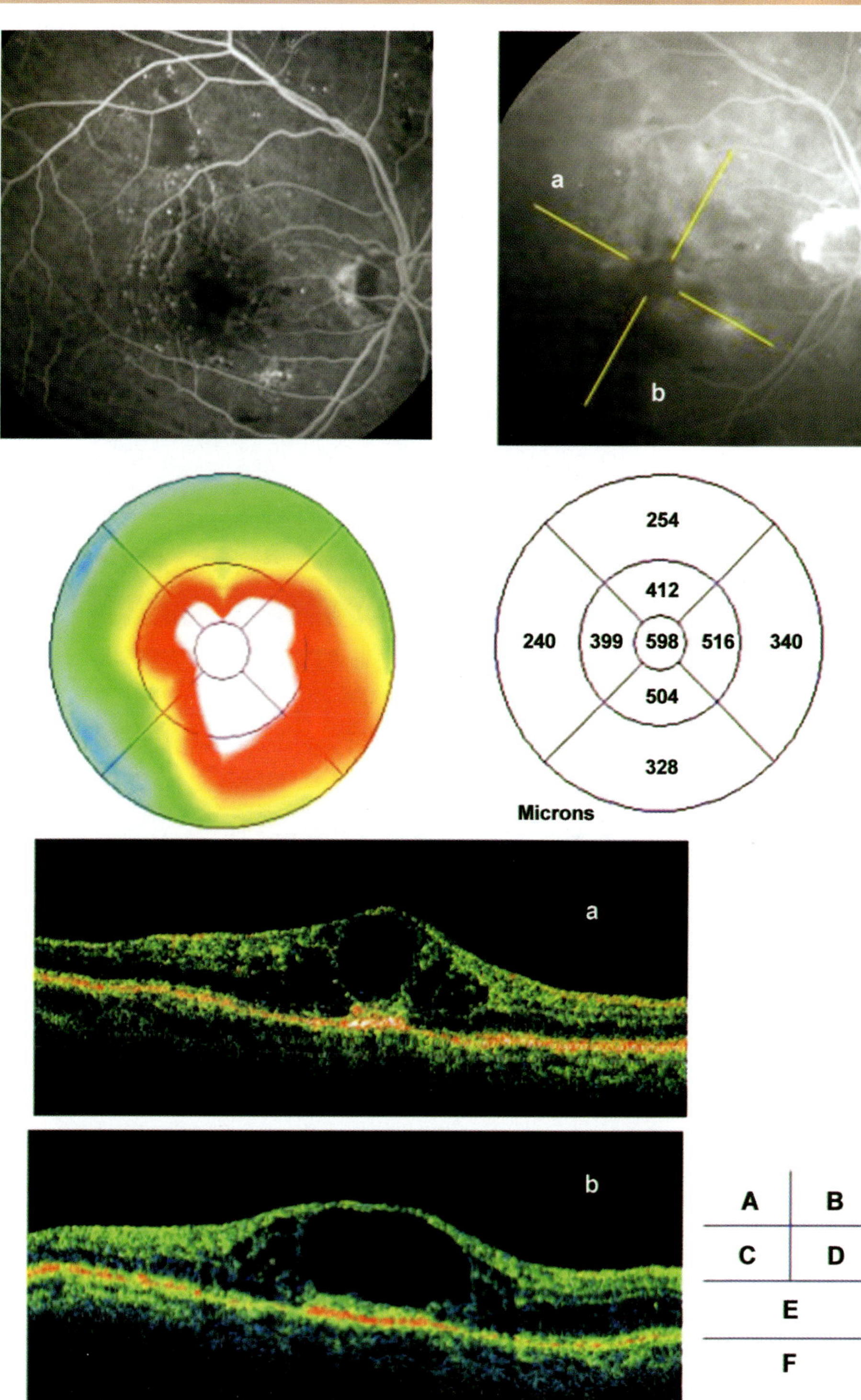

FIGURES 1.12A to F: Severe cystoid macular edema in severe nonproliferative diabetic retinopathy. (A) Fluorescein angiography, early phase, showing areas of capillary non-perfusion. (B) Fluorescein angiography, late phase, showing cystoid macular edema (lines a and b refer to the direction of the linear scans below). (C and D) Retinal thickness maps; color map shows diffuse macular thickening. Central macular thickness has increased to 598 µm. (E) 6 mm scan (a): a large central foveal cyst is surrounded by smaller cysts, resulting in significant macular thickening. (F) 6 mm scan (b) ; on a perpendicular scan, the central cyst seems larger. The visual acuity of this eye is 20/125 (Prof Alain Gaudric MD, France).

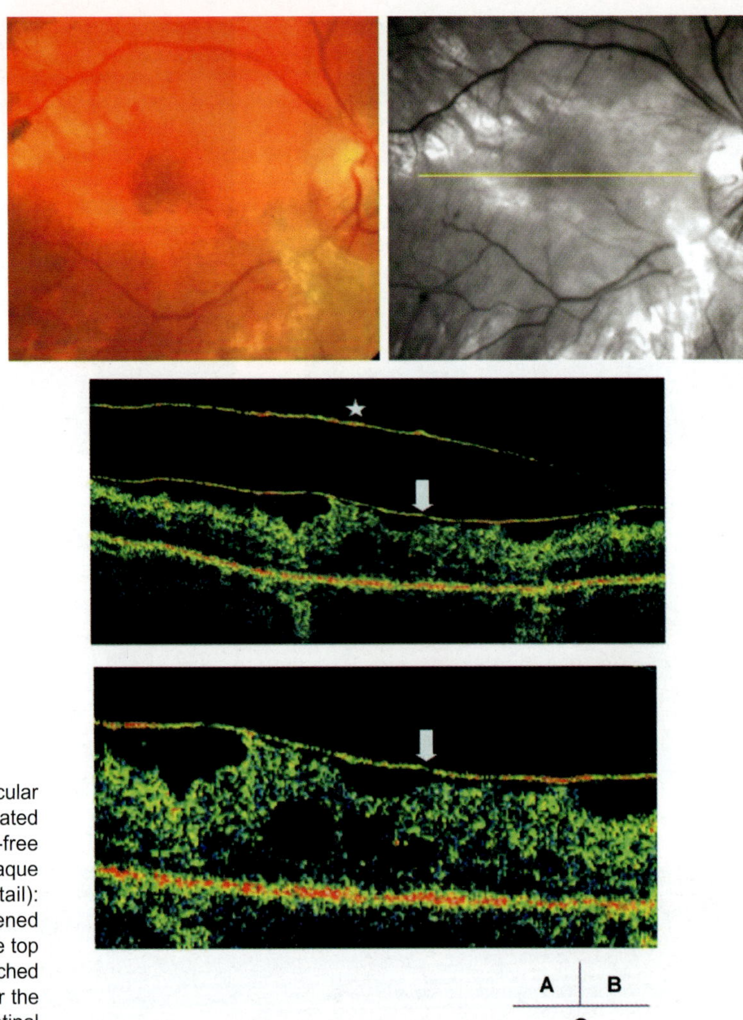

FIGURES 1.13A to D: Epiretinal membrane and diabetic macular edema, in an eye with proliferative diabetic retinopathy treated by panretinal photocoagulation. (A and B) Color and red-free photographs showing retinal folds in the macula and an opaque epiretinal membrane near the optic disk. (C and D) (Detail): Horizontal retinal scan showing cystic changes in a thickened folded retina. An epiretinal membrane (arrow) adheres to the top of the retinal folds. The posterior hyaloid (star) is partially detached from the retina but adheres to the epiretinal membrane near the disc. Visual acuity is 20/200. Pars plana vitrectomy and epiretinal peeling might improve vision, depending on the amount of damage to the macula caused by long-standing macular edema (Prof Alain Gaudric MD, France).

Stratus OCT-3 has enhanced epiretinal membrane visibility. Macular edema may also be combined with an epiretinal membrane (Figures 1.13A to D).

Posterior Hyaloid

The posterior hyaloid is only visible on OCT when it is partly or slightly detached from the retinal surface. As OCT-3 has a 4 mm deep field, a posterior hyaloid detachment from the retinal surface of more than 2 mm may not be visible if the retinal scan is in the center of the box. Lowering the scan to the bottom of the box may enable a detached posterior hyaloid to be visualized 3 to 3.5 mm above the retinal plane.

There are two reasons why the posterior hyaloid may be not visible on OCT scans: [26]

a. either it is completely attached to the retinal surface, or

b. it is completely detached and too far from that surface.

When the posterior hyaloid is not visible at the surface on an OCT scan, it is necessary to ascertain, from the fundus biomicroscopy whether or not the Weiss ring is detached, in order to determine the status of the vitreomacular junction. Optical coherence tomography is especially useful for detecting incomplete or shallow detachments of the posterior hyaloid, which previously were not usually detectable.

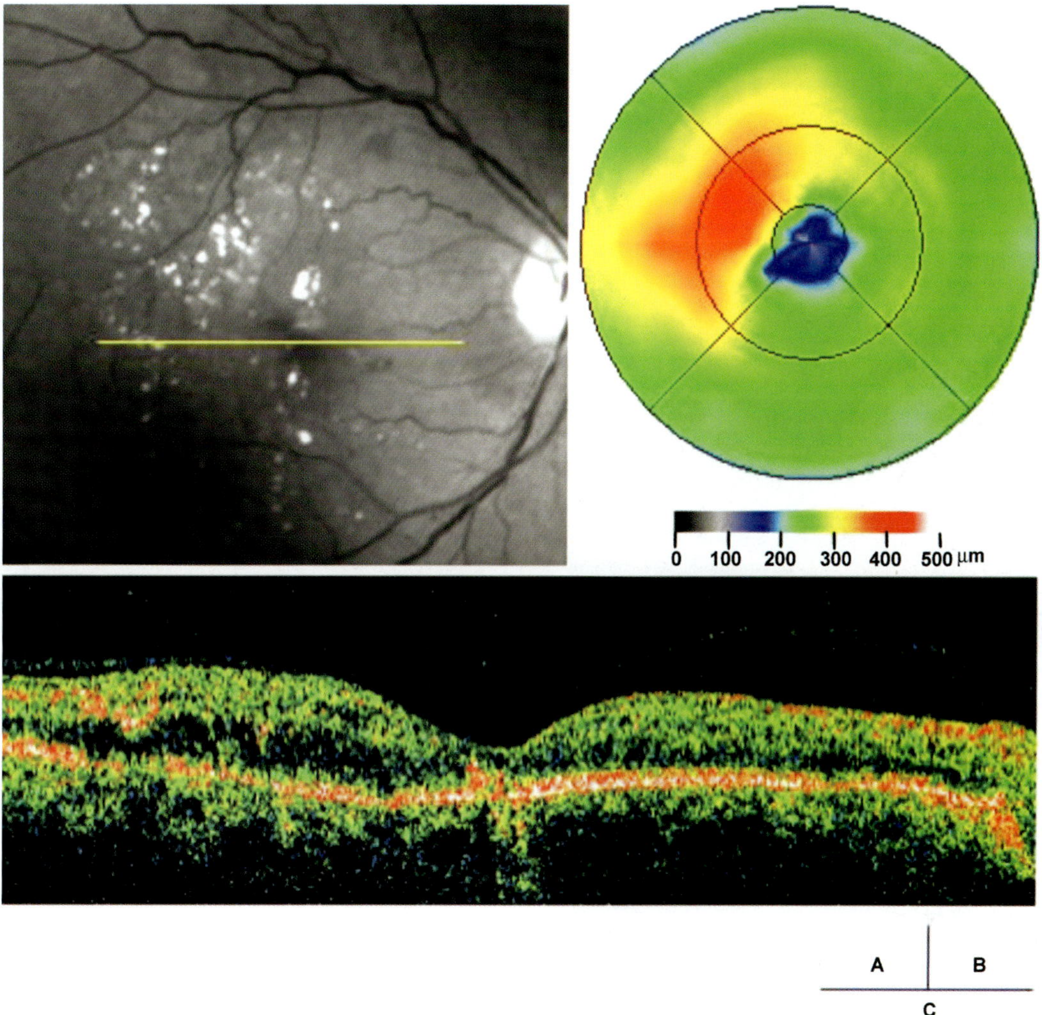

FIGURES 1.14A to C: Partial posterior hyaloid detachment in a case of moderate macular edema. (A) Red-free photograph shows hard exudates encroaching on the fovea. (B) Retinal macular map shows that central average thickness is still normal. (C) Horizontal retinal scan showing persistence of the foveal pit and thickening of the temporal part of the macula. The posterior hyaloid is partly detached from the macular surface, more nasally than temporally; it is thin and displays low reflectivity. This partial detachment has not caused any deformation of the fovea (Prof Alain Gaudric MD, France).

Perifoveolar Vitreous Detachment with a Normal Posterior Hyaloid

In about half the cases of diabetic macular edema, the posterior hyaloid is detached from the retinal surface in the perifoveolar area but remains attached to the foveolar center. This configuration gives the posterior hyaloid its typical double convexity on cross sectional scans (Figures 1.14A to C).[26] In a three-dimensional image, this biconvex appearance would correspond to a posterior hyaloid detachment over the posterior pole, whose limit would describe a circle concentric to the temporal vessels and tangent to the optic disk. Such detachment would exhibit umbilication at its center due to vitreofoveolar adherence. This appearance is not different from the initial stages of posterior vitreous detachment, described in healthy subjects,[37] and shown in fellow eyes of eyes with idiopathic macular holes.[38] However, it may result in increased thickness of a pre-existing macular edema.[39]

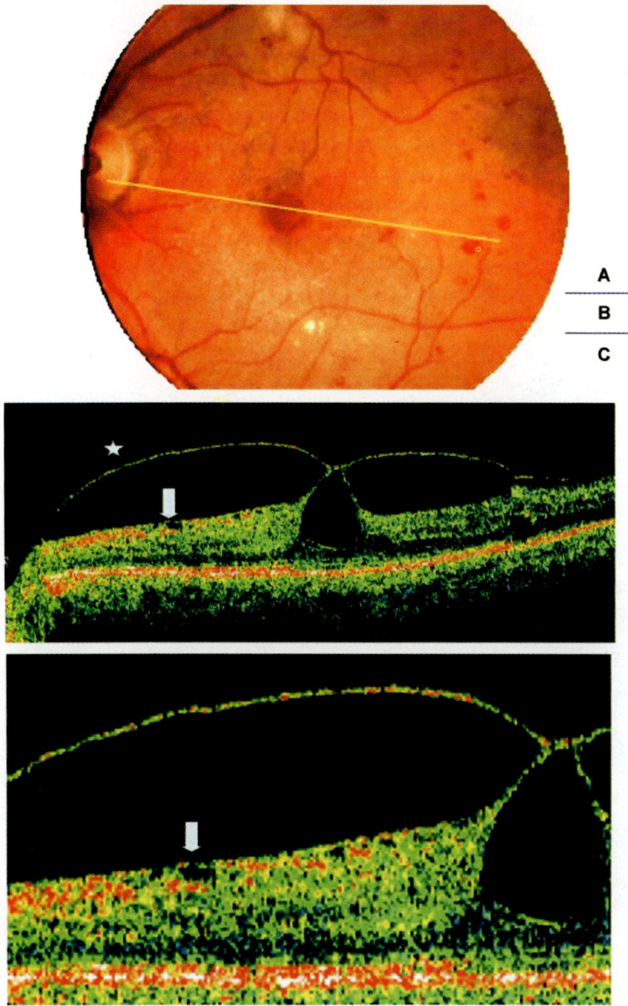

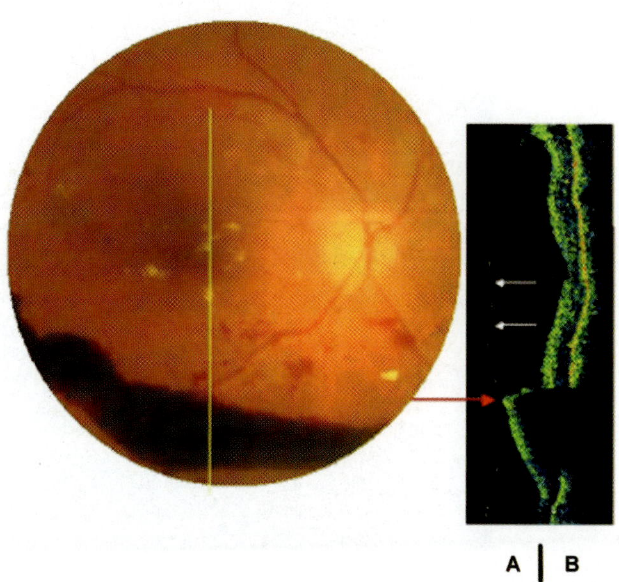

of the posterior hyaloid is unclear. Posterior hyaloid traction may also be combined with an epiretinal membrane which causes or increases macular thickening.[26]

Pre-retinal Hemorrhage

Pre-retinal hemorrhages may completely mask the underlying features (Figures 1.16A and B). On the contrary, intraretinal hemorrhages are rarely visible on OCT scans, as their reflectivity is weak. [26]

FIGURES 1.16A and B: Preretinal hemorrhages in proliferative diabetic retinopathy. (A) Color fundus photograph showing a preretinal hemorrhage. (B) Optical coherence tomography scan shows the horizontal level of the hemorrhage, limited by the posterior hyaloid (white arrows) (Prof Alain Gaudric MD, France).

FIGURES 1.15A to C: Tractional diabetic macular edema in an eye with severe non-proliferative diabetic retinopathy. (A) Color fundus photography showing what looks like a hole in the macula, surrounded by a glistening reflex. Numerous intraretinal hemorrhages are present. (B) 9 mm retinal scan showing an incompletely detached, thick, hyper-reflective posterior hyaloid (arrow) still attached to the optic disc, the foveal center, and the border of the posterior pole. An epiretinal membrane is also present, and adheres to the retinal surface, causing small superficial retinal folds (arrow). See detail in (C). The hole-like appearance on fundus photography is in fact due to the presence of a large foveal cyst. Visual acuity is still 20/50, but only pars plana vitrectomy can preserve or improve vision in this case (Prof Alain Gaudric MD, France).

Lamellar Hole

Lamellar hole may be the end stage of long-standing macular edema with central cyst, combined with vitreomacular traction (Figures 1.17A to C). In rare cases, full thickness macular hole may even occur as an end stage of cystoid macular edema combined with vitreous traction. [26]

Perifoveolar Vitreous Detachment with a Thick Posterior Hyaloid

In rare cases, the partially detached posterior hyaloid looks much thicker and more hyper-reflective than usual. It is also less curved and often straight and taut over the macular area.[35,36] In other cases however, it may retain its biconvexity (Figures 1.15A to C). The reason for this thickening

Tractional Macular Edema

Optical coherence tomography provides a static representation of the macular profile. Once the posterior hyaloid is detached from the macula except for the foveolar center, the last step is the avulsion of the adhesion

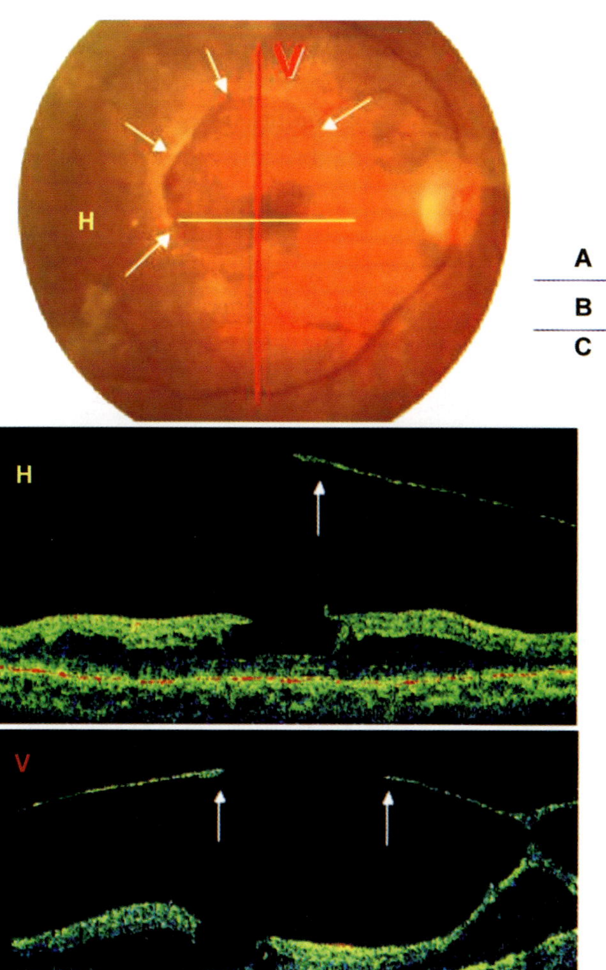

FIGURE 1.17: A macular lamellar hole resulting from macular edema and vitreomacular traction. (A) Color fundus photograph showing a hole in the thick detached posterior hyaloid (arrows). H and V indicate respectively the directions of the horizontal and vertical retinal scans. (B) Horizontal 6 mm retinal scan showing a lamellar macular hole in a thickened macula. Note the partially detached thickened posterior hyaloid (arrow). (C) 9 mm vertical retinal scan showing a lamellar hole in the partially detached posterior hyaloid (arrows), which is still attached to the inferotemporal retinal vein. The lamellar hole probably occurred during the posterior hyaloid detachment (Prof Alain Gaudric MD, France).

to the center, resulting in a change in the profile of the posterior hyaloid from biconvex to dome shape. In diabetic macular edema it is difficult to interpret images showing a change in the posterior hyaloid profile as evidence of significant traction on the macula. A thick, hyper-reflective, taut posterior hyaloid does usually indicate vitreomacular traction. The combination of a hyper-reflective, thick posterior hyaloid adhering to an

elevated foveal center and convex slopes of the thickened macula is strongly suggestive of tractional diabetic macular edema.[26]

RETINAL MAP ANALYSIS

There are two kinds of retinal map analysis which provide complementary information:

Color Map

This gives a topographic representation of retinal thickness calculated from the values measured on each linear scan, so that the values between two linear scans are extrapolated and not measured. [26]

Mean Thickness Map

This gives the average retinal thickness in each of the 9 different sectors of the macula. Average sectorial retinal thickness is calculated from the measures constituting the linear scans. The pattern of the 9 different sectors of the macular map for which the average retinal thickness is measured was modeled on the macular edema pattern of the Early Treatment of Diabetic Retinopathy Study (ETDRS), and is therefore well suited to the assessment of diabetic macular edema. Mean foveal thickness refers to the average of retinal thickness values in the central 1000 microns central disk, and central foveal thickness refers to the average of 6 values of retinal thickness at the intersection of the six radial scans. [26]

The color map shows small variations in each sector and gives semi-quantitative indications of local retinal thickness by means of a color code. The mean thickness map gives the average retinal thickness values of each sector.

It has been shown with Stratus OCT-3 that mean retinal thickness measurement is highly reliable and reproducible in the different areas of OCT mapping, both in normal subjects and in diabetic patients with macular edema.[40,41] Several methods have been proposed to assess the variations in sectorial mean thickness.[42,43] Accuracy of retinal thickness measurement is according to ETDRS zone. Retinal thickness in each zone is calculated as the average of the values measured on the portions of axis passing through that zone. There is also a good correlation between OCT and fluorescein angiography for the detection of areas of leakage.[26]

TREATMENT FOR DIABETIC MACULAR EDEMA

Laser Photocoagulation

Laser photocoagulation of diabetic macular edema is usually based on fundus biomicroscopy, which shows the areas of retinal thickening, and on fluorescein angiography, which shows the leaky microvascular anomalies. Optical coherence tomography mapping is an adjunct to fundus photograph, or fluorescein angiography, for detecting the areas to treat. It might replace fluorescein angiography in the follow-up of photocoagulation. [26]

Pars Plana Vitrectomy

Pars plana vitrectomy is used to treat both tractional and non-tractional diabetic macular edema. The benefit of pars plana vitrectomy for tractional macular edema is widely accepted. The role of OCT in distinguishing tractional from non-tractional diabetic macular edema is essential, although the signs of vitreomacular traction (a hyper-reflective, thickened posterior hyaloid adhering to the top of the macular edema, whose shape is altered by the traction) are not completely accepted. [26]

Intravitreal Drugs

The use of intravitreal drugs (corticosteroids or anti-VEGF) has increased the use of OCT for monitoring the effect of these treatments and helping to reach decisions regarding retreatment. These intravitreal drugs indeed exert a favorable effect on the hydration of the retina, especially of the posterior pole. Their effect in reducing macular thickness or volume precedes the improvement of visual acuity. Conversely, a recurrence of macular thickening often precedes visual acuity impairment. In these cases OCT mapping is a useful indicator of the anatomic efficacy of the drug (Figures 1.18A to G). It has also been shown that measurement of macular thickness by OCT may serve as a pharmacodynamic criterion for non-invasive assessment of the pharmacokinetics of intravitreal triamcinolone. [26,44]

RETINAL ARTERY OCCLUSION

Retinal artery occlusion is relatively common etiology for sudden vision loss in aged adults. The embolization and thrombosis are the common cause of artery obstruction.[45,46] The neuronal cells in the inner retina become edematous during the first few hours after artery occlusion. The intracellular swelling accounts for the whitening or opacification of the affected retina observed by ophthalmoscopically. The retinal opacification usually resolves within 4 to 6 weeks.

OPTICAL COHERENCE TOMOGRAPHY

Optical coherence tomography images of ischemic retina due to central retinal artery occlusion and branch retinal artery occlusion correlate with the histopathological findings of acute retinal ischemia. The affected area demonstrates increased thickness and reflectivity in the inner retina. The marked difference from retinal edema due to other retinal vascular disease such as retinal vein occlusion or diabetic maculopathy is lack of areas or cystic spaces of low reflectivity due to fluid accumulation. This difference probably correlates with the histopathological findings that retinal edema in arterial occlusion is in the intracellular space instead of extracellular space. After the resolution of retinal cloudy edema inner retina becomes atrophic and thin, which is a characteristic of OCT finding of chronic central retinal artery occlusion and branch retinal artery occlusion (Figures 1.19A to F and 1.20A to C).[45]

RETINAL ARTERY MACROANEURYSM

The retinal artery macroaneurysm is fusiform or round dilation of retinal arteriole in the posterior pole. The macroaneurysm generally affects a patient older than sixties, who is usually associated with hypertension and arteriosclerotic cardiovascular diseases. The patient with macroaneurysm is asymptomatic if there is no complication in the macular area, but becomes symptomatic when the macroaneurysm complicates retinal edema, exudation and hemorrhage.

OPTICAL COHERENCE TOMOGRAPHY

The retinal artery macroaneurysm may be associated with vitreous, preretinal, intraretinal, subretinal hemorrhage,

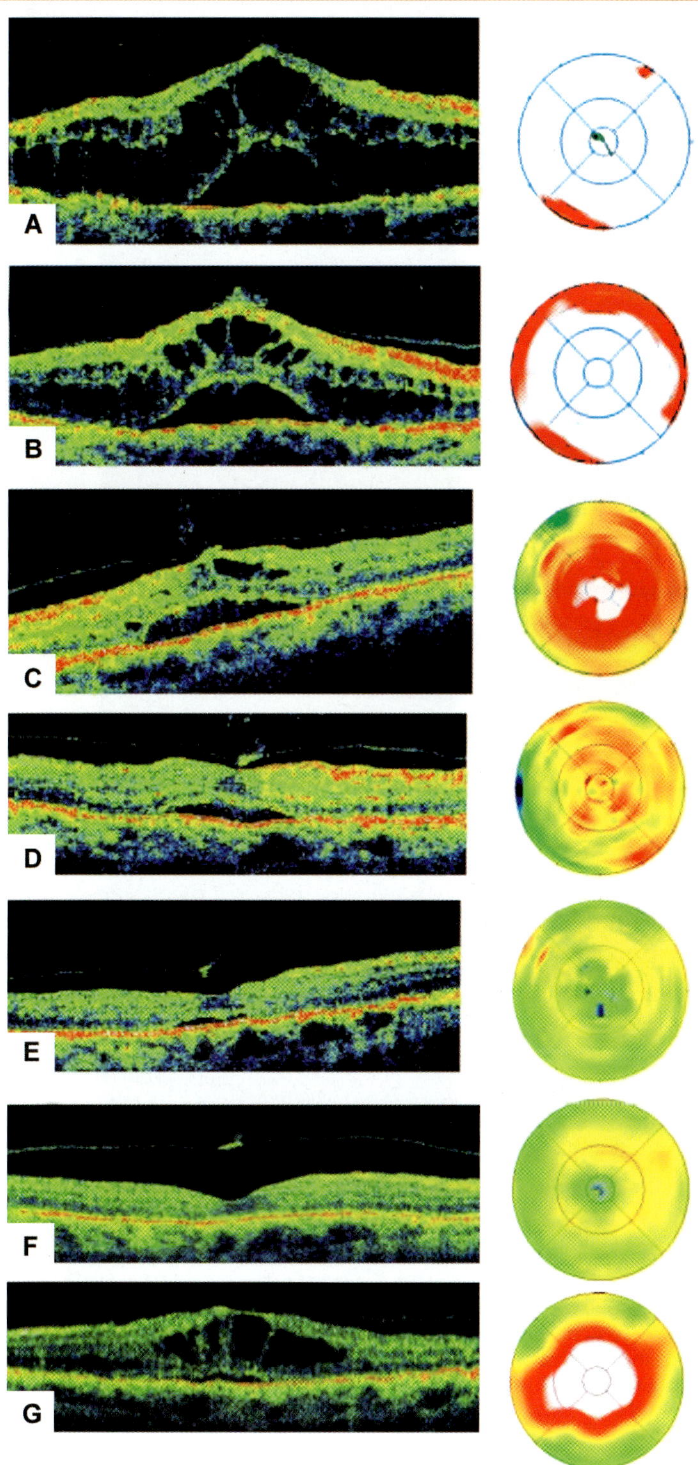

FIGURES 1.18A to G: Evolution of diffuse cystoid macular edema after injection of 4 mg intravitreal triamcinolone acetonide. (A) Severe cystoid macular edema, with foveal detachment before injection. Right color fundus photograph. visual acuity: 20/400. Contor average thickness: 805 µm. (B) Two days after intravitreal triamcinolone acetonide: Center average thickness: 767 µm. (C) Seven days after intravitreal triamcinolone acetonide: Center average thickness: 477 µm. (D) Two weeks after intravitreal triamcinolone acetonide: Center average thickness: 314 µm. (E) Three weeks after intravitreal triamcinolone acetonide: Center average thickness: 264 µm. (F) Two months after intravitreal triamcinolone acetonide: Center average thickness is now almost normal (225 µm). Foveal detachment has progressively stabilized. The posterior hyaloid is detached from the macular surface. Visual acuity has improved to 20/100. (G) Five months after intravitreal triamcinolone acetonide: macular edema has recurred; Center average thickness: 633 µm. VA: 20/400 (Prof Alain Gaudric, MD, France).

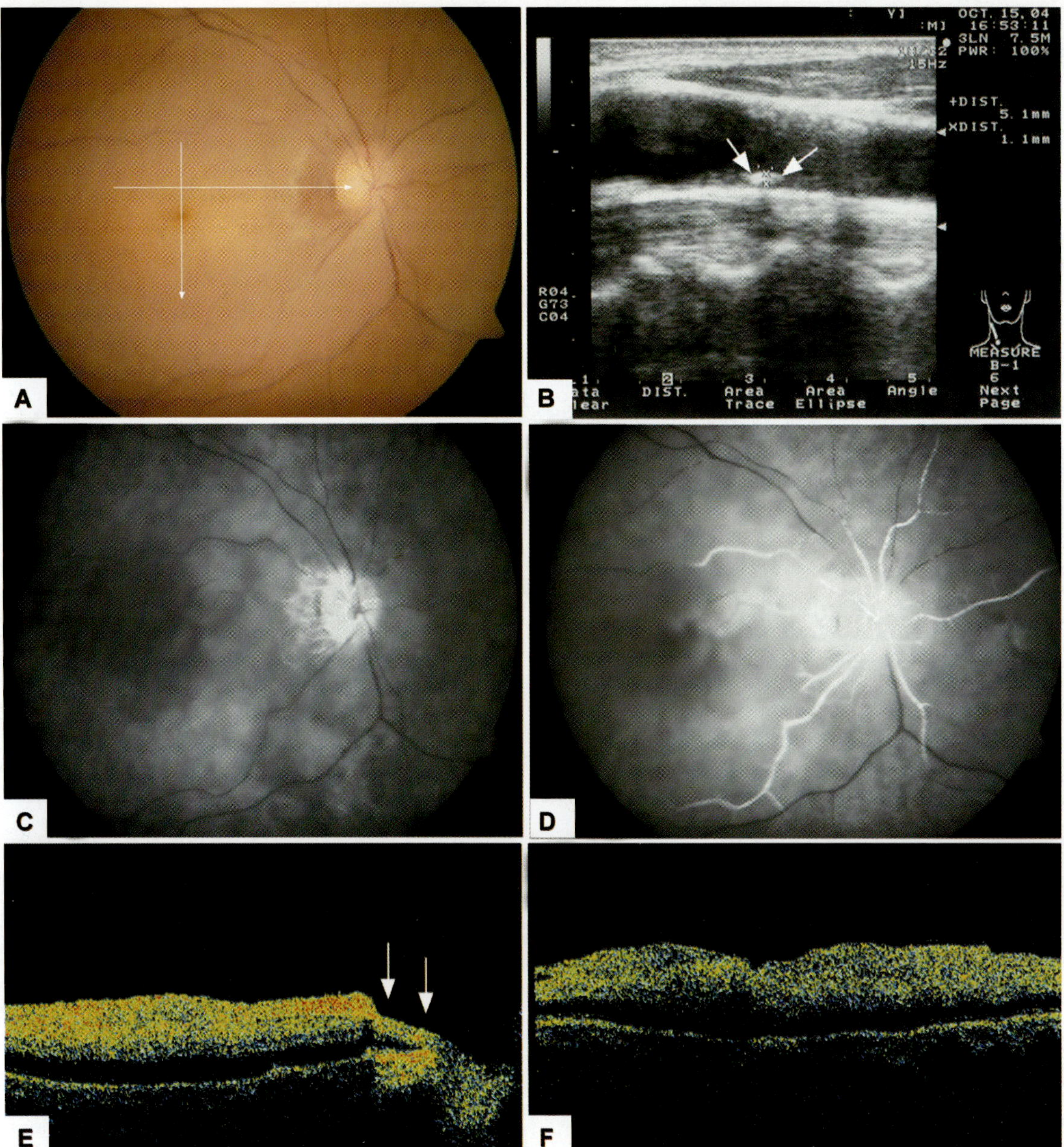

FIGURE 1.19: (A) Fundus photograph. Whitening or opacification as a result of retinal intracellular edema in the posterior pole is significant with cilioretinal arteries sparing one-fourth the papillomacular bundle. (B) A longitudinal echogram of right internal carotid artery demonstrates the atherosclerotic plaque (*arrow*) which may be the origin of the embolus in the central retinal artery. (C) Fluorescein angiogram, 23.4 seconds after injection. Cilioretinal arteries are evident. (D) Fluorescein angiogram, 1 minute and 16 seconds. (E) A vertical OCT scan shows enhanced reflectivity with mild increase of inner retinal thickness without cystic spaces of low reflectivity due to fluid accumulation. (F) A horizontal OCT scan demonstrates cilioretinal arteries sparing in papillomacular bundle (*arrows*) (Keisuke Mori MD, Japan).

or combined. Optical coherence tomography provides an *in vivo* direct visualization of intraretinal pathology with unprecedented resolution if the hemorrhage is posterior to the retina. Intraretinal morphological alterations associated with the macroaneurysm are commonly retinal edema and exudation. Optical coherence tomography demonstrates retinal edema associated with the macroaneurysm as diffuse retinal thickening and elevation with cystic spaces of low reflectivity as a result of fluid accumulation. Hard exudates

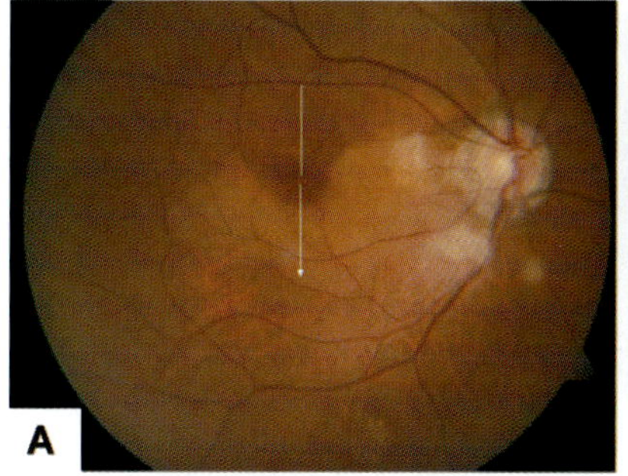 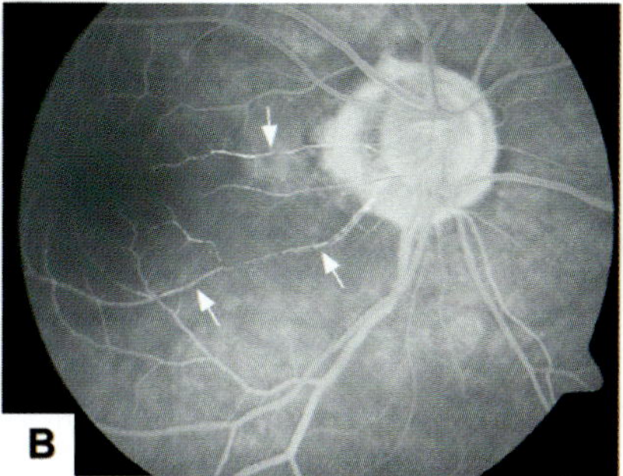 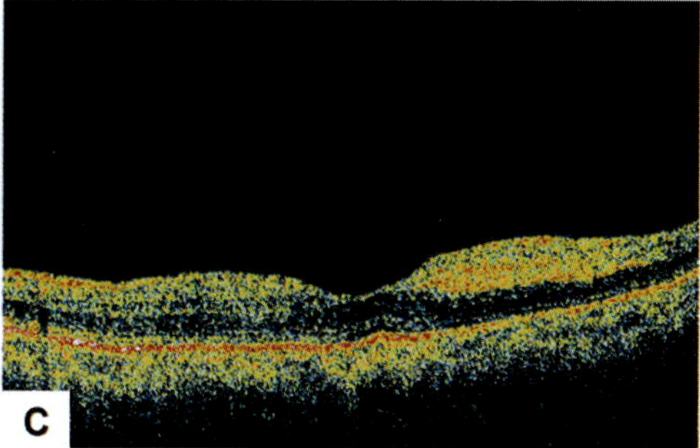

FIGURES 1.20A to C: (A) Fundus photograph. Retinal cloudy swelling is present in the distribution of the occluded artery running through inferior macula. (B) Fluorescein angiogram, 8 minutes and 20 seconds. Note segmentation or box carrying of the blood column in the occluded inferior branch (*arrows*). (C) A vertical OCT scan. The inferior retina with increased reflectivity and thickness (*arrowheads*) contrast with normal superior retina (Keisuke Mori MD, Japan).

are highly backscattering, usually shown as small high reflective dots or areas with shadow of deeper retinal structures. Optical coherence tomography provides information of location in layers of these pathologies (Figures 1.21A to E and 1.22A to F). Cystic space of fluid accumulation and retinal exudation is generally located in the inner and outer plexiform layers. Optical coherence tomography provides follow-up information of these pathologies response to therapeutic interventions.

If the hemorrhage is anterior to the retina, the details of retinal structure are masked by high backscattering of hemorrhage. The preretinal hemorrhage sometimes merges imperceptibly with the retina. Optical coherence tomography can occasionally distinguish hemorrhages beneath internal limiting membrane from posterior hyaloid since the internal limiting membrane tends to be more reflective than the posterior hyaloid.[47]

RETINAL VEIN OCCLUSION

BRANCH RETINAL VEIN OCCLUSION

Branch retinal vein occlusion (BRVO) occurs when blood flow through a branch of the central retinal vein is interrupted. The severity of ocular morbidity from this disease varies greatly depending on the location and extent of the occlusion as well as the development of complications such as macular edema, epiretinal membrane, neovascularization of the disk and elsewhere, traction retinal detachment, and vitreous hemorrhage. A BRVO may cause acute painless vision loss if the vein occlusion is large and/or affecting the macula, or may be asymptomatic if the involved branch is small or more

peripheral. Clinical findings include sectoral venous dilation and tortuosity accompanied by intraretinal hemorrhage and macular edema, usually distal to an arteriovenous crossing that marks the site of occlusion (Figure 1.23). Over time, the hemorrhage and edema may resolve, and the ophthalmoscopic findings may be subtle.

The common adventitial sheath at the crossing site of the branch artery and branch vein may play a role in the pathogenesis of the BRVO. At this site, atherosclerosis causes thickening and hardening of the arterial wall which compresses the underlying vein. The turbulence caused at the crossing may lead to clot formation and occlusion of the branch vein. The venous blood stagnates, and the increasing pressure in the arterial system causes the thinner, weaker veins to break and bleed in the affected distribution. As the blood column slows, it leads to decreased arterial perfusion of the retina. This can lead to retinal ischemia in the distribution of the affected artery. The vitreous may also play a role in compression of susceptible arteriovenous crossing sites.[48]

CENTRAL RETINAL VEIN OCCLUSION

Central retinal vein occlusion (CRVO) is a retinal vascular condition that may cause significant ocular morbidity. It commonly affects men and women equally and occurs predominantly in persons over the age of 65 years. Younger individuals who present with a clinical picture of a CRVO may have an underlying inflammatory etiology. Central retinal vein occlusion classically presents

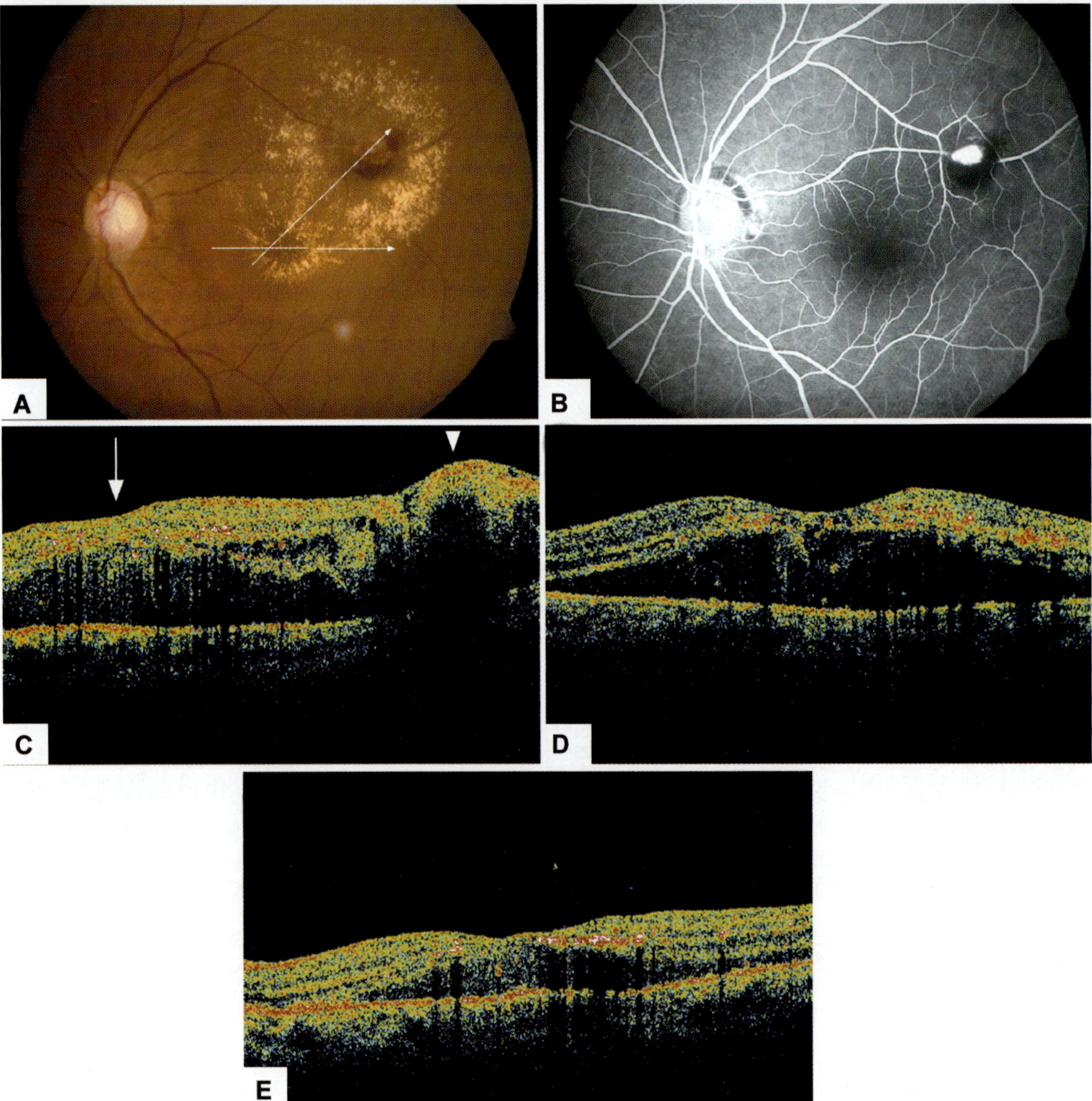

FIGURES 1.21A to E: (A) Fundus photograph before laser shows an arterial macroaneurysm along the arteriole superotemporal to the fovea, complicating retinal edema and exudation. (B) Fluorescein angiogram, 32 second after injection. (C) An oblique OCT scan (5 mm) crossing the macroaneurysm (*arrowhead*) and the parafovea (*arrow*) demonstrates diffuse retinal thickening and elevation with cystic spaces of low reflectivity as a result of fluid accumulation. Small high reflective dots, representing intraretinal exudation, located at the level corresponding to outer plexiform layer. (D) A horizontal OCT scan crossing fovea delineates serous retinal detachment with intraretinal exudation. (E) A macular horizontal cross-sectional image one month after the treatment depicts decreased retinal edema and relative increase of intraretinal exudation (Keisuke Mori MD, Japan).

with acute painless loss of vision in the affected eye. Intraretinal hemorrhages and dilated/tortuous retinal veins in all four quadrants are the hallmark of CRVO. The hemorrhages radiate from the optic nerve head and may result in the classic "blood and thunder" appearance. Optic nerve head swelling, cotton-wool spots, and macular edema are also present to varying degrees. A CRVO is classified by the Central Vein Occlusion Study (CVOS) based on the perfusion status of the retina as determined by fluorescein angiography. A non-perfused or ischemic CRVO has 10 or more disk areas of retinal capillary non-perfusion on fluorescein angiography.

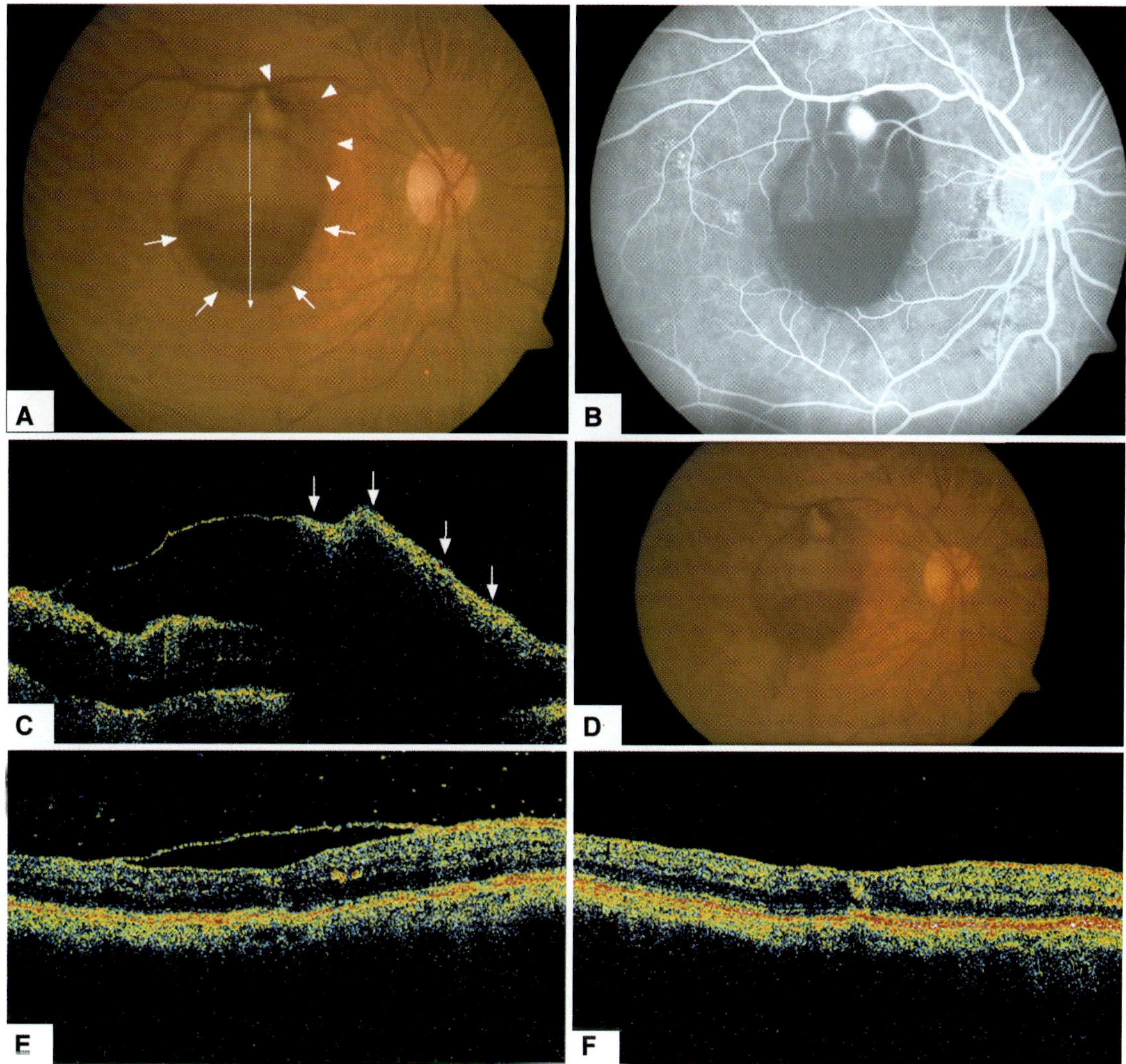

FIGURES 1.22A to F: (A) Fundus photograph before the treatment shows an arterial macroaneurysm along the arteriole superotemporal to the fovea, complicating preretinal (*arrowheads*) and subretinal (*arrows*) hemorrhages. (B) Fluorescein angiogram demonstrates hyperfluorescence of the macroaneurysm. (C) A vertical OCT scan delineates preretinal hemorrhage as a dome-shaped, highly elevated, highly reflective zone beneath the internal limiting membrane (*arrows*). The detail of retinal structure of inferior macula is masked by high backscattering of hemorrhage. (D) Fundus photograph immediately after Nd: YAG laser membranotomy. Vertical OCT cross-sections 7-day (E) and 2-month (F) after the treatment. Please notice rapid clearing of premacular hemorrhage. However, mild foveal edema with intraretinal exudation is delineated by OCT (Keisuke Mori MD, Japan).

Generally, these eyes display more intraretinal hemorrhage, as well as retinal and disk edema, than perfused CRVOs.[48]

OPTICAL COHERENCE TOMOGRAPHY

The gold standard for evaluating macular edema has been fluorescein angiography. More recently, OCT has become an important tool in the management of eyes with macular edema due to branch or central retinal vein occlusion. Optical coherence tomography has demonstrated the ability to detect macular edema that is not appreciable by ophthalmoscopy or fluorescein angiography in various disease processes, including retinal vein occlusion.[49-52] It can also better define the axial distribution of fluid that is observed as thickening of the macula on exam (Figures 1.24A to J and 1.25A to E).[48,51]

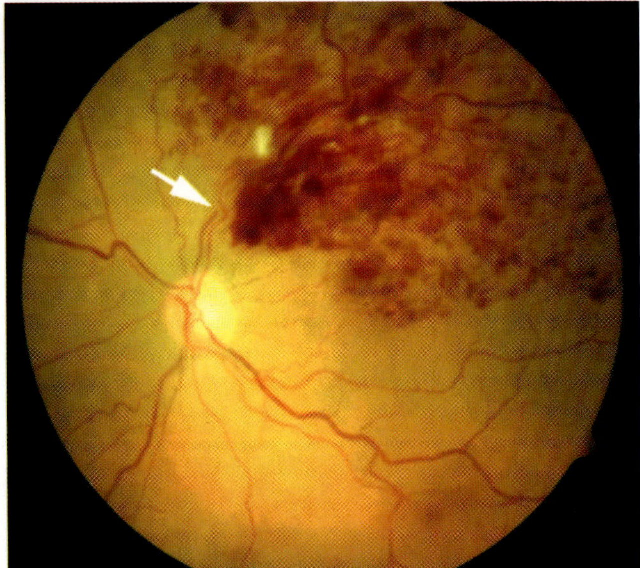

FIGURE 1.23: Branch retinal vein occlusion: Intraretinal hemorrhages and cotton-wool spots distal to an arteriovenous crossing *(arrow)* (Sharon Fekrat MD, USA).

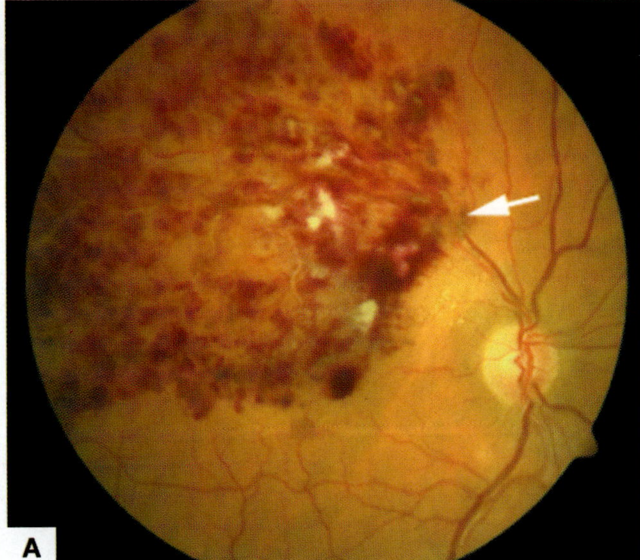

FIGURE 1.24A

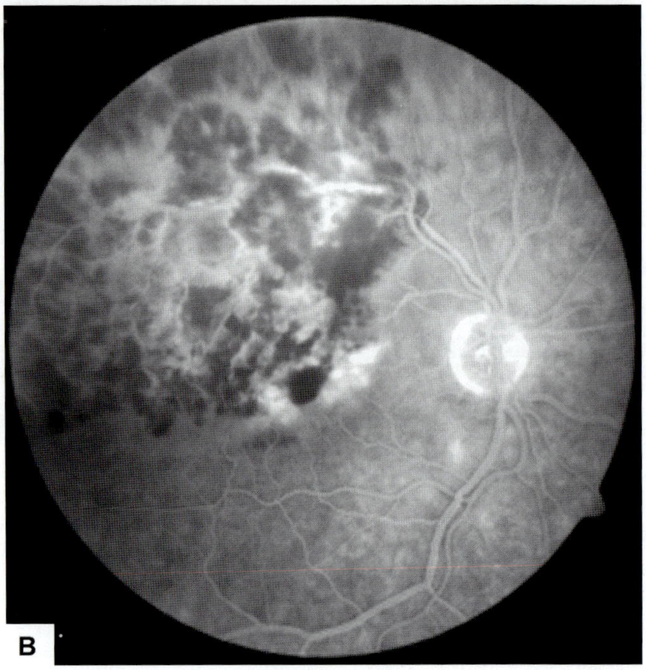

Serous retinal detachment has been reported as an under recognized cause of visual morbidity in eyes with retinal venous occlusive disease, contributing to photoreceptor atrophy from prolonged serous detachment of the fovea. Seventy-one percent of eyes with BRVO have an accompanying serous foveal retinal detachment with or without overlying cystoid macular edema.[50]

Better definition of the anatomy with OCT may allow treatment to be directed at contributing causes for the visual dysfunction. Individuals with macular edema and/or serous foveal retinal detachment may be initially treated with a more conservative approach, such as an intravitreal steroid injection. Optical coherence tomography findings of a concurrent mechanical cause such as an associated epiretinal membrane or traction on the disk may lead to an earlier surgical intervention.[48]

Optic disk traction is a recently recognized finding associated with ischemic CRVO.[53] Optical coherence tomography can determine the configuration of the traction as well as accompanying subretinal fluid better than biomicroscopy. Earlier intervention may be indicated to prevent optic atrophy due to disk traction and secondary changes in laminar flow through the peripapillary blood vessels or retinal atrophy due to prolonged detachment of the macula.[53]

FIGURE 1.24B

Optical coherence tomography plays a major part in monitoring the response to treatment interventions in eyes with retinal vein occlusion. It allows the ophthalmologist to directly follow and assess the response after treatment of macular edema, associated epiretinal membrane, or optic disk traction.[54] Macular thickness can be measured by serial volumetric analysis, and the retinal cross sections

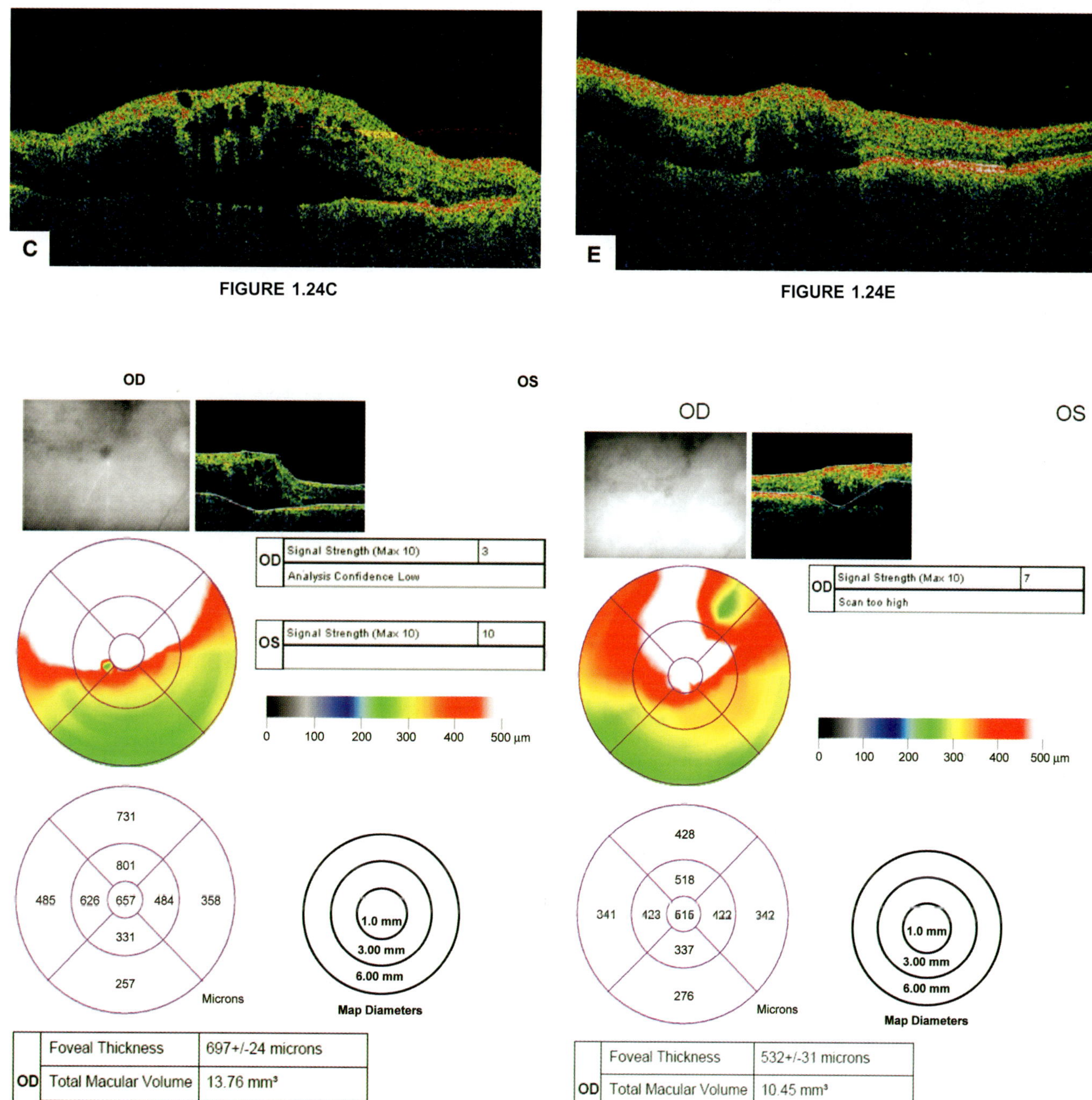

C
FIGURE 1.24C
E
FIGURE 1.24E
OD
OS
OD
Signal Strength (Max 10)   3
Analysis Confidence Low
OS
Signal Strength (Max 10)   10
0 100 200 300 400 500 µm
731
801
485 626 657 484 358
331
257
Microns
1.0 mm
3.00 mm
6.00 mm
Map Diameters
OD
Foveal Thickness   697+/-24 microns
Total Macular Volume   13.76 mm³
Scans used   1, 2, 3, 4, 5, 6
D
FIGURE 1.24D
OD
OS
OD
Signal Strength (Max 10)   7
Scan too high
0 100 200 300 400 500 µm
428
518
341 423 616 422 342
337
276
Microns
1.0 mm
3.00 mm
6.00 mm
Map Diameters
OD
Foveal Thickness   532+/-31 microns
Total Macular Volume   10.45 mm³
Scans used   1, 2, 3, 4, 5, 6
F
FIGURE 1.24F

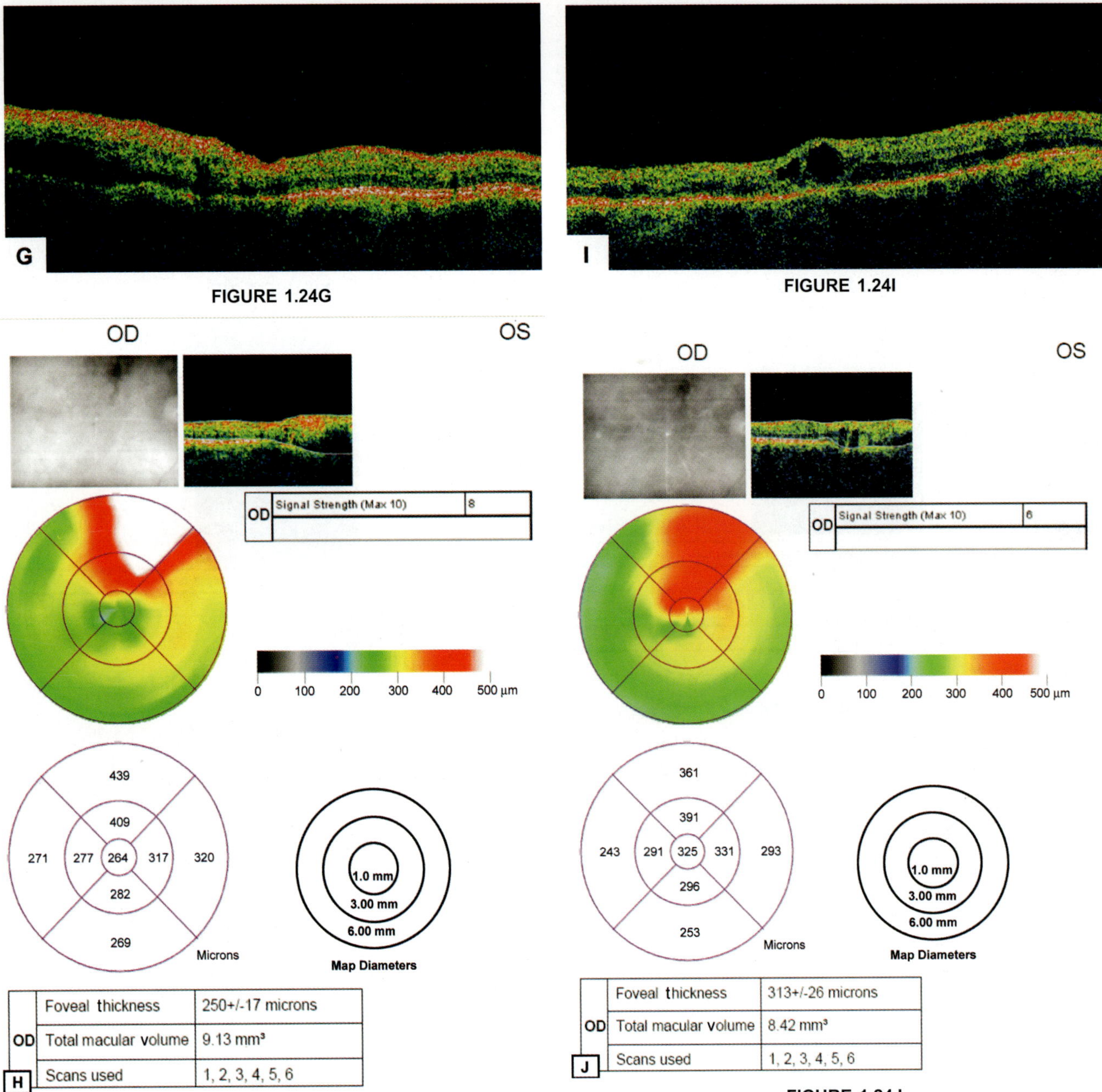

OD	Foveal thickness	250+/-17 microns
	Total macular volume	9.13 mm³
H	Scans used	1, 2, 3, 4, 5, 6

FIGURE 1.24H

OD	Foveal thickness	313+/-26 microns
	Total macular volume	8.42 mm³
J	Scans used	1, 2, 3, 4, 5, 6

FIGURE 1.24J

FIGURES 1.24A to J: A 52-year-old man with a history of hypertension and coronary artery disease presented with five weeks of decreased vision OD. The visual acuity was 20/250 OD and the patient described an inferonasal visual field defect. Examination revealed a BRVO along the superotemporal arcade (A) with characteristic intraretinal hemorrhages, venous tortuosity and cotton-wool spots distal to an arteriovenous crossing (arrow). Areas of capillary non-perfusion were seen on fluorescein angiography (B). Optical coherence tomography demonstrated cystoid macular edema and accompanying serous retinal detachment (C). The foveal thickness was 697±24 microns, and the total macular volume was 13.76 mm³ (D). An intravitreal triamcinolone acetonide (4 mg) injection was performed. One week after injection the visual acuity improved to 20/100, and an OCT of the macula along the 270° meridian (E) showed resolution of the serous fluid and a marked decrease in foveal thickness, measuring 532±31 microns, and total macular volume, 10.45 mm³ (F). One month post injection the visual acuity was still 20/100 and the OCT (270° meridian) demonstrated further resolution of the cystoid macular edema (G). The macular thickness map also showed a decrease in foveal thickness, 250 ±17 microns, and total macular volume, 9.13 mm³ (H). At 3 months post-injection the vision had declined to 20/160 and the OCT showed recurrent cystoid macular edema (I). The foveal thickness was increased, 313±26 microns, however the total macular volume was decreased, 8.42 mm³, attributable to improvement in the edema between the 3 mm and 6 mm rings in the superior quadrant (J) (Sharon Fekrat MD, USA).

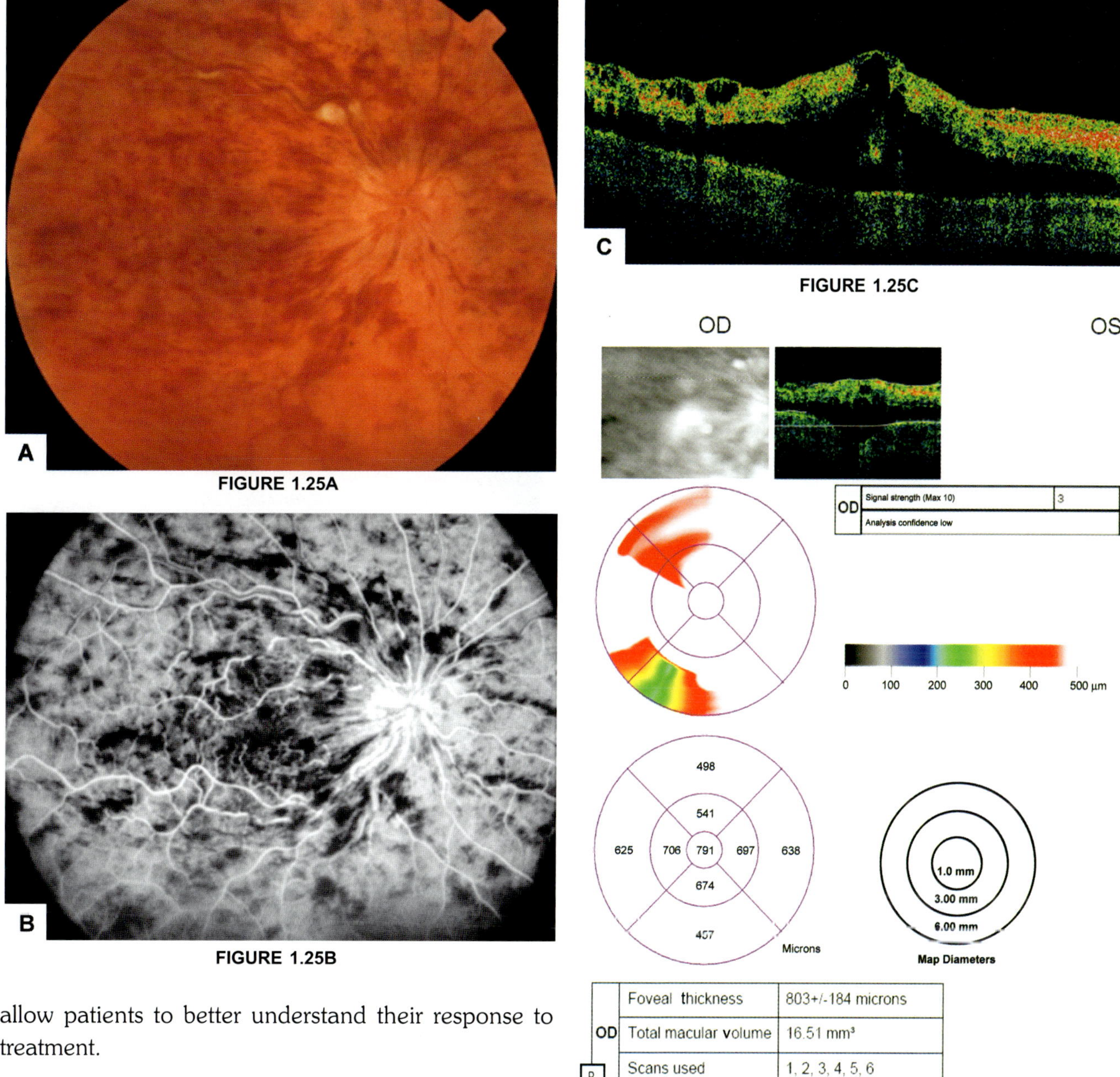

FIGURE 1.25A

FIGURE 1.25B

FIGURE 1.25C

FIGURE 1.25D

allow patients to better understand their response to treatment.

JUXTAFOVEAL TELANGIECTASIAS

Retinal vascular telangiectasias which occur near the fovea have been designated parafoveal or juxtafoveal telangiectasis, and those which are believed idiopathic have been divided into three groups. Group 1 telangiectasias occur unilaterally in middle aged patients and generally cause minimal decrease in vision and are readily identifiable on clinical examination. Group 2 patients have symmetric bilateral involvement by occult telangiectasias

that progress to affect the visual acuity more profoundly. Group 3 patients have central loss of visual acuity in both eyes from occlusive idiopathic telangiectasias in association with varied systemic diseases or central nervous system vasculopathy. These idiopathic conditions are considered non-hereditary and must be differentiated from other secondary causes of telangiectasias including diabetic retinopathy, carotid occlusive disease, branch

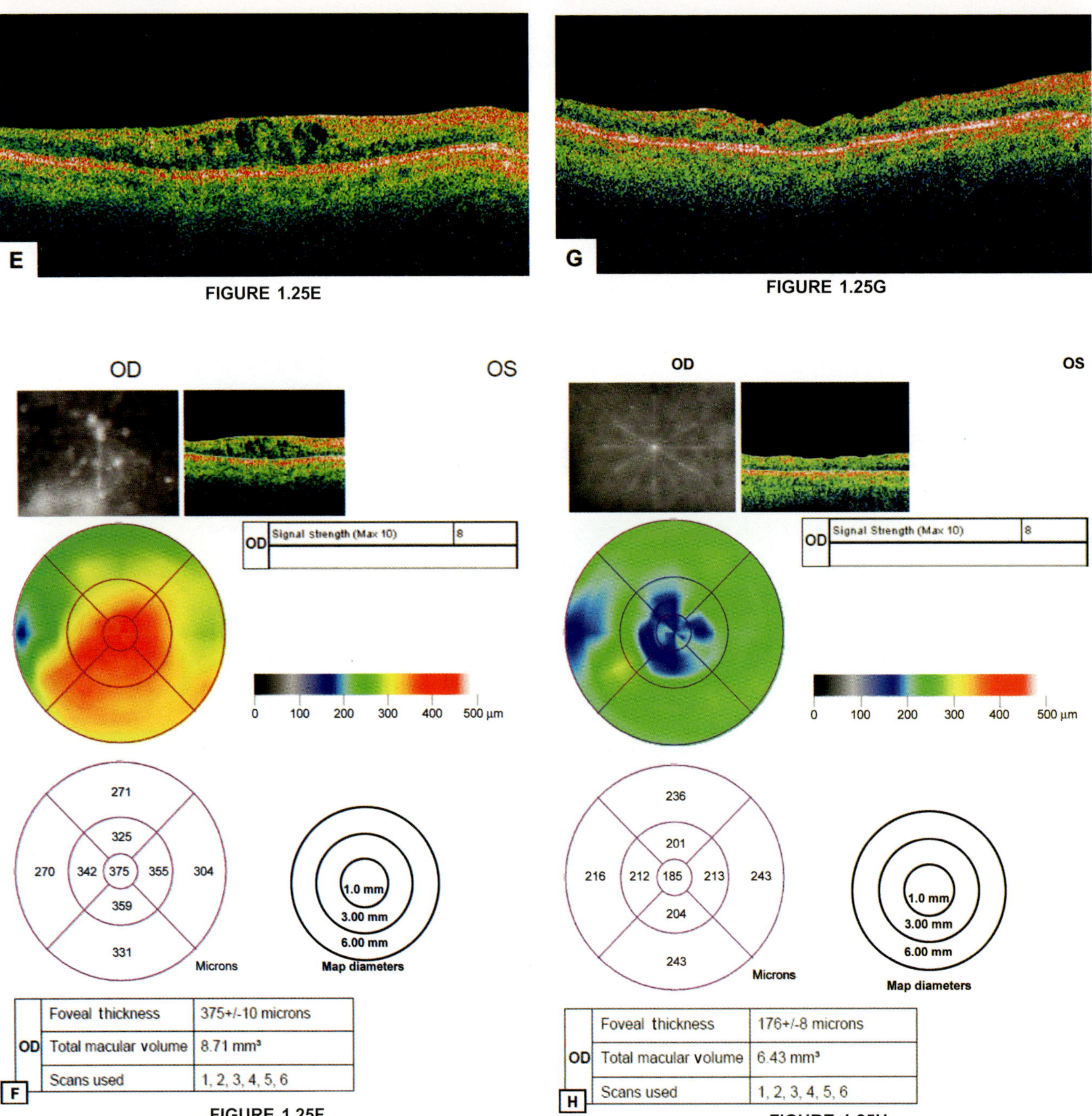

OD	Foveal thickness	375+/-10 microns
	Total macular volume	8.71 mm³
F	Scans used	1, 2, 3, 4, 5, 6

FIGURE 1.25F

OD	Foveal thickness	176+/-8 microns
	Total macular volume	6.43 mm³
H	Scans used	1, 2, 3, 4, 5, 6

FIGURE 1.25H

FIGURES 1.25A to H: A 46-year-old man presented with a visual acuity of 20/125 and dilated/tortuous vessels with retinal hemorrhages in all four quadrants (A). Fluorescein angiography showed a perfused CRVO without any neovascularization (B). The OCT scan through the fovea along the 5° meridian demonstrated cystoid macular edema and subfoveal fluid (C) with a foveal thickness of 803±184 microns and total macular volume of 16.51 mm³ (D). Over the next 11 months intravitreal triamcinolone acetonide (4 mg) was injected twice without improvement in cystoid macular edema or visual acuity. Pars plana vitrectomy combined with radial optic neurotomy and intravitreal triamcinolone acetonide was performed. Four months after surgery, the best corrected visual acuity improved to 20/64. An OCT (5° meridian) demonstrated resolution of the subretinal fluid and improvement in the macular edema (E) with a foveal thickness of 375±10 microns and total macular volume 8.71 mm³ (F). An epiretinal membrane had developed (E) and the patient underwent a second vitrectomy procedure to remove the membrane. Five months after vitrectomy and epiretinal membrane peel, the best corrected visual acuity was 20/40, and the OCT confirmed the absence of the epiretinal membrane with improved edema (G) and a foveal thickness of 176±8 microns and a total macular volume of 6.43 mm³ (H) (Sharon Fekrat MD, USA).

retinal vein occlusion, radiation retinopathy, Eales' disease and sickle cell maculopathy.

Gass and Blodi[55] modified the categorization into three groups with two subgroups each. In group 1A, patients develop mild decrease in visual acuity from 20/25 to 20/40 in one eye secondary to a one to one and a half disk areas of retinal telangiectasias in the temporal half of the macula. These telangiectasias will hyperfluoresce early and leak later. A circinate pattern of hard exudates is generally present and cystoid macular edema may develop. Patients in group 1B complain of metamorphopsia and mild blurring of vision secondary to a small area of capillary telangiectasias encompassing approximately 2 clock hours of the foveolar avascular zone. These telangiectasias will also hyperfluoresce but exhibit minimal leakage.

The most common form of idiopathic juxtafoveal telangiectasia is the group 2A. This form generally progresses to one of five well-described stages. Patients are typically in their fifties or sixties. In the first stage, the patient is asymptomatic and reveals no remarkable findings on biomicroscopy. Angiography reveals hyperfluorescence consistent with minimal capillary dilation and late staining of the temporal fovea (Figures 1.26 and 1.27). In the second stage, the temporal aspect of the macula takes on a grayish discoloration. Development of right angle venules into outer layers of the retina is the hallmark of stage 3. Stage 4 is characterized by retinal pigment epithelium hyperplasia and migration anteriorly along the right angle venules. Finally, in stage 5, a subretinal choroidal neovascular membrane develops in the areas of retinal pigment epithelium hyperplasia. Half of all group 2A patients will have yellow refractile deposits on the inner surface of the retina and 5% will have a "yellow spot" over the fovea.

Two siblings comprise group 2B. They developed subretinal choroidal neovascular membranes with angiographically demonstrated telangiectasias and graying of the temporal macula but no right angle venules or retinal pigment epithelium hyperplasia.

Patients in groups 3A and 3B develop occlusive juxtafoveal telangiectasias in association with systemic disease and neurological vasculopathy, respectively. In group 3A, the loss of vision is fairly sudden and clinical

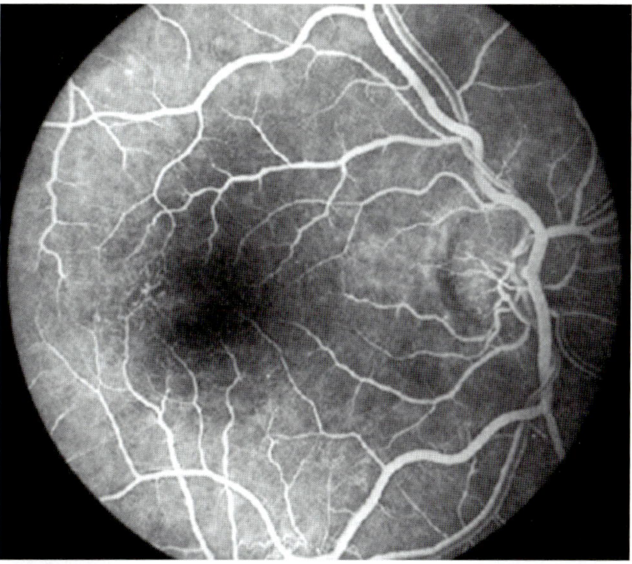

FIGURE 1.26: Laminar venous phase revealing multiple small telangiectatic structures in group 2A patient (Judy E Kim MD, USA).

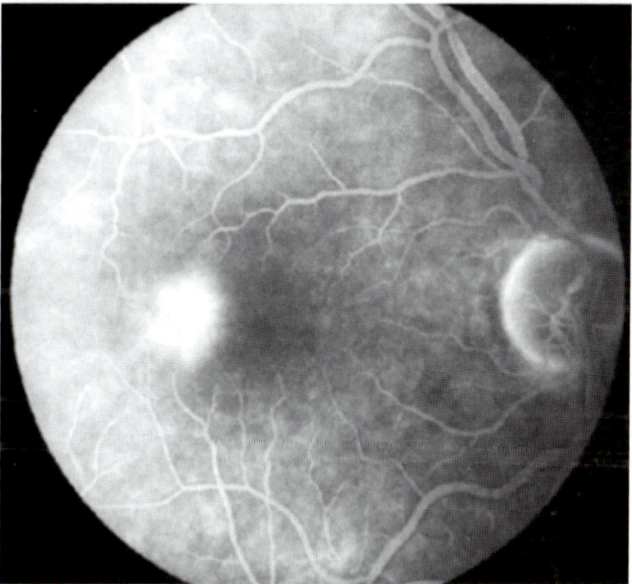

FIGURE 1.27: Late leakage at the temporal aspect of the fovea in group 2A patient (Judy E Kim MD, USA).

findings include occlusion of the perifoveal capillaries and central whitening of the macula. Telangiectasias develop as sequelae to the occlusive event and must be differentiated from radiation retinopathy, diabetic retinopathy and sickle cell retinopathy. Patients in this subgroup have varied associated systemic conditions including myeloproliferative disorders, polycythemia and ulcerative colitis. Group 3B patients also suffer from an obliteration of the perifoveal capillaries leading to central visual loss. In these patients, there are often neurological findings including diminished deep tendon reflexes and optic atrophy.

OPTICAL COHERENCE TOMOGRAPHY

Optical coherence tomography imaging of the central macula has recently been applied to patients with juxtafoveal telangiectasis group 2A.[56] These typically show well demarcated areas of nonreflective clear spaces within the retina at or near the fovea. These spaces can occur at different levels of the retina and are usually elongated (Figure 1.28). They most likely represent the lumens of telangiectactic vessels, being imaged at different "cuts" depending on the OCT scan line orientation. In a sense, what we are imaging is similar to that already described in a diagram form by Gass in his atlas, where he described presumed anatomic changes in the development of acquired juxtafoveal telangiectasia involving the deep retinal plexus. These cavities may represent areas of fluid accumulation.[57] Interestingly, despite significant late leakage noted on fluorescein angiogram, the macula is thickened only minimal to moderate degree. In some cases, there is thinning of the central retina recorded on OCT. Furthermore, there is lack of large cystoid changes seen on OCT images, unlike that of macular edema due to other retinal conditions, such as diabetic retinopathy or vein occlusions. In the eyes with lipid exudates associated with juxtafoveal telangiectasia, OCT demonstrates focal areas of intraretinal high reflectivity.[56]

In stage 4 eyes, there are areas of high reflectivity that correspond to retinal pigment epithelium migration. They block the light reflection and cast a shadow over the outer

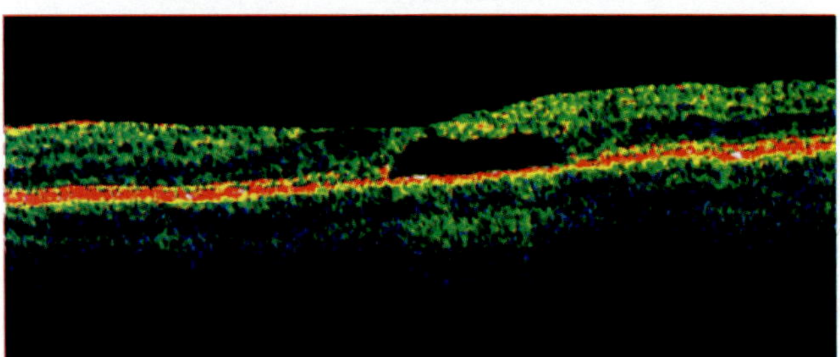

FIGURE 1.28. Spaces of low reflectivity in central fovea of group 2A patient. Note two such spaces in different layers of the retina (Judy E Kim MD, USA).

retinal layers and choroid. In stage 5 eyes, OCT images reveal changes that are consistent with presence of CNV. The CNV appears as a highly reflective mass with thickening along the retinal pigment epithelium signal. They are commonly above the retinal pigment epithelium and under the retina, consistent with the type 2 CNV described by Gass. Subretinal fluid may or may not be present on OCT, despite leakage from CNV seen on fluorescein angiogram.[56]

Due to the proximity of the group 2A telangiectasias to the fovea, treatment options have been limited and no firm guidelines have been established. Focal laser treatment has been performed in some cases to the areas of leakage seen on fluorescein angiogram, but the treatment benefit appears to be limited. Although there is a case report on the benefit of intravitreal triamcinolone acetonide injection for macular edema associated with juxtafoveal telangiectasis, further confirmation is needed in the future. For CNV associated with juxtafoveal telangiectasia, it is generally felt that those lesions closest to the foveal avascular zone should not receive thermal laser ablation so as to avoid a foveal burn and subsequent central scotoma. Photodynamic therapy alone or photodynamic therapy combined with intravitreal triamcinolone may be beneficial for treatment of choroidal neovascular membranes secondary to juxtafoveal telangiectasia. [56]

CENTRAL SEROUS CHORIORETINOPATHY

Central serous chorioretinopathy (CSR) is a condition that typically occurs in males around the age of 40 years, and is characterized by neurosensory detachment of the macula. It can present as the acute form which is classically unilateral and characterized by one or more focal leaks at the retinal pigment epithelium level on fundus fluorescein angiography. The neurosensory detachment contains clear subretinal fluid, but may be cloudy or have subretinal fibrin in some cases. It is typically self limiting and may not lead to a gross visual deficit after resolution. The chronic form, believed to be due to diffuse retinal pigment epithelium disease occurs in the older age group and is usually bilateral. It presents with diffuse retinal pigment epithelium atrophic changes, varying degrees of subretinal fluid, pigmentary alterations and flask shaped retinal pigment epithelium tracks.

ACUTE CENTRAL SEROUS CHORIORETINOPATHY

a. Thickening of the neurosensory layer at the macula with detachment.
b. Presence of retinal pigment epithelial detachment. Isolated small pigment epithelial detachment may be seen in the fellow eyes of patients with CSR.
c. Combination of both. This is seen in active CSR. The pigment epithelial detachment may be small or large and corresponds to the site of leakage on fundus fluorescein angiography (Figures 1.29 to 1.32).

Presence of moderately high reflective mass bridging the detached neurosensory retina and retinal pigment epithelium may be seen in eyes with subretinal fibrin.[58]

CHRONIC CENTRAL SEROUS CHORIORETINOPATHY

a. Presence of foveal atrophy or thinning.
b. Cystoid changes at the fovea.[58]

ASSOCIATED FINDINGS/ COMPLICATIONS

a. Rips of the retinal pigment epithelium.
b. Choroidal neovascularization.[58]

OPTICAL COHERENCE TOMOGRAPHY

Diagnosis of the Disease

Optical coherence tomography can aid in the diagnosis of the disease. Detection of neurosensory detachments can be of special use in conditions where fluorescein angiography may be contraindicated but the clinical suspicion is high.[58]

Following the Progress of the Disease

The neurosensory thickening as well as elevation is seen to reduce with resolution of the disease either spontaneously, after laser photocoagulation or photodynamic therapy.[58]

Prediction of Visual Acuity Recovery

Prediction of visual acuity recovery after macular reattachment may be made depending on the optical coherence tomography of the outer plexiform layer.[58]

Explanation of Poor Visual Acuity Recovery

Optical coherence tomography can provide an explanation for poor visual recovery in the presence of apparent resolution—may detect shallow persistent neurosensory detachment at the fovea, foveal atrophy or cystoid changes at the fovea. [58-65]

AGE-RELATED MACULAR DEGENERATION

The International community in a published classification has identified two phases in age-related macular degeneration (AMD): age-related maculopathy including all type of drusen and retinal pigment epithelium disturbances and age-related macular degeneration including the exudative (or neovascular) form and the atrophic form (with extra or juxtafoveal atrophic patches). Fluorescein angiography remains the gold standard for diagnosis and distinction of these two forms. Leakage is the key symptom of CNV in the exudative form.

Optical coherence tomography provides useful information about quantification of retinal thickness and accumulation of fluid in between or within the retinal layers. In addition, in selected cases, OCT may identify the presence of neovascular membrane, fibrous tissue or vitreoretinal adherence or traction. OCT could become a useful tool for follow-up with or without treatment.[66]

AGE-RELATED MACULOPATHY

Soft Drusen

Soft drusen are considered the most significant marker of the initial stage of age-related maculopathy. Modification in their aspect is an indicator of the risk of developing CNV. Hard drusen are considered as a sign of beginning of ageing, usually not detectable on OCT possibly due to their small size.[66]

Clinically, their shape is irregular, their size larger than 63 microns with indistinct margins, and fairly pale color. The largest drusen are usually situated closest to the fovea, while smaller soft drusen and hard drusen remain in the outer macula.

On OCT, soft drusen are easily recognized as localized multiple elevation of the hyper-reflective band of the retinal pigment epithelium-Bruch's membrane-

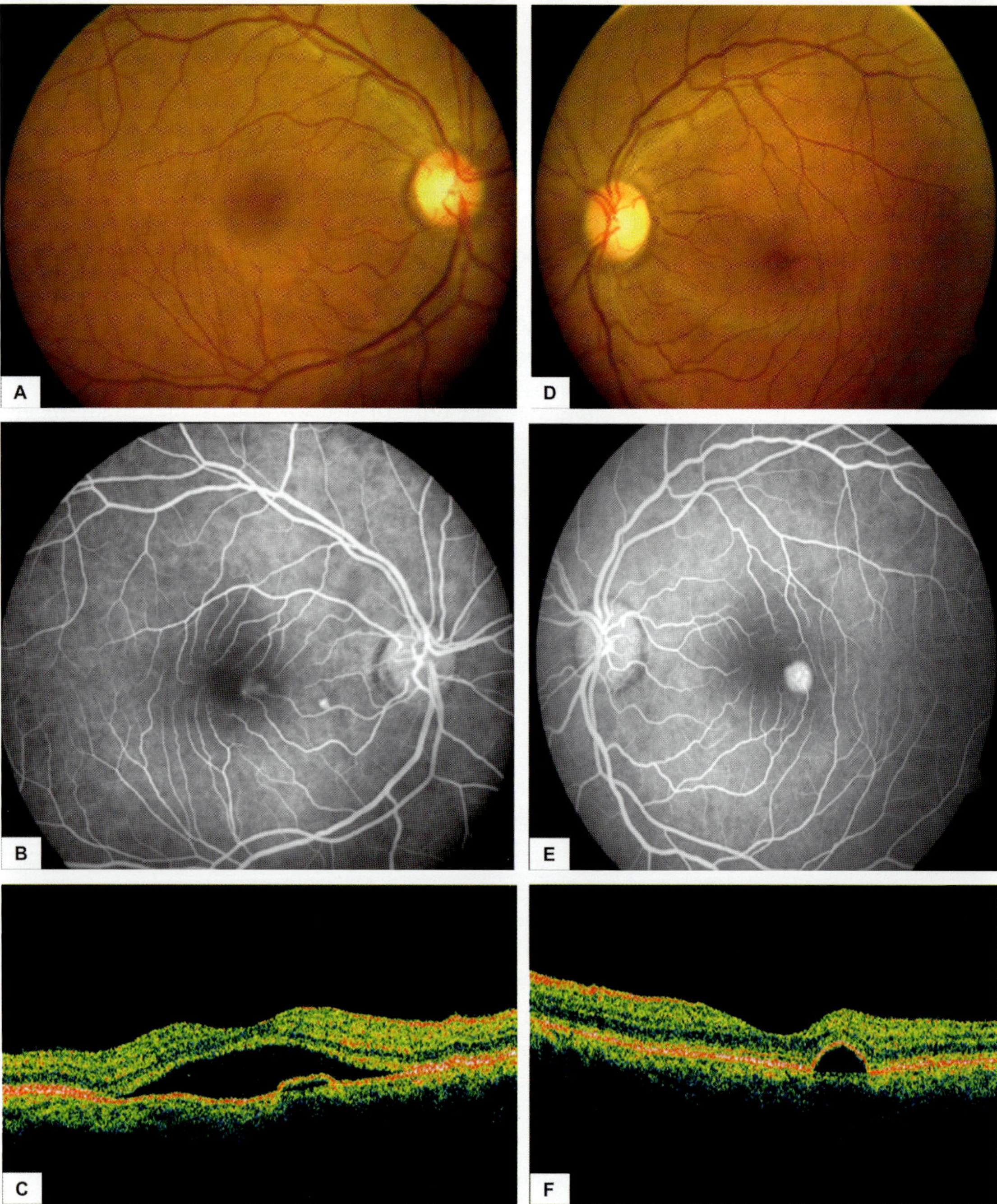

FIGURES 1.29A to F: Clinical photograph, fundus fluorescein angiogram and OCT images of the right eye of a young lady with acute centra serous retinopathy. Note the neurosensory detachment at the macula (A) with a small point leak nasal to the fovea (B). The OCT image – line scan in the horizontal meridian shows a neurosensory elevation of the macula and a small pigment epithelial detachment just nasal to the fovea. This corresponds to the leak on fluorescein angiography (C). (D to F) The asymptomatic fellow eye of the same patient showing a small pigment epithelial detachment temporal to the fovea. Note the absence of a neurosensory elevation on the OCT (Muna Bhende MS, India).

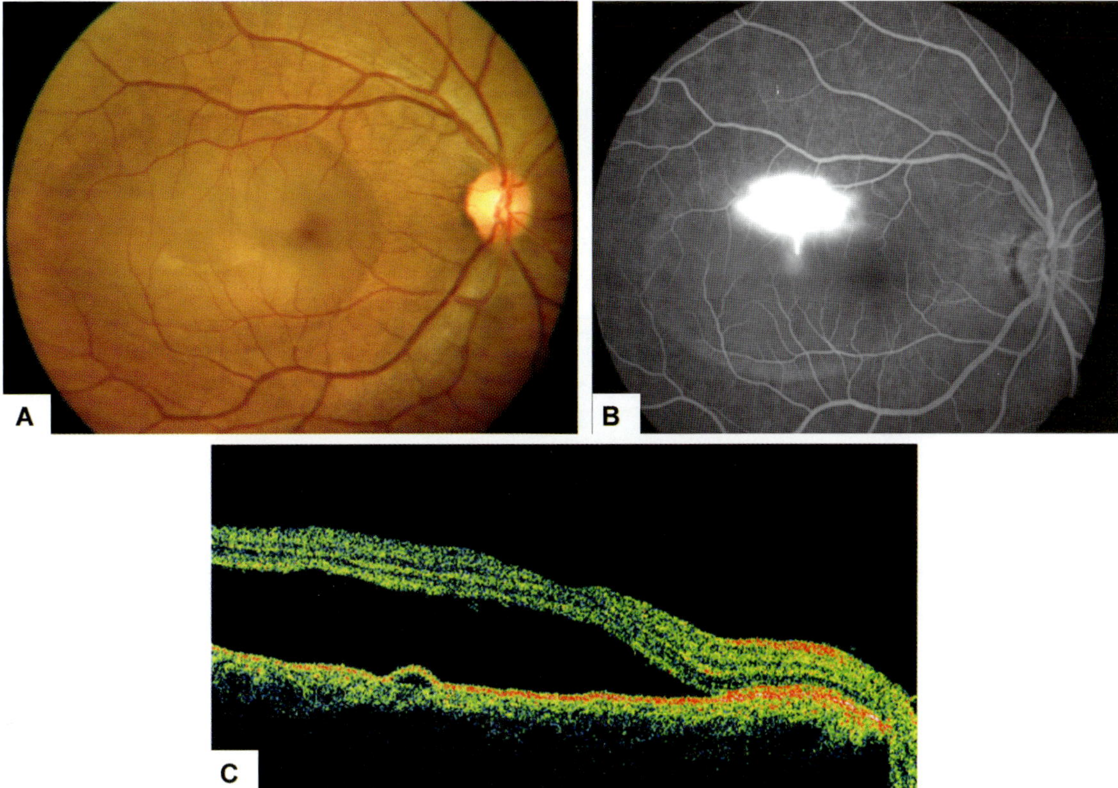

FIGURES 1.30A to C: The right eye of a young male with drop in vision of three months duration. The color photograph (A) shows a serous detachment of the macula. Fluorescein angiography shows a classical smoke stack leak of CSR (B). The OCT image (C) taken in the horizontal meridian through the area of leak on fluorescein angiography shows a large neurosensory elevation with a small elevation of the retinal pigment epithelium corresponding to the site if leak (Muna Bhende MS, India).

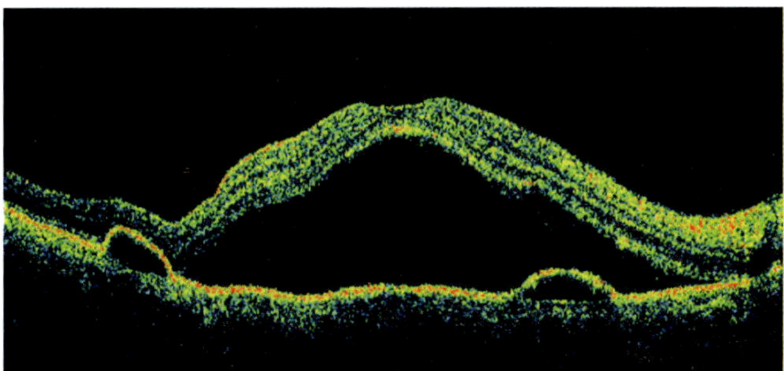

FIGURE 1.31: OCT image of a patient with acute central serous retinopathy showing a highly elevated neurosensory retina at the macula and two small pigment epithelial detachments (Muna Bhende MS, India).

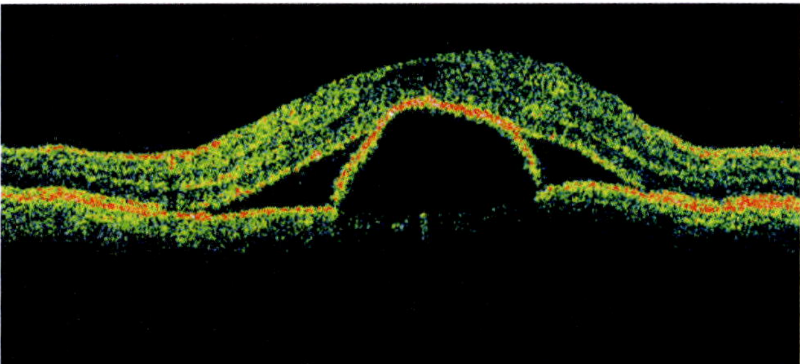

FIGURE 1.32: OCT image of a patient with a neurosensory elevation at the macula and a large serous pigment epithelial detachment under the fovea. These large pigment epithelium detachments can sometimes develop into acute tears or rips of the retinal pigment epithelium and cause sudden severe visual loss (Muna Bhende MS, India).

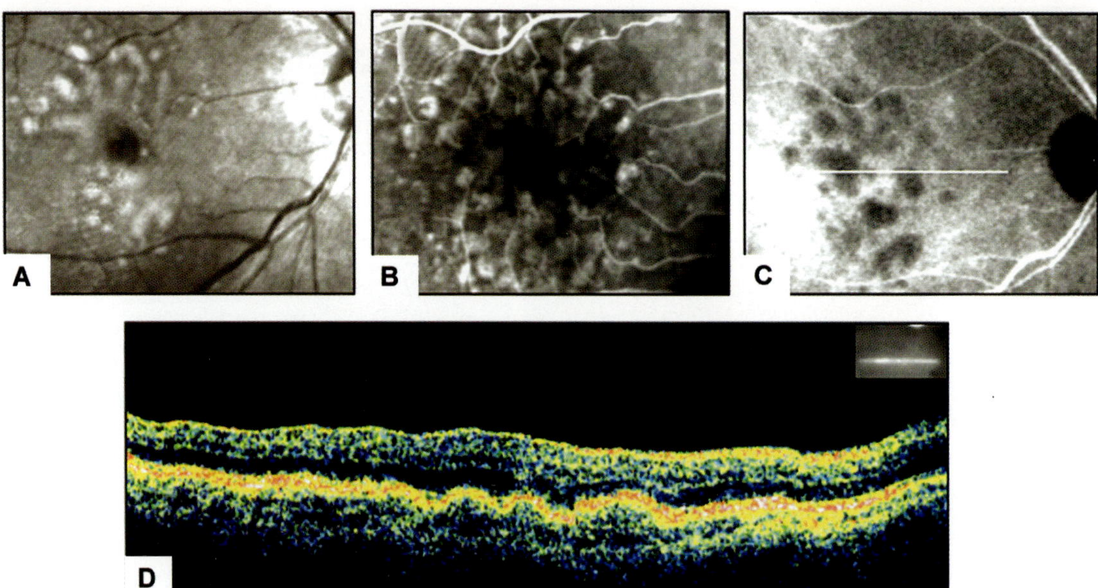

FIGURES 1.33A to D: Soft drusen. (A) Red-free photograph: Numerous macular soft drusen partially confluent. (B) FA: Late-staining drusen. (C) SLO-ICG-A: Late phase: Soft drusen of various sizes, small or large, and confluent, persistent in the late phase. (D) OCT: Corrugated iron like elevations of the retinal pigment epithelium-Bruch's membrane complex, with no shadowing towards the choroid (Prof Gisele Soubrane MD, France).

choriocapillaris complex. During progression of the disease, their elevation might increase in size, in height and become confluent or indistinct. Drusen themselves have moderate reflectivity (green in color), with no shadowing backwards to choroid. There is neither any subretinal nor intraretinal fluid accumulation. The different retinal layers remain normally organized (Figures 1.33A to D). A normal morphology of the overlying neurosensory retina with no change in thickness of the sensory retina and with conservation of the parallelism of the different reflective bands is observed.

The natural history of soft drusen is variable. They become progressively larger and confluent, of irregular shape (Figures 1.34A to D).[66]

ATROPHIC AGE-RELATED MACULAR DEGENERATION

Geographic Atrophy

Dry (atrophic, non-neovascular) age-related macular degeneration is one of the two main clinical types of AMD of equal incidence than wet AMD. Atrophic AMD is characterized by progressive loss of central vision due to loss of retinal pigment epithelium cells with atrophy of the choriocapillaris and death of central photoreceptors. Atrophic AMD is also defined by the absence of exudation and neovascularization.

Geographic atrophy may result of a number of possible manifestations (Figures 1.35A to D and 1.36A to G):

- Presence, extension, and progressive coalescence of small areas of atrophy of the retinal pigment epithelium and the overlying photoreceptors.
- Drusen regression resulting into small atrophic areas initially isolated and perifoveal, gradually enlarging around the fovea. The central sparing may persist for variable time.
- Atrophy secondary to a retinal pigment epithelium tear with retraction of the retinal pigment epithelium.
- Flattening of elevated retinal pigment epithelium and disappearance of any accumulated material (fluid or drusenoid pigment epithelium detachment or pseudo-vitelliform dystrophy).

Clinically, hypopigmentation or depigmentation of the retinal pigment epithelium with clear-cut areas of atrophy, with or without pigmentary migration and drusen, may be seen on biomicroscopic examination, depending on

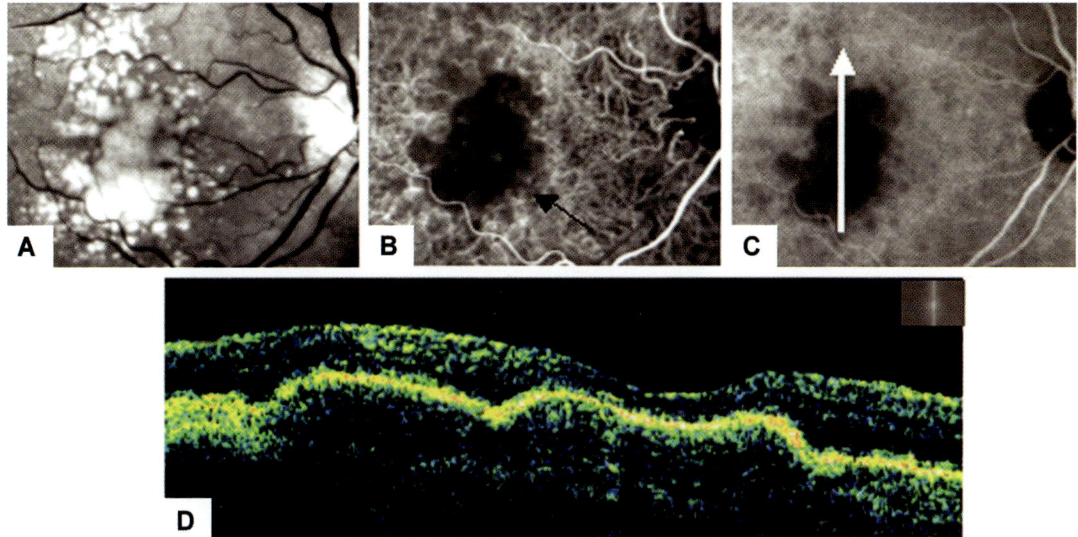

FIGURES 1.34A to D: Confluent soft drusen. (A and B) Red-free photograph and FA: Confluent drusen or moderate drusenoid pigment epithelial detachment, relatively well demarcated and surrounded by many drusen small or large. No signs of CNV. (C) SLO-ICG: The confluent drusen are dark and well delimited. Neither hyperfluorescence nor signs of the presence of CNV are evident at this stage. (D) OCT: Irregular elevation of the retinal pigment epithelium band due to larger confluent drusen, with no shadowing toward the choroid (Prof Gisele Soubrane MD, France).

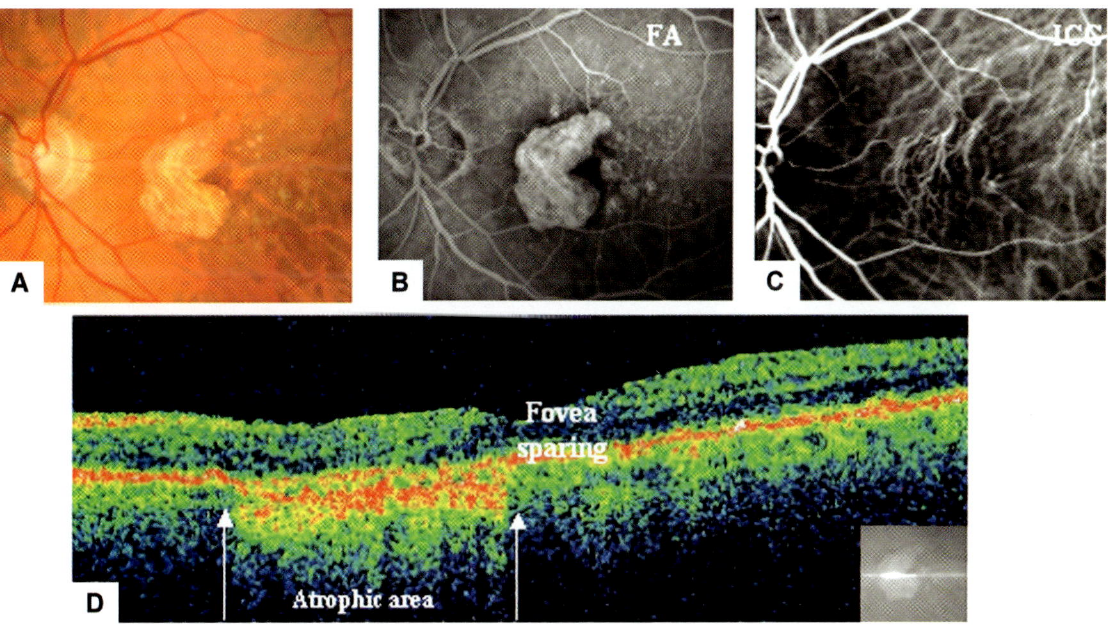

FIGURES 1.35A to D: Atrophic AMD with foveal sparing. (A) Color: Extensive, irregular, discolored, and well-demarcated area in the nasal part of the macula, with sparing of the temporal zone, which contains drusen. The preserved xanthophyll pigment in the foveal center appears dark. (B and C) FA and ICG-A: Progressive abnormal hyperfluorescence of the atrophic area (window defect), sparing the foveal center. On ICG-A, enhanced visibility of choroidal vessels in the atrophic area, with fewer branches. (D) OCT: Hyper-reflective band extending toward the choroid with retinal thinning throughout the atrophic area (Prof Gisele Soubrane MD, France).

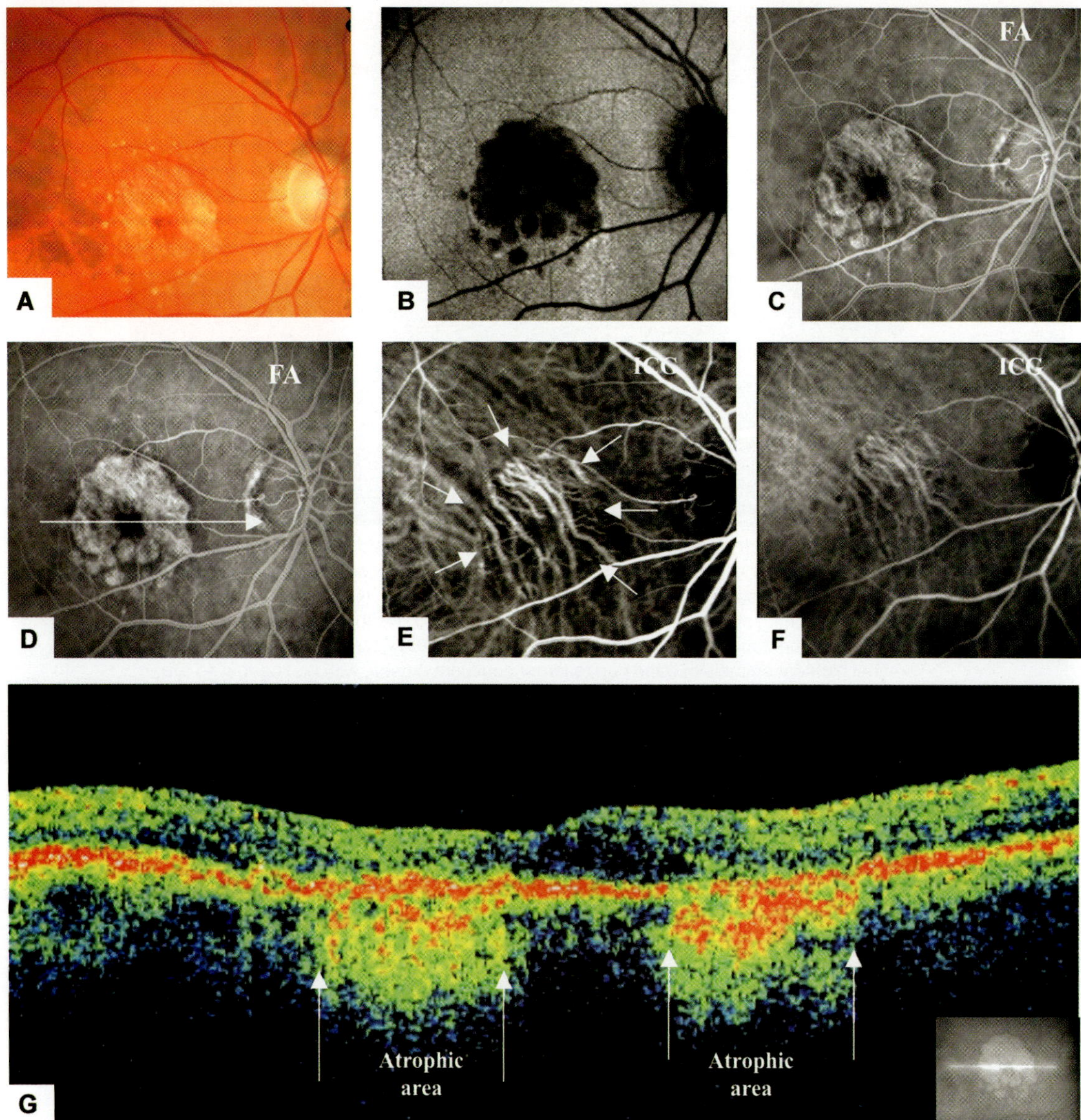

FIGURES 1.36A to G: Geographic atrophy with foveal sparing. (A and B) Color and auto-fluorescence demonstrate a perifoveal, beagle-like, slightly irregular but well-demarcated discolored area. In its center, a small, darker area of preserved xanthophyll pigment is seen. Absence of auto-fluorescence of all the atrophic area. (C and D) On FA, progressive hyperfluorescence and window defect with central sparing. Several soft drusen can be seen in the inferior region. (E and F) ICG angiography: Large choroidal vessels cross the area of atrophy. (G) OCT: Throughout the atrophic area, hyper-reflectivity extending deep toward the choroid with retinal thinning. The central area, which is spared, presents abnormal retinal pigment epithelium-Bruch's membrane band with back shadowing at this level (Prof Gisele Soubrane MD, France).

the extent and location of the lesions. Loss of visual acuity initially moderate may become severe.

On OCT, an atrophic area manifests as:

- A decrease in thickness of the neurosensory retina
- A disappearance of the hyporeflective band corresponding to the photoreceptors
- An increased hyper-reflectivity of the retinal pigment epithelium-Bruch's membrane-choriocapillaris extending back toward the underlying choroid.

The atrophic lesion may be of varying extent with clear-cut limits. When the central macula is involved, the foveal depression is flattened and the neurosensory retina progressively thinned confirms the existence of retinal pigment epithelium atrophy observed with the other imaging methods. [66]

Exudative Age-related Macular Degeneration

Optical coherence tomography is of major interest in exudative maculopathy in providing on one hand, indirect signs, strongly suggestive of leaking vessels and, on the other hand, direct signs of CNV.

The indirect signs, difficult to visualize on fluorescein angiography but obvious on OCT scans include:

- Increase in retinal thickness due to accumulation of either subretinal or intraretinal fluid
- Decrease or even disappearance of the foveal depression
- Detachment of the neurosensory retina
- Detachment of the retinal pigment epithelium (serous, hemorrhagic or fibrovascular) resulting sometimes in a retinal pigment epithelium tear.

The direct signs due to choroidal new vessels themselves are well-imaged on fluorescein angiography but discrete on OCT and require a precise analysis of perfectly focused sections. OCT scans are best oriented by the features observed on fluorescein and indocyanine green angiography. Optical coherence tomography will confirm the CNV and will precise the topography of the new vessels, their exact extent, their relation with the retinal pigment epithelium and the neurosensory retina and their degree of activity. The indications for treatment are based on confrontation of imaging techniques. [66]

A. Classic Choroidal Neovascularization

The classic form of CNV is the typical variant of exudative AMD. It requires urgent treatment. There are several treatment options (direct laser photocoagulation, photodynamic therapy with verteporfin and intravitreal anti-angiogenic drugs). These treatments need very close follow-up. Imaging techniques and OCT are particularly useful for the best management.

Clinically, reduction of visual acuity and metamorphopsia are highly suggestive of CNV and fundus examination reveals characteristic exudative changes (fluid, hemorrhages, and lipids).

On OCT, active classic CNV will be disclose direct and indirect exudative symptoms:

The direct signs are not always clearly defined corresponding to the dimension, location, shape and the stage of progression of CNV.

Typically, classic CNV disclose as a hyper-reflective, fusiform area of thickening, above and adjacent to the retinal pigment epithelium usually separated by a thin less reflective band. The shadowing underneath the retinal pigment epithelium towards the choroid is usually marked (Figures 1.37A to C).

The indirect exudative signs associate increase of thickness of the sensory retina due to intra-retina fluid accumulation (Figures 1.38A to C), flattening of the foveal depression. Conversely, the eventual persistence of the foveal depression provides additive landmarks for the exact location and extension of the CNV detachment and elevation of the neurosensory retina may be associated without or with cystic spaces. Retinal pigment epithelium

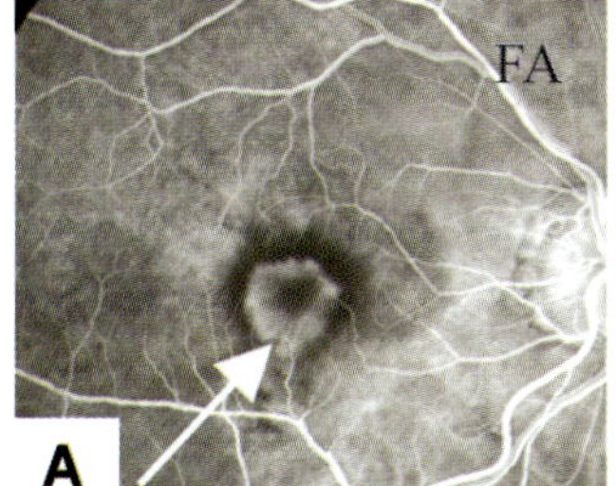
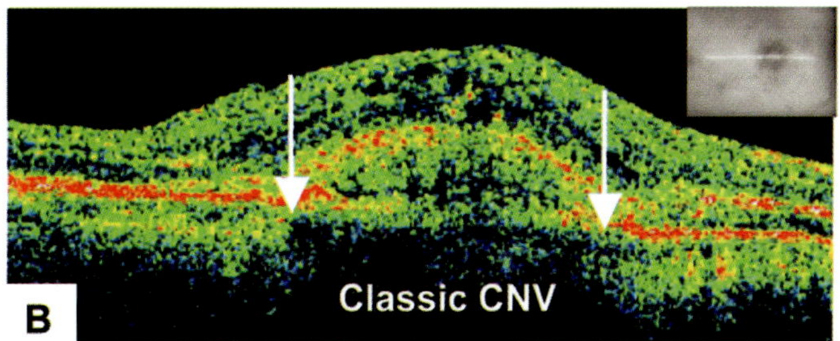
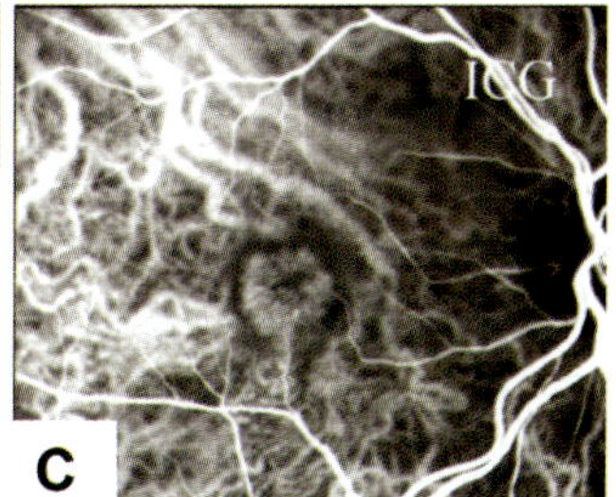

FIGURES 1.37A to C: Recent-onset typical classic CNV. (A) FA: Small (one disc diameter) "cartwheel"-shaped hyperfluorescence (white arrow) surrounded by hyper-pigmented ring (black arrow),that will be masqued by late leakage. (B) OCT: Intraretinal fluid accumulates and forms cystic spaces in the sensory retina. Classic CNV presents as a hyper-reflective band anterior to the RPE, separated by a less reflective area and inducing posterior shadowing in the area between the arrows. (C) ICG-A: Rapid filling of the CNV with late staining (hyperfluorescence). The aspect is similar to that of the image seen on FA but on late-phase ICG, there is minimal leakage (Prof Gisele Soubrane MD, France).

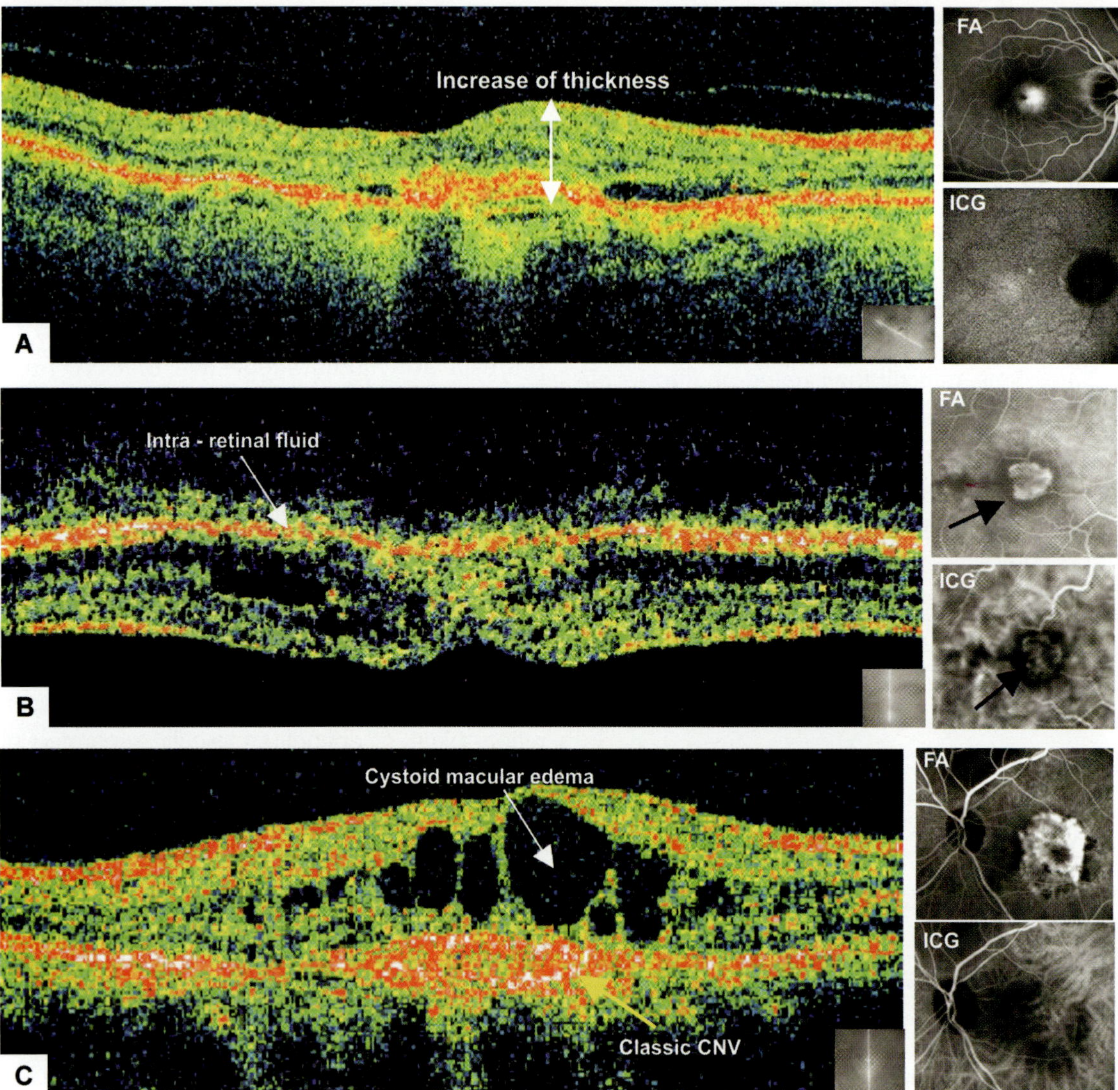

FIGURES 1.38A to C: Exudative AMD, indirects signs. (A) Increase of thickness and intraretinal fluid accumulation with small juxtafoveal intraretinal cyst. (B) Progressive flattening of foveal depression associated with intraretinal fluid accumulation and increase of thickness of the sensory retina. (C) Accentuated increase of thickness of the sensory retina associated with cystoid macular edema and large foveal cyst (Prof Gisele Soubrane MD, France).

detachment (serous or hemorrhagic) may be present if classic CNV are associated with occult CNV.

- The exudative reaction may be accentuated and elevated in active classic CNV or usually more limited as spontaneous fibrosis progressively develops.

The correlation between the presence and absence of leakage in fluorescein angiography, degree of perfusion in indocyanine green and amount of intra- or subretinal fluid in OCT give very useful information for the best management during follow-up.

The OCT features are complementary to those of fluorescein angiography and indocyanine green for selection of treatment options and their evaluation. The location of classic CNV in relation to the center of the fovea is an essential factor for treatment indication. Immediately after laser photocoagulation, after photodynamic therapy (PDT) with verteporfin or after transpupillary thermotherapy, OCT discloses a moderate to major intraretinal accumulation of fluid. This rapid response is due to either the breakdown of the external retinal barrier, or

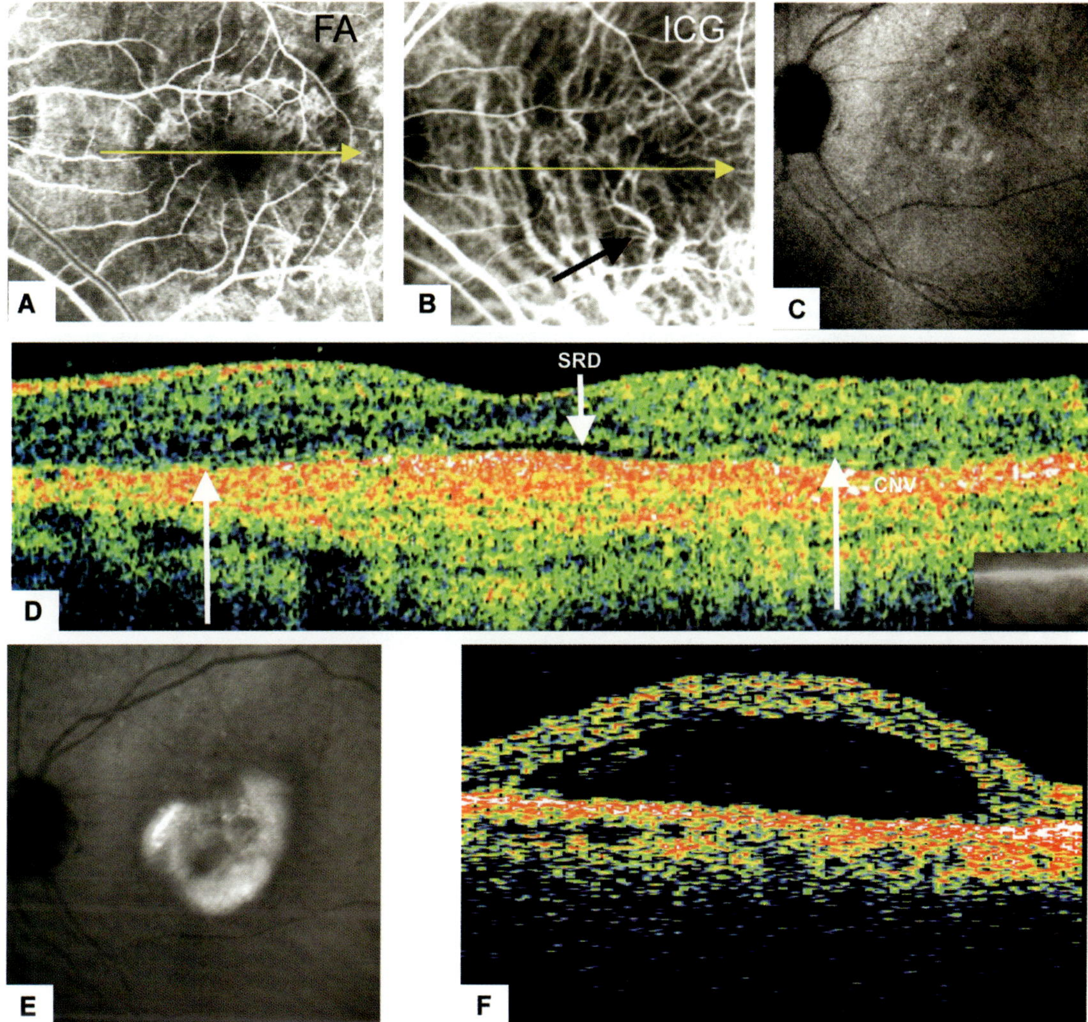

FIGURES 1.39A to F: Classic CNV, before PDT: Extensive (4 disc area), longstanding CNV. (A) FA: The contour of the CNV is outlined by fluorescein filling. The blocked hypofluorescence of the center is due to xanthophyll pigment. (B,C) ICG-A: Well-delineated CNV, with rapid wash-out and draining vessels at 5 o'clock (black arrow). Late staining. (D) OCT: Hyper-reflective fusiform area (long arrows) anterior to the RPE but separated by a (poorly visible) less reflective area. Note the thin band of overlying serous retinal detachment (small arrow). (E, F) Thirty min after PDT, ICG-A and OCT: massive leakage of ICG at distance (Prof Gisele Soubrane MD, France).

to retinal necrosis, or to inflammatory reaction, or to all of these mechanisms. Progressively the acute response will resolve. Four weeks after PDT meticulous analysis of the presence (or disappearance) of subretinal and intraretinal fluid might be of clinical relevance for indication of retreatment (Figures 1.39 and 1.40).[66]

B. *Occult Choroidal Neovascularization*

Occult CNV is the most frequent type of CNV in AMD (60% to 85%). The term "occult" emphasizes that this type of CNV is difficult to visualize, analyze, and localize on fluorescein angiography. The essential advantage of indocyanine green angiography is that it allows detection and localization of the occult CNV nearly always, analysis of the filling and staining pattern of the neovascular network and degree of activity of CNV. [66]

Occult CNV has a variable natural history, with different presentation and progression:

- The initial stage might be almost asymptomatic for many months or years (which explains why it was initially called "dormant" CNV). It is evidenced during follow-up mostly in second eyes as a late staining

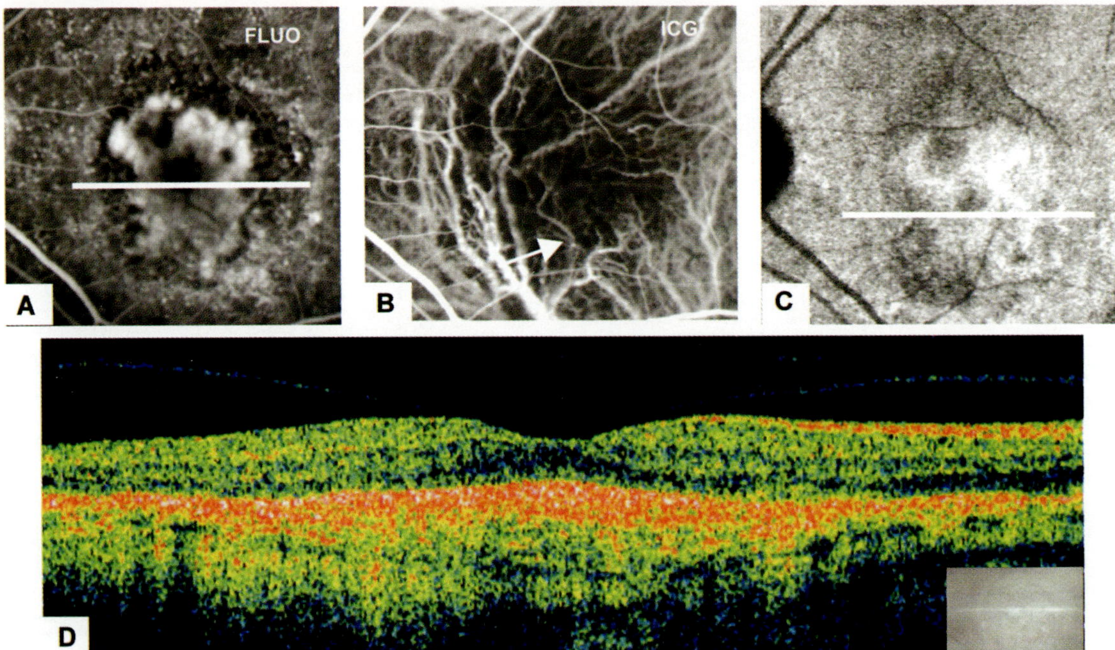

FIGURES 1.40A to D: Same case after 3 PDT sessions. (A) FA: Progressive fibrosis and retraction of the CNV edges, which become concave at the periphery. Absent or minimal leakage and persistence of the hypofluorescent (hyperpigmented ?) ring surrounding the CNV edges. (B and C) ICG-A: Practically no filling of the CNV (arrow). Late hyperfluorescent staining of fibrosis. (D) OCT: The fibrosis appears as a fusiform, hyper-reflective area, merged with the retinal pigment epithelium. No subretinal fluid accumulation (Prof Gisele Soubrane MD, France).

plaque on indocyanine green angiography (Figures 1.41A to D).

- The symptomatic phase will result either from slow progression with deterioration of visual acuity, metamorphopsia, accumulation of lipids and enlargement of the lesion (Figures 1.42A to D) or from sudden acute episodes of exacerbation (sometimes as subretinal hematoma) the development of a serous pigment epithelium detachment is an alternative way of progression to a fibrovascular pigment epithelium detachment and a large disciform scar.

- In addition, classic CNV proliferate within the occult CNV and may result in various combinations (Figures 1.43A to D) (predominantly or minimally occult).

Early diagnosis is thus essential, as the treatment of advanced occult CNV remains extremely difficult, despite considerable recent progress in this area. [66]

Typical Occult Choroidal Neovascularization

On fluorescein angiography, the occult CNV have poorly demarcated boundaries in the early and mid phase frames with late leakage from an undetermined source in the late phase frames (type II of the MPS classification). When progressing, hemorrhages, lipids and growth of the neovascular lesion will occur.

On SLO ICG, most are converted into a well defined network, filling early and encircled by a hypofluorescent halo. Progressively during the sequence, the fluorescence of the net decreases until the inversion phase of indocyanine green angiography where the CNV are barely visible on the background choroidal fluorescence. However, if the amount of fibrosis tissue is more important than the neovascular component, the typical late staining of the plaque will be evident. The association with a retinal pigment epithelium elevation (more or less accentuated) is frequent and detectable on SLO indocyanine green angiography. [66]

On OCT, direct signs of neovascularization are difficult to confirm in this initial stage but can visualize the presence of a hyper-reflective thickened band confounded with the retinal pigment epithelium usually irregular and sometimes fusiform (cigar-like) with shadowing towards

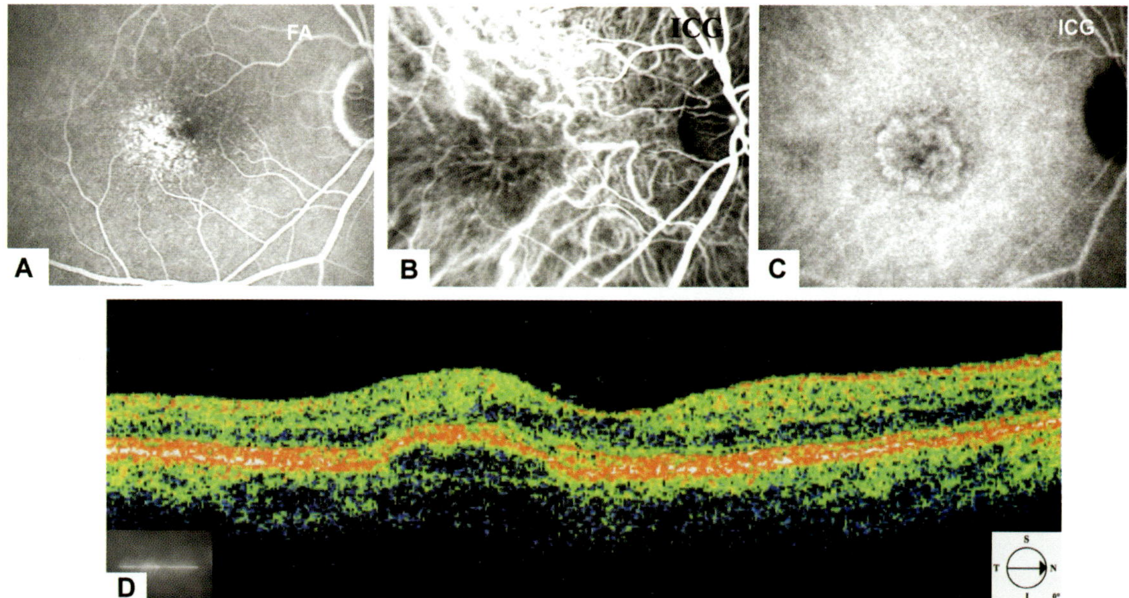

FIGURES 1.41A to D: Typical occult CNV. Initial stage. VA: 20/25. (A) FA: Stippled, poorly demarcated hyperfluorescence (arrow) with pinpoints and leakage suggestive of occult CNV. (B, C) SLO ICG-A: A 1.5 DD CNV delineated from the early phase, with late hyperfluorescence and a dark halo. This membrane is centered on the fovea. The occult CNV on FA is "converted" into a well-defined CNV network, entirely localized. (D) OCT: Slight elevation and increase of thickness of the sensory retina and the retinal pigment epithelium with moderate shadowing (Prof Gisele Soubrane MD, France).

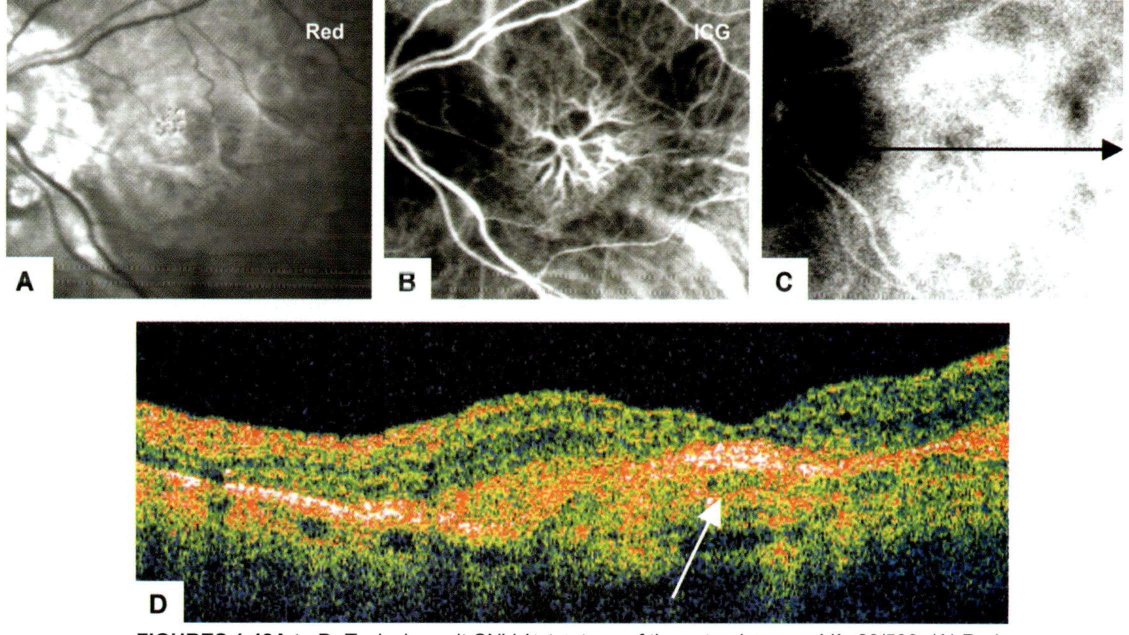

FIGURES 1.42A to D: Typical occult CNV. Late stage of the natural course. VA: 20/500. (A) Red-free photograph: Extensive fibrotic lesion with a mature neovascular network. Note the relative atrophy in the central region. (B and C) SLO ICG-A: *In the early phase*, rapid filling of the central, large-caliber neovascular network, contrasting with the peripheral vessels of the lesion small and rarefied. *In the late phase*, progressive hyperfluorescent staining of the entire fibrous lesion with minimal late leakage. (D) OCT: Absence of fluid accumulation. A large, hyper-reflective subfoveal zone, corresponding to the fibrous tissue, is obvious in the central zone (arrow). Note the relative thinning of the central sensory retina (Prof Gisele Soubrane MD, France).

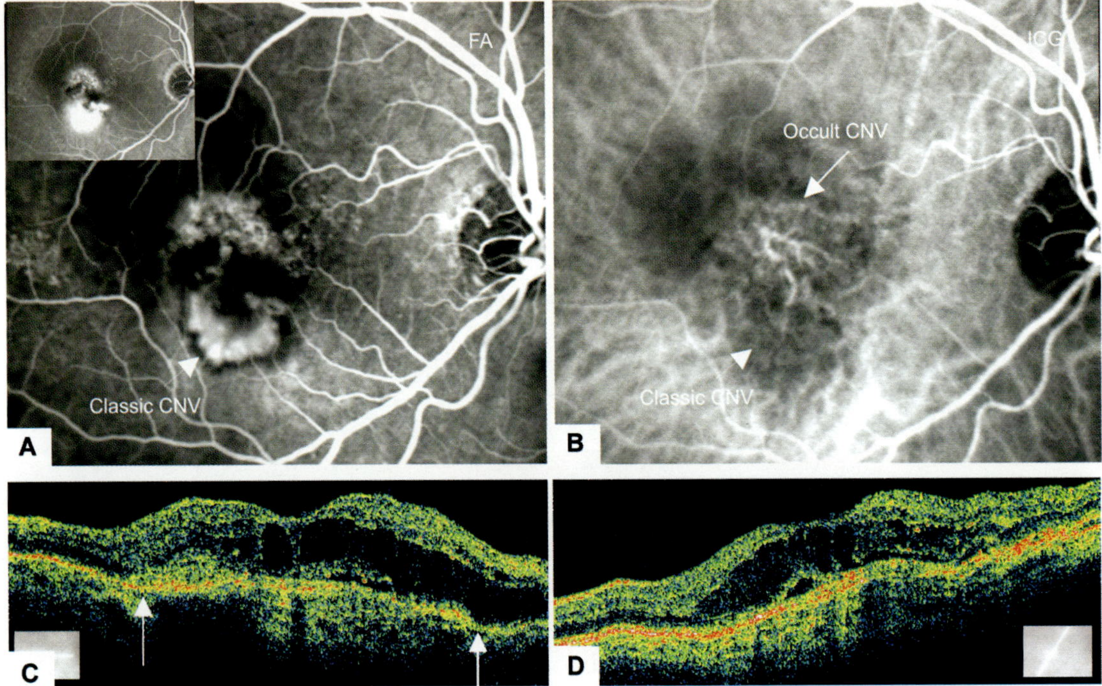

FIGURES 1.43A to D: Typical occult CNV: progression to ingrowth of classic CNV. VA: 20/80. (A) FA: Recent and rapid progression of an active classic CNV (arrow). (B) ICG-A: Well-defined occult CNV network in the upper part of the lesion. Rapid wash-out of the classic component (arrow). (C, D) OCT: Marked exudative reaction with cystoid edema (Prof Gisele Soubrane MD, France).

the choroid in the corresponding area. In a number of eyes a small and limited elevation of the retinal pigment epithelium might be underlying the hyper-reflectivity of the CNV.

The indirect signs are less prominent at this early stage. Subretinal and/or intraretinal accumulation of serous fluid with or without intraretinal cystoid edema confirms the presence of exudation from the CNV. Optical coherence tomography can also demonstrate a limited retinal pigment epithelium detachment, in the vicinity of the hyper-reflective CNV. [66]

During post-treatment follow-up, OCT provides important information about the persistence of active CNV or about the healing processes and eventual development fibrosis. Fibrotic scarring is usually evidenced by the absence of fluid and the presence of a dense, hyper-reflective zone extending posterior towards the choroid often associated to cystic spaces. [66]

Fibrovascular Pigment Epithelium Detachment
The current clinical classification of pigment epithelium detachment is based on biomicroscopic and stereoscopic analysis as well as on fluorescein angiography, indo-

cyanine green angiography, and OCT. Different types of pigment epithelium detachment secondary to AMD may be recognized:

- Avascular serous pigment epithelium detachment: extremely rare or transient in AMD (1%) (usually in young adults).
- Drusenoid pigment epithelium detachment: due to progressive confluence of soft drusen. Drusenoid pigment epithelium detachment usually remains avascular for a long time.
- Fibrovascular pigment epithelium detachment is a subgroup of occult CNV.
- Hemorrhagic pigment epithelium detachment: complication of typical occult CNV or associated with idiopathic choroidal vasculopathy
- Serous pigment epithelium detachment associated with CNV.

Fibrovascular pigment epithelium detachment is one of the common forms of exudative AMD, also recognized as type I occult CNV in the Macular Photocoagulation Study classification. It is an advanced form of occult CNV in AMD often associated with typical occult CNV that

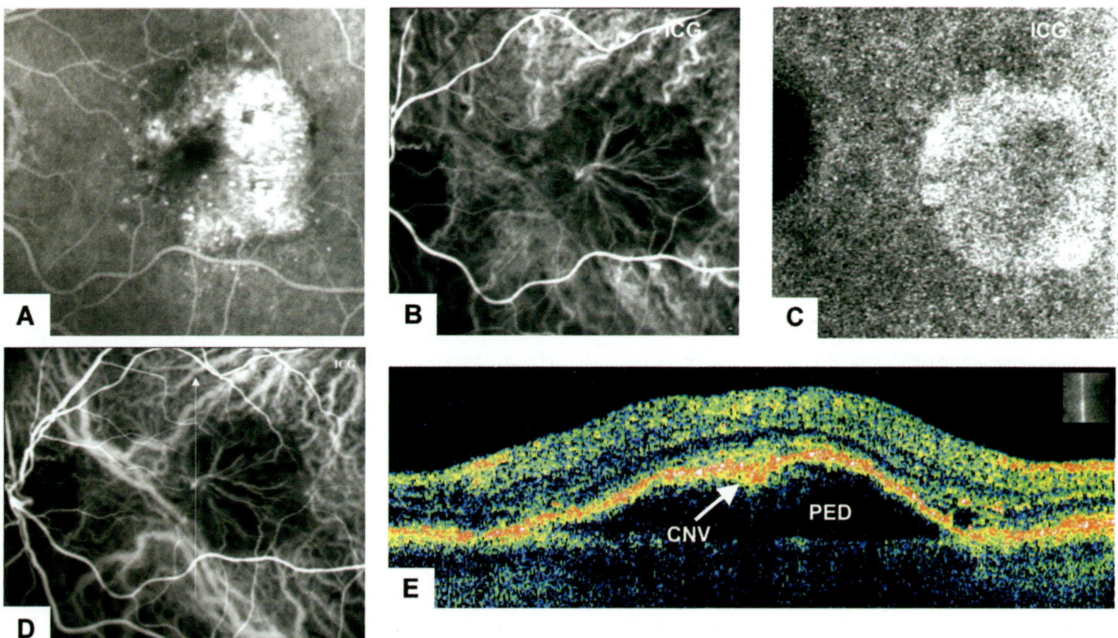

FIGURES 1.44A to E: Fibrovascular PED. Medium-sized lesion (2.5 DD). VA: 20/100. (A) FA: Irregular stippled (pinpoints) hyperfluorescence with late leakage predominant in temporal of the macula. (B to D) SLO ICG-A: The CNV is converted into an extensive network with central feeding vessels resolving in multiple branches. This network contrasts against a hypofluorescent round area representing the elevated retinal pigment epithelium. A well-demarcated hyperfluorescent plaque is observed in the very late phase (inversion phase). (E) OCT: The fibrovascular PED is evidenced on OCT examination, with an associated hyper-reflective zone related to CNV (arrow) (Prof Gisele Soubrane MD, France).

might precede its clinical detection. Decrease in vision and guarded prognosis is the main risk of fibrovascular pigment epithelium detachment.

On fluorescein angiography, an irregular elevation of the retinal pigment epithelium appears as stippled hyperfluorescence, with boundaries that are often poorly demarcated, and fluorescein leakage into the late phase of the angiogram are the characteristic features of fibrovascular pigment epithelium detachment.

On indocyanine green angiography, the occult CNV are mostly converted into a lacy network that will progressively invade the entire pigment epithelium detachment and even extend at distance.

Optical coherence tomography can distinguish a fibrovascular pigment epithelium detachment is slightly hyper-reflective. The elevated retinal pigment epithelium is highly hyper-reflective possibly due to the different focus plane. A thicker hyper-reflectivity notch appended on the choroidal side of the elevated retinal pigment epithelium might represent CNV (Figures 1.44A to E). [66]

Serous Retinal Pigment Epithelium Detachment and Occult Choroidal Neovascularization

Occult CNV associated with serous retinal pigment epithelium detachment (frequently termed "vascularized pigment epithelium detachment") is a severe clinical form of AMD. Exudation originates mainly from CNV (usually occult CNV) and plays a major role in the development of serous pigment epithelium detachment associated with AMD.

Clinical features reveal elevation of the retinal pigment epithelium that is usually well demarcated and accentuated by a light-reflex. The association with a retinal detachment, more or less accentuated is often detected.

Fluorescein angiography demonstrates the features of pigment epithelium detachment with early, progressive, uniform, bright hyperfluorescence and late pooling of fluorescein dye into the pigment epithelium detachment. The CNV may reveal as a more intense hyperfluorescent area. However, CNV may not always be distinguished within the bright hyperfluorescence of pigment epithelium detachment. The retinal pigment epithelium detachment may be observed with various clinical patterns; either the CNV is beneath or contiguous or even remote to the retinal pigment epithelium detachment, or the entire pigment epithelium detachment may be hemorrhagic, masking the CNV. In the later cases, CNV associated with fibrosis can extend into the entire area of the pigment epithelium detachment with subsequent high risk of eventual retinal pigment epithelium tear. [66]

Indocyanine green angiography reveals additional angiographic features of vascularized pigment epithelium detachment:

- With the traditional fundus camera, the serous component of the pigment epithelium detachment is seen as a well-demarcated, grayish, isofluorescent area that obscures the underlying choroidal vessels.
- With the SLO, the serous component of the pigment epithelium detachment remains dark and hypofluorescent throughout the entire angiographic sequence. Its shape and contour are well delineated until the very late phase (inversion phase).
- The hyperfluorescence of choroidal neovascularization is then, seen clearly against the dark background.

Optical coherence tomography examination provides characteristic imaging of the elevated retinal pigment epithelium in front of an optically empty space without shadowing, regardless of the dimensions and the progressively associated changes during natural history. This technique can distinguish the serous component of the pigment epithelium detachment from organized fibrovascular pigment epithelium detachment. The CNV might be suspected as a hyper-reflective notch attached to the deep face of the elevated retinal pigment epithelium.

The different imaging techniques, will distinguish the various locations of CNV:

- Either extention of varying degrees into the pigment epithelium detachment
- Or secondary to AMD at the margin of the pigment epithelium detachment. The pigment epithelium detachment has developed adjacent to the CNV (pigment epithelium detachment-notch)

- Or CNV within the pigment epithelium detachment. The so-called "hot spot" is a small and very limited lesion that is usually associated with chorioretinal anastomosis. A small juxtafoveal hemorrhage on the border of the foveal avascular zone at the end of a retinal vessel may indicate their presence. On fluorescein angiography, its identification is challenging even if not hidden by hemorrhage.

The SLO indocyanine green angiography allows detection of the anastomosis, showing dilated retinal vessels diving deeply towards the choroidal "hot spot" of occult CNV communication between one or multiple macular retinal vessels (arterial or venous) and the CNV is common and evolving.

On OCT, the elevation of the pigment epithelium detachment is associated with indirect exudative signs. The occult CNV can be suspected at the site of thickened retinal pigment epithelium (Figures 1.45 and 1.46). [66]

IDIOPATHIC EPIRETINAL MEMBRANE

An idiopathic epiretinal membrane usually develops after a partial or complete posterior vitreous detachment. It appears as a translucent membrane over the inner retinal surface in the macular area by ophthalmoscopy or biomicroscopy. Contraction of these membranes may result in various retinal pathologies, such as retinal distortion, increased thickness of the macula with or without increased permeability of retinal vessels, and cystoid macular edema.[67] Optical coherence tomography has become a valuable tool for evaluating the morphological changes caused by an epiretinal membrane.[68]

OPTICAL COHERENCE TOMOGRAPHY

An epiretinal membrane appears as a highly reflective layer on the inner retinal surface, on OCT. Occasionally, the membrane is not diffusely adherent to the retina and appears contracted with wrinkling of the retinal surface. More specifically, the morphological changes of the retina detected on OCT in eyes with epiretinal membranes are: increased retinal thickness, loss of normal foveal contour, and cystoid macular edema.[69,70] Retinoschisis has not been commonly reported, however, OCT-3 can capture

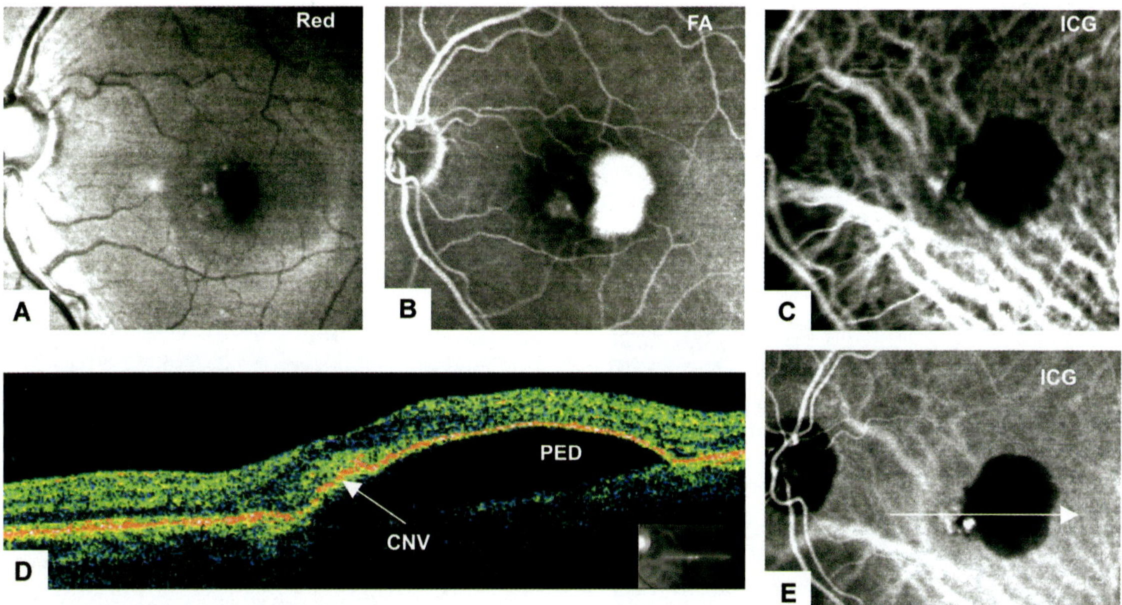

FIGURES 1.45A to E: Occult CNV associated with serous PED within a notched area. (A) Red-free photograph: Recent symptomatic, elevated, round, well-defined PED in the macular region. Note the retinal pigment epithelium changes, without hemorrhage, in the nasal juxtafoveal area. (B) FA: Small localized nasal area of hyperfluorescence demonstrating as progressive, uniform pooling of dye. The PED remains well demarcated, with a notch in the nasal region. The vascular network is undetectable. (C and D) SLO ICG-A: The serous component of the PED is hypofluorescent and remains very dark in the late phase. The PED has a round, regular shape. In the foveal region, a progressive, hyperfluorescent area is seen in the notch at the PED edge, indicating the presence of (occult) CNV (arrow). (E) OCT: Regular smooth bullous retinal pigment epithelium elevation with an optically empty space posteriorly, without shadowing. Note the hyper-reflective area (arrow) corresponding to the occult CNV (Prof Gisele Soubrane MD, France).

this condition not only in the inner layer but also in the outer layer of macular retina.[68]

After removal of the epiretinal membrane by surgery, the mean foveal and parafoveal thicknesses evaluated by OCT are significantly less; however, they are still thicker than the non-affected fellow eyes (Figures 1.47A to F).[68]

SECONDARY EPIRETINAL MEMBRANE AND MACULAR PSEUDOHOLES

Secondary epiretinal membranes are associated with a number of other ocular disorders, including limited form of proliferative vitreoretinopathy, retinal vascular diseases, intraocular inflammatory disorders, ocular trauma, all types of ocular surgeries and other diseases with blood retinal barrier breakdown.[71-74] Epiretinal membranes of differing pathogenesis have different characteristics. Epiretinal membranes occasionally induce retinal distortion that creates macular pseudoholes. Continuous contraction of epiretinal membranes may induce appearance of pseudohole to change from round or oval to slit like, but usually vision decrease is limited.[75] Visual prognosis of eyes with macular pseudoholes is generally good since foveal structure is unaffected. Optical coherence tomography provides useful information for understanding the pathology of macular pseudoholes.[76]

OPTICAL COHERENCE TOMOGRAPHY

Optical coherence tomography demonstrates epiretinal membranes as thin, highly reflective bands anterior to the retina.[76] Morphological characteristics of epiretinal membranes have been identified that allowed their separation into two distinct groups; those with focal points of attachment to the retina and those with global adherence to the retina.[77] Majority of epiretinal membranes (approximately 70%) are globally adherent to the retina.[77,78] The remaining eyes have focally adherent epiretinal membranes. Occasionally OCT cannot distinguish between the epiretinal membrane and the

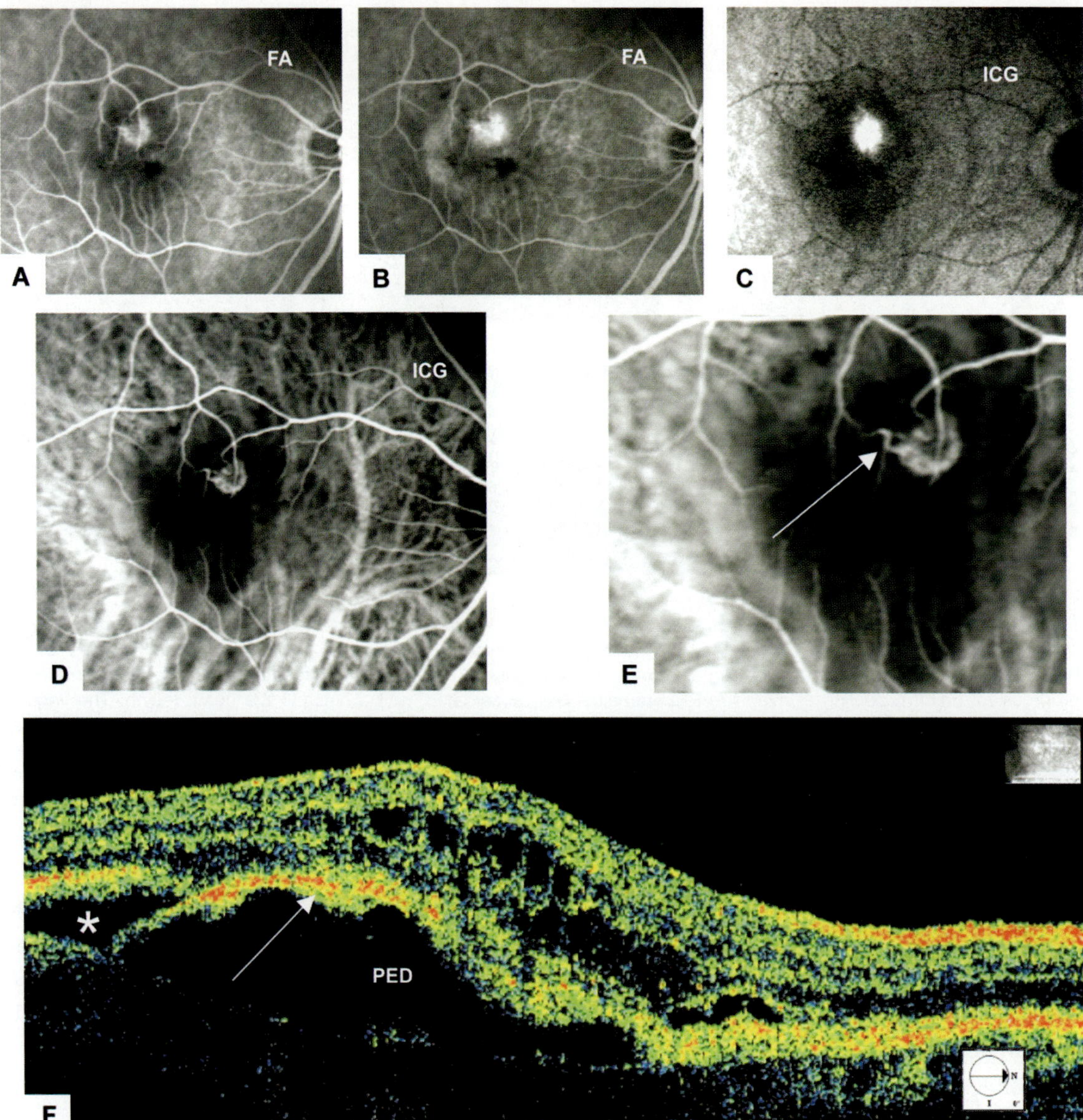

FIGURES 1.46A to F: Vascularized PED with chorioretinal anastomosis. VA: 20/50. (A and B) FA: Three-month history of symptoms. Juxtafoveal "hot spot" with lacy pattern of classic CNV and leakage "in contact" with the retinal vessels. (C to E) SLO ICG-A: Dilated macular retinal artery and venules are "diving" into the deep, lacy clearly demonstrated on the enlarged view (E) (arrow); late leakage is seen. (F) OCT: Extensive PED associated with a limited serous retinal detachment (asterix) and intra-retinal fluid accumulation with cystic spaces. Note the irregular, thinned RPE except in the hyper-reflective zone associated with the CNV (arrow) (Prof Gisele Soubrane MD, France).

anterior surface of the retina if the epiretinal membrane is globally adherent to the retina. Discriminating features are: a difference in contrast between the epiretinal membrane (higher reflectivity) and the retina (lower reflectivity) and the appearance of a membrane tuft or edge contiguous with the retinal surface.[77,78] When correlated to clinical pathogenesis, secondary epiretinal membranes are more likely to be characterized by focal retinal adhesion than are idiopathic epiretinal membranes. Idiopathic epiretinal membranes tend to be globally adherent. The majority of eyes with macular pseudoholes are associated with globally adherent membranes.[76]

An OCT image of fovea with secondary epiretinal membrane typically demonstrates diffuse thickening with

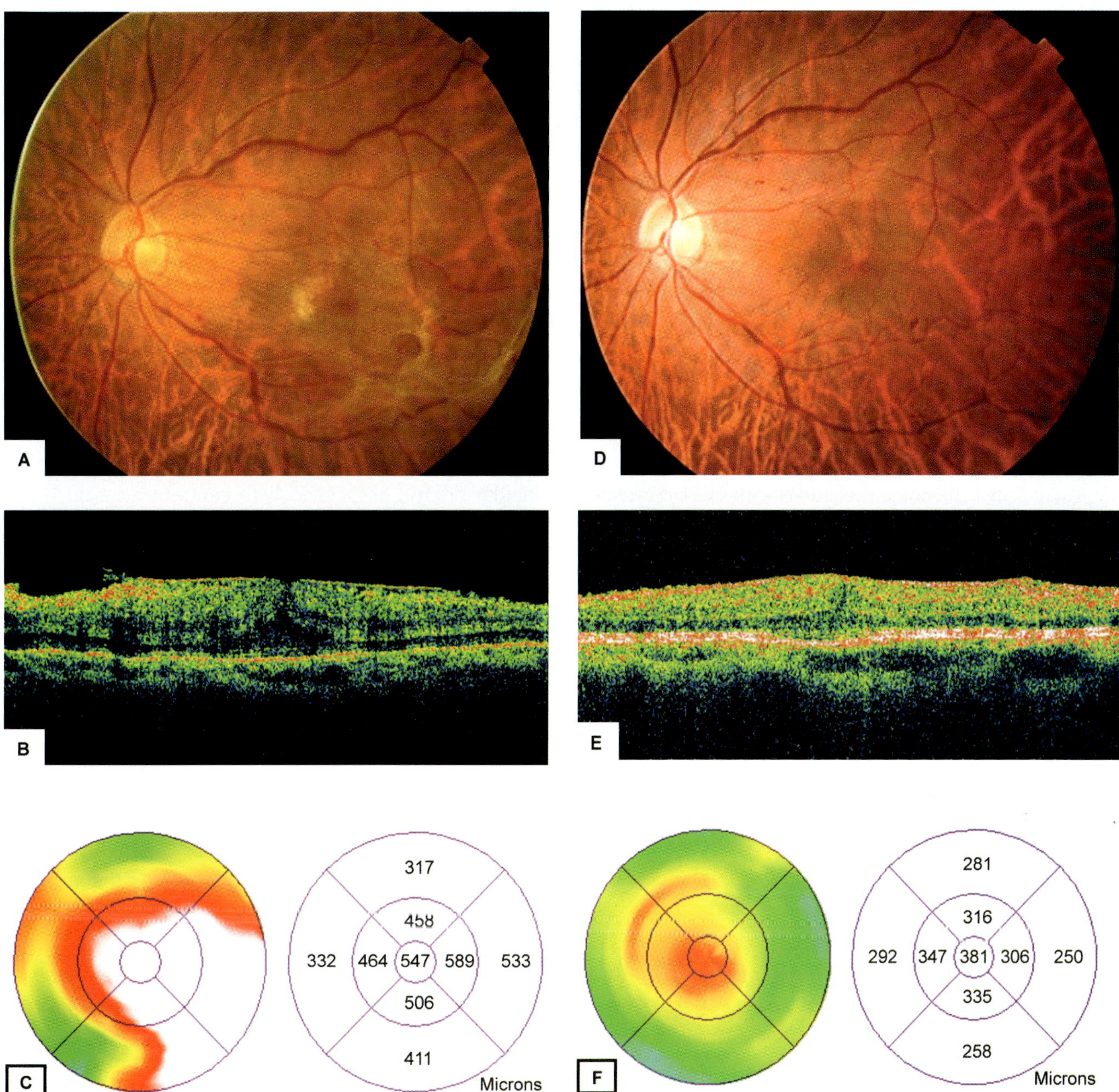

FIGURES 1.47A to F: (A) Preoperative fundus photograph. An epiretinal membrane can be seen mainly in the temporal parafoveal area. The foveal retina is slightly pulled toward the temporal epiretinal membrane. The arcade vessels, especially the inferior vessels, are also pulled toward the membrane. (B) Preoperative OCT image from a 5 mm vertical scan over the macula. Macular edema can be seen. An epiretinal membrane is observed as a bright yellowish line on the surface of the macular retina. No large cystic space can be seen in the macular edema. The foveal thickness is 532 μm. (C) Preoperative OCT map. Macular thickening is identified at the location corresponding to the epiretinal membrane. The diameters of circles are 1, 3, and 6 mm. (D) Postoperative fundus photograph 3 months after surgery. The epiretinal membrane has been completely removed. Slight hemorrhage that occurred during the epiretinal membrane peeling can still be observed. The arcade vessels and fovea are not under tension. (E) Postoperative OCT map 3 months after surgery. An epiretinal membrane is not present, however a moderate macular thickening still remains. The foveal thickness is 407μm. (F) Postoperative OCT map 3 months after surgery. Macular edema has improved (Hiroko Terasaki MD, Japan).

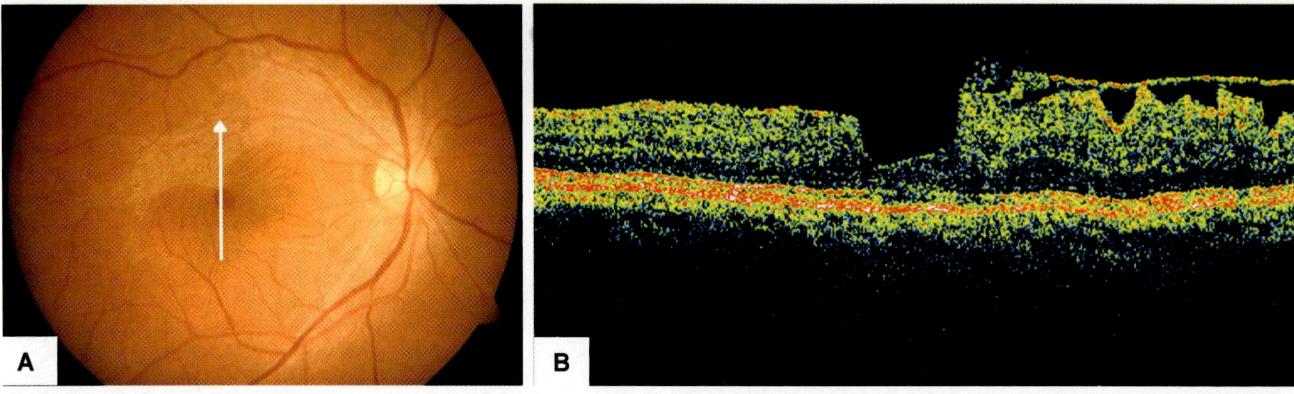

FIGURES 1.48A and B: (A) Fundus photograph shows macular pseudohole surrounded by retinal striae and dense epiretinal membrane superior to fovea. (B) An OCT scan delineates the epiretinal membrane as a highly reflective band focally adherent to the inner retinal surface superior to fovea. The foveal pit encounter is wide and steep with thin fovea at the base, representing macular pseudohole (Keisuke Mori, MD, Japan).

loss of foveal pit. In idiopathic epiretinal membranes mean central macular thickness measured with OCT correlates with visual acuity (Figures 1.48A and B).[77]

Optical coherence tomography provides beneficial information in monitoring surgical removal of epiretinal membrane and decrease of intraretinal edema after vitreous surgery. The foveal pit reappears occasionally in successful cases. However, preoperative and postoperative mean macular thickness do not correlate with postoperative vision, thus indicating that preoperative macular thickness is not predictive of postoperative visual outcome.[81]

Optical coherence tomography is also beneficial in distinguishing macular pseudoholes from ophthalmoscopically similar-appearing lesions such as macular holes, macular lamellar holes, and macular cysts.[76] Typical OCT configuration of macular pseudohole is the contour of the foveal pit, a thickening of the macular edges, a steeper foveal pit contour and the presence of normally reflective retinal tissue at the base of the pseudohole.[77,79]

VITREOMACULAR TRACTION SYNDROME

Macula is one of the regions of physiological vitreoretinal adhesions. In cases with incomplete posterior vitreous detachment persistent vitreomacular traction results in morphological distortion of macula, termed vitreomacular traction syndrome.[80,81] Vitreoretinal attachment in vitreomacular traction syndrome may vary from a broad area around the optic nerve and macula to narrow foveal zone with vitreous strands attachment. Macular distortion

induced persistent macular traction results in cystoid macular edema associated with central vision decrease and metamorphopsia.

Therapeutic intervention for these three clinical categories is vitreous surgery releasing retinal traction by removal of epiretinal membrane and posterior vitreous cortex.[76]

OPTICAL COHERENCE TOMOGRAPHY

Vitreoretinal attachment in vitreomacular traction syndrome may vary from a broad area around the optic nerve and macula to narrow foveal zone with a perifoveal vitreous detachment and focal adhesion to the fovea. Optical coherence tomography demonstrates vitreomacular tractional force due to membrane adherent to macula with attachment of the posterior hyaloid, inducing significant retinal elevation and edema. Optical coherence tomography is also useful in demonstrating anatomic response after surgery for vitreomacular traction syndrome (Figures 1.49A to G).[76,82]

IDIOPATHIC MACULAR HOLE

Idiopathic macular holes represent a retinal defect involving the fovea. Most macular holes are idiopathic, however up to 9% are traumatic and some may be associated with chronic cystoid macular edema.[83]

The pathogenesis of macular hole formation can be paralleled by optical coherence tomography with minor modification. Optical coherence tomography is able to demonstrate changes in the vitreomacular interface not

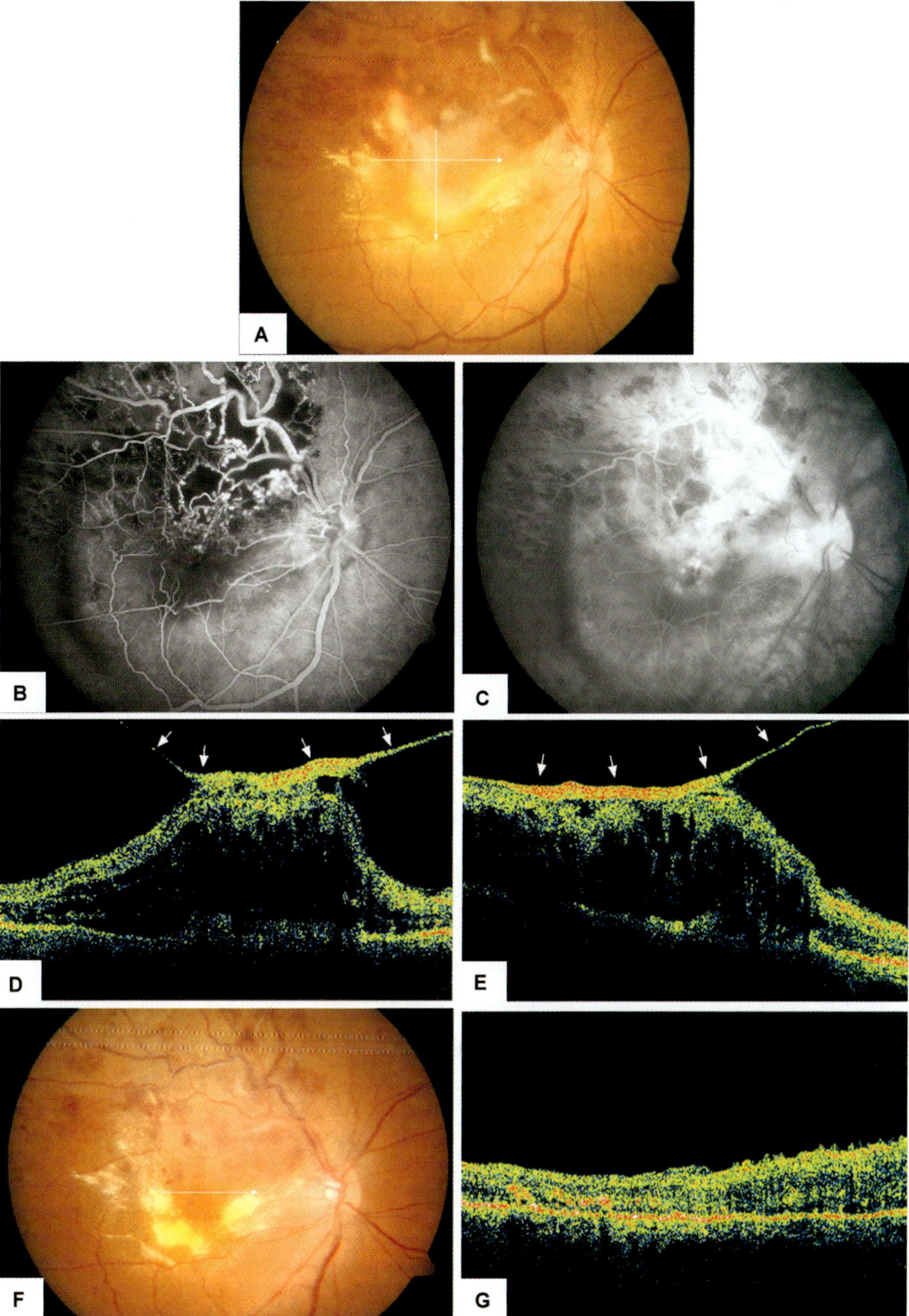

FIGURES 1.49A to G: (A) Fundus photograph before surgery demonstrates advanced branch retinal vein occlusion with glistening epiretinal fibrosis. Fluorescein angiograms of early (B) and late (C) phases demonstrate capillary occlusion and intensive vascular leakage. Horizontal (D) and vertical (E) cross sectional OCT images show dense membrane adherent to macula with attachment of the posterior hyaloid (*arrows*). The vitreomacular tractional force induces significant retinal elevation and edema. (F) Fundus photograph one-month after vitreous surgery. (G) A vertical OCT scan demonstrates release of macular traction, resolution of macular edema, relative increase of intraretinal exudation and significant reduction of retinal thickness (Keisuke Mori, MD, Japan).

visible with biomicroscopy. For example, OCT can demonstrate adherence of the vitreous to the fovea which has previously been described in histologic studies.[84,85] On OCT images, most early stage macular holes have been found to have a separation of the posterior perifoveal vitreous from the retina. A convexity of the posterior hyaloid face has been demonstrated with perifoveal separation and continued attachment at the foveola, disk and peripheral to the foveal region.[86,87] This creates a convex trampolining or tenting effect, which causes a combination of anteroposterior and tangential traction (oblique traction), resulting in macular hole formation. This force is concentrated on the foveola, particularly during eye movement.[83] Posterior vitreous detachment starting in the perifoveal region has been confirmed by anatomical studies,[88] ultrasonography, and biomicroscopy.[89,90]

OPTICAL COHERENCE TOMOGRAPHY

Optical coherence tomography images provide excellent visualization of the earliest stages of macular hole formation and demonstrate the anatomy more clearly than biomicroscopy.[83]

The OCT images show that the initial traction on the macula, as described by Gass,[91,92] is concentrated at the foveola, but with earlier separation of the vitreous from the fovea. Optical coherence tomography has demonstrated perifoveal posterior vitreous detachment in patients with early macular holes.[93] Perifoveal posterior vitreous detachment surrounding a focal area of vitreofoveal adhesion has also been demonstrated in premacular hole lesions.[94]

The staging of macular holes with OCT differs from that originally proposed by Gass.[83] Optical coherence tomography has allowed the proposal of a new staging scheme while maintaining certain conventions to allow this staging system to supplement, rather than replace, the biomicroscopic staging (Figure 1.50).[95] This convention is important for allowing comparison of previously published reports and future studies.

Optical coherence tomography of stage 1 holes reveals foveal splitting rather than foveolar detachment (Figure 1.51). On OCT images, a pseudocyst is formed and may be observed prior to a yellow spot being visible with biomicroscopy. Optical coherence tomography has shown retinal tissue at the base of the pseudocyst in stage 1A and B holes.[96] Optical coherence tomography has documented the progression to a stage 1B hole as this pseudocyst enlarges and extends to the retinal pigment epithelium. In addition to being imaged with OCT, these pseudocysts have also been described with biomicroscopic examination and confirmed with both scanning laser ophthalmoscopy as well as retinal thickness analysis.[97,98]

In distinction to biomicroscopic staging, OCT demonstrates perifoveal posterior vitreous detachment with continued adhesion at the foveola in the early stages of macular hole formation. This finding has been confirmed with ultrasonography patients with stage 1 or 2 macular holes (without opercula).[99]

Full-thickness stage 2 macular holes, less than 400 microns in diameter, result from partial or complete unroofing of the pseudocyst present in a stage 1B holes (Figure 1.52). In this stage, the posterior hyaloid face may remain attached to the roof of the pseudocyst or it may result in operculation which remains contiguous with the posterior hyaloid face. These two different forms of stage 2 holes (OCT staging) are easily differentiated with OCT imaging. This distinction is important as they may have a different natural course and/or respond differently to intervention. The classification of stage 2 holes has been subdivided: stage 2A has continued attachment of the flap to the retina and stage 2B is operculated. This new classification maintains the convention set forth by the Gass classification scheme of stage 2 holes being less than 400 microns and stage 3 being greater than in or equal to 400 microns in diameter. This is important as the conventional method has been utilized in several publications on the natural course and surgical intervention utilizing biomicroscopy and OCT for follow-up. It is important to note that former papers on OCT findings in macular holes have referred to the hole with the attached flap as stage 2 and the operculated hole as stage 3.

Stage 2 holes (OCT staging) may have posterior hyaloid which remains adherent the incompletely detached roof of the pseudocyst. This tissue has the same reflectivity on OCT as retinal tissue and in continuous with the retina prior to separation. Ezra and associates suggested that

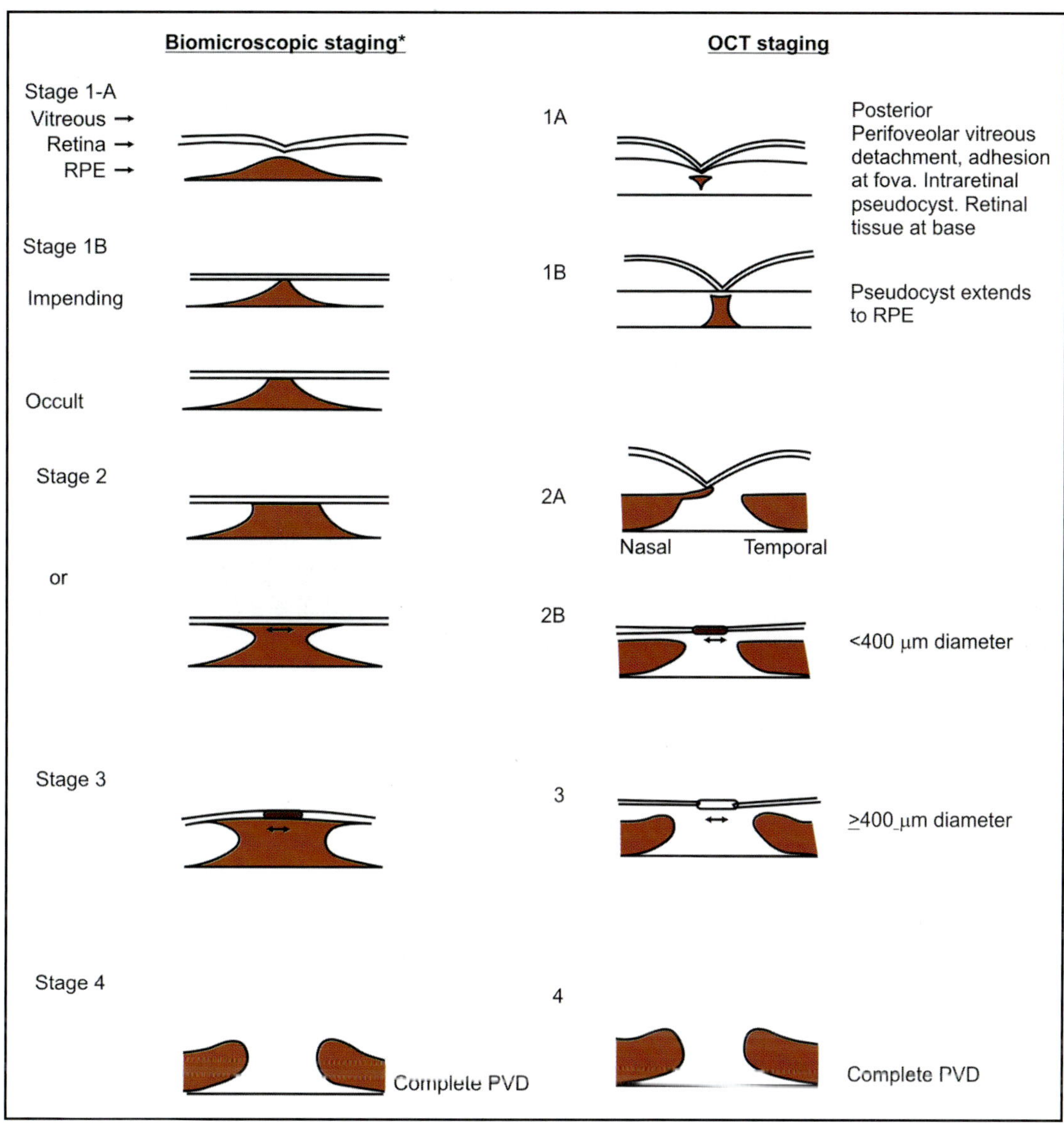

FIGURE 1.50: Illustration of biomicroscopic and OCT staging of macular holes.

Biomicroscopic staging (Gass JDM. Am J Ophthalmol 1995)

Stage 1A: Yellow spot, foveal dehiscence, posterior hyaloid attached to internal limiting membrane
Stage 1B: Yellow ring, lateral spread of photoreceptors
Stage 2: Full thickness macular hole, can opener tear or pseudooperculum, <400 μm diameter
Stage 3: Full thickness macular hole, pseudooperculum, ≥400 μm diameter
Stage 4: Full thickness macular hole with complete posterior vitreous detachment

OCT Staging

Stage 1A: Partial thickness pseudocyst with perifoveal posterior vitreous detachment
Stage 1B: Full thickness pseudocyst with roof
Stage 2A: Full thickness macular hole with partial opening of the roof, focal vitreous attachment to flap
Stage 2B: Full thickness operculated macular hole, traction to retina released
Stage 3: Full thickness operculated macular hole, traction released, ≥400 μm diameter
Stage 4: Full thickness macular hole with complete posterior vitreous detachment, vitreous face may or may not be evident on OCT.

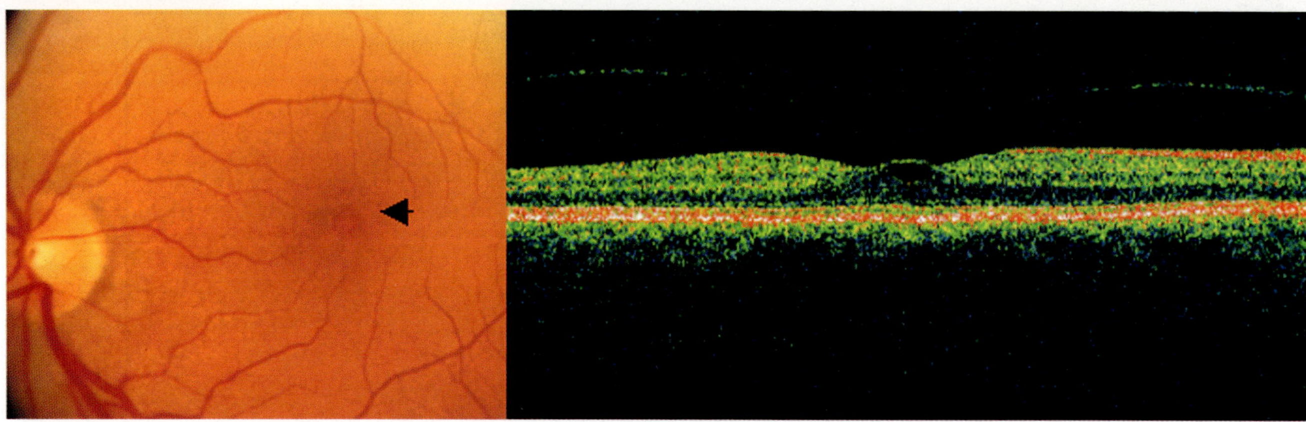

FIGURE 1.51: Stage 1A macular hole. OCT highlights perifoveolar posterior vitreous detachment with continued foveolar adherence and obliquely oriented tractional forces. Retinal tissue remains at the base of the pseudocyst (Michael S. Ip MD, USA).

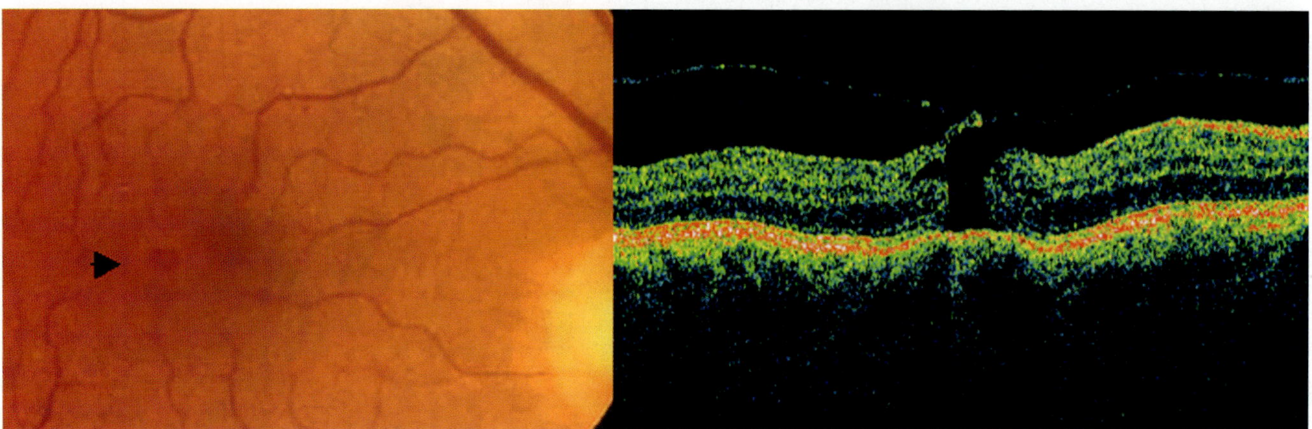

FIGURE 1.52: Stage 2A macular hole. The roof of the pseudocyst is torn which continues to have traction exerted by the vitreous attachments.

this tissue may indeed be retinal tissue. This has now been confirmed though immunohistochemical studies. Up to two-thirds of intraoperative specimens consist of cone photoreceptors, glial cells, and internal limiting membrane rather than a vitreous condensation.[83,100]

On OCT, a stage 3 hole (Figure 1.53) appears to have thickening of the retina with intraretinal cystoid spaces. In contrast to the Gass classification where the posterior hyaloid is attached in the perifoveal region, OCT reveals that in many cases the retinal traction has been released as the posterior perifoveal hyaloid face is completely separated and can be visualized anterior to the hole. The posterior hyaloid may or may not be visualized on OCT images of stage 4 holes (Figure 1.54) depending on whether it has moved too far anteriorly for imaging. A complete posterior vitreous detachment can be confirmed with biomicroscopy and ultrasonography when the vitreous face is not imaged on OCT.[83]

In summary, the significant differences in the Gass' biomicroscopic and the OCT classification of macular hole stages are:[83, 99]

1. The finding of obliquely oriented focal foveolar attachment of the posterior hyaloid face with surrounding vitreomacular separation demonstrated on OCT in distinction to the tangential traction proposed by Gass.

2. Formation of a pseudocyst with retinal tissue at the base of stage 1A holes versus the foveolar dehiscence proposed by Gass as an initial event in macular hole formation, and

3. Subdivision of stage 2 holes into two distinct anatomical appearances, which may respond differently to intervention.

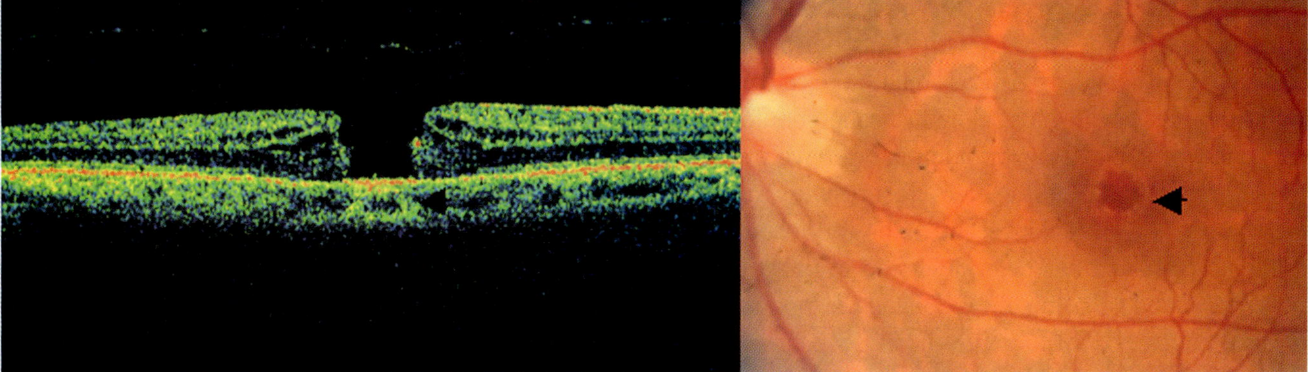

FIGURE 1.53: Stage 3 macular hole. The retinal elements have separated apart and the retina has thickened. An operculum is attached to the visible posterior hyaloid face (Michael S. Ip, MD, USA).

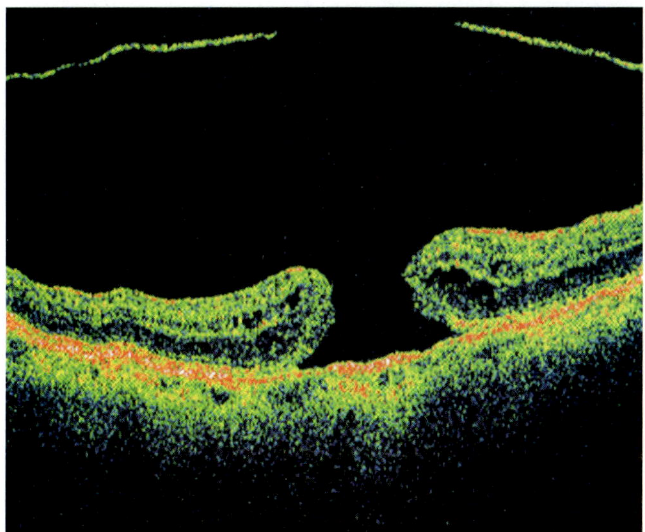

FIGURE 1.54: Stage 4 macular hole. The posterior hyaloid face is detached off the surface of the retina.

Implications on Treatment

Optical coherence tomography has improved both our understanding of the pathogenesis and staging of macular holes. Preoperative OCT can assist in the staging of macular holes and is useful in discussing surgical prognosis with patients. In addition, the images obtained with OCT can be used to enhance patient education in obtaining informed consent for surgery and in demonstrating the results of surgical intervention.[83]

Optical coherence tomography is an excellent modality for imaging premacular hole lesions and their potential progression to full thickness macular holes. Optical coherence tomography may be helpful in identifying those patients who have already developed a central hyaloid detachment and would subsequently be at reduced risk of developing a macular hole versus those who have an attachment and are at continued risk.[83]

Optical coherence tomography can also provide information concerning the risk of developing a macular hole within an individual eye because OCT delineates the anatomy in more detail than biomicroscopy. [83]

Measurements of macular hole diameter with OCT have been correlated with surgical results. There is an increased closure rate with stage 2 versus stage 3 and 4 holes.[101-103] Late reopening of the macular hole after anatomical closure was seen only in holes which measured greater than 400 microns. Based on this, it has been concluded that the preoperative hole diameter on OCT was predictive of the immediate postoperative closure rate and the rate of late reopening. Preoperative hole size is a prognostic factor for hole closure and vision outcome and indicated that the best correlation with the biomicroscopic appearance was the diameter of the hole measured at its narrowest point on OCT.[104]

Successfully repaired macular holes have been subdivided into three patterns based on OCT configuration: the U-type with normal foveal contour, the V-type with steep foveal contour and the W-type with a foveal defect of the neurosensory retina. Theses patterns have also be shown to correlate with postoperative visual acuity (U>V>W).[105]

Optical coherence tomography allows for subdivision of stage 2 macular holes into those with an elevated flap of retinal tissue with continued adherence of the posterior vitreous face and those in which an operculum or pseudo-operculum has already formed which may have implications for treatment. Patients who continue to have an adhesion may benefit from more limited surgical intervention than those who have already had a spontaneous resolution of traction but yet continue to have an open macular hole. Successful hole closure with minimal vitrectomy and dissection of this adhesion followed by fluid gas exchange has been described in patients who have continued adhesion, the OCT stage 2A appearance. Optical coherence tomography has also been used to demonstrate a gas injection induced separation of vitreofoveolar adhesion that resulted in closure of a stage 2A macular hole. [106-108] Peeling of the internal limiting membrane during the standard surgical procedure may improve macular hole closure rates. [109,110] Based on OCT findings, it is possible that this may be of greater necessity in patients who have a OCT stage 2B hole or larger rather than in patients with stage 2A holes in which more limited surgery is likely to be successful. [83]

Visualization of the retinal structures through intraocular gas or silicone oil with OCT is possible. Macular hole closure can be confirmed, by OCT, after surgery has been reported within 24 hours through gas.[111] Although early anatomical hole closure on OCT does not necessarily indicate complete healing, such evaluations may eventually assist investigators in determining the optimum length of time for prone positioning in the postoperative period. Optical coherence tomography images of closed macular holes confirm the centripetal repositioning of photoreceptors in successful surgery and mimic the histopathologic appearance of closed holes.[83,112]

SURGERY FOR CHOROIDAL NEOVASCULAR MEMBRANE

Choroidal neovascular membrane caused by several diseases such as AMD or myopia is the major cause of legal blindness. Various treatments have been attempted, including photocoagulation, photodynamic therapy, surgical removal of CNV, macular translocation and anti-VEGF aptamer. [113-133]

Surgical removal of subfoveal CNV might be effective for classic or predominantly classic CNV. The results of submacular surgery trial show a possibility of improvement of vision by surgical removal of CNV associated with ocular histoplasmosis. [117]

OPTICAL COHERENCE TOMOGRAPHY

The macula in eyes with CNV is characterized by serous retinal detachment, subretinal hemorrhage, macular edema, or serous, hemorrhagic, or fibrovascular pigment epithelial detachment. Optical coherence tomography shows the morphological images consistent with the characteristics of these changes. [134-136]

Surgical Removal of Choroidal Neovascular Membrane

Although surgical removal of subfoveal CNV may not be effective, surgical removal of juxtafoveal CNV could achieve a better visual outcome. Optical coherence tomography shows the elevation of retinal reflection and the hyper-reflective area below the retina at the macula, which is consistent with CNV resulting from AMD. After the surgery, the elevation of the retina reflection at the macula decreases and the retinal reflective thickness may be reduced, because of the reduction of macular edema (Figures 1.55A to F). [137]

Macular Translocation

Macular translocation with 360-degree retinotomy (Figures 1.56A to E) and limited macular translocation (Figures 1.57A to F) may be effective for cases with either type of CNV, classic or occult CNV. The fovea is relocated on healthier retinal pigment epithelium after macular translocation, either in macular translocation with 360-degree retinotomy or limited macular translocation. Therefore, in OCT images, the nearly normal retinal reflection is onto normal retinal pigment epithelium reflective band without the reflective lesion representing CNV or pigment epithelial detachment after the surgeries. The elevation of the reflection before the surgeries due to CNV, pigment epithelial detachment, or serous retinal detachment, may be bearing down on the almost normal retinal pigment epithelium reflection. Macular translocation with 360-degree retinotomy can achieve a large movement of the fovea and the CNV may not be seen on the same image of OCT including the fovea.

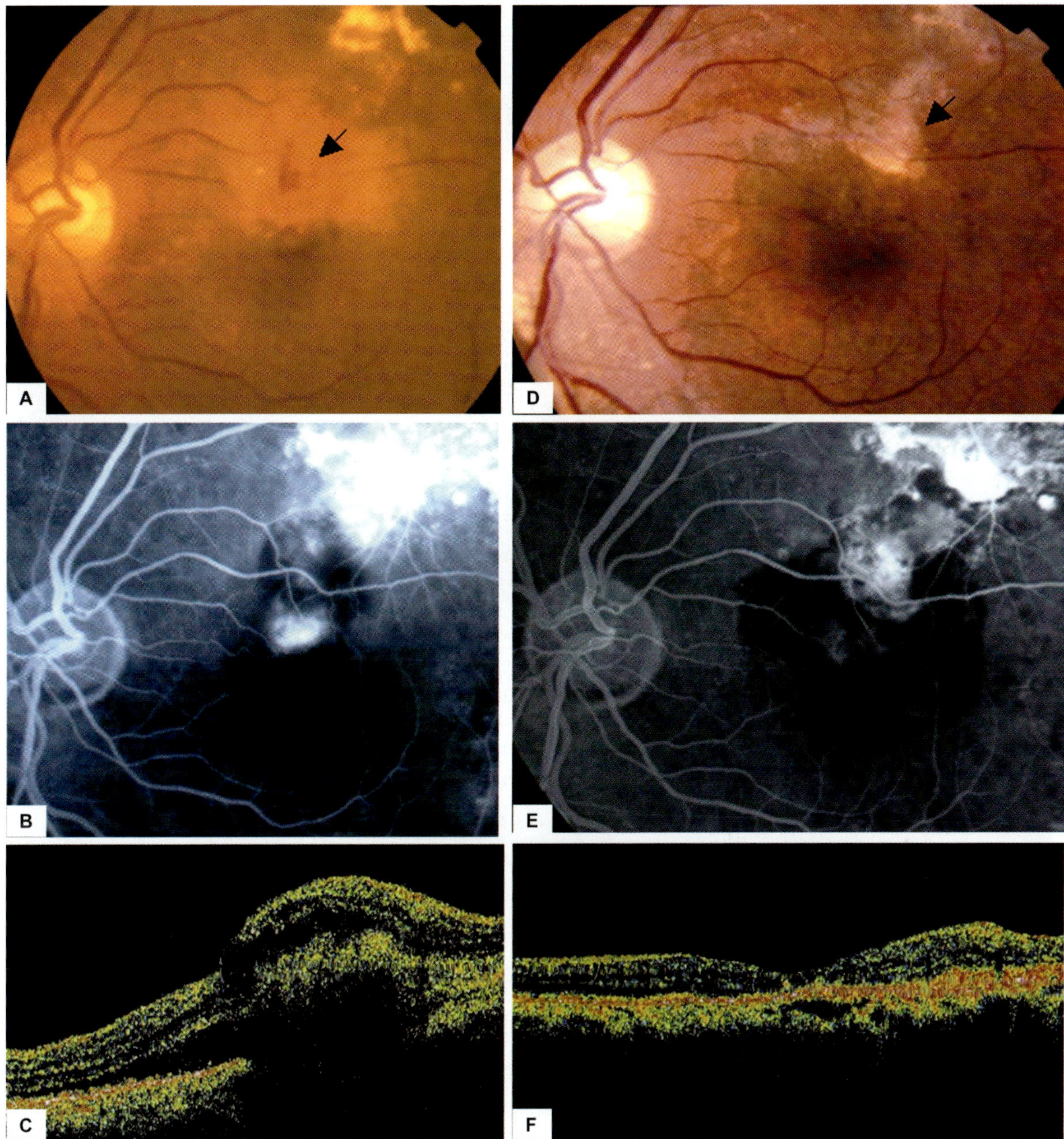

FIGURES 1.55A to F: (A) Fundus photograph of a classic CNV. An elevated subretinal lesion superior to the fovea with a small subretinal hemorrhage is revealed. (B) Fluorescein angiography of the same case. Early fluorescein angiogram shows a hyperfluorescent lesion at the juxtafoveal area which leaked more in the later phases consistent with classic CNV. (C) A vertical OCT image. A hyper-reflective region under the retinal reflectivity which is corresponding to the CNV is detected. Interestingly, the CNV located under the fovea in the OCT image while it located juxtafoveally in fluorescein angiography. The retinal pigment epithelium reflectivity is not clearly shown. The thickness of the CNV is 650 µm. The fovea has reduced intraretinal optical reflectivity which is caused from retinal edema and the thickness of the fovea is 300 µm. (D) Fundus photograph 6 months after surgical removal of CNV combined with cataract surgery. An atrophic area where CNV existed is shown. (E) Fluorescein angiography at early phase exhibits a window defect at the location of the CNV which have been probably caused from the damage of the retinal pigment epithelium when the CNV was removed. (F) A vertical OCT image. OCT reveals no CNV reflection and the clearly reduced elevation of the retina. The thickness of the retinal reflectivity reduces to 110 µm and the foveal decompression is recovered. Reflectivity of retinal pigment epithelium-choroid complex at area where CNV existed is increased. This high reflectivity is probably caused by scar formation (Prof Yasuo Tano MD, Japan).

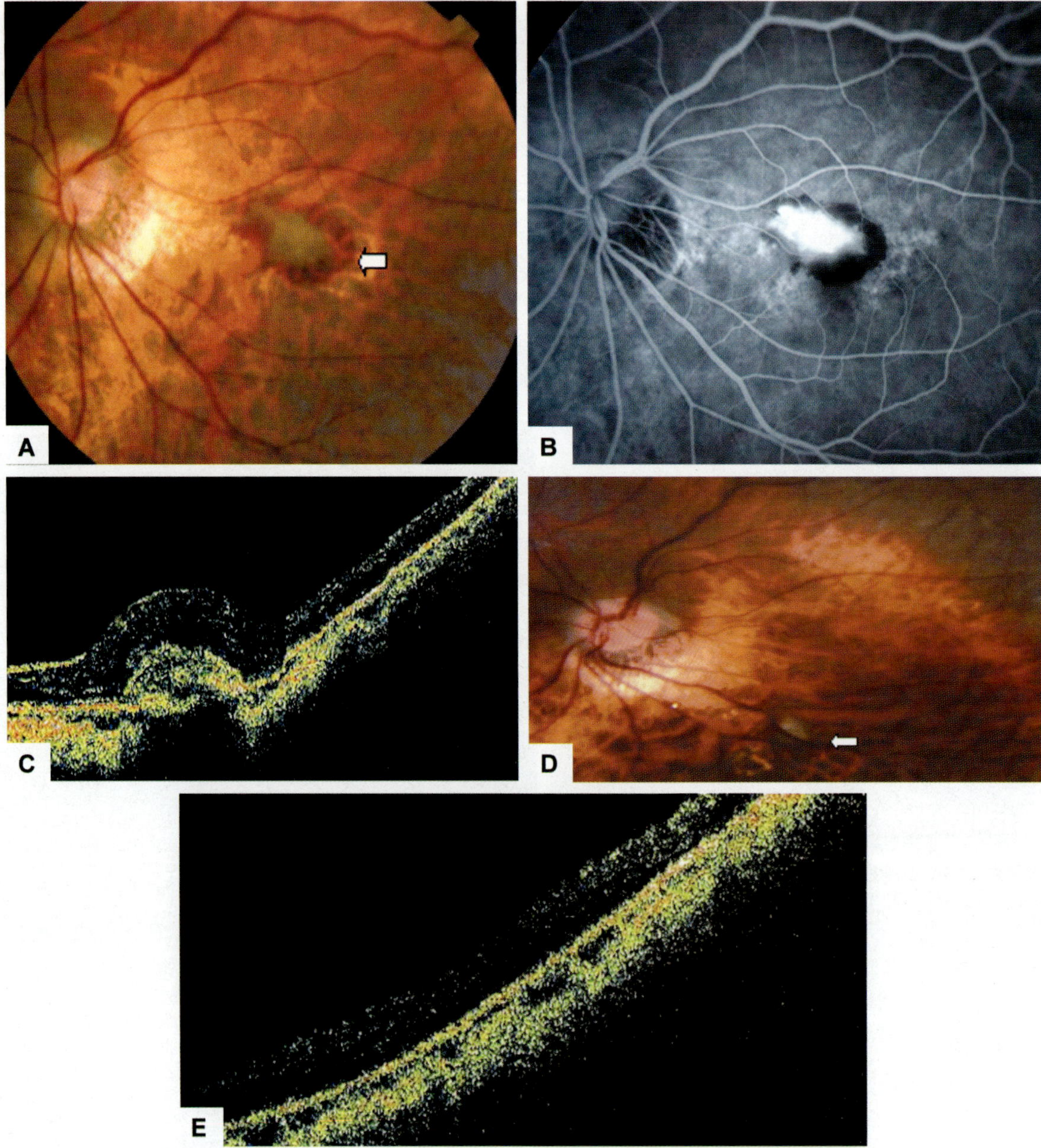

FIGURES 1.56A to E: (A) A round gray lesion with subretinal hemorrhage at the fovea. (B) Early phase fluorescein angiography. The early angiographic image reveals a well-defined area of hyperfluorescence. (C) A vertical OCT image. Optical coherence tomography shows an elevation of the retinal reflectivity and hyper-reflective lesion under the retina which is corresponding to a CNV. The thickness of the CNV is approximately 330 μm and the thickness of the swollen fovea is 360 μm. (D) Fundus photograph 12 months shows the rotation of the retina by approximately 40-degrees after macular translocation with 360-degree retinotomy. (E) A vertical OCT image. Optical coherence tomography shows no elevation of the retinal reflectivity. The decompression of the fovea is recovered and the thickness of the retina is reduced to 200 μm. The reflectivity of the retinal pigment epithelium and choroid under the new fovea is normal (Prof Yasuo Tano MD, Japan).

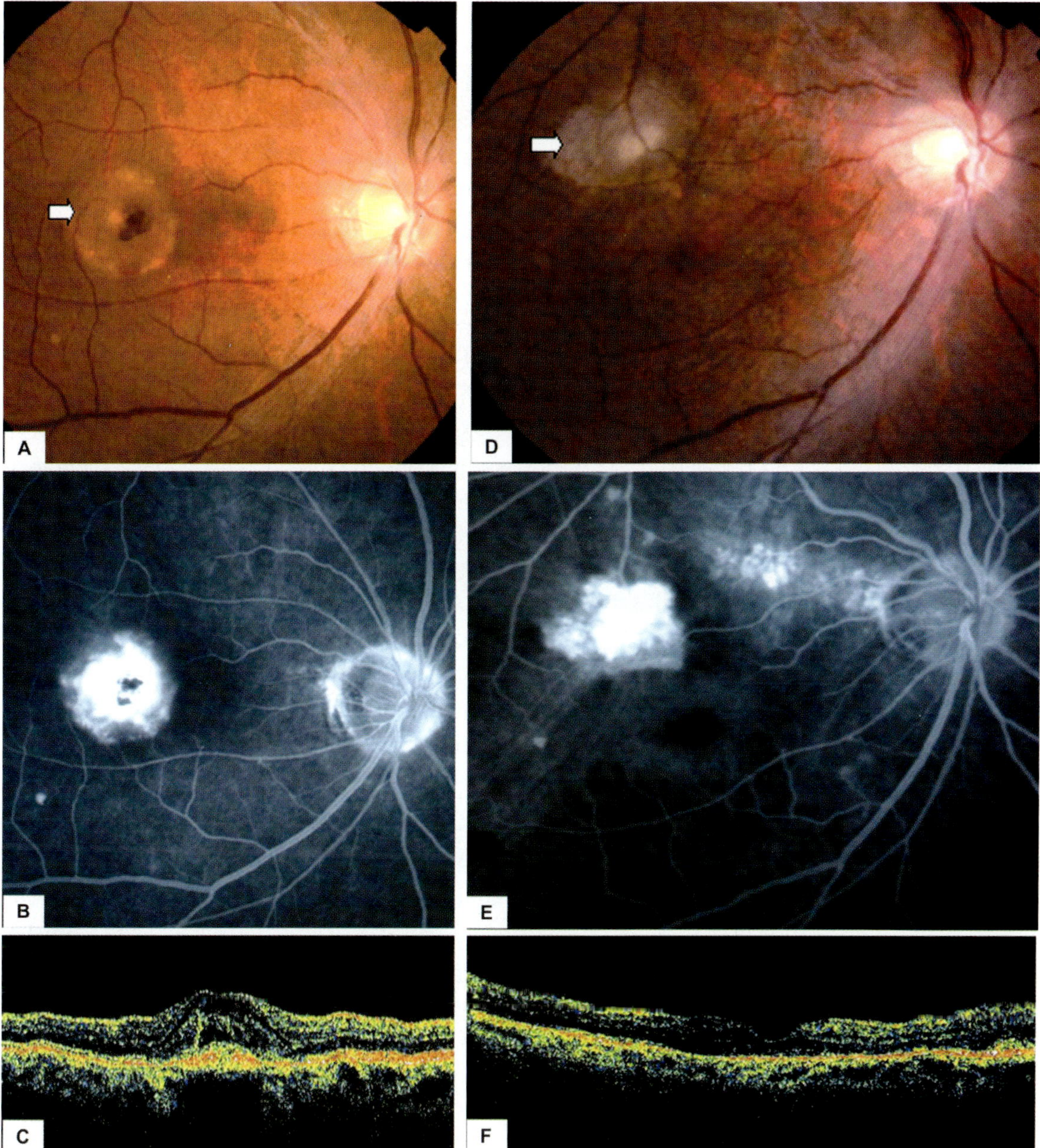

FIGURES 1.57A to F: (A) Fundus examination shows a well-defined round yellowish lesion at the fovea and subretinal hemorrhage. (B) Fluorescein angiogram shows early hyperfluorescence and late staining. This is a classic CNV. (C) A vertical OCT image shows a hyper-reflective region which is corresponding to the CNV under the retinal reflectivity. The thickness of the CNV is 170 μm. The retina is swollen and its thickness is measured 370 μm. (D) Fundus photograph 3 months after limited macular translocation. It reveals that the fovea is slightly moved to the area inferiorly to the CNV. (E) Fluorescein angiography. Fluorescein angiogram also shows the movement of the fovea inferiorly to the CNV. (F) A vertical OCT image after the surgery. OCT shows a hyper-reflective region which is corresponding to the CNV under the retinal reflectivity. The location of the fovea is moved toward inferiorly to the one measured preoperatively. The thickness of the foveal reflectivity is reduced to 125 μm, and there is an obvious foveal contour (Prof Yasuo Tano MD, Japan).

On the other hand, the fovea is moved less than 1 disk diameter after limited macular translocation. Therefore, OCT usually detects CNV or other lesions at the same image of OCT including the fovea after the surgery. [137]

After these surgeries, foveal contour may be recovered. Some cases that show cystoid macular edema detected by fluorescein angiography may not show cystoid space in OCT images postoperatively. [138] The newly located macula, or the macula after the CNV removal, may have slight macular edema or subretinal fluid and OCT is effective to detect them as the hyporeflective space. In the follow-up period, enlargement of CNV involving the new fovea may develop after limited translocation. Recurrence of CNV also may be observed in the eyes in which CNV is removed during the surgeries. Optical coherence tomography is also useful to monitor them. [137]

MACULA AFTER RETINAL DETACHMENT SURGERY

In some cases of rhegmatogenous retinal detachment especially those with shallow retinal detachment, the diagnosis of retinal detachment and the estimation of its extension is difficult. It is also difficult to determine whether retinal reattachment is achieved after retinal reattachment surgery when there is minimal residual subretinal fluid. [139-142]

OPTICAL COHERENCE TOMOGRAPHY

In retinal detachment, there is an accumulation of subretinal fluid between the neurosensory retina and retinal pigment epithelium. This pathology was determined from experimental retinal detachment in an animal model. [143] Histopathologic study of retinal detachment is not applicable to *in vivo* studies, especially in acute retinal detachment cases. Optical coherence tomography is a highly advantageous technique for in vivo studies. With OCT, subretinal fluid is observed as a low- to non-reflective layer between two highly-reflective layers, [144] the neurosensory retina and the retinal pigment epithelium (Figures 1.58A to D). Each border of the subretinal fluid is so distinct that differential diagnosis from retinal edema is relatively easy. This OCT finding of subretinal fluid is sometimes called 'optically clear space'. [139]

The detached neurosensory retina has specific characteristics. [145] The OCT findings of detached neurosensory retina are normal (40%), intraretinal separation (28%), and intraretinal separation with an undulated outer layer (32%). Patients with intraretinal separation and undulation have poor visual acuity. Patients with a highly detached retina also had severely impaired vision. Intraretinal separation is rapidly resolved after successful retinal reattachment surgery. [146]

TREATMENT

The main surgical procedure to repair retinal detachment is scleral buckling and vitrectomy, depending on the case specifics and the surgeon's experience. Optical coherence tomography is useful to disclose a slight elevation of the neurosensory retina in cases with very shallow retinal detachment. It is sometimes difficult to diagnose shallow retinal detachment in a highly myopic eye with severe macular atrophy because of the low contrast between the detached retina and the retinal pigment epithelium. In such cases, shallow retinal detachment can be detected clearly with OCT. [139]

MONITORING

In cases of macula-off rhegmatogenous retinal detachment, the macula is as observed with ophthalmoscopy to be flat after successful retinal reattachment surgery. Pre- and postoperative OCT provides useful information in rhegmatogenous retinal detachment cases. Soon after surgery, some macula-off retinal detachment cases have a completely reattached macula with no subretinal fluid detected with OCT. [139]

On the other hand, OCT can detect even a small amount of residual subretinal fluid, which is difficult to determine using ophthalmoscopy postoperatively. Acute macula-off rhegmatogenous retinal detachment has a favorable postoperative visual recovery, even if there is residual subretinal fluid at the macula. A longer duration of macula-off retinal detachment might influence the degenerative changes of the neurosensory retina and result in a poor visual prognosis. Whether this accumulation of residual subretinal fluid influences postoperative visual recovery is not clear, [140-142] therefore follow-up

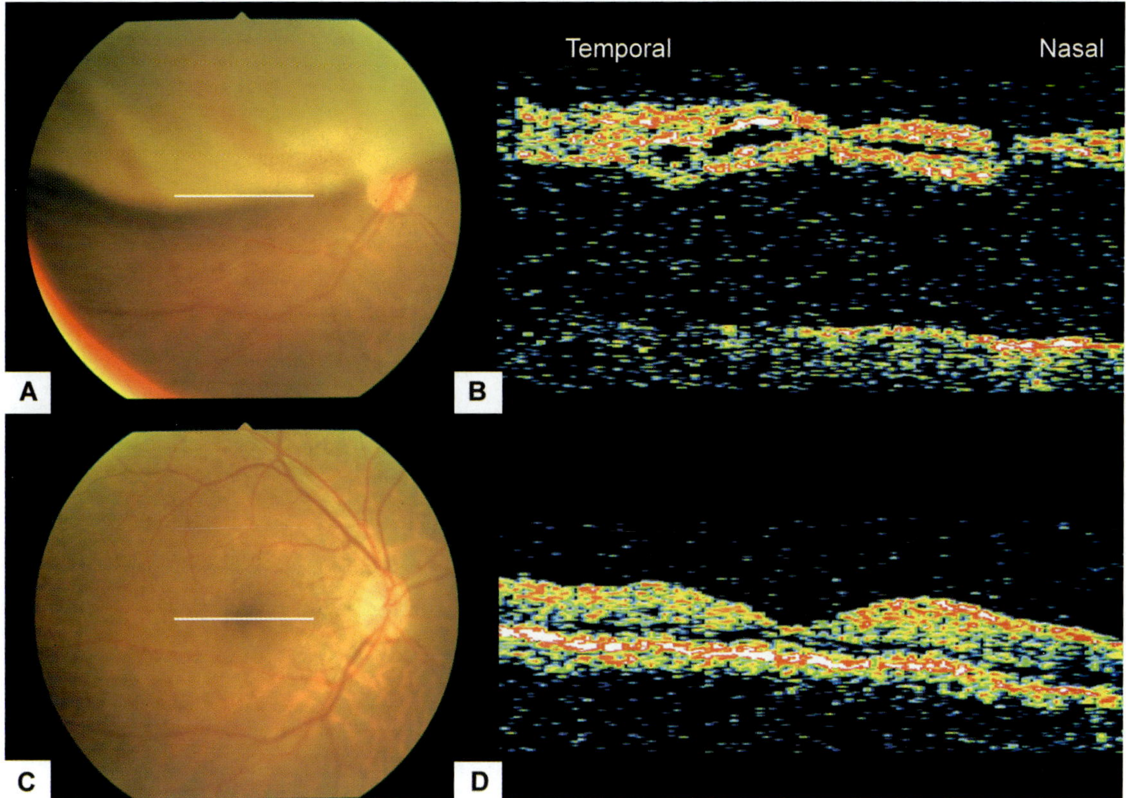

FIGURES 1.58A to D: The right eye with macula-off rhegmatogenous retinal detachment. Preoperative visual acuity was 0.3 with a refractive error of −1 diopters. (A) Preoperative fundus photograph. (B) Preoperative OCT image. Retinal elevation and intraretinal separation around the fovea were observed. (C) Postoperative fundus photograph. Two weeks after scleral buckling, the macula was completely reattached and visual acuity was 0.6. (D) OCT image 2 weeks after operation. The neurosensory retina was completely reattached and the intraretinal clear space observed preoperatively had disappeared (Takayuki Baba MD, Japan).

examination with OCT is important. Residual subretinal fluid can take over 1 year to be absorbed completely after successful scleral buckling surgery. [139]

Rarely, after successful retinal detachment surgery with no postoperative subfoveal fluid confirmed by OCT, a very small amount of subfoveal fluid accumulation occurs during the postoperative period (Figures 1.59A to F). In such cases, there is no subjective visual acuity loss or decreased vision. The reason for the subfoveal fluid recurrence is unknown. The migration of subretinal fluid in the peripheral retina might contribute to this phenomenon. [139]

Apart from rhegmatogenous retinal detachment involving the macula, subretinal fluid at the macula is postoperatively detected in some cases of retinal detachment with a preoperatively spared macula. [147]

Cystoid macular edema occurs after retinal reattachment surgery. Macular detachment, increased duration of macular detachment, cryotherapy, and pseudophakia are suspected risk factors of cystoid macular edema. [148] The OCT image of cystoid macular edema after retinal detachment surgery is characterized by increased retinal thickness and multiple small intraretinal clear spaces. The OCT image of an intraretinal cyst is similar to that of cystoid macular edema of diabetic maculopathy or uveitis. [149]

Subclinical subfoveal fluid is often detected with OCT after scleral procedures in macula-off rhegmatogenous retinal detachment. After vitrectomy with fluid-gas exchange in such retinal detachment cases, complete foveal reattachment can be confirmed with OCT. It is reported to be achieved faster after vitrectomy than after scleral buckling. [139,150]

Focus on Macular Diseases

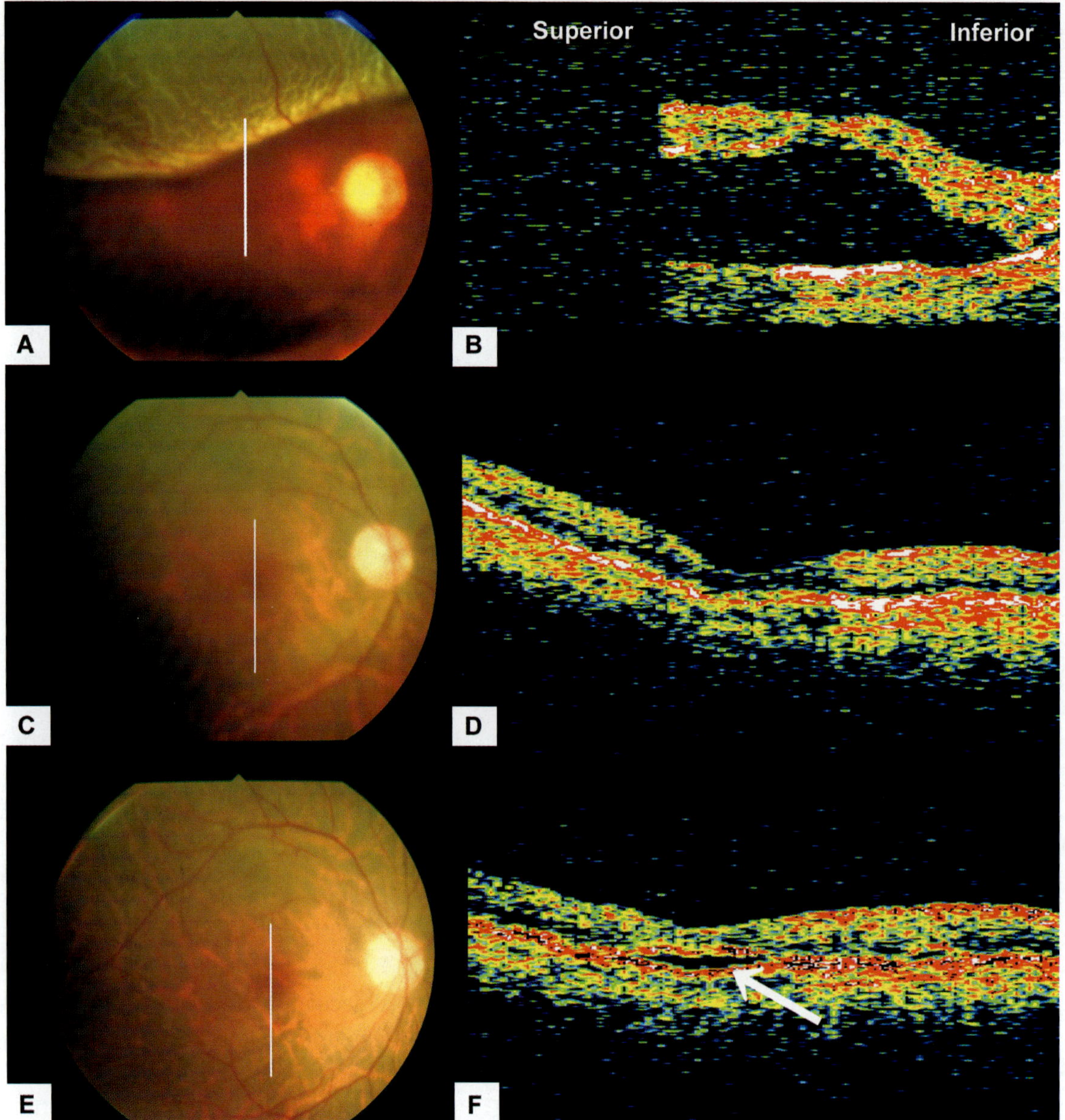

FIGURES 1.59A to F: The right eye with macula-off rhegmatogenous retinal detachment. Preoperative visual acuity was 0.01 with a refractive error of −9 diopters. The duration of macula-off retinal detachment was 2 days. (A) Preoperative fundus photograph. (B) Preoperative OCT image. The retinal detachment involves the macula. The retinal detachment was so bullous that the detached neurosensory retina superior to the macula was out of range. (C) Fundus photograph 1 month after scleral buckling. The macula was reattached and visual acuity was 0.7. (D) OCT image 1 month after operation. The subretinal clear space observed preoperatively had disappeared. Foveal configuration was almost normal. (E) Fundus photograph 3 months after operation. No subretinal fluid was observed ophthalmoscopically and visual acuity was 0.7. (F) OCT image 3 months after operation. A very limited subretinal clear space emerged at the subfoveal (arrow) (Takayuki Baba MD, Japan).

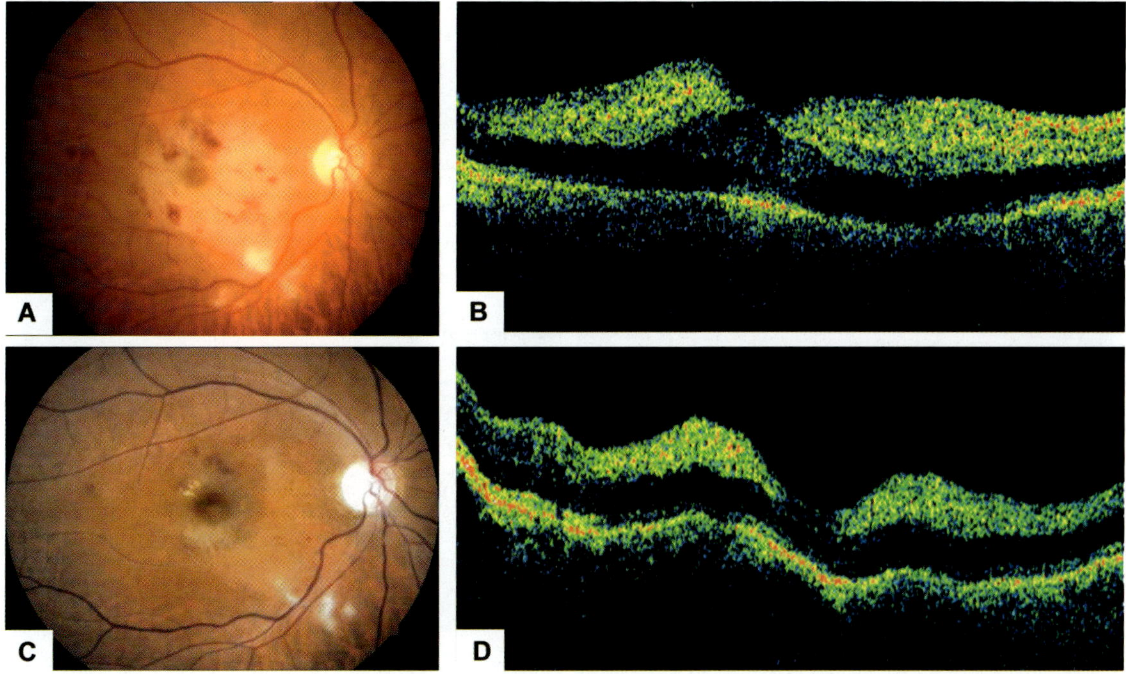

FIGURES 1.60A to D: (A) Fundus photograph of the right eye (day 1) showing macular edema, and retinal hemorrhages. (B) Fundus photograph (month 3) of right eye showing resolved macular edema, retinal hemorrhages and few cotton wool spots. (C) OCT macular thickness map scan (day 1) showing macular edema, with elevation of neurosensory retina, and accumulation of hyper-reflective material under the neurosensory retina. (D) OCT macular thickness map scan (month 3) showing partial resolution of macular edema, hyper-reflective ischemic retina and loss of normal alternate layers of hyper-reflectivity (Pradeep Venkatesh MD, India).

MACULAR INFARCTION

Retinal toxicity in the form of macular infarction is a well established complication of intravitreal aminoglycosides especially gentamicin and amikacin. It usually manifests as pale retinal edema with retinal and preretinal hemorrhages.[151] Experimental studies shown lamellar lysosomal inclusions in the retinal pigment epithelium as the earliest finding in such cases.[152] A subepithelial accumulation of amorphous and granular material, consistent with the morphologic features of hard drusen, and staining positively with periodic acid-Schiff, has also been reported.[152]

Ischemic retina has been shown to exhibit hyper-reflectivity on OCT.[153] In addition to this; fresh infarction may also show macular edema, with elevation of neurosensory retina, and accumulation of hyper-reflective material under the neurosensory retina[151] (Figures 1.60A to D).

SOLAR RETINOPATHY

Solar retinopathy is characterized by visual distortion in patients with history of sun gazing or exposure to solar eclipse. Viewing of sun results in damage to the outer retinal layers. Fundus examination usually reveals a central yellow spot in early period after injury. Later this yellow spot is replaced by small sharply red lesion or a hypopigmented lesion with irregular margins. Fundus fluorescein angiography is usually unremarkable; but occasionally it may show window defect in the area of the lesion (Figures 1.16A to D).[151]

OPTICAL COHERENCE TOMOGRAPHY

Optical coherence tomography is helpful in delineating the exact site of injury *in vivo* in these eyes. Both early and late damage can be picked up with OCT.[151]

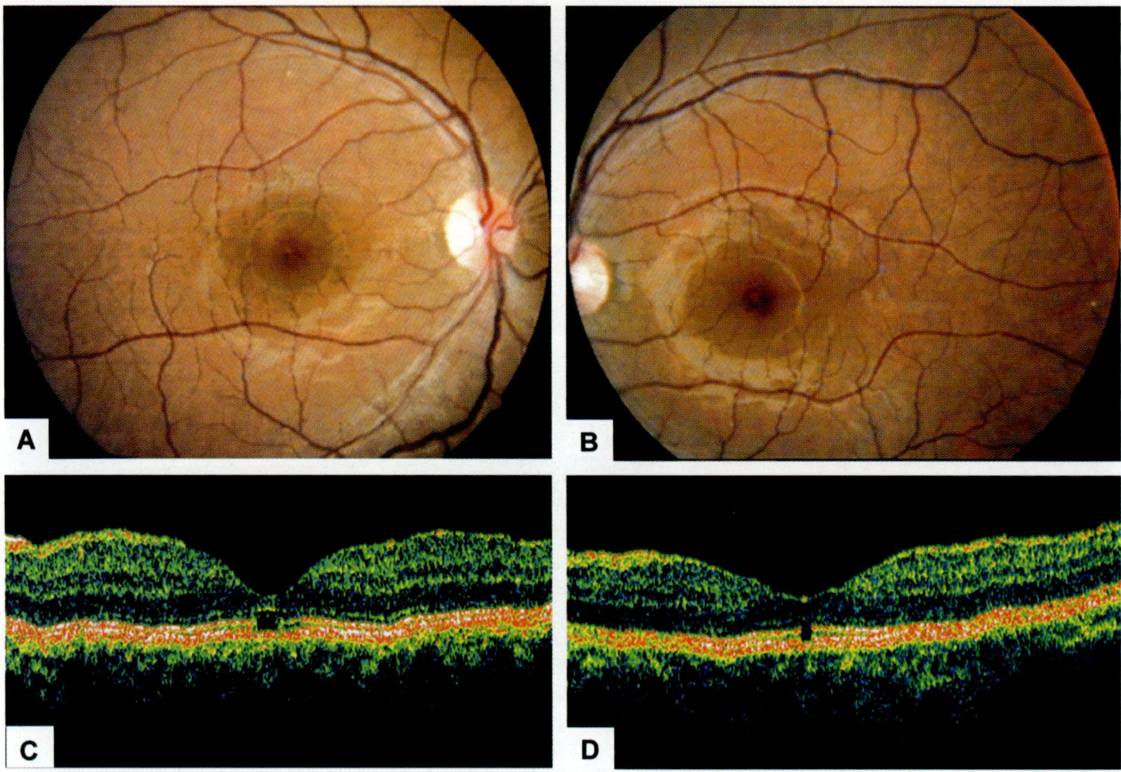

FIGURES 1.61A to D: (A and B) Fundus photographs of bilateral late solar retinopathy showing hypopigmeted lesions (outer lamellar macular hole) in both eyes. (C and D) OCT line scan showing optically clear area in the macular area corresponding to focal defect in retinal pigment epithelium and outer segment of retinal photoreceptors (Pradeep Venkatesh MD, India).

Early Changes

OCT demonstrates hyper-reflectivity in all the foveal layers 48 hours after watching the solar eclipse. These changes generally disappear within a period of one week to one month.[154]

Late Changes

OCT in eyes with chronic solar retinopathy demonstrates selective retinal pigment epithelium and photoreceptor damage. Optical coherence tomography findings correlate well with the histological studies in solar retinopathy eyes.[155-157] Optical coherence tomography shows a normal and preserved foveal contour. A small hyporeflective/ optically clear space is seen in the foveal region in the area corresponding to the outer photoreceptors and retinal pigment epithelium. [155-157] The remaining retinal pigment epithelium is usually normal. A small area of hyper-reflectivity immediately adjacent to the clear area has also been described. [157] These findings represent the damaged photoreceptors and retinal pigment epithelium and may account for the visual complaints.

BERLIN'S EDEMA

Commotio retina is characterized by acute retinal opacification and whitening following blunt trauma. A mild commotio retina present with transient visual loss and usually settles spontaneously with minimal sequelae. However, more severe cases may be associated with permanent visual loss. [151]

In acute stage there is disruption of the outer segments of photoreceptors. This is followed by its phagocytosis by retinal pigment epithelium. Retinal pigment epithelium cells migrate onto retina by next 48 hours to reach the inner plexiform layer or the ganglion cell layer. Thus retinal pigment epithelium may present as multilayered, disorganized structure on the Bruch's membrane with atrophy of outer segment seen as overlying neurosensory atrophy. [151]

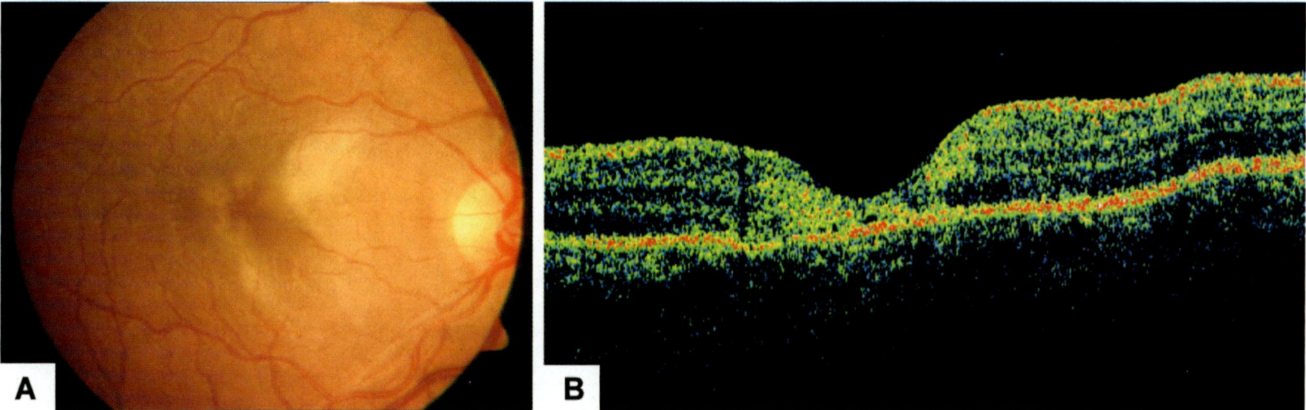

FIGURES 1.62A and B: (A) Fundus photograph showing pale retinal opacification with macular edema; (B) OCT scan showing altered reflectivity in the area of photoreceptor outer segment with increased reflectivity in inner retina representing the migrated retinal pigment epithelium cells (Pradeep Venkatesh MD, India).

Optical coherence tomography is an effective tool in identifying post-traumatic retinal edema with definitive objectivity. Apart from the increase in the thickness of the involved area OCT shows other retinal alterations like changes in the reflectivity and contour of various retinal layers. Optical coherence tomography findings depend on the severity and the duration of commotio retinae.[158,159] Severe cases with extensive photoreceptor disruption show optically clear spaces in the area corresponding to the photoreceptors.[158] The major site of retinal trauma on OCT appears to be at the level of the photoreceptor outer segment/retinal pigment epithelium interface. These changes generally disappear within few weeks. Delayed observation with OCT in these cases may demonstrate moderate increase in the reflectivity in the area corresponding to the photoreceptors probably representing the migrated retinal pigment epithelial cells with disorganized overlying neurosensory retina (Figures 1.62A and B). Studies have shown that the OCT images are consistent with histological changes in commotio retinae which include fragmentation of photoreceptor outer segments and damaged cell bodies.[151,158,159]

SUBHYALOID HEMORRHAGE

Vitreous hemorrhage is not infrequently encountered after ocular trauma. Occasional subhyaloid hemorrhage may also occur.

Hemorrhage results in high reflectivity with shadowing of the underlying layers in the OCT image. The shadowing is more severe with subhyaloid hemorrhage which is thick and dense. Optical coherence tomography may be useful in differentiating subhyaloid hemorrhage from sub-internal limiting membrane hemorrhage (Figures 1.63A and B).[151]

TRAUMATIC MACULAR HOLE

Macular hole may result from trauma.

OPTICAL COHERENCE TOMOGRAPHY

Optical coherence tomography demonstrates the detailed topography of traumatic macular hole (Figures 1.64A and B). Various characteristics like elevation of the hole edges, cystoid changes at the margins, hole size, and changes at the base of the hole and associated retinal pigment epithelium changes can be better evaluated with OCT. Depending on the duration of trauma, the hole may exhibit elevated edges with cystoid changes in recent trauma. Optical coherence tomography of old macular holes usually demonstrate flat edges with associated neurosensory atrophy.[151]

PSEUDOPHAKIC MACULAR EDEMA

Incidence of postoperative cystoid macular edema has gone down with advent of phacoemulsification and better medical care. However, it may still be encountered

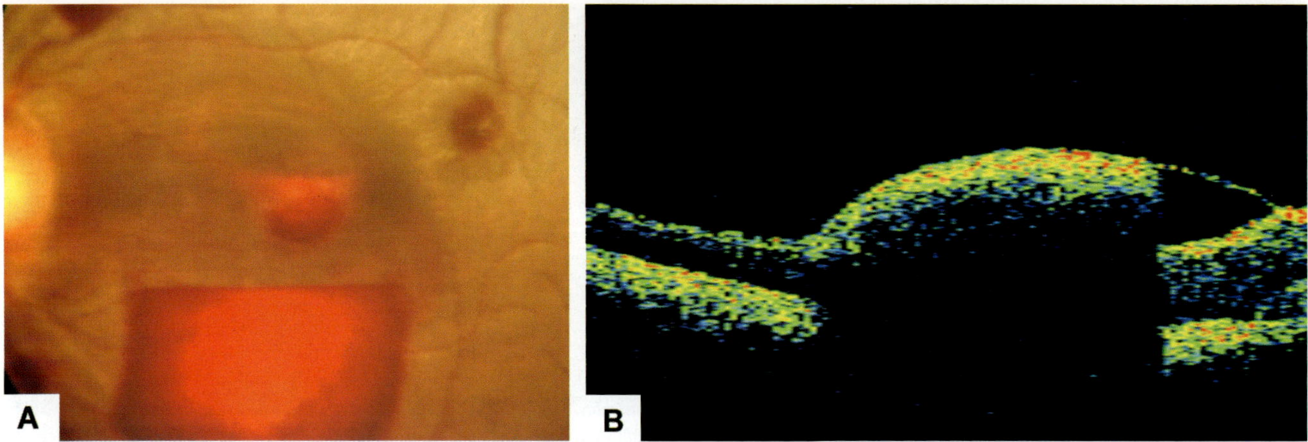

FIGURES 1.63A and B: (A) Fundus photograph showing boat shaped hemorrhage with retinal hemorrhages; (B) OCT scan showing a sub-internal limiting membrane collection of blood seen as increased reflectivity and posterior shadowing (Pradeep Venkatesh MD, India).

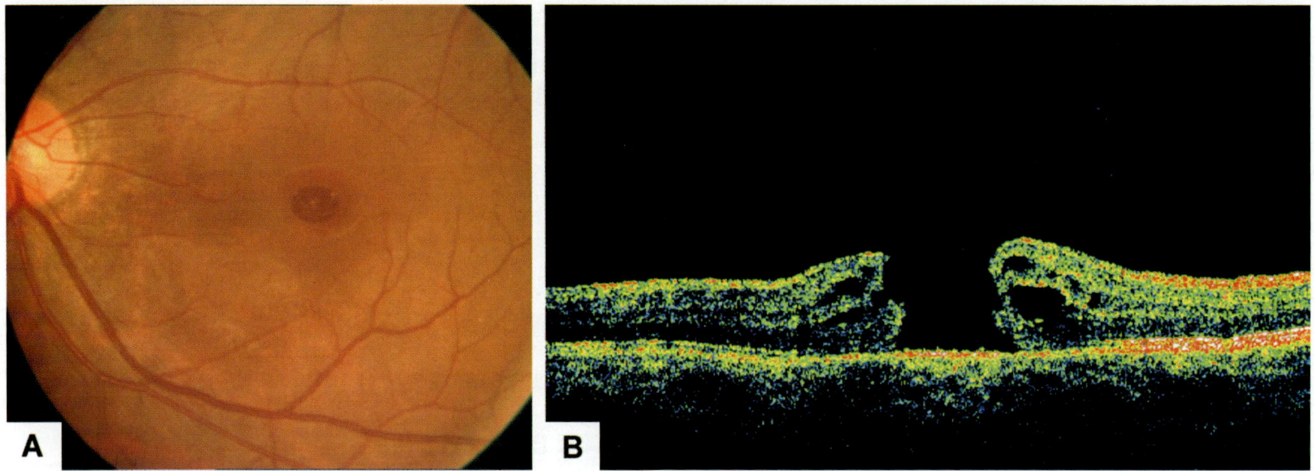

FIGURES 1.64A and B: (A) Fundus photograph showing a full thickness macular hole; (B) OCT scan showing full thickness macular hole with cystoid changes at the edge (Pradeep Venkatesh MD, India).

following an intraocular surgery, and cataract extraction still remains the most common cause for postoperative cystoid macular edema. The diagnosis of cystoid macular edema is based on fundus examination and confirmed by fluorescein angiography.[151]

OPTICAL COHERENCE TOMOGRAPHY

Optical coherence tomography has a very important application in evaluation and management of patients with cystoid macular edema of varied origin.[160,161] Optical coherence tomography is a very effective modality for confirmation of cystoid macular edema with distinct advantages of being a noninvasive and a quick technique.[151]

Cystoid macular edema is seen as intraretinal cystic cavities which are optically clear or possess very low reflectivity and associated increased macular thickness. Retinal pigment epithelium enables exact quantitative assessment of macular edema in terms of increased macular thickness and volume parameters. These parameters can be used to decide the mode of treatment and also to monitor the effect of intervention with good precision (Figures 1.65A A to C).[160,161]

MYOPIC FOVEOSCHISIS

Myopic foveoschisis was first reported as a macular detachment without a retinal hole specific to high

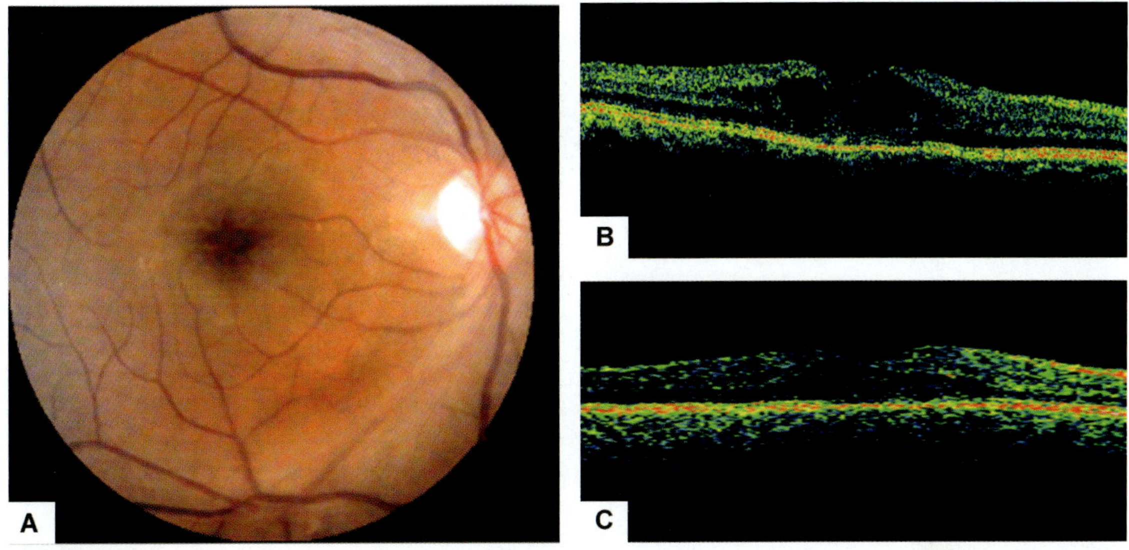

FIGURES 1.65A to C: (A) Fundus photograph showing postoperative cystoid macular edema; (B) OCT scan showing increased macular thickness with cystoid cavities; (C) marked resolution of cystoid space with decrease in macular thickness following subTenon tricort injection (Pradeep Venkatesh MD, India).

myopia.[162] Myopic foveoschisis is not a retinal detachment but a foveal detachment with retinoschisis around the fovea.[163-170]

Myopic foveoschisis is specific to high myopia, which generally is defined as a refractive error greater than −8.0 diopters.[162] The chief complaints at presentation include visual loss, metamorphopsia, relative central scotoma, or all of these; however, some patients can be asymptomatic. The incidence of myopic foveoschisis has been reported to be 10% of highly myopic patients with posterior staphyloma.[171]

Optical coherence tomography is an essential tool for diagnosing myopic foveoschisis.[162]

There are several subtypes of myopic foveoschisis based on retinal morphology including the presence of either a foveal detachment, a lamellar hole, or a macular hole (Figures 1.66A to D).[164,170] Spontaneous resolution, probably resulting from posterior vitreous detachment may occur[172] but is very rare.

OPTICAL COHERENCE TOMOGRAPHY

The mechanism by which myopic foveoschisis develops still remains controversial.[162] Tractional force of the epiretinal membrane may cause myopic foveoschisis. Optical coherence tomography has provided more information and indicated that different subtypes of myopic foveoschisis may have processes specific to their development. For instance, local posterior vitreous detachment at the posterior retina as well as a preretinal strand between the edge of the macular hole and the posterior vitreous surface often are observed in myopic foveoschisis in which a macular hole develops. This indicates that a macular hole associated with myopic foveoschisis may develop as the result of posterior vitreous detachment, which generates anteroposterior traction and consequent retinal tearing at the fovea. Another possible mechanism is retinal vascular traction on the retina. After vitrectomy performed to treat myopic foveoschisis, retinal microfolds form gradually after the surgery. These microfolds are oriented horizontally. Only OCT can detect them. OCT-ophthalmoscope identifies the precise location of the microfolds and shows that they coincide with the retinal arterioles (Figures 1.66A to D). The microfolds seem to be generated by inward traction of the vessels due to axial length elongation, and intraoperative internal limiting membrane peeling might have disclosed the potent tractional force of these vessels. Microfolds are present even in patients with high myopia who did not undergo surgery. Thus, myopic foveoschisis might be a multifactorial disease.[162,173]

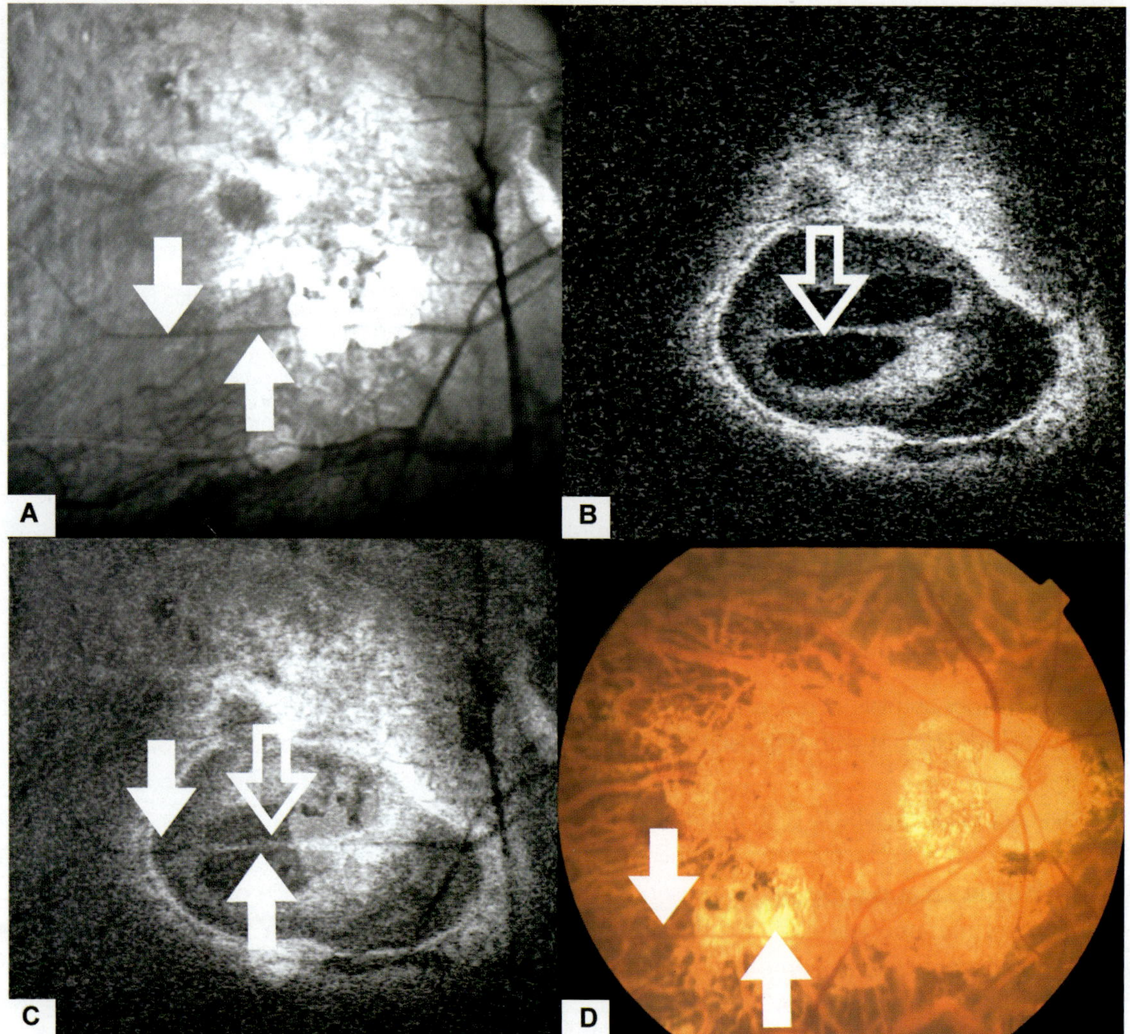

FIGURES 1.66A to D: Optical coherence tomography-ophthalmoscopy identifies the exact location of the retinal microfolds. (A) A scanning laser ophthalmoscope (SLO) image and (B) A C-scan image showing linear retinal microfolds. (C) The C-scan image was overlaid onto SLO image that pinpoints the location on the retina. (D) The retinal microfolds coincide exactly with the retinal arterioles. Closed arrows in (A), (C), and (D) indicate retinal arteriole and open arrows in (B) and (C) retinal microfold (Prof Yasuo Tano MD, Japan).

Vitrectomy, including removal of the vitreous cortex, internal limiting membrane peeling, and gas tamponade, is a useful treatment to achieve foveal reattachment and consequent visual improvement if the fovea is detached.[162] After surgery; OCT typically shows that foveal detachment gradually resolves over time. Foveal detachment completely resolves soon after surgery in some cases; however, other cases can take longer than 6 months to resolve (Figures 1.67A to C). Although there is a risk of macular hole formation even after surgery, 80 to 90% of patients have improved visual acuity. The surgery usually results in stabilization of the fixation point in scanning laser ophthalmoscope microperimetry, indicating that retinal function has improved.

There is a risk that a macular hole may enlarge after surgery in cases in which the hole is small (early hole).[174] These detachments can be treated with additional long-term gas tamponade or another vitrectomy. [162]

OPTIC NERVE HEAD PIT

Optic nerve head pits are associated with various retinal changes. Most of the retinal changes are temporal to the

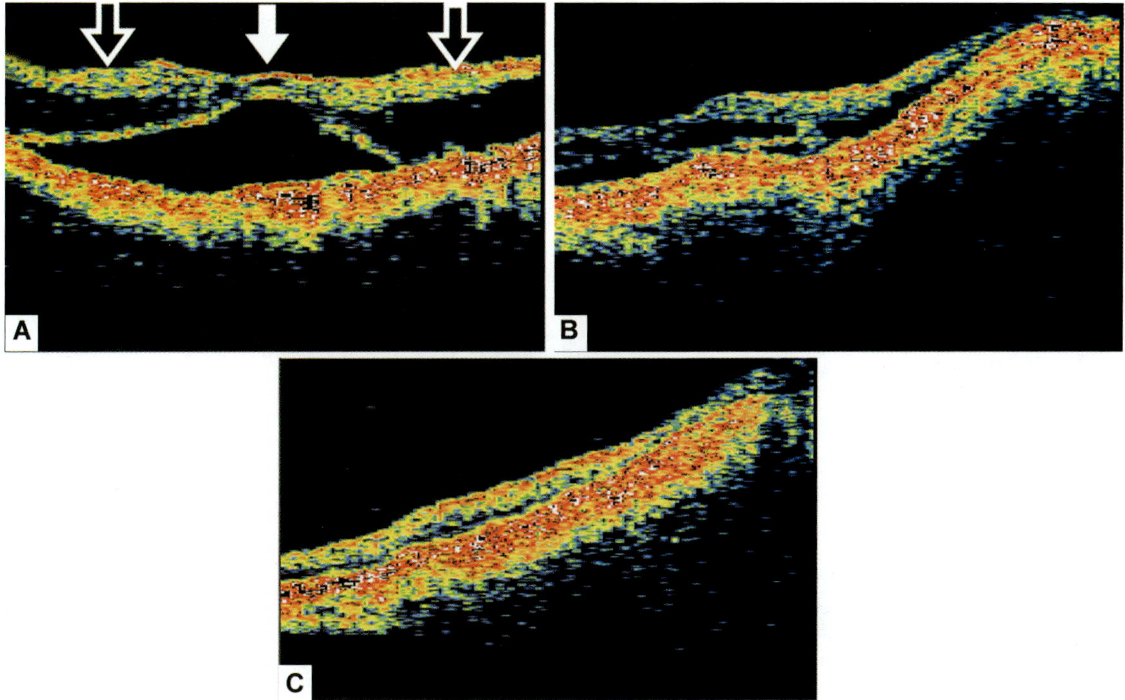

FIGURES 1.67A to C: Time course of the retinal morphologic changes after vitrectomy for myopic foveoschisis. (A) Foveal detachment (closed arrow) and retinoschisis surrounding the retina (open arrows) are observed preoperatively. (B) One month after vitrectomy that included removal of the vitreous cortex, internal limiting membrane peeling, and gas tamponade, the amount of subretinal fluid has decreased; however, the foveal detachment remains. (C) Six months postoperatively, respectively, the retinal detachment has decreased further; and finally the retina is reattached completely (Prof Yasuo Tano MD, Japan).

disk, located between the temporal vascular arcade. Thirty percent of these patients develop maculopathy that may include schisis like cavity in the macula, macular detachment and lamellar or full thickness macular hole.[175] It has been suggested that fluid from the vitreous leaks through the optic pit to fill the retinal and the subretinal space.[175,176] It has also been observed that retinal elevation associated with optic disk pit resists gas compression unlike pneumatic displacements of rhegmatogenous detachments.[177,178]

OPTICAL COHERENCE TOMOGRAPHY

Optical coherence tomography allows enhanced visualization of retinal changes in these eyes revealing the collection of fluid at several distinct levels of retina (Figures 1.68A to E).[177-180] Optical coherence tomography may reveal a connection between the optic nerve pit and schisis cavity in the inner retinal layers. Bridging retinal elements may also be identified on OCT. It also demonstrates the deep and superficial breaks apart from the schisis cavity. Studies have shown its useful application especially in clinically suspected pseudomacular holes where OCT may reveal a foveal schisis or a lamellar macular hole.[178,181]

Lincoff and associates [177] showed that OCT images provide a detailed understanding of the pathogenesis of macular changes associated with optic disk pit. They observed that pneumatic displacement of the outer layer detachment is associated with improvement in central visual acuity; however, it is temporary as the OCT revealed

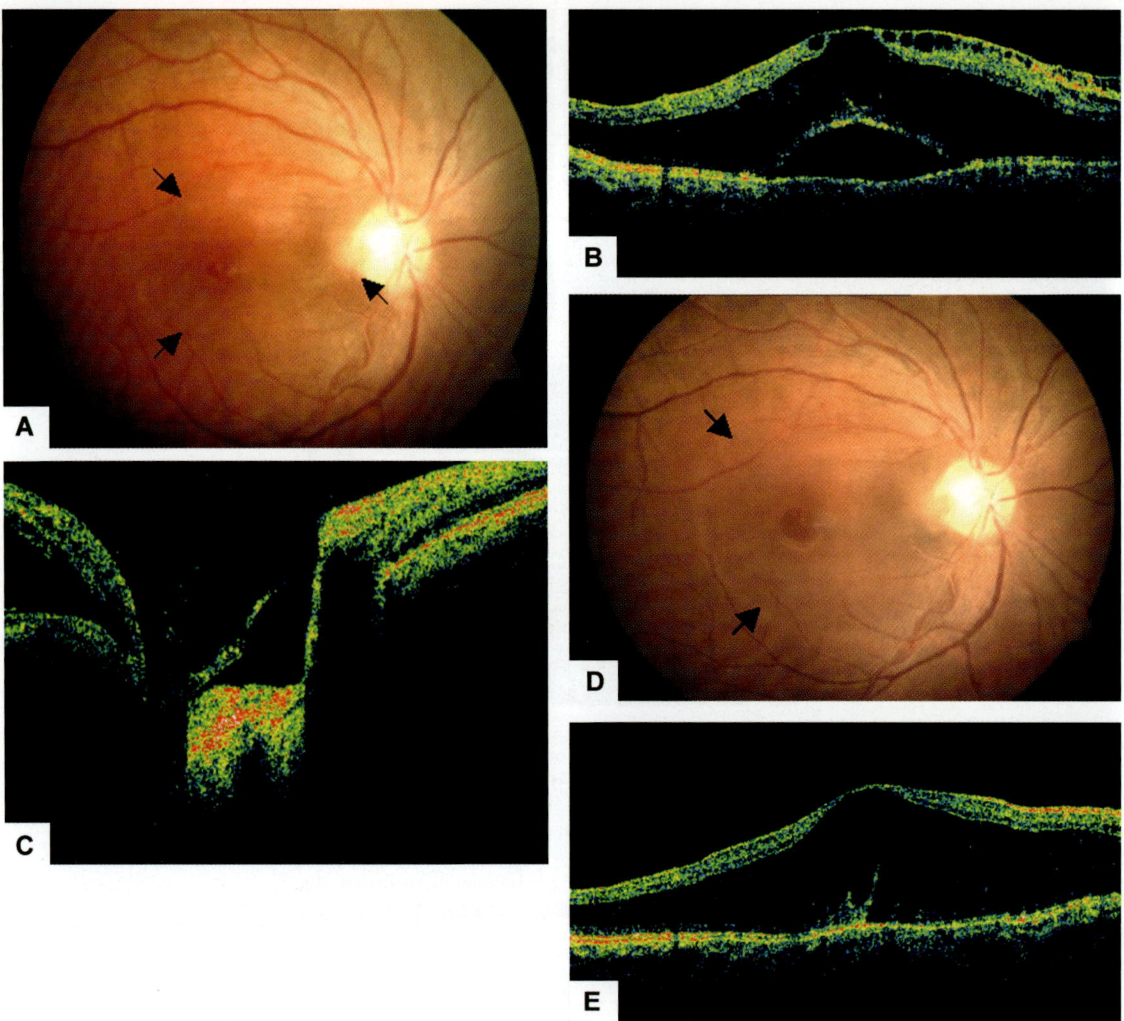

FIGURES 1.68A to E: (A) Fundus photograph showing optic disk pit with macular schisis. (B) OCT line scan through the macular area showing splitting in the outer retinal layer with faint bridging tissue traversing the schisis cavity along with submacular fluid collection. (C) OCT line scan of the optic disk showing defect in the area corresponding to the pit. (D) Post-laser (3 weeks) fundus photograph showing decrease in the height of macular detachment and schisis. (E) Post-laser (3 weeks) macular scan showing persisting schisis cavity with resorption of subretinal fluid (Pradeep Venkatesh MD, India).

that the inner layer separation or the schisis cavity persists thus providing a conduit for the continuous flow of fluid from the pit to the subretinal space. Persistence of the schisis cavity may be responsible for the frequent failure of laser photocoagulation at the edge of optic disk to create a barrier for the fluid egress from the pit.

Optical coherence tomography also has a useful application in postoperative evaluation and monitoring the reabsorption of submacular fluid in these eyes after a vitrectomy-laser-gas procedure or macular buckling.[177-180]

Optical coherence tomography demonstrated a schisis cavity with splitting of outer retinal layers. A concurrent subretinal collection of fluid creating a bilaminar structure may be observed on OCT. An area suggesting the connection between the pit and the schisis cavity may also be seen. This area appears to be the pathway allowing the passage of fluid into the retinal stroma. Some patients may demonstrate foveal central thinning and or a full thickness macular hole; whereas, others may present with macular retinoschisis without any subretinal fluid collection.

RETINAL AND CHOROIDAL INFLAMMATION

Inflammations of the posterior segment can be grouped into two major categories depending on their most common anatomic features: retinitis and choroiditis. Inflammatory conditions may present with focal, multifocal or diffuse involvement. Infectious involvement is seen more commonly in the retina and choroid than in the anterior segment. In most cases the blood-retinal barrier is compromised leading to leakage and fluid accumulation, such as detachment of the choroid, retinal pigment epithelium and retina. Some cases present with typical pathological findings in funduscopy such as toxoplasmosis, but plenty of cases in early stages make a clear diagnosis difficult by funduscopy only.[181-190]

OPTICAL COHERENCE TOMOGRAPHY

The biomicroscopic examination and the fluorescein angiography of the central fundus regions may not be sufficient, in some cases, to exactly locate lesions, estimate their extent, differentiate lesions of the fovea, observe membranes and follow the results of medical or surgical treatment.

Fluorescein angiography is two-dimensional where perfusion is visualized; however, the nerve fiber layer, pathologic epiretinal structures and the posterior vitreous cannot be observed. A clear-cut assignment to retinal layers is often not possible.[191]

Linear scans produced by the OCT are an adjunctive means to:

- Demonstrate the morphology of retinal layers
- Visualize merging structures
- Localize edema, detachments, membranes, scars, and
- Quantify the extent and changes of pathological lesions.[181]

Inflammatory diseases of the retina are often accompanied by opaque ocular media due to corneal decompensation, complicated cataracts and vitreous opacities. In those cases the light beam of OCT may not reach the region of interest, particularly the retina and choroid. Therefore a sufficient amount of media clarity is mandatory for an OCT examination.[181-190]

- In inflammatory diseases, OCT detects fluids in or beneath the retina or choroid associated with

detachment of the sensory retina, cystoid macular edema, diffuse macular edema and detachment of the retinal pigment epithelium, and allows a precise anatomical localization and quantification (Figures 1.69A to C). Complications of inflammatory disease of the retina and choroid are persistent macular edema, epiretinal membrane, choroidal neovascularization and scar formation.[181]

Optical coherence tomography provides additional information in acute and chronic inflammation: Fluid accumulation in different layers is dominating in the former; the incidence of sequelae is predominant in the latter.[181]

Acute Inflammation

- Cystoid macular edema
- Detachment of sensory retina
- Detachment of retinal pigment epithelium

Chronic Inflammation

- Cystoid macular edema
- Epiretinal membrane
- Choroidal neovascularization (Figures 1.70A to D)
- Scar formation.

Since the sequelae of the treatment of intraocular inflammations may sometimes be more detrimental than the disease itself, indications for therapy should rely on definite features. These features qualify the OCT for use in precisely defined intraocular inflammations when indications for:

- Cytotoxic treatment
- Laser surgery
- Pars plana vitrectomy
- Epiretinal membrane peeling, and
- Excision of subretinal neovascular membrane, are sought.[181]

TYPES OF INFLAMMATION

Choroiditis

In choroiditis clear media are found due to lacking cellular vitreous infiltration. In acute stages the creamy whitish lesions present in OCT as focal convex thickening of the retinal pigment epithelium and underlying structures with

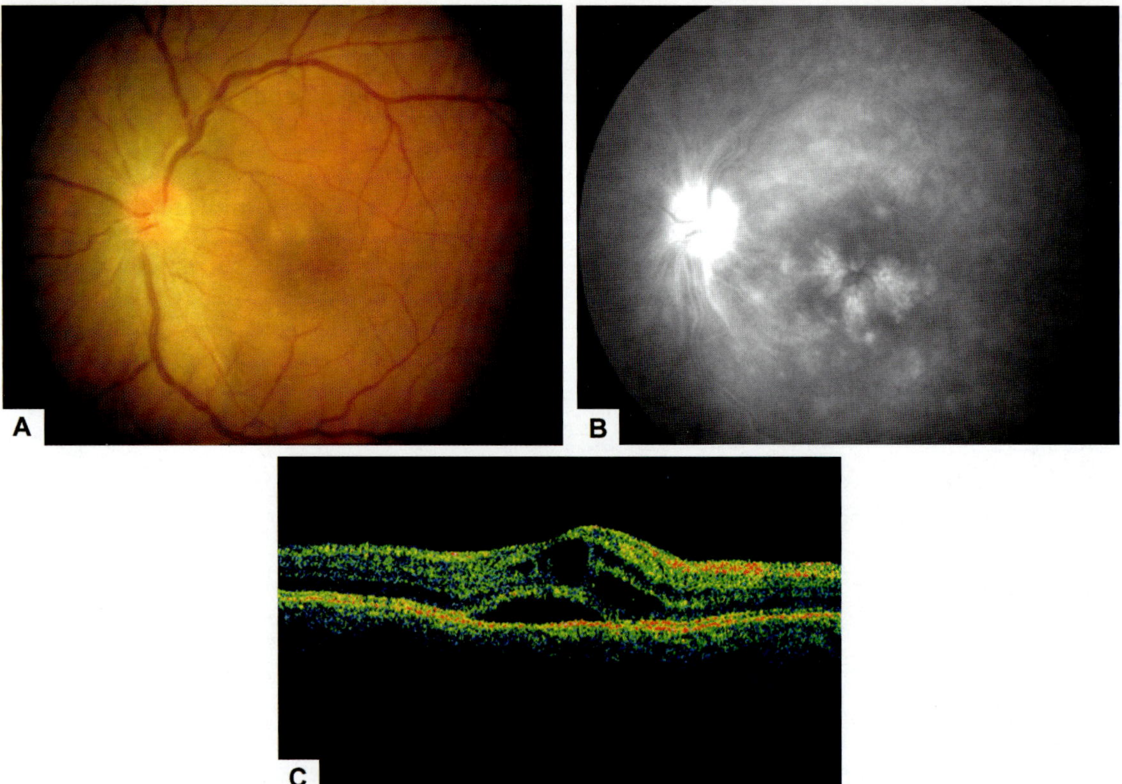

FIGURES 1.69A to C: (A and B) Fundus photograph and fluorescein angiography of the left eye revealing cystoid macular edema and a typical flower petal pattern on late phase angiogram. There is no obvious pooling of dye suggestive of neurosensory detachment. (C) OCT not only confirms the presence of cystoid macular edema (thick arrow), but also detects a subtle neurosensory detachment (thin arrow) in the left eye (Jyotirmay Biswas MS, India).

enhanced light transmission into deeper layers in some cases. Only in extensive and acute inflammation a simultaneous sensory detachment is found (Figures 1.71 to 1.74). Treatment regimens can be changed depending on the amount of subretinal fluid.[181]

Serpiginous Choroiditis

In chronic serpiginous choroiditis, funduscopy reveals a serpiginous choroidal atrophy and hypertrophy of retinal pigment epithelium. In OCT a focal enhancement of backscatter in underlying tissue like in geographic atrophy or laser scars can be seen.[181]

Retinochoroiditis (Toxoplasmosis)

Active lesions in toxoplasmosis can be distinguished from scars by OCT. Vitreous inflammatory cell infiltrates, posterior vitreous detachment, and granulomas at the posterior vitreous layer are visualized.

In acute stage of toxoplasmosis the white retinal infiltration shows a bright reflective inner retinal layer and a thickening of the retina. Due to the backscatter of the nerve fiber layer the underlying outer retinal layers appear optically empty. The predominant infiltration of the nerve fiber layer is consistent with the histological finding of destruction of nerve fibers in retinal infiltration due to toxoplasmosis, therefore called a retinochoroiditis. The retina is thickened in this area. Depending on the clinical stage, focal or general vitreous infiltration is found. In late scar formation the typical findings of scars are visualized by OCT: focal thinning of the retina, thickening of the retinal pigment epithelium and choriocapillaris and in various degrees an enhanced transmission into deeper

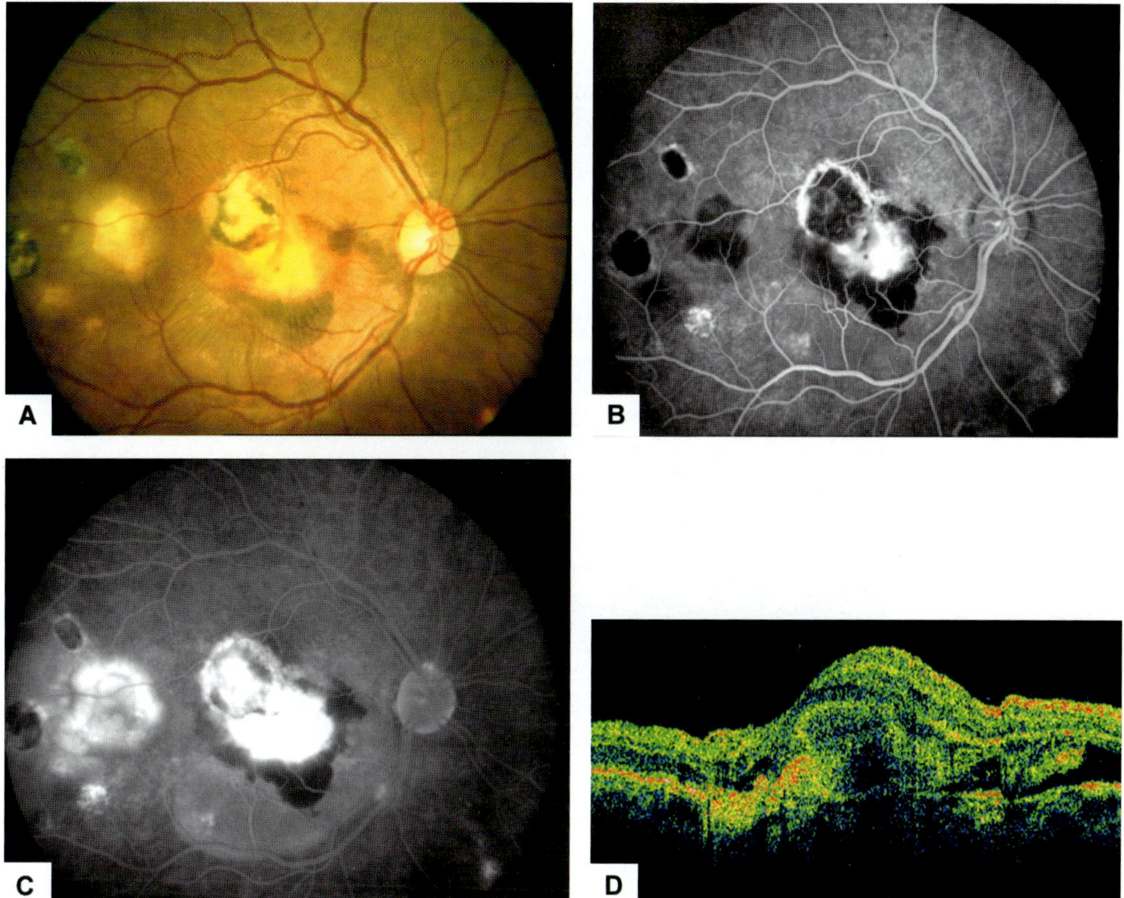

FIGURES 1.70A to D: (A) Fundus photograph of the right eye shows choroidal neovascular membrane. (B,C) Fluorescein angiography reveals a classic choroidal neovascular membrane in the right eye (early and late phase). (D) OCT line scan shows areas of disrupted retinal pigment epithelium with increases hyper-reflectivity from the outer retinal layers with adjacent hyporeflective areas suggesting of the presence of intraretinal fluid. These findings are consistent with classic choroidal neovascular membrane (Jyotirmay Biswas MS, India).

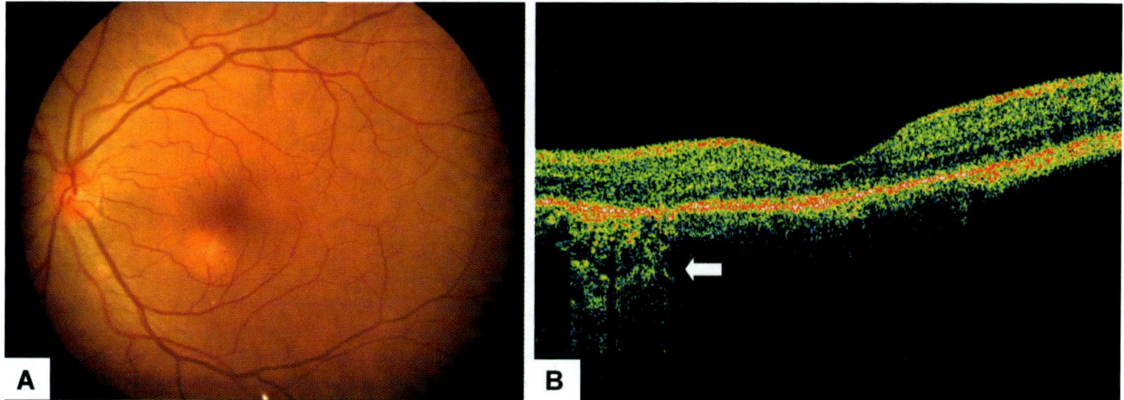

FIGURES 1.71A and B: (A) Fundus photograph shows a focal choroiditis lesion. (B) OCT line scan passing through the lesion shows lesions beneath the retinal pigment epithelium with few areas of moderate backscatter (Jyotirmay Biswas MS, India).

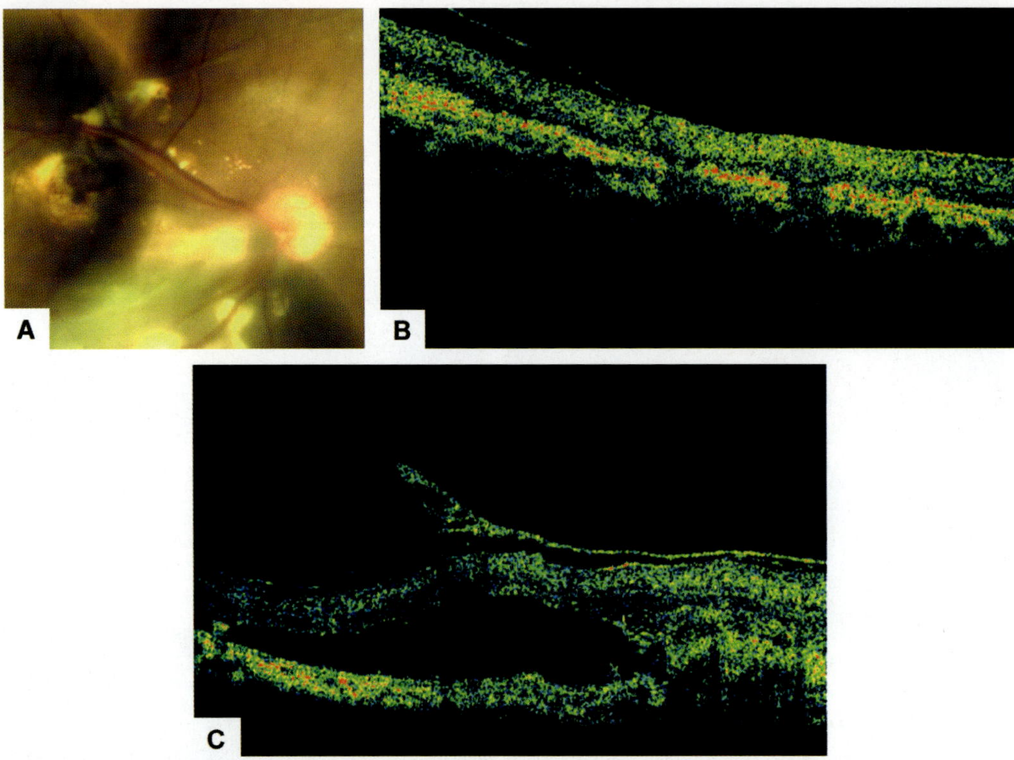

FIGURES 1.72A to C: (A) Fundus photograph showing healed tuberculous choroiditis. (B,C) OCT line scans passing through different lesions showing scars and neurosensory detachment (Jyotirmay Biswas MS, India).

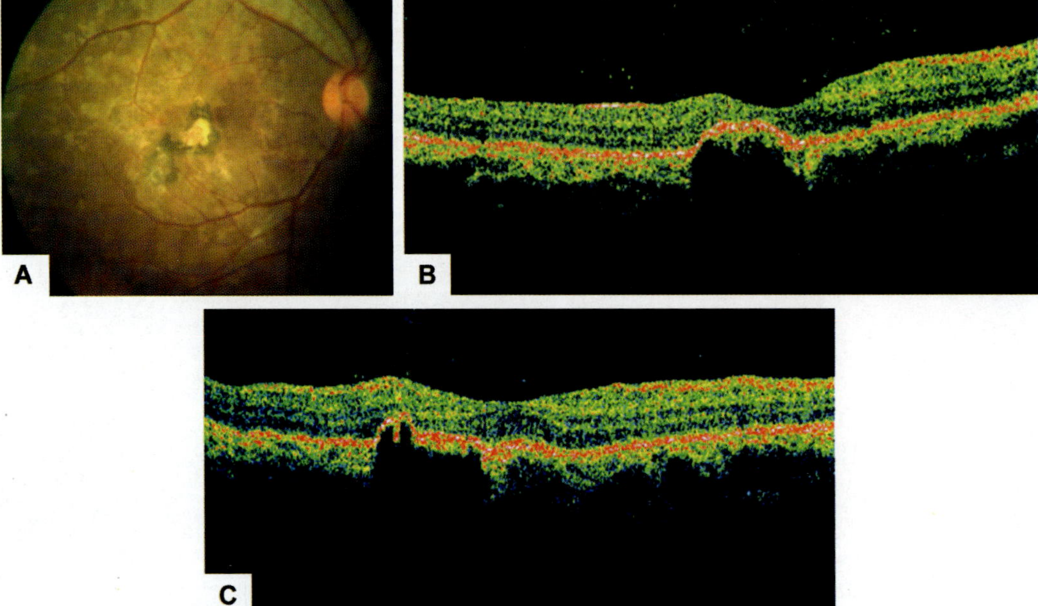

FIGURES 1.73A to C: (A) Fundus picture of the right eye shows healed choroiditis lesions with subretinal gliosis and scarring at the posterior pole. (B, C) OCT line scan passing through the lesions and the scar shows hypertrophied and irregular retinal pigment epithelium layer and overall thinning of the retina. Also seen are scars beneath the retinal pigment epithelium (Jyotirmay Biswas MS, India).

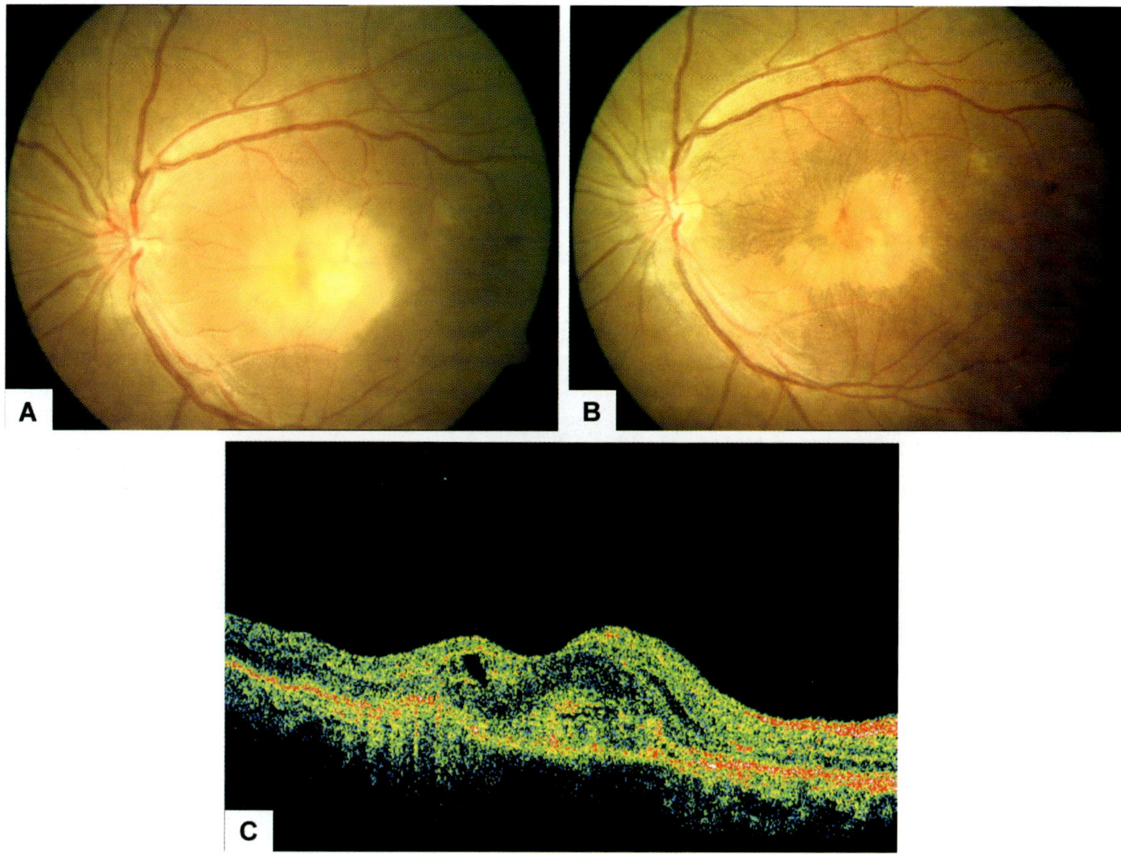

FIGURES 1.74A to C: Fundus examination shows a large choroidal granuloma at the posterior pole. (B) Fundus photograph shows healed choroiditis with subretinal scarring and choroidal neovascularisation. (C) OCT scan passing through the scar showing retinal pigment epithelium hypertrophy with intraretinal cyst and fibrovascular complex and disrupted retinal pigment epithelium at few points (Jyotirmay Biswas MS, India).

layers. The effectiveness of medical treatment (antibiotic drugs and/or high-dose corticosteroids) is obviated by OCT monitoring showing the resolution of vitreous infiltrates and macular edema. [181]

Retinal Vasculitis

Cystoid macular edema is the prominent pathological findings by OCT. In most cases the CME detected by OCT reveal a far more extensive lesion than biomicroscopy or fluorescein angiography would have suggested (Figures 1.75A and B). The medical treatment based on the OCT may be more aggressive. [181]

Neuroretinitis

The most common finding in neuroretinitis is a diffuse thickening of the retina. In rare cases a higher backscatter due to hard exudates within the sensory retina may occur. [181]

Vogt-Koyanagi-Harada Syndrome

Vogt-Koyanagi-Harada (VKH) syndrome is a rare systemic disease involving various melanocyte-containing organs. Bilateral uveitis associated with cutaneous, neurologic, and auditory abnormalities characterizes this syndrome (Figures 1.76A to D).

Two patterns of serous retinal detachments can occur in VKH; namely, a true serous detachment and a cystic space with intraretinal fluid accumulation in the outer retina. A true serous retinal detachment occurs in 69% patients and 40% have intraretinal fluid accumulation with no associated serous retinal detachment. [191] A true detachment has a lenticular optical empty space in the

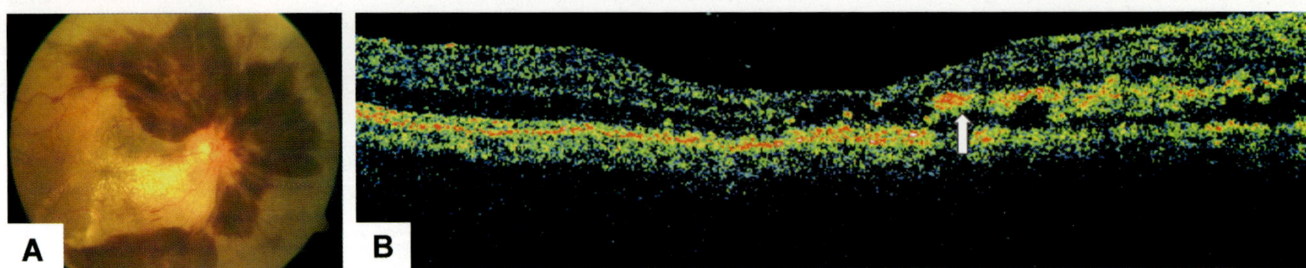

FIGURES 1.75A and B: (A) Fundus photograph shows hemorrhages, macular fan and areas of vasculitis. (B) OCT line scan of the right macula shows hyper-reflective areas suggestive of hard exudates (Jyotirmay Biswas MS, India).

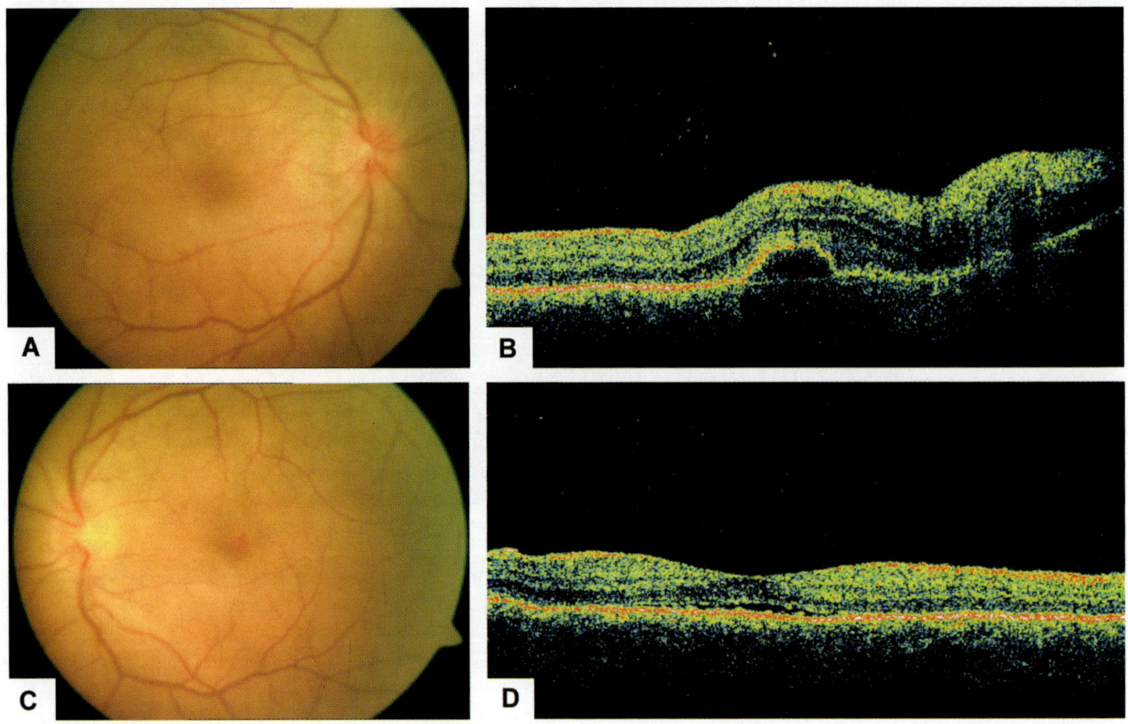

FIGURES 1.76A to D: (A) Fundus picture of the right eye shows settled retinal detachment with few areas of pigment epithelial detachment. (B) OCT scan reveals pigment epithelial detachment. (C) Fundus picture of the left eye shows normal posterior pole. (D) OCT scan of the left eye shows a subtle neurosensory detachment at the fovea (Jyotirmay Biswas MS, India).

subretinal space. The outer surface being clearly demarcated forms a sharp angle with the retinal pigment epithelium. The subretinal space does not contain reflective dots or reflective tissue on the retinal pigment epithelium. Intraretinal fluid accumulation has cystoid spaces generally delineated by surrounding retinal tissue and has a thin reflective layer on the retinal pigment epithelium. The intraretinal cystoid space has highly reflective dots.

Sympathetic Ophthalmia

Sympathetic ophthalmia is a bilateral granulomatous panuveitis that occurs after either surgery or penetrating trauma to one eye. The traumatized eye is called the exciting eye and the non-injured eye is called the sympathizing eye.

Optical coherence tomography is extremely sensitive in identifying neurosensory retinal elevation because of the distinct difference in optical reflectivity between

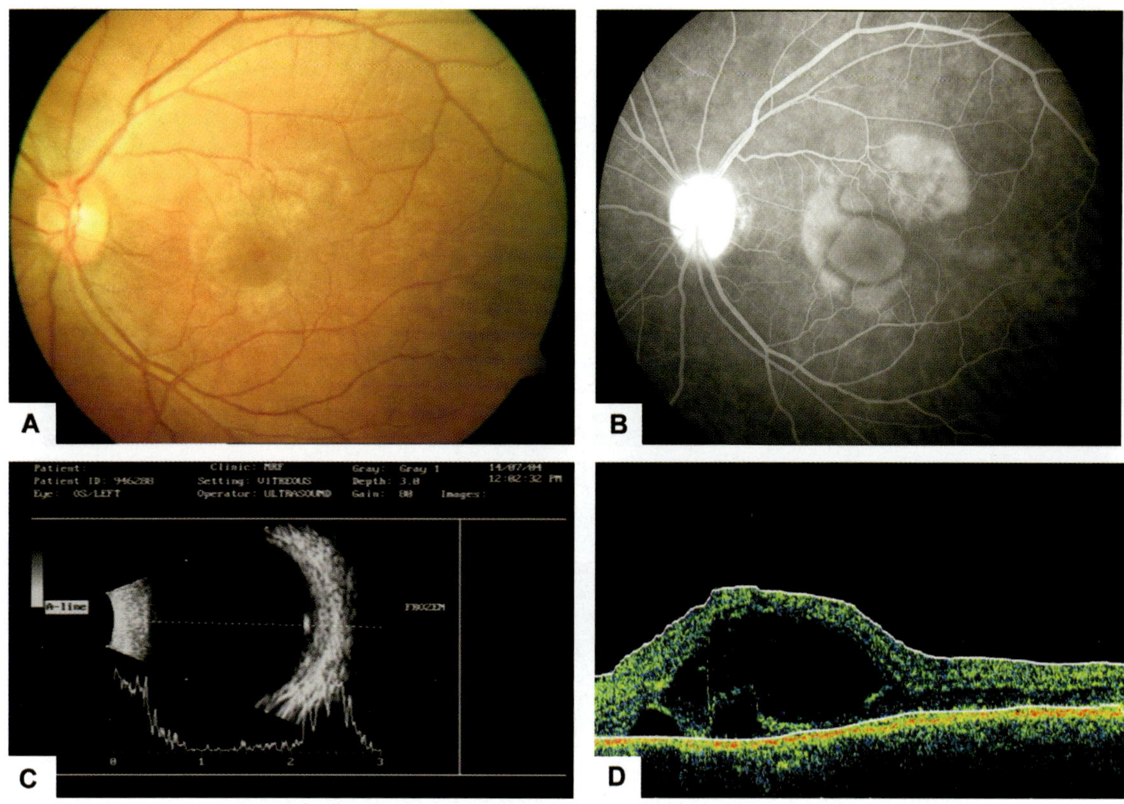

FIGURES 1.77A to D: (A) Fundus photograph of the left eye showing multiple pockets of fluid at the posterior pole. (B) Fluorescein angiogram of the left eye showing pooling of the dye. (C) B-scan of the left eye showing a shallow retinal elevation and choroidal thickness was 1.5 mm. (D) OCT scan of the left showing multiple neurosensory detachments at the macula (Jyotirmay Biswas MS, India).

photoreceptors and underlying retinal pigment epithelium/choriocapillaris. In patients with retinal detachment, OCT can detect the presence of shallow subretinal fluid or cystoid macular edema that may be difficult to identify by other methods, confirming a macula-involving retinal detachment (Figures 1.77A to D).

In the acute phase, the fluorescein angiogram typically demonstrates multiple hyperfluorescent sites of leakage at the level of the retinal pigment epithelium which persist during the venous phase. In severe cases, these foci may coalesce with pooling of dye beneath areas of exudative retinal detachment. The sites of early blocked fluorescence generally correspond to the clinically observed Dalen Fuchs nodules.

Posterior Scleritis

Posterior scleritis presents with protean manifestations. It can rarely be confused with central serous retinopathy, VKH and tumor. Ultrasound and fluorescein angiography play an important role in the diagnosis of posterior scleritis (Figures 1.78A to C).

GENERAL FINDINGS IN INFLAMMATORY DISEASE OF RETINA AND CHOROID IN OCT

- OCT demonstrated three different patterns of macular edema in uveitis: detachment of the sensory retina (20%), diffuse macular edema (55%) and cystoid macular edema (25%). Cystoid fluid accumulation of cystoid macular edema was located predominantly in the outer retinal layer. Patients with cystoid macular edema had significantly greater retinal thickness and worse visual acuity. [181] The sensitivity of OCT for detecting cystoid macular edema compared with fluorescein angiography is 96% and OCT specificity is 100%. In 40% of uveitis patients an epiretinal membrane may be found on OCT. Choroidal neovasculari-

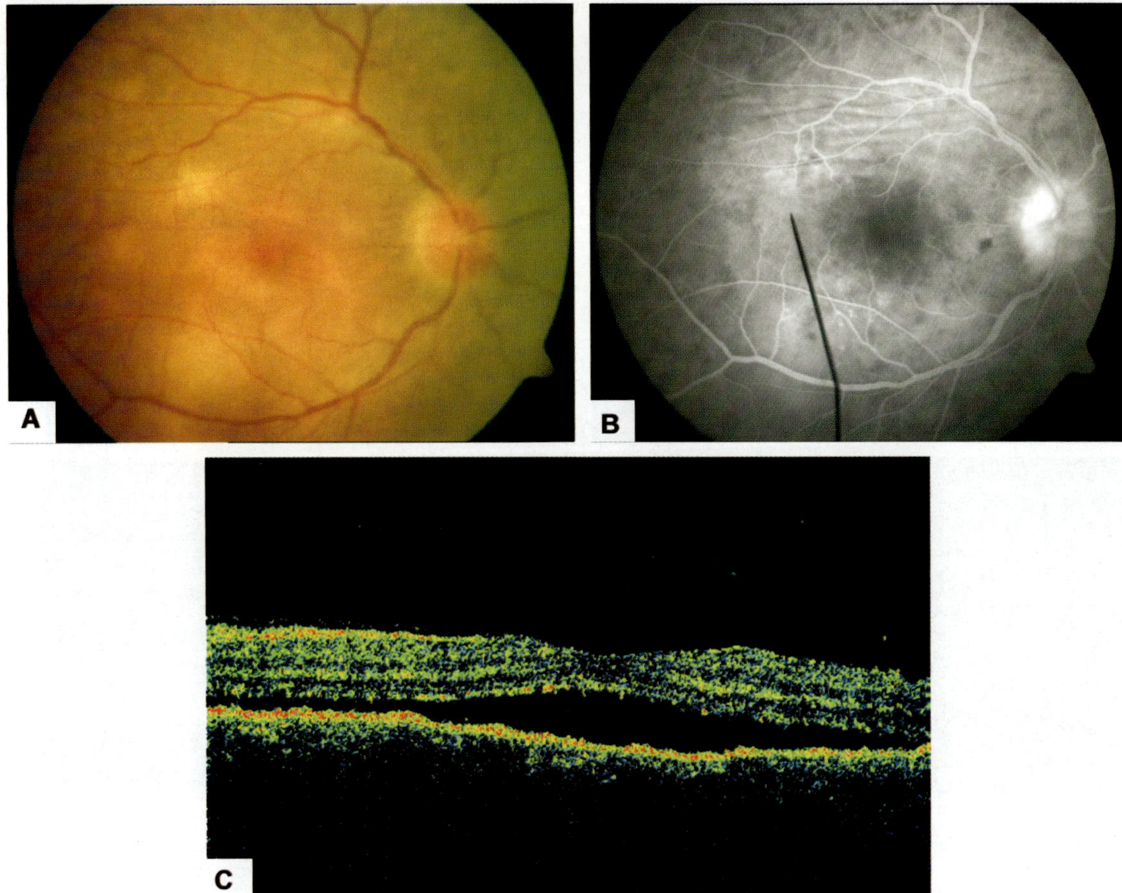

FIGURES 1.78A to C: (A) Fundus lesions suggestive of pockets of fluid and choroidal folds. (B) Fluorescein angiography shows multi-hyperfluorescent spots. (C) OCT scan shows a neurosensory detachment along with cystoid macular edema (Jyotirmay Biswas MS, India).

sation may follow various inflammatory diseases. The extent and localization to the fovea including fluid accumulation can be visualized by OCT for decision-making strategies. In the OCT, scar formation in presumed ocular histoplasmosis syndrome or toxoplasmosis is similar to a chorioretinal atrophic scar after laser treatment or in geographic atrophy. [181]

Indications for laser or surgical treatment depend primarily on clinical features, and the localization in relation to the macula. Fluorescein angiography shows a mapping of the retinal perfusion with leakage but no relation to retinal layers. [181]

Since optical coherence tomography is a non-invasive, non-contact imaging modality, which produces high-resolution cross-sectional images of the ocular fundus helping to identify the morphology of intraocular tissue layers, distinct advantages of the OCT compared to fluorescein angiography can be demonstrated.

OCT evaluation in uveitis may be useful in following conditions:

- Cystoid macular edema
- Epiretinal membranes
- Granulomas
- Detachment of the retinal pigment epithelium or the sensory retina
- Choroidal neovascularization
- Subretinal membranes.

None of the chorioretinal inflammatory diseases present a typical and unique pathognomonic finding in OCT. Inflammation is due to a breakdown of the blood-retinal barrier and causes fluid accumulation in various layers (retina, retinal pigment epithelium). Therefore OCT will visualize in most cases the fluid accumulation following structural changes. Due to the light transmission into deeper layers, the clear-cut visualization of OCT is better in the inner layers and deteriorating toward the outer layers and deeper structures, such as choroid. Optical coherence tomography helps in indicating treatment and surgical intervention, in visualizing structural changes and relation to the merging structures:

- Direct visualization of inflammation (e.g. toxoplasmosis)
- Visualization of sequelae (e.g. epiretinal membrane)

Treatment indications in uveitis patients utilizing the OCT as the main diagnostic tool are membrane peeling, subretinal membrane excision and vitrectomy, laser coagulation and aggressive medical treatment including cytotoxic agents. These observations indicate that the OCT seems to be the most appropriate device to precisely localize secondary CNV and allow decision-making for a surgical strategy. The effectiveness of anti-inflammatory treatment and the surgical outcome can be objectively monitored. This makes the OCT an additional instrument for the visualization of inflammatory processes and sequelae in the central fundus. [181]

INTRAOCULAR TUMORS

There are several types of tumors that can occur in the posterior segment of the eye.[192-194] They are generally classified based on the main tissue involved. The spectrum of tumors in each tissue varies. The differentiation of these tumors is made primarily by indirect ophthalmoscopy.[192]

Ancillary testing with fundus fluorescein angiography, indocyanine green angiography, ultrasonography, OCT, color Doppler testing, magnetic resonance imaging, computed tomography, and fine needle aspiration biopsy can assist in confirming the diagnosis. [192]

Optical coherence tomography provides cross sectional imaging of the retina and retinal pigment epithelium primarily, and deeper tissues, including the choroid and sclera, show poorer resolution. With this in mind, OCT of retinal and retinal pigment epithelium tumors show good resolution whereas OCT of choroidal tumors show only superficial information of the choroidal tumor, but more extensive information of the overlying retina and retinal pigment epithelium. [192]

CHOROIDAL TUMORS

Choroidal Nevus

Choroidal melanocytic nevus is a benign tumor that is seen with increasing frequency in the latter decades of life. It is estimated that between 4% to 6% of caucasians manifest a uveal nevus.[195] It can occur in the iris, ciliary body, or choroid, and is most frequent in the posterior choroid. Choroidal nevus varies in size from a fraction of a millimeter to several millimeters in base. The degree of pigmentation can extend from dark brown to slate gray to completely yellow, or amelanotic. Overlying degenerative changes of the retina and retinal pigment epithelium can occur with the most common being drusen, retinal pigment epithelial atrophy and hyperplasia, and clumped orange pigment. [192]

Most choroidal nevi are less than 2 mm in thickness. It is often difficult to differentiate those nevi that are near 2 mm in thickness from small choroidal melanoma. Risk factors predictive of small melanoma have been identified and include tumor thickness greater than 2 mm, overlying orange pigment, associated subretinal fluid, symptoms of flashes, floaters, or blurred vision, and location of the mass at the optic disk. [192,196-198] The presence of three or more of these five risk factors imparts greater than 50% risk that the tumor will grow, a sign of malignant melanoma.[192]

Choroidal nevus is poorly imaged on OCT due to its location deep in the choroid; however, the overlying retina can show several alterations (Figures 1.79A and B). Specific OCT findings of the choroidal nevus are limited to its anterior surface with minimal information deeper within the mass. These findings included increased thickness of the retinal pigment epithelium/choriocapillaris layer and optical qualities within the anterior portion of the nevus of hyporeflectivity (62%), iso reflectivity, and hyperreflectivity. Hyporeflectivity may also be observed. Optical coherence tomography is more sensitive in the detection of related retinal edema, subretinal fluid, retinal thinning, photoreceptor attenuation, and retinal pigment epithelium detachment.[192]

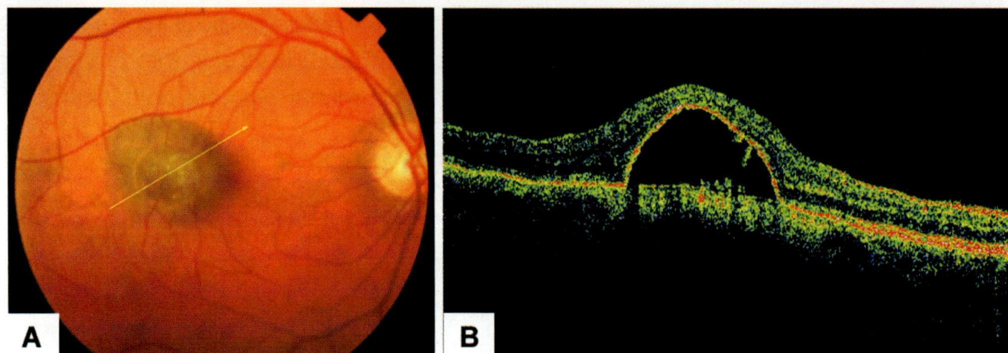

FIGURES 1.79A and B: (A) Pigmented choroidal nevus shows overlying retinal pigment epithelium detachment outlined with subtle orange pigment. (B) Optical coherence tomography shows obvious overlying retinal pigment epithelium detachment with debris in the subpigment epithelial space (Jerry A, Shields MD, Carol L Shields MD, USA).

The findings on OCT of retinal edema, retinal pigment epithelium alterations, photoreceptor loss, and retinal pigment epithelium detachment are related to chronic retinal degeneration and suggest a stable, chronic choroidal nevus. Presence of subretinal fluid and photoreceptor preservation suggests a more acute situation and potentially a more active lesion with risk for growth into melanoma.[192,199]

Choroidal Melanoma

Malignant melanoma of the choroid is uncommon, found in 6 persons per million population.[193,194,200,201] Melanoma usually grows as a localized elevated mass protruding toward the vitreous cavity on its inner aspect and limited by the sclera on its outer aspect. Occasionally, it will grow into a mushroom configuration or grow horizontally as a diffuse, flat lesion.[202] As the tumor grows it may become associated with widespread changes in the overlying retinal pigment epithelium including atrophy and degeneration, clumped orange pigment, serous retinal pigment epithelium detachment, sensory retinal detachment, sensory retinal infiltration or erosion, cystoid retinal edema, and occasionally hemorrhage.[192]

Choroidal melanoma, in general, is poorly imaged on OCT. However, detection of overlying subretinal fluid by OCT could be important in confirming the suspicion of melanoma in eyes with borderline small or intermediate size tumors.[199] This confirms the previous clinical observations that presence of subretinal fluid is a risk factor for eventual growth of the tumor.[196-198] The OCT findings of subretinal fluid might have a predictive value in identifying choroidal melanocytic tumors that are likely to grow.[192,199]

Optical coherence tomography can detect intraretinal edema before it is visually symptomatic or clinically appreciable. Optical coherence tomography is useful in monitoring resolution of radiation-induced macular edema following therapy with laser photocoagulation or intravitreal triamcinolone acetonide (Figures 1.80A to C). The long term effects of intravitreal triamcinolone for radiation maculopathy are not known, but monitoring of the macular edema with OCT is informative and provides an objective guideline for documentation of treatment results.[192]

Choroidal Metastasis

Cancer metastatic to the choroid is probably more common than generally realized.[193,194,203] It typically originates from breast carcinoma or lung carcinoma. Choroidal metastases can be unilateral and unifocal or bilateral and multifocal. The bilateral lesions are related to breast carcinoma in nearly 70% of cases.[195] Lung carcinoma metastasis is usually unifocal. Most choroidal metastases occur posterior to the equator of the fundus in the macular or paramacular regions. It generally appears as a flat or slightly elevated amelanotic lesion with poorly discernible margins. Scattered clumps of brown pigment can be seen over the lesion, which

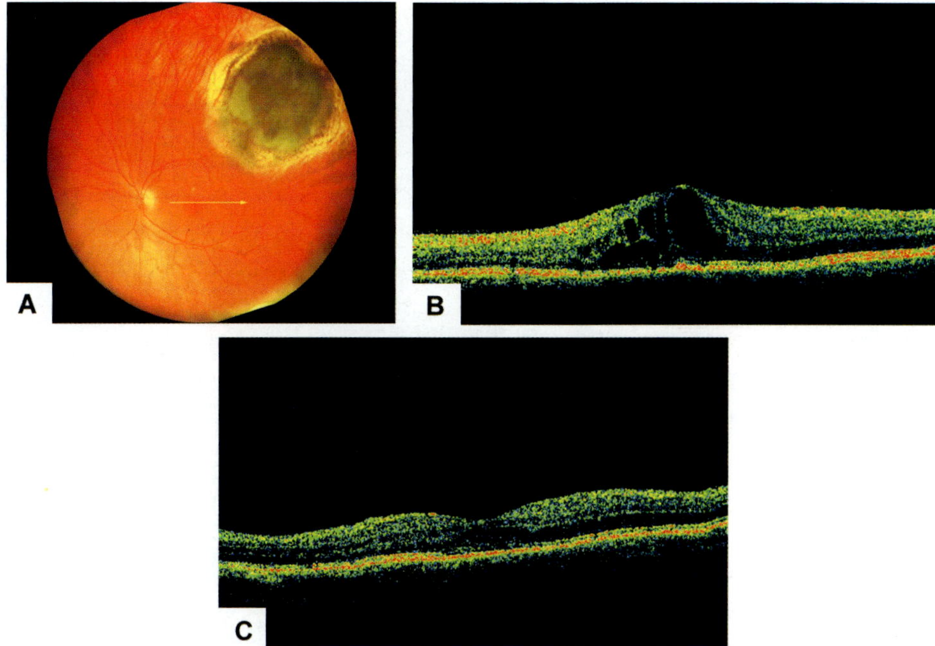

FIGURES 1.80A to C: (A) Twelve months following plaque radiotherapy for a choroidal melanoma, tumor regression was achieved but radiation maculopathy was noted. (B) At that time, OCT revealed cystoid macular edema of 446 microns and intravitreal triamcinolone acetonide was injected. (C) Four months after injection, the foveal anatomy was restored with foveal thickness of 207 microns (Jerry A, Shields MD, Carol L, Shields MD, USA).

correlates histopathologically with lipofuscin pigment within macrophages at the level of the retinal pigment epithelium. Overlying retinal pigment epithelium changes and sensory retinal detachment can accompany these lesions. [192]

Like other choroidal tumors, choroidal metastasis is not well imaged by OCT, but the overlying retinal and retinal pigment epithelial changes can be illustrated. Optical coherence tomography can depict overlying subretinal fluid, retinal pigment epithelial hyperplasia, retinal pigment epithelial detachment, and clumps of orange pigment. Resolution of subretinal fluid on OCT can be documented following therapy of the metastasis (Figures 1.81A to D). [192,204]

Choroidal Hemangioma

Choroidal hemangioma is considered a hamartomatous vascular tumor and is usually not clinically detectable until the second or third decade of life. [193,194,205-207] This lesion appears typically as a round or oval, slightly elevated, orange-colored tumor. Classically, choroidal hemangioma occurs in the posterior pole. [205] It usually exhibits slow enlargement in early life and by young adulthood it can develop overlying atrophic changes in the retinal pigment epithelium, cystoid degeneration of the sensory retina, and sensory retinal detachment. [192]

On OCT, choroidal hemangioma is imaged with poor resolution of the mass itself. The mass appears to be optically reflective at its anterior surface with little detail deeper into the choroidal mass. On the other hand, OCT is quite beneficial for imaging the overlying retina and ascertaining the reason for visual loss. Visual loss occurs due to subretinal fluid, intraretinal edema, chronic photoreceptor loss, induced hyperopia, tilt of the fovea on the elevated mass as well as long-standing related amblyopia. Newly active choroidal hemangioma shows

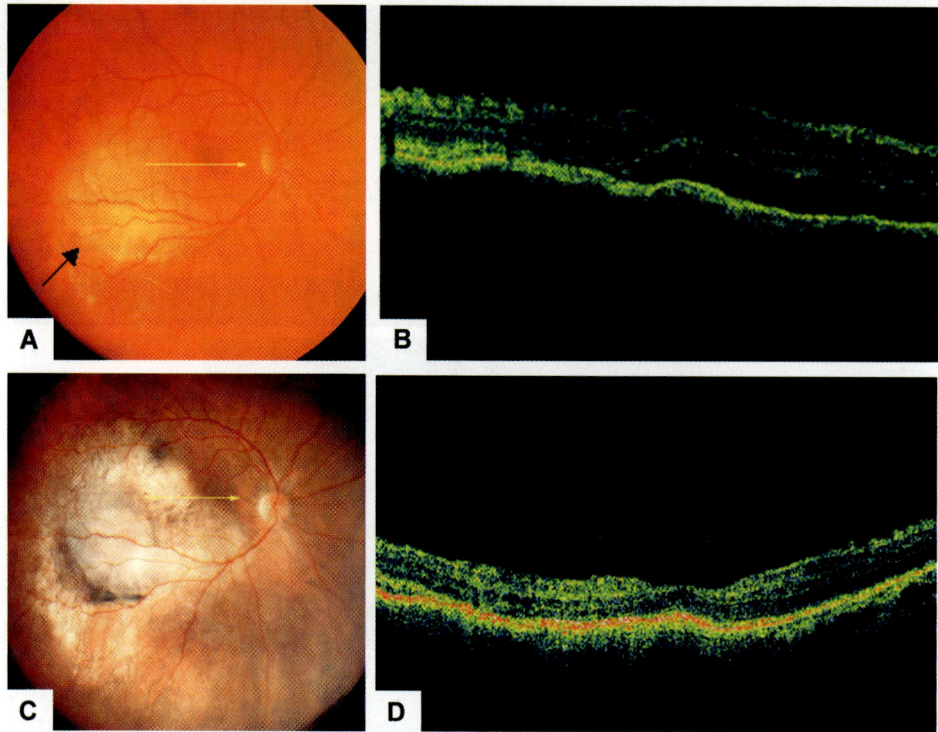

FIGURES 1.81A to D: (A) Amelanotic choroidal metastasis in the foveal region produced subretinal fluid. (B) Optical coherence tomography before therapy demonstrates subfoveal fluid. (C) Following 9 months of hormonal therapy, the choroidal metastasis regressed. (D) Following 9 months of hormonal therapy, the subretinal fluid regressed (Jerry A, Shields MD, Carol L, Shields MD, USA).

subretinal fluid and preserved photoreceptor layer with minimal intraretinal edema. Chronically leaking choroidal hemangioma displays additional photoreceptor attenuation and overlying intraretinal edema and even bullous retinoschisis. When a tumor is discovered with newly active or chronic features causing visual loss, treatment is advised. Options for treatment include laser photocoagulation, transpupillary thermotherapy, application of a radiation plaque, and most recently, photodynamic therapy. Optical coherence tomography is an important tool in depicting resolution of subretinal fluid and foveal edema following therapy. This is especially helpful for those eyes that receive photodynamic therapy for management of choroidal hemangioma as the subretinal or intraretinal fluid generally resolves rapidly and parallels return of visual acuity (Figures 1.82A to D). [192,208]

Choroidal Osteoma

Choroidal osteoma is a benign intraocular tumor comprised of mature bone that typically replaces the full thickness choroid. This tumor classically manifests as an orange-yellow plaque deep to the retina in the juxtapapillary or macular region. [209,210] It most often occurs as a unilateral condition in teen-aged or young adult females. Unfortunately, the etiology and pathogenesis of this tumor is poorly understood. Despite its benign histopathology, it can compromise visual acuity. [211] Since this condition typically occurs in otherwise healthy young patients, most can anticipate experiencing one or many of these outcomes. [192]

The OCT, features of choroidal osteoma include preservation of the inner retinal layers with atrophy of the outer layers, especially the photoreceptor layer of the retina. Often subretinal fluid or separation of the neurosensory retina from the excavation underlying choroidal tumor is noted. The retinal pigment epithelium layer is indistinct as both the calcified tumor and retinal pigment epithelium layer appear as one layer of bright signal. [212,213] Abrupt elevation of the choroidal tumor at its margin, dense optical reflectivity, and complete

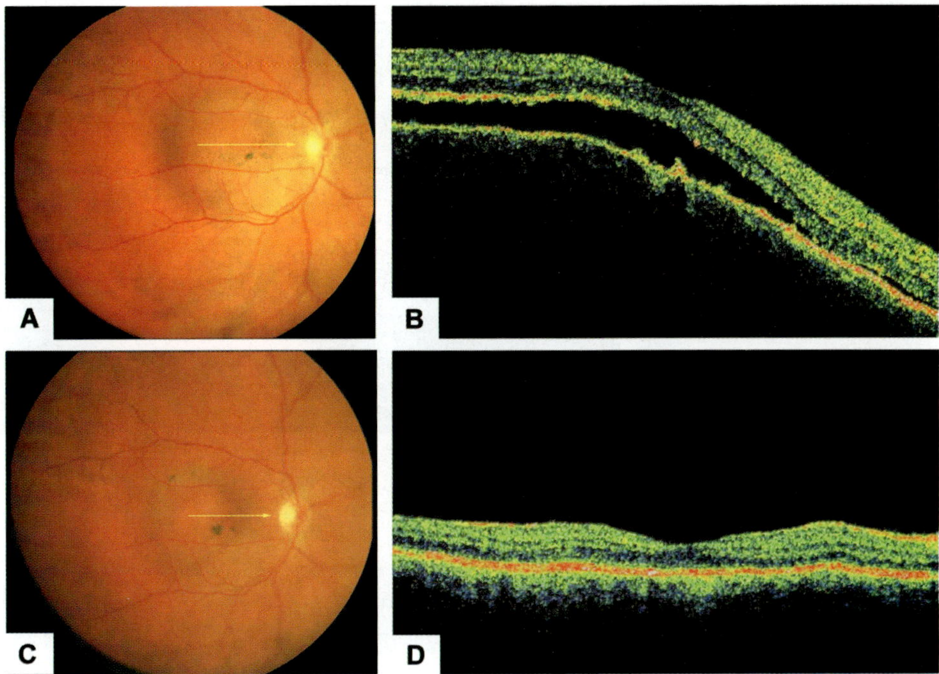

FIGURES 1.82A to D: (A) Subfoveal choroidal hemangioma with overlying subretinal fluid. (B) Subretinal fluid and focal retinal pigment epithelial hyperplasia is documented on OCT. (C) Following photodynamic therapy, the tumor has regressed. (D) Following photodynamic therapy, the subretinal fluid resolved on OCT (Jerry A, Shields MD, Carol L, Shields MD, USA).

shadowing are characteristic of the choroidal osteoma. Areas of elevation and excavation can be found (Figures 1.83A and B). In the areas of osteoma decalcification, where the lesion clinically appears atrophic and white, there is mild transmission of light through the tumor, whereas in areas where the osteoma is calcified and appears orange, light transmission is blocked and more complete shadowing is noted. [192,213]

LESIONS OF THE RETINAL PIGMENT EPITHELIUM

The lesions affecting the retinal pigment epithelium which will be discussed in this section are congenital hypertrophy of the retinal pigment epithelium, congenital simple hamartoma of the retinal pigment epithelium, and combined hamartoma of the retinal pigment epithelium and retina. [192,214]

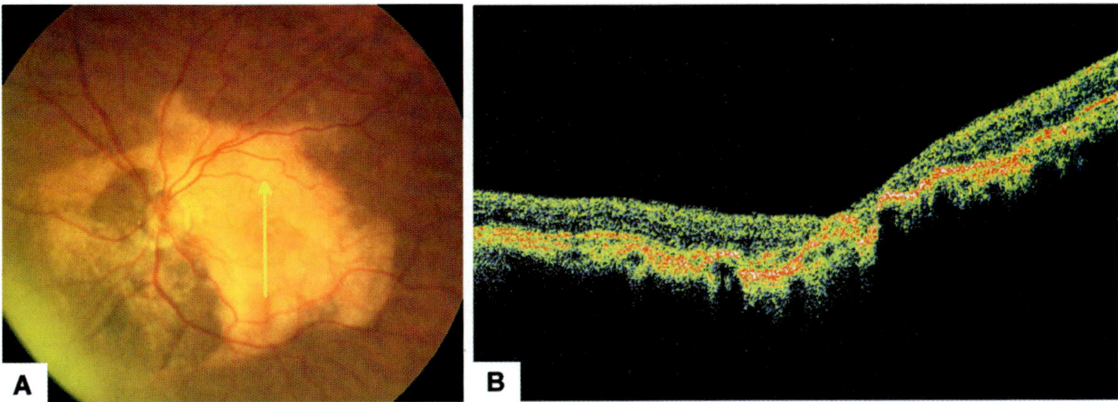

FIGURES 1.83A and B: (A) Panoret™ image shows calcified circumpapillary choroidal osteoma. (B) Optical coherence tomography demonstrates preservation of the inner retinal layers but loss of photoreceptor layer of the retina overlying the irregular choroidal mass. The slightly nodular appearance to the retinal pigment epithelium layer could represent retinal pigment epithelial hyperplasia or irregular surface of the choroidal osteoma (Jerry A, Shields MD, Carol L, Shields MD, USA).

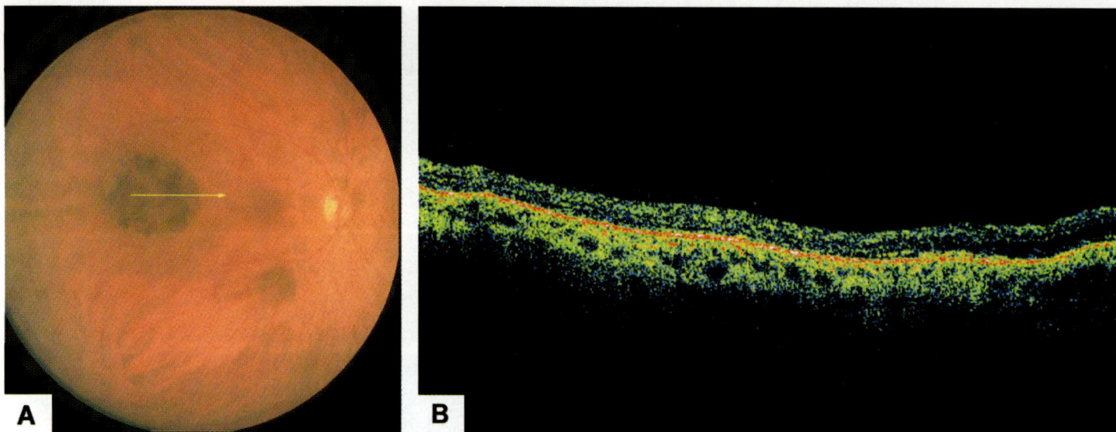

FIGURES 1.84A and B: (A) Panoret™ image shows CHRPE temporal to the fovea. (B) Optical coherence tomography shows slight thickening and increased reflectivity of the retinal pigment epithelium layer with thinned overlying retina and loss of photoreceptors in the region of the flat CHRPE. Note the normal adjacent retina with lucent photoreceptor layer (Jerry A, Shields MD, Carol L, Shields MD, USA).

Congenital Hypertrophy of the Retinal Pigment Epithelium

Congenital hypertrophy of the retinal pigment epithelium (CHRPE) is a flat, heavily pigmented benign lesion that varies in diameter from 1 to several mm and may be found anywhere in the fundus (Figures 1.84A and B).[215] This lesion displays sharp margins that may be associated with a surrounding clear halo, which, in turn, is surrounded by a halo of pigmentation. Patchy round areas of hypo pigmentation within the central portion of the lesion are termed lacunae. Slight growth of CHRPE over many years has been documented.[193,194,215] Histopathologically, these lesions represent hypertrophy of the retinal pigment epithelium with the enlarged retinal pigment epithelial cells containing large round melanosomes. Rarely, adenoma or adenocarcinoma can develop within CHRPE.[216]

By OCT, CHRPE shows slight increased thickness of the retinal pigment epithelium layer with slight shadowing deep to the lesion. The overlying retina is thinned and there is loss of the photoreceptor layer. This tumor is typically difficult to image by OCT as it is usually located in the peripheral fundus.[192]

Congenital Simple Hamartoma of the Retinal Pigment Epithelium

Simple hamartoma of the retinal pigment epithelium is an uncommon, presumed congenital lesion that has been recognized to have characteristic ophthalmoscopic, angiographic, and OCT features.[192,217,218] On clinical examination, this circumscribed benign tumor appears as a small black mass in the macular region measuring a mean of 0.8 mm in basal dimension and 1.6 mm thickness, involving full thickness retina and protruding into the vitreous. Minimally dilated retinal vessels feeding the mass and mild retinal traction can be noted. The lesion blocks fluorescence on angiography and often manifests a ring of staining around the small tumor. There is only one report in the literature on the OCT of this tumor and the features included an abruptly elevated, dome-shaped, optically dense mass protruding from the retina into the vitreous cavity, with complete shadowing of the deeper levels (Figures 1.85A and B).[192,219]

Combined Hamartoma of the Retina and Retinal Pigment Epithelium

The combined hamartoma of the retina and retinal pigment epithelium represents a disorganized proliferation of glial and vascular elements of the retina along with retinal pigment epithelial cells.[219] It is generally associated with vitreoretinal interface disturbance and retinal folds or striae. While most commonly found adjacent to the disk, it can also occur in the macula or mid periphery.[192]

The combined hamartoma of the retinal pigment epithelium and retina shows many interesting findings on OCT. Thickened retinal mass with a hyper-reflective

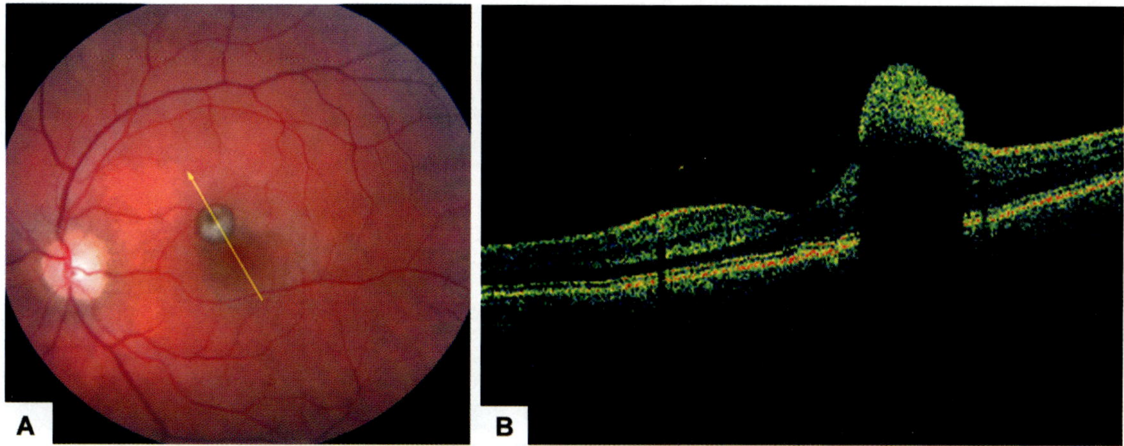

FIGURES 1.85A and B: (A) The hamartoma appears as a small black mass in the foveal retina. (B) On OCT, the mass shows a domed, reflective appearance protruding into the vitreous cavity with abrupt shadowing of deeper tissues and barely sparing the foveola (Jerry A, Shields MD, Carol L, Shields MD, USA).

(high backscatter) surface and deep shadowing have been observed.[220] A distinct epiretinal membrane with secondary retinal folds and has also been observed. Additional findings on OCT included full thickness retinal disorganization in all cases. The adjacent retina was normal in architecture and seemed to gradually thicken into the disorganized tissue. Tractional component from the epiretinal membrane or epiretinal component secondary to the retinal tumor may be the cause for distorted retinal findings. [192,221]

TUMORS OF THE RETINA AND OPTIC DISK

Capillary Hemangioma

Retinal capillary hemangioma is a vascular hamartoma that may involve the optic disk and/or retina.[193,194,222-224] When associated with similar lesions of the central nervous system, it is called von Hippel-Lindau syndrome.[193,222-224] Retinal capillary hemangioma located away from the disk is usually associated with one or more feeding arteries and draining veins. Lipid exudation in the macula and retinal detachment are common accompanying manifestations. At the disk the tumor may occur as an inner retinal (endophytic) or deep retinal (exophytic) juxtapapillary lesion. It appears as reddish-orange tumor of variable size, ranging from less than 1 mm to several mm in diameter. Intraretinal and subretinal lipid exudation may extend into the macula, even if the tumor rests in the far periphery. [192]

With OCT, retinal capillary hemangioma displays thickening and disorganization of the retinal layers. The lesion is optically dense due to multiple interfaces of the diffuse capillary channels within the vascular mass. Slight shadowing of deeper tissues is often seen. Optical coherence tomography is most beneficial in detecting subretinal fluid, intraretinal edema, and preretinal fibrosis in the macular region that can accompany retinal capillary hemangioma (Figures 1.86A to C). Chronic cases with intraretinal edema can manifest with a cystoid appearance and even the appearance of retinoschisis. Chronic subretinal fluid shows thinning of the photoreceptor layer. Optical coherence tomography is used to monitor the response to therapy with resolution of the macular subretinal fluid and edema. Epiretinal component could be secondary to the retinal tumor.[192]

Cavernous Hemangiomas

Cavernous hemangioma of the retina or optic nerve is an uncommon tumor that appears as dark grape-like lesion in the sensory the retina.[193,194,222,223] It can vary in size from a few vascular clusters to larger lesions 10 to 15 mm in diameter. Intraretinal and subretinal exudation is not generally associated with this lesion although occasionally vitreous hemorrhage can occur. There is occasionally a familial tendency, with an autosomal dominant pattern of inheritance in which cases intracranial and cutaneous hemangiomas can be present.

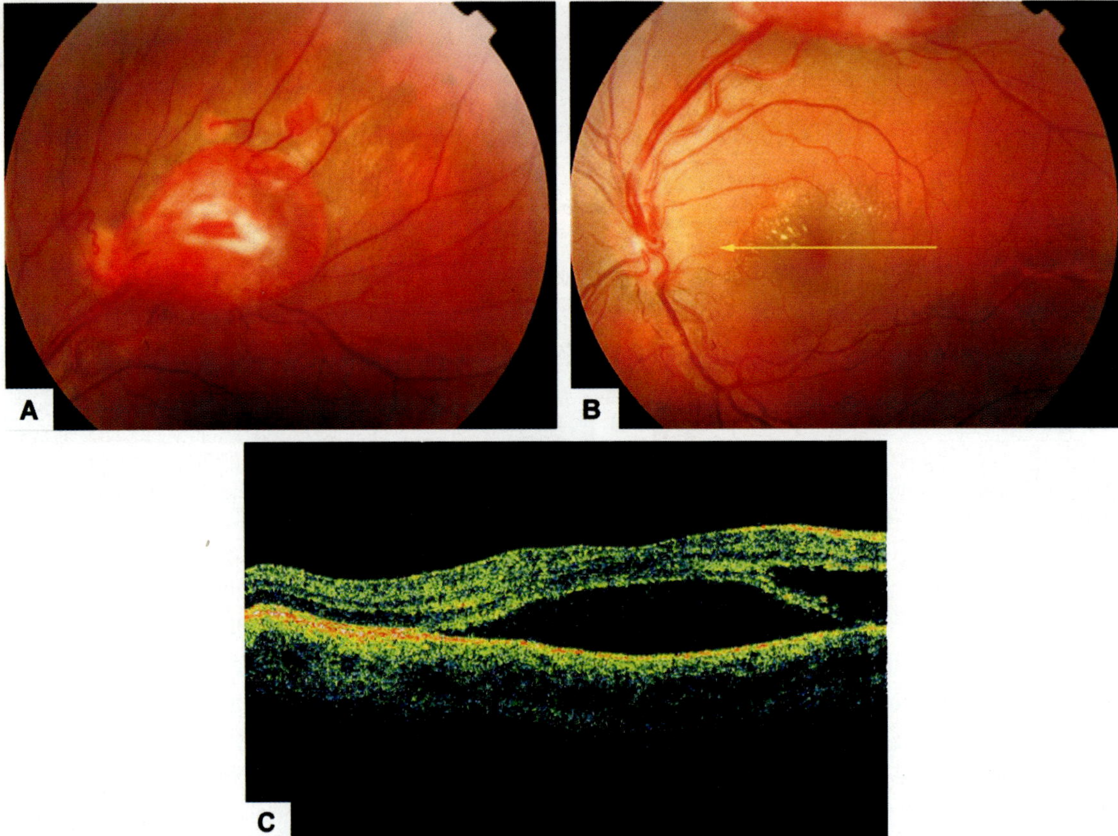

FIGURES 1.86A to C: Retinal capillary hemangioma. (A) Multiple hemangiomas are noted along the superotemporal vascular arcade. (B) Macular exudation and edema from the hemangiomas are shown. (C) Optical coherence tomography shows subretinal fluid in the foveal region and intraretinal edema in the perifoveal area (Jerry A, Shields MD, Carol L, Shields MD, USA).

The tumor is relatively stable and rarely shows true growth. Histopathologically, it is characterized by a cluster of thin-walled dilated veins that replace the normal architecture of the retina or optic nerve head.[192]

Optical coherence tomography of retinal cavernous hemangioma shows an optically dense mass with a lobulated surface. Preretinal fibrosis from chronic vitreous hemorrhage can be seen. If the aneurysms are large, a cystic appearance might be suggested on OCT; however, the anterior reflectivity might cause shadowing and blunt the visibility of deeper levels.[192]

Racemose Hemangioma

The retinal racemose hemangioma is actually a congenital-arteriovenous malformation that can be a simple communication or a complex array of intertwining vessels.[193,194,223,224] The involved vessels are dilated, tortuous, and often more numerous than in the normal eye. Visual function can be normal, and spontaneous hemorrhage rarely occurs. Branch retinal vascular obstruction is a concern at the site of crossing of the large angiomatous vessels.[225] When this arteriovenous malformation is associated with similar midbrain, mandibular, maxillary or pterygoid fossa lesions, it is called the Wyburn-Mason syndrome. With OCT, the racemose hemangioma appears as a relatively large intraretinal cystic mass due to the dilated vessels. Rarely, surrounding retinal changes of retinal atrophy, edema, and hemorrhage can be found[192] (Figures 1.87A to D).

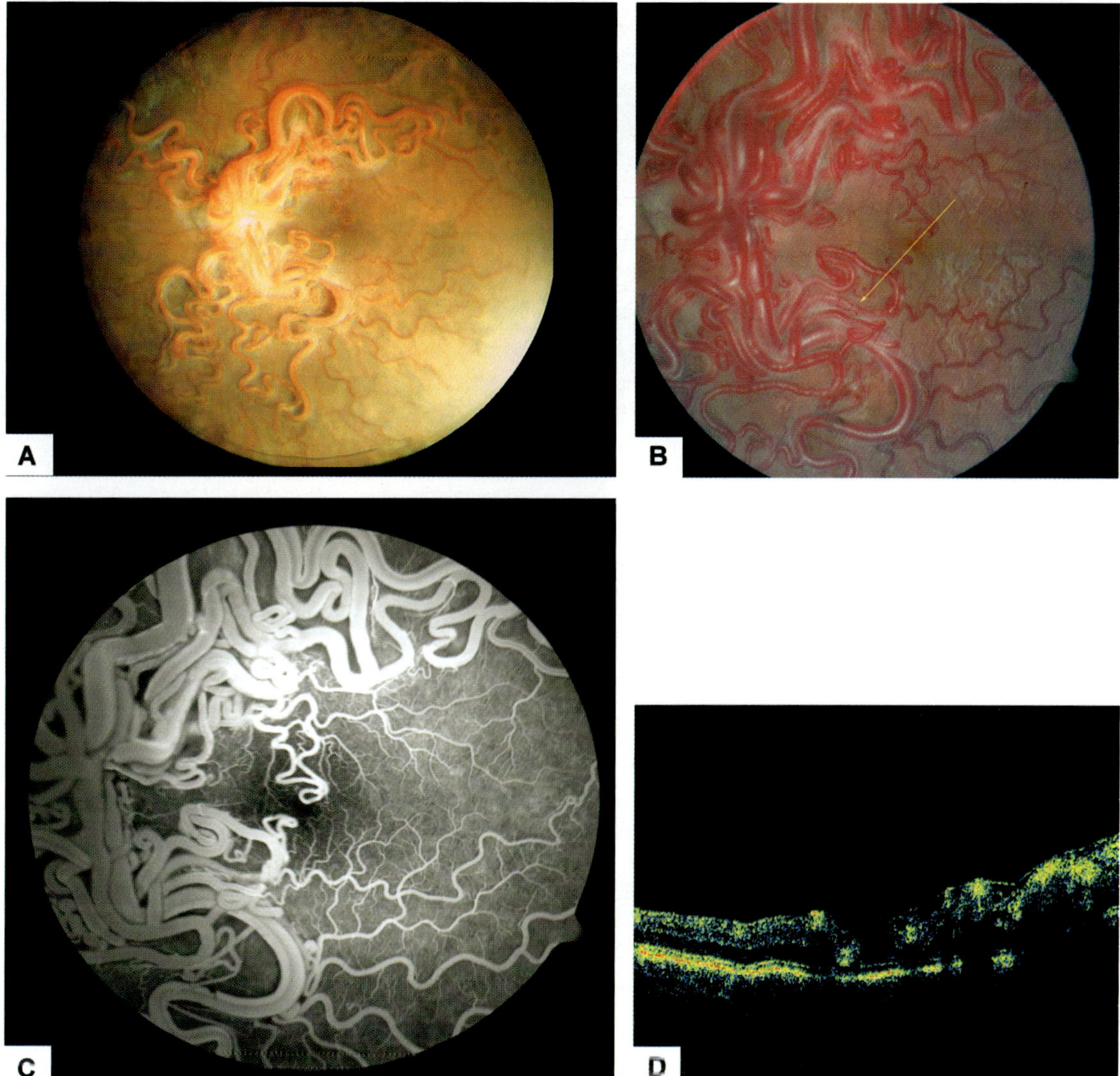

FIGURES 1.87A to D: Retinal racemose hemangioma. (A) Panoret™ image showing snake-like configuration of the arteriovenous malformation. (B)The mass obscures a view of the optic disk. (C) Fluorescein angiography demonstrates the non-leaking, widely dilated vessels. (D) OCT shows irregularity to the retinal surface from the large caliber vessels and shadowing of the deeper structures. There is a faint epiretinal membrane (Jerry A, Shields MD, Carol L, Shields MD, USA).

Astrocytic Hamartoma of the Retina

Astrocytic hamartoma is a retinal lesion typically seen in patients who have tuberous sclerosis.[193,194,222,223] It occurs in the superficial retina or optic disk as a white, round or oval, elevated mass with occasional intralesional calcification imposing a mulberry-like appearance. Mild associated retinal traction can be found. The astrocytic hamartoma is frequently multiple and, despite its white color, is usually highly vascularized. It carries minimal growth potential. Histopathologically, it is usually composed of fibrillary astrocytes, although a giant cells variant is occasionally seen.[192]

With OCT, retinal astrocytic hamartoma shows gently sloping irregular surface overlying an optically dense, disorganized mass replacing the retinal architecture. If there is calcification within the astrocytic hamartoma, then the reflectivity of the mass is high and deep shadowing is noted[192] (Figures 1.88A and B).

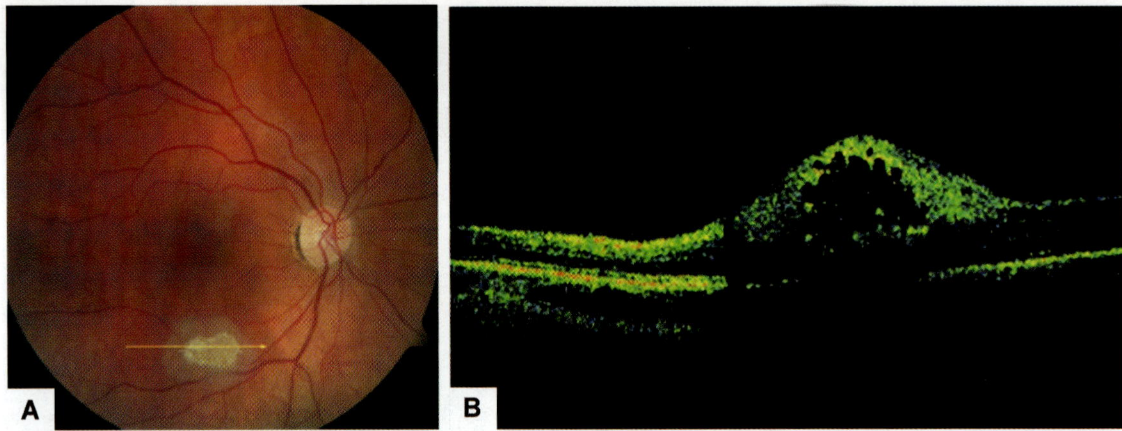

FIGURES 1.88A and B: Retinal astrocytic hamartoma. (A) A calcified retinal astrocytic hamartoma is noted inferior to the macula. (B) Optical coherence tomography shows an intraretinal mass with anterior homogeneous appearance but with deeper "moth eaten" appearance and abrupt reflectivity and shadowing consistent with nodules of calcification (Jerry A, Shields MD, Carol L, Shields MD, USA).

Retinoblastoma

Retinoblastoma is the most common intraocular malignancy of childhood.[192-194,226,227] This tumor grows in either an endophytic or exophytic pattern. The endophytic retinal mass usually has a vascular, cauliflower appearance with scattered tumor nodules along the inner retinal surface and in the vitreous cavity. In the exophytic form there is marked prominence of the vasculature of the tumor and the overlying retina. Histopathologically, retinoblastoma is composed of well differentiated to undifferentiated neuroblastic cells, with scanty cytoplasm, and sometimes characteristic rosettes. [192]

During the very early phases of the fluorescein angiogram, vascular hyperfluorescence is evident from the large vessels which course throughout this cellular tumor. As the study continues, there is leakage from the tumor vasculature causing an increasing hyperfluorescence diffusely within the mass. On OCT, retinoblastoma shows an optically dense appearance with shadowing of the deep tissues. Intralesional calcification can cause higher internal reflectivity (backscattering) and denser shadowing posterior to the tumor. There is abrupt transition of the normal retinal architecture to the retinal mass. If the mass is intraretinal, full thickness retina is

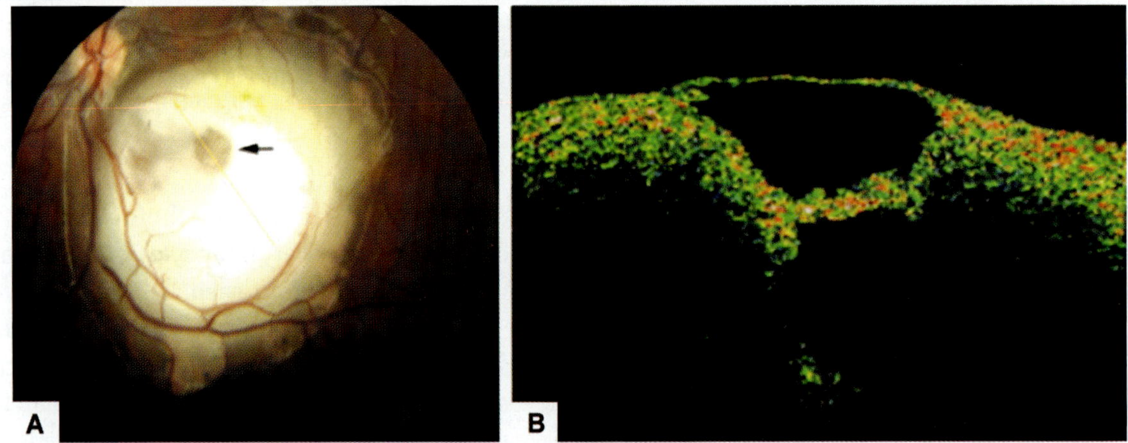

FIGURES 1.89A and B: Retinoblastoma. (A) Retinoblastoma with cavities (arrow) was found in a 4-year-old girl. (B) Optical coherence tomography shows a dense homogeneous retinal mass with cavities anteriorly (Jerry A, Shields MD, Carol L, Shields MD, USA).

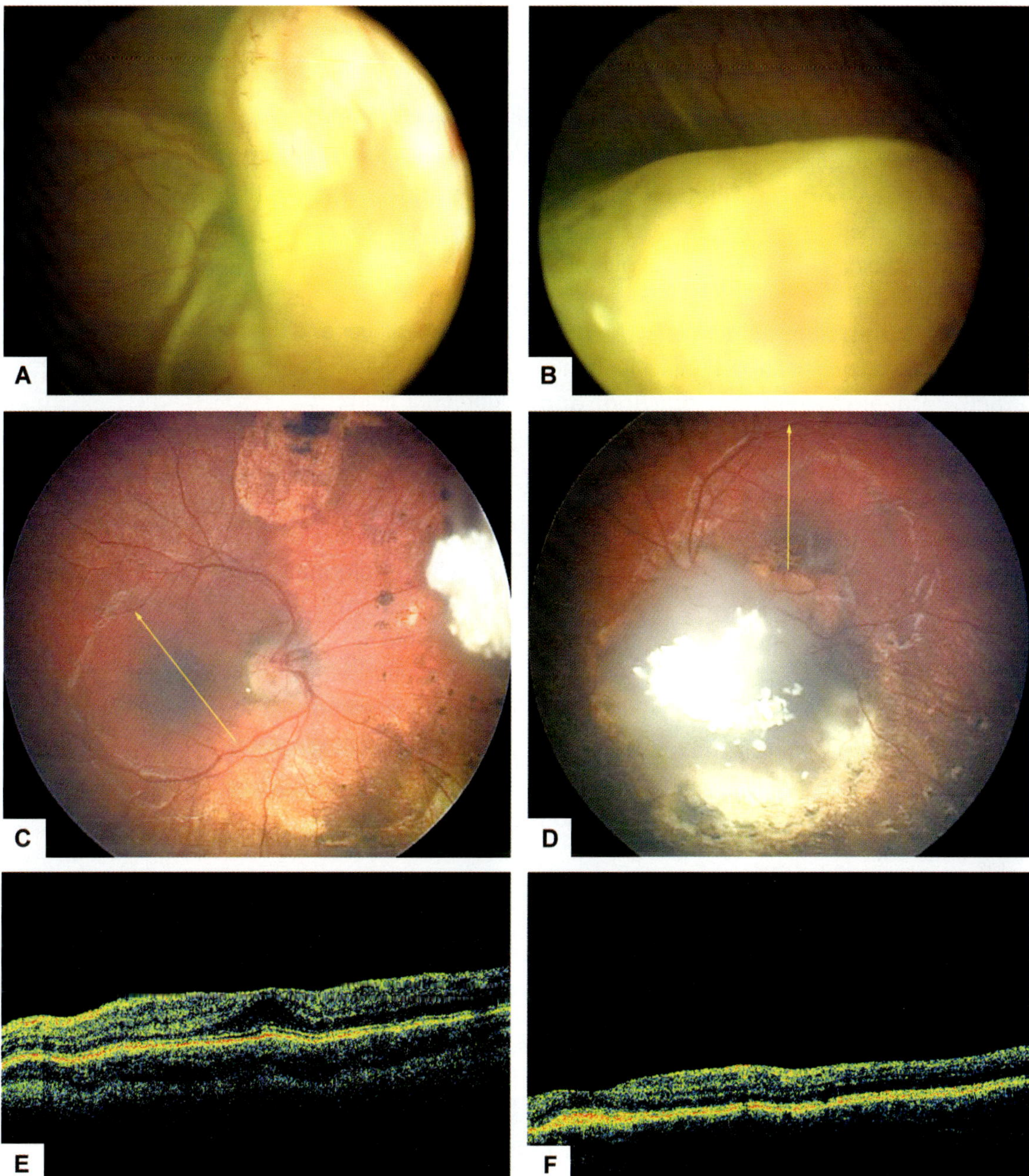

FIGURES 1.90A to F: Retinoblastoma. (A) Advanced retinoblastoma with total retinal detachment in the right eye. (B) Advanced retinoblastoma with total retinal detachment in the left eye. (C) Following chemoreduction and thermotherapy, the tumors regressed and the retina flattened in the right eye. (D) Following chemoreduction and thermotherapy, the tumors regressed and the retina flattened in the left eye. (E) Six years following stable regression, OCT of the right eye shows normal macular architecture without edema or subretinal fluid but with blunted foveal depression. (F) Six years following stable regression, OCT of the left eye shows normal superotemporal macular architecture without edema or subretinal fluid and with normal foveal depression, but with retinal pigment epithelial thickening (Jerry A, Shields MD, Carol L, Shields MD, USA).

involved (Figures 1.89A and B). An endophytic retinoblastoma may be difficult to image due to overlying vitreous seeds. An exophytic tumor shows retinal detachment overlying the neoplasm. In rare cases, intraretinal empty cavities can be visualized and these are usually found in well differentiated portions of the tumor (Figures 1.90A to F). Optical coherence tomography is a useful test in monitoring reasons for visual loss following treatment of retinoblastoma. Causes for visual loss include retinal atrophy, retinal edema, persistent retinal detachment, optic disk edema or atrophy, macular tumor scar, cataract, corneal dryness and scarring, and amblyopia. In some instances, eyes with total retinal detachment from retinoblastoma have recovered complete function of the retina both clinically and anatomically, confirmed on OCT (Figures 1.90A to F).[192,228]

MELANOCYTOMA OF THE OPTIC NERVE

Melanocytoma is a heavily pigmented benign tumor that is usually located on the optic disk.[192-194,229] It can vary in size from less than 1 disk diameter to a much larger lesion extending into the overlying vitreous and adjacent retina and choroid. Histopathologically, it is composed of large pigmented melanocytes found near the region of the lamina cribrosa.

Because of the heavily pigmented cells, this lesion shows hypofluorescence throughout fluorescein angiogram. On OCT, melanocytoma is found to occupy the anterior portion of the optic nerve in a sessile or dome-shaped fashion (Figures 1.91A and B). There is disorganization of the normal optic nerve features. Shadowing of deeper tissues is present. The mass often spills over into and under the adjacent retina. By OCT, the retinal involvement appears as optically dense material in the nerve fiber layer and the choroidal involvement appears as slight elevation of the choroid, sometimes with subretinal fluid.[192]

Optical coherence tomography is a useful technique for imaging the primary and secondary effects of intraocular tumors. It is most suited for information regarding tumors of the retina and retinal pigment epithelium. Information regarding details of choroidal tumors is currently limited due to lack of penetration of the light into the choroid. Optical coherence tomography is especially helpful in imaging the retina following treatment of intraocular tumors and provides important information on the reasons for visual acuity change.[192]

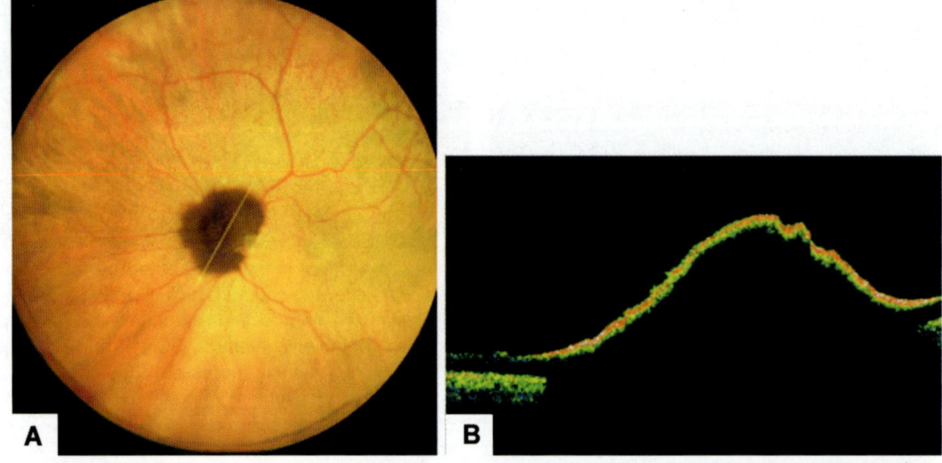

FIGURES 1.91A and B: Optic disk melanocytoma. (A) Panoret™ image shows the darkly pigmented optic nerve mass with adjacent retinal infiltration. (B) Optical coherence tomography shows a thin, delicate, echogenic line delineating the anterior aspect of the melanocytoma with abrupt and complete shadowing behind, obscuring all details of the optic nerve and adjacent retina (Jerry A, Shields MD, Carol L, Shields MD, USA).

REFERENCES

1. Brezinski ME, Tearney GJ, Bouma B, et al. Optical biopsy with optical coherence tomography. Ann N Y Acad Sci 1998; 9:838:68-74.
2. Huang D, Swanson EA, Lin CP, et al. Optical coherence tomography. Science 1991; 254:1178-81.
3. Fujimoto JG, Brezinski ME, Tearney GJ, et al. Optical biopsy and imaging using optical coherence tomography. Nat Med 1995; 1:970-2.
4. Fercher AF, Roth E. Ophthalmic laser interferometry. In: Müller GJ, (Ed): Optical Instrumentation for Biomedical Laser Applications. Belllingham, Wash: SPIE; 1986; 658:48-51.
5. Fercher AF. Optical coherence tomography. J Biomed Opt 1996; 1:157-73.
6. Hee MR, Izatt JA, Swanson EA, et al. Optical coherence tomography of human retina. Arch Ophthalmol 1995; 113:325-32.
7. Youngquist RC, Carr S, Davies DEN. Optical coherence domain reflectometry: a new optical evaluation technique. Opt Lett 1987; 12:158-60.
8. Takada K, Yokohama I, Chida K, Noda J. New measurement system for fault location in optic waveguide devices based on an interferometrc technique. Appl Opt 1987; 26:1603-10.
9. Huang D, Wang J, Lin CP, Puliafito CA, Fujimoto JG. Micron-resolution ranging of cornea and anterior chamber by optical reflectometry. Lasers Surg Med 1991; 11:419-25.
10. Swanson EA, Izatt JA, Hee MR, et al. In vivo retinal imaging by optical coherence tomography. Opt Lett 1993; 18:1864-66.
11. Huang D, Swanson EA, Hee MR, et al. Optical coherence tomography. Science 1991; 254:1178–81.
12. Swanson EA, Huang D, Hee MR, et al. High-speed optical coherence domain reflectometry. Opt Lett 1992; 17:151-3.
13. Hee MR, Huang D, Swanson EA, Fujimoto JG. Polarization-sensitive low coherence reflectometer for birefringence characterization and ranging. J Opt Soc Am B 1992; 9:903-8.
14. Olsen T. The accuracy of ultrasonic determination of axial length in pseudophakic eyes. Acta Ophthalmol (Copenh). 1989; 67:141-4.
15. Bamber JC, Trstam M. Diagnostic ultrasound. In Webb S (Ed): The Physics of Medical Imaging. Philadelphia: Adam Hilger. 1988;319-88.
16. Puliafito CA, Hee MR, Lin CP, et al. Imaging of macular diseases with optical coherence tomography. Ophthalmology 1995; 102:217-29.
17. Fujimoto JG, Brezinski ME, Tearney GJ, et al. Optical biopsy and imaging using optical coherence tomography. Nat Med 1995; 9:970-2.
18. Jaffe GJ, Caprioli J. Optical coherence tomography to detect and manage retinal disease and glaucoma. Am J Ophthalmol 2004; 137:156-69.
19. Hee MR, Puliafito CA, Duker JS, et al. Topography of diabetic macular edema with optical coherence tomography. Ophthalmology 1998; 105:360–70.
20. Pires I, Bernardes RC, Lobo CL, et al. Retinal thickness in eyes with mild non proliferative retinopathy in patients with type 2 diabetes mellitus: comparison of measurements obtained by retinal thickness analysis and optical coherence tomography. Arch Ophthalmol 2002; 120:1301–6.
21. Polito A, Shah SM, Haller JA, et al. Comparison between retinal thickness analyzer and optical coherence tomography for assessment of foveal thickness in eyes with macular disease. Am J Ophthalmol 2002; 134:240–51.
22. Neubauer AS, Priglinger S, S. Ullrich S, et al. Comparison of foveal thickness measured with the retinal thickness analyzer and optical coherence tomography. Retina 2001; 21:596–601.
23. Konno S, Akiba J, Yoshida A. Retinal thickness measurements with optical coherence tomography and the scanning retinal thickness analyzer. Retina 2001; 21:57–61.
24. H. Sanchez-Tocino H, Alvarez-Vidal A, Maldonado MJ, et al. Retinal thickness study with optical coherence tomography in patients with diabetes. Invest Ophthalmol Vis Sci 2002; 43;1588–94.
25. Antcliff RJ, Stanford R, Chauhan DS, et al. Comparison between optical coherence tomography and fundus fluorescein angiography for the detection of cystoid macular edema in patients with uveitis. Ophthalmology 2000; 107:593–9.
26. Gaudric A, Massin P, Erginay A. Diabetic macular edema. In: Saxena S, Meredith TA (Ed): Optical Coherence Tomography in Retinal Diseases. New Delhi: Jaypee Medical Publishers, 2006;45-82.
27. Yamamoto S, Yamamoto T, Hayashi M, Takeuchi S. Morphological and functional analyses of diabetic macular edema by optical coherence tomography and multifocal electroretinograms. Graefes Arch Clin Exp Ophthalmol 2001; 239.96-101.
28. Antcliff RJ, Marshall J. The pathogenesis of edema in diabetic maculopathy. Semin Ophthalmol 1999; 14:223-32.
29. Puliafito CA, Hee MR, Lin CP, et al. Imaging of macular diseases with optical coherence tomography. Ophthalmology 1995; 102:217-29.
30. Otani T, Kishi S, Maruyama Y. Patterns of diabetic macular edema with optical coherence tomography. Am J Ophthalmol 1999; 127:688-93.
31. Yamamoto T, Hitani K, Tsukahara I, et al. Early postoperative retinal thickness changes and complications after vitrectomy for diabetic macular edema. Am J Ophthalmol 2003; 135:14-9.
32. Catier A, Tadayoni R, Paques M, et al. Optical Coherence Tomography characterization of macular edema according to various etiology. Am J Ophthalmol 2005 (In press).
33. Otani T, Kishi S. Tomographic findings of foveal hard exudates in diabetic macular edema. Am J Ophthalmol 2001; 131:50-4.

34. Imai M, Iijima H, Hanada N. Optical coherence tomography of tractional macular elevations in eyes with proliferative diabetic retinopathy. Am J Ophthalmol 2001; 132:81-4.

35. Kaiser PK, Riemann CD, Sears JE, Lewis H. Macular traction detachment and diabetic macular edema associated with posterior hyaloidal traction. Am J Ophthalmol 2001; 131: 44-9.

36. Massin P, Duguid G, Erginay A, et al. Optical coherence tomography for evaluating diabetic macular edema before and after vitrectomy. Am J Ophthalmol 2003; 135:169-77.

37. Uchino E, Uemura A, Ohba N. Initial stages of posterior vitreous detachment in healthy eyes of older persons evaluated by optical coherence tomography. Arch Ophthalmol 2001; 19:1475-9.

38. Ito Y, Terasaki H, Suzuki T, et al. Mapping posterior vitreous detachment by optical coherence tomography in eyes with idiopathic macular hole. Am J Ophthalmol 2003; 35: 351-5.

39. Gaucher D, Tadayoni R, Erginay A, et al. Optical coherence tomography assessment of the vitreoretinal relationship in diabetic macular edema. Am J Ophthalmol 2005 (In press).

40. Browning DJ, Fraser CM. Intraobserver variability in optical coherence tomography. Am J Ophthalmol 2004; 138:477-79.

41. Goebel W, Kretzchmar-Gross T. Retinal thickness in diabetic retinopathy: a study using optical coherence tomography (OCT). Retina. 2002; 22:759-67.

42. Browning DJ, Fraser CJ. Regional patterns of sight-threatening diabetic macular edema. Am J Ophthalmol 2005; 140:117-24.

43. Chan A, Duker JS. A standardized method for reporting changes in macular thickening using optical coherence tomography. Arch Ophthalmol 2005; 123:939-43.

44. Audren F, Tod M, Massin P, et al. Pharmacokinetic-pharmacodynamic modeling of the effect of triamcinolone acetonide on central macular thickness in patients with diabetic macular edema. Invest Ophthalmol Vis Sci 2004; 45:3435-41.

45. Mori K. Retinal artery occlusion and retinal arterial macro-aneurysm. In Saxena S, Meredith TA (Ed): Optical Coherence Tomography in Retinal Diseases. New Delhi: Jaypee Brothers Medical Publishers, 2006;99-101.

46. Yanoff M, Fine BS. Ocular Pathology: A Text and Atlas. 3rd ed. Philadelphia, PA: JB Lippincott 1989; pp 383-400.

47. Mori K. Retinal artery occlusion and retinal arterial macro-aneurysm. In Saxena S, Meredith TA (Eds): Optical Coherence Tomography in Retinal Diseases. New Delhi: Jaypee Brothers Medical Publishers, 2006; pp 102-7.

48. See RF, Fekrat S. In Saxena S, Meredith TA (Eds): Optical Coherence Tomography in Retinal Diseases. New Delhi: Jaypee Brothers Medical Publishers, 2006; pp 83-97.

49. Apushkin MA, Fishman GA, Janowicz MJ. Monitoring cystoid macular edema by optical coherence tomography in patients with retinitis pigmentosa. Ophthalmology 2004; 111:1899-1904.

50. Spaide RF, Lee JK, Klancnik JK, Jr., Gross NE. Optical coherence tomography of branch retinal vein occlusion. Retina. 2003; 23:343-7.

51. Antcliff RJ, Stanford MR, Chauhan DS, et al. Comparison between optical coherence tomography and fundus fluorescein angiography for the detection of cystoid macular edema in patients with uveitis. Ophthalmology 2000; 107:593-9.

52. Kang SW, Park CY, Ham DI. The correlation between fluorescein angiographic and optical coherence tomographic features in clinically significant diabetic macular edema. Am J Ophthalmol 2004; 137:313-22.

53. Rumelt S, Karatas M, Pikkel J, et al. Optic disc traction syndrome associated with central retinal vein occlusion. Arch Ophthalmol 2003; 121:1093-7.

54. Ip MS, Kumar KS. Intravitreous triamcinolone acetonide as treatment for macular edema from central retinal vein occlusion. Arch Ophthalmol 2002; 120:1217-9.

55. Gass JDM, Blodi B. Idiopathic juxtafoveal retinal telangiec-tasis: update of classification and follow-up study. Ophthalmology 1993;100;1536-46.

56. Hamilton R, Kim JE, Spaide RF. Juxtafoveal telangiectasis. In Saxena S, Meredith TA (Eds): Optical Coherence Tomography in Retinal Diseases. New Delhi: Jaypee Brothers Medical Publishers, 2006; pp 131-6.

57. Cruz-Villegas V, Puliafito C, Fujimoto JG. Retinal Vascular Diseases. Optical Coherence Tomography of Ocular Diseases, 2nd ed. Thorofare, NJ. SLACK Incorporated, 2004; pp 103-56.

58. Bhende M, Nair BK. Central serous chorioretinopathy. In Saxena S, Meredith TA (Eds): Optical Coherence Tomography in Retinal Diseases. New Delhi: Jaypee Brothers Medical Publishers, 2006; pp 137-44.

59. Hee MR, Puliafito CA, Wong C, et al. Optical coherence tomography of central serous chorioretinopathy. Am J Ophthalmol 1995; 120:65-74.

60. Wang M, Sander B, Lund-Andersen H, Larsen M. Detection of shallow detachments in central serous chorioretinopathy. Acta Ophthalmol Scand 1999; 77:402-5.

61. Iida T, Hagimura N, Sato T, Kishi S. Evaluation of central serous chorioretinopathy with optical coherence tomography. Am J Ophthalmol 2000; 129:16-20.

62. Wang MS, Sander B, Larsen M. Retinal atrophy in idiopathic central serous chorioretinopathy. Am J Ophthalmol 2002; 133:787-93.

63. Iida T, Yannuzzi LA, Spaide RF, et al. Cystoid macular degeneration in chronic central serous chorioretinopathy. Retina 2003; 23:1-7.

64. Montero JA, Ruiz-Moreno JM. Optical coherence tomography characterisation of idiopathic central serous chorioretinopathy. Br J Ophthalmol 2005; 89:562-4.

65. Piccolino FC, de la Longrais RR, Ravera G, et al. The foveal photoreceptor layer and visual acuity loss in central serous chorioretinopathy. Am J Ophthalmol 2005; 139:87-99.

66. Soubrane G, Coscas G. Age-related macular degeneration and choroidal neovascularization. In Saxena S, Meredith TA (Eds): Optical Coherence Tomography in Retinal Diseases. New Delhi: Jaypee Brothers Medical Publishers, 2006, pp 109-30.

67. Gass JD. Stereoscopic Atlas of Macular Diseases: Diagnosis and Treatment, 4th edition. St. Louis: Mosby. 1997; pp 938-51.

68. Terasaki H, Ito Y. Idiopathic epiretinal membranes. In Saxena S, Meredith TA (Eds): Optical Coherence Tomography in Retinal Diseases. New Delhi: Jaypee Brothers Medical Publishers, 2006; pp 145-52.

69. Mavrofrides EC, Rogers AH, Truong S, et al. Vitreoretinal interface disorders. In Optical Coherence Tomography of Ocular Diseases, Second edition. Thorofare, Slack. 2004; pp 57-77.

70. McDonald HR, Johnson RN, Ai E, Schatz H. Macular Epiretinal Membrane. In Ryan SJ (Ed). Retina St. Louis: Mosby. 2001; pp 2531-46.

71. Mcdonald HR, Shatz H, Johnson RN. Introduction to epiretinal membrane. In Ryan S (Ed.) Retina. St. Louis: Mosby. 1994; pp 1819-25.

72. Tannenbaum, HL, Schepens CL, Elzeneiny I, Freeman HM. Macular pucker following retinal detachment surgery. Arch Ophthalmol 1970; 83: 286-93.

73. Wise GN. Congenital preretinal macular fibrosis. Am J Ophthalmol 1975; 79:363-5.

74. Lobes LA Jr, Burton TC. The incidence of macular pucker after retinal detachment surgery. Am J Ophthalmol 1978; 85:72-7.

75. Gass JDM. Stereoscopic Atlas of Macular Diseases: Diagnosis and Yreatment. St. Louis: Mosby, 1987.

76. Mori K. Secondary epiretinal membrane, macular pseudoholes and vitreomacular traction syndrome. In Saxena S, Meredith TA (Eds): Optical Coherence Tomography in Retinal Diseases. New Delhi: Jaypee Brothers Medical Publishers, 2006; pp 153-62.

77. Wilkins JR, Puliafito CA, Hee MR, et al. Characterization of epiretinal membrane using optical coherence tomography. Ophthalmology 1996; 103:2142-51.

78. Mori K, Gehlbach PL, Sano A, et al. Comparison of epiretinal membranes of differing pathogenesis using optical coherence tomography. Retina 2004; 24: 57-62.

79. Massin P, Allouch C, Haouchine B, et al. Optical coherence tomography of idiopathic macular epiretinal membranes before and after surgery. Am J Ophthalmol 2000; 130: 732-39.

80. Smiddy WE, Michels RG, Glaser BM, de Bustos S. Vitrectomy for macular traction caused by incomplete vitreous separation. Arch Ophthalmol 1988; 106:624-28.

81. Margherio RR, Trese MT, Margherio AR, Cartright K. Surgical management of vitreomacular traction syndromes. Ophthalmology 1989; 96:1437-45.

82. Carpineto P, Ciancaglini M, Aharrh-Gnama A, et al. Optical coherence tomography imaging of surgical resolution of bilateral vitreomacular traction syndrome related to incomplete posterior vitreoschisis: a case report. Eur J Ophthalmol 2004; 14: 438-41.

83. Ip MS, Grage-Feldman M. Idiopathic macular hole. In Saxena S, Meredith TA (Eds): Optical Coherence Tomography in Retinal Diseases. New Delhi: Jaypee Brothers Medical Publishers, 2006; pp 163-78.

84. Grignolo A. Fibrous components of the vitreous body. Arch Ophthalmol 1952; 47:760-74.

85. Eisner G. Clinical anatomy of the vitreous. In Jakobiec FA (Ed): Ocular Anatomy, Embryology, and Teratology. Philadelphia: Harper & Row Publishers 1982; 413-7.

86. Hee MR, Puliafito CA, Wong C, et al. Optical coherence tomography of macular holes. Ophthalmology 1995; 102:748-56.

87. Puliafito, CA, Hee MR, Lin CP, et al. Imaging of macular diseases with optical coherence tomography. Ophthalmology 1995; 102:217-9.

88. Foos RY. Vitreoretinal juncture; topographical variations. Invest Ophthalmol 1972; 11:801-8.

89. Kakehashi A, Schepens CL, Trempe CL. Vitreomacular observations, II: data on the pathogenesis of idiopathic macular breaks. Graefes Arch Clin Exp Ophthalmol 1996; 234:425-33.

90. Kim JW, Freeman WR, Azen SP, et al., for the Vitrectomy for Macular Hole Study Group. Prospective randomized trial of vitrectomy or observation for stage 2 macular holes. Am J Ophthalmol 1996; 121:605-14.

91. Gass JDM. Idiopathic senile macular hole: its early stages and pathogenesis. Arch Ophthalmol 1988; 106:629-39.

92. Gass JDM. Reappraisal of biomicroscopic classification of stages of development of a macular hole. Am J Ophthalmol 1995; 119:752-9.

93. Gaudric A, Haouchine B, Massin P, et al. Macular hole formation: new data provided by optical coherence tomography. Arch Ophthalmol 1999; 117:744-51.

94. Haouchine B, Massin P, Gaudric A. Foveal pseudocyst as the first step in macular hole formation: a prospective study by optical coherence tomography. Ophthalmology 2001; 108:15-22.

95. Altaweel, M and Ip, M. Macular hole: improved understanding of pathogenesis, staging, and management based on optical coherence tomography. Semin Ophthalmol 2002; 18:58-66.

96. Azzolini C, Patelli F, Brancato R. Correlation between optical coherence tomography data and biomicroscopic interpretation of idiopathic macular hole. Am J Ophthalmol 2001; 132:348-55.

97. Tolentino FI, Schepens CL, Freeman HM. Vitreoretinal Disorders: Diagnosis and Management, Philadelphia: WB Saunders Co. 1976; pp 400-12.

98. Asrani S, Zeimer R, Goldberg M, et al. Serial optical sectioning of macular holes at different stages of development. Ophthalmology 1998; 105:66-77.

99. Johnson MW, Van Newkirk MR, Meyer KA. Perifoveal vitreous detachment is the primary pathogenic event in idiopathic macular hole formation. Arch Ophthalmol 2001; 119:215-22.

100. Ezra E, Fariss RN, Possin DE, et al. Immunocytochemical characterization of macular hole opercula. Arch Ophthalmol 2001; 119:223-231.

101. Ryan EH Jr, Gilbert HD. Results of surgical treatment of recent-onset full-thickness idiopathic macular hole. Arch Ophthalmol 1994; 112:1545-53.

102. Ip MS, Baker BJ, Duker JS, et al. Anatomical outcomes of surgery for idiopathic macular hole as determined by optical coherence tomography. Arch Ophthalmol 2002; 120:29-35.

103. Freeman WR, Azen SP, Kim JW, et al. For the Vitrectomy for Treatment of Macular Hole Study Group. Vitrectomy for the treatment of full-thickness stage 3 or 4 macular holes: results of a multicentered randomized clinical trial. Arch Ophthalmol 1997; 115:11-21.

104. Ullrich S, Haritoglou C, Gass C, et al. Macular hole size as a prognostic factor in macular hole surgery. Br J Ophthalmol 2002; 86:390-3.

105. Imai M, Iijima H, Gotoh T, et al. Optical coherence tomography of successfully repaired idiopathic macular holes. Am J Ophthalmol 1999;128:621-7.

106. Spaide RF. Macular hole repair with minimal vitrectomy. Retina. 2002, 22:183-6.

107. Costa RA, Cardillo JA, Morales PH, et al. Optical coherence tomography evaluation of idiopathic macular hole treatment by gas-assisted posterior vitreous detachment. Am J Ophthalmol 2001; 132:264-6.

108. Chan CK, Wessels IF, Friedrichsen EJ. Treatment of idiopathic macular holes by induced posterior vitreous detachment. Ophthalmology 1995; 102:757-67.

109. Smiddy WE, Feuer W, Cordahl G. Internal limiting membrane peeling in macular hole surgery. Ophthalmology 2001; 108:1471-8.

110. Brooks HL Jr. Macular hole surgery with and without internal limiting membrane peeling. Ophthalmology 2000; 107:1939-49.

111. Kasuga Y, Arai J, Akimoto M, et al. Optical coherence tomography to confirm early closure of macular holes. Am J Ophthalmol 2000;130:675-6.

112. Madreperla SA, Geiger GL, Funata M, et al. Clinicopathologic correlation of a macular hole treated by cortical vitreous peeling and gas tamponade. Ophthalmology 1994; 101:682-6.

113. Macular Photocoagulation Study Group. Laser photocoagulation of subfoveal neovascular lesions in age-related macular degeneration. Results of a randomized clinical trial. Arch Ophthalmol 1991; 109:1220-31.

114. Hawkins BS, Bressler NM, Miskala PH, et al. Submacular Surgery Trials (SST) Research Group. Surgery for subfoveal choroidal neovascularization in age-related macular degeneration: ophthalmic findings: SST report no. 11. Ophthalmology 2004; 111:1967-80.

115. Bressler NM, Bressler SB, Childs AL, et al. Submacular Surgery Trials (SST) Research Group. Surgery for hemorrhagic choroidal neovascular lesions of age-related macular degeneration: ophthalmic findings: SST report no. 13. Ophthalmology 2004; 111:1993-2006.

116. Brindeau C, Glacet-Bernard A, Coscas F, et al. Surgical removal of subfoveal choroidal neovascularization: visual outcome and prognostic value of fluorescein angiography and optical coherence tomography. Eur J Ophthalmol 2001; 11:287-95.

117. Hawkins BS, Bressler NM, Bressler SB, et al; Submacular Surgery Trials Research Group. Surgical removal vs observation for subfoveal choroidal neovascularization, either associated with the ocular histoplasmosis syndrome or idiopathic: I. Ophthalmic findings from a randomized clinical trial: Submacular Surgery Trials (SST) Group H Trial: SST Report No. 9. Arch Ophthalmol 2004; 122:1597-1611.

118. Machemer R, Steinhorst UH. Retinal separation, retinotomy, and macular relocation: II. A surgical approach for age-related macular degeneration? Graefes Arch Clin Exp Ophthalmol 1993; 231:635-41.

119. Ninomiya Y, Lewis JM, Hasegawa T, Tano Y. Retinotomy and foveal translocation for surgical management of subfoveal choroidal neovascular membranes. Am J Ophthalmol 1996; 122:613-21.

120. Fujikado T, Ohji M, Hayashi A, et al. Anatomic and functional recovery of the fovea after foveal translocation surgery without large retinotomy and simultaneous excision of a neovascular membrane. Am J Ophthalmol 1998; 126:839-42.

121. Wolf S, Lappas A, Weinberger AW, Kirchhof B. Macular translocation for surgical management of subfoveal choroidal neovascularizations in patients with AMD: first results. Graefes Arch Clin Exp Ophthalmol 1999; 237:51-7.

122. Eckardt C, Eckardt U, Conrad HG. Macular rotation with and without counter-rotation of the globe in patients with age-related macular degeneration. Graefes Arch Clin Exp Ophthalmol 1999; 237:313-25.

123. Cekic O, Ohji M, Hayashi A, et al. Foveal translocation surgery in age-related macular degeneration. Lancet 1999; 354(9175):340.

124. Lewis H, Kaiser PK, Lewis S, Estafanous M. Macular translocation for subfoveal choroidal neovascularization in age-related macular degeneration: A prospective study. Am J Ophthalmol 1999; 128:135-46.

125. de Juan E Jr, Vander JF. Effective macular translocation without scleral imbrication. Am J Ophthalmol 1999; 128:380-2.

126. Lewis H. Macular translocation with choriosceral outfolding: a pilot clinical study. Am J Ophthalmol 2001; 132:156-63.

127. Ohji M, Fujikado T, Kusaka S, et al. Comparison of three techniques of foveal translocation in patients with subfoveal choroidal neovascularization resulting from age-related macular degeneration. Am J Ophthalmol 2001; 132:888-96.

128. Tano Y. Pathologic myopia: Where are we now? Am J Ophthalmol 2002; 134:645-60.
129. Kamei M, Tano Y, Yasuhara T, et al. Macular translocation with chorioscleral outfolding: 2-year results. Am J Ophthalmol 2004; 138:574-81.
130. Treatment of age-related macular degeneration with photodynamic therapy (TAP) Study Group. Photodynamic therapy of subfoveal choroidal neovascularization in age-related macular degeneration with verteporfin: one-year results of 2 randomized clinical trials—TAP report 1. Arch Ophthalmol 1999; 117:1329-45.
131. Treatment of age-related macular degeneration with photodynamic therapy (TAP) Study Group. Photodynamic therapy of subfoveal choroidal neovascularization in age-related macular degeneration with verteporfin: two-year results of 2 randomized clinical trials—TAP report 2. Arch Ophthalmol 2001; 119:198-207.
132. Treatment of age-related macular degeneration with photodynamic therapy (TAP) Study Group. Verteporfin therapy of subfoveal choroidal neovascularization in age-related macular degeneration with verteporfin: additional information regarding baseline lesion composition's impact on vision outcomes—TAP report No. 3. Arch Ophthalmol 2002; 120:1443-54.
133. Verteporfin In Photodynamic Therapy Study Group. Verteporfin therapy of subfoveal choroidal neovascularization in age-related macular degeneration: two-year results of a randomized clinical trial including lesions with occult with no classic choroidal neovascularization-Verteporfin in photodynamic therapy report 2. Am J Ophthalmol 2001; 131:541-60.
134. Hee MR, Baumal CR, Puliafito CA, et al. Optical coherence tomography of age-related macular degeneration and choroidal neovascularization. Ophthalmology 1996; 103:1260-70.
135. Puliafito CA, Hee MR, Schuman JS, et al. Macular degeneration. In Puliafito CA, Hee MR, Schuman JS, Fujimoto JG (Eds): Optical Coherence Tomography of Ocular Diseases. New Jersey: SLACK incorporated 1996; pp 187-246.
136. Giovannini A, Amato G, Mariotti C, Scassellati-Sforzolini B. Optical coherence tomography in the assessment of retinal pigment epithelial tear. Retina 2000; 20:37-40.
137. Sakguchi H, Ohji M, Kamei M, Tano Y. Surgery for choroidal neovascular membrane. In Saxena S, Meredith TA (Eds): Optical Coherence Tomography in Retinal Diseases. New Delhi: Jaypee Brothers Medical Publishers, 2006; pp 179-90.
138. Terasaki H, Ishikawa K, Suzuki T, et al. Morphologic and angiographic assessment of the macula after macular translocation surgery with 360-degree retinotomy. Am J Ophthalmol 2003; 110: 2403-8.
139. Baba T. Macula after retinal detachment surgery. In Saxena S, Meredith TA (Eds): Optical Coherence Tomography in Retinal Diseases. New Delhi: Jaypee Brothers Medical Publishers, 2006; pp 191-202.
140. Hagimura N, Iida T, Suto K, Kishi S. Persistent foveal retinal detachment after successful rhegmatogenous retinal detachment surgery. Am J Ophthalmol 2002; 133: 516-20.
141. Wolfensberger TJ, Gonvers M. Optical coherence tomography in the evaluation of incomplete visual acuity recovery after macula-off retinal detachments. Graefes Arch Clin Exp Ophthalmol 2002;240:85-9.
142. Baba T, Hirose A, Moriyama M, Mochizuki M. Tomographic image and visual recovery of acute macula-off rhegmatogenous retinal detachment. Graefes Arch Clin Exp Ophthalmol 2004; 242:576-81.
143. Machemer R. Experimental retinal detachment in the owl monkey. II. Histology of retina and pigment epithelium. Am J Ophthalmol 1968; 66:396-410.
144. Ip MS, Garza-Karren C, Duker JS et al. Differentiation of degenerative retinoschisis from retinal detachment using optical coherence tomography. Ophthalmology 1999; 106:600-5.
145. Hagimura N, Suto K, Iida T, Kishi S. Optical coherence tomography of the neurosensory retina in rhegmatogenous retinal detachment. Am J Ophthalmol 2000; 129:186-90.
146. Theodossiadis PG, Georgalas IG, Emfietzoglou J, et al. Optical coherence tomography findings in the macula after treatment of rhegmatogenous retinal detachments with spared macula preoperatively. Retina 2003; 23:69-75.
147. Sabates NR, Sabates FN, Sabates R, et al. Macular changes after retinal detachment surgery. Am J Ophthalmol 1989; 108:22-9.
148. Antcliff RJ, Stanford MR, Chauhan DS, et al. Comparison between optical coherence tomography and fundus fluorescein angiography for the detection of cystoid macular edema in patients with uveitis. Ophthalmology 2000; 107:593.
149. Wolfensberger TJ. Foveal reattachment after macula-off retinal detachment occurs faster after vitrectomy than after buckle surgery. Ophthalmology 2004; 111: 1340-43.
150. Baba T, Hirose A, Kawazoe Y, Mochizuki M. Optical coherence tomography for retinal detachment with a macular hole in a highly myopic eye. Ophthalmic Surg Lasers Imaging 2003; 34:483.
151. Venkatesh P, Garg S, Soni P. Miscellaneous retinal disorders. In Saxena S, Meredith TA (Eds): Optical Coherence Tomography in Retinal Diseases. New Delhi: Jaypee Brothers Medical Publishers, 2006, pp 363-78.
152. Tabatabay CA, D'Amico DJ, Hanninen LA, Kenyon KR. Experimental drusen formation induced by intravitreal aminoglycoside injection. Arch Ophthalmol 1987; 105:826-30.
153. Gupta V, Gupta A, Dogra MR. Retinal vascular occlusions. In: Gupta V, Gupta A, Dogra MR (Eds): Atlas: Optical Coherence Tomography of Macular Disorders. Jaypee New Delhi. First edition 2004; pp103-5.
154. Bechmann M, Ehrt O, Thiel MJ et al. Optical coherence tomography findings in early solar retinopathy. Am J Ophthalmol 2000; 84:546-7.

155. Jorge R, Costa RA, Quirino LS et al. Optical coherence tomography in patients with late solar retinopathy. Am J Ophthalmol 2004;137:1139-42.

156. Garg S, Martidis A, Nelson ML, Sivalingam A. Optical coherence tomography of chronic solar retinopathy. Am J Ophthalmol 2004; 137:351-4.

157. Kaushik S, Gupta V, Gupta A. Optical coherence tomography findings in solar retinopathy. Ophthalmic Surg Lasers Imaging 2004; 35:52-5.

158. Ismail R, Tanner V, Wiliamson S. Optical coherence tomography imaging of severe commotio retinae and associated macular hole. Br J Ophthalmol 2002; 86: 473-4.

159. Meyer CH, Rodrigues EB, Mennel S. Acute commotion retinae determination by cross-sectional Optical coherence tomography. Eur J Ophthalmol 2003; 13:816-8.

160. Hee MR, Puliafito CA, Wong C, et al. Quantitative assessment of macular edema with optical coherence tomography. Arch Ophthalmol 1995; 113:1019-29.

161. Nelson ML, Martidis A. Managing cystoid macular edema after cataract surgery. Curr Opin Ophthalmol 2003; 14:39-43.

162. Ikuno Y, Tano Y. Myopic foveoschisis. In Saxena S, Meredith TA (Eds): Optical Coherence Tomography in Retinal Diseases. New Delhi: Jaypee Brothers Medical Publishers, 2006; pp 203-10.

163. Takano M, Kishi S. Foveal retinoschisis and retinal detachment in severely myopic eyes with posterior staphyloma. Am J Ophthalmol 1999; 128:472-6.

164. Benhamou N, Massin P, Haouchine B, et al. Macular retinoschisis in highly myopic eyes. Am J Ophthalmol 2002; 133:794-800.

165. Kanda S, Uemura A, Sakamoto Y, Kita H. Vitrectomy with internal limiting membrane peeling for macular retinoschisis and retinal detachment without macular hole in highly myopic eyes. Am J Ophthalmol 2003; 136:177-80.

166. Kobayashi H, Kishi S. Vitreous surgery for highly myopic eyes with foveal detachment and retinoschisis. Ophthalmology 2003; 110:1702-7.

167. Ikuno Y, Sayanagi K, Ohji M, et al. Vitrectomy and internal limiting membrane peeling for myopic foveoschisis. Am J Ophthalmol 2004; 137:719-24.

168. Bando H, Ikuno Y, Choi JS, et al. Ultra structure of internal limiting membrane in myopic foveoschisis. Am J Ophthalmol 2005; 139:197-9.

169. Matsumura N, Ikuno Y, Tano Y. Posterior vitreous detachment and macular hole formation in myopic foveoschisis. Am J Ophthalmol 2004; 138:1071-3.

170. Ikuno Y, Gomi F, Tano Y. Potent retinal arteriolar traction as a possible cause of myopic foveoschisis. Am J Ophthalmol 2005 (In press).

171. Baba T, Ohno-Matsui K, Futagami S, et al. Prevalence and characteristics of foveal retinal detachment without macular hole in high myopia. Am J Ophthalmol 2003; 135:338-42.

172. Polito A, Lanzetta P, Del Borrello M, Bandello F. Spontaneous resolution of a shallow detachment of the macula in a highly myopic eye. Am J Ophthalmol 2003; 135:546-7.

173. Sayanagi K, Ikuno Y, Gomi F, Tano Y. Retinal vascular microfolds in highly myopic eyes. Am J Ophthalmol 2005 (In press).

174. Ikuno Y, Tano Y. Early macular holes with retinoschisis in highly myopic eyes. Am J Ophthalmol 2003; 136:741-4.

175. Gass JDM. Serous detachment of the macula secondary to optic disc pits. Am J Ophthalmol 1969;67:821-41.

176. Lincoff H, Lopez R, Kreissig I, et al. Retinoschisis with optic nerve pit. Arch Ophthalmol 1988;109:61-7.

177. Lincoff H, Kreissig I. Optical coherence tomography of pneumatic displacement of optic pit maculopathy. Br J Ophthalmol 1998;82:367-72.

178. Rutledge BK, Puliafito CA, Duker JS, et al. Optical coherence tomography of macular lesion associated with optic nerve pits. Ophthalmology 1996;103:1047-53.

179. Konno S, Akiba J, Sato E, et al. Optical coherence tomography in successful surgery of retinal detachment associated with optic nerve head pit. Ophthalmic Surg Lasers 2000;31:236-39.

180. Bechmann M, Mueller AI, Gandorfer A, et al. Macular hole surgery in eye with a optic pit. Am J Ophthamol 2001;132: 263-4.

181. Hassenstein A, Schaudig U, Richard G. Inflammatory diseases of the retina and choroid: an overview. In Saxena S, Meredith TA (Eds): Optical Coherence Tomography in Retinal Diseases. New Delhi: Jaypee Brothers Medical Publishers, 2006; pp 291-302.

182. Markomichelakis NN, Halkiadakis I, Pantelia E, et al. Patterns of macular edema in patients with uveitis: qualitative and quantitative assessment using optical coherence tomography. Ophthalmology 2004; 111:946-53.

183. Antcliff RJ, Stanford MR, Chauhan DS, et al. Comparison between optical coherence tomography and fundus fluorescein angiography for the detection of cystoid macular edema in patients with uveitis. Ophthalmology 2000; 107:593-9.

184. Hee MR, Puliafito CA, Wong C, et al. Quantitative assessment of macular edema with optical coherence tomography. Arch Ophthalmol 1995; 113:1019-29.

185. Wilkins JR, Puliafito CA, Hee MR, et al. Characterization of epiretinal membranes using optical coherence tomography. Ophthalmology 1996; 103:2142-51.

186. Hee MR, Baumal CR, Puliafito CA, et al. Optical coherence tomography of age-related macular degeneration and choroidal neovascularization. Ophthalmology 1996; 103:1260-70.

187. Puliafito CA, Hee MR, Lin CP, et al. Imaging of macular diseases with optical coherence tomography. Ophthalmology 1995; 102:217-29.

188. Hee MR, Puliafito CA, Wong C, et al. Optical coherence tomography of central serous chorioretinopathy. Am J Ophthalmol 1995; 120:63-74.

189. Hassenstein A, Bialasiewicz AA, Richard G. Optical coherence tomography in uveitis patients. Am J Ophthalmol 2000; 130:669-70.

190. Walter A, Bialasiewicz AA, Hassenstein A, et al. Optical coherence tomography imaging in ocular inflammations. In: Süveges I, Follmann P. (eds.): Proc. XIth Congress of the Eur Soc Ophthalmology, Bologna, Monduzzi Editore, 1997; pp 1583-5.

191. Maruyama Y, Kishi S. Tomographic features of serous retinal detachment in Vogt-Koyanagi Harada syndrome. Ophthalmic Surg Lasers Imaging 2004; 35:239-42.

192. Shields CL, Materin MA, Shields JA. Ocular oncology. In Saxena S, Meredith TA (Eds): Optical Coherence Tomography in Retinal Diseases. New Delhi: Jaypee Brothers Medical Publishers, 2006; pp 251-70.

193. Shields JA, Shields CL. Intraocular Tumors: A Text and Atlas. Philadelphia: WB Saunders, 1992.

194. Shields JA, Shields CL. Atlas of Intraocular Tumors. Philadelphia, Lippincott Williams and Wilkins, 1999.

195. Sumich P, Mitchell P, Wang JJ. Choroidal nevi in a white population: the Blue Mountains Study. Arch Ophthalmol 1998; 116: 645-50.

196. Shields C, Shields JA, Kiratli H, et al. Risk factors for growth and metastasis of small choroidal melanocytic lesions. Ophthalmology 1995; 102:1351-61.

197. Shields CL, Cater JC, Shields JA, et al. Combination of clinical factors predictive of growth of small choroidal melanocytic tumors. Arch Ophthalmol 2000; 118:360-64.

198. Shields CL, Demirci H, Materin MA, et al. Clinical factors in the identification of small choroidal melanoma. Can J Ophthalmol 2004; 39:351-57.

199. Espinoza G, Rosenblatt B, Harbour JW. Optical coherence tomography in the evaluation of retinal changes associated with suspicious choroidal melanocytic tumors. Am J Ophthalmol 2004; 137: 90-95.

200. Shields JA, Shields CL, Donoso LA. Management of posterior uveal melanomas. Surv Ophthalmol 1991; 36:161-95.

201. Shields CL, Shields JA. Recent developments in the management of choroidal melanoma. Curr Opin Ophthalmol 2004; 15:244-51.

202. Shields CL, Shields JA, DePotter P, et al. Diffuse choroidal melanoma: Clinical features predictive of metastasis. Arch Ophthalmol 1996; 114:956-63.

203. Shields CL, Shields JA, Gross N, et al. Survey of 520 uveal metastases. Ophthalmology, 1997; 104:1265-76.

204. Manquez ME, Shields CL, Karatza EC, Shields JA. Regression of choroidal metastases from breast carcinoma using aromatase inhibitors. Arch Ophthalmol (In press).

205. Shields CL, Honavar SG, Shields JA, et al. Circumscribed choroidal hemangioma. Clinical manifestations and factors predictive of visual outcome in 200 consecutive cases. Ophthalmology 2001; 108:2237-48.

206. Mashayekhi A, Shields CL. Circumscribed choroidal hemangioma. Curr Opin Ophthalmol 2003; 14:142-49.

207. Shields JA, Shields CL, Materin MA, et al. Changing concepts in management of circumscribed choroidal hemangioma. The 2003 J. Howard Stokes Lecture, part 1. Ophthalmic Surg Lasers 2004; 35:383-93.

208. Shields CL, Materin MA, Marr BP, et al. Resolution of advanced cystoid macular edema following photodynamic therapy of choroidal hemangioma. Ophthalmic Surg Laser Imaging (In press).

209. Gass JD, Guerry RK, Jack RL, Harris G. Choroidal Osteoma. Arch Ophthalmol 1978; 96:428-35.

210. Shields CL, Shields JA, Augsburger JJ. Choroidal osteoma. Surv Ophthalmol 1988; 33:17-27.

211. Aylward GW, Chang TS, Pautler SE, Gass JD. A long-term follow-up of choroidal osteoma. Arch Ophthalmol 1998; 116:1337-41.

212. Ide T, Ohguro N, Hayashi A, et al. Optical coherence tomography patterns of choroidal osteoma. Am J Ophthalmol 2000; 130:131-34.

213. Fukasawa A, Iijima H. Optical coherence tomography of choroidal osteoma. Am J Ophthalmol 2002; 133:419-21.

214. Shields JA, Shields CL, Gunduz K, Eagle RC Jr. Neoplasms of the retinal pigment epithelium. The 1998 Albert Ruedemann Sr. Memorial Lecture. Part 2. Arch Ophthalmol 1999; 117:601-08.

215. Shields CL, Mashayekhi A, Ho T, et al. Solitary congenital hypertrophy of the retinal pigment epithelium: Clinical features and frequency of enlargement in 330 patients. Ophthalmology 2003; 110:1968-76.

216. Shields JA, Shields CL, Singh AD. Acquired tumors arising from congenital hypertrophy of the retinal pigment epithelium. Arch Ophthalmol 2000; 118:637-41.

217. Shields CL, Shields JA, Marr BP, et al. Congenital simple hamartoma of the retinal pigment epithelium. A study of five cases. Ophthalmology 2003; 110:1005-11.

218. Shields CL, Materin MA, Karatza E, Shields JA. Optical coherence tomography (OCT) of congenital simple hamartoma of the retinal pigment epithelium. Retina. 2004; 24:327-328.

219. Schachat AP, Shields JA, Fine SL, et al, the Macula Society Research Committee. Combined hamartomas of the retina and retinal pigment epithelium. Ophthalmology 1984; 91:1609-14.

220. Ting TD, McCuen BW 2nd, Fekrat S. Combined hamartoma of the retina and retinal pigment epithelium: Optical coherence tomography. Retina 2002; 22:98-101.

221. Stallman JB. Visual improvement after pars plana vitrectomy and membrane peeling for vitreoretinal traction associated with combined hamartoma of the retina and retinal pigment epithelium. Retina 2002; 22:101-04.

222. Shields JA, Shields CL. Tumors of the retina and optic disc. In Regillo CD, Brown GC, Flynn HW Jr (Eds): Vitreoretinal Disease. The Essentials. New York: Thieme Medical Publisheres, Inc, 1999; pp 439-54.

223. Shields CL, Shields JA. Phakomatoses. In Regillo CD, Brown GC, Flynn HW Jr (Eds): Vitreoretinal Disease. The Essentials.

New York: Thieme Medical Publisheres, Inc, 1999; pp 377-90.

224. Singh AD, Shields CL, Shields JA. Major review: Von Hippel-Lindau disease. Surv Ophthalmol 2001; 46:117-42.

225. Shah GK, Shields JA, Lanning R. Branch retinal vein obstruction secondary to retinal arteriovenous communication. Am J Ophthalmol 1998; 126:446-48.

226. Shields CL, Shields JA. Recent developments in the management of retinoblastoma. J Ped Ophthalmol Strabismus. 1999; 36:8-18.

227. Shields CL, Meadows AT, Leahey AM, Shields JA. Continuing challenges in the management of retinoblastoma with chemotherapy. Editorial. Retina (In press).

228. Shields CL, Materin MA, Shields JA. Restoration of foveal anatomy and function following chemoreduction for bilateral retinoblastoma with total retinal detachment. Arch Ophthalmol (In press).

229. Shields JA, Demirci H, Mashayekhi A, Shields CL. Melanocytoma of the optic disc in 115 cases. The 2004 Samuel Johnson Memorial Lecture. Ophthalmology 2004; 111:1739-46.

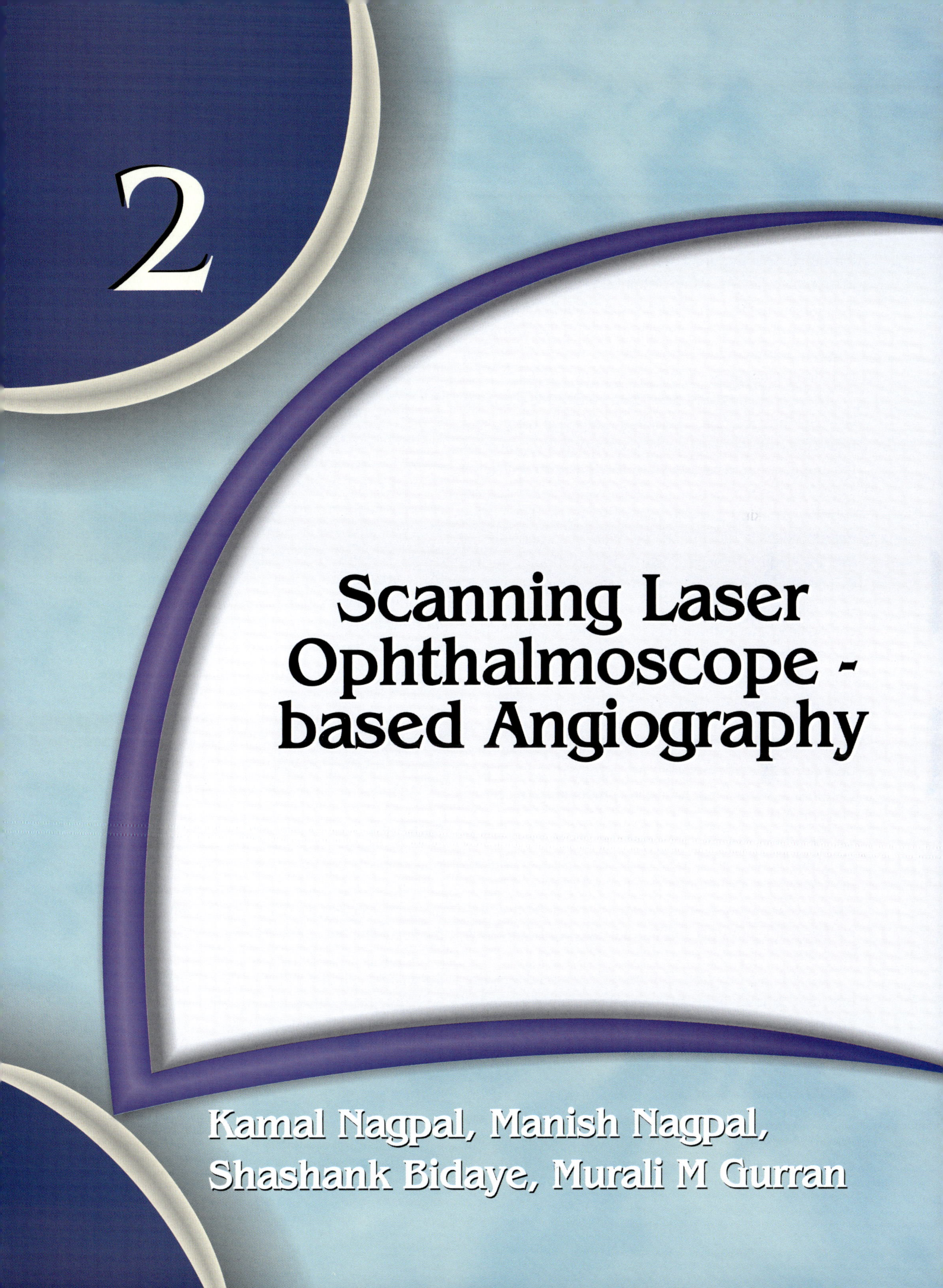

Scanning Laser Ophthalmoscope - based Angiography

Kamal Nagpal, Manish Nagpal,
Shashank Bidaye, Murali M Gurran

INTRODUCTION

While imaging the fundus, both the illuminating and reflected beams need to pass through the same aperture, the pupil. This frequently leads to requirement of high illumination levels, often intolerable by the subject. Secondly, in order to visualize the different structures present in the various layers of the retina, tomographic imaging is imperative. These are the major challenges in retinal imaging.

These problems have been countered by the scanning laser ophthalmoscope. The retina is scanned with a low power, narrow laser beam in such a way that most of the papillary area is available for the reflected light. Therefore the intensity of the illuminating beam can be kept low, making it more acceptable for patients. The reflected light is descanned, detected by a photodiode and the digitized image is stored in a computer. In the Confocal Scanning Laser Ophthalmoscope (cSLO) a small pinhole is placed in front of the photodiode on a conjugate plane to the retina. By moving the pinhole it is possible to select light reflected from different focal planes in the retina and so produce tomographic images. Thus, 3D images can be produced. Due to these features, the cSLO has had a major impact on research in ophthalmology. In this review we intend to diskuss the principles, performance and applications of this instrument, particularly its use in combined fluorescence angiography.

The cSLO, a relatively new imaging technique has the property of providing optical sections through the use of confocal optics.[1,2] One can obtain three dimensional aspects of structures which would otherwise be invisible owing to the contrast degrading effects of overlying elements.[3-8]

In 1980, a group from Boston, USA, created a device that used a laser light source to illuminate the fundus and produce an image of it on a television monitor. They described this device as the Flying Spot TV ophthalmoscope.[3] The scanning laser ophthalmoscope as it was later termed provides a high quality image of the fundus using less than 1/1000 of the light necessary to illuminate the fundus with conventional light ophthalmoscopy.[7] During image acquisition, only one point on the fundus is illuminated at any one time. The laser sweeps across the fundus in a raster-like fashion so that a piece-by-piece image of the fundus is built up on the monitor. [4,9-14]

In addition, because the SLO only illuminates a small area of the fundus at any one time, only a small amount of the patient's pupil—normally about 0.9 mm is used for illumination, allowing the rest of it to be available for light collection. This is quite different from conventional indirect ophthalmoscopy, where almost the whole pupil is used for illumination, while about 1/10th of the pupil is used for viewing. This implies that pupil dilation is not always necessary when acquiring fundal images with the SLO.[15] The acquisition time is very much reduced. However, the problem of contrast, as the whole thickness of laser beam from various layers is captured persists. This was answered when Webb modified his instrument based on confocal principle, in 1987, which increased the contrast and quality. This was named "Confocal Scanning Laser Ophthalmoscope" the CSLO.[9] Several modifications later, the principle is still the same.[16-20] In essence, a large leap was made since Jackman and Webster photographed first retinal image in live eye in 1886.[21] While fundus cameras made many procedures, like fluorescein angiography and indocyanine green angiography possible, the images lacked the quality to support ICGA. Thus it did not gain much popularity until recently with the availability of cSLO.[22-28]

PRINCIPLE

The color of the fundus is characterized by mixture of reflected wavelengths. The mixture is determined by the amount of light reflected at various reflecting surfaces in the eye. Different retinal structures are more easily viewed at different wavelengths of light. Therefore, by varying the wavelength of laser light, different fundal features may be highlighted. Short wavelength light is predominantly reflected by the retinal layers, and is used to view macular pigmentation and arcuate fiber bundles.[9,10,11,23,29] As the wavelength increases, it becomes easier to see the retinal and choroidal vessels in those eyes without heavy pigmentation. With wavelengths of 600 nm or above, there is a large increase in light penetration, and the choroidal vasculature becomes apparent in darkly pigmented fundi. It has been shown that near-infrared imaging is well suited for investigating subretinal structures.[30,31]

The SLO utilizes a combination of three lasers at appropriate wavelengths to form a color image, which is analogous to the formation of color television images using red, green, and blue phosphors. The lasers used are 790, 820 and 488 nm. Each of the three beams are aimed and detected through the same set of optics. These beams can be used individually or in combination. The beam is swept horizontally and line by line vertically across the retina using a rotating polygon mirror and galvanometer-driven mirror respectively. Thus a 20 microns moving spot is swept across the retina to form a rectangular raster.[9-12]

Because only one point of the retina is illuminated and imaged at any time, scattering is avoided and contrast enhanced. The average power of laser light used is 2 mW. The scanning beam illuminates each area point ($10 \mu \times 10 \mu$) for only 0.1 to 0.7 microseconds. The reflected light passes through the scanning optics until it is separated from the incident light path by a partially reflecting mirror. The reflected light then passes through a confocal barrier which consists of a pin-hole. Finally, the light is collected by the light detecting unit, Avalanche Photo Diode. A computer digitizes the signal from Avalanche photo diode, assigning each point a number. This assignment of brightness point by point goes on continuously as the SLO produces a stream of point brightness measurements. From these, a two-dimensional image is constructed electronically. This signal is digitized and stored.[9-11]

CONFOCAL PRINCIPLE

The contrast of a fundus image is determined by the amount of reflected light picked up by the detector. If the detector picks up all the light reflected by the fundus, the image produced will have poor contrast and show little detail. To improve the contrast and resolution of the SLO, the confocal mode is used. In this mode, only light which is reflected from the focal plane of the laser is detected by the photo detector. Light which is reflected or scattered by other retinal layers is ignored. This is in

contrast with conventional ophthalmic imaging, where objects outside the plane of interest contribute to the image, degrading the quality of the image of the object of interest.[4]

Confocality of the system is achieved by placing a pinhole in front of the detector, which is conjugate to the laser focus. It aids toward increasing the spatial resolution, by suppression of light from planes anterior and posterior to the plane of interest and restraining the scattered light. This increases the contrast and minimizes unwanted reflexes. The size of the pinhole determines the degree of confocality, such that a small pinhole aperture will give a highly confocal image. By passing the reflected light through pinhole, the point of illumination is only 250 microns thick. Thus, the image produced is a narrow optical section of the area of fundus under investigation. Also, it facilitates focus on a particular plane, i.e. inner retina, mid retina, outer retina, retinal pigment epithelium-Bruchs membrane complex, choriocapillaries, etc. Acquisition of images in up to 64 consecutive focal planes to a depth of 8 mm is possible. The result is a dramatic 3D image series, with axial resolution of 250 μm.[4,9-12,32]

COMMERCIALLY AVAILABLE CONFOCAL SCANNING LASER OPHTHALMOSCOPES

The first widely used SLO was the Rodenstock device which provided facilities for confocal imaging, fluorescein angiography and indocyanine green angiography, and psychophysical measurements such as microperimetry.[20,32,33] These used a variety of lasers of different wavelengths to give realtime videoimages. In comparison with photographic techniques, the spatial resolution of videoimages is inherently lower. This is because the horizontal scan lines which make up the image are limited to approximately 600 compared with the equivalent of 4000 or more for photographs. The mechanical limitations of the spinning polygon mirror mean that this limit will not be easily improved. Despite this limit the confocal optics of the SLO can result in improved resolution compared with photographs because it allows optical sectioning, and so the contrast degrading effects of structures above or below the depth of interest can be reduced. The depth resolution can be of the order of several hundred micrometers. In this way small vessels or other structural detail obscured by the scattering of neural tissue in the optic nerve can be seen and some of the contrast degrading effects of ocular media opacities can be bypassed.[32-34]

HEIDELBERG RETINAL ANGIOGRAPHY

Heidelberg Retinal Angiography (HRA2) has a smaller, more powerful camera than the original HRA and is easier to manipulate. The HRA2's main advantages over conventional imaging are its image quality, dynamic capabilities, and efficiency. Compared to both the original HRA and fundus cameras, the HRA2 takes higher-resolution images, which means better definition and greater detail. With fluorescein, the HRA2 enables physicians to see details just 5 μm in size—three times smaller than the 15 μm details visible with a fundus camera image—and all in an image that is just 1536 $\times$ 1536 pixels with a 30° field of view. Fundus cameras with much larger image sizes cannot match this resolution. HRA2's images require less storage space.[34]

Because the HRA2 suppresses scattered light, it can resolve to 5 μm per pixel, compared to the fundus camera's 15 to 18 μm per pixel. Indocyanine green angiography performed with the HRA2 provides greater chorioretinal detail than ordinary fundus camera indocyanine green angiography because of both reduced light scatter and the HRA2 laser's particular sensitivity to the indocyanine green dye, lacking the fuzzy, diffuse quality of indocyanine green angiography images from fundus cameras.[36-43] The HRA2 also takes images in up to 64 consecutive focal planes to a depth of 8 mm, which produces a 3D image series that can aid physicians in evaluating choroidal melanoma. In terms of field of view, the HRA2 is narrower than the conventional fundus camera. Fundus cameras are generally capable of 45° or 50°, 30° or 35°, and 20°, whereas the HRA2's fields of view are 30°, 20°, and 15°.[5-7,32,33] Users can create 60° photomontages using an automated feature or make 120° photomontages manually with the system's automatic mosaic image construction feature and increase it to 150° by combining this feature with the accessory Staurenghi Wide Field lens.[44,60]

One disadvantage of the HRA systems is their lack of color imaging, which facilitates angiogram interpretation.[45-47]

DYNAMIC ANGIOGRAPHY

The HRA systems offer still-frames and full-motion indocyanine green angiography—a significant advantage over the fundus camera's static—only indocyanine green angiography, which is not informative and fast enough (a may be collected frame every 3 seconds). For choroidal studies, the first 6 seconds are important. Infrared imaging, with extremely high resolution, and realtime video of the vessels filling, imparts the detailed information for circulation studies.[12,48,49] Simultaneous fluorescein angiography and indocyanine green angiography not only saves time, but also aids the diagnosis by helping the correlation of the choroidal pathology on the indocyanine green angiogram with the fluorescein angiogram's retinal landmarks.[50,51]

ADDITIONAL IMAGING MODES

In addition to its fluorescein and indocyanine green angiography imaging capabilities, the HRA2 also offers several noninvasive imaging modes, including blue-reflectance and infrared-reflectance imaging.[10] Blue-reflectance imaging may be valuable for viewing details of the ocular nerve fiber layer, but it requires a clear media without cataracts. Noninvasive imaging with barely visible infrared reflectance light is suitable for viewing the fundus of an extremely light-sensitive patient such as a child, as well as for viewing through a cataract, visualizing a choroidal nevus, or evaluating the retinal pigment epithelium. With the HRA2, users can view these images simultaneously with fluorescein or indocyanine green angiography. Unlike the original HRA, the HRA2 also provides autofluorescence imaging to help physicians confirm diagnoses of macular holes, pseudo-vittelliform lesions, retinal pigment epithelium atrophy, central serous chorioretinopathy, and Best's disease. This modality may also aid the study of Stargardt's dystrophy when users employ the normal fluorescein angiography setting without injecting fluorescein. Patients without cataracts get the best imaging.[19,52-55]

CLINICAL ADVANTAGES

Realtime angiography helps location of feeder vessels and choroidal neovascularization (CNV) associated with macular degeneration. The resolution and dynamicity of images illustrates circulation in the large and small vessels that feed CNV complexes, including their filling up and then draining, which is a rapid process, using the rapid frame rate to capture that circulation. In comparison, a fundus camera requires physicians to compare still images captured as far as 1 or 2 seconds apart. Thus it gives deep understanding into choroidal vasculature.[56,57]

High speed indocyanine green angiography is required to identify the choroidal involvement with CNV for photodynamic therapy (PDT). Feeder vessel treatment implies treatment of a lesion by sealing off the blood supply with a tiny laser spot. In the past, the entire lesion had to be cauterized, destroying the retina in the process. Although the HRA2 is particularly useful for locating and treating feeder vessels, it also helps physicians differentiate retinal angiomatous proliferation from CNV, which promotes early diagnosis and treatment. It can even help distinguish recurrence from persistence after laser therapy. In addition to offering patients better clinical outcomes, the low light levels used in HRA systems make examinations much more comfortable. The retinal light exposure required for the HRA2 is only about 1% of that needed with a photographic system, and without a bright flash and lag time between consecutive images, the system minimizes patient eye movement.[56,57]

EASE OF USE

The HRA systems have touch-screen displays, enabling the photographer to switch quickly from one mode to the next. The overall ergonomics and ease of use have been much improved for the HRA2, which has been designed to support software and firmware upgrades and Heidelberg add-ons to grow along with the user's needs.[10]

MAJOR ADVANTAGES OF HEIDELBERG RETINAL ANGIOGRAPHY

Major advantages of HRA2 are listed below:[5-7,12-14,45,46,60]

1. High resolution.
2. Confocality: This results in enhanced image contrast, detail and sharpness.
3. Low light intensity (low retinal irradiance): The retinal light exposure required for angiography on the HRA2 is only about 1% of the exposure necessary with a photographic system, so it is much safer for patients.
4. Low light exposure: This is more comfortable to patients and is especially useful in children.
5. Immediate results: The images are acquired in less than a second.
6. Good images in small pupils: This is especially important for diabetics because they typically do not dilate very well and account for a large number of patients seen in the retina clinic. This is a tremendous advantage compared to imaging with standard fundus cameras because the contrast and detail on these patients are far better.
7. Good images in media opacities.
8. Minimal stray light.
9. Highest image contrast and detail.
10. The monochromacy of the laser allows for a barrier filter with less than 0.01% transmittance at the excitation wavelength, compared with the 0.5% overlapping of excitor and barrier filter used in the fundus camera.
11. High 'signal to noise' ratio.
12. The cSLO allows evaluation of CNV during the early phase of the indocyanine green angiography study, which is apparently not feasible using the camera-based systems.
13. Realtime recording facilitates recognition of feeder vessels and enables detection of small capillaries within CNV.
14. Rapid acquisition rates permit evaluation of many images during the filling and transit phase, especially of choroids.
15. Ability to readily view the elevation of optic nerve in patients with optic disk swelling, especially with mild elevation, in whom ophthalmoscopic findings can be subtle.
16. Simultaneous fluorescein and indocyanine green angiography, with dynamic high speed angiography.

17. Stereo and wide field imaging is possible.
18. 3D scanning.
19. Infrared and blue reflectance images are possible.
20. Autofluorescence.
21. Visualization of retinal vessels even in late phases.
22. Easy practical operation.
23. Optical section images.

DISADVANTAGES OF HEIDELBERG RETINAL ANGIOGRAPHY

Despite the recent advances, one of the limitations of SLO images has been the lack of realistic color in the images. Important information such as pallor of the disk or subtle aspects of the color appearance of drusen, diabetic retinopathy and other fundus features are lost with SLO imaging. Although the depth resolution and the resistance to contrast degrading effects provide an advantage over conventional imaging, the lack of color is a severe handicap. Also, inherent difference in lateral resolution common to all SLOs in comparison with color photography is a problem. In addition, each laser emits at a single wavelength while the photographic method in combination with the white light flash gives a broad spectral response. As a consequence some differences could arise in comparing subtle color rendition. In particular, with yellowing of the lens, the short wavelength blue laser could contribute a reduced blue component in comparison with the photographic method. The main shortcomings may be enumerated as under:[10,46,47]

1. Disturbing central artifacts from the corneal surface cause hindrance in the red-free and infrared modes. These may be eliminated by introducing a polarization filter in the optical pathway.
2. Precise focusing in simultaneous fluorescein and indocyanine green mode is only possible for either the fluorescein or indocyanine green angiography due to chromatic aberrations and the different wavelengths used for two, which account for an approximate 2.5D difference.
3. High resolution mode is not available for simultaneous angiography recordings.
4. Inability to consistently image the periphery.
5. The images need to be stored in CDs, because of the large sizes.

6. Low resolution: 768 × 768 pixels, as compared to 1000 × 1000 pixels in fundus cameras, although confocality improves the image quality.
7. Current SLOs are mounted on a fixed stage and are not portable. This design does not easily accommodate all patients, especially young children or anesthetized patients.
8. Color imaging is not possible.
9. High cost.

DESCRIPTION OF THE INSTRUMENT[10,58,59]

Hardware

The hardware consists of:

A. The camera device: The laser scanning camera is the core of HRA. It contains the three-dimensional scanning system, the detector and the main part of the electronics. It is mounted on a special camera mount which also contains the headrest for the patient. The camera mount is designed so that the measuring position on the ocular fundus can be selected by rotating the camera around two orthogonal axes.

B. Interactive touch panel as a central control unit: The following features can be controlled with the help of this unit:

- Light intensity
- Sensitivity control
- Field of view (scan size): 15, 20 or 30 degrees
- Scan depth control
- Optical focus adaptation
- Focus range
- Imaging modes
    1. Fluorescein angiography
    2. Indocyanine green angiography
    3. Green reflectance
    4. Infra-red reflectance
    5. Fluorescein and indocyanine green angiography , simultaneous
    6. Fluorescein angiography + infra-red reflectance, simultaneous
    7. Indocyanine green angiography + infrared reflectance, simultaneously.
- Type of images
    - Still photo
    - Realtime movie

C. A box containing the laser source of 488 nm: For fluorescein angiography excitation and blue reflectance

D. A box containing diode laser sources (790 and 820 nm): For indocyanine green excitation and infrared reflectance, respectively.

Software

The software used is Heidelberg eye explorer, which has the following image acquisition options:
- Continuous mode
- Single image acquisition mode
- Stereo pairs
- Confocal image sequence with a variable scan depth and automated alignment.

Laser Safety

The instrument emits visible and invisible laser light. The HRA is a class I laser system, with no safety hazard. To guarantee the safety of the user and the patient at all times, a limit has been imposed on the maximum period of time for which the laser beam can be switched on. If exceeded, the screen shows the message: 'laser safety, laser timed out'. Image acquisition is automatically interrupted and can only be continued after a specified waiting period (about 30 minutes). However, this is rare during normal use of the instrument.

Fixation

In patients with severe visual impairment in the fellow eye that disables the use of an external fixation target. Although the internal fixation targets can be easily visualized in presence of infrared laser light, patients may have problems visualizing these targets in the red free and fluorescein angiography mode.

The quality of image is proportional to 'signal-to-noise" ratio. This ratio is increased by a factor of square-root of the number of images averaged, i.e. averaging more than 9 images will increase the signal to noise ratio in the generated mean image by a factor of 3.

COMBINED FLUORESCENCE ANGIOGRAPHY

Fluorescence angiography is close to mandatory for diagnosis and management of a large number of retinal disorders. It allows visualization of the retinal and choroidal vasculature. Fluorescein angiography is valuable in accurate imaging of the retinal circulation. It allows identification of leakage of the small fluorescein molecule in pathological states affecting the retinal vasculature. Its inherent limitations toward imaging of the choroidal circulation led to development of infrared angiography using indocyanine green dye, which was introduced approximately 20 years ago.[61,62]

Biophysically different (Table 2.1, Figures 2.1 and 2.2) from the fluorescein molecule, it delineates the choroidal

Table 2.1: Properties of sodium fluorescein and indocyanine green	
Sodium fluorescein	*Indocyanine green*
Crystalline hydrocarbon with molecular weight of 376 Dalton	Tricarbocyanine dye molecule with molecular weight of 775 Dalton
Absorbs light energy between 465 and 490 nm (blue spectrum) and fluoresces between 520 and 530 nm (green-yellow spectrum)	Absorbs at 790 nm and emits at 835 nm (near infrared)
Approximately 60-80% protein bound, with >20% free to diffuse through the choriocapillaris	98% bound to plasma proteins, so cannot diffuse through the choriocapillaris
The liver and kidneys eliminate it within 24 hours from the body, though traces may be found in the body for up to a week after the injection	Rapidly eliminated by the liver rapidly removes it, through the enterohepatic circulation. No significant staining of normal ocular tissue noted
Retinal pigment epithelium and choroid absorbs 60-75% of blue green light, resulting in poor transmission of fluorescence and reduced visualization through overlying hemorrhage, fluid, lipid and pigments.	Only about 20-30% or infrared is absorbed by the pigment epithelium and being a longer wavelength, it has more penetration. This allows visualization through the overlying opacities.

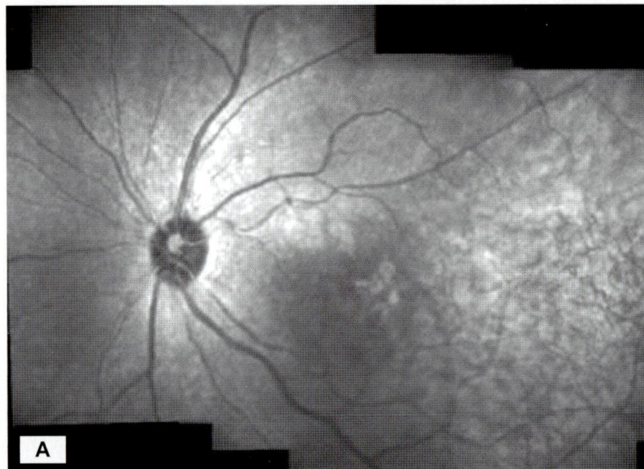

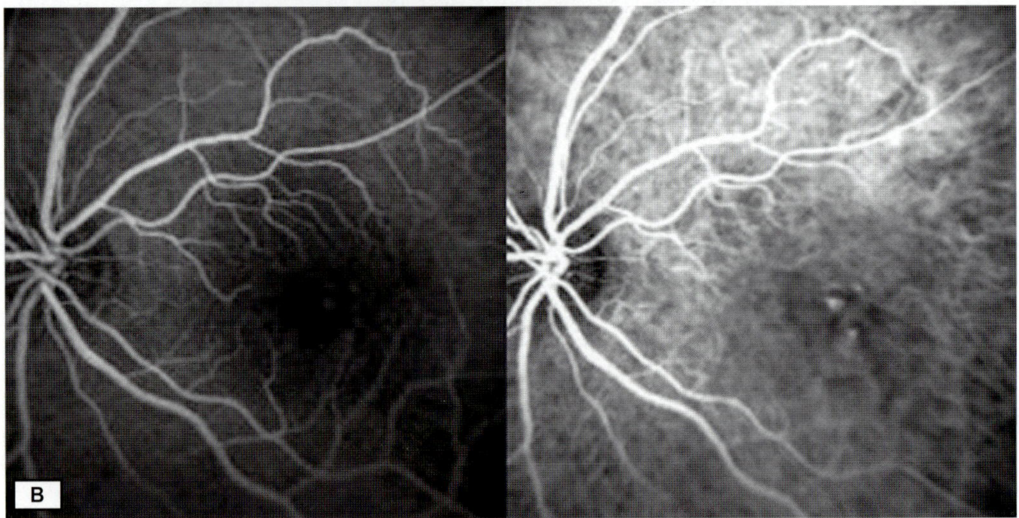

FIGURES 2.1A and B: Age-related macular degeneration. (A) Infrared photograph shows a macular lesion. (B) Simultaneous fluorescein angiography and indocyanine green angiography. Hyperfluorescent leaking spots, not apparent on fluorescein angiography are much better visualized in indocyanine green angiography.

circulation in a better way. The dye absorbs and emits light in the near-infrared spectrum, allowing better penetration through the retinal pigment epithelium and extraneous absorbing material such as exudates, hemorrhages, etc. Secondly, this molecule is larger (molecular weight, 775 D versus 332 D for fluorescein) and more protein-bound in plasma, so it does not leak from the choriocapillaris (which leads to obscuration of choroidal vessels), as sodium fluorescein dye normally does. Clinically, the obvious differences in the appearance of the two dyes in the fundus are the appearance of the "black macula" and the diffuse "background staining" obscuring visualization of the deeper choroidal vessels, as observed by fluorescein molecule and are precluded in indocyanine green angiography.

Because of the properties mentioned above, the role of indocyanine green angiography in the retinal diagnostic armamentarium, particularly for studying the normal choroidal circulation, and conditions like central serous chorioretinopathy, choroidal tumors, and age-related macular degeneration with CNV, especially occult forms, is obvious. However, since its inception a couple of decades ago, indocyanine green angiography has been saddled with technical snags, which challenged the practicality of the procedure. To begin with, indocyanine green angiography was performed with infrared

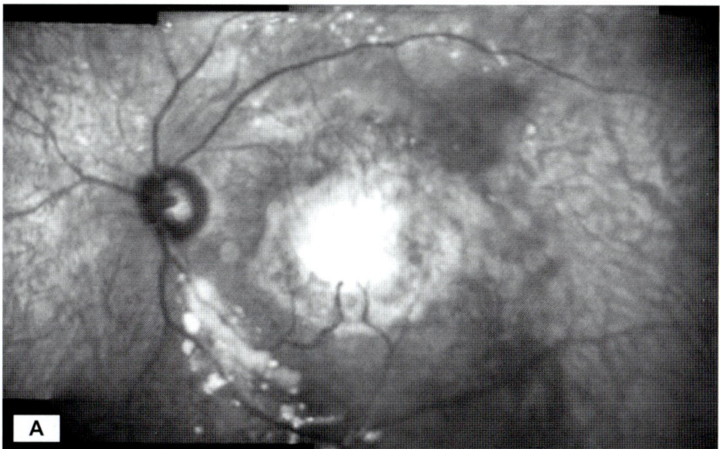

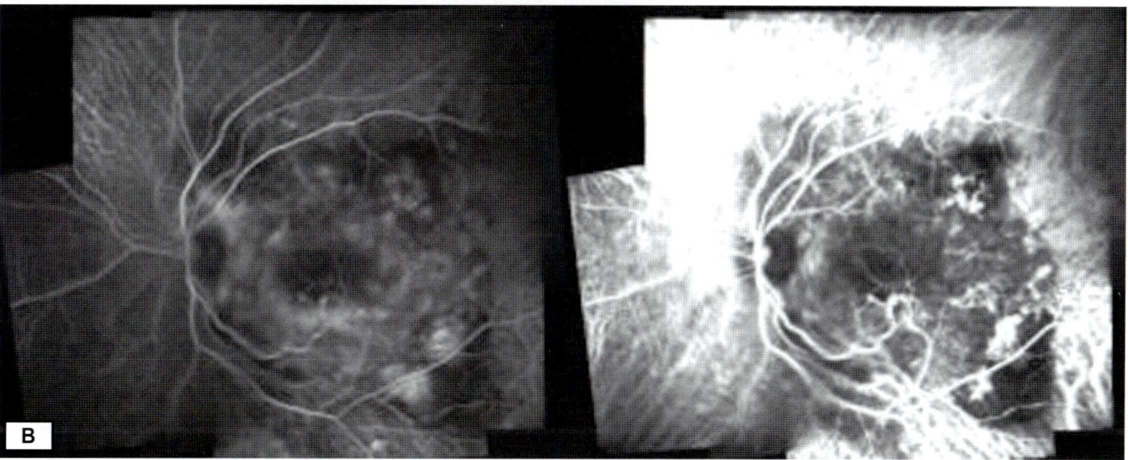

FIGURES 2.2A and B: Age-related macular degeneration with choroidal neovascularization. (A) Infrared reflectance photograph shows a large, occult macular lesion. (B) Simultaneous fluorescein angiography and indocyanine green angiography. Hyperfluorescent leaking spots, not apparent on fluorescein angiography are much better visualized. The hyperfluorescent area of fluorescein angiography corresponds to the membrane in indocyanine green angiography. Indocyanine green angiography delineates focal hot spots much better.

photographic film. However, the poor sensitivity of film coupled with the relatively weak fluorescence properties of the dye caused this method to be abandoned. However, contemporary technological advances and adaptations in fundus cameras, digital videocameras equipped with barrier-interference filters and scanning laser ophthalmoscopes have facilitated fluorescein and indocyanine green imaging. Simultaneous angiography with fluorescein and indocyanine green dyes, using a complex multispectral fundus camera, with limited image quality was reported in 1973.[63] In 1993, another approach used a modified fundus camera, the filters of which were changed during angiography to allow

sequential fluorescein and indocyanine green angiography after simultaneous injection of both dyes.[51] Bischoff and associates[64] in 1995 reported on a modification of a scanning laser ophthalmoscope for simultaneous fluorescein and indocyanine green angiography. By using an argon laser in addition to the diode laser for indocyanine green angiography, as well as suitable filters for detecting fluorescence emission, this scanning laser ophthalmoscope allows for simultaneous fluorescein and indocyanine green angiography. These efforts have rendered indocyanine green angiography a truly valuable adjunct for fluorescein angiography.

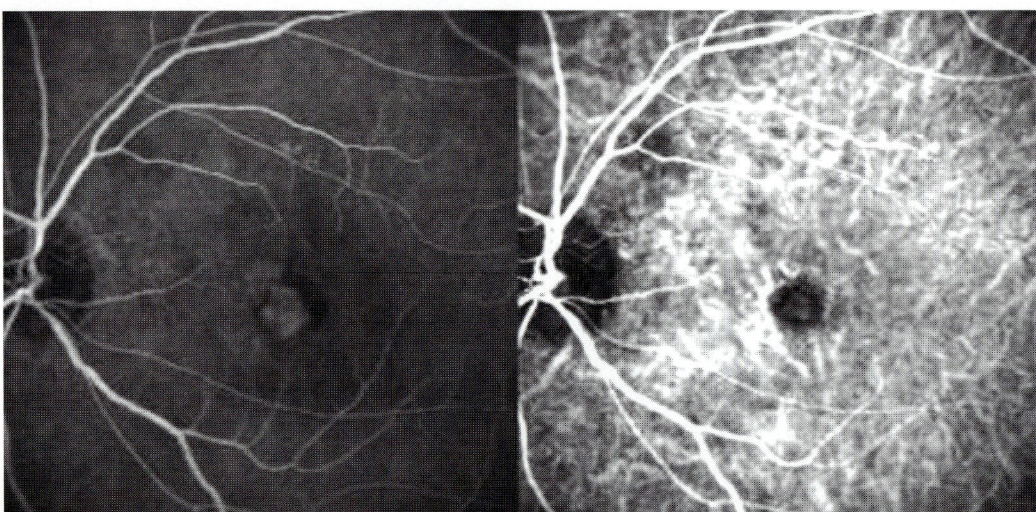

FIGURE 2.3: Simultaneous fluorescein angiography and indocyanine green angiography in classic choroidal neovascularization. In such cases fluorescein angiography is sufficient, and indocyanine green angiography does not reveal any further information.

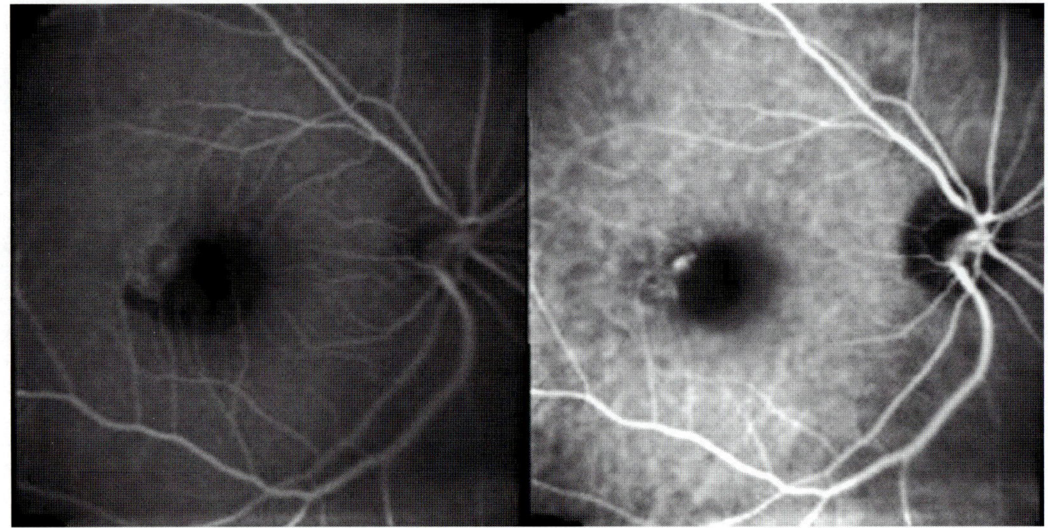

FIGURE 2.4: Simultaneous fluorescein angiography and indocyanine green angiography image revealing diffuse leak on fluorescein angiography shows a localized hot spot in the indocyanine green angiography.

COMBINED FLUORESCEIN ANGIOGRAPHY AND INDOCYANINE GREEN ANGIOGRAPHY

It is known that both studies are needed for diagnosis and localization in difficult cases. Single combined intravenous injection of fluorescein and indocyanine green dyes can be used to get both images, which can be done sequentially or simultaneously. Sequential imaging involves a single injection, followed by fluorescein angiography photos followed by indocyanine green angiography photos. Simultaneous imaging entails a single injection after which simultaneous acquisition of fluorescein angiography and indocyanine green angiography images is carried out. It needs a special system with both fluorescein and indocyanine green excitation systems, which is possible with HRA (Figures 2.1 to 2.21).

The most obvious advantage of truly simultaneous imaging is the negation of the possibility that one of the

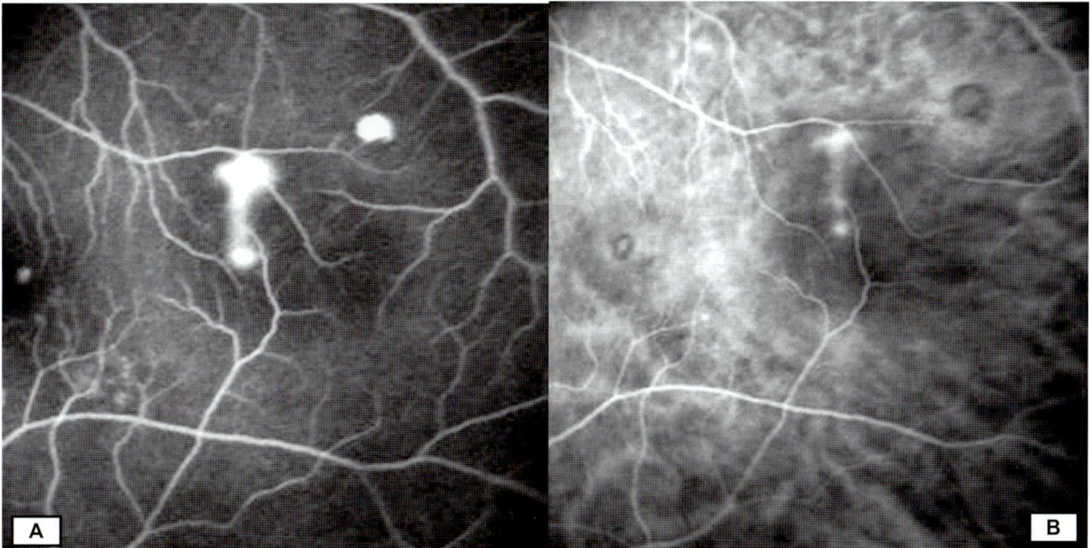

FIGURES 2.5A and B: (A) Fluorescein photograph showing a smoke stack leak and a near by area of pigment epithelial detachment. (B) Indocyanine green angiography reveals generalized choroidal and pigment epithelial changes as compared to the fluorescein angiography.

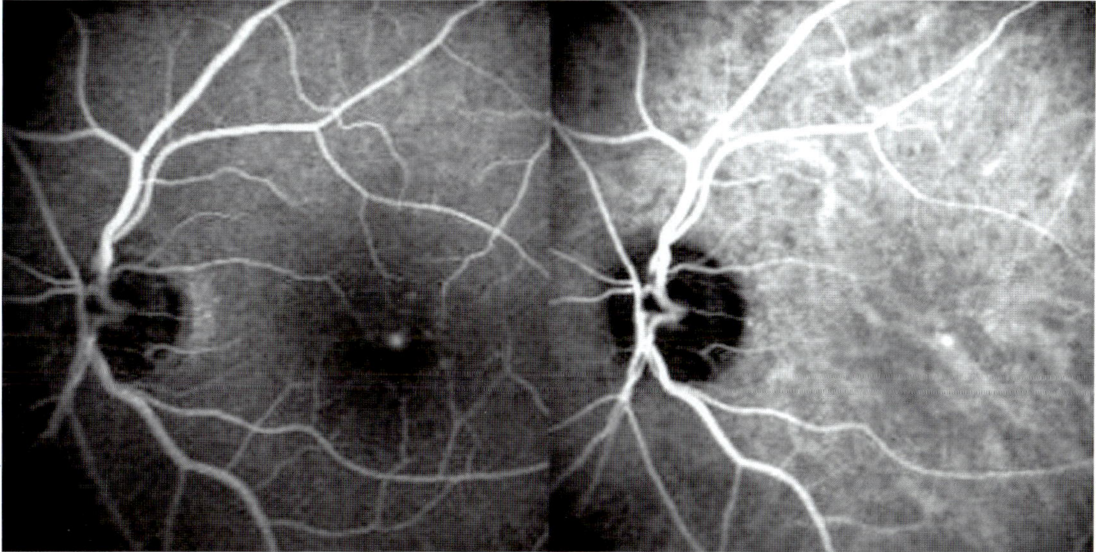

FIGURE 2.6: Simultaneous fluorescein angiography and indocyanine green angiography in which indocyanine green angiography reveals generalized and diffuse pigmentary changes suggesting a more generalized pathology.

angiograms is of higher quality as compared to the other, which may lead to difference in visualization of pathological states. The potential reasons that one study might be of better or of differing quality as compared to the other include differences in centering, patient movement, continuous eye movements, focus, exposure, blinking, and other factors.[65] These factors decrease the significance of the relative differences between the two films. An exact overlap of the transit of the two dyes despite the ever variable external factors is only possible if the images are acquired simultaneously.

The other significant advantage of simultaneous angiography technique is the time sequence correlation.[66] Both the dyes are injected and therefore imaged simultaneously. Therefore the physiological differences in their distribution and circulation through the eye are easily

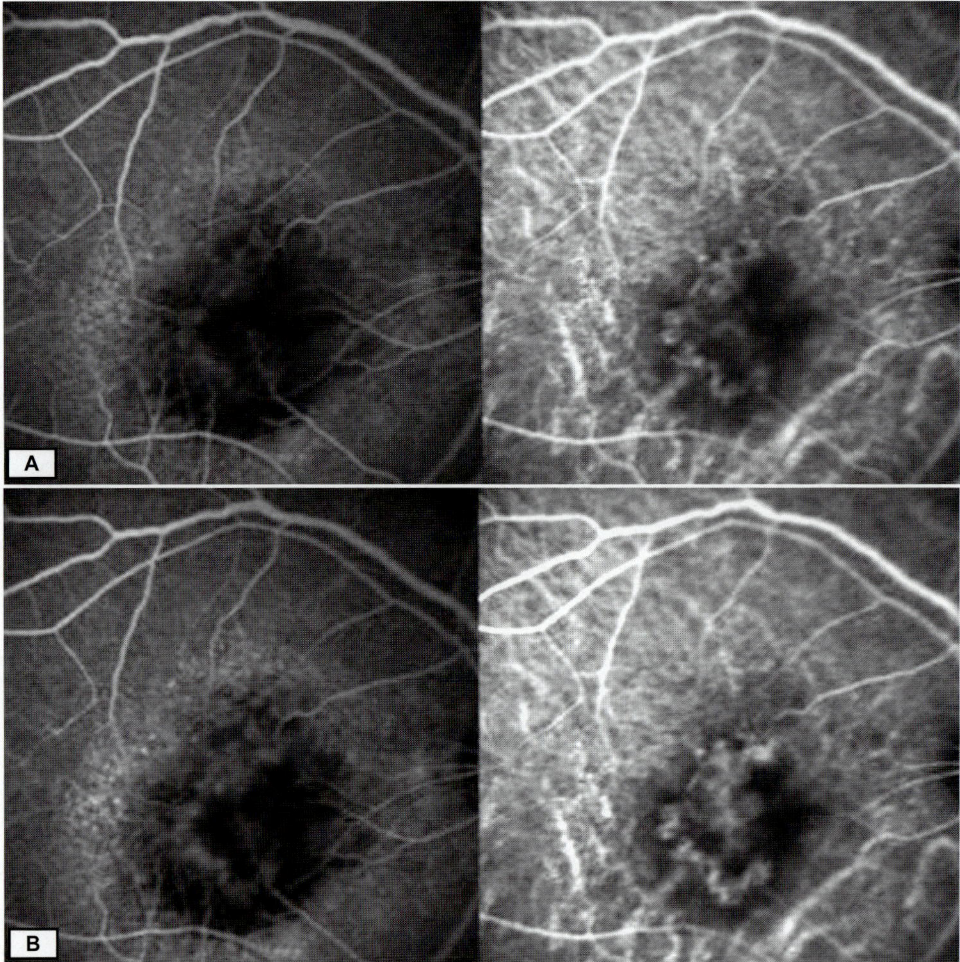

FIGURES 2.7A and B: (A) Early phase of simultaneous fluorescein angiography and indocyanine green angiography, in a case of age-related macular degeneration. Shows lacy network in fluorescein angiography, choroidal neovascular membrane is clearly outlined in indocyanine green angiography with central feeder vessel (umbrella). (B) Feeder vessel has become more prominent in indocyanine green angiography.

diskernable. Furthermore, the differences in response to the pathological states of the retinal and choroidal circulation are made obvious and are readily comparable. Thus the relative value of each type of dye in normal physiology and different disease processes become apparent, which is relevant both for clinical and research purposes.

The final advantage is that of efficiency.[66] With a single injection and one photographic session which lasts up to 10 minutes, the whole study is completed. The time required to perform the entire study is considerably shorter than first performing a fluorescein study, reviewing it, and subsequently performing the indocyanine green study.

Patient compliance and the investigators ease are noteworthy.

Technical disadvantages of the SLO system include the lack of wide-angle possibilities and the inherent difference between digital and film-based fluorescein angiograms, which may be significant in special cases. Some loss of resolution is expected, when videorecording is compared with single photographic frames. However, the additional information provided by the moving pictures in a videoangiogram, provides dynamic information about the choroidal and retinal filling patterns and pathological states. Investigation is possible at low retinal irradiance and offers high-contrast digital images.

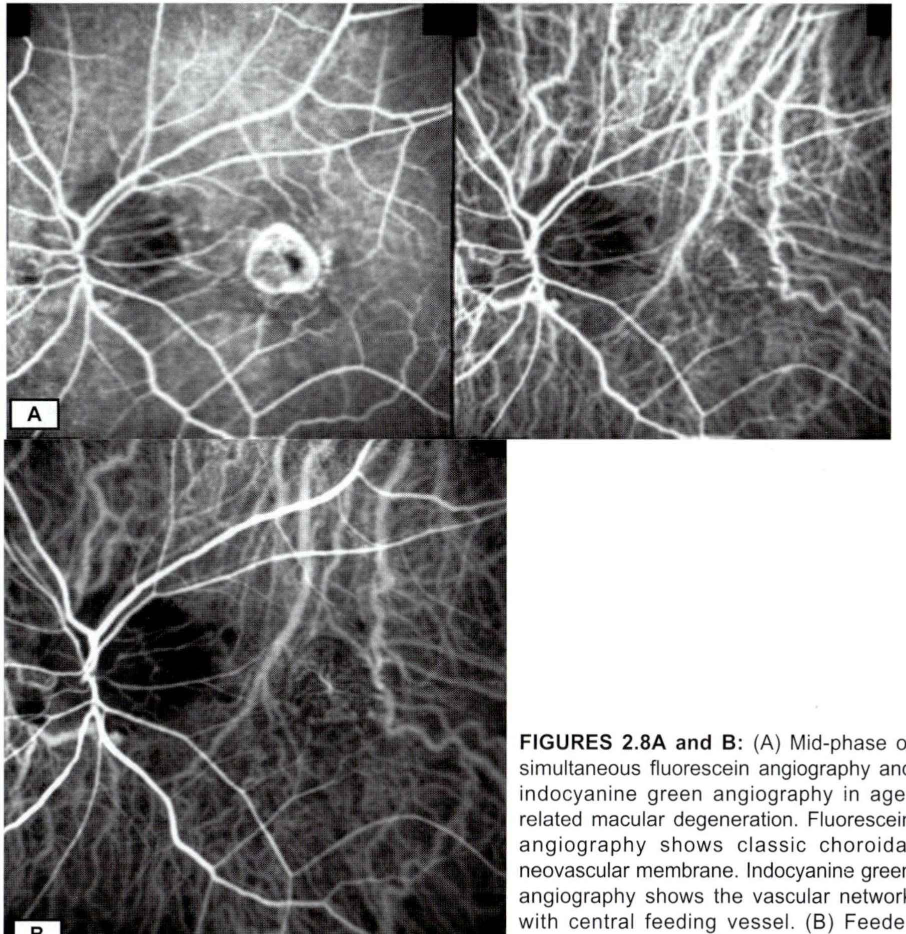

FIGURES 2.8A and B: (A) Mid-phase of simultaneous fluorescein angiography and indocyanine green angiography in age-related macular degeneration. Fluorescein angiography shows classic choroidal neovascular membrane. Indocyanine green angiography shows the vascular network with central feeding vessel. (B) Feeder vessel is very well seen in this image.

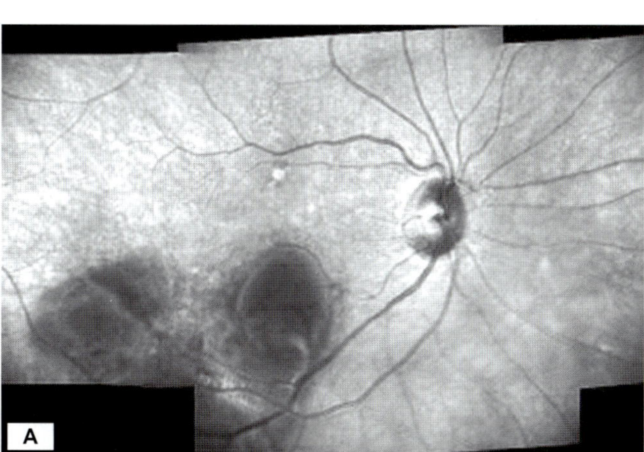

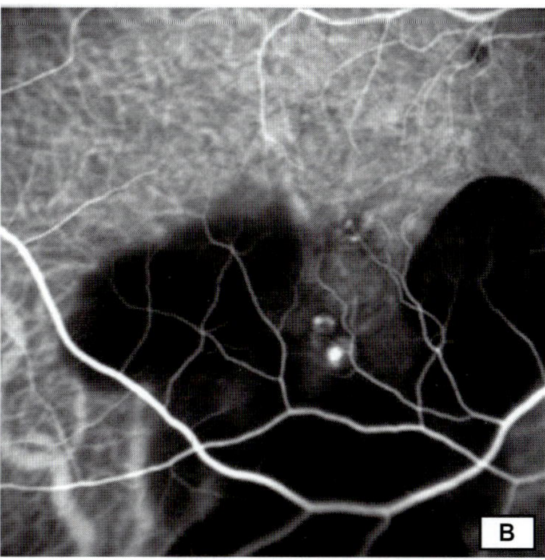

FIGURES 2.9A and B: (A) Infrared photograph showing hemorrhagic patches in a case of idiopathic polypoidal choroidal vasculopathy. (B) Mid phase of indocyanine green angiography shows few choroidal hyperfluorescent areas in a polypoidal fashion.

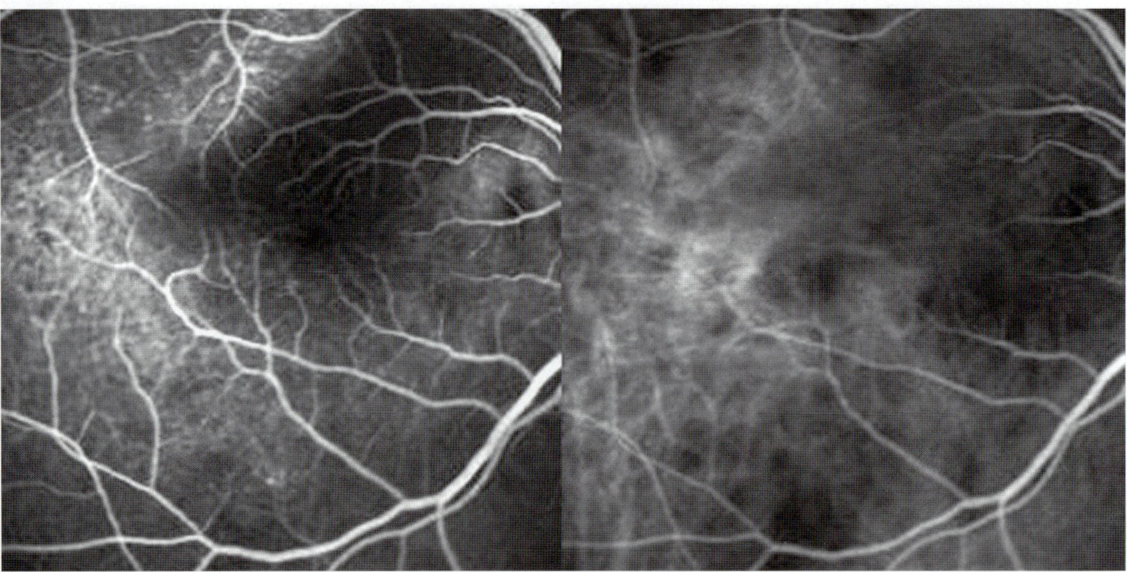

FIGURE 2.10. Fluorescein angiography shows mottled hyper fluorescence and indocyanine green angiography shows areas of choroidal hypoperfusion in a case of posterior scleritis.

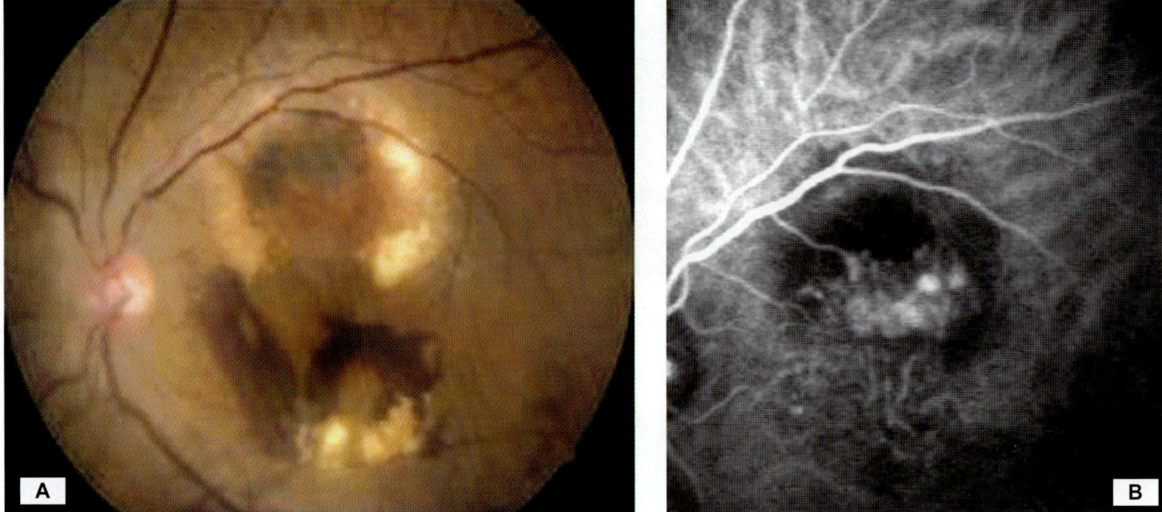

FIGURES 2.11A and B: (A) Large serous and hemorrhagic collections in idiopathic polypoidal choroidal vasculopathy. (B) Choroidal polyps seen in indocyanine green angiography.

CONFOCAL SCANNING LASER OPHTHALMOSCOPE FOR FLUORESCEIN ANGIOGRAPHY

The cSLO provides information, which is valuable both in terms of horizontal and temporal resolution.[66] Advantages of the scanning laser ophthalmoscope include the ability to use an excitation light that scans each point of the retina in a raster like fashion for only 0.1 to 0.7 microseconds allowing intense excitation, thus providing a stronger emission signal which is detected and electronically coded for subsequent image composition on a computer screen.[65] Due to the sensitivity of the instrument, up to 70% of the photons exiting the eye are detected. The illumination levels are safe and tolerable and imaging is possible through small pupils and through hazy media. The rate of imaging is 20 to 30 frames per second, which is superior to digital imaging systems. The

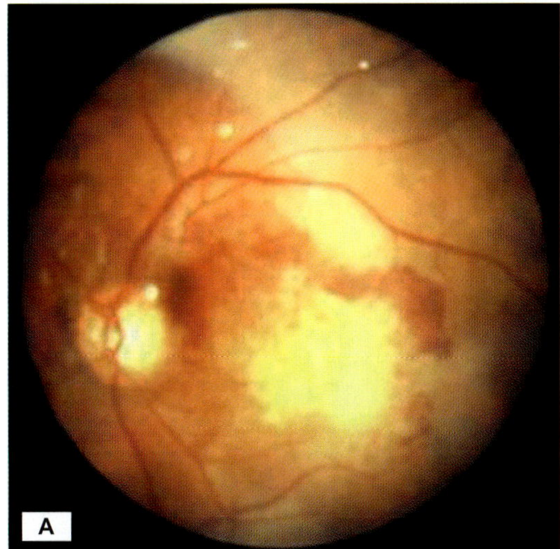

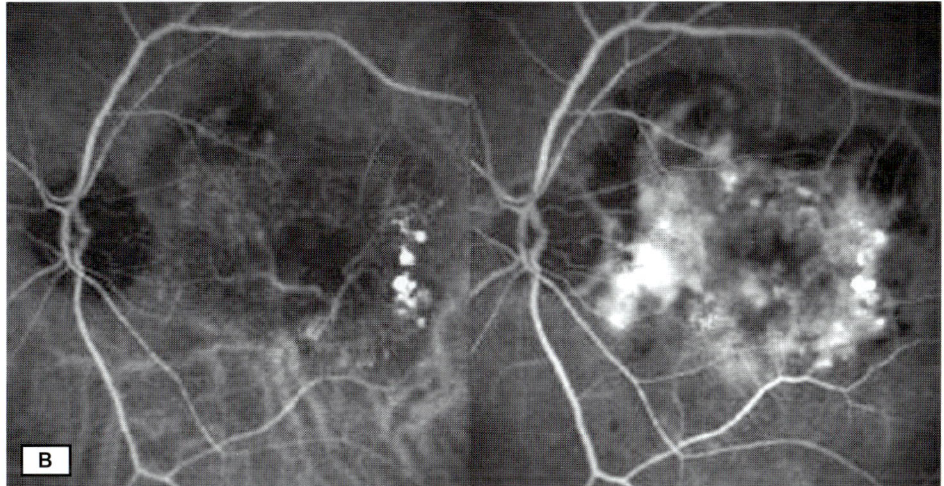

FIGURES 2.12A and B: (A) Large subretinal lesion. (B) Fluorescein angiography showing diffuse leak on and around lesion, choroidal polyps seen on indocyanine green angiography.

ability to view multiple or video-rate images provides more information than single frames, because greater detail of the dyes in the transit phases and leakage patterns are obtained. Stereoscopic imaging is also possible using scanning laser ophthalmoscope. Further, by optically isolating the image plane, tomographic information and higher contrast is possible. Unlike conventional imaging, in which out-of-focus objects appear blurred, confocal imaging allows for diskrimination between out-of-focus objects. Thus, scattered light and light originating from out-of-focus structures is suppressed and a greater image contrast is obtained. Furthermore, the depth location of subretinal neovascular membranes by scanning at different planes of focus is feasible.

Detection of fundus autofluorescence is possible. Acquisition of red-free and infrared fundus photographs, as well as storing all images digitally so that any image can be recalled or transported at any time or location without any loss of image quality are the other considerable advantages of the cSLO. The use of a computer affords flexibility in image storage and processing.

MECHANISM OF FLUORESCENCE ANGIOGRAPHY WITH CONFOCAL SCANNING LASER OPHTHALMOSCOPE

By using an argon laser in addition to the diode laser for indocyanine green angiography, as well as suitable filters for detecting fluorescence emission, the scanning laser ophthalmoscope allows for simultaneous fluorescein

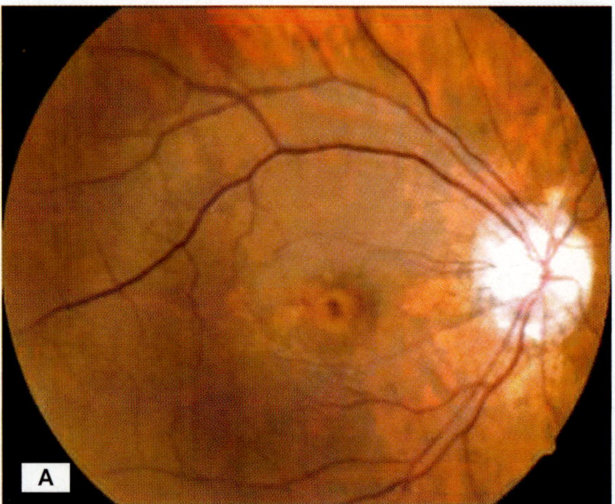

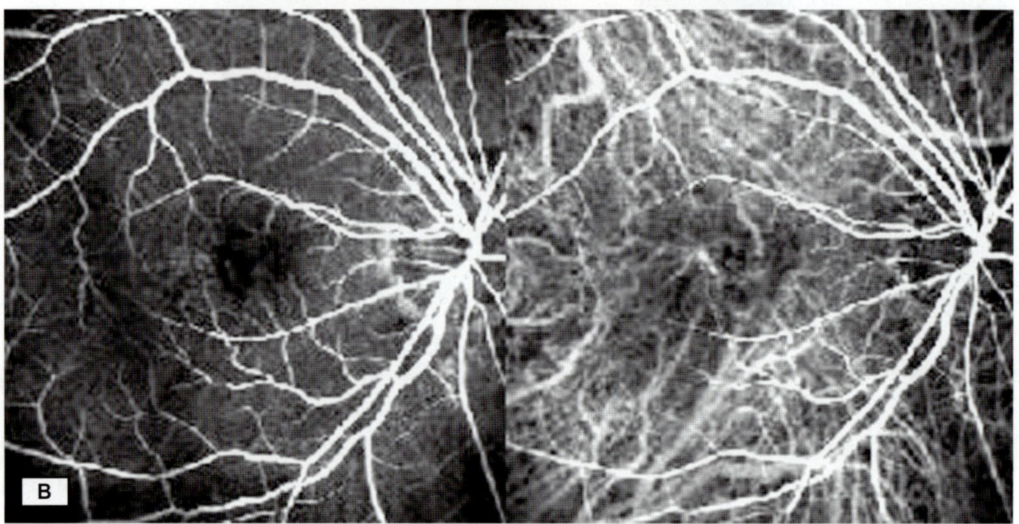

FIGURES 2.13A and B: (A) Subretinal lesion. (B) Combined fluorescein angiography and indocyanine green angiography revealing feeding channels on indocyanine green angiography.

and indocyanine green angiography. The confocal scanning laser ophthalmoscope (Heidelberg Retina Angiograph, Heidelberg Engineering Inc, Heidelberg, Germany) uses 2 laser light sources with 3 wavelengths for scanning fundus illumination. An argon-ion laser (488 nm and 514 nm wavelength) is used to provide red-free photographs (green, 514 nm) and blue light was used for excitation during fluorescein angiograms (blue, 488 nm). The second is a diode laser (795 nm wavelength) that provides illumination to excite the indocyanine green dye, which fluoresces at 835 nm. Maximal retinal irradiance at 30 degrees was 0.2 mW/cm^2 for the argon laser and 1.6 mW/cm^2 for the diode laser, well below the limits established by the American National Standards Institute and other international standards.[11] Two scanning mirrors provide the horizontal and vertical scanning directions. The illumination beam has a diameter of 3 mm, and the full aperture of the dilated or undilated eye is used to collect light from the posterior pole. The field of view can be variable. The confocal detection unit employs a small (400 microns) pinhole aperture to suppress light originating from below or above the focal plane.[67]

For simultaneous fluorescein angiography and indocyanine green angiography, the laser radiation is deflected by means of a resonant scanner so that the two are done quasi-simultaneously. The infrared laser is guided onto each line scan, and the blue radiation is

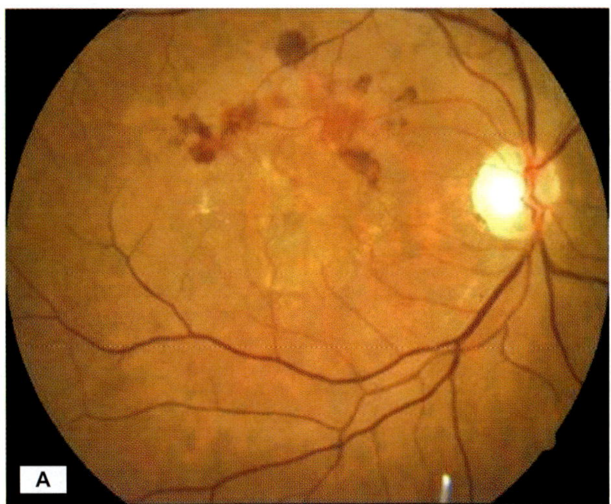

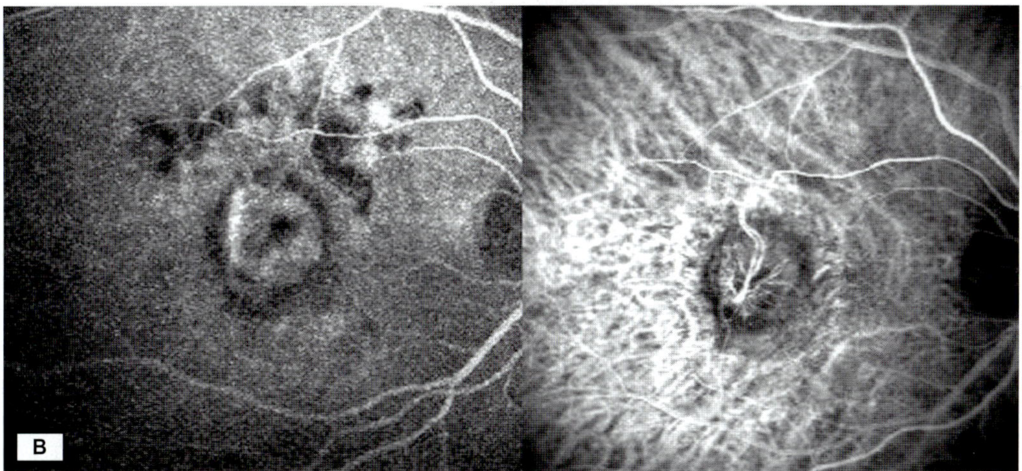

FIGURES 2.14A and B: (A) Choroidal neovascular membrane in age-related macular degeneration. (B) Fluorescein angiography showing staining and leakage of membrane, indocyanine green angiography reveals feeding arteriole and venule of membrane.

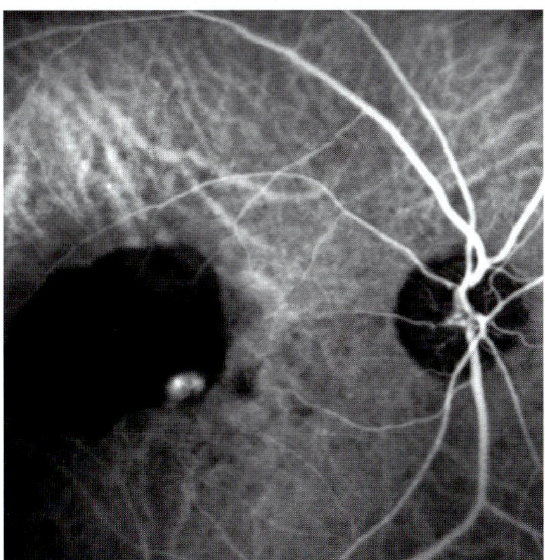

FIGURE 2.15: Hot spot visualized on indocyanine green angiography.

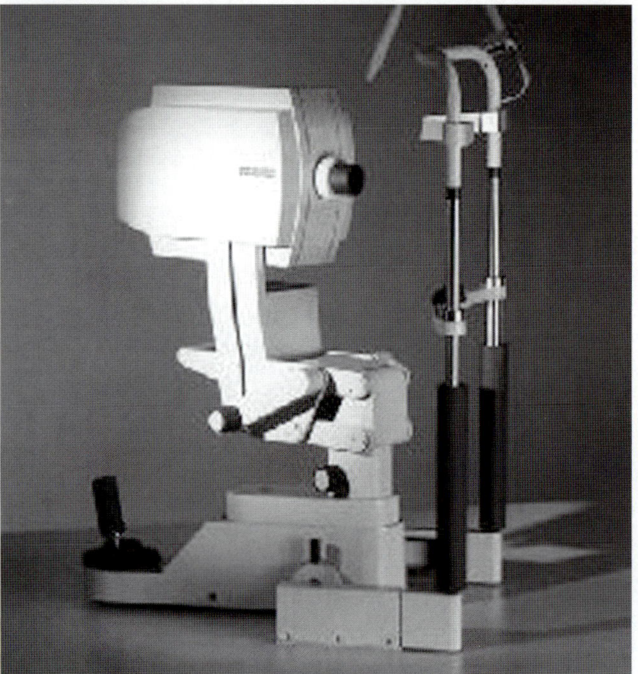

FIGURE 2.16: The Heidelberg retinal angiography camera.

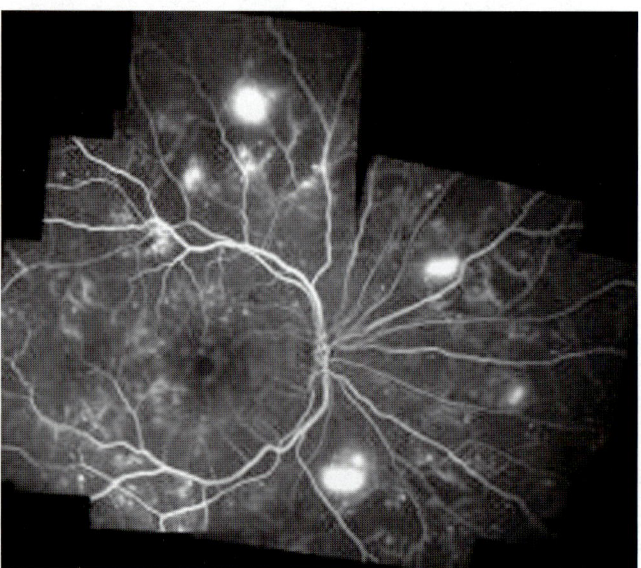

FIGURE 2.17: Collage of proliferative diabetic retinopathy.

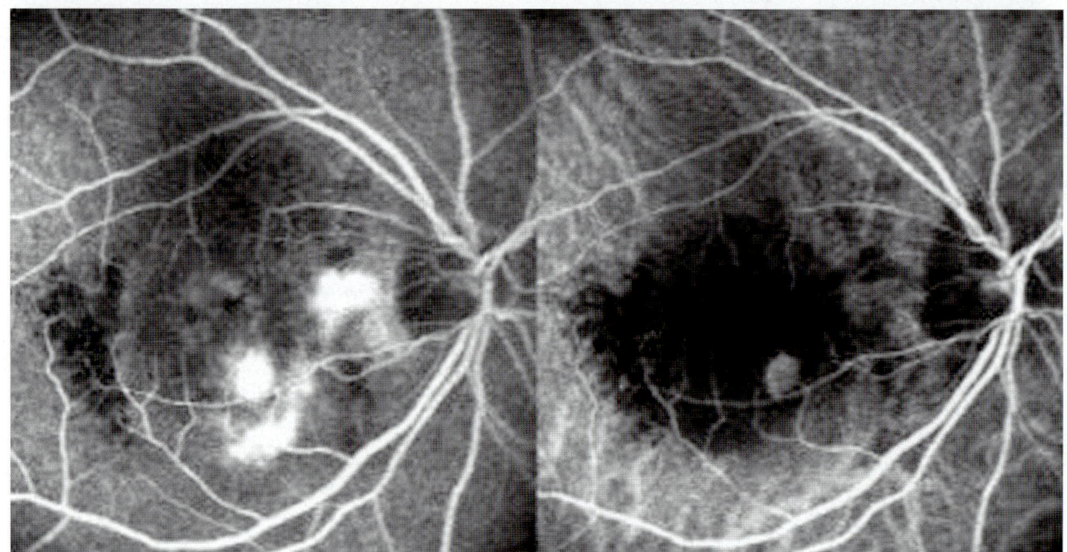

FIGURE 2.18: Hot spot identified on the indocyanine green angiography on the right is clearly identified as compared to the diffuse leakage seen on fluorescein angiography on the left.

applied during the return movement of the scanning mirror. Images are digitized up to the rate of 20 frames per second with the time separation between corresponding lines of the 2 angiograms being in the order of 0.1 milliseconds. Each frame contains 256 pixels vertically and 256 pixels horizontally and 8 bit per pixel intensity quantitation. During examination, both fluorescein angiography and indocyanine green angiography angiograms are displayed simultaneously on the monitor. The images are stored digitally in the RAM of the computer during acquisition and subsequently transferred onto the hard disk.

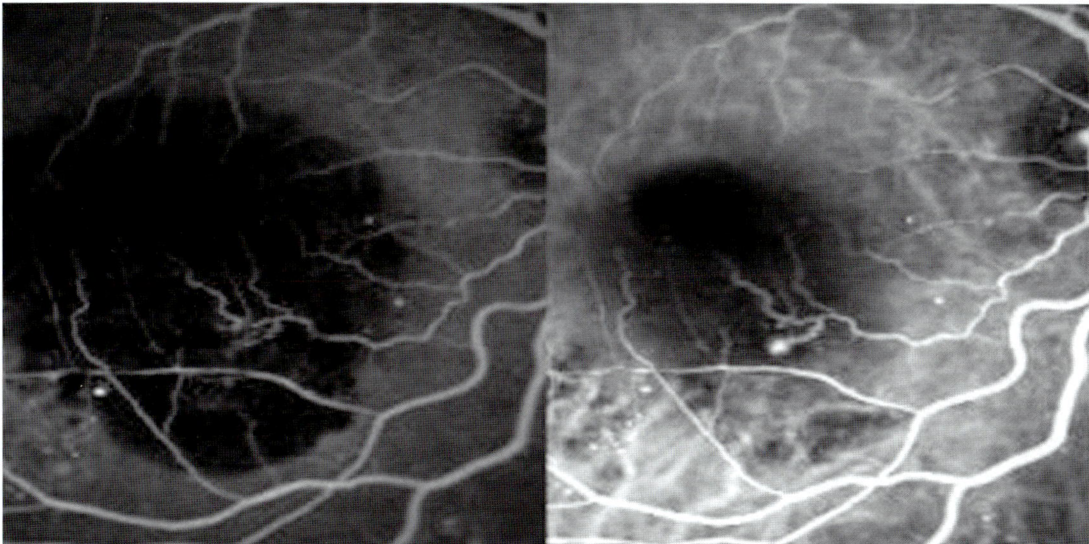

FIGURE 2.19: Intense hot spot on the right indocyanine green angiography picture is a macroaneurysm which has lead to subretinal blood collection, resulting in blocked fluorescence on the fluorescein angiography on the left, as a differential diagnosis to choroidal neovascular membrane.

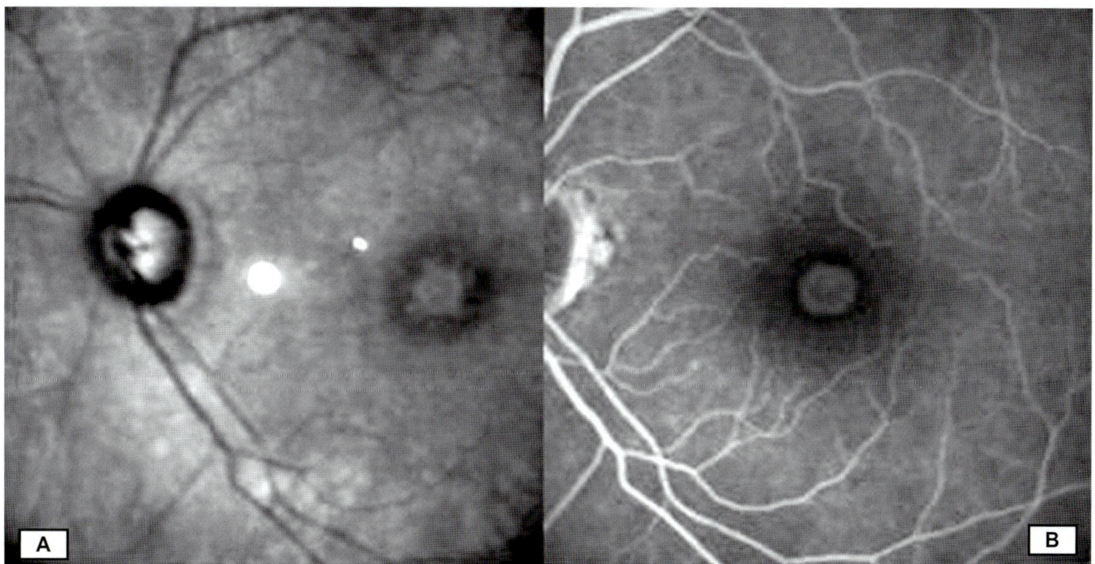

FIGURES 2.20A and B: (A) Autofluorescence of macular hole and (B) True fluorescence of macular hole.

The light intensity during simultaneous fluorescein angiography and indocyanine green angiography is balanced by independently adjusting detector sensitivity for fluorescein fluorescence and laser power for inducing indocyanine green fluorescence. The laser used for indocyanine green angiography is working at up to 2 mW radiation power, where as the laser power for fluorescein angiography is fixed to 300 microW. In simultaneous acquisition, every horizontal scan line is illuminated with the two lasers, one after the other, while the same detector electronics is used for both lines. The light detecting unit is Avalanche Photo Diode, which is approximately three times more sensitive to 788 nm compared to 488 nm. Because of the increased light power for indocyanine green and higher sensitivity of the detector system, indocyanine green angiography pictures are typically

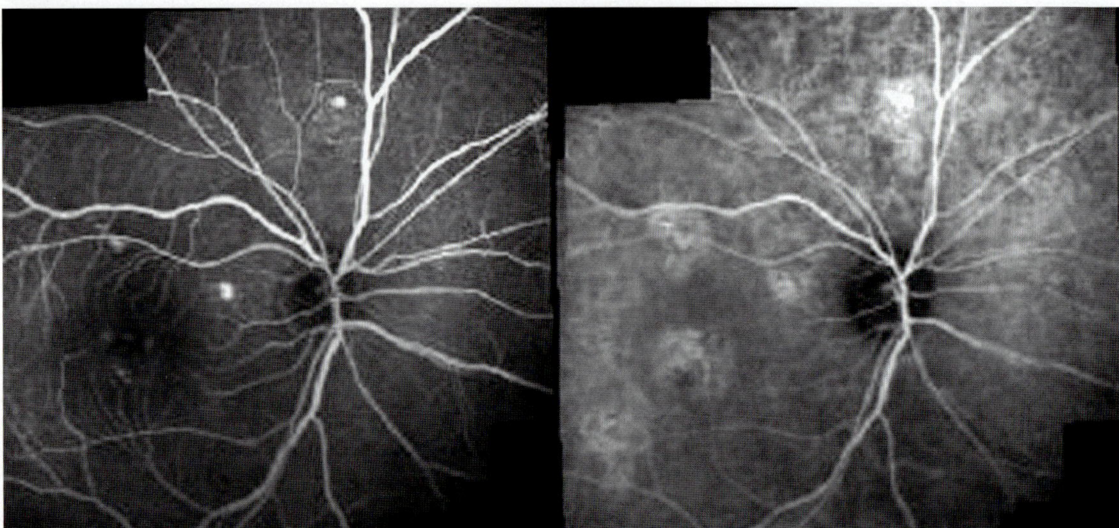

FIGURE 2.21: In a patient having central serous retinopathy, the indocyanine green angiography picture on the right reveals much wider areas of pigmentary alterations as compared to the corresponding fluorescein angiography picture on the left.

brighter than fluorescein angiography images. To acquire both images with proper brightness, the detector sensitivity is adjusted to the fluorescein angiography images, whereas the brightness of the indocyanine green angiography images is adjusted by diminishing the laser power for indocyanine green.

DISADVANTAGES OF SIMULTANEOUS FLUORESCEIN ANGIOGRAPHY AND INDOCYANINE GREEN ANGIOGRAPHY[10]

1. A focus difference (approximately 2.5 D) between fluorescein angiography and indocyanine green angiography scans occurs, which results from chromatic aberrations and different wavelengths used for fluorescein angiography and indocyanine green angiography.
2. Precise focusing is only possible for either the fluorescein angiography or indocyanine green angiography.
3. The high-resolution mode is not available for simultaneous recordings.
4. A single allergic event during the course of such a study would pose a perplexing problem for the clinician, who has to judge which of the two agents (or if both) are involved.

PROCEDURE OF SIMULTANEOUS FLUORESCEIN ANGIOGRAPHY AND INDOCYANINE GREEN ANGIOGRAPHY

It is recommended to use larger pupil sizes in imaging applications where axial resolution is desired. The target eye, the eye which has to be given preference in angiography is determined. In monocular pathologies, i.e. central retinal vein occlusion, that eye is targeted. In binocular pathologies, i.e. diabetic retinopathy, the eye in which activity (macular edema) is expected, is targeted. The usual parameters used are low intensity, focus 0, field 30 degrees.

Various authors have advised various dye dosages. We administer 2 ml of 25% sodium fluorescein (equal to 500 mg), along with 25 mg indocyanine green dye. Two ml is injected intravenous. The mixture of both dyes in a single syringe is not associated with precipitation.

SEQUENCE OF IMAGE TAKING

To begin with, infrared reflectance photographs are taken. Then the camera is focused on the area of interest (usually posterior pole) of the target eye. The dye mixture is injected as a bolus. Simultaneous fluorescein angiography, indocyanine green angiography mode is selected. Once the dye appears at the disk, continuous (series/movie) mode is started, till the memory is full (usually 60 seconds). Subsequently, the mode is changed to still images, which are taken continuously for few minutes. Fifteen-degree images of the macula are taken. Images beyond 20 minutes are usually not necessary. The HRA images can be given in the form of a compact disk or printouts to the patient.

REFERENCES

1. Mainster MA, Webb RH, Timberlake GT, Hughes GW. Scanning laser ophthalmoscopy. Clinical applications. Ophthalmology 1982; 89: 852-57.
2. Scheider A. Neue Verfahren Zur Darstellungund Messung der Aderhautzirkulation mit indozyanin Grun. Folia Ophthalmol 1990; 15: 283.
3. Webb RH, Hughes GW, Pomerantzeff O. Flying spot TV ophthalmoscope. Appl Opt. 1980; 19:2991-97.
4. Nasemann J, Muller M. Scanning laser angiography. Berlin, Federal Republic of Germany, Quintessenz Verlag, 1990; pp 63-80.
5. Wolf S, Toonen H, Arend O, et al. Zur Quantifizierung der retinalen Kapillardurchblutung mit Hilfe des scanning laser ophthalmoscopes. Biomed Tech Berlin 1990; 35:131.
6. Scheider A, Schroedel C. High resolution indocyanine green angiography with a scanning laser ophthalmoscope. Am J Ophthalmol 1989; 108:458.
7. Klingbeil U, Plesch A, Rappl W, Wutz H. Ophthalmic image acquisition and analysis system. Proceedings of the International Society for Optical Engineering 1988; 1001:310.
8. Plesch A, Klinbeil U. Optical characteristics of a scanning laser ophthalmoscope. Proceedings of the International Society for Optical Engineering. 1989; 1161:390.
9. Webb RH, Hughes GW, Delori FC. Confocal scanning laser ophthalmoscope. Appl Opt 1987; 26:1492-99.
10. Jorzik JJ, Bindewald A, Dithmar S, Holz FG. Digital simultaneous fluorescein angiography and indocyanine green angiography autofluorescence and red-free imaging with a solid state laser based confocal scanning laser ophthalmoscope. Retina. 2005; 25:405-16.
11. The Laser Institute of America. American National Standard for the safe use of lasers. Toledo, OH: The Institute; 1993 (ANSI Z 136.1-1993).
12. Scheider A, Kaboth A, Neuhauser L. Detection of subretinal neovascular membranes with indocyanine green angiography and an infrared scanning laser ophthalmoscope. Am J Ophthalmol 1992; 113:45-51.
13. Mikelberg FS, Wijsman K, Schulzer M. Reproducibility of topographic parameters obtained with the Heidelberg retinal tomography. J Glaucoma. 1993; 2:101-3.
14. Bartsch DU, Weinreb RN, Zinser G, Freeman WR. Confocal scanning infrared laser ophthalmoscopy for indocyanine green angiography. Am J Ophthalmol 1995; 120:642-51.
15. Donnelly WJ, Roorda A. Optimal pupil size in the human eye for axial resolution. J Opt Soc Am A Opt Image Sci Vis 2003; 20:2010-15.
16. Freeman WR, Bartsch DU, Mueller AJ. Simultaneous indocyanine green angiography and fluorescein angiography using a confocal scanning laser ophthalmoscope. Arch Ophthalmol 1998; 116:455-63.
17. Girkin CA, McGwin G Jr, Long C, et al. Subjective and objective optic nerve assessment in african-americans and whites. Invest Ophthalmol Vis Sci 2004; 45:2272-78.
18. Bindewald A, Jorzik JJ, Roth F, Holz FG. Confocal scanning laser ophthalmoscope digital fundus autofluorescence imaging. Ophthalmologe 2005; 102:259-64.
19. Ruckman VA, Fitzke FW, Bird AC. Distribution of fundus autofluorescence with a scanning laser ophthalmoscope. Br J Ophthalmol 1995; 79:407-12.
20. Freeman WF. Simultaneous indocyanine green and fluorescein angiography using a confocal scanning laser ophthalmoscope. Arch Ophthalmol 1998; 116:455-63.
21. Jackman WT, Webster JD. On photographing the retina of the living human eye. The Philadelphia Photographer 1886; 23:340-41
22. Squirrell D, Dinakaran S, Dhingra S, et al. Oral fluorescein angiography with the scanning laser ophthalmoscope in diabetic retinopathy: a case controlled comparison with intravenous fluorescein angiography. Eye.2005; 19:411-17.
23. Sharp PF, Manivannan A. The scanning laser ophthalmoscope. Phys Med Biol 1997; 42:951-66.
24. Novotny HR, Alvis DL. A method of photographing fluorescence in circulating blood in the human retina. Circulation 1961; 24:82-86.
25. Rabb MF, Burton TC, Schatz H, Yannuzi LA. Fluorescein angiography of the fundus: A schematic approach to interpretation. Surv Ophthalmol 1978; 22:387-403.
26. Guyer DR, Puliafito CA, Mones JM et al. Digital indocyanine green angiography in chorioretinal disorders. Ophthalmology 1992; 99:287-91.
27. Yannuzi LA, Slakter JS, Sorenson JA, et al. Digital ICG videoangiography and choroidal neovascularization. Retina 1992; 12:191-223.
28. Scheider A, Kaboth A, Neuhauser L. The detection of subretinal neovascular membranes with indocyanine green and an infrared scanning laser ophthalmoscope. Am J Ophthalmol 1992; 113:45-51.
29. Webb RH, Hughes GW. Scanning laser ophthalmoscope. IEEE Trans Biomed Eng 1981; 28:488-92.
30. Elsner AE, Burns SA, Weiter JJ, Delori FC. Infrared imaging of subretinal structures in the human ocular fundus. Vision Res 1996; 36:191-205.
31. Staurenghi G, Aschero M, La Capria A, et al. Visualization of neovascular membranes with infrared light without dye injection by means of scanning laser ophthalmoscope. Arch Ophthalmol 1996; 114:365.
32. Schneider U, Kuck H, Inhoffen W, Kreissig I. Fundus-controlled microperimetry with the scanning laser ophthalmoscope in macular diseases. Klin Monatsbl Augenheilkd 1993; 203:212-18.

33. Rudolph G, Kalpadakis P, Ehrt O, et al. Scanning laser ophthalmoscope multifocal electroretinography and microperimetry in patients with Stargardt's disease. Ophthalmologe 2003; 100:720-26.

34. Scheider A, Schroedel C. Indocyanine green angiography. First results with a scanning laser ophthalmoscope. ARVO abstracts. Supplement to Invest. Opthalmol Vis Sci Philadelphia, 1990(S);462.

35. Kelly JP, Weiss AH, Zhou Q et al. Imaging a child's fundus without dilation using a handheld confocal scanning laser ophthalmoscope. Arch Ophthalmol 2003; 121:391-96.

36. Yoneya S, Noyori K. Improved visualization of the choroidal circulation with indocyanine green angiography. Arch Ophthalmol 1993; 111:1165-6J.

37. Yannuzi LA, Rohrer KT, Tindel LJ, et al. Fluorescein agiography complication survey. Ophthalmology 1986; 93:611-17.

38. Arnold JJ, Quaranta M, Soubrane G, et al. Indocyanine green angiography of drusen. Am J Ophthalmol 1997; 124:344-56.

39. Spaide RF. Fluorescein angiography. Diseases of the Retina and Vitreous. Philadelphia: WB Saunders Co, 1999; pp 29-38.

40. Tittl MK, Slakter JS, Spaide RF, et al. Indocyanine green videoangiography. Diseases of the Retina and Vitreous. Philadelphia, WB Saunders Co. 1999; pp 29-38.

41. Bartsch DU, Weinreb RN, Zinser G, Freeman WR. Confocal scanning infrared laser ophthalmoscopy for ICGA. Am J Ophthalmol 1995; 120; 642-51.

42. Dithmar S, Holz FG, Bellman C, Volcker HE. Confocal scanning laser indocyanine green angiography of neovascularization. Ophthalmology 1997; 94:343-47.

43. Freeman WR, Bartsch DU, Mueller AJ et al. Simultaneous indocyanine green angiography and fluorescein angiography using a confocal scanning laser ophthalmoscope. Arch Ophthalmol 1998; 116:455-63.

44. Staurenghi G. Scanning laser ophthalmoscope and angiography with a Wide-Field contact lens system. Arch Ophthalmol 2005;123:244-52.

45. Manivannan A, Sharp PF, Phillips RP, Forrester JV. Digital fundus imaging using a scanning laser ophthalmoscope. Physiol Meas 1993; 14:43-56.

46. Sharp PF, Manivannan A. The scanning laser ophthalmoscope-a review of its role in bioscience and medicine. Phys Med Biol 2004;49:1085-96.

47. Manivannan A, Kirkpatrick JN, Sharp PF, Forrester JV. Novel approach towards color imaging using a scanning laser ophthalmoscope. Ophthalmology 1998; 82:342-45.

48. Wolf S, Remsky A, Elsner AE, et al. Indocyanine green video angiography in patients with age-related macular degeneration related retinal pigment epithelial detachments. Ger J Ophthalmol 1994; 3:224-27.

49. Guyer DR, Yanuzi LA, Slakter JS, et al. Digital indocyanine green video angiography of occult choroidal neovascularization. Ophthalmology 1994;101:1727-35.

50. Flower RW, Hochheimer BF. A clinical technique and apparatus for simultaneous angiography of the separate retinal and choroidal circulations. Invest Opthalmol Vis Sci 1973;12;248-61.

51. Miller K. Protocols for the efficacious use of indocyanine green/sodium fluorescein angiography. J Ophthalmic Photography 1993;15:63-64.

52. Bellman C, Holz FG, Schapp O, et al. Topography of fundus autofluorescence with a confocal scanning laser ophthalmoscope. Ophthalmologe 1997;94:385-91.

53. Holz FG, Bellman C, Margaritidis M, et al. Patterns of increased in vivo FAF in the junctional zone of geographic atrophy of the retinal pigment epithelium associated with age-related macular degeneration. Graefes Arch Clin Exp Ophthalmol 1999;237:145-52.

54. Holz FG. Autofluorescence imaging of the macula. Ophthalmology 2001;98:10-18.

55. Spaide RF. Fundus autofluorescence and age related macular degeneration. Ophthalmology 2003; 110:292-99.

56. Staurenghi G, Orzalesi N, La Capria A, Aschero M. Laser treatment of feeder vessels in subfoveal choroidal neovascular membranes: a revisit using dynamic indocyanine green angiography. Ophthalmology. 1998;105:2297-05.

57. Coscas F, Stanescu D, Coscas G, Soubrane G. Feeder vessel treatment of choroidal neovascularization in age-related macular degeneration. J Fr Ophthalmol 2003; 26:602-08.

58. Kirkpatrick JN, Manivannan A, Gupta AK, et al. Fundus imaging in patients with cataract: role for a variable wavelength scanning laser ophthalmoscope. Br J Ophthalmol 1995;79:892-99.

59. HRA brochure: Product manual. Heidelberg Engineering. Heidelberg, Germany.

60. Rivero ME, Bartsch DU, Otto T, Freeman WR. Automated scanning laser ophthalmoscope image montages of retinal diseases. Ophthalmology 1999;106:2296-2300.

61. Flower RW, Hochheimer BF. Clinical infrared absorption angiography of the choroid. Am J Ophthalmol 1972; 73:458-98.

62. Bischoff P, Flower RW. Ten years experience with choroidal angiography using indocyanine green dye: a new routine examination or an epilogue? Doc Ophthalmol 1985; 60:235-91.

63. Flower RW, Hochheimer BF. A clinical technique and apparatus for simultaneous angiography of the separate retinal and choroidal circulations. Invest Ophthalmol Vis Sci. 1973; 12:248-261.

64. Bischoff PM, Niederberger HJ, Torok B, Speier P. Simultaneous indocyanine green and fluorescein angiography. Retina 1995;15:91-99.

65. Freeman WR, Bartsch DU, Mueller AJ, et al. Arch Ophthalmol 1998; 116:455-63.

66. Bischoff PM, Niederberger HJ, Torok B, Speiser P. Retina 1995;15:91-99.

67. Holz FG, Bellmann C, MD, Rohrscheider K, et al. Simultaneous confocal scanning laser fluorescein and indocyanine green angiography. Am J Ophthalmol 1998;125:227-36.

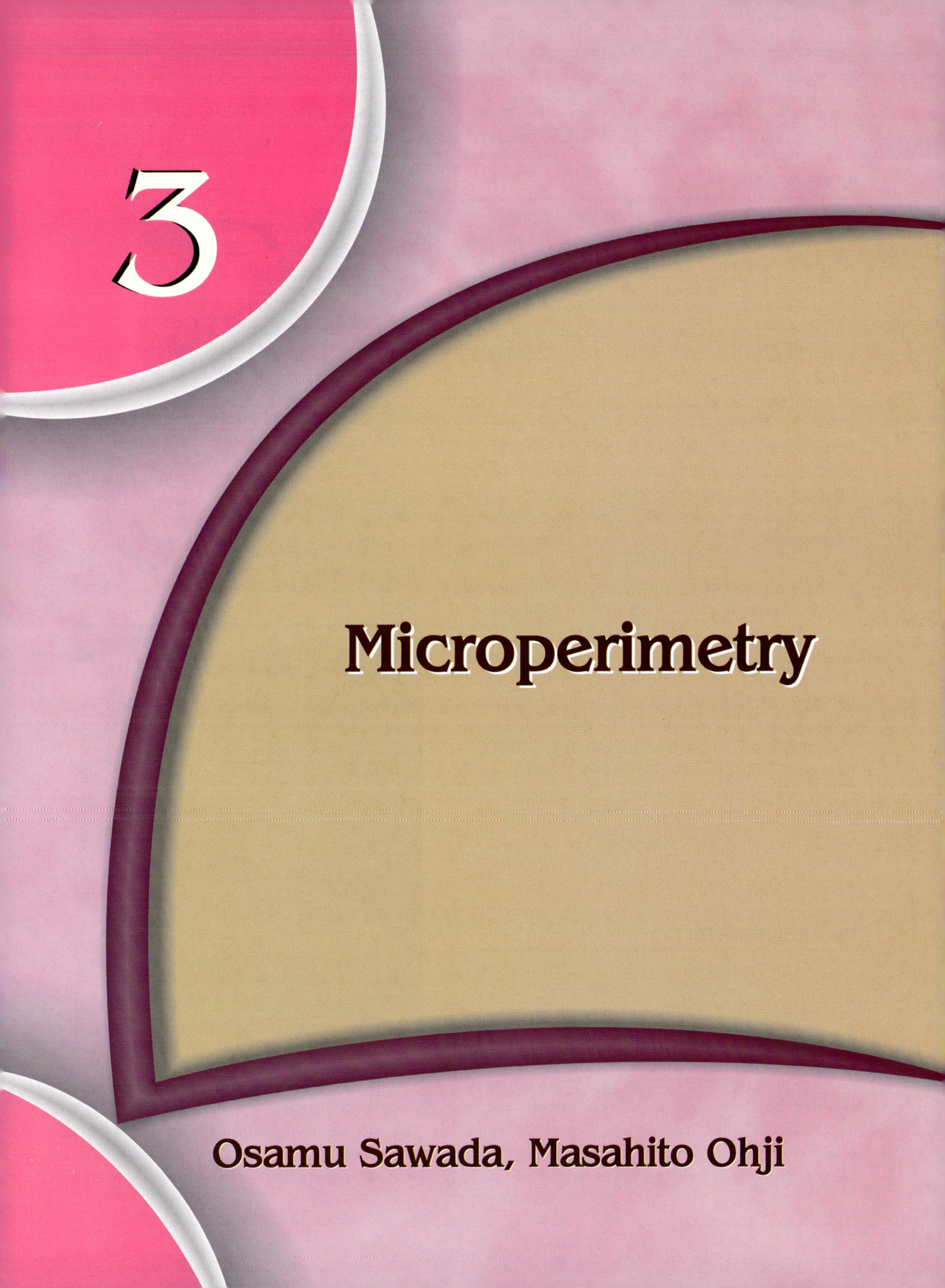

Microperimetry

Osamu Sawada, Masahito Ohji

INTRODUCTION

Many diseases cause blindness and visual disturbance, especially macular diseases. Diseases such as macular degeneration, macular edema secondary to retinal vein occlusions and diabetic maculopathy are the most important causes. Visual acuity is the gold standards of visual function examination. Unfortunately, visual acuity is insufficient to quantify in detail the visual function in patients with macular diseases.

Automated full-threshold static perimetry has been established in clinical practice to reveal and quantify functional defects of the visual field, but it is difficult to obtain adequate evaluation in patients with macular disease because of unstable fixation.

To evaluate correctly the correlation between retinal pathologies and functional defects, microperimetry has been developed into clinical use, providing a simultaneous observation of the fundus and a correction for eye movements during the perimetric examination. For years, the scanning laser ophthalmoscope[1-4] (SLO, Rodenstock, Germany) was the only commercial available microperimeter. But it had a manual control limitation including lack of real-time fundus tracking and narrow field of view of only 33 × 22 degrees. Recently, a new instrument named the microperimeter 1 (NIDEK Technologies, Italy) has been introduced. The MP1 allows fundus perimetry in a larger field with automated full-threshold perimetry software. Furthermore, real-color fundus image acquisition is possible, and an overlay of the perimetric findings onto the fundus image is also possible.

THE MICROPERIMETER 1

The microperimeter 1 is a new automatic fundus-related perimetry, with which fixation and retinal date are superimposed on a color fundus photograph (Figures 3.1 to 3.5).

The microperimeter 1 uses infrared light to generate real time, non-mydriatic 45° images of retina displayed on a monitor during the examination. Infrared light is used to ensure patient comfort and corporation. A full color digital image is captured at the beginning or end of the examination. Fundus camera includes a correction

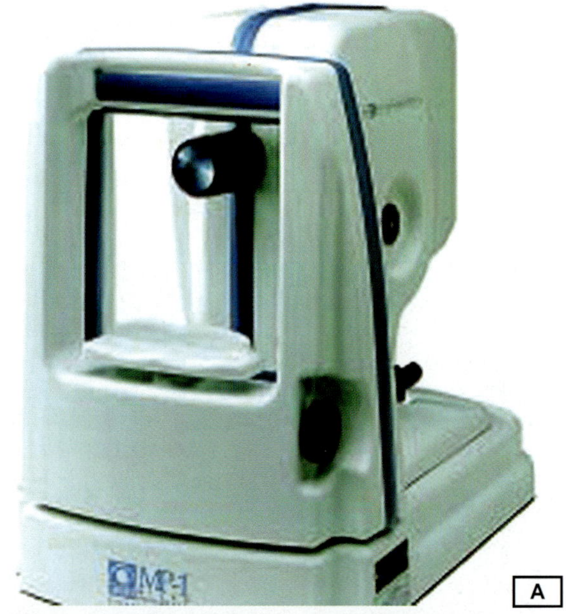

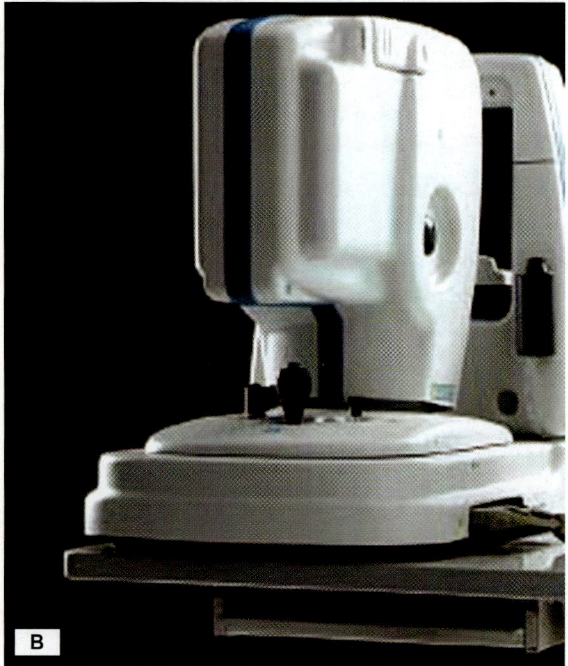

FIGURES 3.1A and B: Microperimeter 1

system for patients with refractive errors (range from −12.5 to +16 diopters).

The microperimeter 1 includes an automated eye tracking system to compensate eye movements. At first an infrared camera tracks a reference frame and an area

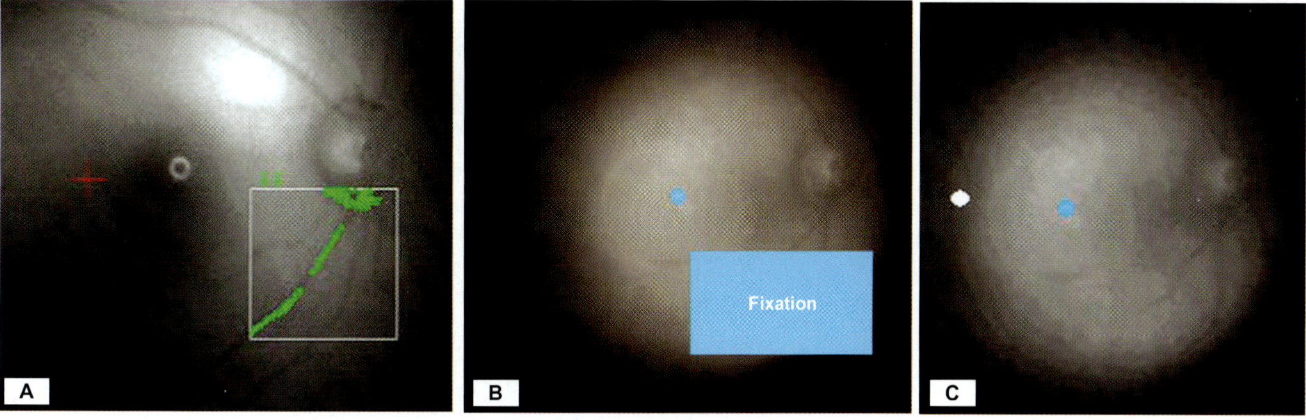

FIGURES 3.2A to C: The autotracking system. (A) The specific position is memorized. (B and C) Automated tracking system is used to correct eye movement. The relative position in an eye is displayed.

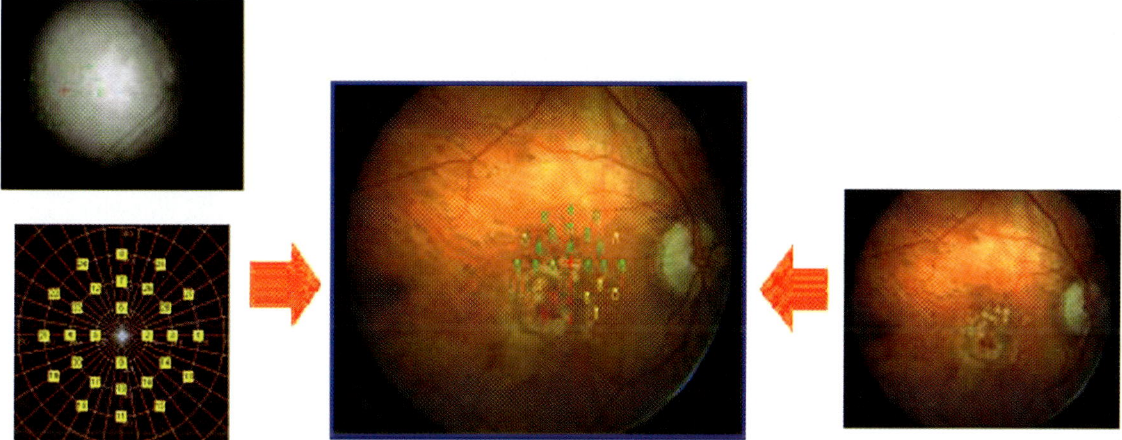

FIGURE 3.3. Superimposed visual field data and color photograph

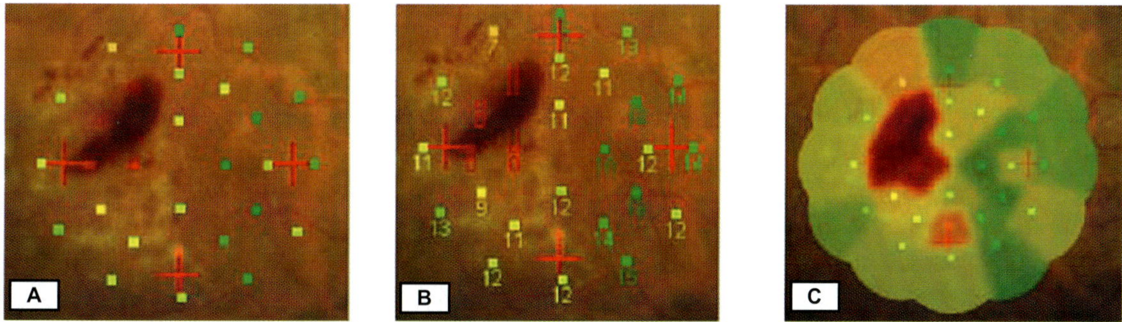

FIGURES 3.4A to C: Map display. (A) Symbolic map, (B) Numerical map, (C) Interpolated color map

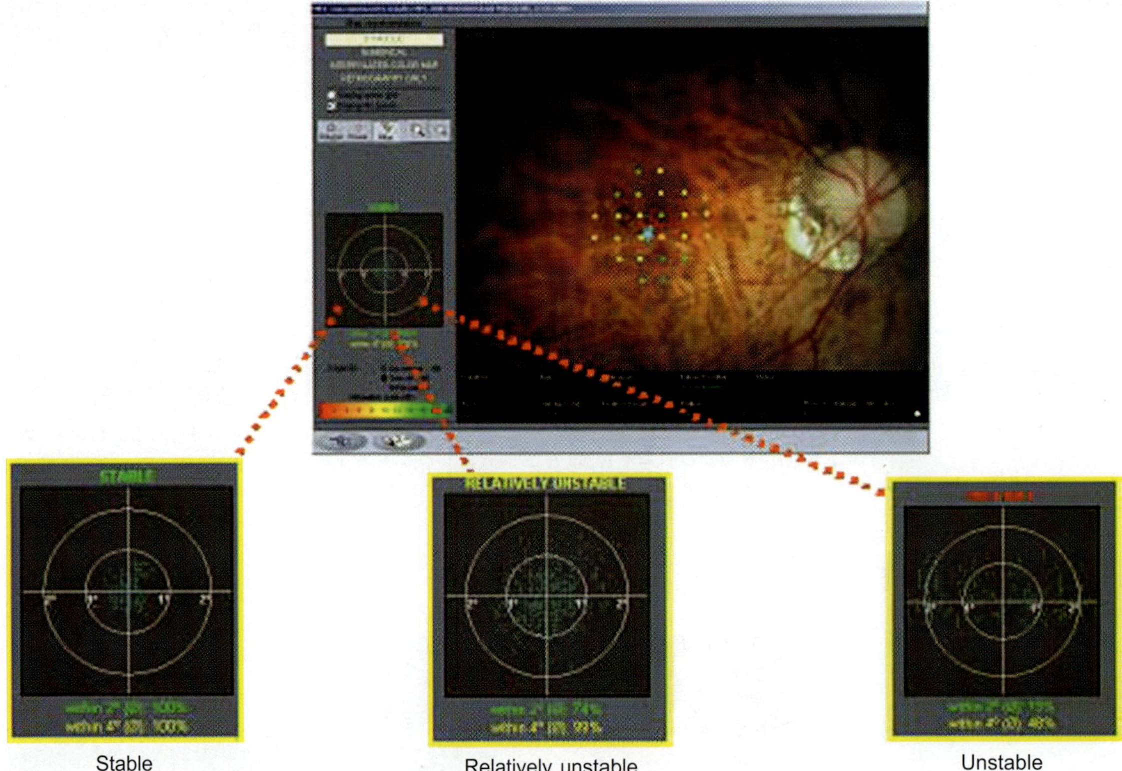

Stable   Relatively unstable   Unstable

FIGURE 3.5: Fixation analysis

of interest is defined. During examination, any eye movement is detected by image acquisition with 25 frames per second. The autotracking system including high-speed tracking software calculates horizontal, vertical and rotational shifts relative to a reference frame and reflects the stimulus position on the display corrected according to the actual location of the fundus.

The microperimeter 1 performs microperimetry using selectable target strategies and programmable parameters by examiners. The microperimeter 1 uses a liquid crystal display to project stimuli. Stimulus intensity can be set on 1 (0.1 log) step scale from 0 to 20 dB, where 0 dB represents the brightest luminance of 400 asb (127 candles/square meter). Stimulus size can be set by the examiner, from I to V of Goldmann standard perimeter. The fixation target, set at 100 asb, can be varied in size and sharp (a cross or a ring are commended for patients with central fixation, four crosses or a large ring for patients with paracentral fixation) according to the patient's visual acuity and macula scotoma.

The microperimeter 1, accurately overlays data from perimetry and fundus photography. Then, the Micro Perimeter 1 makes it possible to combine and cross-analyze the visual field defects and visible structural pathologies on the fundus.

COMPARISON WITH OTHER INSTRUMENTS

Springer and associates [5] reported on comparison with conventional threshold perimetry, the Octopus 101 perimetry. This report indicates that the microperimeter 1 provides reproducible differential light threshold values with a systematic difference of 11.4 to 18.3 dB compared with conventional static perimetry using the Octopus 101. With a larger difference in the lower part of the visual field, differential light sensitivity values in the microperimeter 1 are comparable to the threshold values obtained with the Octopus 101 using a correction factor of 11.4 to 18.3 dB according to stimulus location. With regard to fixation control, fixation analysis and surveillance with the microperimeter 1 is far superior to the Octopus 101, because *eye movement* is directly monitored, and compensated. Fundus perimetry such as the microperimeter 1 provides advantages of an exact documentation of actual test location on the retina and a real-time correction of *eye movements*.

Rohrschneider and associates [6] reported on comparison between the microperimeter 1 and the SLO. According to this report, both instruments enable detection of sensitivity loss of the central visual field and an analysis of fixation behavior during examination. The major drawbacks of the microperimeter 1 are the low quality of black-and-white infrared images, which has to use a high level of infrared illumination to achieve a satisfying contrast between retinal vessels and the fundus for the autotracking system, and the possibility to miss defining a specific test grid on base of the fundus image. However, with realtime fundus tracking and color visualization of the fundus, the microperimeter 1 microperimetry, as an automated fundus perimetric examination, provides comparable results to the SLO.

CONCLUSION

The MP1 is useful as a microperimetry to detect visual field defect combined with color fundus photographs.

The microperimeter 1 is an excellent instrument in performance to combine visible pathology of the fundus from fundus photography with visual field defects obtainable from fundus-controlled perimetry. Additionally, the *eye* tracking system makes it possible to determine location and stability of fixation accurately.

REFERENCES

1. Rohrschneider K, Bultmann S, Gluck R, et al. Scanning laser ophthalmoscope fundus perimetry before and after laser photocoagulation for clinically significant diabetic macular edema. Am J Ophthalmol 2000; 129:27-32.
2. Mori F, Ishiko S, Kitaya N, et al. Use of scanning laser ophthalmoscope microperimetry in clinically significant macular edema in type 2 diabetes mellitus. Jpn J Ophthalmol 2002; 46:650-55.
3. Varano M, Scassa C, Capaldo N, et al. Development of macular pseudoholes: a 36-month period of follow-up. Retina 2002; 22:435-42.
4. Ergun E, Maar N, Radner W, et al. Scotoma size and reading speed in patients with subfoveal occult choroidal neovascularization in age-related macular degeneration. Ophthalmology 2003; 110:65-69.
5. Springer C, Bültmann S, Völker HE, et al. Fundus perimetry with the micro perimeter 1 in normal individuals. Ophthalmology 2005; 112:848-54.
6. Rohrschneider K, Springer C, Bültmann S, et al. Microperimetry-comparison between the microperimetry 1 and scanning laser ophthalmoscope-fundus perimetry. Am J Ophthalmol 2005; 139:125-34.

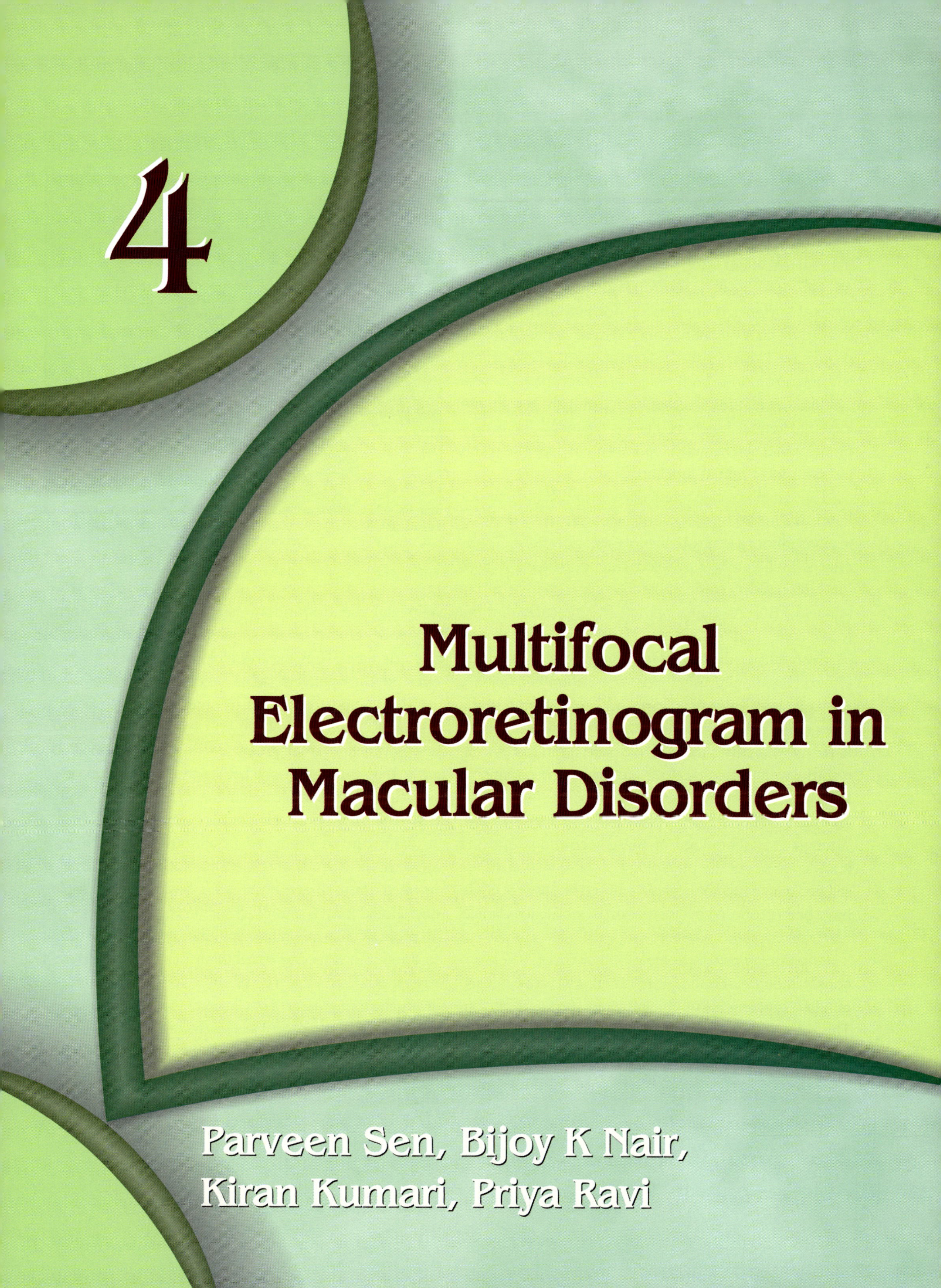

Multifocal Electroretinogram in Macular Disorders

Parveen Sen, Bijoy K Nair,
Kiran Kumari, Priya Ravi

INTRODUCTION

The electroretinogram (ERG) is an electrical potential generated by the retina in response to a flash of light. It is an excellent tool for studying retinal function objectively.[1,2] It can be recorded noninvasively from the corneal surface. It consists of positive and negative waveforms that originate from different stages of retinal processing. However, the ERG response to a flash of light is a mass response from retinal photoreceptors as well as the other retinal cells. It does not provide insight into localized retinal function. Hence the need for a new protocol that can stimulate various areas separately and evaluate focal retinal function.

The multifocal electroretinogram (mfERG) allows for functional retinal field mapping by concurrently deriving responses from a large number of retinal locations. Recording is done in a light adapted state. In general, it gives local information comparable to cone responses in the full-field ERG. An abnormal mfERG indicates that the foveal cones and/or bipolar cell layers are dysfunctional.

Erich Sutter[3] developed the method of the multifocal electroretinography using cross-correlation with binary m-sequences Sutter and Tran in 1992,[4] described the topography of the first order kernel of the multifocal ERG in human subjects. Electrical responses from the eye are recorded with a corneal electrode just as in conventional ERG recording, but the special nature of the stimulus and analysis produce a topographic map of ERG responses. Though the technology of these recordings and the knowledge about the physiology of these responses are still evolving basic guidelines for usage of this procedure have been proposed by International Society for Clinical Electrophysiology of Vision.[5]

The display usually contains either 61 or 103 hexagons, although 241 and 509 hexagons have been used in a few experiments to obtain higher spatial resolution. The display is scaled so that each hexagon stimulates approximately the same number of receptors. Since the cone density is higher toward the centre the hexagons are smaller (Figure 4.1).

Though the overall effect is of a randomly flickering screen each hexagon flashes individually according to

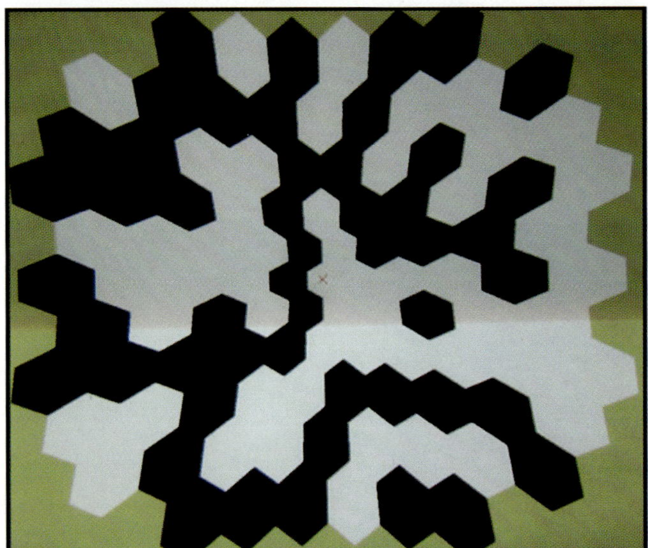

FIGURE 4.1: Showing geometry of 103-hexagonal stimulus with central fixation cross.

a special pseudo-random sequence known as an m-sequence. On an average, only half of them are on at any one time. Thus the overall luminance of the screen over time is relatively stable (equiluminant).

The tracings of the mfERG are not direct electrical responses from a local region of retina. The mfERG waveforms are a mathematical extraction of signals. By correlating the continuous ERG signal with the on or off phases of each stimulus element, the focal ERG signal associated with each element is calculated.[6]

Data can be displayed in various ways such as a topographic 3D response density plots, group averages or trace arrays. Trace array is the basic mfERG display and should form a part of all standard display protocols. To properly interpret mfERGs in the clinic, it is important to know the response distribution in the normal retina as well as its intersubject variability. At photopic luminance levels, the topography of the first order multifocal response derived from a normal subject resembles a smooth surface with a prominent central peak.[7,8] When data are collected under identical conditions, the factors affecting reproducibility and intersubject variability are (a) the ability of the subject to fixate and (b) noise contamination due to blinks or eye movements.[9]

WAVEFORMS

NOMENCLATURE OF PEAKS

The typical waveform of the first order response or first order kernel (K1) mfERG response is a biphasic wave (Figure 4.2). There is an initial negative deflection followed by a positive peak. There may be a second negative deflection after the peak. These are labeled N1, P1 and N2 respectively. There is some homology between this waveform and the conventional ERG photopic waveform, but they are not identical. Thus the designations 'a wave' and 'b wave' is not recommended.

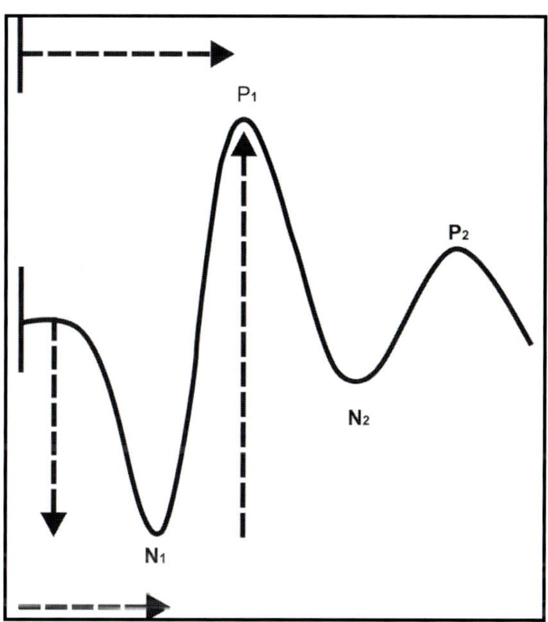

FIGURE 4.2: Nomenclature of mf ERG wave waveform
Amplitude recordings:
Amplitude of N1: From the baseline TO the trough of the first negative wave
Amplitude of P1: From the trough of N1 TO the peak of P1.

CELLULAR ORIGIN

Various studies in humans have shown that the origin of the N1 wave is from the same cells of the retina which give rise to the a-wave of the full-field cone ERG, and the origin of the P1 wave is from the same cells of the retina which give rise to the cone b-wave and oscillatory potentials. However, the cellular origin and the physiology of these waveforms are still not clear. Hence a direct correlation between the mfERG waveform and cone ERG should not be made.

STIMULUS

The stimulus source used in recording a mfERG is generally delivered by a cathode ray tube (CRT) with frame frequency of 75 Hz. Other devices are also used such as LCD projectors, LED arrays and scanning laser ophthalmoscopes. The luminance of the stimulus elements on the CRT screen should be 100 to 200 cd/m^2 in the lighted state and <1 cd/m^2 in the dark state. This means that the mean screen luminance during testing will be 50 to 100 cd/m^2.[5]

STIMULUS PATTERN

The hexagonal stimulus pattern is so designed that it compensates for local differences in cone density across the retina. Thus, in a standard protocol the central hexagons are smaller than the more peripheral ones. It subtends a visual angle of 20 to 30 degrees on either side of fixation. Commercial mfERG instruments use an m-sequence to control the order of flicker of the stimulus elements (between light and dark). This sequence is recommended for routine testing. Different sequences, or the inclusion of global light or dark frames, are used for specialized testing. [10] Contrast between the lighted and darkened stimulus elements should be 90% or greater. The background region of the CRT (beyond the area of stimulus hexagons) should have a luminance equal to the mean luminance of the stimulus array.

FIXATION TARGETS

Stable fixation is essential to obtain reliable mfERG recordings.[11] Central fixation dots or crosses are available with most stimulus programs. They should cover as little as possible of the central stimulus element to avoid diminishing the response (but may need enlargement for low vision patients).

RECORDING EQUIPMENT

AMPLIFIERS AND FILTERS

An alternating current (AC) amplifier is used with a gain of 100,000 or 200,000. The bandpass filter of 3 to 300 Hz or 10 to 300 Hz removes extraneous electrical noise while preserving waveforms of interest.

Signal analysis is done digitally.

ARTIFACT REJECTION

Because blinks and other movements can distort the recorded waveforms, there are 'artifact rejection' programs to eliminate some of the obvious peaks or drifts from being added to the cumulative recording. Artifact rejection is often used to 'clean up' a record, but should not in general be applied multiple times to smoothen up the plot.[12]

DISPLAY OPTIONS

Trace arrays. All commercial multifocal software programs can produce an array of the mfERG traces from different regions of the macula. This is the basic mfERG display and should be a part of all standard display protocols. This must be referred to for diagnosis in clinical setting.

GROUP AVERAGES

Software programs can average together the mfERG responses from any defined area of the retina. This can be helpful for comparing quadrants, hemiretinal areas, or successive rings from center to periphery. This helps to look at the distribution pattern of the disease. It is the distribution, which helps, in differential diagnosis of various maculopathies.

TOPOGRAPHIC (3D) RESPONSE DENSITY PLOTS

These plots show the overall signal strength per unit area of retina (combining N and P components) in a 3-dimensional figure. This gives the clinician an instant overview of the retinal pathology. These 3D plots however incorporate both negative and positive deflections, so waveform information is lost and noise can be enhanced.[13] It is recommended that 3D plots not be used by themselves to display mfERG data; they should always be accompanied by a corresponding trace array.

KERNELS

For most of the clinical work only first order kernels are considered.

CLINICAL PROTOCOL

PUPILS

The pupils should be fully dilated and pupil size should be noted. The cornea should be anesthetized.

ELECTRODES

Recording Electrodes

Electrodes that contact the cornea or bulbar conjunctiva are recommended for mfERG recording. Most commonly used electrodes include Burian-Allen contact lens electrode and the DTL electrode. Contact lens electrodes provide the highest amplitude and most stable recordings; such electrodes should be centrally transparent with an optical opening as large as possible, and incorporate a device to hold the lids apart. The amplitudes recorded with the DTL electrodes are smaller though the patient comfort and cooperation is more. The signal-to-noise-ratio is better with Burian-Allen electrodes. Poor or unstable electrode contact is a major cause of poor quality records. Care should be taken to make sure that the contact lens of the Burian-Allen electrode is clear to allow good vision and refraction. In addition, the optics of Burian-Allen electrodes may cause more stray light than the cornea alone as well as prismatic effects if the contact lens does not fit perfectly.[5] The corneal surface is protected with a non-viscous, non-irritating and non-allergenic ionic conductive solution.

Reference Electrodes

Burian Allen electrode has reference electrode incorporated into the contact lens-speculum assembly ('bipolar electrodes'). This is the most stable configuration electrically. Alternatively, electrodes can be placed near each orbital rim temporally as a reference for the corresponding eye. The forehead has also been used as a reference electrode site.

Ground Electrodes

A separate skin electrode should be attached to an indifferent point and connected to ground. Typical locations are on the forehead or ear.

PATIENT POSITIONING

Subjects should sit comfortably in front of the screen or instrument. The viewing distance will vary with screen size, in order to control the area (visual angle) of retina being stimulated.

FIXATION MONITORING

Since good fixation is essential, fixation should be monitored in some fashion, either by direct observation of the patient or by the use of monitoring instrumentation. Eye movements can alter the optimal corneal electrode position, produce electrical artifacts, or allow blockage of light by the electrode or eyelid. Patients who cannot see a fixation target may be given a larger fixation target.

REFRACTION

Lenses are typically placed in a holder positioned in front of the eye. Because lenses alter the relative magnification of the stimulus, the viewing distance must be adjusted to compensate for the same. Also care must be taken to avoid inducing a ring scotoma with a plus lens.[14] Both monocular and binocular recording is possible. Binocular recording allows good fixation but signals can be altered by decentration of either eye.

ADAPTATION

Subjects should be in ordinary room light for 15 minutes before testing, assuming no prior exposure to bright sun or fundus photography. Longer adaptation may be needed after such exposure. A previous full-field ERG with photopic recordings is acceptable as long as the exposure (especially flicker) was not unusually prolonged.

ROOM ILLUMINATION

Room lights should be on, and ideally produce illumination at the subject close to that of the stimulus screen.

RECORDING SEQUENCE

Stimulus Geometry

Size 20 to 30 degrees of visual angle on either side of fixation.

Number of elements: Most often elements used are 61 or 103, 241 and 509 elements are used for more critical localization.

Duration of recording: Total time is typically about 4 min for 61 elements, or 8 min for 103 elements. The overall recording time is divided into shorter segments (e.g. 15 to 30s). This allows the patient to rest in between. Also a poor record can be discarded without losing the entire data.

The choice of stimulus array and recording time is a trade-off between the stability of recording and the topographic resolution of the data. Large stimulus elements, e.g. 61 give signals with less noise, but small areas of retinal dysfunction can be missed.

Smaller stimulus elements, e.g. 103 will show more accurately the outline of dysfunctional areas, but require longer recording time to obtain an acceptable signal to noise ratio. Large elements with a short recording time are easier for patients and suitable for a general overview of macular function. Very small elements such as a 241-hexagon array may sometimes be needed for accurate tracking of functional defects (Figures 4.3 to 4.6).

MfERG AND NOISE

It has been found that the signal-to-noise ratio was better with less spatial resolution, with higher retinal illuminance, i.e. dilated pupils compared to recordings in miosis, and with longer recording times.[15] Higher spatial resolution of 241 hexagons in the 30-degree field size may reduce the response amplitude so that some responses may lie within the noise level. Low retinal illuminance may again lead to smaller responses, a lower signal-to-noise ratio. The use of very high retinal illuminances may induce an increased contribution of stray light. Theoretically, the longer the recording time, the higher is the quality of the derived responses. But practically, it can decrease the concentration and cooperation of the patients with the duration of the examination. To improve the quality of the recordings, the recording session should be subdivided into several segments.

MfERG AND REFRACTIVE ERROR

In a study the N1, P1, and N2 amplitudes were significantly correlated with the severity of myopia in adult subjects.[16,17] The response amplitudes of N1, P1, and N2 decreased as the dioptric power of myopia increased. The severity of myopia was also significantly correlated with N1, P1, and N2 implicit times in adults with myopia (Figures 4.7A and B).

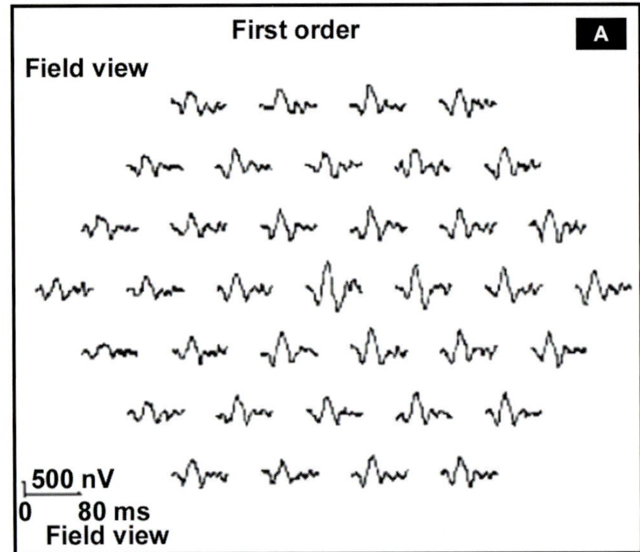

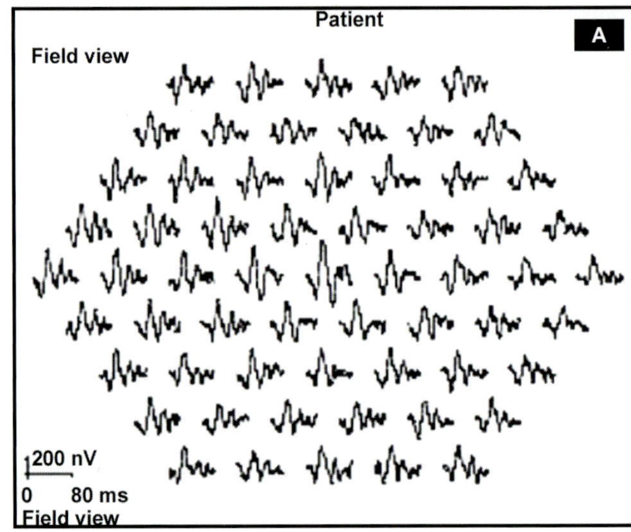

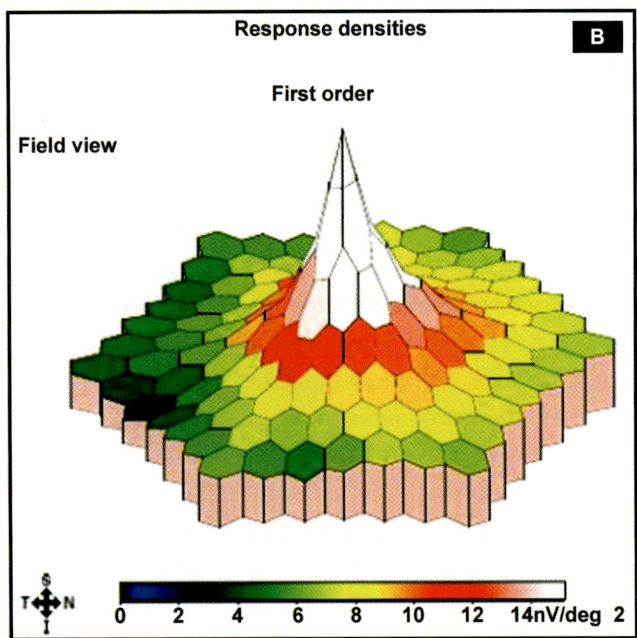

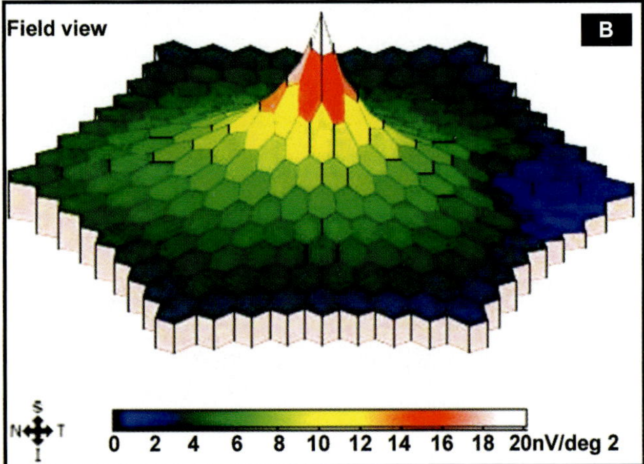

FIGURES 4.4A and B: (A) Trace array of the 61 mfERG responses. (B) Three-dimensional plot of the response density of 61 mfERG responses.

FIGURES 4.3A and B: Multifocal ERG of a normal subject. (A) Trace array of the 37-mfERG responses of the first order kernel. (B) Three-dimensional plot of the response density of the 37 mfERG response.

MfERG AND AGING

Each localized response in mfERG shows a significant aging effect most commonly in N1P1 amplitude. The average decline of the response, was approximately 5% per decade, varying from 3.3% (peripherally) to 7.5% (perifoveally). [18,19] The decline was significantly higher for the superior than for the inferior retina for amplitude parameters. Increases in P1 implicit time have also been seen. The relative rate of change with age was similar for the nasal and the temporal retina. Information about changes in discrete retinal areas with age should make the mfERG more useful in quantitatively monitoring progression of retinal disease.

CLINICAL APPLICATIONS

Multifocal Erg has revolutionized clinical electrophysiology. This technique has provided insight into the mechanisms of retinal disease. As in the case of the full-field ERG, the ganglion cells contribute relatively little

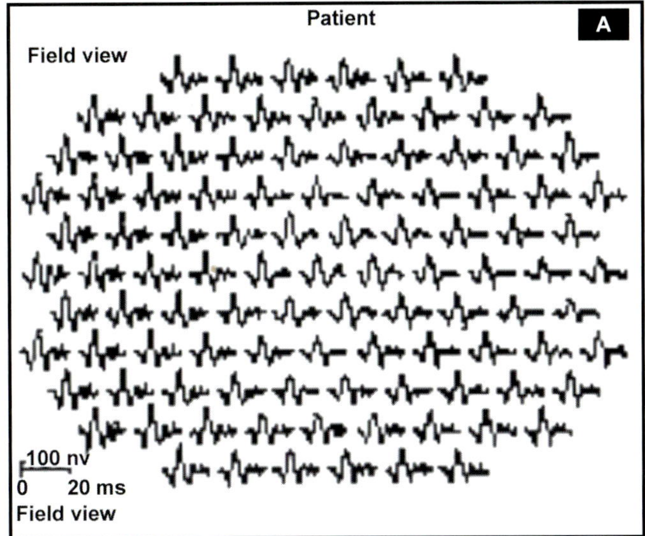

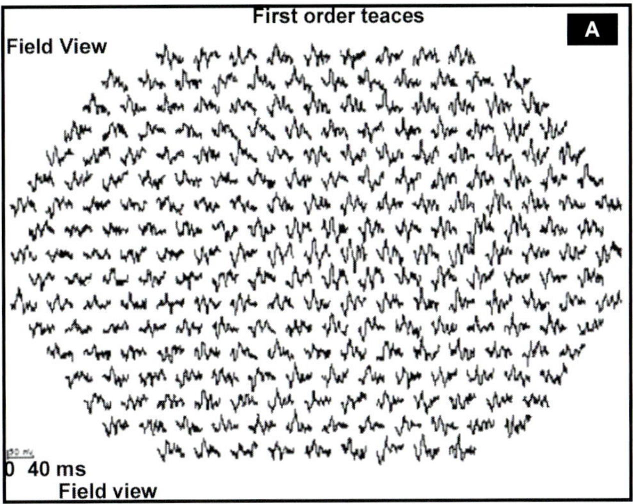

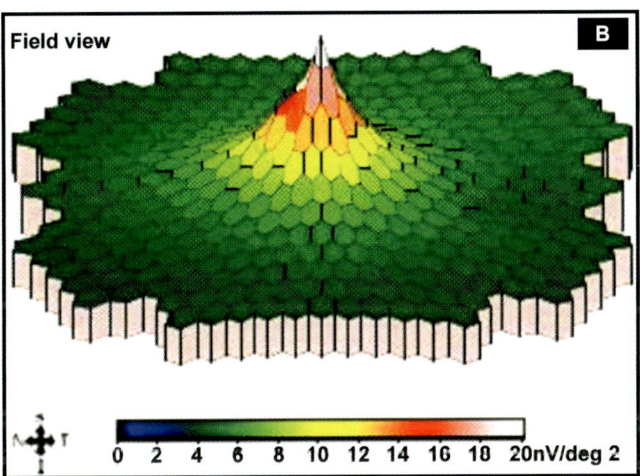

FIGURES 4.5A and B: (A) Trace array 103 multifocal ERG responses, (B) Three-dimensional plot of the response densities.

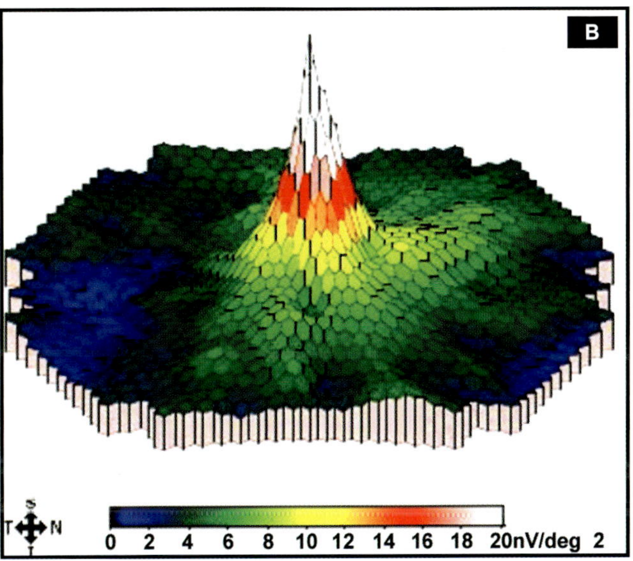

FIGURES 4.6A and B: (A) Trace array of the 241 mfERG responses. (B) Three-dimensional plot of the response density of 241 mfERG responses.

to the response. The mfERG is particularly valuable in cases where the fundus appears normal, and it is difficult to distinguish whether it is a disease of the outer retina or that of the optic nerve, which is responsible for the subnormal vision. Since ganglion cells do not contribute much to mfERG responses an abnormal mfERG points towards an outer retinal pathology.[20]

In contrast to a single response using focal ERG or pattern ERG the mfERG indicates not only a central loss of function in maculopathies but also allows a detailed description of the extent of the lesion. This helps in distinguishing between various macular diseases. Hence the mfERG can also help differentiate amongst outer retinal diseases, to follow the progression of retinal diseases, and, with the addition of the mfVEP, to differentiate between organic and nonorganic causes of visual loss.[21]

The implicit time of the mERG responses, not amplitude, has been found to be the more sensitive measure of damage in degenerative diseases of the receptors. The MfERG findings of few retinal diseases are given below.

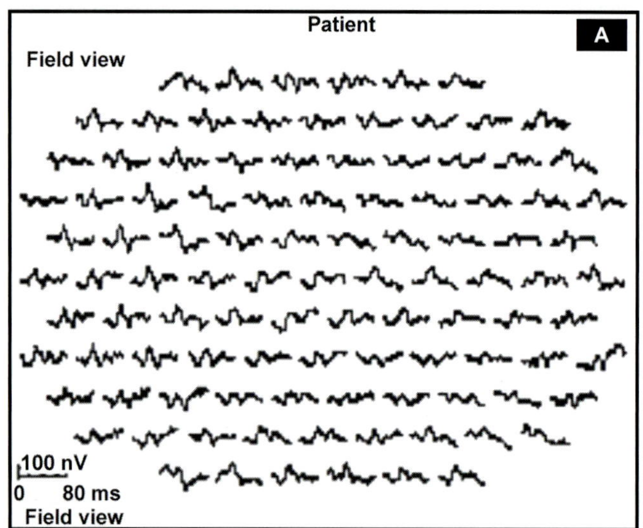

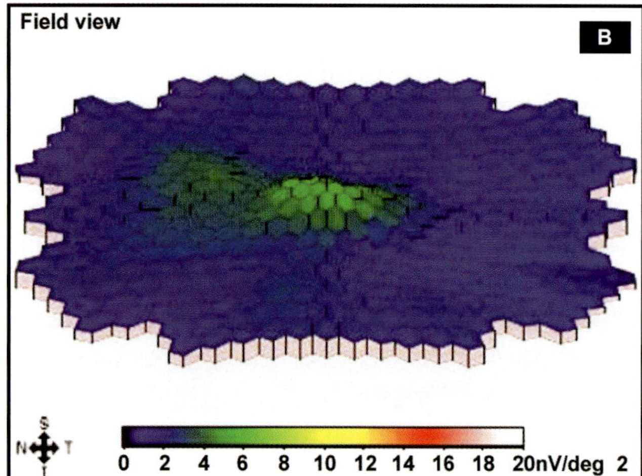

FIGURES 4.7A and B: Data of a patient with pathological myopia with myopic macular degeneration. (A) Trace array of the right eye. (B) Three-dimensional plot of response density showing generalized depression of responses.

MACULOPATHIES

In the maculopathies the central responses are lost or markedly diminished surrounded by normal or at least clearly recordable response. This leads to a crater or volcano like appearance in the three-dimensional plot of response density. The loss of central activity can be found in all kinds of maculopathies as in age-related macular degeneration (AMD), vitelliform maculopathies, macular holes, juvenile retinoschisis, central serous retinopathy and others. Differences may occur in the extent of the central lesion in different diseases. For example, in early stages of Stargardt's maculopathy or chloroquine retinopathy the responses may be diminished most markedly in the ring of 2–7 degree eccentricity leaving a discernable response in the fovea.[22, 23]

RETINITIS PIGMENTOSA

The principle finding in retinitis pigmentosa is a diminished central response surrounded by ERGs, which are hardly discernable from noise. Patients with retinitis pigmentosa who have a preserved central island of vision may have a discernable foveal response even when Ganzfeld ERG is extinguished (Figures 4.8A and B).[24] In segmental or perivenous retinitis pigmentosa the responses are lost in the affected regions.

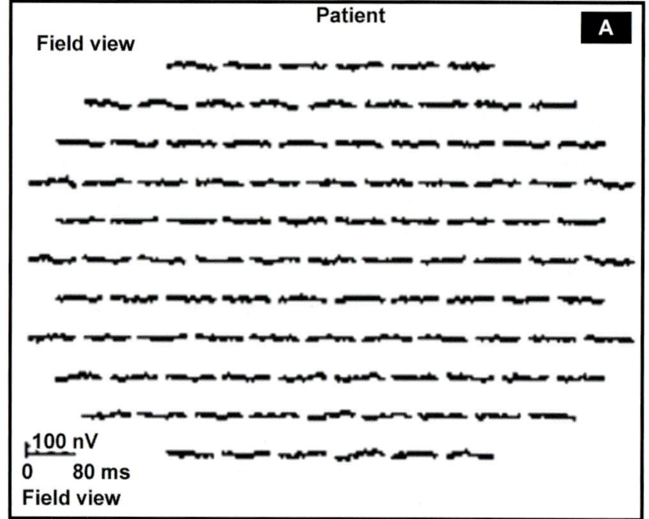

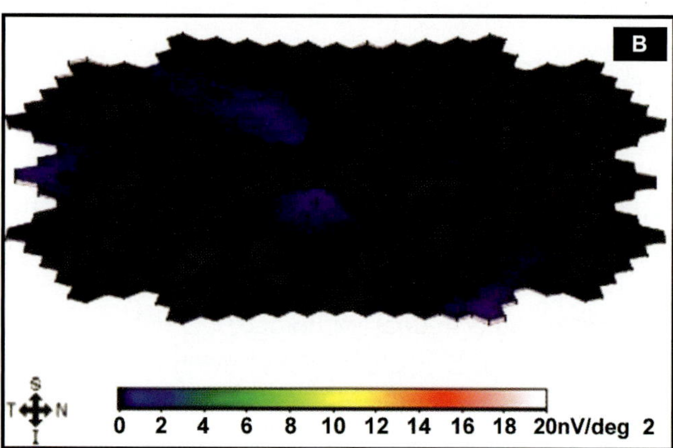

FIGURES 4.8A and B: Example of mfERG responses of a 63-year-old patient with retinitis pigmentosa. (A) Trace array. (B) Three dimensional response density plot showing extinguished responses.

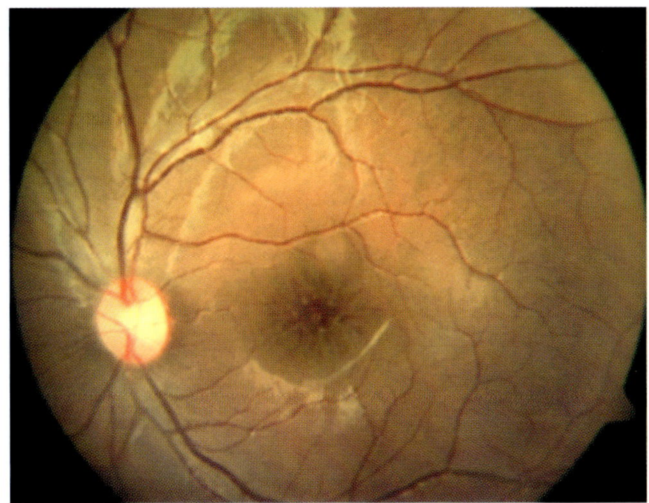

(A) Fundus photograph showing a tapetal reflex with cartwheel like appearance at the fovea suggestive of foveal schisis.

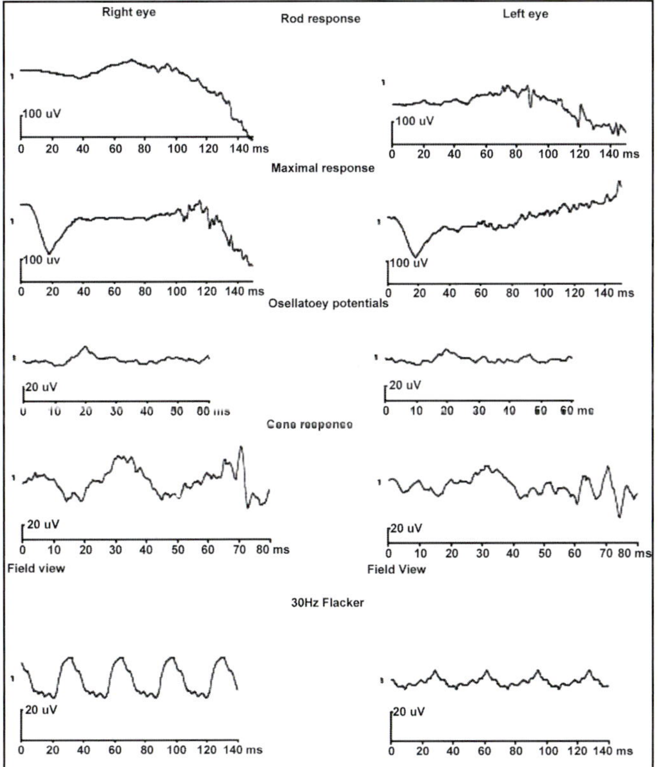

(B) Full-field ERG with negative waveform in the combined response; both rods AND cone responses are reduced.

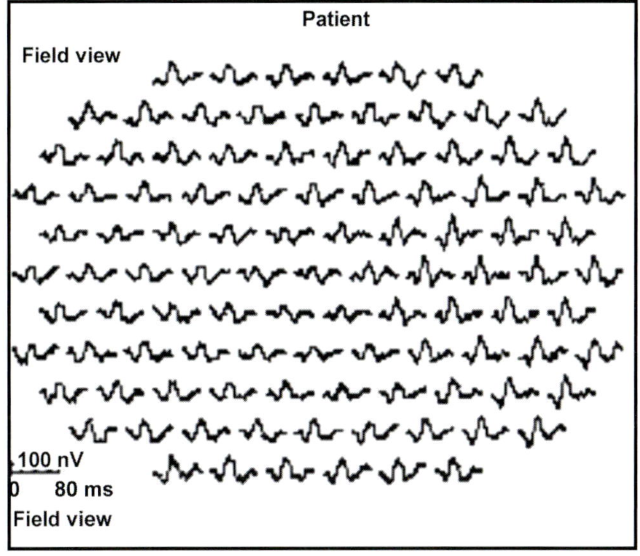

(C) Trace array of the same patient showing reduced P1/N1 ratio of central responses.

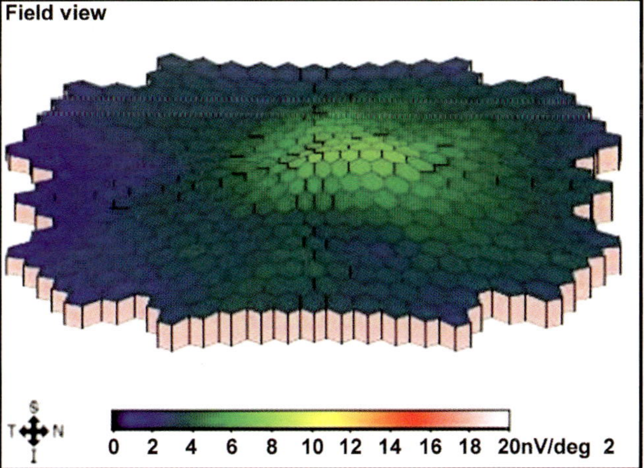

(D) Three-dimensional response density plot showing reduction of central peak amplitude.

FIGURES 4.9A to D: Example of mf ERG responses left eye of a 12-year-old boy with X-linked retinoschisis.

X-LINKED JUVENILE RETINOSCHISIS

The trace array and 3D topography of multifocal ERG shows multi-area amplitude decrease with absence or reduction of central peak amplitude in patients with retinoschisis. The P1/N1 ratio of multifocal ERG average response densities in six-ring retinal regions was different from the b/a ratio of Ganzfeld ERG.[25] The multifocal ERG and Ganzfeld ERG each has its advantage in the diagnosis of retinoschisis (Figures 4.9A to D).

STARGARDT'S MACULOPATHY AND CONE DYSTROPHY

Stargardt's disease is characterized by a normal full-field ERG and reduced responses in mfERG. In a series of 101 eyes with Stargardt's maculopathy the electrophysiological changes were restricted to the macula (up to 7 degrees) in only 7 eyes while in 56 eyes alterations were found out to 12 degrees and even more peripheral in 24 eyes.[22] The combination of small fundus changes and central defect in the multifocal ERG is observed both in cases of foveal cone dystrophy and early stages of Stargardt's macular dystrophy. In cone dystrophies, however, the multifocal ERG-responses across the entire retina are markedly decreased or lost (Figures 4.10 and 4.11).

VITELLIFORM MACULAR DYSTROPHY

MfERG can detect focal retinal dysfunction in vitelliform macular dystrophy, which would not be apparent in the full field ERG. In contrast to other macular disorders, amplitudes rather than implicit times seem to be affected in the MfERG of vitelliform macular dystrophy (Figures 4.12A to D). [26]

CENTRAL SEROUS CHORIORETINOPATHY

Decrease in amplitudes as well as increase in the implicit time of mfERG responses is seen in central serous retinopathy. In a study by Suzuki and associates [27] the multifocal ERG amplitudes were significantly reduced at the first attack of central serous retinopathy in all patients compared with the values in the normal controls. Multifocal ERG latencies of the patients significantly increased compared with normal controls, for P1 (P < 01) and N2 (P < 01). After the resolution of retinal detachment, although the multifocal ERG amplitudes increased markedly, they did not improve to the normal level during the follow-up period (4-23 months). Persistent functional impairment of the retina was found by multifocal Ergs in patients with central serous retinopathy even after the resolution of sub retinal fluid. A topographical analysis of the multifocal ERG is useful in the clinical observation of central serous retinopathy (Figures 4.13A to D).

EPIMACULAR MEMBRANE

The electrical retinal response densities in the foveal and the perifoveal area are commonly decreased in patients with idiopathic epimacular membranes. The electrical retinal response density of these areas gradually improved after peeling of the epimacular membrane. This improvement can continue even 6 months after the operation. [28]

MACULAR HOLE

In patients with macular holes Szlyk and associates[29] and Moschos and associates[30] could not only demonstrate a decrease of central responses preoperatively but also that those responses might increase after surgical treatment. Multifocal ERG can therefore serve as a measure for the success of a therapeutic intervention.

AGE-RELATED MACULAR DEGENERATION AND CHOROIDAL NEOVASCULAR MEMBRANE

Multifocal ERG is a useful tool for the clinical follow-up of choroidal neovascular membrane (Figures 4.14A to C). It offers interesting non-subjective data of retinal sensitivity of patients with macular diseases treated with photodynamic therapy.[31, 32] In addition we obtained a central retinal sensitivity map where we were able to evaluate the extent and depth of retinal damage. Electrophysiological testing in AMD has also been used recently to evaluate the efficacy and safety of newer anti-VEGF (Vascular Endothelial Growth Factor) drugs being used intravitreally.[33]

MULTIFOCAL ERG IN DRUG TOXICITIES

Various drugs are known to be retinotoxic. Many drugs can provoke a bull's eye maculopathy. Most of them will

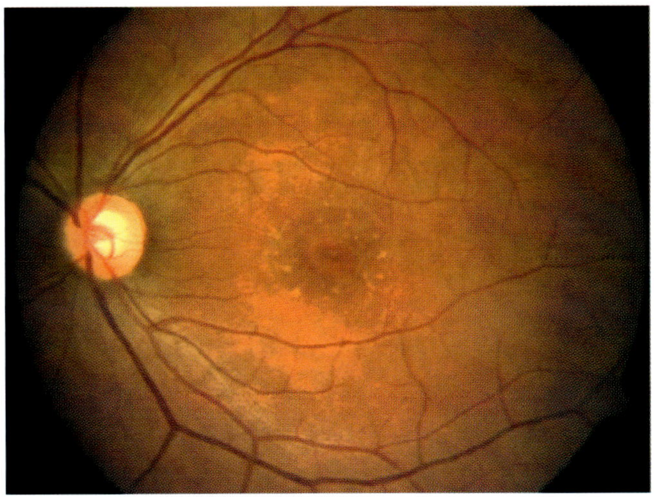

(A) Fundus photograph of the left eye showing metal beaten appearance of the macula with a few flecks.

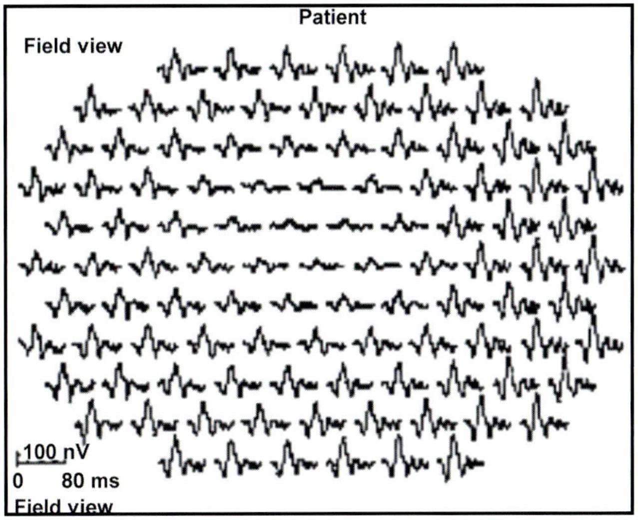

(C) Trace array showing reduced central responses AND near normal peripheral responses.

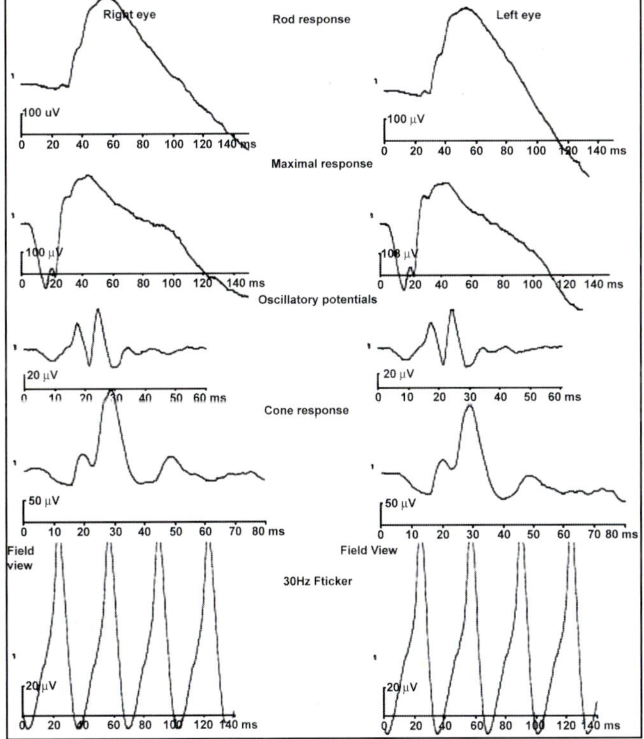

(B) Normal full field ERG.

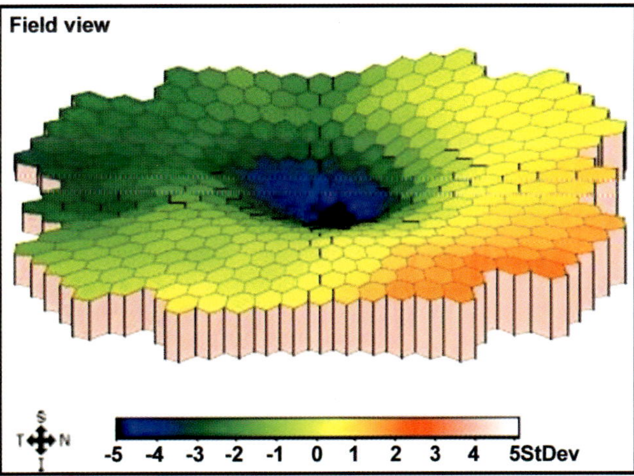

(D) Three dimensional response density plot showing typical volcano or crater like appearance.

FIGURES 4.10A to D: Example of the left eye of a 30-year-old female with a vision of 20/200 N18 in both eyes in Stargardt's macular dystrophy.

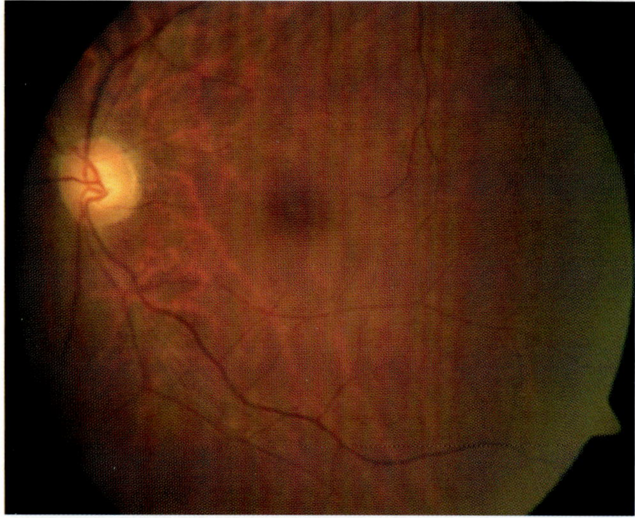

(A) Fundus photograph of the right eye showing mild temporal disk pallor, AND mild arteriolar attenuation. Macula appears unremarkable.

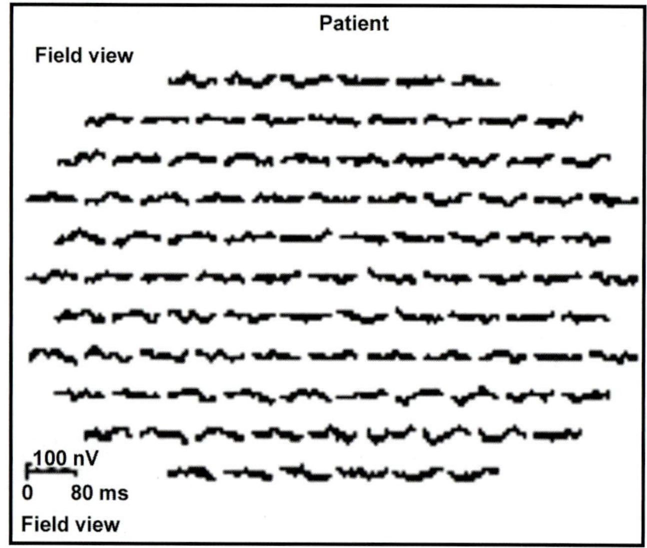

(C) Trace array showing reduced central AND peripheral responses.

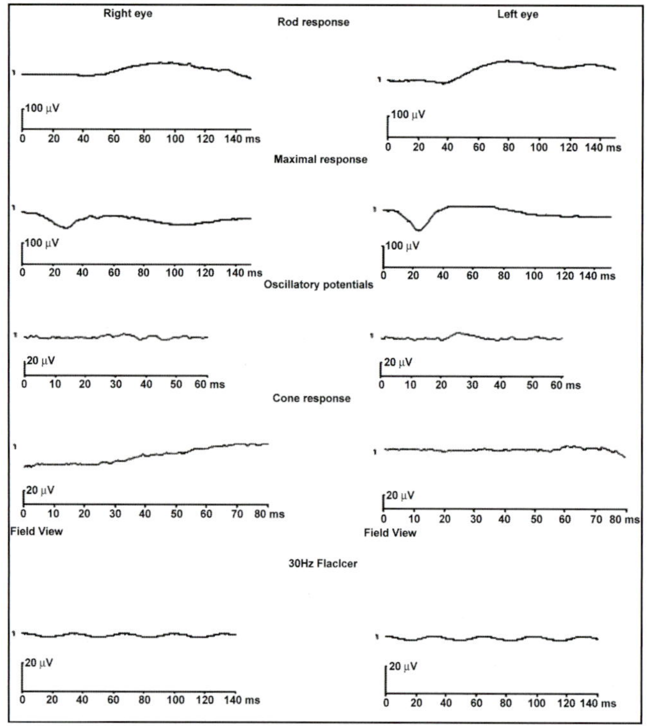

(B) Full-field ERG subnormal rod AND cone responses.

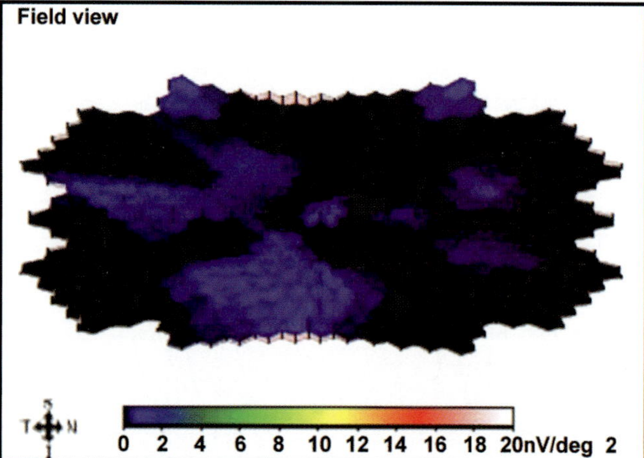

(D) Three-dimensional response density plot does not show a crater like appearance. Generalized reduction of responses is seen.

FIGURES 4.11A to D: Example of the left eye of a 59-year-old male with cone dystrophy.

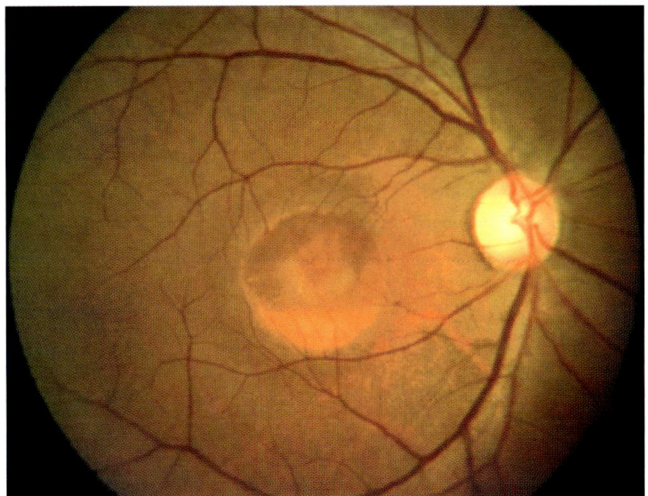

(A) Fundus photograph of the right eye showing pseudohypopyon stage of vitelliform disease.

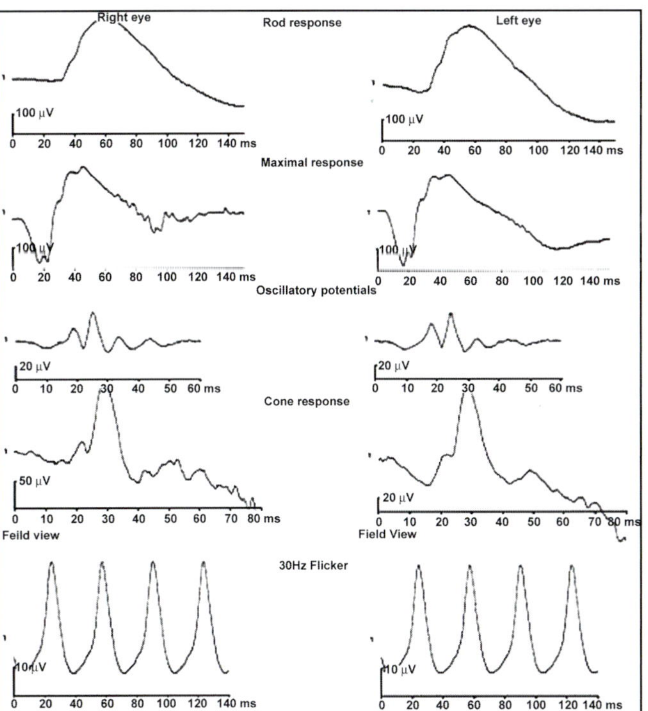

(B) Normal full field ERG.

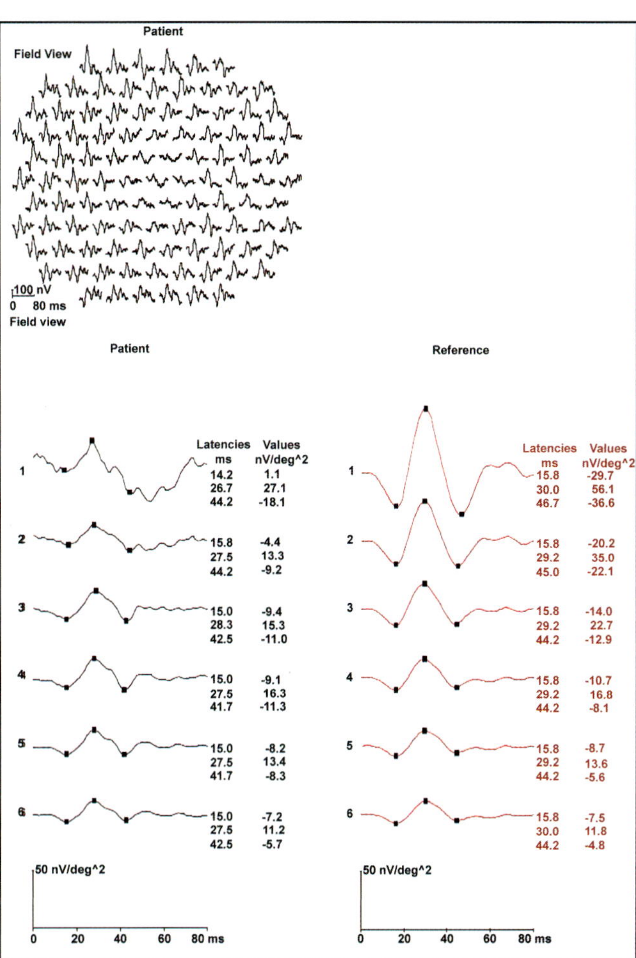

(C) Trace arrays with ring averages in response density scaling showing remarkably reduced amplitudes especially in the central two rings. Implicit times appear normal.

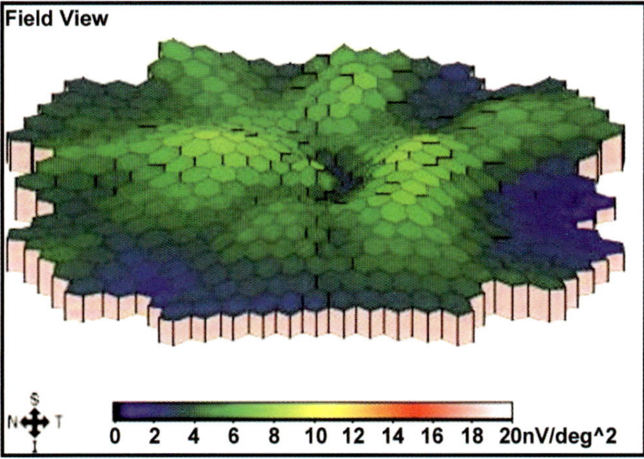

(D) Three-dimensional response density plot showing multiarea amplitude decrease.

Figures 4.12A to D: Example of right eye a 44-year-old man with vitelliform macular dystrophy.

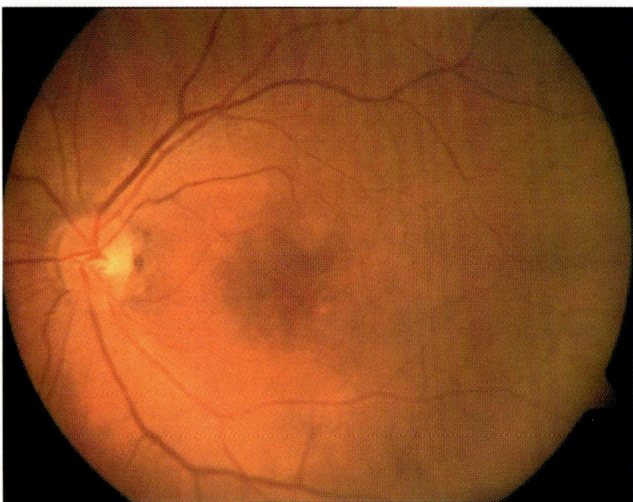

(A) Fundus photograph of the left eye showing resolving central serous retinopathy.

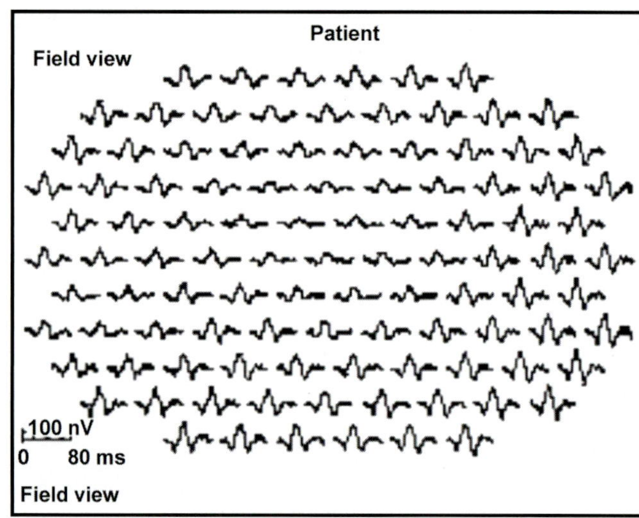

(C) Trace arrays showing subnormal response more in the central than in periphery.

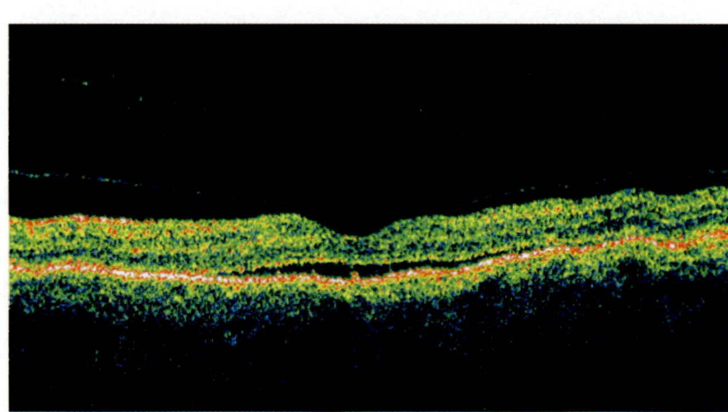

(B) Optical coherence tomography showing minimal subretinal fluid.

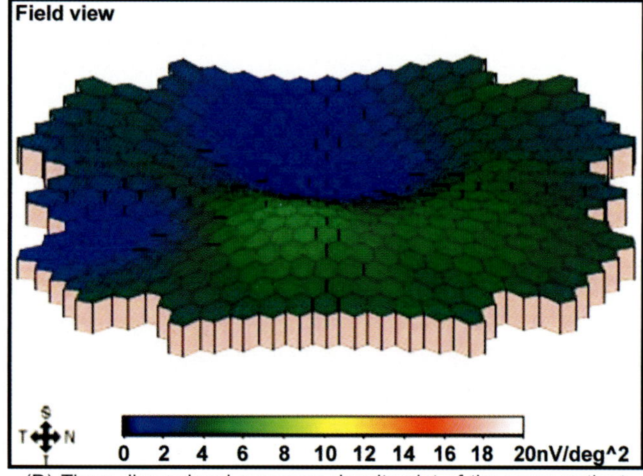

(D) Three-dimensional response density plot of the same patient.

FIGURES 4.13A to D: Example of left eye a 68-year-old man of central serous retinopathy with a vision of 20/30.

cause a widespread damage in the late stages. Early damage is usually restricted to the macula and hence may not be easily picked up on full-field ERG. It is important to diagnose this early damage because the toxicity of the drugs may be reversible at this stage and a permanent visual impairment can be prevented.

Hydroxychloroquine and Chloroquine

These are commonly used for rheumatoid arthritis and systemic lupus erythematosus and rheumatoid arthritis. Chloroquine is the more toxic of the two. It is no longer the drug of choice because of its retinotxicity. Long-term hydroxychloroquine use may also be associated with mfERG abnormalities. The mfERG appears to detect retinal physiological change earlier than visual acuity testing, color vision testing, or Amsler grid testing can.[34-36] The mfErg complements perimetry. It provides important evidence for hydroxychloroquine toxicity. Toxicity due to hydroxychloroquine can cause reduced amplitudes as well as increased implicit times. Multifocal ERG objectively demonstrates depression of signals in the perifoveal region in visually symptomatic patients with

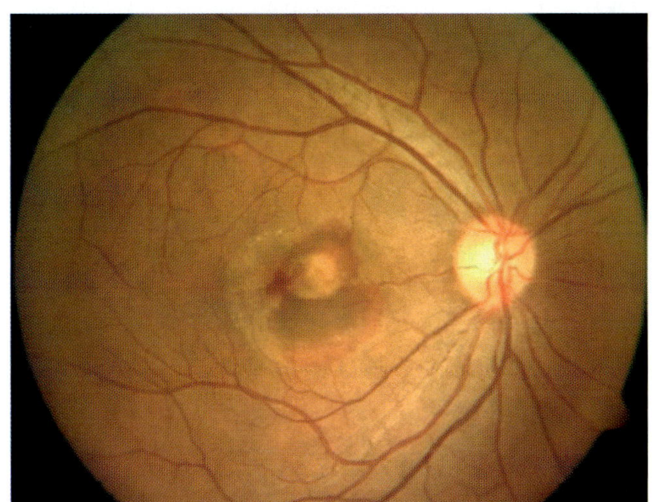

(A) Fundus photograph of the right eye showing well defined classic subfoveal choroidal neovascular membrane.

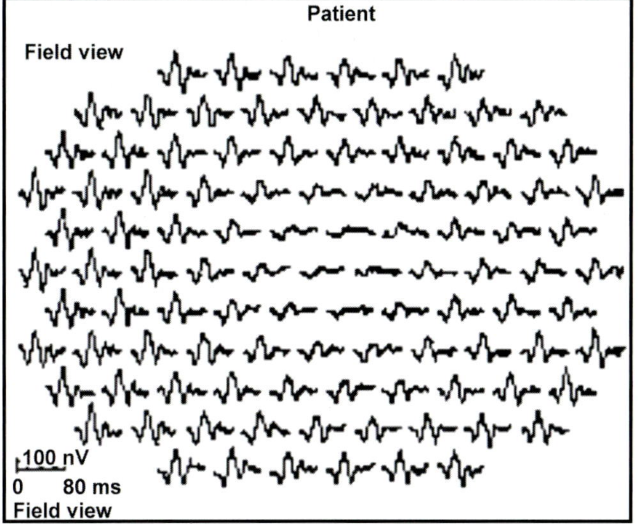

(B) Trace arrays showing reduced central amplitude AND normal responses in the periphery.

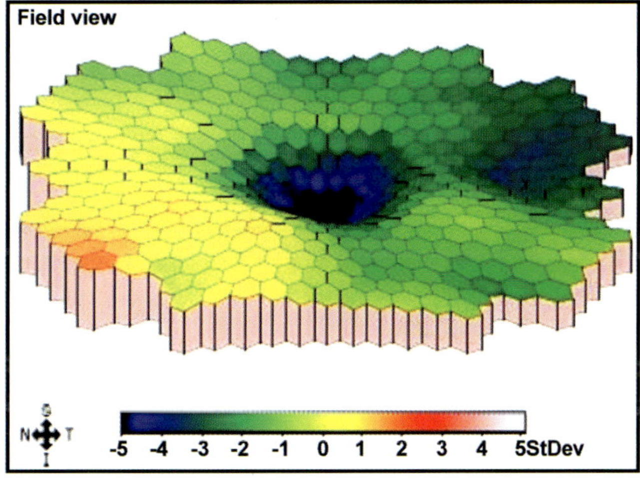

(C) Three dimensional response density plot of the same patient.

FIGURES 4.14A to C: Example of 40-year-old male with a visual acuity of 20/120 with choroidal neovascular membrane.

long-term hydroxychloroquine use. Even patients with normal visual acuity and no fundus abnormalities can have abnormal results (Figures 4.15A to D). There were 4 patterns of abnormal mfERG amplitude change observed: (i) paracentral loss, (ii) foveal loss, (iii) peripheral loss, and (4) generalized loss. Response densities can improve after termination of hydroxychloroquine.[37]

Other drugs that have been documented to show irregularities on mfERG include deferoxamine[38] and ethambutol.[39] The N1 amplitudes have been seen to be significantly lower in the ethambutol treated patients than in the control group. Ethambutol is possibly toxic to the retina, and not only the optic nerve. The multifocal ERG may be of value to diagnose and monitor patients taking ethambutol.

VASCULAR DISORDERS, DIABETIC RETINOPATHY AND RETINAL INFLAMMATIONS

Vascular disorders, diabetic retinopathy and inflammatory retinal diseases may deferentially affect inner and mid-retinal layers and are frequently associated with a break-down of the blood-retinal barrier and consecutive retinal

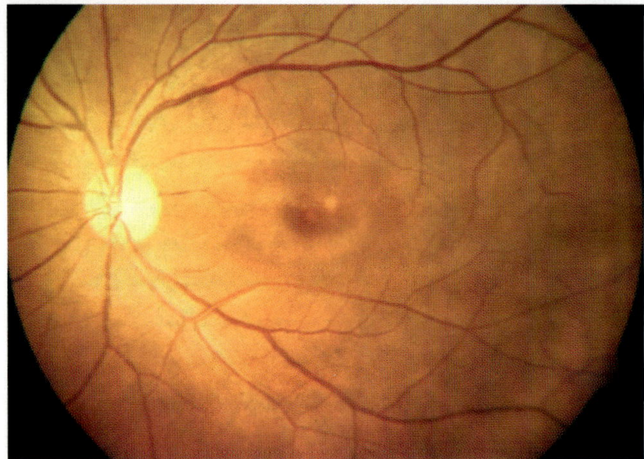

(A) Fundus photograph of the left eye showing few retinal pigment epithelium alterations at the macula.

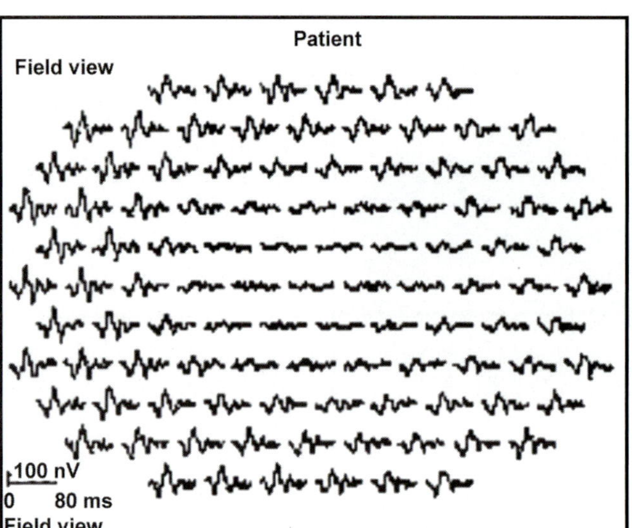

(B) Trace arrays showing reduced central responses.

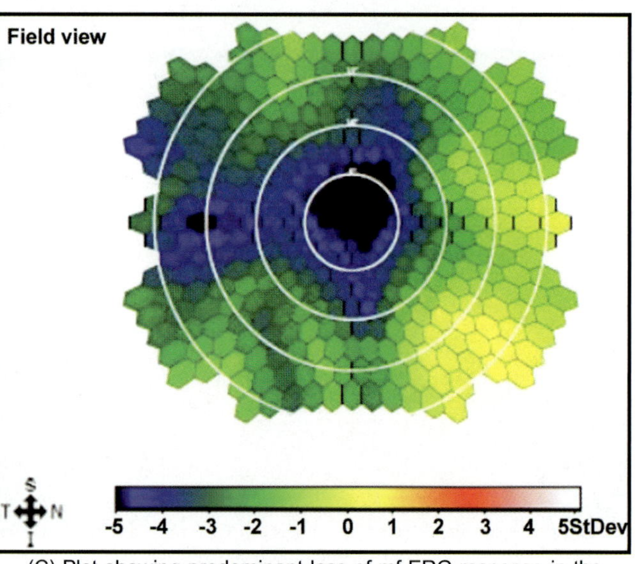

(C) Plot showing predominant loss of mf ERG response in the central 10 degrees.

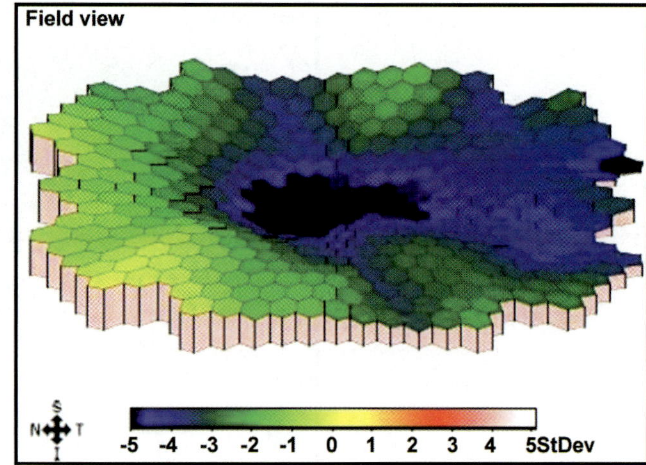

(D) Three-dimensional response density plot of the same patient with markedly reduced foveal responses.

FIGURES 4.15A to D: Example of a 36-year-old female on hydroxychloroquine for rheumatoid arthritis for the last 4 years. Patients visual acuity was 20/20 both eyes.

edema. In central venous occlusion an overall decrease of mfERG amplitude in the entire test field is seen, although the loss of macular activity is more pronounced. There are also delays in implicit times. Retinal edema in different diseases can also lead to implicit time delays of up to 40 ms, similar to those seen in receptor dystrophies like retinitis pigmentosa.[40] Wide Field-mfERG may be a more sensitive indicator of the underlying disease affecting the retina in eyes with central retinal vein occlusion and may have a role in the clinical setting. Hemicentral retinal vein occlusion[41] and branch retinal vein occlusion[42] also have shown reduced amplitude and increased implicit times on mfERG corresponding to the area of occlusion.

CYSTOID MACULAR EDEMA

The mfERG is a promising tool to evaluate the visual function in different areas at retinal posterior pole for the patients with cystoid macular edema. Marked delay in timing is also found in patients with cystoid macular edema due to intermediate uveitis and in regions with exudation due to diabetic retinopathy. The response densities of N1 wave are better analysis index for cystoid macular edema.[43]

In diabetic retinopathy response components like the nonlinear second order kernel and the ERG to low constrast [10] are decreased in early stages.

This is just the beginning of our understanding of the multifocal ERG. It has got various applications. Many new examination protocols and analysis programs are being devised which will further our understanding and open new horizons in ophthalmology.

REFERENCES

1. Riggs LA. Electroretinography. Vis Res 1986; 26:1443-59.
2. Plant GT. Recent advances in the electrophysiology of visual disorders. Curr Opin Ophthalmol 1995; 6:54-9.
3. Sutter EE. Imaging visual function with the multifocal m-sequence technique. Vis Res 2001; 41:1241-55.
4. Sutter EE, Tran D. The field topography of ERG components in man—I. The photopic luminance response. Vis Res 1992; 32:433-46.
5. Marmor MF, Hood DC, Keating D, et al. Guidelines for basic multifocal electroretinography (mfERG). Doc Ophthalmol 2003; 106:105-15.
6. Keating D, Parks S, and Evans A. Technical aspects of multifocal ERG recording. Doc Ophthalmol 2000; 100: 77-98.
7. Hood DC, Seiple W, Holopigian K, et al. A comparison of the components of the multi-focal and full-field ERGs. Visual Neuroscience 1997; 14:533-44.
8. Verdon WA, Haegerstrom-Portnoy G. Topography of the multifocal electroretinogram. Doc Ophthalmol 1998; 95:73-90.
9. Parks S, Keating D, Evans A, L, et al. Comparison of repeatability of the multifocal electroretinogram and Humphrey perimeter. Doc Ophthalmol 1997; 92:281-89.
10. Shimada Y, Li Y, Bearse MA, et al. Assessment of early retinal changes in diabetes using a new multifocal ERG protocol. Br J Ophthalmol 2001; 85: 414-19.
11. Chisholm JA, Keating D, Parks S, et al. The impact of fixation on the multifocal electroretinogram: Doc Ophthalmol 2001; 102:131-39.
12. Nagatomo A, Nao-i N, Maruiwa F, et al. Multifocal electroretinograms in normal subjects. Jpn J Ophthalmol 1998; 42:129-35.
13. Jiang F, Huang S, Luo G, et al. The measurement of multifocal electroretinography. Yan Ke Xue Bao 2001; 17:217-19.
14. Palmowski AM, Berninger T, Allgayer R, et al. Effects of refractive blur on the multifocal electroretinogram. Doc Ophthalmol 1999; 99: 41-54.
15. Kretschmann U, Bock M, Gockeln R, et al. Clinical applications of multifocal electroretinography. Doc Ophthalmol 2000; 100:99-113.
16. Luu CD, Lau AM, Lee SY. Multifocal electroretinogram in adults and children with myopia. Arch Ophthalmol 2006; 124:328-34.
17. Kawabata H, Adachi-Usami E. Multifocal electroretinogram in myopia. Invest Ophthalmol Vis Sci 1997; 38:2844-51.
18. Tzekov RT, Gerth C, Werner JS. Senescence of human multifocal electroretinogram components: A localized approach. Graefes Arch Clin Exp Ophthalmol 2004; 242:549-60.
19. Nabeshima T. The Effects of Aging on the Multifocal Electroretinogram. Jpn J Ophthalmol 2001; 45:114-15.
20. Hood DC, Odel JG, Chen CS, et al. The multifocal electroretinogram. J Neuroophthalmol 2003; 23:225-35.
21. Hood DC, Zhang X. Multifocal ERG and VEP responses and visual fields: comparing disease-related changes. Doc Ophthalmol 2000;100:115-37.
22. Kretschmann U, Seeliger MW, Ruether K, et al. Multifocal electroretinography in patients with Stargardt's macular dystrophy. Br J Ophthalmol 1998; 82:267-75.
23. Kellner U, Kraus H, Foerster MH. Multifocal ERG in chloroquine retinopathy. In Hubsch S, Graf M (Eds). Foveal Cone Dystrophy: Diagnostic Ranking of the Multifocal Electroretinogram: Klin Monatsbl Augenheilkd 2002;219: 370-72.
24. Granse L, Ponjavic V, Andreasson S. Full-field ERG, multifocal ERG and multifocal VEP in patients with retinitis pigmentosa and residual central visual fields. Acta Ophthalmol Scand 2004; 82:701-6.
25. Huang S, Wu D, Jiang F, et al. The multifocal electroretinogram in X-linked juvenile retinoschisis. Doc Ophthalmol 2003;106:251-55.
26. Palmowski AM, Allgayer R, Heinemann-Vernaleken B, et al. Detection of retinal dysfunction in vitelliform macular dystrophy using the multifocal ERG (MF-ERG). Doc Ophthalmol 2003;106:145-52.
27. Suzuki K, Hasegawa S, Usui T, et al. Multifocal electro-retinogram in patients with central serous chorioretinopathy. Jpn J Ophthalmol 2002; 46:308-14.
28. Papaspirou A, Theodossiadis G. Assessment of macular function by multifocal electroretinogram before and after epimacular membrane surgery. Retina 2001;21:590-95.
29. Szlyk JP, Vajaranant TS, Rana R, et al. Assessing responses of the macula in patients with macular holes using a new system measuring localized visual acuity and the mfERG. Doc Ophthalmol 2005;110:181-91.
30. Moschos M, Apostolopoulos M, Ladas J, et al . Multifocal ERG changes before and after macular hole surgery: Doc Ophthalmol 2001;102:31-40.
31. Ruther K, Breidenbach K, Schwartz R, et al. Testing central retinal function with multifocal electroretinography before

and after photodynamic therapy. Ophthalmologe. 2003;100:459-64.

32. Jiang L, Jin C, Wen F, et al. The changes of multifocal electroretinography in the early stage of photodynamic therapy for choroidal neovascularization. Doc Ophthalmol 2003;107:165-70.

33. Maturi RK,Bleau LA,Wilson DL. Electrophysiological findings after intravitreal bevacizumab(Avastin) treatment. Retina 2006;270-74.

34. Moschos MN, Moschos MM, Apostolopoulos M, et al. Assessing hydroxychloroquine toxicity by the multifocal ERG Doc Ophthalmol 2004;108:47-53.

35. So SC, Hedges TR, Schuman JS, et al. Evaluation of hydroxychloroquine retinopathy with multifocal electroretinography. Ophthalmic Surg Lasers Imaging 2003; 34:251-58.

36. Tzekov RT, Serrato A, Marmor MF. ERG findings in patients using hydroxychloroquine. Doc Ophthalmol 2004;108: 87-97.

37. Maturi RK, Yu M, Weleber RG. Multifocal electroretino-

graphic evaluation of long-term hydroxychloroquine users. Arch Ophthalmol 2004;122:973-81.

38. Schmidt D, Finke J. Bull's-Eye Maculopathy with Deferoxamine treatment. Klin Monatsbl Augenheilkd. 2004; 221:204-09.

39. Behbehani RS, Affel EL, Sergott RC, et al. Multifocal ERG in ethambutol associated visual loss. Br J Ophthalmol 2005; 89:976-82.

40. Dolan FM, Parks S, Keating D, et al. Multifocal electro-retinographic features of central retinal vein occlusion Invest Ophthalmol Vis Sci 2003;44:4954-59.

41. Dolan FM, Parks S, Keating D, et al. Wide field multifocal and standard full field electroretinographic features of hemi retinal vein occlusion. Doc Ophthalmol 2006; 112:43-52.

42. Ohshima A, Hasegawa S, Takada R, et al. Multifocal electroretinograms in patients with branch retinal artery occlusion. Jpn J Ophthalmol 2001; 45:516-22.

43. Wu D, Jiang F, Liang J, et al. Multifocal electroretinogram in cystoid macular edema. Yan Ke Xue Bao. 2003; 19:253-56.

5

Fluorescein Angiography and Indocyanine Green Angiography in Macular Disorders

Muna Bhende, Arun Bhargava, Arindam Chakravarti

INTRODUCTION

Fluorescein angiography and indocyanine green (ICG) angiography play a significant role in the management of various macular disorders. This chapter introduces the reader to some of the important acquired, non-inflammatory retinal disorders involving the macula, where fluorescein angiography and ICG imaging is important.[1-5]

FLUORESCEIN ANGIOGRAPHY

The application of fluorescein angiography in the diagnosis of ocular disease is based on two fundamental properties displayed by sodium fluorescein, i.e. luminescence and fluorescence.

Luminescence occurs when energy in the form of electromagnetic radiation is absorbed at one frequency and re-emitted at another. The decay that occurs when the electrons shift back into the original state can be in the visible spectrum and this is called luminescence. With continuous excitation of electrons, fluorescence is produced.

Sodium fluorescein is a compound that is excited in the blue range of the spectrum (465-490 nm) and emits light in the green-yellow range (520-530 nm).

After intravenous injection of the dye, the blue light of the fundus camera is used to excite the fluorescein molecules within the eye, and the emitted light passes back through a green filter to be processed and displayed.

The passage of the dye through the circulation results in typical patterns or phases on the fluorescein angiogram. The angiogram is initially devoid of any fluorescence, this is followed 10 seconds later by the bright patchy choroidal fluorescence which in turn is followed by the retinal arterial phase 2 seconds later and the arteriovenous phase. Maximum fluorescence is seen about 20 to 30 seconds after injection and most of the dye empties out after 3 to 5 minutes. Fluorescein dye leaks freely from the choriocapillaries but does not cross the retinal capillary endothelial cells, hence is useful in studying abnormalities of the retinal circulation rather than the choroidal circulation.

Abnormalities on the fluorescein angiogram can be either decreased fluorescence (hypofluorescence) or increased fluorescence (hyperfluorescence). These can be due to abnormalities in blood flow or due to lesions that affect the normal pattern of fluorescence.

The macula has certain specific fluorescein angiographic characteristics due to its different structure:

- The presence of the capillary free zone or the foveal avascular zone about 400 to 500 μ in diameter
- Absence of choroidal fluorescence in the macula due to greater density of the retinal pigment epithelium and the presence of xanthophyll in the outer retinal layers
- Increased density of choroidal melanocytes in darkly pigmented individuals which obscures choroidal fluorescence

Fluorescein angiography is the gold standard where study of abnormalities of the retinal vasculature is required and also in most cases of abnormal choroidal vasculature.[1-5]

INDOCYANINE GREEN ANGIOGRAPHY

Indocyanine green angiography was developed to overcome some of the limitations of fluorescein angiography, i.e. poor transmission through media haze and poor visualization of the choroidal circulation.

Indocyanine green is a water soluble tricarbocyanine dye that absorbs light in the near infra red range of 790 to 805 nm and emits light at 770 to 835 nm. This activity permits visualization of abnormalities through blood, pigment and lipid. After intravenous injection the dye is 98% protein bound, 80% of which is to globulins. This allows less dye to escape from the choriocapillaris and thus permits enhanced visualization of the choroidal circulation.

Specific areas where ICG angiography is useful are occult CNV, polypoidal choroidal vasculopathy, chorioretinal inflammatory disorders, choroidal tumors and some cases of central serous chorioretinopathy. [1-5]

DIABETIC MACULOPATHY

Macular edema is one of the major causes of visual loss in diabetic patients, the others being proliferative diabetic retinopathy and optic neuropathy. Diabetic macular edema (DME) can be focal, diffuse, ischemic or mixed.[6-11]

Clinically significant macular edema (CSME) is defined as macular edema with one of the following characteristics:[8,9]

- Thickening of the retina at or within 500 microns of the foveal center
- Hard exudates 500 microns or less from the center of the fovea, with associated retinal thickening
- Areas of retinal thickening at least one disk area in size, at or within one disk diameter of the foveal center

The diabetic macular edema disease severity scale classified diabetic maculopathy into the following two major levels, with subcategories for diabetic macular edema

- Diabetic macular edema absent : No retinal thickening or hard exudates in posterior pole
- Diabetic macular edema present: Some retinal thickening or hard exudates in posterior pole

If diabetic macular edema is present, it can be categorized as follows:

- *Mild Diabetic Macular Edema*
  Some retinal thickening or hard exudates in posterior pole but distant from the macula
- *Moderate Diabetic Macular Edema*
  Retinal thickening or hard exudates approaching the center of the macula but not involving the center
- *Severe Diabetic Macular Edema*
  Retinal thickening or hard exudates involving the center of the macula.

CLINICAL FEATURES

- **Focal maculopathy** results from exudative leakage from a single microaneurysm or a cluster of them forming a well demarcated area of retinal thickening. Hard exudates usually surround these lesions in a circular pattern (Figures 5.1A to C).
- **Diffuse maculopathy** results from a generalized breakdown of the blood retinal barrier leading to leakage from microaneurysms, capillaries and arterioles throughout the posterior pole. Hard exudates are less common and the edema is usually chronic. Diffuse maculopathy may be associated with thickened, taut posterior hyaloid. This should be differentiated from macular edema related to vitreomacular traction (Figures 5.1D to F).

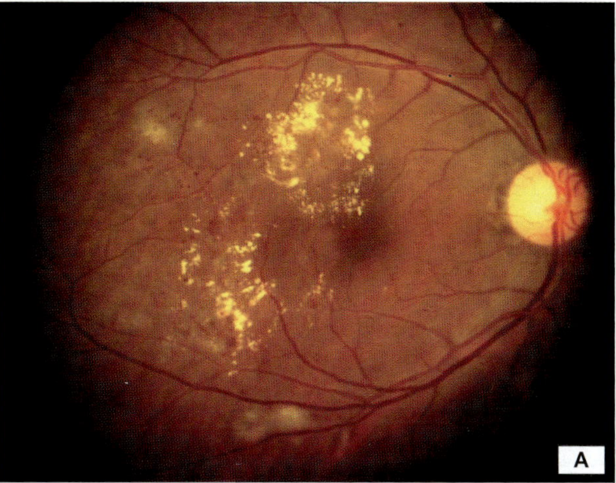
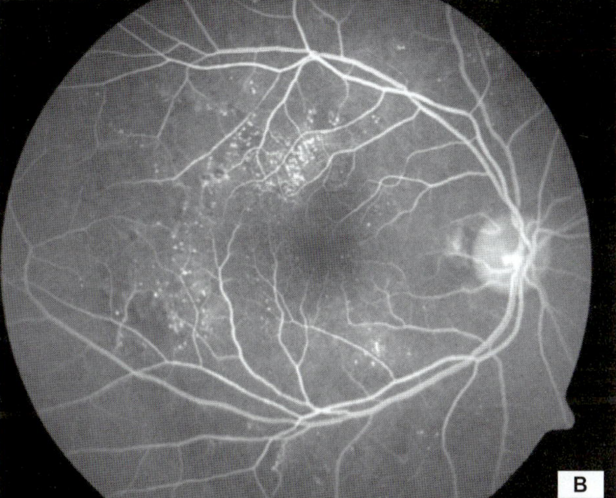
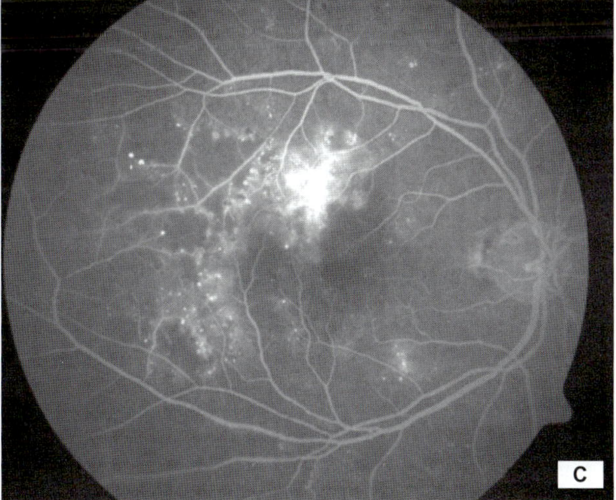

FIGURES 5.1A to C: Focal Diabetic Macular Edema. Clinical picture showing circinate rings of hard exudates surrounding microaneurysms. The hard exudates are seen to encroach on the foveal center. Fundus fluorescein angiography shows leakage from dot like microaneurysms clusters superotemporal to the macula.

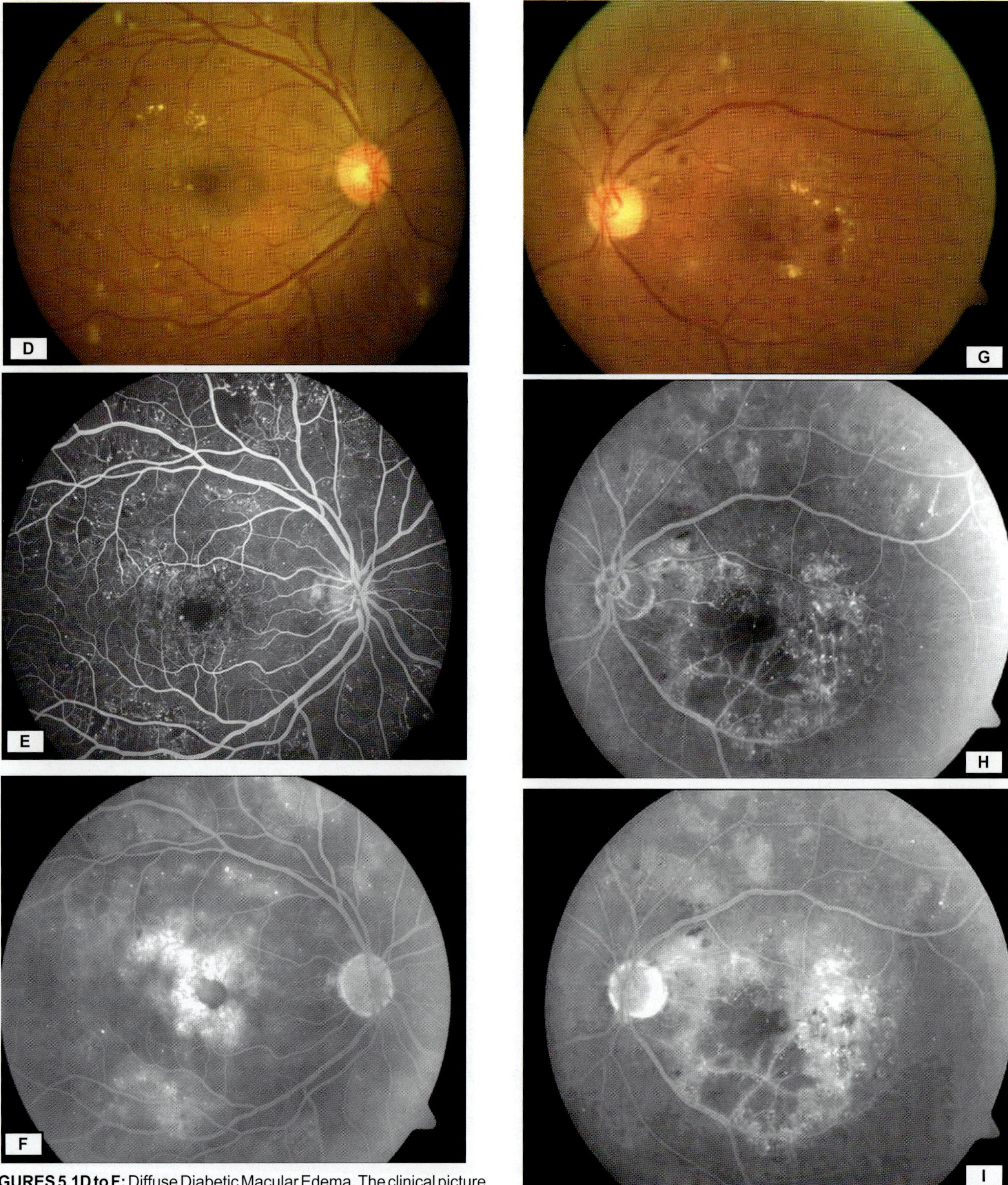

FIGURES 5.1D to F: Diffuse Diabetic Macular Edema. The clinical picture shows a few hard exudates, a large microaneurysm close to the fovea and a large cystic space at the fovea. Fundus fluorescein angiography shows dilated perifoveal capillaries and a few microaneurysms. The late frame shows the petalloid appearance of cystoid macular edema. Also note the honeycomb pattern of hyperfluorescence corresponding to cystoid edema away from the fovea.

FIGURES 5.1G to I: Ischemic Diabetic Macular Edema. The clinical picture shows a few hemorrhages at the macula and hard exudates superotemporal to the fovea. Few laser spots are seen. Fundus fluorescein angiography shows an enlarged, distorted foveal avascular zone with areas of capillary dropout inferiorly. Leaking microaneurysms are seen superotemporal to the fovea.

- **Ischemic maculopathy** is typically described as a washed out featureless macula with no exudates. Sclerosed macular vessels may be seen (Figures 5.1G to I),
- **Cystoid macular edema** can occur.

TREATMENT

- Optimal glycemic and hypertensive control
- Management of dyslipidemia
- Laser photocoagulation
- Vitreous surgery
- Pharmacologic treatment

FLUORESCEIN ANGIOGRAPHY

Fluorescein angiography is not for diagnosis of CSME[7-9]

- Fluorescein angiography is a guide to focal treatment
- Detection of capillary non perfusion is possible
- Diagnosis of diffuse macular edema is possible
- Plan for re-treatment can be made.

Fluorescein angiography reveals the following:

- Diskrete lesions: Micro aneurysms, intraretinal microvascular abnormalities, pruned capillaries that leak fluorescein
- Diffuse lesions: Diffuse leaking capillaries, areas of capillary non perfusion
- Flower petal pattern of cystoid macular edema
- Enlarged distorted foveal avascular zone that causes visual disability once it exceeds 100 microns in diameter.

DRY AGE-RELATED MACULAR DEGENERATION

HARD DRUSEN (FIGURES 5.2A TO C)

Clinical Features

- Hard drusen are not visible clinically until they are 30 to 50 μ in size
- They appear as yellow deposits lying deep to the retina; usually clustered at the posterior pole
- They play a significant role in the evolution of age-related macular degeneration (AMD)
- They are almost a common finding after the fifth decade of life.

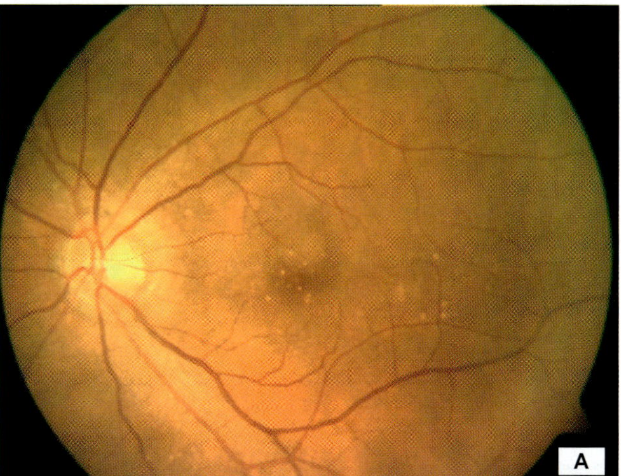
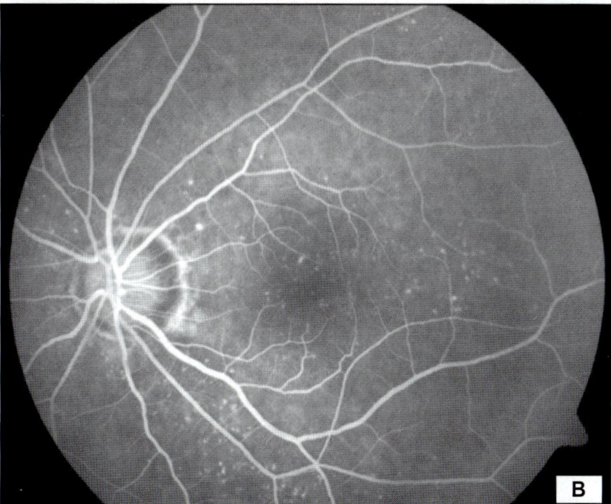
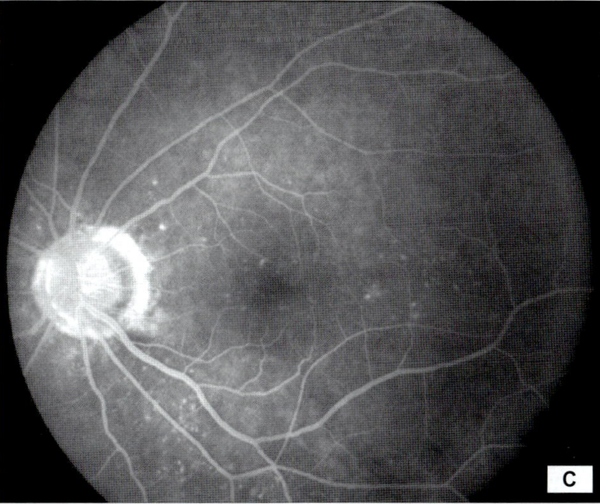

FIGURES 5.2A to C: Hard drusen. Note the yellow diskrete lesions at the posterior pole. On fundus fluorescein angiography these appear as hyperfluorescent dots, more numerous than apparent clinically. In the late phase, they are seen to fade away with the background fluorescence.

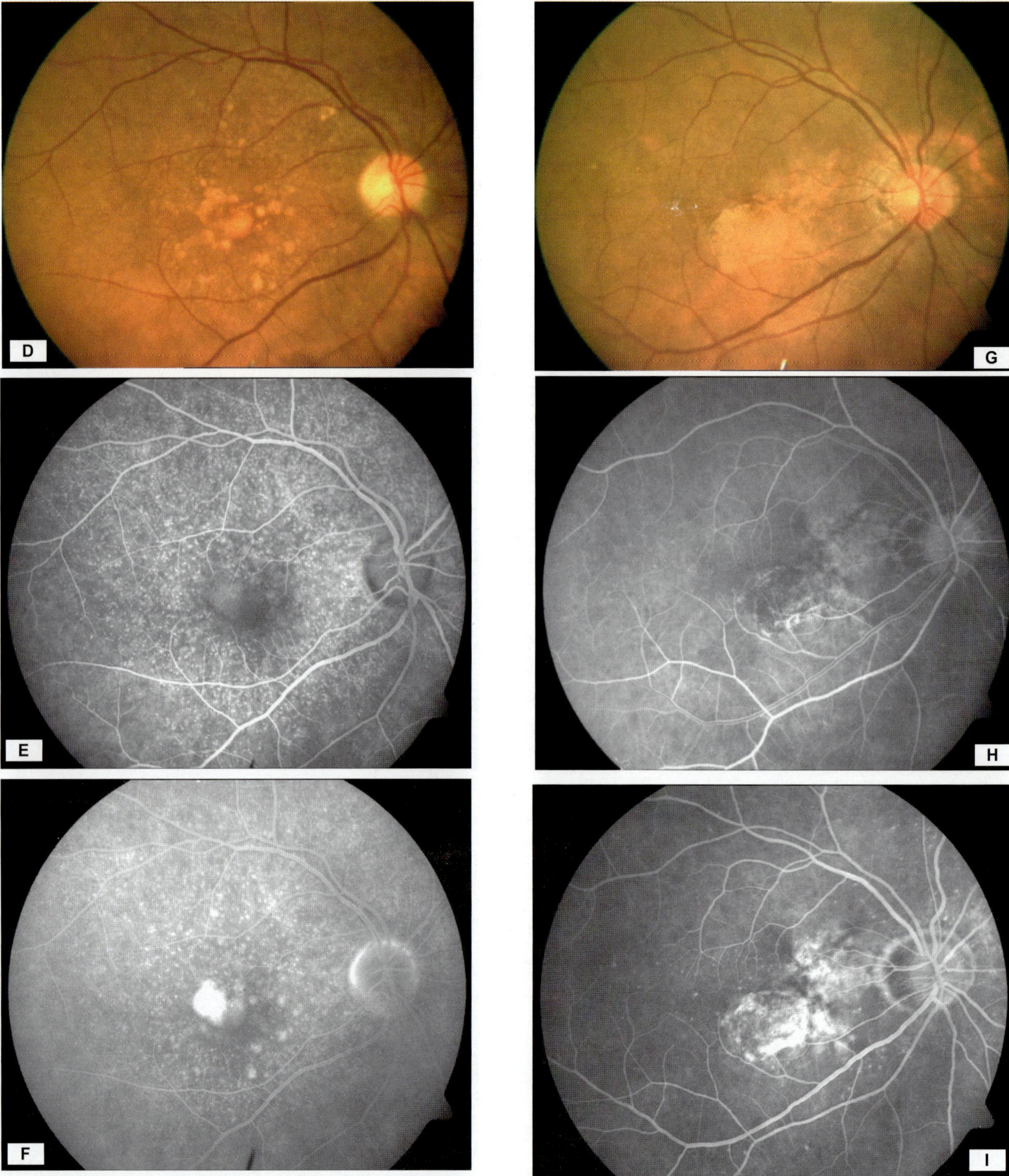

FIGURES 5.2D to F: Soft drusen. Clinical picture showing large, confluent soft drusen at the macula with surrounding hard drusen. Fundus fluorescein angiography shows faint hyperfluorescence of the soft drusen compared to the bright hyperfluorescence of the hard drusen. The late phase shows asymmetric staining of the drusen at the foveal center and faint staining of the other soft drusen.

FIGURES 5.2G to I: Geographic atrophy. Clinical picture shows a well demarcated area of geographic atrophy and hard drusen. Fundus fluorescein angiography shows prominence of the large choroidal vessels within the area of atrophy and staining in the late phase. Hyperfluorescence of the hard drusen is also seen.

Fluorescein Angiography

Following features may be present:[12-14]
- Bright hyperfluorescence in the mid venous phase
- Persistent through the middle and late phases
- Fade away soon after the background choroidal fluorescence
- Transmission defects due to overlying retinal pigment epithelium atrophy
- Drusen are more numerous than those seen clinically.

SOFT DRUSEN (FIGURES 5.2D TO F)

Clinical Features

- Soft drusen may be divided into granular, fluid and membranous subtypes
- The granular type has a coarse appearance with a crescentic or sinuous shape
- The fluid type or drusenoid pigment epithelial detachment can evolve into an avascular serous pigment epithelial detachment. This includes drusen over 500μ in size. Symptoms include mild distortion when the drusenoid pigment epithelial detachment is under or close to the foveal center. Hyperpigmentation may occur on the surface indicating its long standing nature
- Membranous subtype is associated with a high risk of choroidal neovascularization (CNV). This subtype clinically appears paler and shallower than the yellow hard drusen.

Fluorescein Angiography

Following features may be present:
- Hyperfluorescence is faint and seen in the later phases
- Drusenoid pigment epithelial detachments show faint late hyperfluorescence with hypofluorescent figures in of overlying hyperpigmentation. This gives them a lobulated appearance the area.
- Membranous drusen show later and less hyperfluorescence than the hard drusen.

GEOGRAPHIC ATROPHY (FIGURES 5.2G TO I)

Clinical Features

- Geographic atrophy is the end result of non neovascular or atrophic AMD

- It may be either related to or independent of drusen
- This accounts for 12 to 25% of severe visual loss in eyes with AMD
- It is seen as sharply delineated zones of atrophy of the retinal pigment epithelium and choriocapillaries through which the choroidal vessels are better visualized
- There is a relatively low risk of developing CNV.

Fluorescein Angiography

Fluorescein angiography is not a diagnostic tool for geographic atrophy.

Following features may be present:
- Delayed choroidal perfusion
- Hyperfluorescence in the mid phases which fades with the background choroidal fluorescence.

WET AGE-RELATED MACULAR DEGENERATION

Choroidal neovascularization is the major cause of severe visual loss in AMD and forms the bulk of the lesions included under wet AMD. Symptoms include loss of vision, scotomas and metamorphopsia.[1-5]

Choroidal neovascularization can be classified based on the lesion composition:[14,15]
- Predominantly classic CNV (Figures 5.3A to C): 50% or more of the lesion is composed of classic CNV
- Minimally classic CNV (Figures 5.3D to F): Less than 50% of the lesion is classic CNV
- Occult (Figures 5.3G to M): There is no classic component within the lesion

Based on the location, they can be classified as subfoveal, juxtafoveal, extrafoveal and juxtapapillary.

CLINICAL FEATURES

- Choroidal neovascularization appears as a greenish gray subretinal lesion
- Associated subretinal fluid and/or cystoid macular edema may be present
- Subretinal or sub retinal pigment epithelium hemorrhage may be present
- Retinal pigment epithelium detachments may occur which may be serous, hemorrhagic or mixed

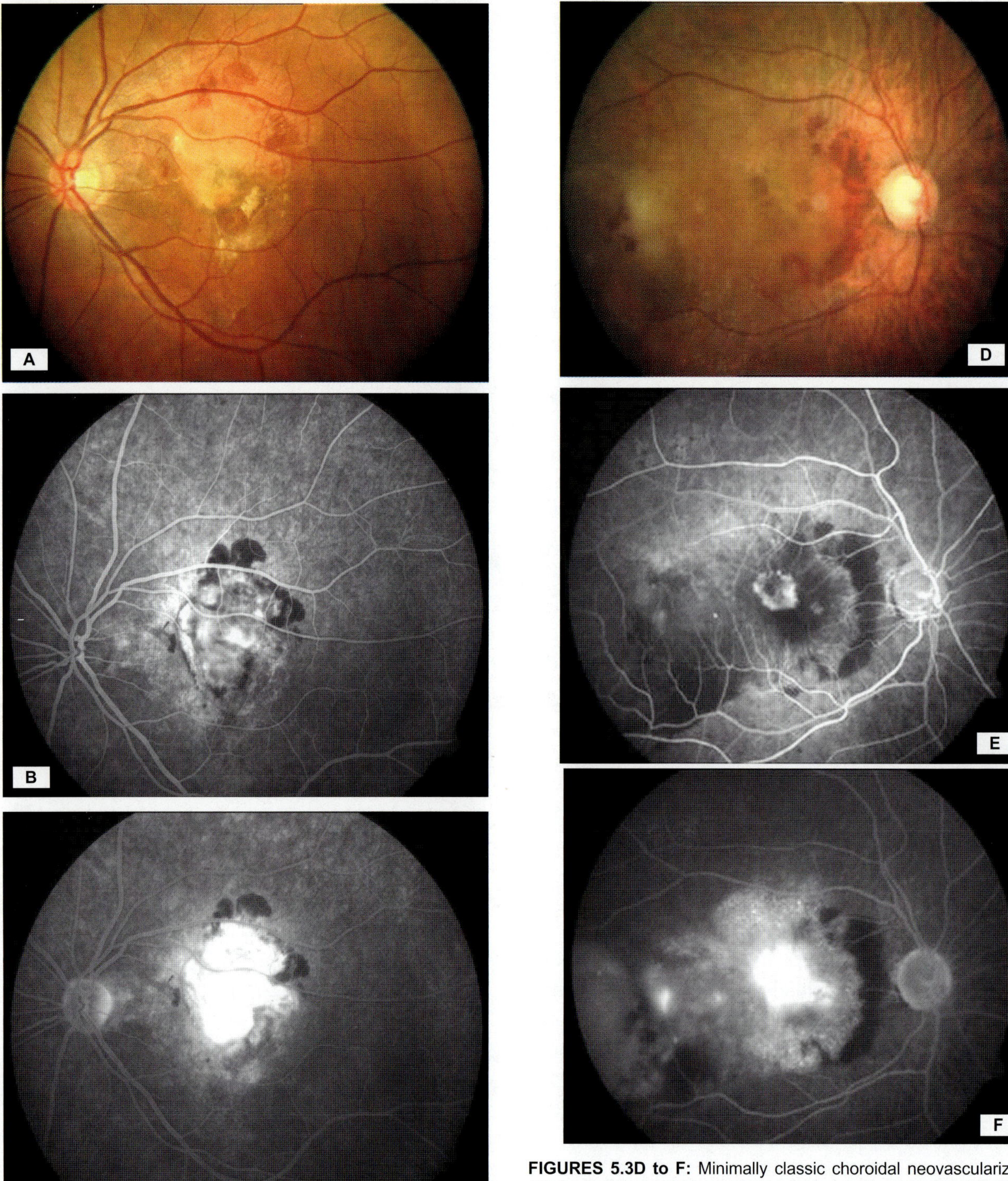

FIGURES 5.3A to C: Predominantly classic choroidal neovascularization. Clinical picture shows a greenish yellow subretinal lesion with hemorrhage. Scarring at the inferior aspect is seen. Fundus fluorescein angiography shows early hyperfluorescence of the lesion with late leakage. The entire extent of the membrane is seen from the early phase.

FIGURES 5.3D to F: Minimally classic choroidal neovascularization. Clinical picture shows a large lesion with subretinal fluid and hemorrhage. A smaller yellowish area is seen just above the foveal center. Fundus fluorescein angiography shows a small classic choroidal neovascularization. The late phase image shows mottled hyperfluorescence over a much larger extent, along with pooling of dye in the temporal aspect of the lesion. The classic component occupies less than 50% of the entire lesion; hence it is referred to as a minimally classic choroidal neovascularization.

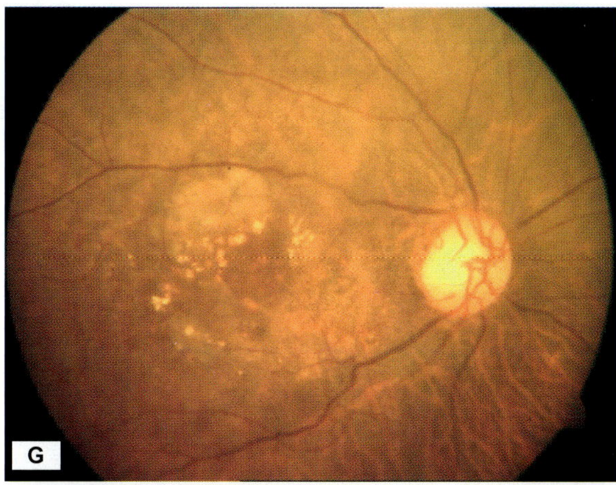

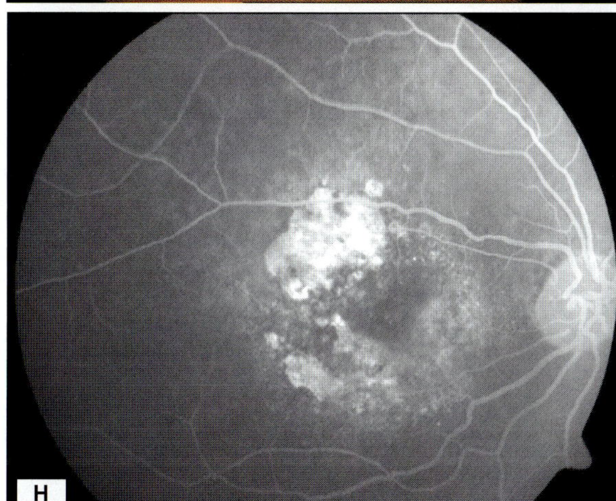

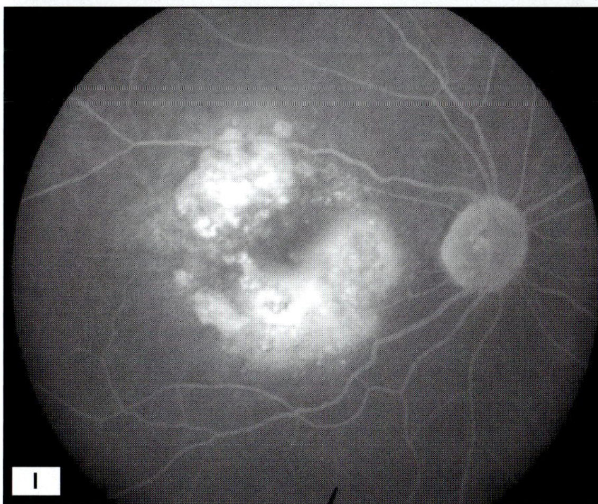

FIGURES 5.3G to I: Occult choroidal neovascularization. Clinical picture showing an ill defined macular lesion. Few hard drusens are seen with areas of geographic atrophy temporal to the fovea. The area nasal to the fovea shows irregular elevation of the RPE and a few hard exudates. Fundus fluorescein angiography shows hyperfluorescence in the area corresponding to the area of drusen and geographic atrophy. Hyperfluorescent dots are seen in the area of RPE irregularity. The late phase shows increase in hyperfluorescence in this area suggesting an occult choroidal neovascularization.

- Subretinal lipid may be present
- Fibrovascular tissue may be present
- Drusen, and retinal pigment epithelium elevation may be present.

CLASSIC CHOROIDAL NEOVASCULARIZATION

Fluorescein Angiography

- Early, well defined, bright hyperfluorescence
- Late fuzziness of margins with pooling of dye in the overlying subsensory retinal space
- Classically described as a lacy or cartwheel pattern
- Blocked fluorescence may be seen due to blood, pigment or fibrous tissue
- Hyperfluorescence from an associated serous pigment epithelium detachment
- Feeder vessels may be identified.

Indocyanine Green Angiography

- Demonstrates the classic CNV
- May show an associated occult component such as a hot spot
- Mainly used in occult or minimally classic CNV.

OCCULT CHOROIDAL NEOVASCULARIZATION

Occult choroidal neovascularization is more of an angiographic classification. Cases can be divided into two patterns:

a. Fibrovascular pigment epithelial detachment, and
b. Late leakage of an undetermined source.

Fluorescein Angiography

Fibrovascular Pigment Epithelium Detachment

- Irregular elevation of the retinal pigment epithelium with a stippled appearance
- Late staining within the fibrous tissue or pooling of dye within the subretinal space overlying the pigment epithelium detachment.

Late Leakage of an Undetermined Source

- Speckled hyperfluorescence with late pooling of dye in the overlying subretinal space
- No identifiable classic CNV or pigment epithelium detachment in the early phases
- Boundaries are not well-defined in most cases.

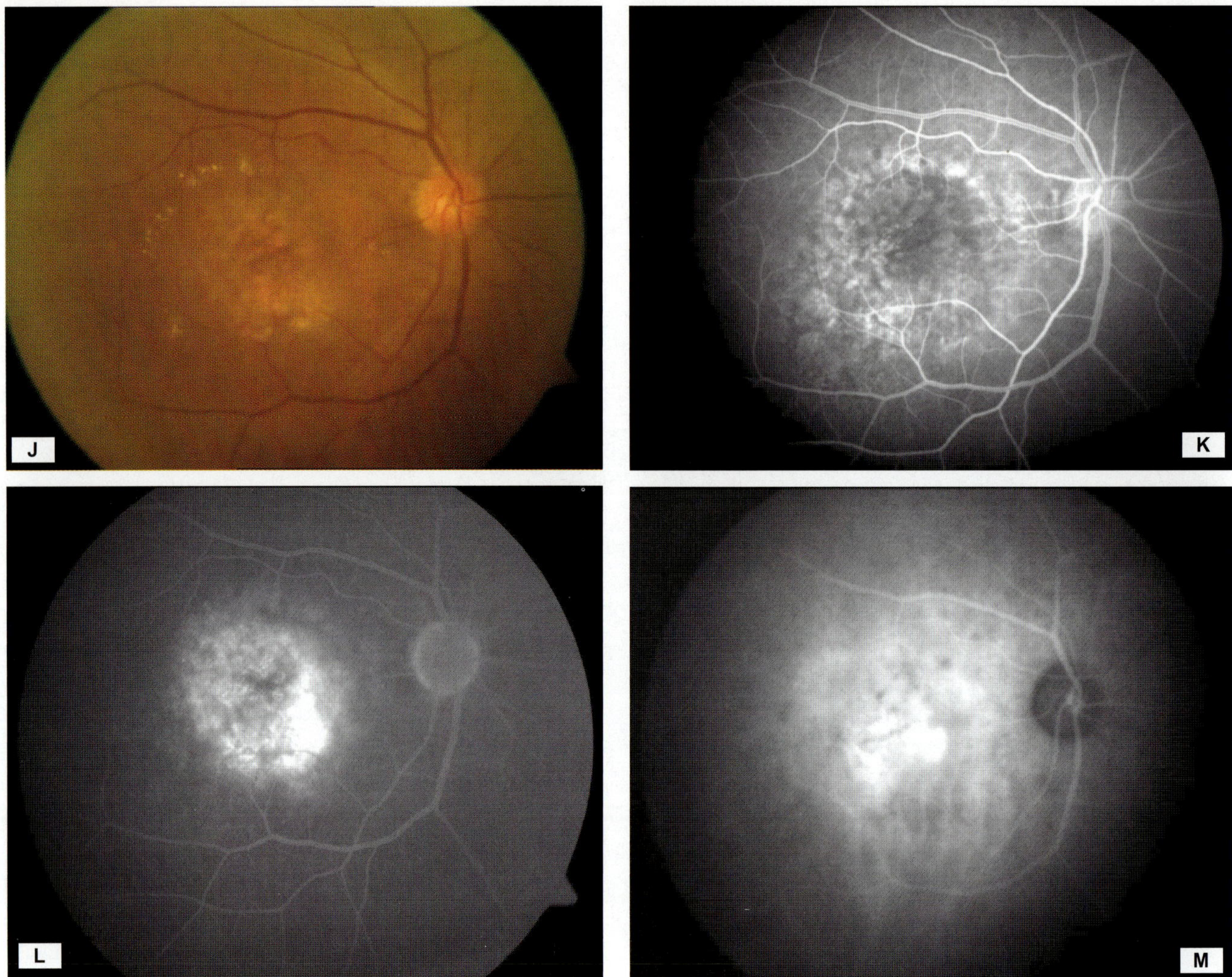

FIGURES 5.3J to M: Occult choroidal neovascularization. Clinical picture shows an area of RPE irregularity at the macula with hard exudates. Fundus fluorescein angiography shows hyperfluorescent areas within the lesion. Late phases show intense hyperfluorescence in the area suggestive of fibrovascular PED. Late phase ICG shows a plaque like lesion in the central part with a hot spot nasal to it.

Indocyanine Green Angiography

- Plaque—a distinct area of late hyperfluorescence > 1 disk area in size
- Hot spot—a focal area of intense hyperfluorescence seen in the mid phase and persisting even after the dye has left the circulation. This is < 1 disk area in size.
- Combination of the two.

RETINAL ARTERY MACROANEURYSM

Retinal artery macroaneurysm is a round or fusiform dilatation of the retinal arterioles within the first three orders of bifurcation. There is a strong association with hypertension and arteriosclerotic vascular disease.[1-5]

CLINICAL FEATURES (FIGURES 5.4A TO F)

- Retinal artery macroaneurysm occurs in the sixth to seventh decade of life
- It may be seen on routine examination
- Commonest presenting symptom is acute visual loss
- Superotemporal vessel is most often involved
- Most frequent clinical sign is a shallow serous detachment with a circinate ring of lipid exudates around the macroaneurysm

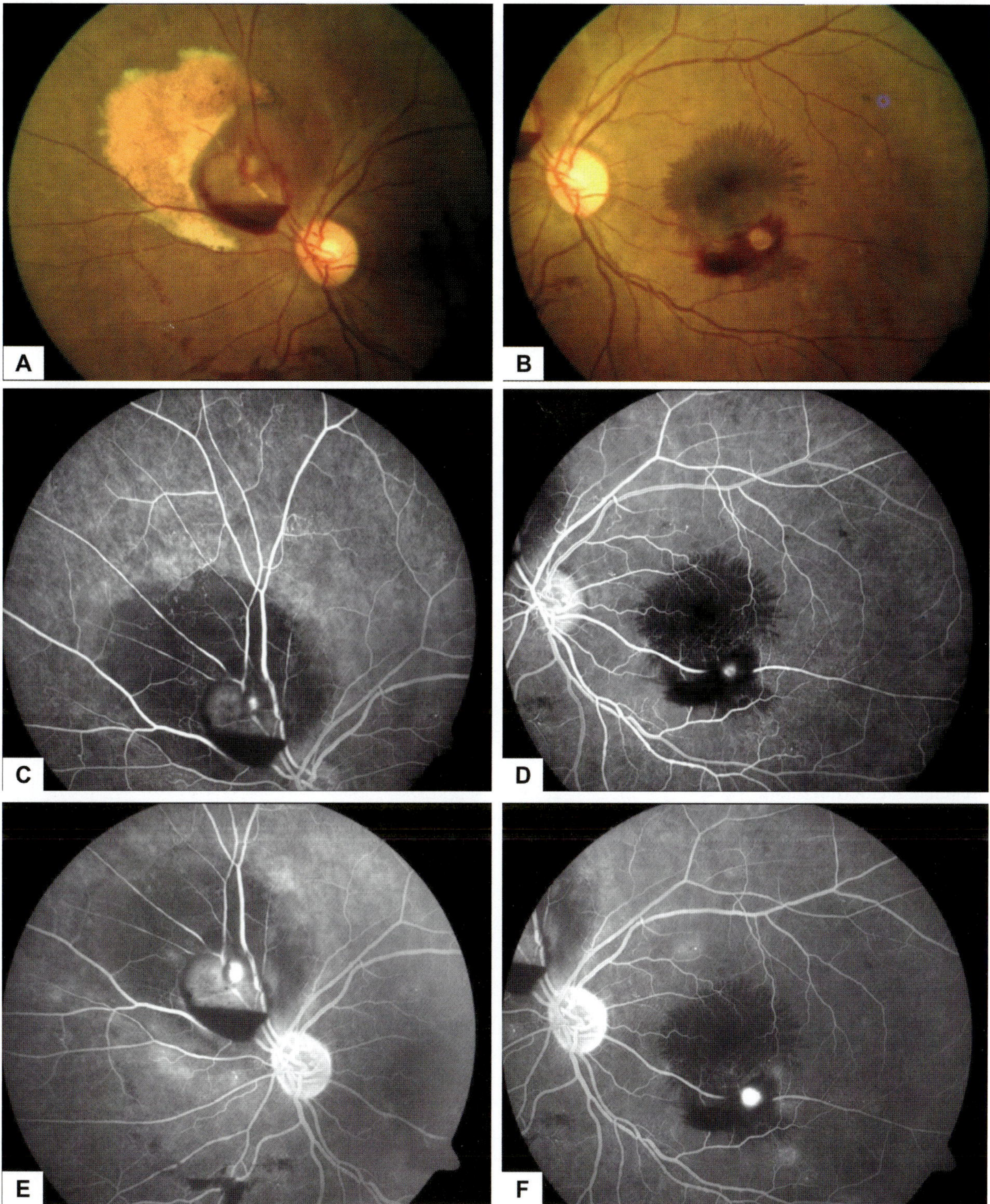

FIGURES 5.4A to F: Retinal artery macroaneursym in a patient with aortoarteritis. Clinical pictures show the lesions superonasal to the disk and inferior to the fovea. Note the varying levels of hemorrhage associated with the lesion. Sclerosis of the adjacent vessel is seen. Fundus fluorescein angiography shows hyperfluorescence in the area of the macroneurysm which increases in intensity in the late phase.

- Hemorrhage in all planes of the retina can be observed intraretinal, subretinal as well as vitreous hemorrhage.

TREATMENT

- Most cases resolve spontaneously with thrombosis and fibrosis
- Direct thermal laser to leaking macroaneurysms causing lipid exudation or serous detachment
- Pneumatic or surgical displacement of subretinal hemorrhage due to a bleeding macroaneurysm
- Laser hyaloidotomy in case of subhyaloid hemorrhage
- Vitrectomy is useful in case of vitreous hemorrhage sufficient to obscure retinal details.

FLUORESCEIN ANGIOGRAPHY

- Typically fluoresces completely in the early phases with late leakage
- Partial or complete lockage of fluorescence may occur due to hemorrhage
- Alteration in the caliber of the involved arteriole may be seen.

INDOCYANINE GREEN ANGIOGRAPHY

- It may be useful in demonstrating the lesion in the presence of hemorrhage.

COATS' DISEASE

Coats' disease is an idiopathic condition characterized by telangiectatic and aneurysmal retinal vessels with subretinal exudation (Figures 5.5A and B). Recently a genetic mutation of CRB1 gene has been linked to the disease. Two-thirds of patients present before 10 years with complaints of poor vision, strabismus and leucocoria.[1-5]

CLINICAL FEATURES

- Coats' disease is characterised by localized lipid rich yellow subretinal exudates
- Vascular anomalies like sheathing, telangiectasia, tortuosity, and aneurysmal dilatation are present

- The vascular anomalies are usually in the periphery and exudation is predominantly at the posterior pole
- In adult-onset Coats' disease, limited areas of involvement, slower progression of disease and hemorrhage near vascular dilatations are seen.
- Secondary complications like secondary glaucoma or phthisis bulbi may develop.

FLUORESCEIN ANGIOGRAPHY

- Telangiectasia, aneurysms and beading of vessels may be seen giving a "light bulb" appearance
- Zones of capillary nonperfusion are typically surrounded by areas of arteriolar and venular anomalies.

TREATMENT

Treatment is indicated if exudates are extensive and either threaten central visual acuity or produce significant retinal detachment.

Modalities include: photocoagulation, cryotherapy, scleral buckling, subretinal fluid drainage and vitreous surgery.

RETINAL ARTERIAL OCCLUSIONS

Retinal arterial occlusions form one of the true ocular emergencies. Conventionally they can be classified into:[1-5]

1. Central retinal artery occlusion
2. Branch retinal arterial occlusion
3. Cilioretinal artery occlusion
4. Combined central retinal artery and vein occlusion
5. Cotton-wool spot.

CENTRAL RETINAL ARTERY OCCLUSION (FIGURES 5.6A TO D)

Clinical Features

- A history of painless visual loss occurring over few seconds is the most common finding
- Involvement is usually unilateral but a bilateral simultaneous involvement should raise suspicion of cardiac valvular disease, giant cell arteritis and other vascular inflammations
- Profound loss of visual acuity is present
- Relative afferent papillary defect is present

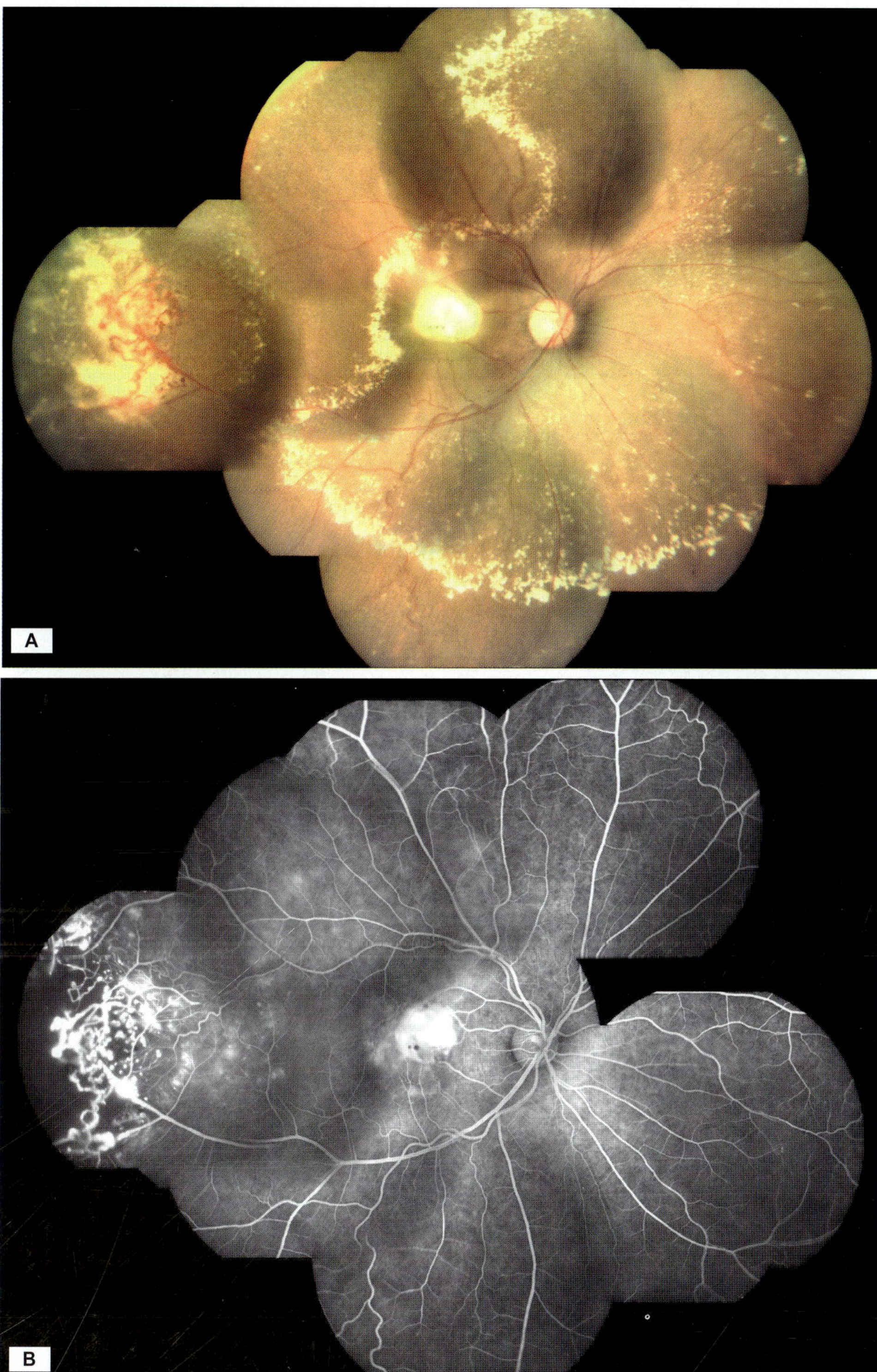

FIGURES 5.5A and B: Coats' disease. Clinical picture shows vascular malformations with exudation in the temporal periphery. A large circinate of exudates is seen in the midperiphery and organized exudates at the macula. Subretinal fluid is seen inferiorly. Fundus fluorescein angiography shows the telangiectatic vessels in the periphery with a light bulb appearance. Areas of capillary non-perfusion and staining of the macular exudate are also seen.

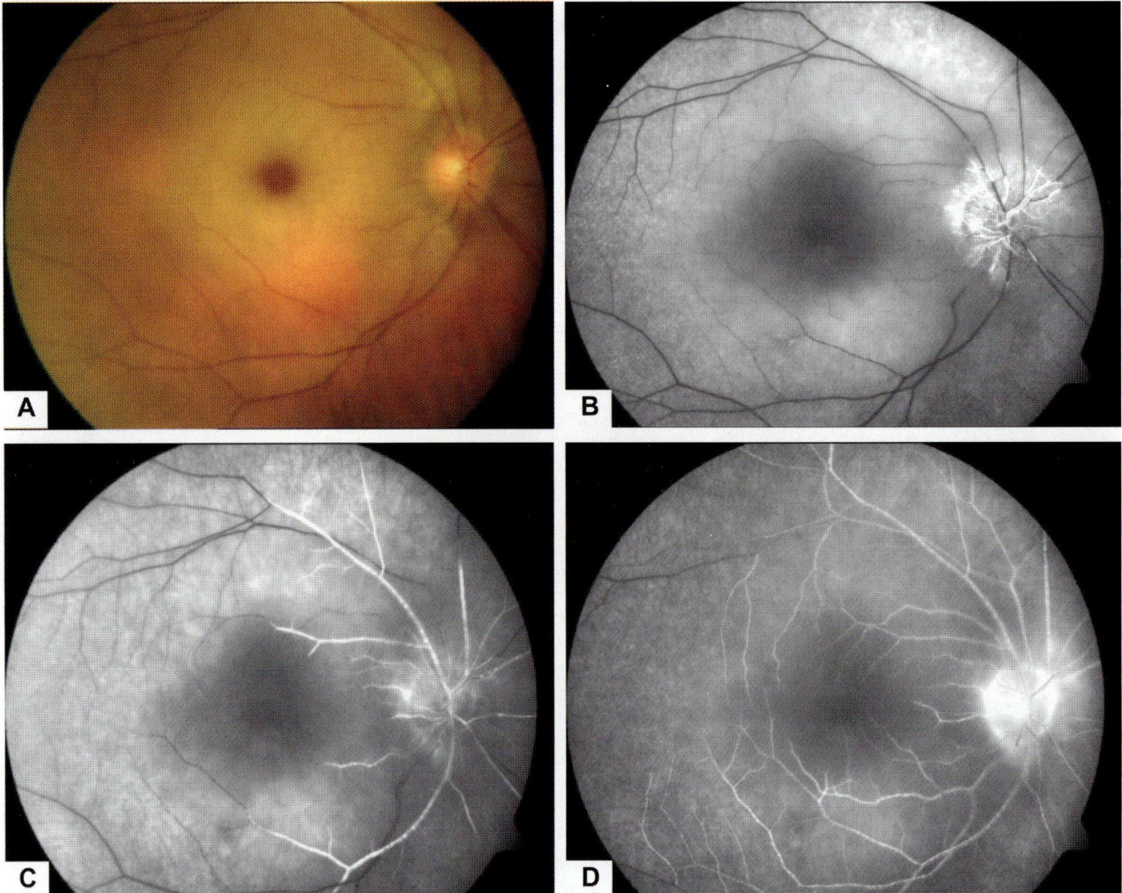

FIGURES 5.6A to D: Central retinal artery occlusion. Clinical picture shows the typical cherry red spot at the macula and broken blood column within the vessels. Fundus fluorescein angiography shows grossly delayed filling of the arterioles which is incomplete even in the late phases.

- Opacified superficial retina which assumes a yellow white appearance is observed
- Cherry red spot is visible at the macula due to the intact choroidal circulation
- Irregular caliber of the retinal vessels with "box carring" of the blood column within the arterioles is seen
- A patent cilioretinal artery that supplies papillomacular bundle may be present. This is seen as an area in the papillomacular bundle with a normal appearance and carries with it a better visual prognosis
- An embolus may be seen within the retinal arterial system, most commonly the Hollenhorst plaque.

Fluorescein Angiography

- Delay in retinal arterial filling, delay in arteriovenous transit time (normal being <11 sec)
- Late staining of optic disk may occur
- Patent cilioretinal artery may be identified.

Other Investigations

- *Electroretinography*
  Electroretinography shows a decreased to absent b wave signifying ischemia of the inner retina.

BRANCH RETINAL ARTERY OBSTRUCTION

Clinical Features

- A localized region of superficial retinal whitening along the distribution of the obstructed retinal vessel is observed
- Temporal vessels are involved more frequently.

Fluorescein Angiography

- Artery to artery collaterals may develop; these are pathognomonic of branch retinal arterial occlusion
- Rarely neovascularization may occur.

CILIORETINAL ARTERY OBSTRUCTION

Cilioretinal artery occlusion is seen clinically in 20% of eyes with arterial occlusion.

Three clinical variants are seen:
- Isolated cilioretinal artery occlusion
- Associated with central retinal vein occlusion
- Associated with anterior ischemic optic neuropathy

Visual prognosis is usually worse when cilioretinal artery occlusion is associated with anterior ischemic optic neuropathy, primarily due to the optic nerve damage.

Clinical Features

- An area of superficial retinal whitening along the course of the vessel is present.

Fluorescein Angiography

- Normally the cilioretinal artery fills concomitantly with the choroidal circulation about 1 to 2 seconds before filling of the retinal arteries. This filling is delayed in case of an occlusion.

RETINAL VEIN OCCLUSIONS

CENTRAL RETINAL VEIN OCCLUSION

Central retinal vein occlusion (CRVO) is a common retinal vascular disorder with propensity for severe visual handicap. The common associations are diabetes, hypertension, cardiovascular disease and glaucoma. Patients are usually over the age of 50 years.[1-5]

Therapeutic options are designed to prevent and treat sight threatening complications such as macular edema and neovascularization. These include systemic work-up, laser, intravitreal steroids, anti-VEGF agents as well as surgical techniques such as radial optic neurotomy and shunt procedures.

Clinical Features

- Patient complains of sudden painless loss of vision

- History of transient visual obscurations with intervening normal periods
- The disease classically presents with decreased vision noticed on getting up in the morning
- It may even be an incidental finding
- Variable visual acuity is present
- Typically a "blood and thunder" appearance with superficial and deep retinal hemorrhages in all four quadrants radiating from the optic disk
- Dilated, tortuous retinal veins are observed
- Disk swelling, soft exudates and macular edema may be present
- Breakthrough vitreous hemorrhage may occur.

With disease progression the following may occur:
- Optociliary shunt vessels on the optic disk
- Neovascularization of the disk, retina, iris and angle
- Persistent macular edema, epiretinal membrane
- Neovascular glaucoma.

Fluorescein Angiography

Fluorescein angiography is not indicated in the early stages as extensive hemorrhages may render the image uninformative.

Fluorescein angiography can categorize CRVO into perfused (Figures 5.7A to C), non-perfused (Figures 5.7D to F) or indeterminate
- Fluorescein angiography demonstrates a delayed filling of the venous system with some degree of delay in arterial filling as well
- Non-perfusion is described as disk diameters of capillary dropout. > 10 DD of dropout indicates a non-perfused or ischemic CRVO, <10 DD indicates a perfused or non-ischemic CRVO and in cases where hemorrhages obscure most findings, it is categorized as indeterminate
- Neovascularization of the disk and retina may be demonstrated
- Collaterals are seen as linking channels between the veins which stain but do not leak as profusely as neovascularization
- Macular edema is seen as a petalloid pattern of late leakage, most often in a perfused or non-ischemic CRVO
- Varying degrees of macular ischemia may be seen.

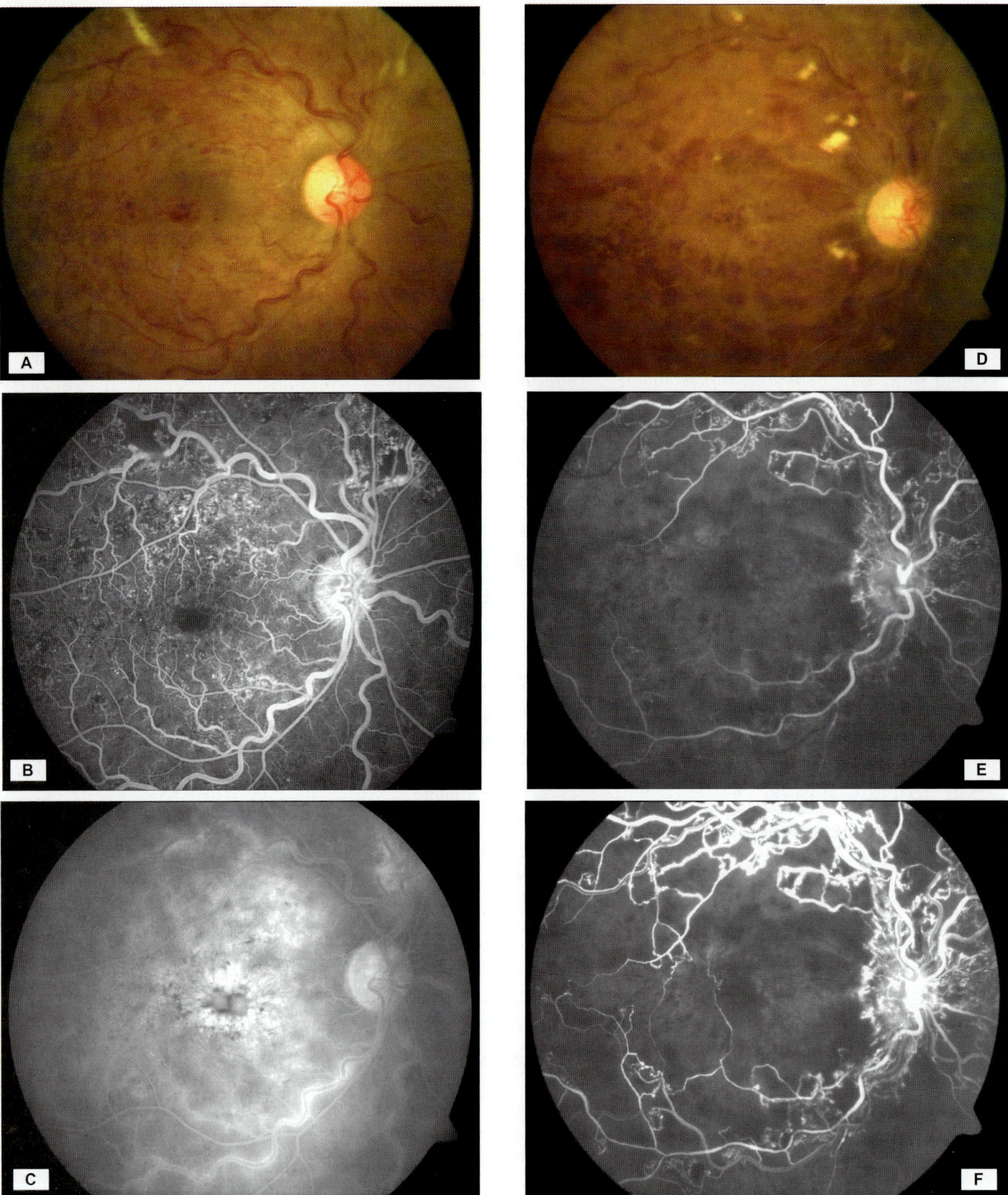

FIGURES 5.7A to C: Non-ischemic central retinal vein occlusion. Clinical picture shows dilated veins, retinal hemorrhages and macular edema. Fundus fluorescein angiography show dilated disk capillaries, two areas of capillary non-perfusion and dilated perifoveal capillaries with late CME. Staining of the veins is seen.

FIGURES 5.7D to F: Ischemic central retinal vein occlusion. Clinical picture shows dilated veins with hemorrhages and cotton-wool spots. Hemorrhages are also seen in the macular area. Fundus fluorescein angiography shows blocked fluorescence, large areas of capillary dropout and collateral formation.

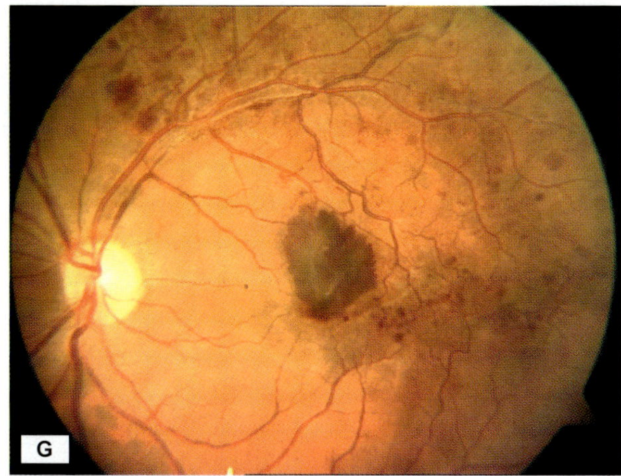

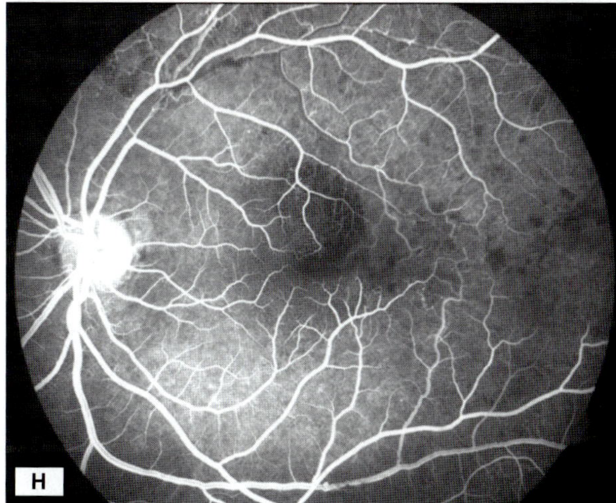

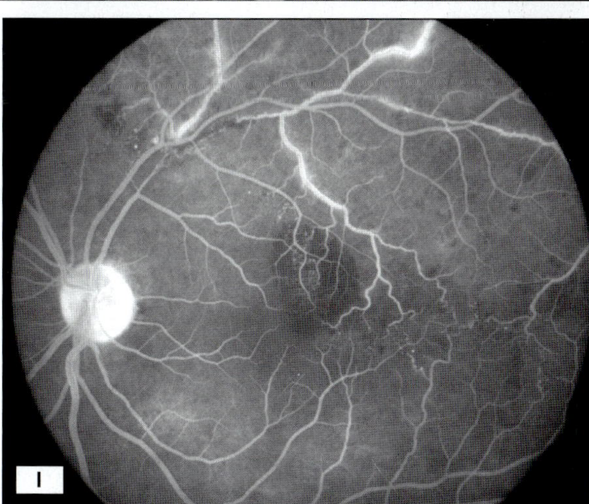

FIGURES 5.7G to I: Branch retinal vein occlusion. Clinical picture showing superotemporal branch retinal vein occlusion with the occluded segment showing sclerosis. Hemorrhages in the involved quadrant and a large hemorrhage in the macula are seen. Fundus fluorescein angiography shows the occluded segment in the mid phases. The late phase image shows collaterals bypassing the occluded segment and staining of the vessel wall.

Other Investigations

- Electroretinography testing
- Visual fields
- Systemic work-up if diabetes, hypertension and cardiovascular disease have been in a patient over the age of 60 years. It is indicated more often in young patients and those with bilateral disease. Investigations are directed toward excluding hypercoagulability states and systemic vascular diseases.

BRANCH RETINAL VEIN OCCLUSION

Branch retinal vein occlusion (BRVO) is a common retinal vascular disease with no gender predilection. It usually occurs at an arteriovenous crossing and most often affects the superotemporal vein (Figures 5.7G to I). Risk factors are similar to those for CRVO. Ages between 60 and 70 years are most often affected.

Treatment is directed toward the vision threatening complications—macular edema and neovascularization. Other causes for vision loss are epiretinal membrane formation, tractional retinal detachment involving the macula and sometimes a combined traction-rhegmatogenous retinal detachment. [1-5]

Clinical Features

- Patient complains of sudden onset loss of vision
- Visual field loss is present
- Segmental distribution of intraretinal hemorrhages is observed
- Dilatation of the involved vein is present
- Cotton-wool spots and hard exudates may be observed
- Macular hemorrhages and/or edema may be present
- Later, one may see sclerosis of the involved vein, neovascularization of the disk and retina in the involved sector.

Fluorescein Angiography

Fluorescein angiography is not useful in the acute phase due to extensive hemorrhages. It is of more value 6 to 8 weeks after the acute episode to detect areas of nonperfusion and neovascularization.

- Delayed arterial and venous filling in the involved segment
- Areas of capillary dropout: > 5 DD is considered to be a non-perfused BRVO
- Collaterals which bypass the obstruction: This indicates a compensatory mechanism
- Neovascularization of the disk or retina: These are indications for sectoral laser photocoagulation
- Macular ischemia or edema: An ischemic macula is unlikely to respond favorably to grid laser photocoagulation.

CENTRAL SEROUS CHORIORETINOPATHY

Central serous chorioretinopathy (CSR) is characterised by idiopathic serous detachment of the macula, seen most commonly in young to middle aged males. It is believed to be due to choroidal hyperpermeability and retinal pigment epithelium dysfunction.[16-21]

It is self limiting with almost normal recovery of vision but has a 50% predilection for recurrence and involvement of the contralateral eye. It results in significant visual impairment in approximately 5% of patients.

Associations with type-A personality and steroid intake have been described.

CLINICAL FEATURES

- Serous retinal detachment at the macula. The subretinal fluid may be clear or turbid with subretinal precipitates or fibrin
- Pigment epithelial detachment either alone or under a serous retinal detachment
- Retinal pigment epithelium atrophic tracks: These are flask shaped and extend inferiorly from the macula. They are indicative of previous episodes of CSR
- Bullous retinal detachments with subretinal fibrin. These usually occur in cases of bilateral disease.

FLUORESCEIN ANGIOGRAPHY

- Demonstrates the point of leak in the retinal pigment epithelium (Figures 5.8A to C)
- Smoke stack leak (Figures 5.8D to F). Here the hyperfluorescence starts as a point and rises upward in an umbrella or inverted smoke stack pattern within the margins of the detachment

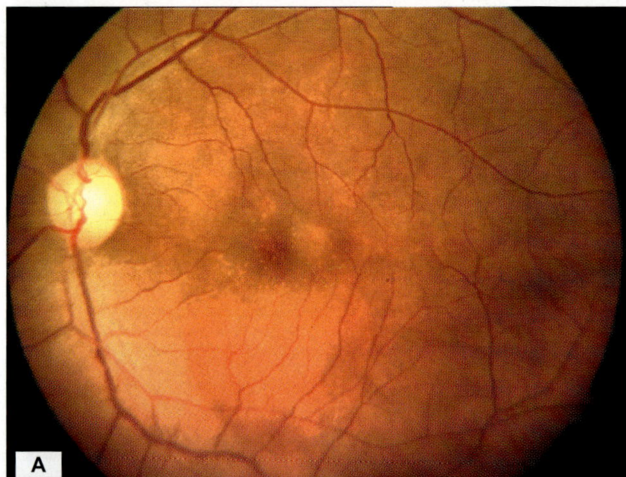
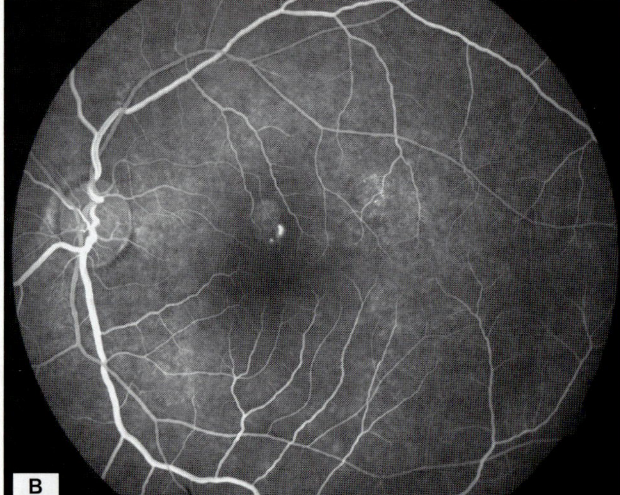
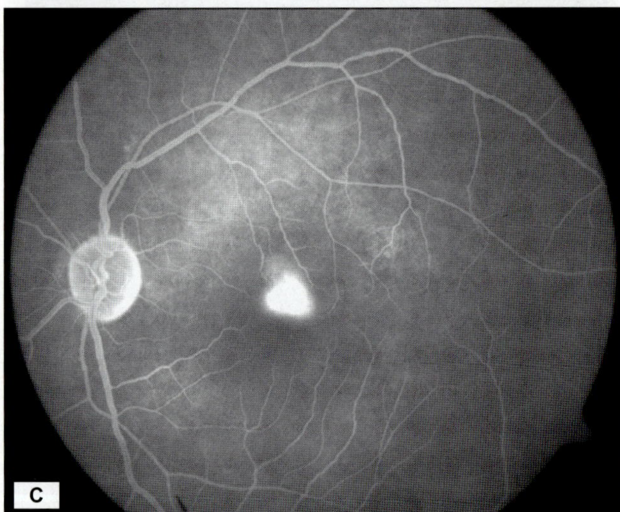

FIGURES 5.8A to C: Central serous retinopathy. Clinical picture shows a serous detachment at the macula with subretinal precipitates. Fundus fluorescein angiography shows a point leak which increases uniformly in all directions in the late phase.

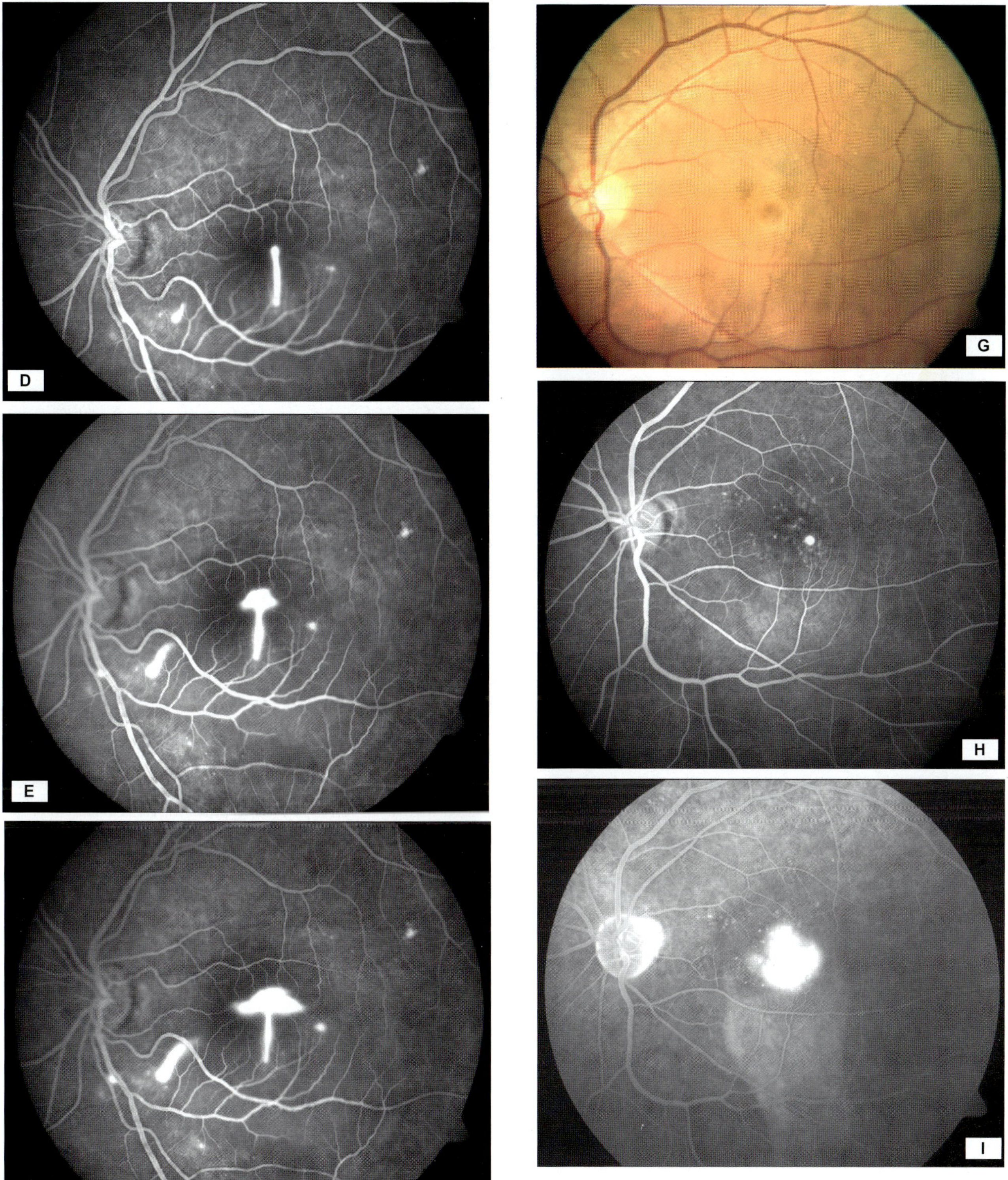

FIGURES 5.8D to F: Smoke stack leaks in central serous retinopathy. Note how the fluorescein dye rises up toward the upper border of the detachment. Two ink blot leaks are also seen.

FIGURES 5.8G to I: Chronic central serous retinopathy with retinal pigment epithelium tracks. Clinical picture shows fibrin at the macula and a flask shaped area of subretinal fluid tracking inferiorly. The point leak is seen to increase in the late phase, and hyperfluoresence in the area of the detachment is seen.

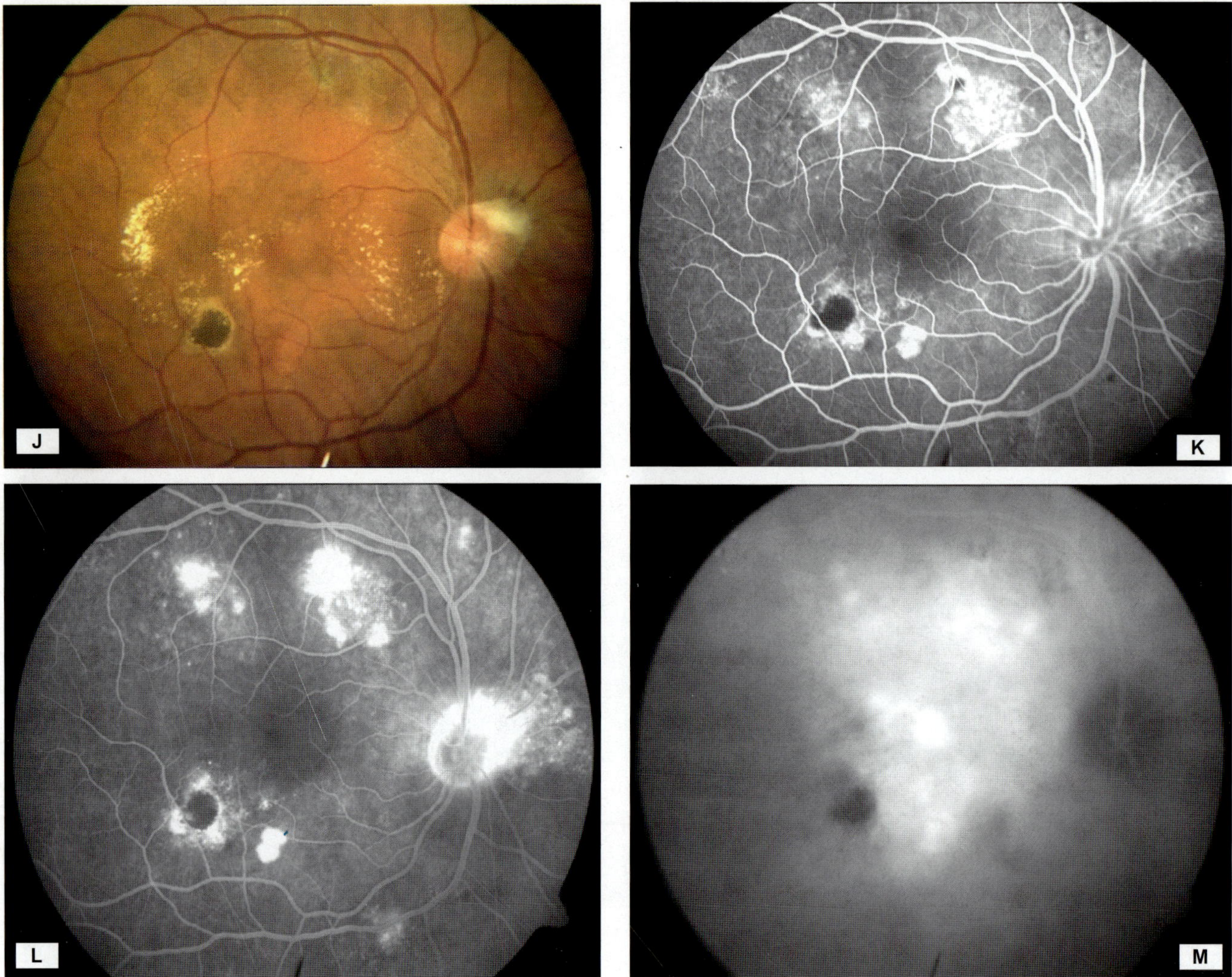

FIGURES 5.8J to M: Central serous retinopathy with multiple leaks. Clinical picture shows subretinal fluid at the macula with hard exudates. Laser marks are seen inferotemporal to the fovea. Fundus fluorescein angiography shows multiple hyperfluorescent spots clustered at the posterior pole but no definite leak. ICG angiography shows multiple hyperfluorescent areas at the posterior pole suggesting a basic pathology in the choroid.

- Ink blot leak (Figures 5.8G to I) where the point leak spreads symmetrically in all directions
- Leaks may be one or multiple
- Often diffuse mottled hyperfluorescence may be seen without a definite leaking point. This is seen in cases of chronic CSR (Figures 5.8J to L)
- Serous pigment epithelial detachments with early hyperfluorescence limited to the margins of the detachment
- Secondary changes such as cystoid macular edema and choroidal neovascular membrane formation may be demonstrated.

INDOCYANINE GREEN ANGIOGRAPHY

- It demonstrates that the primary abnormality is in the choroidal circulation
- It is of particular importance if no definite leak is seen on fluorescein angiography
- Multiple foci of choroidal hyperpermeability (Figure 5.8M) may be seen.
- The area of pigment epithelium detachment is hypofluorescent with a hyperfluorescent halo in the late phase.

PARAFOVEAL TELANGIECTASIS

A group of development retinal vascular disorders characterized by ectasia and incompetence of the parafoveal retinal capillaries. They present with mild to moderate degrees of visual loss. [1-5]

CLINICAL FEATURES

Parafoveal telangiectasis is divided into 3 groups:

Group 1A: Unilateral congenital telangiectasis. It is seen in males around the age of 40. It involves the temporal half of the macula. Visual loss occurs due to macular edema or exudation.

Group 1B: There is unilateral involvement of one clock hour at the edge of the foveal avascular zone.

Group 2A: This is the most common form. Acquired form affects males and females in the middle age. The disease is bilateral and can cause minimal to moderate visual loss due to intraretinal neovascularization. It usually affects the temporal half first. It can be further divided into three stages:
- Stage 1: Minimal or no evidence of capillary dilatation on slit lamp biomicroscopy
- Stage 2 : Faint graying or loss of transparency of the parafoveolar retina
- Stage 3: Dilated and blunted 'right angled' venules
- Stage 4: Stellate foci of intraretinal pigmentation
- Stage 5 : Subretinal neovascularization

Yellowish crystalline deposits in the parafoveolar retina may be seen from stage 2 onward.

Group 2B: Juvenile familial form. It is seen at a younger age and with no evidence of pigmented plaques, right angled venules or retinal deposits.

Group 3A: It is seen in middle age or later in life. Bilateral form is present with telangiectatic capillaries and progressive loss of the juxtafoveal capillary network. Macular changes are similar to sickle cell retinopathy and diabetic retinopathy.

Group 3B: Associated features such as optic atrophy, abnormal deep tendon reflexes and other central nervous system involvement may be present.

INDICATION FOR TREATMENT

Visual loss due to subretinal neovascularization.

TREATMENT

- Thermal laser for extra/ juxtafoveal CNV
- Photodynamic therapy or transpupillary thermo-therapy for juxta/ subfoveal CNV
- Triamcinolone acetonide alone or in combination with PDT. This has also been tried in cases with macular edema and no CNV.

FLUORESCEIN ANGIOGRAPHY

- Early phases show parafoveolar capillary dilatation with late stages showing staining of the parafoveolar area, typically sparing the central fovea (Figures 5.9 A to C).
- Blocked fluorescence in the area of retinal pigment epithelium hyperplasia
- Leakage from CNV (Figures 5.9 D to F) if present. It can have associated cystoid macular edema involving the foveal centre in cases of sub/juxtafoveal CNV.

RETINAL ANGIOMATOUS PROLIFERATION

Retinal angiomatous proliferation (RAP) is a distinct subgroup of neovascular AMD where the initial stages involve angiomatous proliferation within the retina culminating in a retinochoroidal anastomosis. The presence of a demonstrable RAP lesion is a poor prognostic sign when conventional treatment for CNV is considered. [22]

Treatment modalities include photodynamic therapy either alone or in combination with intravitreal steroids.

CLINICAL FEATURES

Stage 1 (Figures 5.10A to D): Intraretinal neovascularization is accompanied by intraretinal hemorrhages and edema.

Stage 2 (Figures 5.10E to H): Subretinal neovascularization is due to the extension of the intraretinal neovascularization into the subretinal space. A serous pigment epithelial detachment may be seen associated with the proliferation.

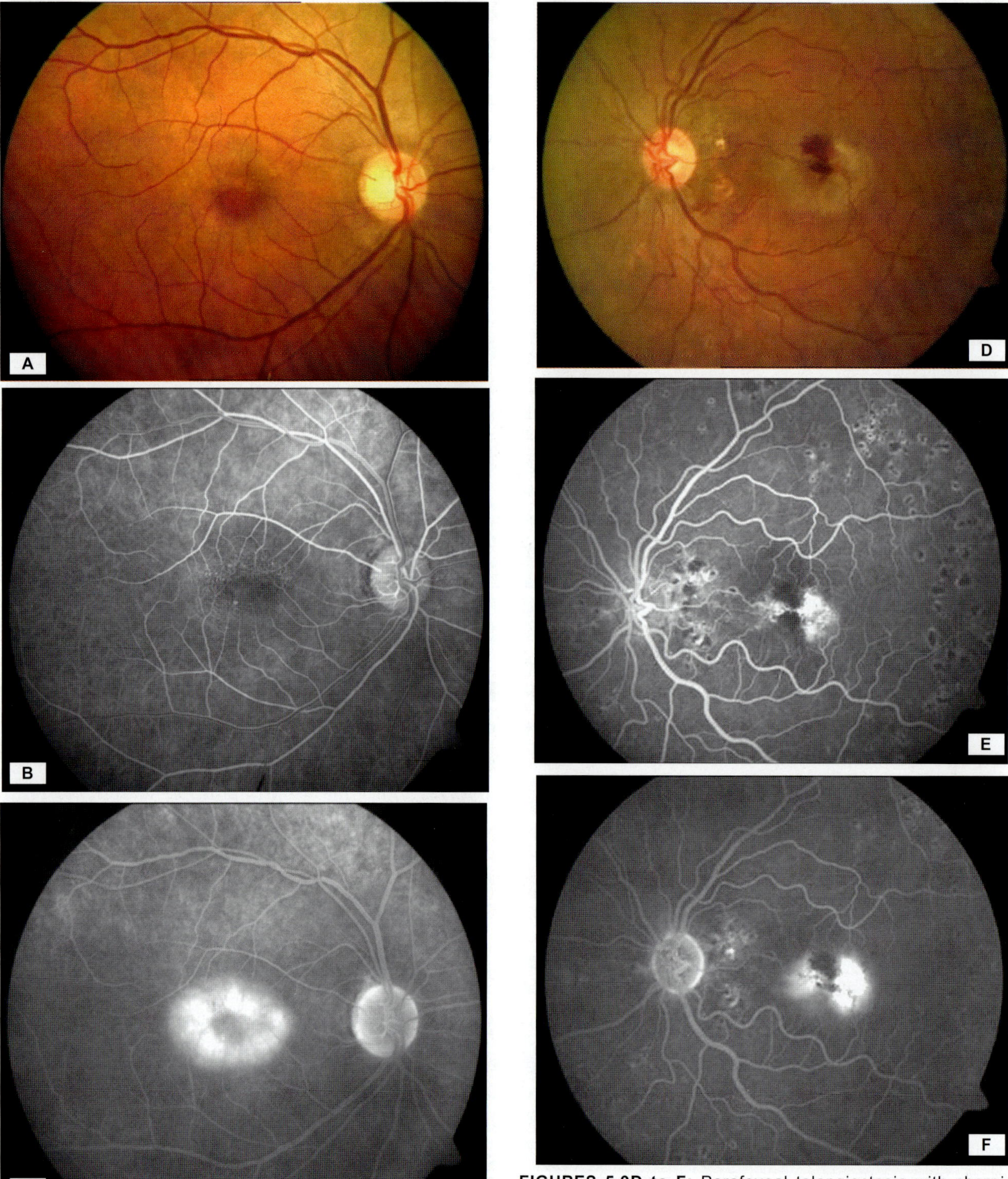

FIGURES 5.9A to C: Parafoveal telangiectasia. Clinical picture shows grayish diskoloration of the parafoveolar retina with glistening deposits and blunt ended venules. Fundus fluorescein angiography shows a dilated parafoveolar network with staining of the area in the late phases.

FIGURES 5.9D to F: Parafoveal telangiectasia with choroidal neovascularization. Clinical picture shows grayish diskoloration of the parafoveal area, along with retinal hemorrhages and a yellow membrane superotemporal to the fovea. Fundus fluorescein angiography shows staining of the parafoveal area with intense hyperfluorescence in the region of the choroidal neovascularization.

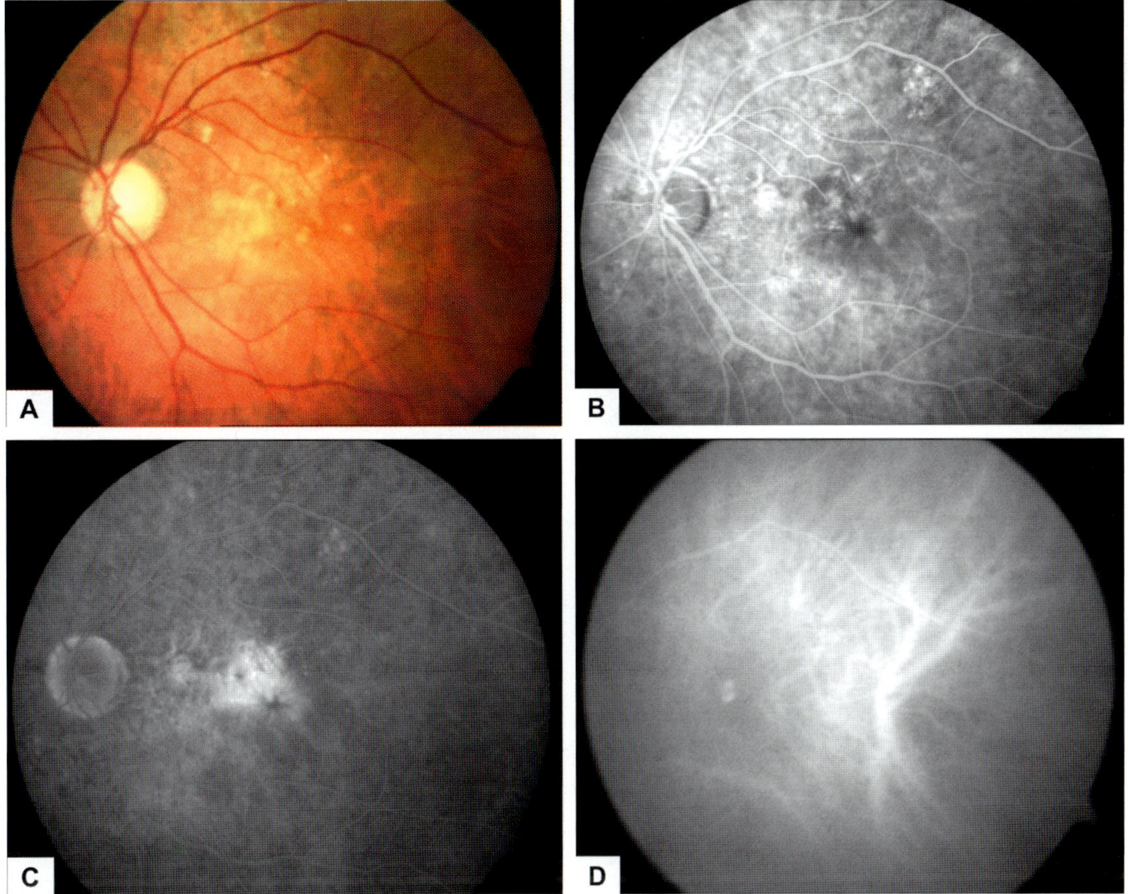

FIGURES 5.10A to D: Retinal angiomatous proliferation lesion-early stage. Clinical picture shows a retinal vessel dipping into the retina superonasal to the fovea. An intraretinal hemorrhage is seen at this point along with RPE changes. Macular edema is also seen. Fundus fluorescein angiography clearly shows the dipping retinal vessel with hyperfluorescence around it indicative of a choroidal neovascularization. The late phase shows cystoid macular edema along with intense leak from the choroidal neovascularization. ICG angiogram shows a spot of bright hyperfluorescence at the site of the lesion.

Stage 3 (Figures 5.10I to L): Clinically evident choroidal neovascular membrane associated with a vascularized pigment epithelium detachment. A retinochoroidal anastomosis is seen as a right angled retinal vessel dipping into the choroid.

FLUORESCEIN ANGIOGRAPHY

Stage 1: Focal area of intraretinal staining with an indistinct border corresponding to the intraretinal neovascularization and edema is present. Cystoid macular edema may be seen.

Stage 2: Fluorescein angiography is less useful and may be misleading. May mimic a minimally classic CNV as there is an area of well defined hyperfluorescence within an area of ill defined hyperfluorescence.

Stage 3: Right angled retinal vessel in case of a retinochoroidal anastomosis is present. A vascularized pigment epithelial detachment may also be seen.

INDOCYANINE GREEN ANGIOGRAPHY

Stage 1: Focal area of intense hyperfluorescence within the retina—"hot spot".

Stage 2: Helpful in making an accurate diagnosis. Hypofluorescence of the serous component of the pigment epithelial detachment with an adjacent hot spot is observed.

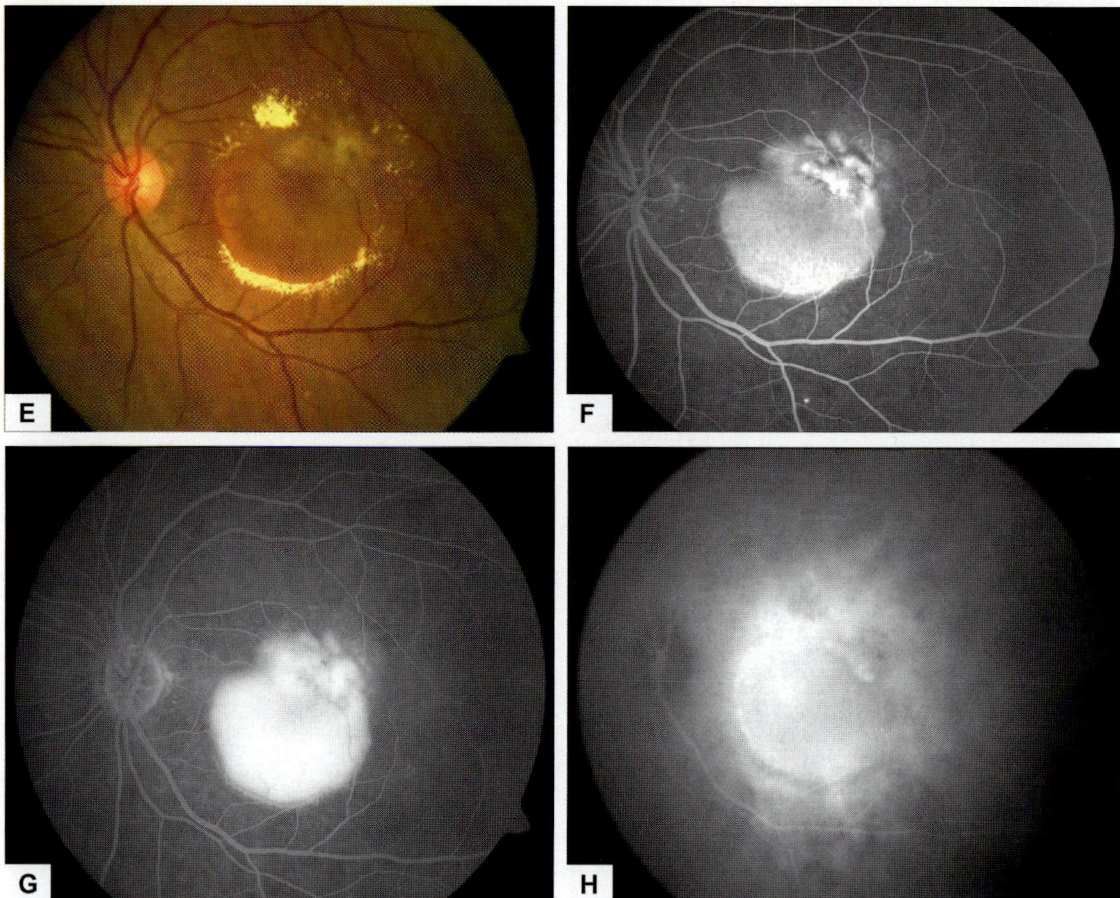

FIGURES 5.10E to H: Retinal angiomatous proliferation lesion. Clinical picture shows a choroidal neovascularization superotemporal to the fovea and a large serous PED adjacent to it. A superficial retinal hemorrhage is seen at the site of the choroidal neovascularization. Hard exudates are seen at the margin of the PED. Fundus fluorescein angiography shows uniform early hyperfluorescence of the PED along with filling of the choroidal neovascularization which causes a fuzzy superior border. ICG shows a hypofluorescent rim of the PED and hyperfluorescence in the area of choroidal neovascularization.

Stage 3: Laminating CNV in the presence of a vascularized pigment epithelial detachment is present.

Retinochoroidal anastomosis may be demonstrated in the late phases.

OPTIC DISK PIT

Optic disk pit is a congenital defect of the optic nerve head. It is believed to be either due to improper closure of the embryonal fissure or to a defect in the primitive epithelial papilla. Visual acuity is usually normal unless there is development of a serous macular detachment.[1-5]

CLINICAL FEATURES

- Single (95%) or multiple optic disk pits may be present
- Optic disk pit appears as a gray or yellowish colored round to oval depression within the optic nerve head
- It is situated commonly on the temporal side and is eccentrically located
- Serous retinal detachment connecting with the margin of the pit and involving the macular area may be present (Figures 5.11A to C)
- Cystic macular changes or macular hole formation may be seen.

FLUORESCEIN ANGIOGRAPHY

- Hypofluorescent area corresponding to the pit in the early phase

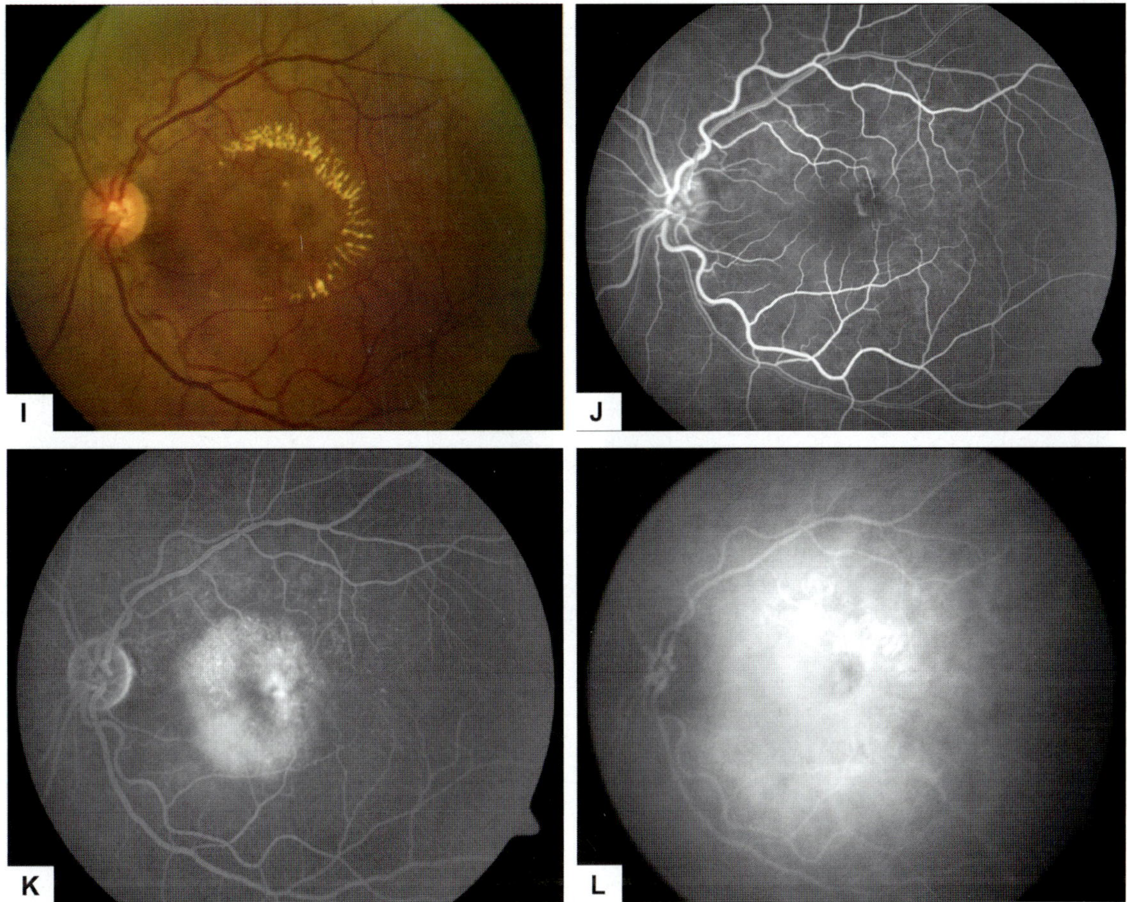

FIGURES 5.10I to L: Retinal angiomatous proliferation lesion. A choroidal neovascularization is seen superotemporal to the fovea with a retinal vessel dipping into the center. This is surrounded by subretinal fluid and exudates. Fundus fluorescein angiography shows the choroidal neovascularization in association with the dipping vessel. The late phase shows a diffuse area of hyperfluorescence corresponding to a fibrovascular PED. ICG shows the choroidal neovascularization along with hypofluorescence in the area of the PED.

- Late hyperfluorescence due to leakage from vessels at the base of the pit
- Faint leakage of dye at the edge of the pit (Figures 5.11D to F) may be seen
- Pooling of dye within the sensory retinal detachment.

TREATMENT

Treatment is indicated in case of serous retinal detachment and modalities include laser to the peripapillary retinal pigment epithelium, pneumatic retinopexy and vitrectomy with oil or gas tamponade.

POLYPOIDAL CHOROIDAL VASCULOPATHY

Polypoidal choroidal vasculopathy (PCV) is a peculiar hemorrhagic disorder of the macula described as both "posterior uveal bleeding syndrome" and "multiple recurrent retinal pigment epithelium detachments in black women".[23-31]

CLINICAL FEATURES (FIGURES 5.12A TO J)

- Dilated choroidal vascular channels are observed
- Terminal orange, bulging polypoid dilatations are observed
- Recurrent subretinal and vitreous hemorrhage may be present
- Relatively minimal fibrous scarring may be present
- Rarely massive vitreous hemorrhage, retinal detachment and secondary glaucoma may occur.

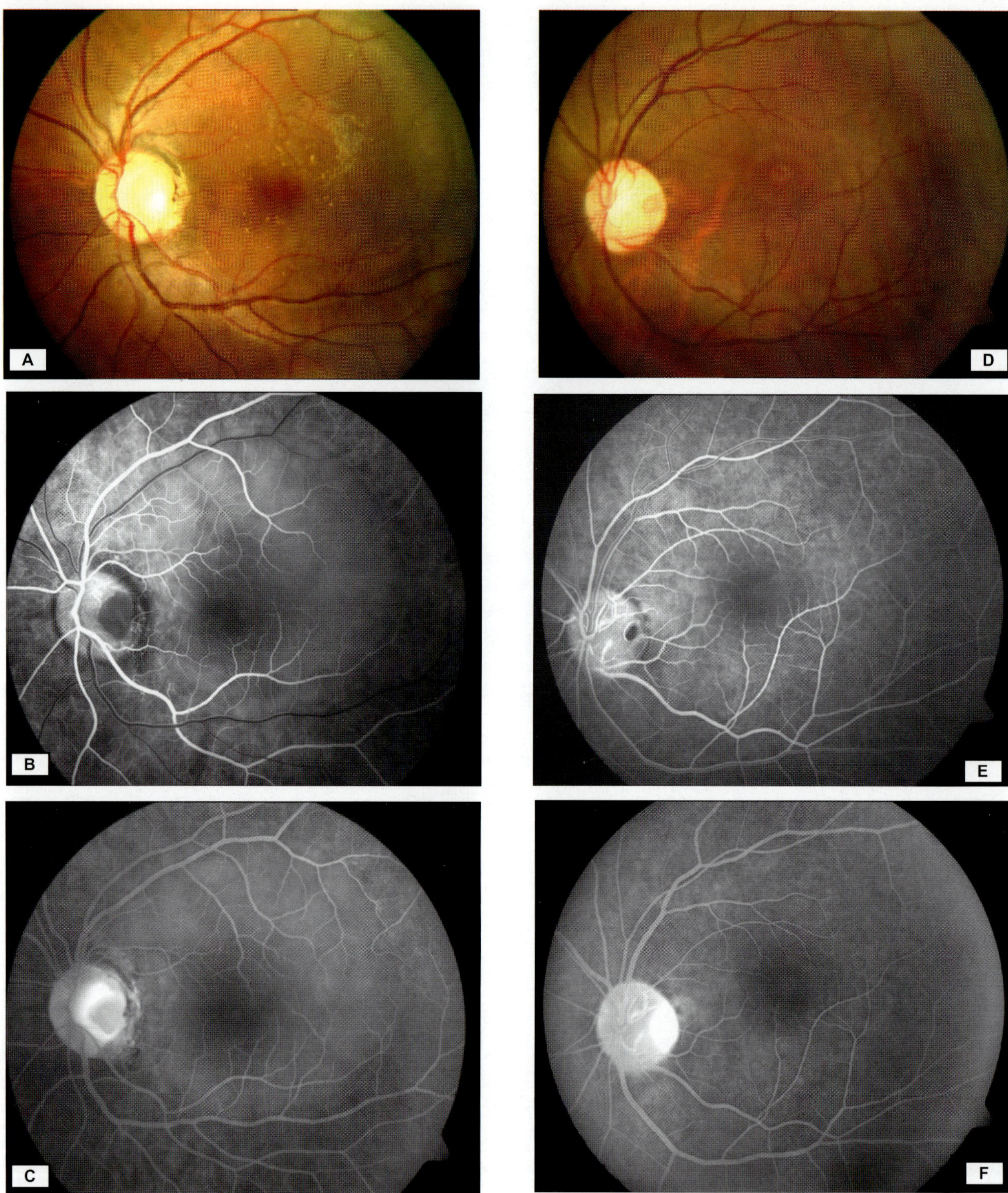

FIGURES 5.11A to C: Optic pit with serous macular detachment. Clinical picture shows an optic pit on the temporal aspect with serous macular elevation. The fluid extends from the edge of the optic disk and shows subretinal precipitates. Fundus fluorescein angiography shows a filling defect in the area of the pit with late staining and pooling of dye in the area of serous detachment.

FIGURES 5.11D to F: Optic pit. Clinical picture shows a small pit on the temporal part of the disk. Cystic macular changes are seen. Fundus fluorescein angiography shows an early filling defect in the region of the pit with late staining. Faint staining with a fuzzy margin is seen at the temporal border of the disk.

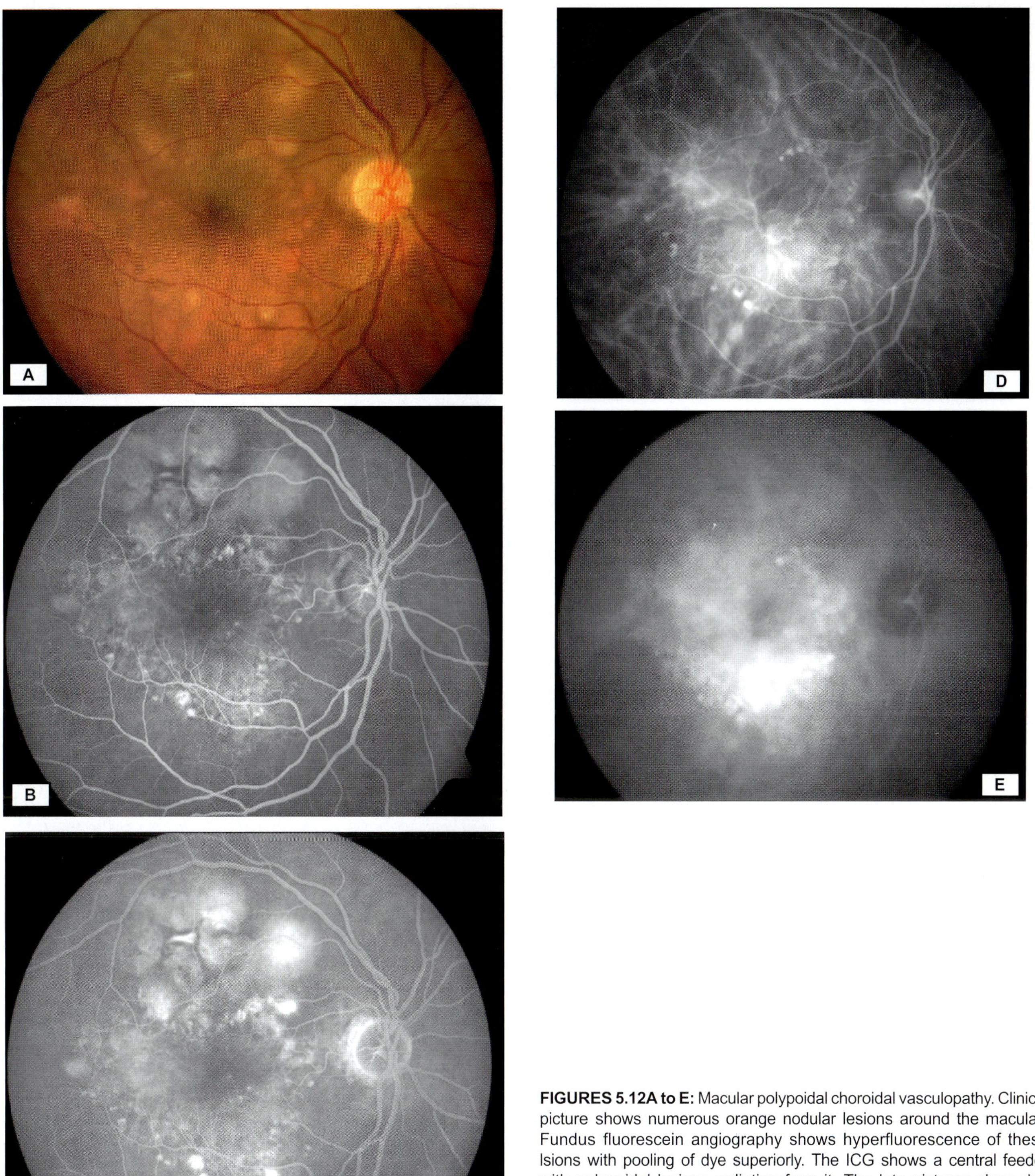

FIGURES 5.12A to E: Macular polypoidal choroidal vasculopathy. Clinical picture shows numerous orange nodular lesions around the macula . Fundus fluorescein angiography shows hyperfluorescence of these lsions with pooling of dye superiorly. The ICG shows a central feeder with polypoidal lesions radiating from it. The late pictures show dye leakage from the abnormal choroidal vessels. Washout of dye with central hypofluorescence of the polyps is seen, especially in the inferior part.

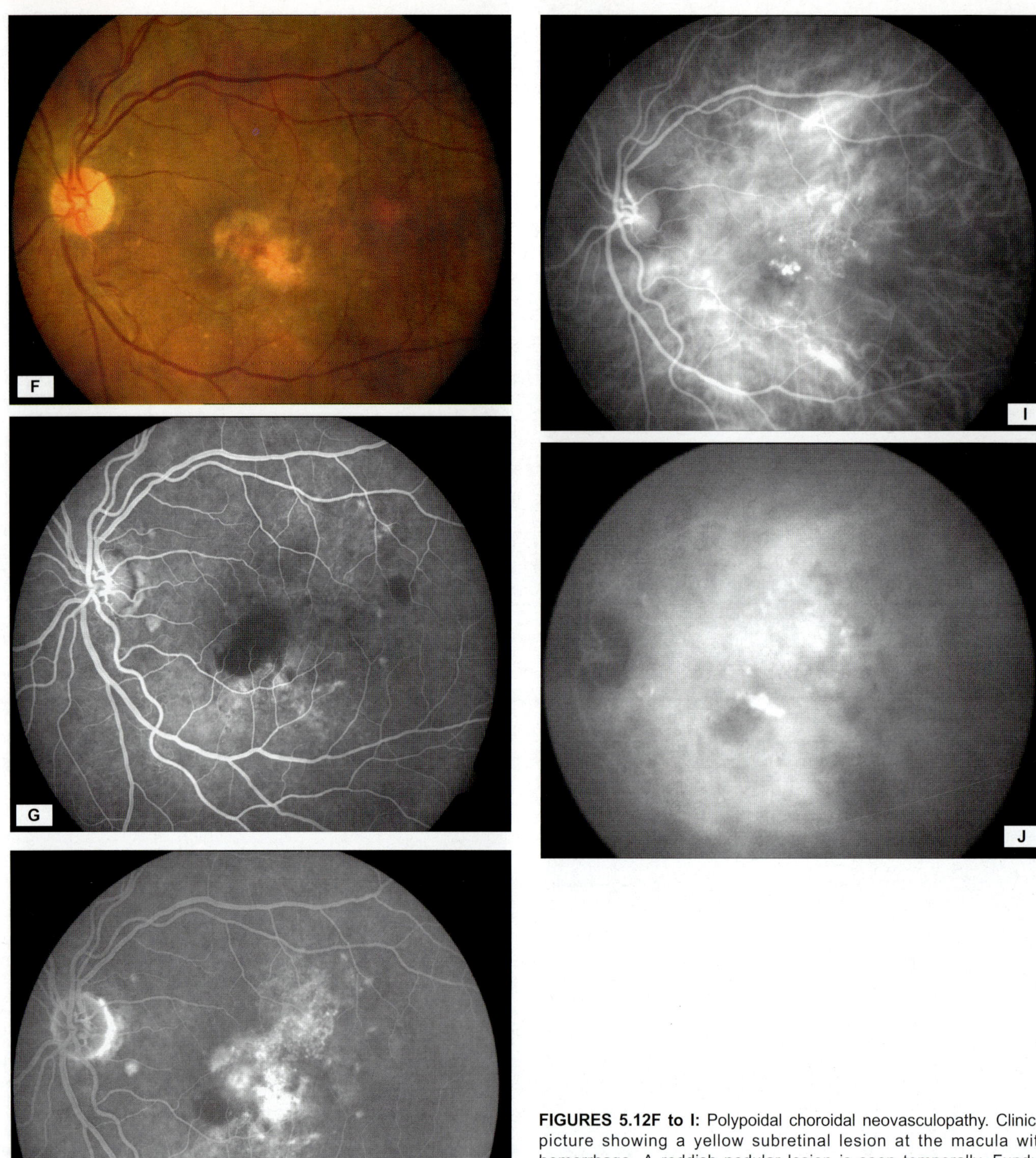

FIGURES 5.12F to I: Polypoidal choroidal neovasculopathy. Clinical picture showing a yellow subretinal lesion at the macula with hemorrhage. A reddish nodular lesion is seen temporally. Fundus fluorescein angiography findings of late mottled hyperfluorescence are suspicious of an occult choroidal neovascularization. ICG angiography shows a polypoidal network at the macula. The late film shows washout of dye from the superior part and late hyperfluorescence of the foveal part.

PATHOLOGY

- Inner choroidal abnormality is present
- Thin walled dilated, aneurysmal vessels of venular origin are observed
- Growth occurs by three mechanisms:
  - Simple vessel hypertrophy
  - Conversion into the advancing edge of a vascular channel
  - Unfolding of a cluster of aneurysmal elements and transformation into enlarging vascular, tubular components.

TYPES

1. Peripapillary
2. Macular
3. Peripheral.

MIMICKING CONDITIONS

1. Central serous retinopathy
2. Choroidal neovascularization
3. Vascular malformations
4. Choroidal tumors
5. Inflammatory conditions.

INDICATIONS FOR TREATMENT

- Serosanguinous detachment causing decreased vision
- Polypoidal CNV
- Vitreous hemorrhage
- Submacular hemorrhage.

TREATMENT

- Observation
- Laser photocoagulation
- Photodynamic therapy/transpupillary thermotherapy
- Indocyanine green dye mediated photothrombosis
- Vitreoretinal surgery.

FLUORESCEIN ANGIOGRAPHY

- Speckled fluorescence resembling an occult CNV.
- Associated pigment epithelial detachment.

INDOCYANINE GREEN ANGIOGRAPHY

- Early phase:
  Distinct network of vessels within the choroidal circulation with surrounding hypofluorescence
  Small hyperfluorescent polyps arising from the larger choroidal vessels
- Mid phase:
  Increase in the size of the polyps
- Late phase:
  Reversal of the pattern of fluorescence with the center of the lesion hypo and the surrounding area hyperfluorescent
  Lesions < 0.5 DD have intense uniform fluorescence
  Internal details may be seen in larger lesions
- Very late phase
  Dye disappearance—"wash out"—in non-leaking lesions
  Persistent hyperfluorescence in leaking lesions.

POSTOPERATIVE CYSTOID MACULAR EDEMA

Postoperative cystoid macular edema (CME) represents one of the most common causes of unexpected decrease in visual acuity after any ophthalmic surgical procedure. Cataract surgery is one of the most common causes of CME (commonly referred to as Irvine – Gass syndrome) but other surgeries like scleral buckling, penetrating keratoplasty, secondary intraocular lens (IOL) implantation, glaucoma filtering surgery, Nd: YAG laser treatment can also lead to it.[1-5]

Cystoid macular edema is more frequently associated with intraoperative complications such as disruption of posterior capsule, vitreous loss, retention of cortical matter, dislocated IOL, inadequate wound closure, etc. Clinically significant CME usually occurs within 4 to 12 weeks of surgery. Clinically significant CME is usually defined as symptomatic decrease in vision whereas chronic CME is defined as persistent decline in visual acuity for more than 6 months.

Treatment is directed towards inflammatory mediators especially prostaglandins and modalities include non-steroidal anti-inflammatory drugs, corticosteroids, carbonic anhydrase inhibitors, Nd: YAG vitreolysis and vitrectomy.

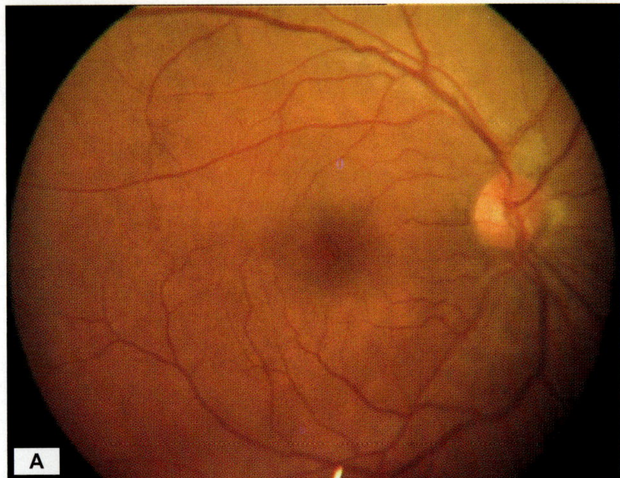

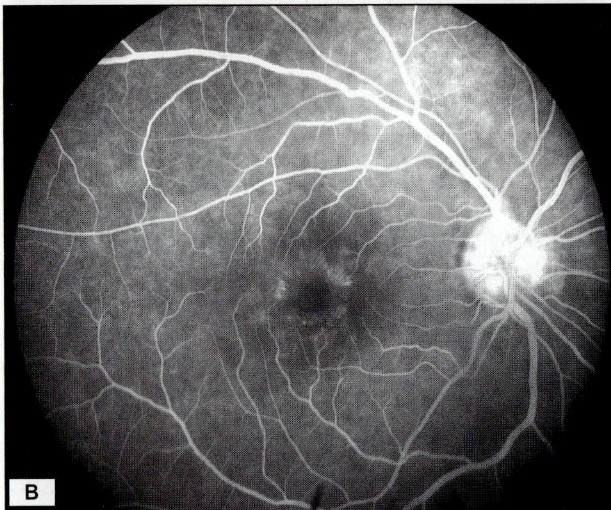

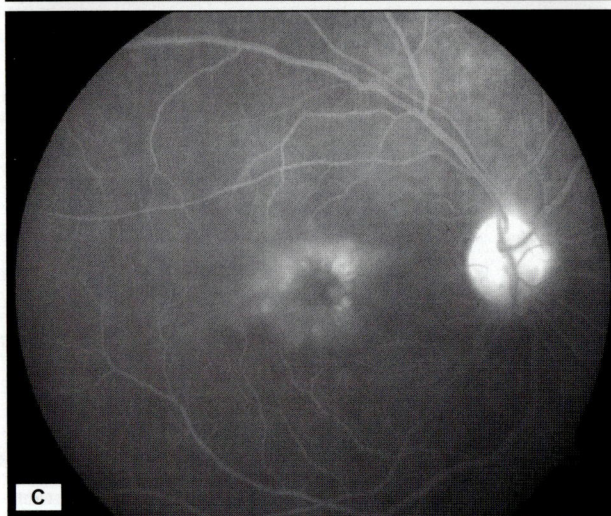

FIGURES 5.13A to C: Postoperative cystoid macular edema. The clinical picture shows mild disk hyperemia and cystoid macular edema. Fundus fluorescein angiography shows dilated perifoveal capillaries with late leakage in a petalloid pattern. The disk shows late leakage.

CLINICAL FEATURES

- Moderate decrease in vision is the commonest complaint
- Vitreous incarceration may be seen at the wound site
- Fundus findings are subtle and are best seen on 78/90 diopters
- The foveal reflex is absent; macula appears thickened with teardrop-like spaces seen best with oblique illumination on slit lamp
- Optic nerve head edema may be present
- In chronic CME, retinal pigment epithelium alterations, lamellar or full thickness macular holes may be seen.

FLUORESCEIN ANGIOGRAPHY

- Fluorescein angiography plays an important role in diagnosing CME. Angiographic CME is defined as CME noted only on angiogram with no clinical findings
- The angiogram is characteristic showing dye leakage in early phases from the parafoveal retinal capillaries (Figures 5.13A to C)
- Late phases of the angiogram demonstrate the classic petalloid pattern of dye leakage with late staining of the optic nerve head.

REFERENCES

1. Schatz, HS, Burton T, Yannuzzi LA, et al, Interpretation of fundus fluorescein angiography. St Louis Mosby-Year Book; 1978.
2. Gass JDM. Stereoscopic Atlas of Macular Disease: Diagnosis and Treatment, 4th Ed. St Louis Mosby-Year Book; 1997.
3. Yannuzzi LA, Flower RW, Slakter JS. Indocyanine Green Angiography. Mosby Year Book, Inc 1997.
4. Guyer DR, Yannuzzi LA, Chang S, et al, Retina-Vitreous-Macula. WB Saunders Company, 1999.
5. Ryan, SJ. Retina 4th Ed. Elsevier, Inc. 2006.
6. Wilkinson CP, Ferris FL 3rd, Klein RE, et al. Global Diabetic Retinopathy Project Group. Proposed international clinical diabetic retinopathy and diabetic macular edema disease severity scales. Ophthalmology 2003; 110:1677-82.
7. Kylstra JA, Brown JC, Jaffe GJ et al. The importance of fluorescein angiography in planning laser treatment of diabetic macular edema. Ophthalmology 1999; 106:2068-73.
8. Early Treatment Diabetic Retinopathy Study Research Group. Fluorescein angiographic risk factors for progression of diabetic retinopathy. ETDRS report number 13. Ophthalmology 1991; 98(5 Suppl):834-40.

9. Early Treatment Diabetic Retinopathy Study Research Group. Classification of diabetic retinopathy from fluorescein angiograms. ETDRS report number 11. Ophthalmology 1991; 98(5 Suppl):807-22.

10. Patz A, Finkelstein D, Fine SL, Murphy RP. The role of fluorescein angiography in national collaborative studies. Ophthalmology 1986; 93:1466-70.

11. Smith RT, Lee CM, Charles HC et al. Quantification of diabetic macular edema. Arch Ophthalmol 1987; 105:218-22.

12. Yannuzzi LA, Hope-Ross M, Slakter JS, et al. Analysis of vascularized pigment epithelial detachments using indocyanine green videoangiography. Retina 1994; 14:99-113.

13. Olsen TW, Feng X, Kasper TJ, et al. Fluorescein angiographic lesion type frequency in neovascular age-related macular degeneration. Ophthalmology 2004; 111:250-55.

14. Friedman SM, Margo CE. Choroidal neovascular membranes: reproducibility of angiographic interpretation. Am J Ophthalmol 2000;130:839-41.

15. Fernandes LH, Freund KB, Yannuzzi LA, et al. The nature of focal areas of hyperfluorescence or hot spots imaged with indocyanine green angiography. Retina 2002; 22:557-68.

16. Yannuzzi LA, Slakter JS, Gross NE, et al. Indocyanine green angiography-guided photodynamic therapy for treatment of chronic central serous chorioretinopathy: a pilot study. Retina 2003; 23:288-98.

17. Spaide RF, Hall L, Haas A, et al. Indocyanine green videoangiography of older patients with central serous chorioretinopathy. Retina 1996; 16:203-13.

18. Slakter JS, Yannuzzi LA, Guyer DR, et al. Indocyanine-green angiography. Curr Opin Ophthalmol 1995; 6:25-32.

19. Piccolino FC, Borgia L. Central serous chorioretinopathy and indocyanine green angiography. Retina 1994; 14:231-42.

20. Kitaya N, Nagaoka T, Hikichi T et al. Features of abnormal choroidal circulation in central serous chorioretinopathy. Br J Ophthalmol 2003; 87:709-12.

21. Cardillo Piccolino F, Eandi CM, et al. Photodynamic therapy for chronic central serous chorioretinopathy. Retina 2003; 23:752-63.

22. Yannuzzi LA, Negrao S, Iida T et al. Retinal angiomatous proliferation in age-related macular degeneration. Retina 2001; 21:416-34.

23. Nakajima M, Yuzawa M, Shimada H, Mori R. Correlation between indocyanine green angiographic findings and histopathology of polypoidal choroidal vasculopathy. Jpn J Ophthalmol 2004; 48:249-55.

24. Ciardella AP, Donsoff IM, Huang SJ, et al. Polypoidal choroidal vasculopathy. Surv Ophthalmol 2004; 49:25-37.

25. Ciardella AP, Donsoff IM, Yannuzzi LA. Polypoidal choroidal vasculopathy. Ophthalmol Clin North Am 2002; 15:537-54.

26. Yannuzzi LA, Freund KB, Goldbaum M, et al. Polypoidal choroidal vasculopathy masquerading as central serous chorioretinopathy. Ophthalmology 2000; 107:767-77.

27. Yannuzzi LA, Wong DW, Sforzolini BS, et al. Polypoidal choroidal vasculopathy and neovascularized age-related macular degeneration. Arch Ophthalmol 1999; 117:1503-10.

28. Moorthy RS, Lyon AT, Rabb MF et al. Idiopathic polypoidal choroidal vasculopathy of the macula. Ophthalmology 1998; 105:1380-85.

29. Yannuzzi LA, Ciardella A, Spaide RF et al. The expanding clinical spectrum of idiopathic polypoidal choroidal vasculopathy. Arch Ophthalmol 1997; 115:478-85.

30. Spaide RF, Yannuzzi LA, Slakter JS, et al. Indocyanine green videoangiography of idiopathic polypoidal choroidal vasculopathy. Retina 1995; 15:100-110.

31. Yannuzzi LA, Sorenson J, Spaide RF, Lipson B. Idiopathic polypoidal choroidal vasculopathy (IPCV). Retina 1990; 10.1-8.

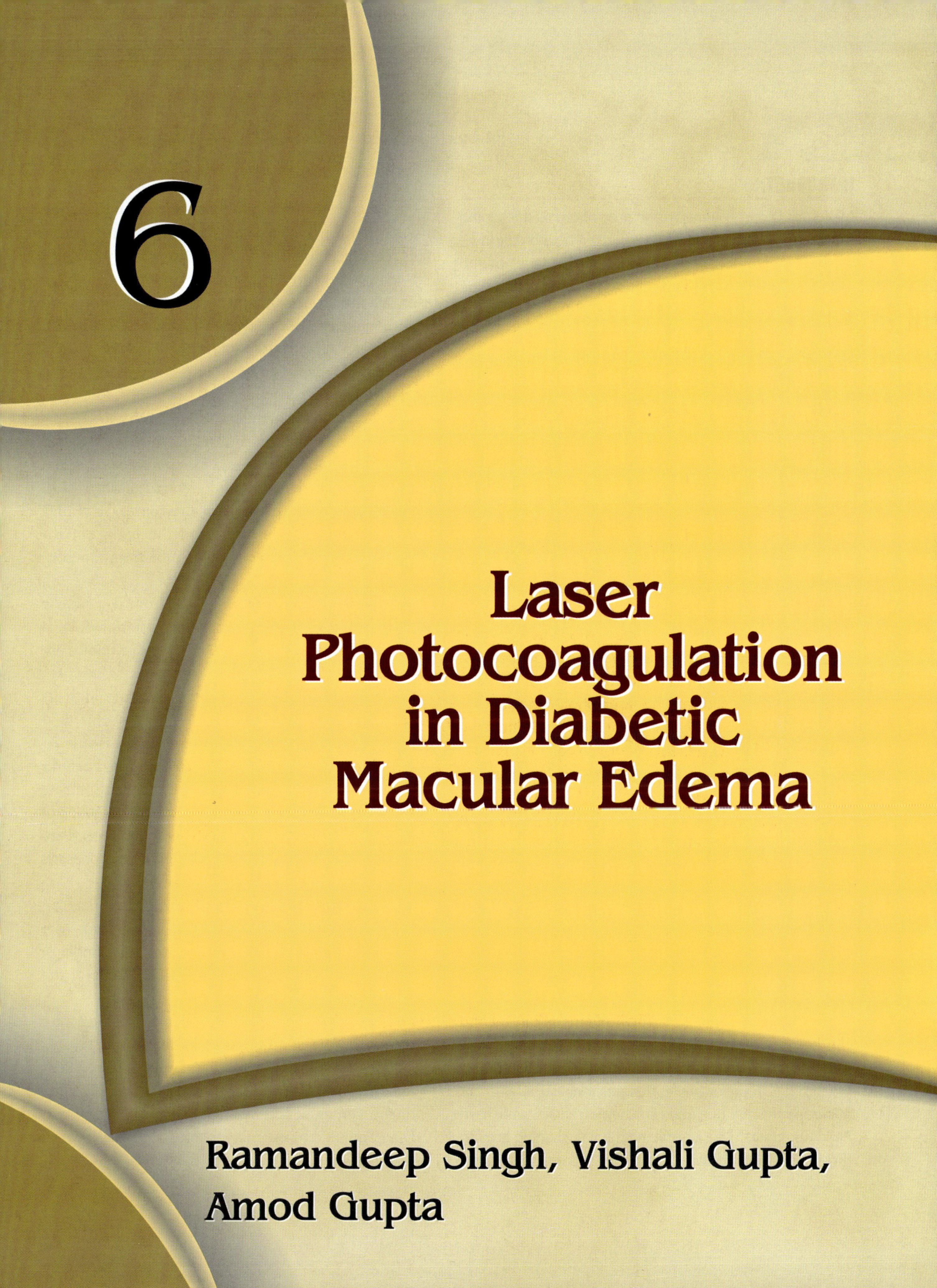

Laser Photocoagulation in Diabetic Macular Edema

Ramandeep Singh, Vishali Gupta,
Amod Gupta

INTRODUCTION

Macular edema is defined as an area of retinal thickening in the region of the macula. It is caused by a breakdown of the inner blood-retinal barrier at the level of the capillary endothelium. Diabetic macular edema is the most common cause of a moderate visual loss among diabetic patients.[1] The prevalence of diabetic maculopathy is more in older onset insulin dependent patients, i.e. NIDDM patients requiring insulin.[2] Diabetic maculopathy can be exudative, ischemic or of a combined nature.[3] The exudative component of maculopathy is amenable to treatment by laser.

Macular edema may be the first symptom of diabetic retinopathy and may be associated with proliferative or non-proliferative (background) retinopathy. Patients can develop diabetic macular edema any time during the course of diabetic retinopathy. As the severity of overall retinopathy increases, the proportion of *eyes* with macular edema also increases: 3% in eyes with mild non proliferative diabetic retinopathy (NPDR), 38% with moderate to severe NPDR, and 71% with proliferative diabetic retinopathy (PDR).[4] However, 50% of the drop in vision can be reduced by laser photocoagulation.

According to the Early Treatment Diabetic Retinopathy Study (ETDRS) all patients with clinically significant macular edema should undergo laser treatment as this reduces the risk of moderate visual loss by around 50%.[5,6] Moderate visual loss was defined by ETDRS as doubling of visual angle, i.e. drop of 15 or more letters on ETDRS charts or drop of 3 or more lines of Snellen equivalent. The ETDRS[7] demonstrated that focal laser photocoagulation for clinically significant macular edema (CSME), reduces the risk of moderate visual loss.

CLINICAL FEATURES

Diagnosis of the diabetic macular edema is clinical and can be done using either a contact lens or one of the high power +78D or +90D non-contact lens. Clinically, the findings in patients with diabetic macular edema are microaneurysms, dot and blot hemorrhages, and hard (lipid) exudates. These result in retinal thickening around the macula and cystic changes in the macula. Lipid exudation occurs from the leaking microaneurysms, which may surround the leaking microaneurysms in the form of a ring, known as circinate retinopathy. Histologically, lipids may accumulate in the outer plexiform retina first followed by scattering in all layers of the retina in severe cases. When exudates occupy the foveal area, they result in permanent visual loss even if the exudates reabsorb after treatment. In advanced stages, there may be atrophy of the pigment epithelium or fibrous changes within the central foveal area.

Macular edema is broadly classified into two groups, i.e. focal macular edema and diffuse macular edema.

Focal macular edema is a localized area of retinal thickening and leakage is predominantly from foci of microaneurysms, seen clearly on fluorescein angiography. The hard exudates derived from the leaky microaneurysms separate the edematous area from the non-edematous area.

Diffuse macular edema occurs from a generally dilated capillary bed throughout the posterior pole. It is a bilaterally symmetrical condition. Hard exudates are less common in this variety.

Certain systemic factors may contribute with its exacerbation and amelioration such as, systemic fluid retention due to cardiovascular or renal disease or systemic hypertension including pre-eclampsia. Features on fluorescein angiography include enhanced visibility of the capillary bed due to either increased caliber of some of the capillaries or widening of the intercapillary spaces. Formation of cystoid spaces in the late phase is more common in diffuse macular edema.

According to ETDRS,[8] diabetic macular edema can be graded into CSME, which is a good indicator for laser photocoagulation. It includes any of the following findings:
1. Retinal thickening at or within 500 microns of the center of the macula.
2. Hard exudates at or within 500 microns of the center of the macula, with adjacent retinal thickening
3. An area or areas of retinal thickening at least 1 disk area in size, part of which is within 1 disk diameter of the center of the macula.

Diagrammatic representation of CSME is shown in Figures 6.1A to C.

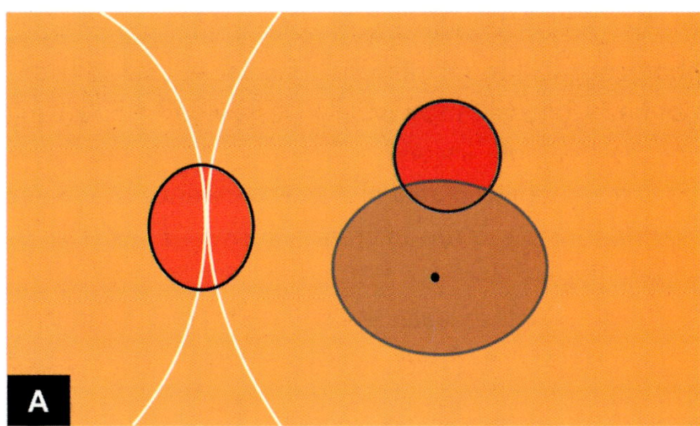

FIGURE 6.1A: Retinal thickening at or within 500 microns of the center of the macula

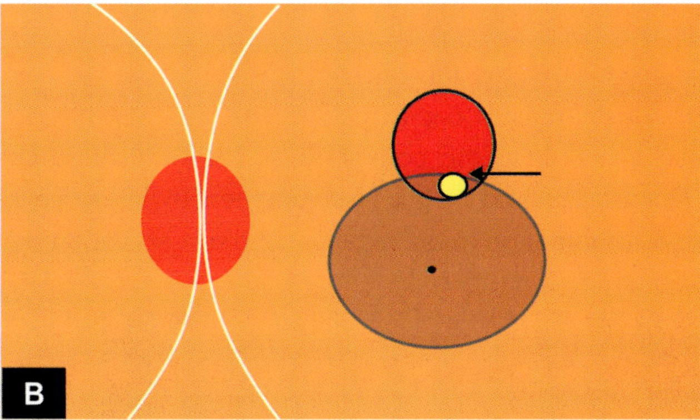

FIGURE 6.1B: Hard exudates at or within 500 microns of the center of the macula (arrow), with adjacent retinal thickening

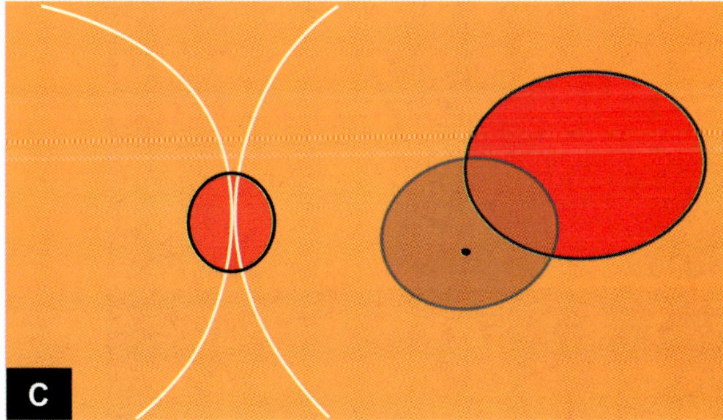

FIGURE 6.1C: An area of retinal thickening at least 1 disk area in size, part of which is within 1 disk diameter of the center of the macula

ANCILLARY TESTING

COLOR STEREOFUNDUS PHOTOGRAPHS

Color stereo photographs at various intervals can be compared to document the disease progression or regression.

FUNDUS FLUORESCEIN ANGIOGRAPHY

Fundus fluorescein angiography aids in the diagnosis and treatment of diabetic macular edema. Fluorescein angiography permits direct visualization of vascular changes i.e. areas of focal leakage from microaneurysms or diffuse leakage of fluid from abnormal capillary dilatation, increased capillary permeability, and areas of capillary non-perfusion. This is used to guide laser therapy when indicated.

Drawbacks to using fluorescein angiography include its invasive nature, expensive equipment, and adverse reactions. Allergic-type reactions to sodium fluorescein have been reported in patients undergoing fluorescein angiography, although the incidence is rare.

In general, the use of fluorescein angiography is limited to determining method of detection of areas amenable to laser photocoagulation in diabetic macular edema.

OPTICAL COHERENCE TOMOGRAPHY

The conventional two-dimensional imaging techniques including fundus photograph and fluorescein angiography give a topographical view of the retina. Optical coherence tomography (OCT) captures reflected light from retinal structures to create a cross-sectional image of the retina, which is comparable to histological sections as seen with a light microscope. On OCT, diabetic macular edema could be differentiated into 5 distinct patterns. These include:

1. Sponge like retina.
2. Cystoid macular edema.
3. Serous retinal detachment.
4. Foveal tractional retinal detachment.
5. Taut posterior hyaloid membrane.

Optical coherence tomography is used in diabetic macular edema for quantitative measurement of macular thickness and subjective analysis of the foveal architecture, which allows a precise and reproducible way to monitor macular edema. Optical coherence tomography is gradually replacing most methods of assessing the treatment response to any treatment modality for diabetic macular edema. Optical coherence tomography also helps us differentiate between tractional and non-tractional varieties of diabetic macular edema.

LASER TREATMENT

The goal of macular laser photocoagulation for diabetic macular edema is to limit vascular leakage through focal laser or grid laser burns. The ETDRS compared outcomes in eyes assigned to either deferral of macular laser photocoagulation or immediate treatment for clinically significant diabetic macular edema.[1] Results showed that laser photocoagulation reduced the risk of vision loss by 50% in patients with CSME. [7]

Argon green (514 nm) and frequency doubled Nd: YAG (532 nm) lasers are the lasers of choice in the management of diabetic macular edema. Green light is absorbed well by melanin and hemoglobin. The closure is believed to be mediated by the thermal effect following absorption of laser radiation by chromophobes in the inner retinal layer. Over next few months, after the closure of leakage areas, the excess fluid begins to reabsorb into the surrounding tissues and eventually the hard exudates will be reabsorbed.

The ETDRS gave the treatment strategy of laser photocoagulation for diabetic macular edema and this has been followed most widely worldwide.[1, 9] Following are the treatable lesions:

1. Discrete points of retinal hyperflourscence or leakage (Most of these are microaneurysms) (Figures 6.2A and B).
2. Areas of diffuse leakage within the retina, i.e. microaneurysms, diffusely leaking retinal capillary bed (Figures 6.3A and B), and
3. Thickened retinal avascular zone (Figures 6.4A and B).

Treatment of the macula ideally is guided by the fluorescein angiography, which helps to detect areas of focal leakage, diffuse leakage from dilated capillary bed and areas of capillary non-perfusion. Local laser treatment for CSME consists of direct focal treatment (Figures 6.2A and B), grid laser treatment to diffuse leaks, or a combination (modified grid) of direct and grid laser treatment (Figures 6.3A and B).

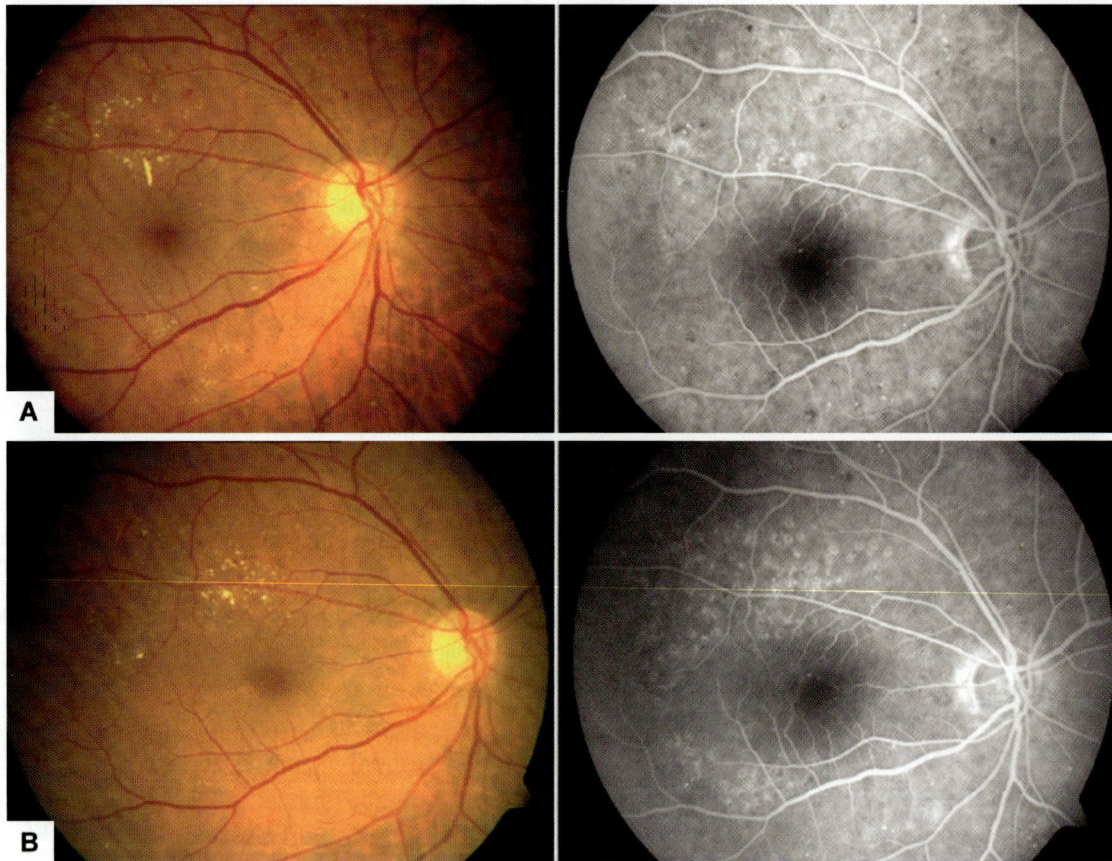

FIGURES 6.2A and B: Focal leaks greater than 500 μ from the center of the macula causing retinal thickness/or hard exudates (A and B; Pre- and post-laser).

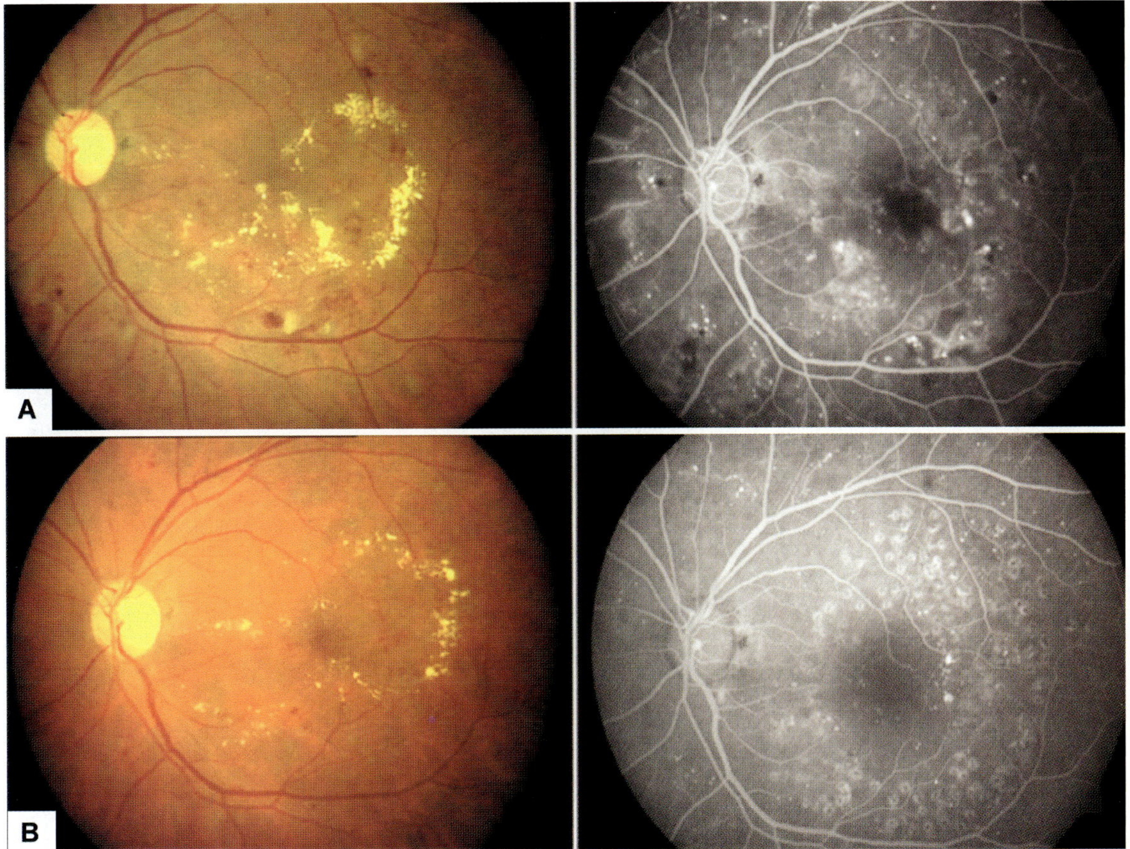

FIGURES 6.3A and B: Areas of diffuse leakage from extensive number of microaneurysms and capillary leak (A and B; Pre- and post-laser).

TECHNIQUE

FOCAL LASER PHOTOCOAGULATION

All focal leaks located between 500 to 3000 μm are treated directly with 50 to 100 μm spots at 0.1 second duration to produce grayish whitening of the micro-aneurysms. Focal lesions located within 300 to 500 μm from the center of the macula are treated if the visual acuity is $\leq$ 20/40 and the clinician believes the laser photocoagulation of these areas will not damage the remaining foveal capillary network.

GRID LASER PHOTOCOAGULATION

All areas of diffuse leakage extending from arcade to arcade are treated with 50 to 200 μm spot size placed one burn width apart, at 0.1 second duration. The laser burns must be at least 500 μm away from the foveal center and 500 μm away from the disk margins. Avascular zones (Figure 6.5), other than the normal avascular foveal zone are also treated. Laser is done in a C-shaped manner within the vascular arcades and avoiding the area of the papillomacular bundle.

A repeat flourescein angiography is to be done at 3 months. Laser for any persisting focal or diffuse leak is augmented accordingly (Figures 6.6A and B).

In case the macular edema still persists one should contemplate other treatment modalities such as intra-vitreal steroid injection or vitrectomy. Some authors suggest grid laser photocoagulation once the edema subsides with intravitreal steroid injection.

SUB-THRESHOLD DIODE LASER IN DIABETIC MACULAR EDEMA

Lee and Olk [10] have shown that subthreshold diode laser

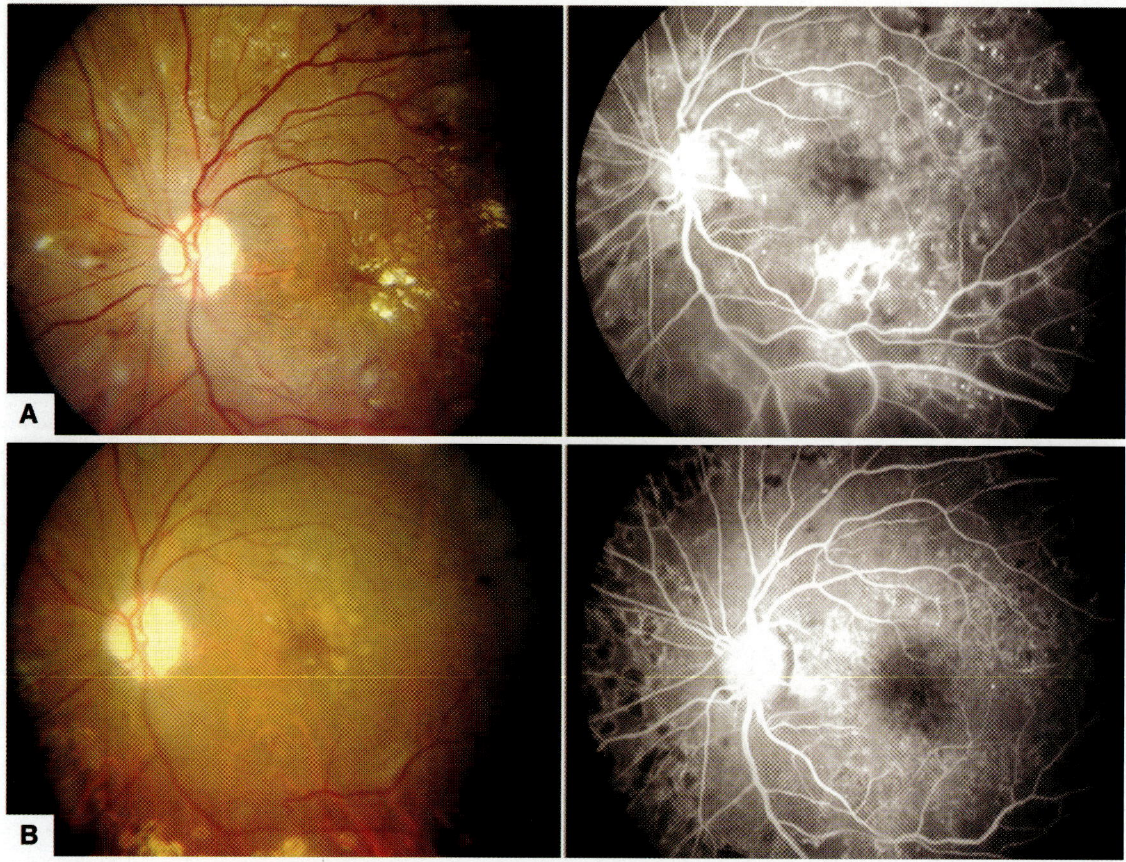

FIGURES 6.4A and B: Thickened retinal avascular zone other than foveal avascular zone (A and B; Pre- and post-laser).

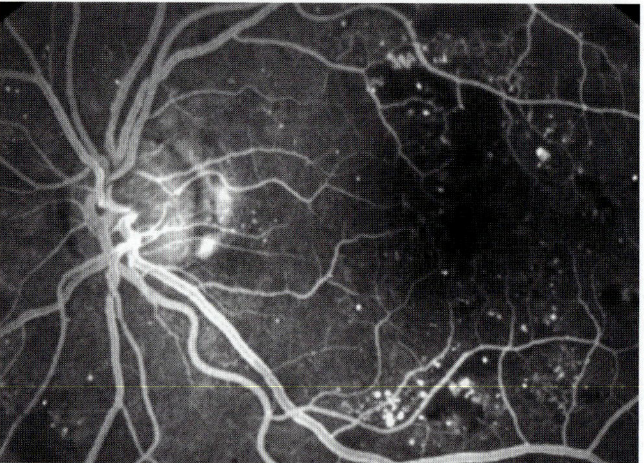

FIGURE 6.5: Enlarged foveal avascular zone.

burns are as effective as creating visible burns in the treatment of macular edema in diabetic maculopathy. In this method, the authors first noted the amount of power needed to produce a visible burn on the nasal retina with the spot size and duration constant at $125\,\mu$ and 200 msec respectively. Subsequently, the duration was reduced to 100 msec and it was then used as the treatment burn parameter. The only disadvantage that they found with this approach is that the macular edema needed a longer duration to resolve.

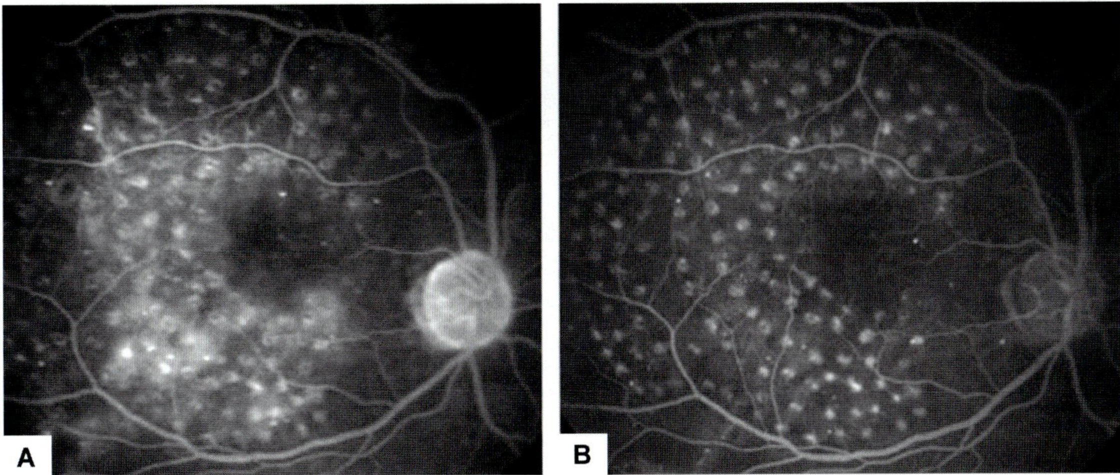

FIGURES 6.6A and B: Laser augmentation (A and B; Pre- and post-treatment).

REFERENCES

1. Early treatment diabetic retinopathy study report no. 1: Photocoagulation of iabetic macular edema. Arch Ophthalmol 1985; 103:1796-1806.
2. Klein R, Barbara EKK, Moss SE, Davis DM, DeMets DL. The Wisconsin Epidemiologic study of diabetic retinopathy IV. Diabetic macular edema. Ophthalmology 1984; 91:1464-74.
3. Mandi D, Conway R, Joseph ELK. Diabetic maculopathies. Diagnosis and treatment. Ophthalmology clinics of North America 1993; 6:213-29.
4. Klein R, Klein BEK, Moss SE. Visual impairment in diabetes. Ophthalmology 1984; 91:1-8
5. Early Treatment Diabetic Retinopathy Study Research Group. ETDRS Report no.1. Photocoagulation for diabetic macular edema. Arch Ophthalmol 1985; 103:1796-1806.
6. Early Treatment Diabetic Retinopathy Study Research Group. ETDRS Report no.4. Photocoagulation for diabetic macular edema. Int Ophthalmol Clinics 1987: 27;265-72.
7. Early Treatment Diabetic Retinopathy Study Research Group. Treatment techniques and clinical guidelines for photocoagulation of diabetic macular edema: Early Treatment Diabetic Retinopathy Study. Report Number 2. Ophthalmology 1987; 84:761–74.
8. Early Treatment Diabetic Retinopathy Study Research Group. Early photocoagulation for diabetic retinopathy. ETDRS report number 9. Ophthalmology 1991; 98:766–85.
9. Lee CM, Olk RJ. Modified grid laser photocoagulation for diffuse macular edema: Long-term visual results. Ophthalmology 1991; 98:1594-1602.
10. Lee CM, Olk RJ. Diabetic Retinopathy: Practical management. 1st ed. Philadelphia, JB Lippincott 1993; 88-93.

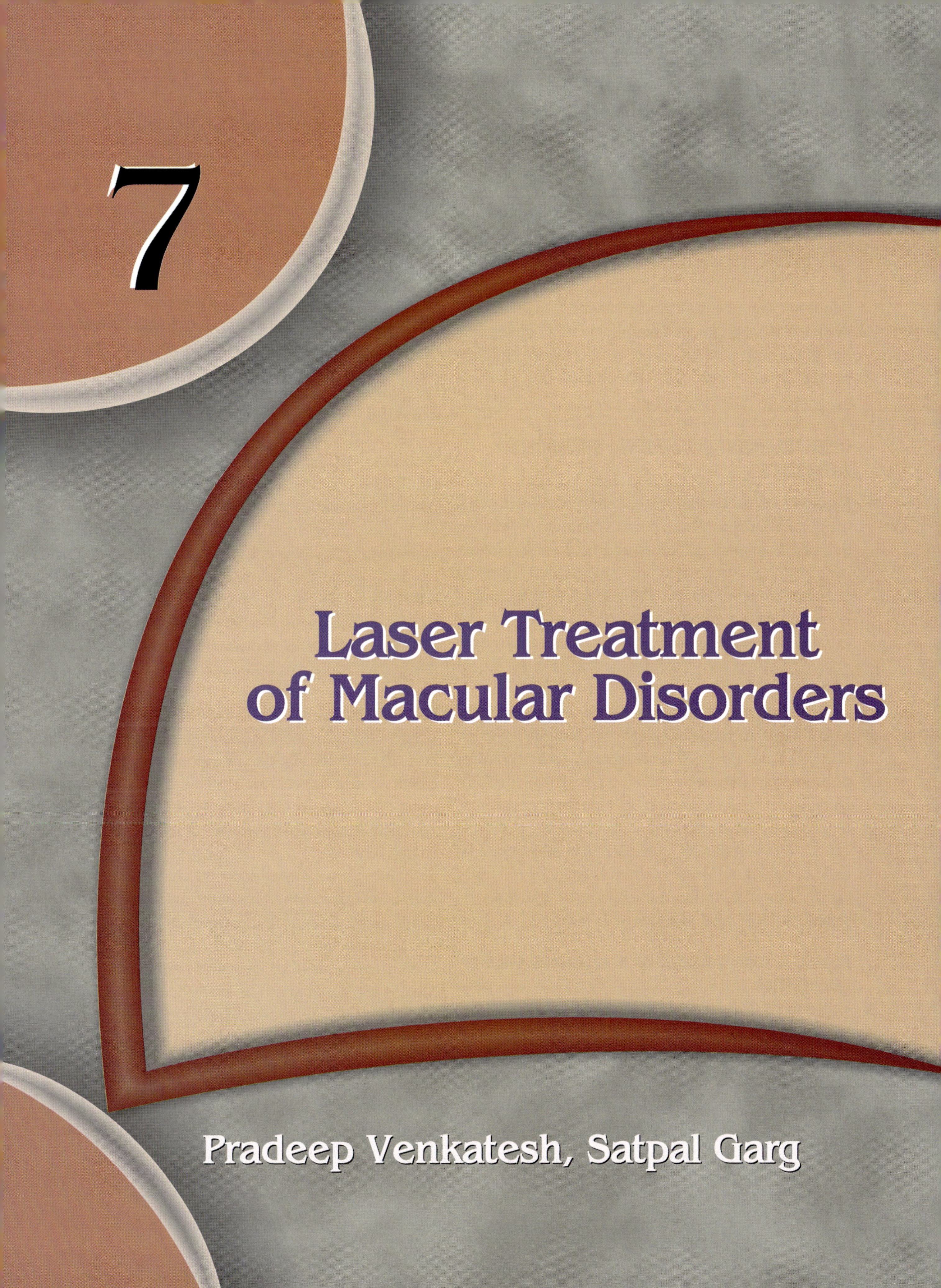

Laser Treatment of Macular Disorders

Pradeep Venkatesh, Satpal Garg

INTRODUCTION

Macular disorders have a propensity to result in visual loss. Some like central serous retinopathy have a favorable natural history while others like diabetic retinopathy lead to significant visual loss. Laser treatment has become an important ingredient in the treatment of most retinal disorders. Though lasers have a high safety index, it is prudent to have clear cut guidelines about when and how to treat these conditions. This chapter provides the guidelines for laser treatment.

LASER TREATMENT IN CHOROIDAL NEOVASCULAR MEMBRANES

Ingrowth of choroidal vessels between the Bruch's membrane and the retinal pigment epithelium or between the retinal pigment epithelium and neurosensory retina is an abnormal occurrence and is designated choroidal neovascularization. Based on the location of the membrane in relation to the foveal center, the ingrowth be extrafoveal, juxtafoveal or subfoveal. When the posterior edge of a choroidal membrane lies beneath the foveal center it is designated subfoveal, when it is between 1μ and 199μ as juxtafoveal and between 200μ and 2500μ as extrafoveal membrane. Apart from age-related macular degeneration there are other conditions in which choroidal neovascular ingrowth may occur. These include pathological myopia, angioid streaks, chorioretinal scar (after choroiditis, laser burn, and cryotherapy), presumed ocular histoplasmosis syndrome and idiopathic choroidal neovascularization. Visual loss from choroidal membranes results from exudative detachment of the macula, subretinal bleed and diskiform scar formation.

CHOROIDAL NEOVASCULARIZATION IN AGE-RELATED MACULAR DEGENERATION

Two forms of age-related macular degeneration (AMD) are recognized, the atrophic type and the exudative type. Although the exudative form of AMD is less common, it accounts for majority of the visual loss. Unlike visual loss from the atrophic type, visual loss from the exudative form may be retarded by early detection and appropriate laser treatment. Patients having subfoveal membranes present with complaints of metamorphopsia and decrease of vision. The natural course of exudative AMD is rapidly detrimental to vision and so does not allow for any delay in treatment. Studies have shown that when the time interval from development of symptoms to presentation is less than 2 weeks, 80% of choroidal membranes are treatable. This decreases to 40 and 10% when the time delay is 2 months and 4 months respectively. Though the overall incidence of subfoveal choroidal neovascularization still remains unknown in age-related macular degeneration, choroidal vascular ingrowth accounts for 90% of the severe, irreversible visual loss.[1-3]

On fundus examination, several manifestations of exudative AMD may be seen, either alone or in conjunction. These lesions include confluent soft drusen, subretinal membrane, serous or hemorrhagic retinal pigment epithelial detachment, subretinal hemorrhage or exudation, retinal pigment epithelial tears and diskiform scarring. When choroidal neovascular membrane (CNV) arises from the edge of a patch of geographic atrophy, signs of retinal pigment epithelial atrophy are also in evidence. Choroidal neovascular membrane may be identified in some patients by yellow-green diskoloration, elevation of the overlying neurosensory retina using a slit beam and by pigment proliferation above the membrane. If the overlying pigment epithelium is atrophic, one may be able to appreciate the subretinal vascular network. Diskiform scar appears as a yellow-white fibrovascular tissue that is usually quite irregular appreciably elevated and there is associated distortion of the overlying retinal architecture.

In a large majority of patients however the choroidal membrane may not be easily evident on fundus biomicroscopy due to the presence of overlying serous retinal detachment or hemorrhage. In such situations several techniques like fluorescein angiography, indocyanine angiography and optical coherence tomography could be employed to detect and localize the membrane or detect overlying fluid accumulation.

Fluorescein angiography is still the most important diagnostic modality in the management of choroidal neovascularization. It is emphasized that the angiogram must not be older than 72 hours for planning laser treatment of these membranes. This is because the vascular ingrowth has a high growth rate (6 to 10μ/ day)

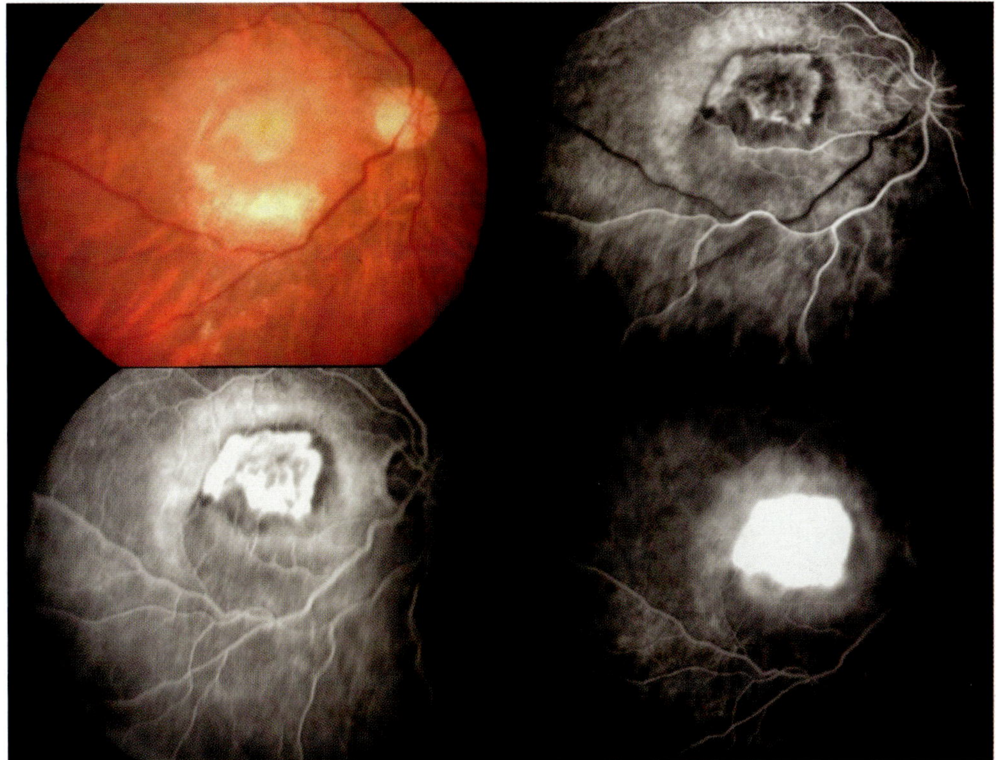

FIGURE 7.1: Classic choroidal neovascular membrane in a patient with exudative age-related macular degeneration. Well-defined neovascular net is clearly visible in the early angiographic frame.

and may rapidly increase in extent.[4-6] Based on fluorescein angiographic features choroidal membranes are classified as classic, occult and mixed lesions. The mixed lesions are further subdivided into predominantly classic and minimally classic lesions. Classic lesions have a characteristic lacy pattern in early phases of the angiogram with leakage in the late phases (Figure 7.1). The margins are well defined except in the late phases when it may become obscured by leakage of the dye. The extent and location of such membranes are easily defined.[7] A well-defined lesion is one in which the entire 360 degrees of the boundaries is well demarcated. If the entire boundary is not well demarcated, then the lesion is poorly defined. The lesion components that can be a hindrance to a full definition of the lesion are blood, hyperplastic pigment, fibrous tissue and retinal pigment epithelial detachments.

Occult membranes include two patterns of hyperfluorescent lesions, fibrovascular pigment epithelial detachments and late leakage of an undetermined source (Figures 7.2A andB). The former usually appears 1 to 2 minutes after injection of the dye and may have either well defined or poorly defined margins. It corresponds to fibrovascular tissue associated with the choroidal neovascularization. The latter is seen in the late phases and the source of leakage cannot be determined by evaluating the early or mid phases of the angiogram. Occult membranes may be more evident if up to 10-minute frames are obtained and studied during fluorescein angiography. Other features that may be evident on fluorescein angiography are blocked fluorescence from subretinal hemorrhage or pigment clumping, fibrovascular or serous pigment epithelial detachments, retinal pigment epithelial tear and drusenoid retinal pigment epithelial detachment. Fluorescein angiography is also necessary during follow-up of a patient who has undergone laser photocoagulation for choroidal neovascularization. Lesions are defined as persistent or recurrent based on the angiography features at 6 weeks and subsequent 3 monthly follow-ups.

Simultaneous or sequential indocyanine green (ICG) angiography may be helpful in defining a choroidal

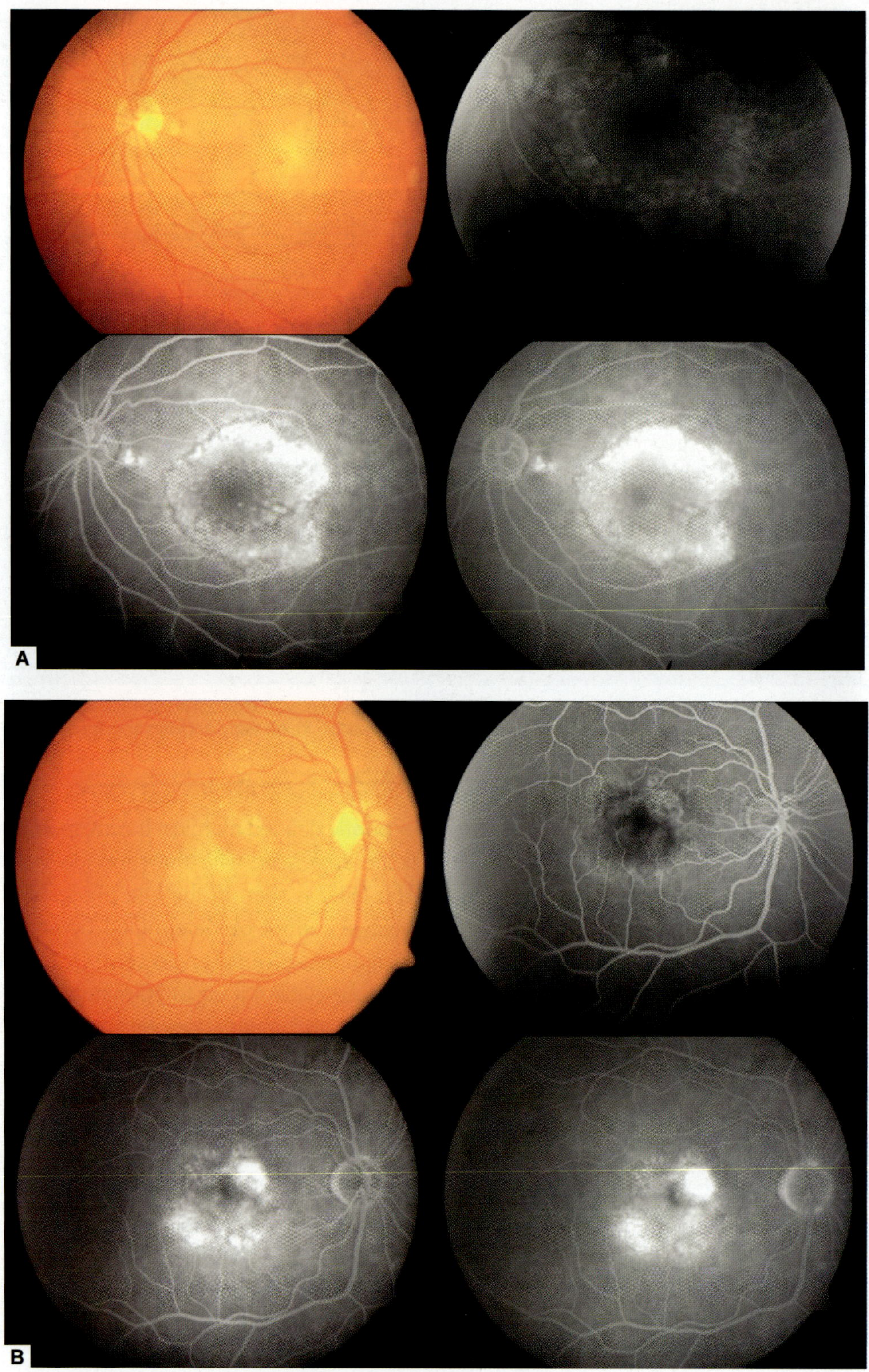

FIGURES 7.2A and B: Fibrovascular pigment epithelial detachment, one subtype of occult choroidal neovascularization (A) and late leakage of unknown origin, the other subtype (B).

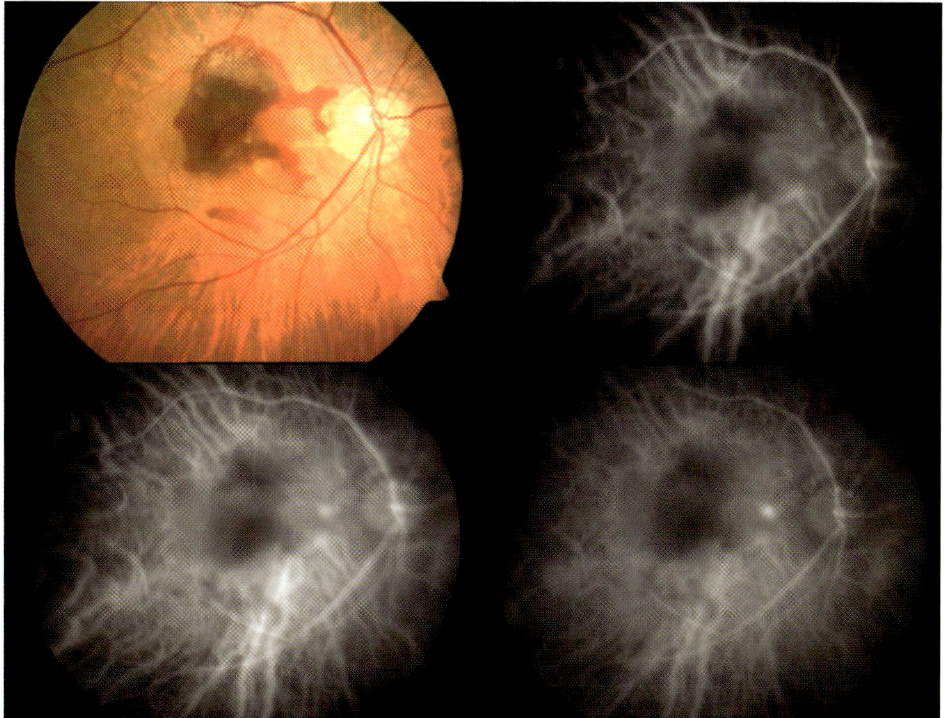

FIGURE 7.3: Indocyanine green angiography showing 'hot-spot' in a patient with choroidal neovascularization and subretinal hemorrhage.

neovascular membrane better in patients with occult neovascular membranes. About one-third of these patients may develop a focal hot spot or plaque lesion on ICG angiography (Figure 7.3).

The ideal treatment in choroidal neovascular membranes would be one that selectively and permanently eradicates the 'ingrowth' without causing any collateral damage to the surrounding normal retina. This objective is yet to be realized. Modalities that destroy the membrane more effectively cause significant collateral damage while those that decrease this damage, result in only transient regression of the membrane. Hence, all available laser modalities have advantages and disadvantages and help in preventing severe visual loss to varying extent.

The goal of treatment is only to reduce the risk of additional visual loss. Restoration of vision occurs only rarely with all modalities of treatment. Hence success is usually defined in terms of stabilization of vision.

Laser modalities that have been more extensively evaluated and which are currently accepted as having varying degrees of benefit are conventional laser therapy, photodynamic therapy and transpupillary thermotherapy. Herein we diskuss conventional laser treatment and provide the rationale and steps of a new technique that has been evaluated and reported by us using the diopexy probe.[8]

Conventional (Direct) Laser Treatment

Direct treatment using conventional laser systems may still be the modality of choice for treating patients with extrafoveal choroidal neovascular membranes. However when this method is used for subfoveal lesions, there are significant limitations and disadvantages. Conventional laser treatment for subfoveal membranes is effective in only a small percentage of cases (10%-15%) that have a well-defined CNV with distinct margins and wherein the size of the membrane is less than 3.5 MPS (Macular Photocoagulation Study) disk areas. The disadvantages of direct laser treatment are several and include an immediate, significant fall in central vision and the evolution of a dense central scotoma. The risk of recurrence following treatment of subfoveal choroidal neovascularization by laser photocoagulation is also high. Nevertheless, studies have shown that the beneficial effect of laser treatment becomes appreciable after a 2-year follow-up period. The MPS study has reported that while 47% of patients with subfoveal CNV who were not treated with laser lost 6 or more lines of visual acuity from baseline, the corresponding figure in the laser treated group was 22% at the end of 3-year follow-up.[9, 10] The MPS also reported treatment benefit following conventional treatment in patients with juxtafoveal, extrafoveal and new subfoveal recurrent choroidal neovascular membranes.[11-14]

Pretreatment evaluation includes slit lamp biomicroscopy, fundus photography, and a good quality fluorescein angiography, not more than 72 to 96 hours old and optical coherence tomography. Patient must be told about the nature of his disease, available treatment options, possible risk-benefit issues and an informed consent must be obtained. The desired result of focal direct photocoagulation is total obliteration of the neovascular membrane.

The membrane is first delimited by moderate intensity non-confluent laser spots extending to atleast $100\mu m$ into the surrounding normal retina. Subsequently, intense confluent burns are applied to the membrane per se until uniform whitening is observed (Figures 7.4 and 7.5). A 532 nm frequency doubled YAG laser, argon blue green or argon green laser can be used. Argon laser is avoided while treating juxtafoveal membranes, as there is higher risk of collateral damage from xanthophyll absorption. A feeder vessel, if present, should also be treated. Most patients can be treated under topical anesthesia. Pressure on the globe during treatment has been reported to improve results and also decrease the risk of laser-induced bleeding.[15] Synopsis of the treatment parameters for direct treatment of choroidal neovascular membranes is depicted in Table 7.1. Thereafter patient is asked to follow-up every 2 to 3 months at least until a year, with a repeat fluorescein angiography at every visit. Avoiding aspirin and lifting of heavy objects until regression of new vessels occur, has been advised by MPS, as these are thought to increase the risk of bleeding.[16] Follow-up angiograms have been advised at 1, 3 and 6 weeks to

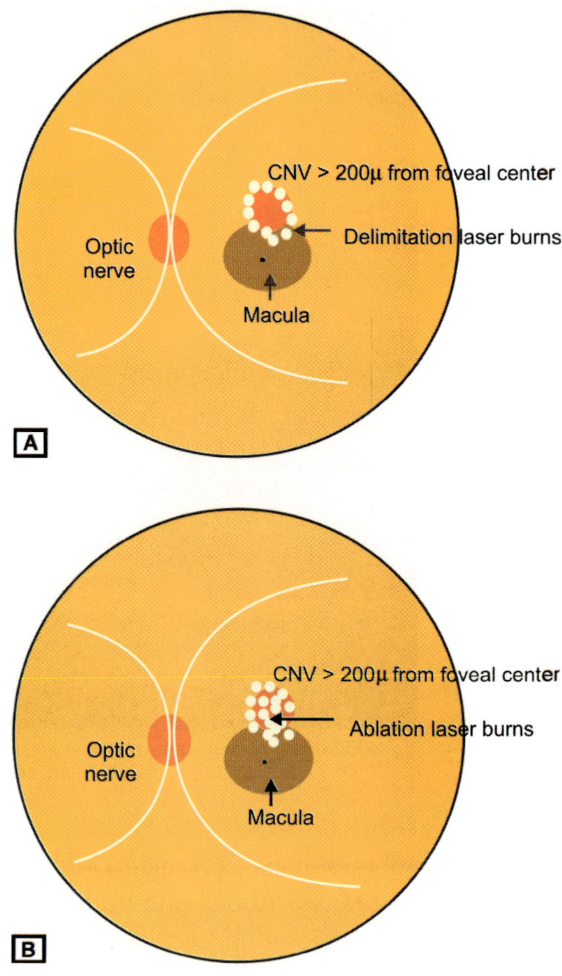

FIGURES 7.4A and B: Diagrammatic representation of treatment technique for managing choroidal neovascularization using conventional laser. The perimeter of the membrane is first demarcated (A) followed by direct laser of the entire membrane (B).

identify incomplete treatment, persistence and new recurrent lesions.[17] Results of conventional laser treatment reported in literature following long-term studies are given in Table 7.2.

Feeder Vessel Treatment

Feeder vessel treatment was advocated by the macular photocoagulation study report. However, identification of such vessels was very rare due to technical limitations inherent in the fluorescein angiographic systems available in the last decade and earlier. With the advent of high speed ICG angiography and good resolution digital

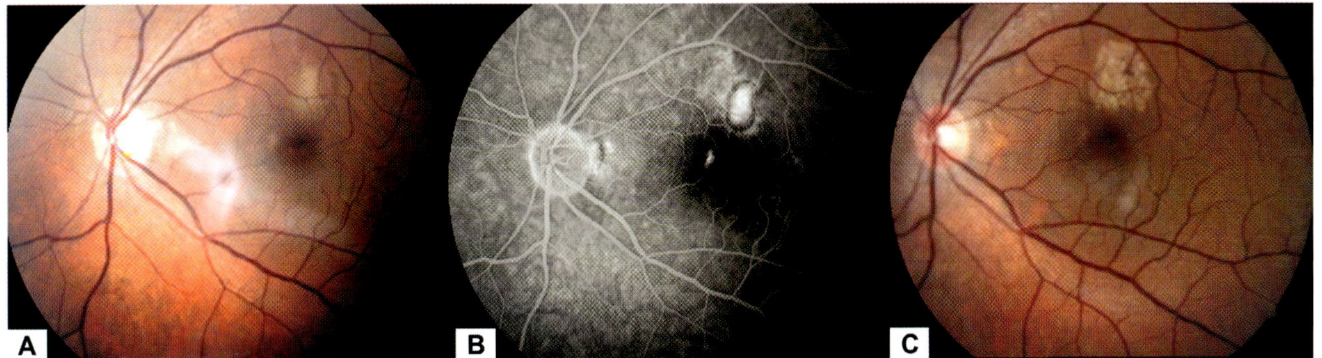

FIGURES 7.5A to C: Pre-laser clinical photograph, late phase angiographic frame and immediate post-laser photograph of a treated extrafoveal choroidal neovascularization using the conventional technique.

Table 7.1: Treatment parameters for focal laser of choroidal neovascular membrane in age-related macular degeneration

Type of CNV	Characteristics	Border	Membrane	Treatment area
Extrafoveal	Spot-size Time Intensity	100μ -200μ 0.1-0.2 sec Moderate	200μ 0.2-0.5 sec Intense	100μ beyond hyperfluorescence on fluorescein angiography
Juxtafoveal	Spot-size Time Intensity	200μ 0.2-0.5 sec Moderate	200μ 0.2-0.5 sec Intense	Confined to hyperfluorescence on fluorescein angiography
Subfoveal	Spot-size Time Intensity	200μ 0.2 sec Intense	200μ 0.2-0.5 sec Intense	Confined to hyperfluorescence on fluorescein angiography

Table 7.2: Results of focal laser treatment of choroidal neovascular membrane in age-related macular degeneration

Extrafoveal CNV

Severe visual loss	No laser	With laser
• 1 year	41%	24%
• 3 years	63%	45%
• 5 years	64%	46%
• Recurrence at 1 year: 75%		

Juxtafoveal CNV: Severe visual loss at 1 year
- No laser   45%
- With laser   31%
- Recurrence at 1 year: 22%

Subfoveal CNV: at 2 years (> 6 line loss)
- No laser   37%
- With laser   20%

monitors, identification of feeder vessels has been reported to become easier.

A feeder vessel is an afferent choroidal arteriole that directly supplies the choroidal neovascular net. Most feeder vessels are about a hundred to 100,000 μ long. Some neovascular nets may have more than one feeder vessel. It is usually visible only for a second or so during circulation of the dye in the initial phases. High speed ICG allows visualization of these vessels as images can be captured at a rate of 30 to 40 frames per second. The learning curve for capture and detection of these vessels has been reported to be about one year for those with no experience in retinal diseases. After one year there is said to be good inter and intra observer reproducibility.[18]

Feeder vessel treatment has been attempted with several available laser wavelengths.[19, 20] Most reported has been with the multi-pulse 810 nm diode laser and microburst yellow laser. After superimposing the feeder vessel image onto a good quality retinal image, a 75 to 200 μ laser spot is placed on an extrafoveal path of the feeder vessel. Multiple pulses are applied for a total of 400 to 1200 pulses. The duration of each pulse is 100 ms and inter-pulse interval is 100 to 200 ms. The laser power varies from 150 to 1000 mW. Authors of this report considered the treatment to be controlled and incremental and hence resulting in minimal collateral damage. They also advice that repeat high speed ICG be performed within 72 hours in case of classic membranes and retreat if complete closure is not detected. During a follow-up of 6 months they found that only 18% of 31 patients treated by feeder vessel method had lost 3 or greater lines of vision compared to double this percent in patients who had not received treatment. Limitations of this method other than the difficulty in detecting feeder vessels are the risk of reperfusion and occurrence of hemorrhages following laser.

Trans-scleral Diode Laser Photocoagulation

Choroidal neovascular membranes may be considered more as an aberrant ingrowth of the choriocapillaris beneath the retinal pigment epithelium and/or into the subretinal space. The initiating factor seems to be a full-thickness dehiscence or breach in the Bruch's membrane. In addition it has been reported that there is a dilatation of the choroidal arteries in the submacular area on choroidal angiography in a significant number of patients with age-related macular degeneration.[21] They also suggested that such rigid, dilated arteries might cause increased pressure in the submacular choriocapillaris, which predisposes to the occurrence of exudative pigment epithelial detachment and choroidal neovascularization.

It is well established that the laser-tissue interaction during photocoagulation is largely pigment dependent and this is true even in the treatment of choroidal neovascular membranes. Hence it is important to know the pattern of pigment distribution within the choroid. Histopathological studies have shown that pigment density in the choroid increases towards the outer choroid and that the primitive choroid (choriocapillaris and medium sized vessels) has little or no pigment.[22] This is certainly a disadvantage in the laser treatment of choroidal neovascular membranes by the conventional trans-retinal route.

The above factors could explain the unsatisfactory results of trans-retinal laser delivery in patients with subfoveal choroidal neovascular membranes. By this route, the retinal pigment epithelium absorbs a large portion of the laser energy with resulting damage to the adjoining outer retina. Due to this there is an immediate and significant decrease in vision following treatment. It has been demonstrated that there is also a concurrent thrombotic occlusion of choriocapillaris following this form of laser delivery.[23] However, it has also been reported that when the laser energy delivered is moderate, there is a gradual repair of choriocapillaris, and within 30 days it is almost normal again as circulation is restored.[24, 25] With intense photocoagulation there is an increased risk of causing breaks in Bruch's membrane that in turn may initiate choroidal neovascularization.[26,27] The above two reasons could possibly explain the high rate of recurrence and failure following the conventional route of laser treatment in patients with subfoveal choroidal neovascular membranes.

Taking the above factors into consideration, we evaluated the safety and effectiveness of transscleral diode laser photocoagulation using the diopexy probe (Figure 7.6) in patients with choroidal neovascular membranes secondary to age-related macular degeneration. We believed that the transscleral route does not cause direct and intense absorption of laser energy by the retinal pigment epithelial cells. Hence, the outer retinal elements are preserved and there would be no immediate and sustained decrease in visual acuity. Experimental studies have indicated that anatomic vascular connections observed on vascular casts cannot provide normal flow rates after occlusion of proximal, adjacent arteries (as

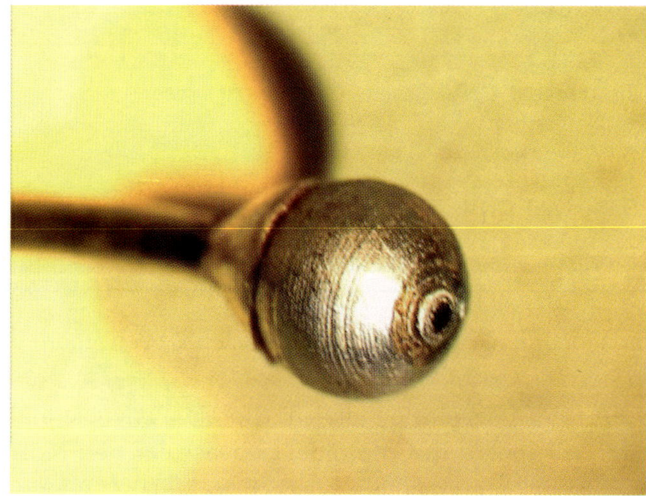

FIGURE 7.6: Diopexy probe used for trans-scleral diode laser photocoagulation of exudative age-related macular degeneration.

occurs by trans-scleral laser delivery) and that functionally, choroidal blood flow is segmented and the precapillary arterioles act as end-arterioles.[28] The destruction of larger, proximal choroidal vessels does cause nonperfusion of large areas of the choroid but it has been reported that the resulting chorioretinal damage is much smaller than expected.[29-31]

In our study, 18 eyes of 18 patients with subfoveal choroidal neovascularization were included for treatment. All patients were treated within 72 hours of obtaining the fluorescein angiogram. Patients were admitted in hospital. Laser was done in operation theatre under aseptic conditions and peribulbar anesthesia. Lateral rectus muscle was bridled after doing a limited peritomy temporally. Intermuscular septa on either side were dissected and then the diopexy probe was introduced. With the laser set to continuous mode a test burn was applied to the temporal retina and the time taken to obtain a visible burn was noted. The probe was then gently guided to the submacular area under indirect ophthalmoscopy control. After this treatment burn was applied to the region of the membrane as determined by site of leakage seen on early phase of fluorescein angiography. To help in localizing the site of leakage during the treatment, the treating surgeon would refer to a large size printout of the early fluorescein angiographic phase of the eye affixed to the operation theatre wall. End point was taken as either appearance of a visible reaction or four times the time taken to obtain the test burn. Accuracy of the spot was established by indirect ophthalmoscopic visualization throughout the treatment period. Conjunctiva was closed with 6-0 vicryl interrupted sutures and subconjunctival gentamicin plus dexamethasone injection given.

At 12 weeks, 81.5% patients showed stabilization (+/– 5 letters) in letter visual acuity score and one patient showed improvement (gain of more than five letters) in letter visual acuity score. Reading speed levels, contrast

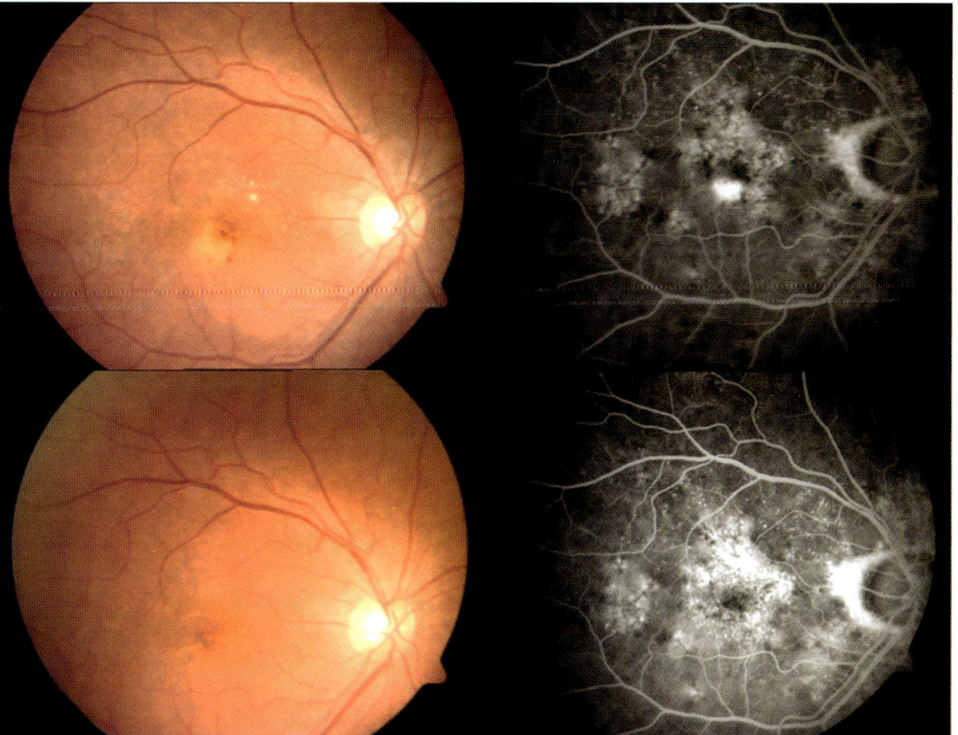

FIGURE 7.7: Pre- and post-laser images of a patient with a small choroidal neovascularization secondary to age-related macular degeneration treated by one session of trans-scleral diode laser photocoagulation. Vision improved from 3/60 (20/400) to 6/24 (20/80). A new membrane was noted at 9 months of follow-up. As newer modalities are now available, the patient chose re-treatment by transpupillary thermotherapy. Response to transpupillary thermotherapy has been poor and the patient has a vision of 2/60 at the most recent follow-up.

requirement were found to be similar to pre laser level at 3 months follow-up. At 12 weeks, moderate fluorescein leakage was seen in 1 eye, minimal leakage was seen in 5 eyes, absence of leakage was seen in 10 eyes and progression was seen in two eyes.[8] Some examples of choroidal neovascular membranes treated using the diopexy probe are shown in Figure 7.7.

Though the outcome of treatment in our clinical trial showed that trans-scleral diode laser treatment has a beneficial effect in curtailing the growth of subfoveal choroidal neovascular membranes there were some limitations. These limitations included, non-randomized nature of the study with no controls, small number of eyes treated, lack of ICG evaluation in all cases and the short follow-up period.

CHOROIDAL NEOVASCULARIZATION FROM NON-AMD ETIOLOGY

Choroidal neovascular membranes may also be seen in patients with myopia, ocular histoplasmosis syndrome, parafoveal telangiectasis, intraocular tumors, angioid streaks, choroidal rupture, and choroidal scars from inflammation or following laser and without any known cause (idiopathic). The same topographic and angiographic patterns probably apply to choroidal membranes in this group of patients as well. Interestingly most of these lesions, unlike in AMD, are usually subfoveal and well defined. Results of controlled trials for non-AMD associated CNV are available for idiopathic cases, myopia and ocular histoplasmosis syndrome only. For most other conditions there are isolated case reports or case series.

Parafoveal Telangiectasis

Parafoveal telangiectasis is dilation of the capillary bed confined predominantly to the parafoveal region and that is congenital/ developmental or acquired in origin. Age at presentation and unilateral or bilateral involvement depends on the type of parafoveal telangiectasis. Most patients do not have any other concurrent ocular or systemic pathology. The commonest type of parafoveal telangiectasis belongs to group 2 (bilateral and acquired). Patients usually present between the 4th-6th decade with blurring or distortion of vision. Some may develop subretinal neovascularization and serous exudation.

Fundus examination reveals subtle to mild dilation of the involved capillaries. The area of involvement may vary from just one clock hour to as large as 1 to 2 disk areas. Right-angled venules draining the area may be present along with hyperplasia of the adjacent retinal pigment epithelium. A few small refractile deposits also may be present. On fluorescein angiography the involved vessels appear dilated and ectatic with absent to minimal leakage in the late phases.

Laser photocoagulation for parafoveal telangiectasis is indicated only in a limited number of patients who develop serous detachment or subfoveal neovascularization as most telangiectasias are situated close to or within the foveal avascular zone.[32, 33] Rarely, patients with type 1 telangiectasis and associated macular edema or lipid exudation may also benefit from grid laser photocoagulation. Prophylactic treatment is not recommended, as they are also known to undergo spontaneous regression. Successful treatment of CNV using transpupillary thermotherapy in a patient with parafoveal telangiectasis is shown in Figure 7.8. Figure 7.9 shows resolution of exudates in a patient with type 1 telangiectasis and 6/12 (20/40) vision following grid laser photocoagulation.

Osseous Choristoma

Osseous choristoma of the choroid, also called choroidal osteoma, is a very rare and unusual form of intraocular ossification. Histopathologically a plaque like bony lesion replaces the choroid in a focal area. Clinically, choroidal osteoma is unilateral in 75% of patients and tends to be located in the peripapillary or juxtapapillary area and may extend into the macular region. The size of the lesion may range from 2 mm to 22 mm and the elevation, 0.5 mm to 2.5 mm. Early in its evolution they may have an orange color similar to a choroidal hemangioma. The most characteristic feature is the double optic nerve sign on ultrasonography. Several complications have been reported in association with choroidal osteoma such as sensory detachment and choroidal neovascular membrane. The latter is said to occur in about a third of patients with choroidal osteoma.[34] Because of thinning and degeneration of the overlying retinal pigment epithelium treating such choroidal neovascular membranes might

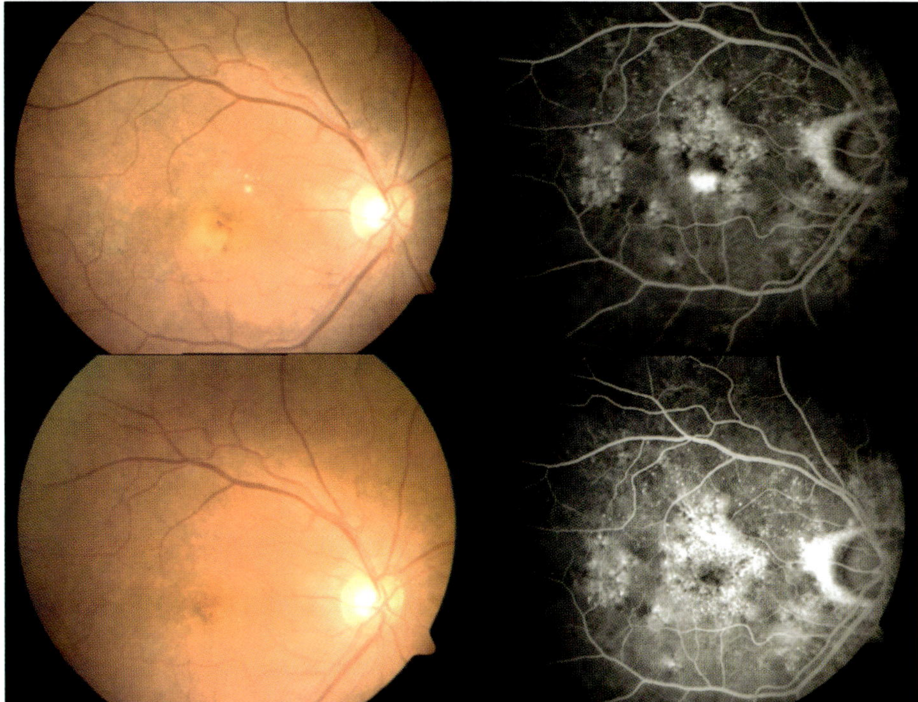

FIGURE 7.8: Pre- and post-treatment images of a patient with subfoveal choroidal neovascularization secondary to idiopathic parafoveal telangiectasis type 2B. Pre-transpupillary thermotherapy vision was counting finger at 1 meter; post-treatment vision has remained 6/18 (20/60) at 12 months follow-up. No recurrence has been observed so far.

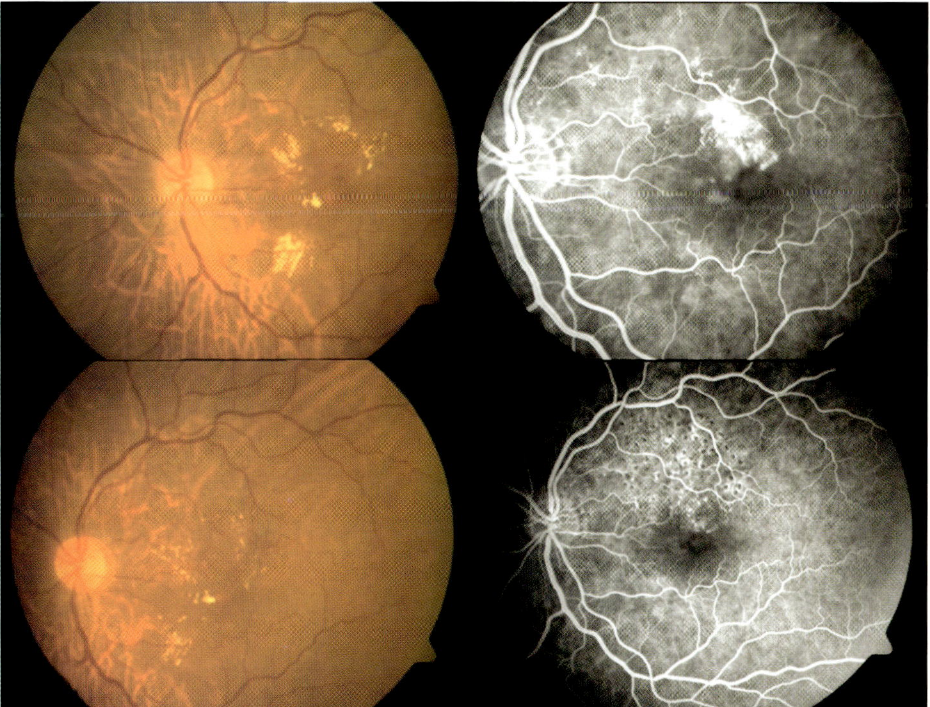

FIGURE 7.9: Pre- and post-treatment images of a patient with parafoveal telangiectasis, type 1B. Decrease in exudation and angiographic leakage is evident post-laser. Vision has stayed 6/9 (20/30).

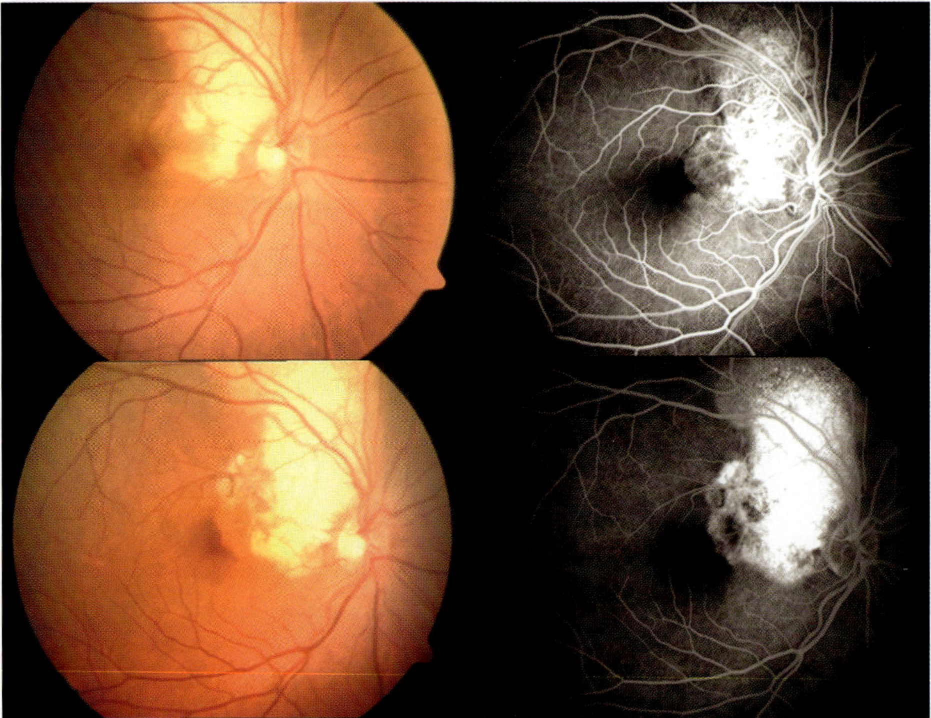

FIGURE 7.10: Pre- and post-treatment images of choroidal neovascularization along the foveal margin of a lady in the fourth decade with choroidal osteoma. Treatment of this juxtafoveal membrane was with conventional 532 nm laser. Pretreatment vision was 6/9 (20/30). Post-treatment vision has remained 6/12 (20/40) at 18 months of follow-up. No recurrence has been observed.

require multiple sessions.[35, 36] Successful treatment of a juxtafoveal CNV in a patient with choroidal osteoma treated using 532 nm laser is shown in Figure 7.10.

Myopia

Myopia may also present with a CNV most commonly involving the macular and peripapillary region. Choroidal neovascularization may give rise to transudate or frank hemorrhage. The hemorrhage per se or hyperplasia of retinal pigment epithelial cells or both may give rise to a dark spot called the Foster-Fuch's spot. Over time, these spots disintegrate and become surrounded by a halo of fundus atrophy. These lesions occur earlier in patients with higher myopic errors and affects 5 to 10% of the myopic population with axial length of 26.5 mm or more.[37] Such a lesion is seen more commonly in females. Unlike choroidal membranes in AMD, in myopia the choroidal membranes are smaller and also leak less profusely (due to loss of choriocapillaris) on fluorescein angiography.

Laser photocoagulation for choroidal membranes in highly myopic eyes has remained ill defined in the absence of large, randomized studies. While some have reported favorable outcome even in the absence of any treatment, others have shown better response following laser treatment.[38, 39] Recurrence is reported to occur in more than half of the treated patients and is said to carry a poor visual prognosis.[40-42] Successful treatment of myopic CNV is shown in Figures 7.11 and 7.12.

Choroidal Rupture

Choroidal rupture is a manifestation of blunt trauma to the eye. The rupture may involve the entire thickness of the choroid or may be partial. In the acute phase immediately after trauma, the rupture may be obscured by a subretinal or localized choroidal bleed. In the resolved stages, choroidal rupture has a typical appearance. Depending on the type of force involved in producing the rupture, there are two types of choroidal rupture: direct and indirect. Direct ruptures are situated anterior to the

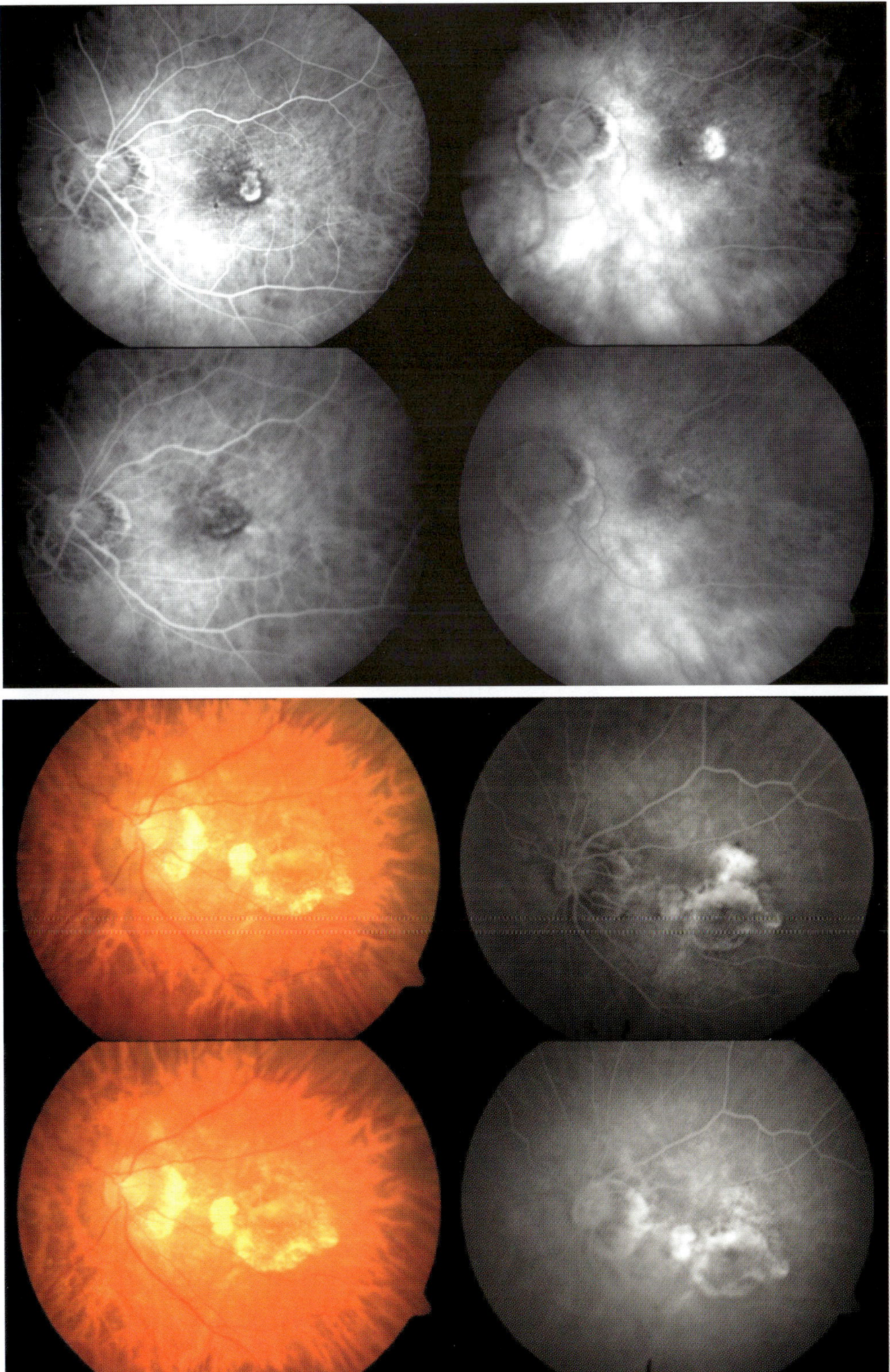

FIGURES 7.11 and 7.12: Pre-treatment images and post-laser photograph of two patients with choroidal neovascularization secondary to myopia. Resolution of choroidal neovascular membrane following transpupillary thermotherapy is evident in both.

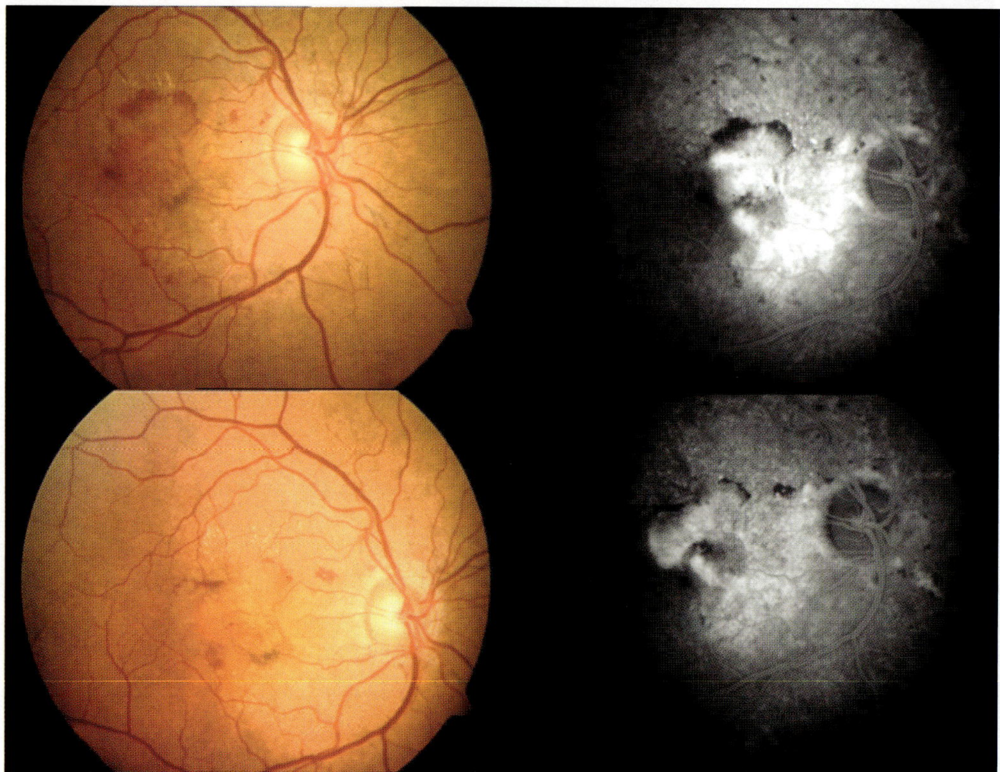

FIGURE 7.13: Development of new choroidal neovascular membrane is evident 6 months after this patient with subfoveal choroidal neovascular membrane secondary to angioid streaks was treated with transpupillary thermotherapy.

equator and are parallel to the ora while indirect ruptures are more common and situated behind the equator. They are usually located in the posterior pole, have a crescentric yellow-white appearance with the concavity towards the disk and a variable width. Choroidal ruptures may result in loss of vision if they involve the fovea. Choroidal neovascularization is a component of the healing process but usually regresses spontaneously without any sequelae. Sometimes however, laser photocoagulation may become necessary.[43-44]

Angioid Streaks

Angioid streaks are ophthalmoscopically visible cracks in the Bruch's membrane. It may be an incidental finding or may be a manifestation of a systemic disease such as pseudoxanthoma elasticum, Ehlers-Danlos syndrome, Paget's disease, senile elastosis and sickle cell disease. They usually develop in the 2nd or 3rd decade and are not seen in children. Ophthalmoscopically they appear as dark brownish-red, irregular streaks surrounding the optic disk and extending radially for a variable distance from there. They may show branching and may closely mimic the large retinal vessels. Angioid streaks may occur in association with other fundus features such as peau de orange appearance, choroidal neovascularization and diskiform macular degeneration. Choroidal neovascularization is reported to occur in 70% of patients with angioid streaks. Successful treatment of CNV in patients with angioid streaks has been reported with conventional laser and photodynamic therapy.[45-48] Appearance of 'new' choroidal neovascular membrane in a patient treated with transpupillary thermotherapy is shown in Figure 7.13. Immediate post-laser photograph of another patient treated with conventional laser is shown in Figure 7.14. Figure 7.15 shows resolution of CNV associated with angioid streaks following conventional laser.

Idiopathic Choroidal Neovascularization

Idiopathic choroidal neovascularization has a clearly documented role of laser in literature.[49, 50] However,

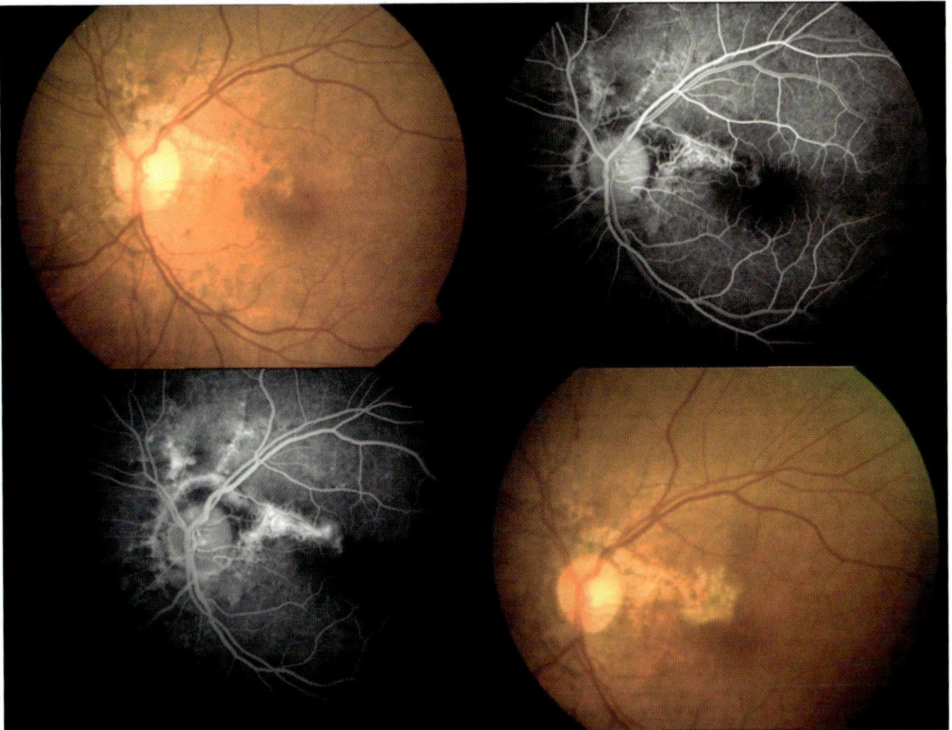

FIGURE 7.14: Pre-treatment images and immediate post-laser photograph of a patient with juxtafoveal choroidal neovascular membrane secondary to angioid streaks.

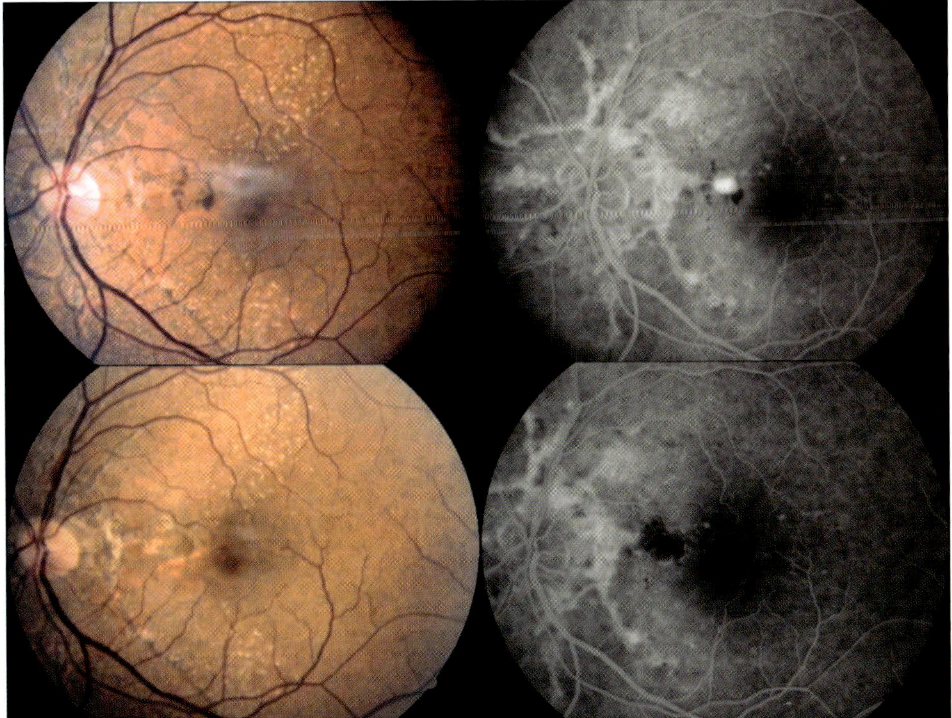

FIGURE 7.15: Resolution of extrafoveal choroidal neovascularization is evident in these pre- and post-laser images of another patient with angioid streaks treated with conventional laser.

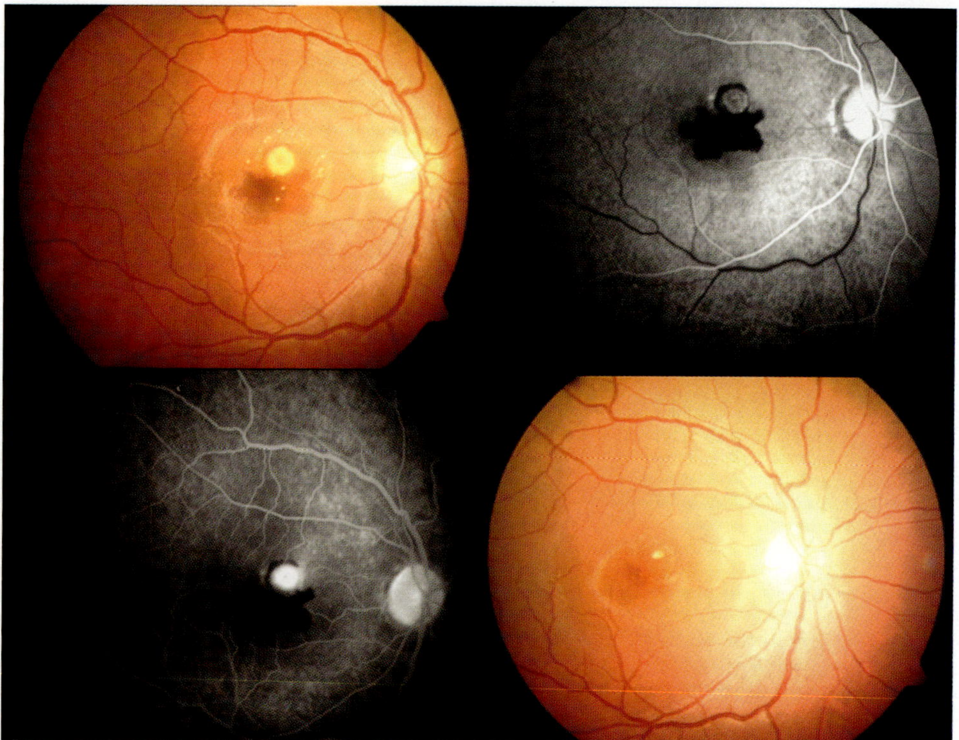

FIGURE 7.16: Resolution of choroidal neovascular membrane following transpupillary thermotherapy can be appreciated in these pre- and post-treatment images of a young patient with idiopathic choroidal neovascular membrane.

caution is recommended in treating and interpreting results of theses studies as they have a more favorable natural history compared to other forms of choroidal neovascularization.[51] Regression of choroidal neovascular membrane following transpupillary thermotherapy is shown in Figure 7.16.

Choroidal Neovascularization Secondary to Several Inflammatory Disorders

Choroidal neovascularization secondary to several inflammatory disorders such as sarcoidosis, toxoplasmosis, syphilis, serpiginous choroidopathy, Vogt Koyanagi Harada's disease and presumed ocular histoplasmosis syndrome, has been reported. [52, 53] Except for presumed ocular histoplasmosis syndrome wherein large trials have been conducted, all others have been reports of single or series of cases.[54] Success with conventional laser has been reported in several of these reports. Adjunctive use of systemic corticosteroids is poorly defined in the management of post-inflammatory choroidal neovascular membranes.

Idiopathic Polypoidal Choroidal Vasculopathy

Idiopathic polypoidal choroidal vasculopathy was first described by Yannuzzi in 1982 and currently several cases of atypical wet AMD are now being recognized as idiopathic polypoidal choroidal vasculopathy following superior imaging provided by ICG angiography.[55, 56] The disease is reported to be more common in women of pigmented races, including Asians. Hypertension is a significant risk factor.[57] Idiopathic polypoidal choroidal vasculopathy usually presents between the 5th and 7th decade and is characterized by typical orange red, branching vascular pattern having bulbous endings with or without associated sero-sanguinous detachment. The usual location is the peripapillary or macular area. Laser photocoagulation is reported to decrease the exudation and risk of hemorrhage. The overall role of laser is however still poorly defined.

Retinal Angiomatous Proliferation

Retinal angiomatous proliferation is a more recently recognized variant of wet AMD wherein neovascular elements bud from within the retina, grow into the subretinal space and may later anastomose with choroidal neovascular elements.[58]

PROPHYLACTIC LASER FOR DRUSEN

Drusen are considered predisposing lesions for the evolution of visually threatening complications in elderly patients. This is more so in patients with large and confluent drusen. Since the advent of laser therapy it has been observed that laser burns applied to the macula cause a decrease in the number and size of drusen.[59, 60] However, the actual benefit of such treatment in reducing the risk of later stages of AMD is still not clear. Some reports have shown definite decrease in the size of drusen but have also cautioned that such treatment may increase the risk of developing choroidal neovascularization. Two randomized trials have evaluated prophylactic treatment outcomes with argon green laser and diode laser in patients with drusen.[61, 62] While both these trials showed drusen reduction, the argon laser study cautioned against the possibility of increased risk of CNV development in treated patients at 3-year of follow-up.

The Complications of Age-related macular degeneration Prevention Trial (CAPT) is an ongoing NEI sponsored, multicentric, prospective, randomized study evaluating the effectiveness and safety of low energy argon green laser burns in patients with at least 10 large drusen in both eyes. One eye is being treated (only by CAPT certified ophthalmologists) and the fellow eye is used as control. The Prophylactic Treatment of AMD Study (PTAMD) is another ongoing trial evaluating the safety and efficacy of sub-threshold diode laser photocoagulation in patients with drusen.

LASER IN RETINAL VEIN OCCLUSION

Occlusion of the retinal venous system occurs more commonly than arterial occlusions. Systemic hypertension is the commonest association and thrombus formation the most likely mechanism.[63] Other factors include compression of the vein by extraluminal factors and inflammation of the vessel wall. Retinal vein occlusions may occur in the elderly (common) as well as in young individuals. Apart from hypertension, other risk factors for retinal venous occlusion are open angle glaucoma, male gender and hyperopic refractive error. Diabetes mellitus does not seem to be an independent risk factor although these occlusions are seen frequently in diabetics. Some of the other associations are cardiovascular and peripheral vascular disease, elevated serum cholesterol and lipids, lupus anticoagulant factor and hyperviscosity syndromes (polycythemia, Waldenstrom's macroglobulinemia). [64]

Venous occlusion of the retina may be incidentally detected or the patient may present with features of a sudden/rapid loss of vision (due to macular hemorrhage, vitreous hemorrhage) or a gradual blurring of vision (macular edema, macular ischemia, tractional detachment of the macula). The ophthalmoscopic appearance is dependent on the severity of occlusion and the size of vessel involved. Common to all is dilation and tortuosity of the vessels and intra-retinal hemorrhages in the corresponding quadrant. Rarely, cotton wool spots and arteriolar narrowing may be seen in severe occlusion of the central retinal vein. Optic disk edema is a common feature in central retinal vein occlusion. In later stages one may find disk and iris neovascularization, neovascularization elsewhere, venous-venous collaterals, opto-ciliary vessels at the disk, fibrous proliferation and traction on the retina.

Although there are several clinical features that help to distinguish ischemic from non-ischemic central retinal vein occlusion (Table 7.3), one criterion for making such a differentiation is fluorescein angiography. The ischemic index is calculated based on the extent of capillary non-perfusion evident on fluorescein angiography. Based on the ischemic index, central retinal vein occlusions into has been classified into three types:

i. Well perfused (42%),
ii. Very ischemic (43%), and
iii. Intermediate (15%).

An eye is considered to be very ischemic if the ischemic index is more than or equal to 50%. Even initially well-perfused eyes should be watched carefully during follow-up as some of these have been reported to become ischemic later on. The patients presenting with recent onset central retinal vein occlusion are classified as

Table 7.3: Differences between ischemic and non-ischemic central retinal vein occlusion

Features	Non-ischemic	Ischemic
Visual acuity	> 6/60	< 6/60
Afferent pupillary defect	< 0.3 log units	> 1.2 log units
Severity of hemorrhage	Not extensive	Extensive
Ischemic index	< 50%	> 50%
Electroretinography (b/a ratio)	> 1.0	< 1.0
Complications (NVI / NVG)*	Rare	Common

*NVI/NVG: Neovascularisation of iris / neovascular glaucoma

ischemic or non-ischemic variety so as to prognosticate and advice regarding follow-up.

A summary on approach to management of patients with branch retinal and central retinal vein occlusion are given in the Flow Charts 7.1 and 7.2 taking into consideration the Branch Vein Occlusion Study (BVOS) and the Central Vein Occlusion Study (CVOS).

MANAGEMENT OF BRANCH RETINAL VEIN OCCLUSION (BRANCH VEIN OCCLUSION STUDY RECOMMENDATIONS)

A high quality fluorescein angiogram depicting the retinal vascular characteristics should be obtained after the intraretinal hemorrhages have cleared (3-6 months). Capillary abnormalities such as macular edema, macular non-perfusion, and large segments of capillary non-perfusion (>5 disk diameters) are defined.

Treatment of Macular Edema

Fluorescein angiography based demonstration of cystoid macular leakage without capillary non-perfusion suggests that macular edema is the cause of visual loss. If the visual acuity is < 20/40 even after 3 months in such patients, which precludes spontaneous improvement seen in a sizeable number of patients, grid laser photocoagulation is advocated. Grid laser is done in the areas of capillary leakage essentially in the same way as that of a diabetic grid laser and is confined only to the area of angiographic

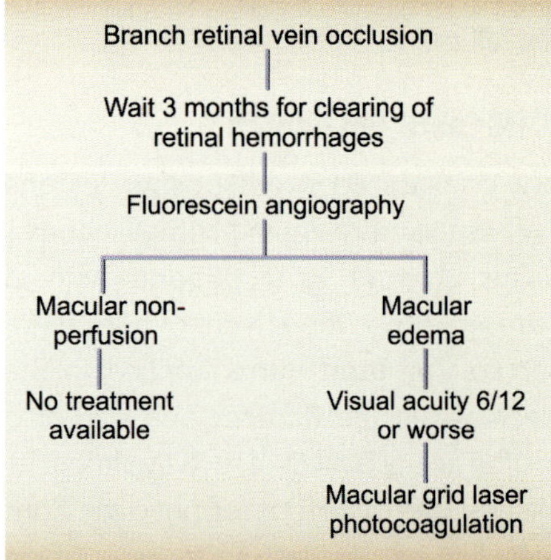

Flow chart 7.1: Algorithm for management of branch retinal vein occlusion

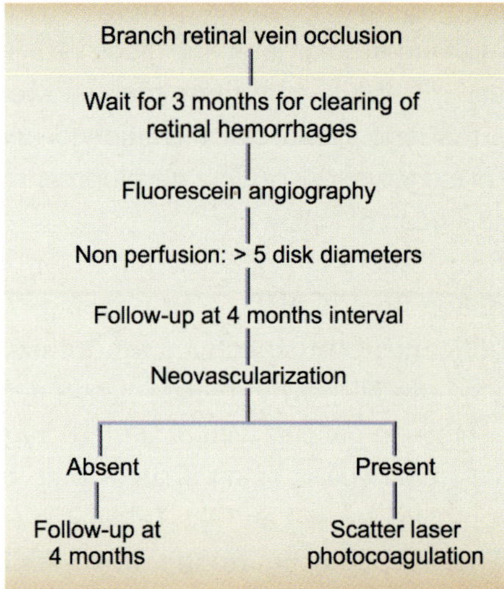

Flow chart 7.2: Algorithm for management of branch retinal vein occlusion

leakage (Figure 7.17). If macular ischemia explains the visual loss, there is no treatment. [65]

Treatment of Neovascularization

Patients showing >5 disk areas of capillary non-perfusion are followed at 4-monthly intervals for development of neovascularization. If new vessels are confirmed, laser photocoagulation in the involved quadrant will suffice. Medium white burns, 200 to 500 μm in diameter spaced one burn width apart, covering the entire area of non-perfusion, beyond two disk diameters from the center

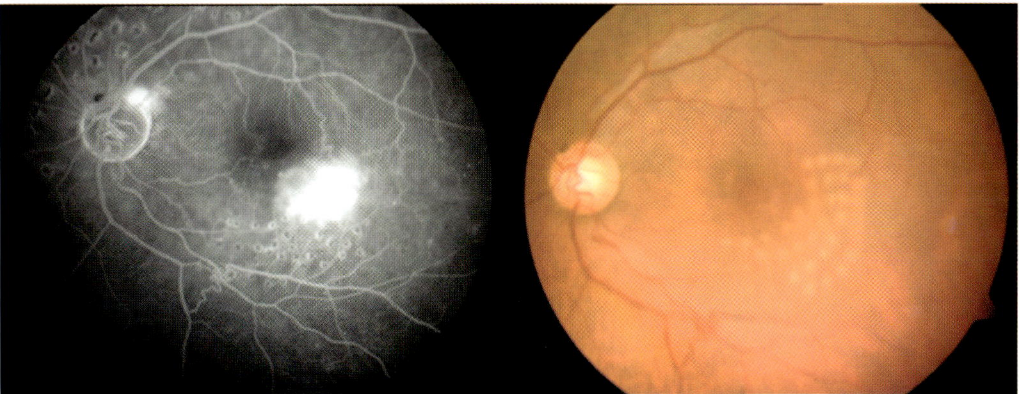

FIGURE 7.17: Immediate post-laser color photograph depicting strengthening of grid laser photocoagulation for persisting macular edema in an elderly patient with branch retinal vein occlusion.

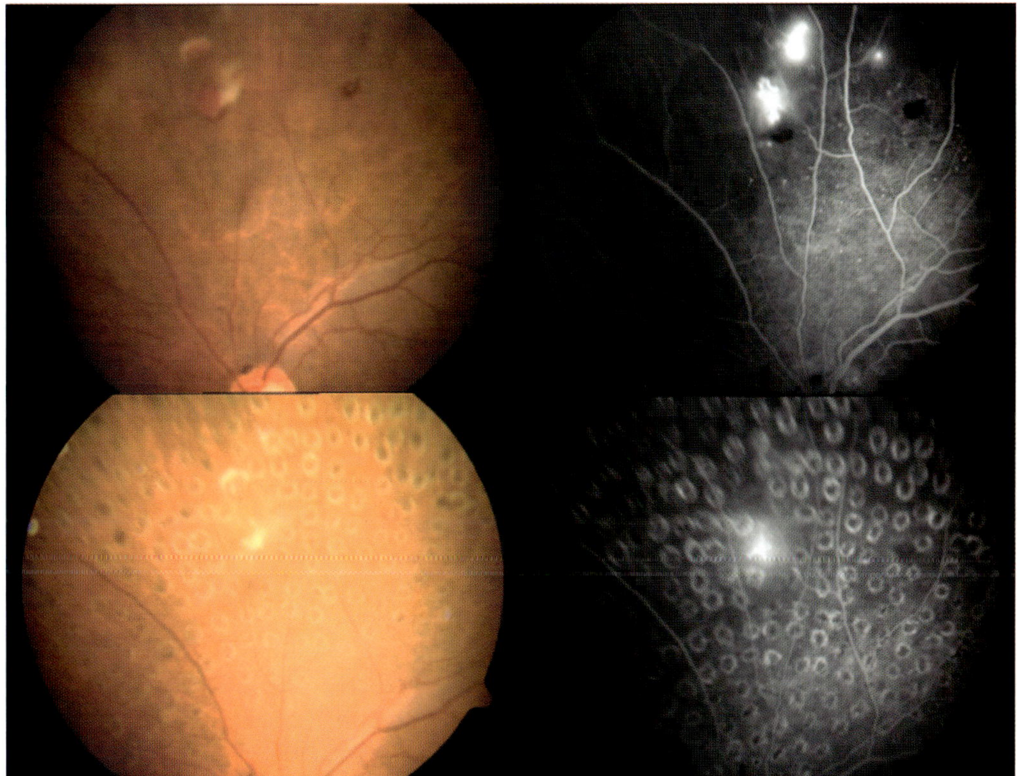

FIGURE 7.18: Pre- and post-laser images of a patient with branch retinal vein occlusion showing regression of new vessels following one session of scatter laser.

of the macula and extending peripherally to the equator is recommended. Regression of neovascularization elsewhere and neovascularization of the disk seen in two different patients with branch retinal vein occlusion is shown in Figures 7.18 and 7.19. The patient with neovascularization of the disk needed panretinal photocoagulation augmentation to achieve regression of neovascularization of the disk. [66]

MANAGEMENT OF CENTRAL RETINAL VEIN OCCLUSION (CENTRAL VEIN OCCLUSION STUDY RECOMMENDATIONS)

Fluorescein angiography for macular edema and retinal non-perfusion is performed at four monthly intervals. Gonioscopy and slit lamp biomicroscopy (in undilated pupil) for angle and iris neovascularization should be performed every one month.[67, 68] Panretinal photocoagulation is performed only if iris or angle new vessels

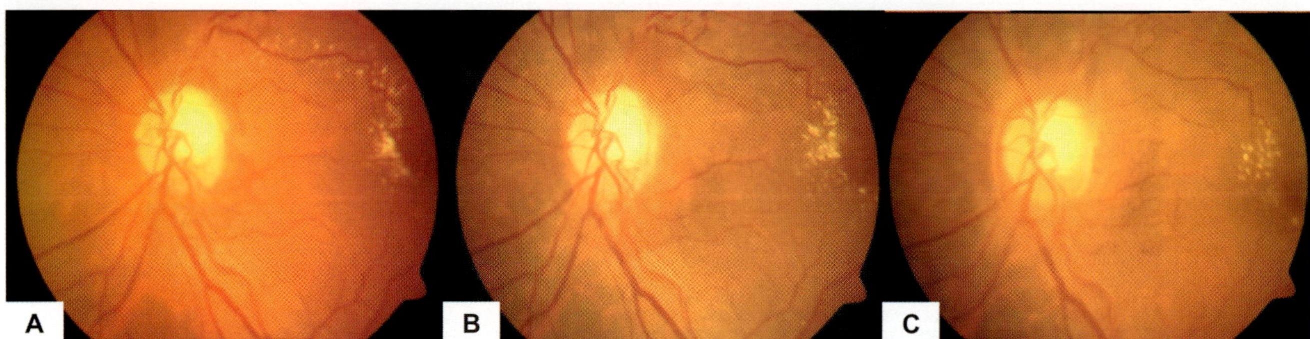

FIGURES 7.19A to C: Neovascularization of the disk in a patient with branch retinal vein occlusion and hypertension (A). Increasing proliferation is evident 3 months after panretinal photocoagulation (B). Signs of regression become evident at the 6 month follow-up after panretinal photocoagulation augmentation (C).

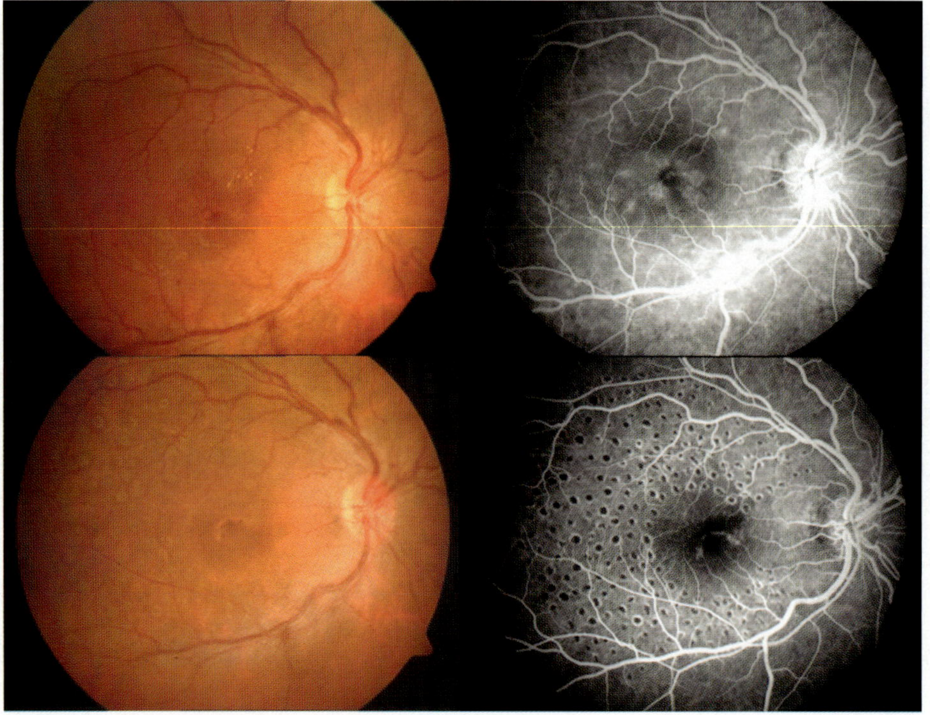

FIGURE 7.20: Resolution of macular edema is visible in these pre- and post-laser images of a young, non-hypertensive patient with central retinal vein occlusion. Visual acuity however remained at the pre-laser value of 6/60 (20/200).

more than 2 clock hours develops.[69] The technique and parameters for scatter laser are as for proliferative diabetic retinopathy. Macular grid for macular edema may not improve central visual acuity although angiographic resolution can be obtained.[70] Patients below 50 years of age and non-hypertensive however may show some benefit. The technique of grid laser is the same as described for diabetic macular edema.

Angiographic resolution of cystoid macular edema is evident in Figure 7.20 following grid laser. Visual acuity however remained unchanged.

Laser-induced Chorioretinal Anastomosis

Earlier experiments had demonstrated the feasibility of creating an anastomosis between a retinal vein and the choroidal circulation. Subsequently, McAllister and associates[71] reported their findings on the role of laser induced chorioretinal anastomosis in patients with non-ischemic form of central retinal vein occlusion. In all 29 patients whom they studied the indication was progressing loss of vision from macular edema. A successful arrest of this progression with subsequent improvement was seen in 33% of cases following chorioretinal anastomosis. The laser used was argon green laser (50 μ spot size, 1.5 to 2.5 W power, 100 msec duration) delivered to a focal spot on a retinal vein located atleast 3 disk diameters away from the disk in the inferotemporal or inferonasal quadrant (to avoid the posterior ciliary arteries and the long ciliary arteries along the horizontal meridian). A small intraretinal or subretinal hemorrhage was seen in all patients (the bleed being controlled by pressure on the contact lens). On an average each patient needed 1.8 sittings and the time for formation of the anastomosis varied from 3 weeks to 7 weeks. They called for larger, randomized controlled trials to further demonstrate the efficacy or otherwise of this treatment option in patients with non-ischemic central retinal vein occlusion.

A few years later, Fekrat and associates[72] reported successful creation of a chorioretinal anastomosis in 38% patients. Patients in whom successful anastomosis is created are said to improve by an average of four lines. More recently long term results with a modified technique have been reported.[73] A serious complication of this procedure is development of choroidal neovascularization, this risk being greater in more ischemic eyes.[74-76] It has been suggested that ideal candidates for laser induced anastomosis procedure are those with vision below 10/200 and have perfused macular edema that does not resolve within four months. Patients with long standing vascular occlusion (more than 3 months) are said to be poor candidates.

LASER IN CENTRAL SEROUS RETINOPATHY

Central serous retinopathy is a relatively benign and self-limited disorder and in most cases the serous detachment resolves spontaneously in about 3 to 4 months. Visual complaints (metamorphopsia, dyschromatopsia, relative scotoma) may however persist for a variable period or remain permanently. Recurrences are not infrequent and are reported to occur in nearly one-half of patients.[77] Prognosis decreases with increase in the number of recurrences and some cases may progress to a stage of chronic retinal pigment epithelium decompensation.[78]

Presently medical therapy has no established role in the management of central serous retinopathy. It is stated here with emphasis that corticosteroids in any form are not recommended and may indeed be a contraindication as they risk increasing the duration and rate of recurrence of this disorder.[79]

Laser photocoagulation is the only well established treatment modality in patients suffering from central serous retinopathy. Treating the leakage site directly with laser (argon green, krypton, diode or frequency doubled YAG laser) hastens resolution of the disease but does not affect the final visual acuity or the recurrence rate.[80-83] Laser photocoagulation has also been reported to be beneficial in patients with multifocal leaks and large detachments and also in some patients with retinal pigment epithelial decompensation. For the latter, grid laser, as for diabetic macular edema has been found useful.[84-86]

Laser treatment has however been reported to result in suboptimal recovery of contrast sensitivity in comparison to cases that resolve spontaneously. Hence, photocoagulation should be undertaken only in the presence of specific indications. The indications for this treatment are a matter of debate. Some of the recommended indications are:

- Patient prefers treatment following proper explanation. This is usually for occupational reasons or in functionally one-eyed patients wherein the quality of work is disturbed
- Angiographic leak persists beyond 3 months (chronic central serous retinopathy)
- In recurrent central serous retinopathy to hasten visual recovery and decrease the risk of chronic retinal pigment epithelial decompensation.

Before proceeding with laser photocoagulation, the following prerequisites should be taken into consideration. The visual acuity must be less than 6/12 (20/40) and there should be a well-defined leakage point on fluorescein angiography that is atleast 500 μ away

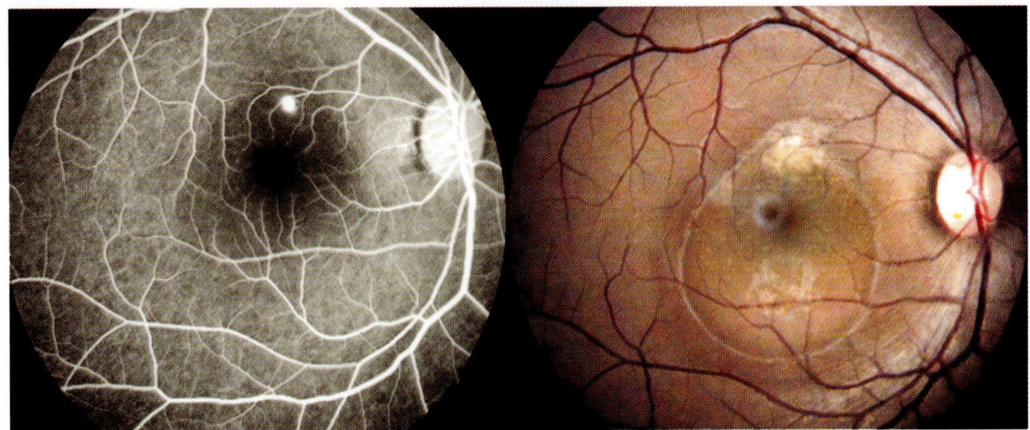

FIGURE 7.21: Fluorescein angiographic image and immediate post-laser photograph in a patient with central serous retinopathy.

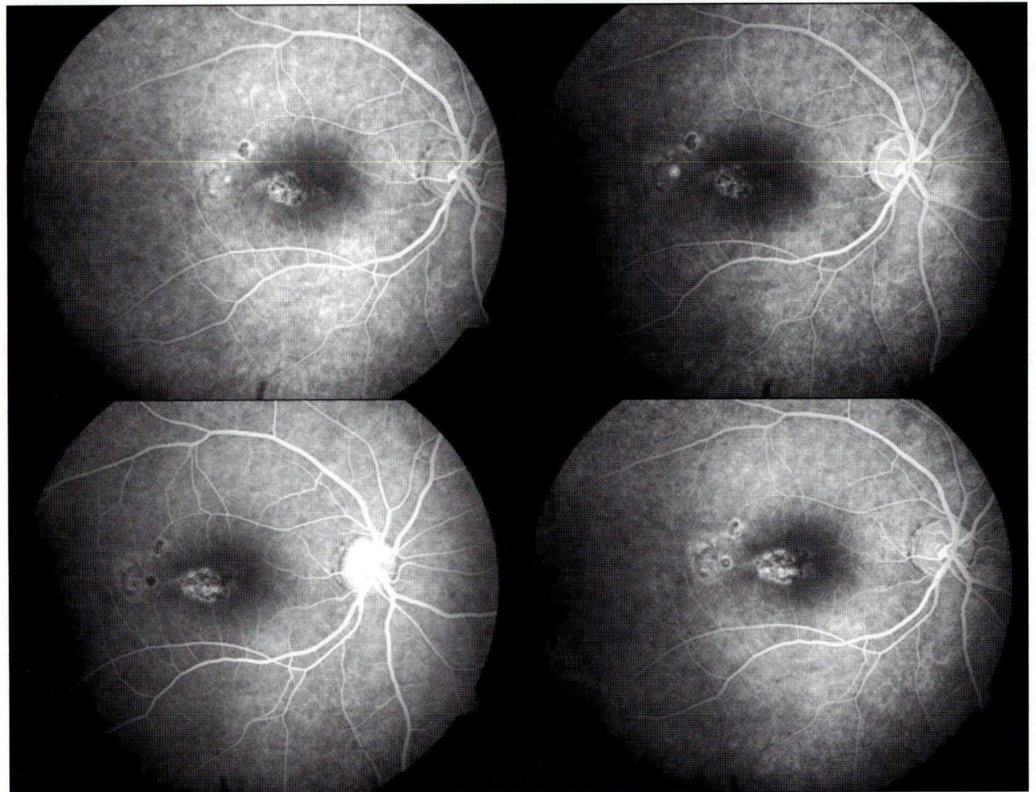

FIGURES 7.22A to D: Pre (A and B) and post-laser (C and D) fluorescein angiographic images of a patient with central serous retinopathy and chronic retinal pigment epithelial decompensation.

from the center of the foveal avascular zone. The preferred technique is direct treatment to the leakage point using 100 to 200 μ spot size, 0.1 to 0.2 second duration, 100 to 200 mW energy. Not more than 3-5 spots are generally required and the end point is mild whitening. Some of the complications that are known to occur, following laser photocoagulation, are foveal burn, traction lines, retinal pigment epithelial tear and secondary choroidal neovascularization when high energy is used.

Resolution of leakage in central serous retinopathy following laser photocoagulation is seen in Figures 7.21 to 7.23.

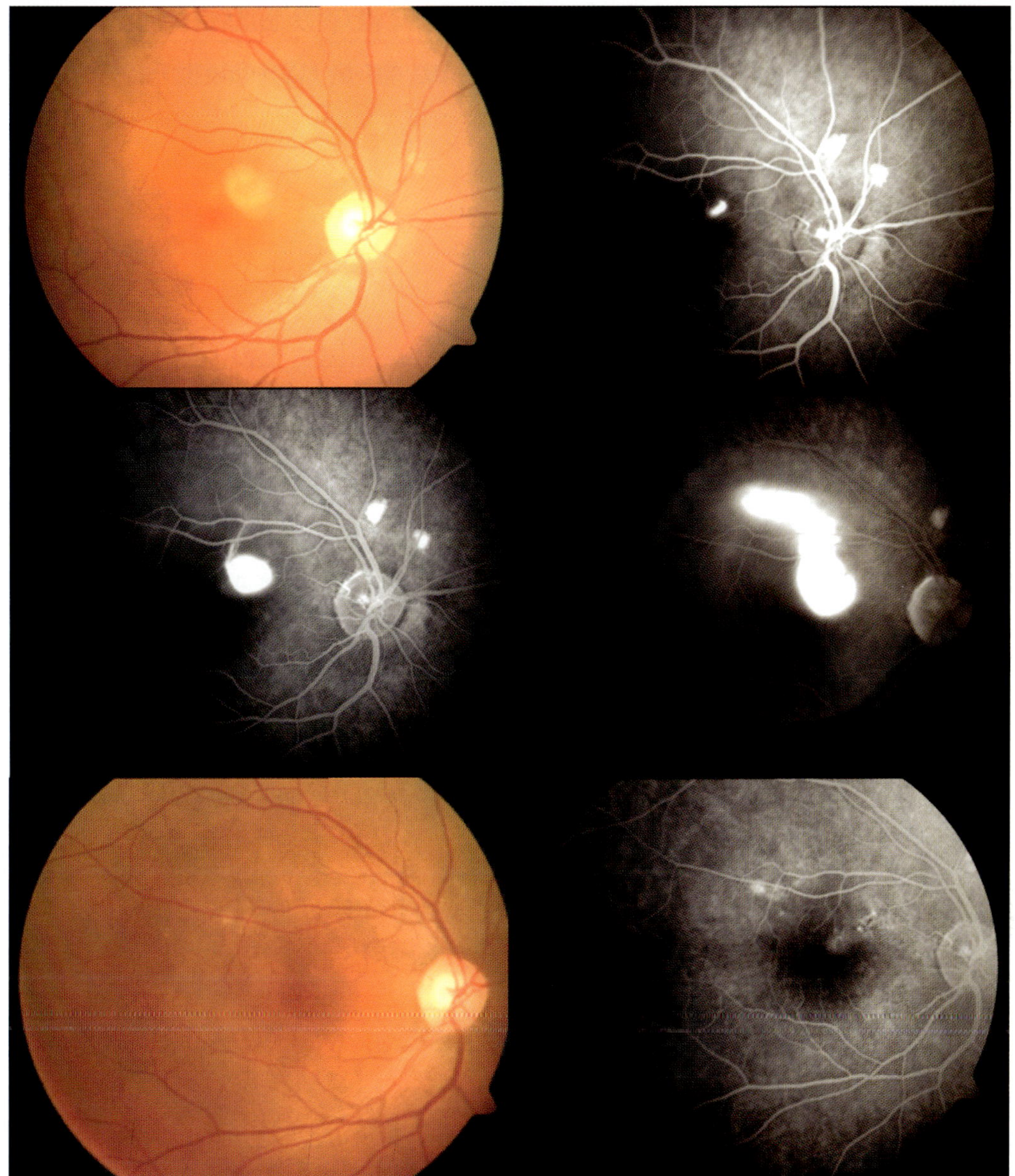

FIGURE 7.23A to F: Pre (A to D) and post-laser (E,F) images showing resolution of active leak following direct laser in a patient with recurrent central serous retinopathy.

Currently, successful treatment of persistent leaks in central serous retinopathy has also been reported using photodynamic therapy and micropulse laser.[87, 88]

LASER IN OPTIC DISK PIT

An optic nerve pit is an excavation of the optic nerve head. They are thought to arise from a defective closure of the embryonic fissure because of their frequent asso-ciation with coloboma of the inferonasal retina, inferior region of the choroid or a large optic nerve head. The size of the pit may vary from very small to very large (nearly involving the entire disk). They are usually situated along the temporal margin (but may also be located in the center), have a grayish color (vary from yellow-black) and well demarcated margins. There may be associated peripapillary chorioretinal changes. Recently association with early renal failure in some of these patients has been reported.[89] Fluorescein angiography is useful in confirming the diagnosis.

Optic disk pits may produce visual field defects and may also lead to a loss of vision due to its propensity to cause a serous detachment of the macula (Kranenburg syndrome). This detachment is thought to result from seepage of fluid vitreous or cerebrospinal fluid across the pit. Others consider it to be a form of schisis within the retinal layers. Serous detachment of the macula has been reported to occur in 40 to 90% of these cases.[90, 91] Though spontaneous resolution of these detachments have been reported, the overall outcome is said to be poor.[92] Hence, early treatment may be indicated in such eyes.

Treatment is indicated only in the presence of an associated serous macular detachment. Laser photocoagulation alone, along the temporal margin of the optic disk pit, was earlier considered to be the only necessary treatment.[93] However, it has been seen that although this treatment may help to flatten the detachment, it does not necessarily lead to an improvement in vision. Currently it is felt that visual results may improve if laser photocoagulation is performed after relieving traction on the pit by posterior vitrectomy and fluid-gas exchange.[94]

Decrease in macular detachment following laser photocoagulation in seen in two patients with optic disk pit (Figure 7.24).

LASER IN RETINAL VASCULAR ANOMALIES

RETINAL ARTERY MACROANEURYSM

Cousins and associates[95] have classified acquired macroaneurysms involving the retinal vasculature into four types. These are typical retinal artery macroaneurysm, retinal venous aneurysms, retinal capillary macroaneurysm and collateral associated macroaneurysm. The last three types of macroaneurysms are more common and may be encountered in diabetic retinopathy, venous occlusive disease, radiation retinopathy, sickle cell disease etc. Retinal artery macroaneurysm is usually an isolated finding with characteristic features. By definition, they are saccular or fusiform dilation of the retinal arteriole involving usually, the first three divisions. Their diameter is more than 125 μ (the upper limit for microaneurysm) but less than 250 μ. They are usually solitary and unilateral but may be multiple in 20% and bilateral in 10%. They usually involve the temporal vessels and are often located at the bifurcations.

Retinal artery macroaneurysms generally occur in elderly women (6th decade) and about 75% of patients have associated systemic hypertension. Clinically two forms of presentation are seen, the acute type and the chronic type.[96, 97] In the acute form, patient presents with a sudden loss of vision (due to retinal or vitreous

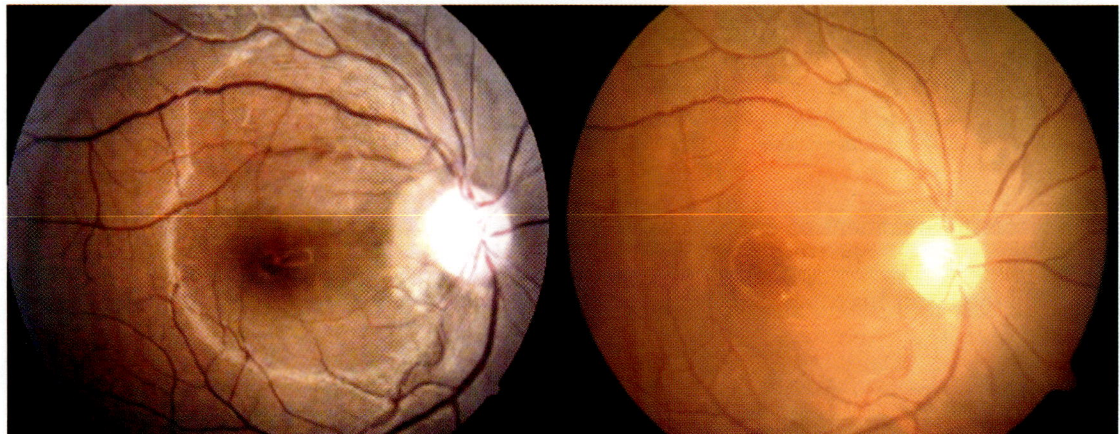

FIGURE 7.24: Immediate post-laser and late follow-up images of a young lady with bilateral optic disk pit and serous detachment in the right eye (shown here). Note flattening of the detachment following laser. No improvement in vision was however observed.

hemorrhage) while in the chronic form they present with a gradual loss of vision due to leakage and exudation into the macular area. The latter is usually diagnosed easily while the former is difficult to diagnose because of two reasons. Firstly, associated hemorrhage during the acute stage obscures visibility of the macroaneurysm and secondly, most resolve spontaneously after the hemorrhage and so may not be easily evident by the time the retinal or vitreous hemorrhage clears. The only characteristic feature during the acute stage is the presence of 'hour-glass' shaped hemorrhage due to simultaneous pre-retinal and subretinal collection of blood. This type of hemorrhage is not seen in all patients however. Fluorescein angiography may be helpful in identifying retinal artery macroaneurysms.

No treatment is recommended for a macroaneurysm with the acute form of presentation as recurrent hemorrhages are not known to occur and the visual recovery is good in most patients without treatment. Occasionally, pars plana vitrectomy may be necessary in patients with non-clearing vitreous hemorrhage. For those presenting with exudation into the macular area one may consider direct or indirect laser photocoagulation of the macroaneurysm if exudation is tending to progress towards the fovea and there is associated decrease in vision.[98] Indirect treatment a spot size of 200 to 300 μ is chosen, power of about 200 mW and duration of 0.2 to 0.5 seconds is set. The laser is focused directly on the macroaneurysm so as to obtain slow and gentle whitening. In indirect treatment, the laser burns are placed around the aneurysm. Branch retinal artery occlusion has been reported as a complication of direct treatment.

CONGENITAL ANEURYSMAL DILATIONS

Congenital aneurysmal dilations involving the retinal vascular system may be classified into the following categories:

- **Leber's multiple miliary aneurysms**: aneurysmal dilations without any subretinal exudation. They are probably a non-progressive or early form of Coats' disease

- **Coats' disease**: multiple aneurysmal dilations with massive subretinal exudation and intraretinal hemorrhages
- **von Hippel's syndrome**: frank retinal arteriovenous malformations with massive subretinal exudation.

All of the above have been collectively designated as the exudative vasculopathies.

Coats' Disease

Whether the term Coats' disease should be referred to include only those cases encountered in childhood (and adolescence) or also those encountered in adults is controversial (adult onset disease: diagnosis after 16 years of age). Analysis of the subretinal fluid in Coats' disease shows the presence of cholesterol crystals.

Ophthalmoscopic examination in Coats' disease reveals varying degree of subretinal exudation and varying forms of vascular anomalies (aneurysmal dilations, telangiectasia, sheathing, tortuosity, neovascular tufts). In severe cases there is an extensive exudative retinal detachment. The vascular anomalies may be missed either because they are very subtle or because they are obscured by the retinal exudation and hemorrhages. Not infrequently, the vascular anomalies are situated peripherally while the exudation is predominantly in the macular region or posterior pole. The disease is usually progressive with periods of quiescence and exacerbations. Pain is a feature only when neovascular glaucoma develops in the end stage of very severe disease. Fluorescein angiography reveals more number of vascular anomalies than that seen by fundus examination and may also demonstrate other signs of a more generalized blood retinal barrier defect such as perivascular leakage, areas of capillary non-perfusion around the areas of vascular anomalies and vascular communicating channels.

Consider treatment early as prospective studies have shown that even small lesions tend to increase in size and severity with time. This increases the risk of visual loss from macular exudation or exudative retinal detachment. Precede treatment by fluorescein angiography to identify all areas of vascular anomalies. If the vascular anomalies are posterior to the equator and there is no exudative detachment direct laser photocoagulation is performed (slit lamp/laser indirect ophthalmoscope). If the vascular anomalies are anterior to the equator and there is no exudative detachment cryotherapy (freeze-refreeze cycle) or laser indirect ophthalmoscope may be effective. If there is an exudative detachment drain subretinal fluid externally (may need to reform the globe) and treat the vascular anomalies using laser photocoagulation or cryotherapy. Single session of laser is rarely successful and most patients need multiple sessions.

Laser is performed by directly treating all aneurysmal dilations.[99, 100] Whitening of the lesions should be the end point. A spot size of 200 to 500 μ is chosen with power setting of about 200 mW and duration of 0.2 to 0.5 seconds. Excessive energy use must be avoided as it can increase the exudation. Some authors have also advocated a grid pattern of laser photocoagulation. Successful treatment allows preservation of vision and prevents complications like neovascular glaucoma.

von Hippel's Syndrome

Capillary hemangioma of the retina is a vascular hamartoma with distinct clinical and angiographic features. These tumors may be situated in the peripapillary region or in the periphery. Peripheral retinal capillary hemangiomas are also called as the von Hippel tumor. The peripapillary tumors may be endophytic or intra-retinal. These tumors are progressive, have feeder vessels, and lead to varying degrees of retinal exudation (circinate retinopathy to exudative retinal detachment). The peripheral tumors, as reported in literature, are said to be minuscule in the early stages (as small as a micro-aneurysm) with no obvious feeder vessels. They are also said to resemble grayish nubbins or telengiectatic vessels in the early stages. With time, the capillary channels proliferate; begin to function as arteriovenous shunts with subsequent formation and dilation of afferent and efferent feeder vessels. Ophthalmoscopically they appear as an orange mass with dilated feeder vessels.

von Hippel-Lindau syndrome is considered as one of the neurocristopathies or phakomatoses with an autosomal dominant inheritance. It is characterized by retinal capillary hemangiomas (the most frequent manifestation), infratentorial (cerebellar, brain stem, spinal cord) hemangioblastomas, renal cell carcinoma and pheochromocytoma.[101] One fourth of patients with von Hippel tumor are said to harbor this syndrome; the risk is said to be higher if the tumor is bilateral or multiple.

Capillary peripheral hemangiomas may lead to visual loss by the ability of the exudates to accumulate preferentially in the macula or by breaching the internal limiting membrane and growing into the vitreous (may simulate neovascularization) and causing subsequent tractional effects and vitreous hemorrhage. These tumors should be treated early (at the time of detection) even in the absence of exudation or large size because they invariably progress and on becoming large are more resistant to treatment. Observation alone is only recommended for those touching the optic nerve head. The treatment of choice is laser photocoagulation, cryotherapy or a combination of the two. Recent reports on the use of transpupillary thermotherapy are also available. Tumors larger than 2.5 disk diameters are extremely resistant to any mode of treatment and carry a poor prognosis.

Direct treatment is employed for small lesions while feeder vessel treatment is indicated for larger lesions. For direct treatment argon green or frequency doubled YAG laser may be used. A large spot (200-500 μ) and long duration (0.2-1.0 seconds) is chosen and power is set so as to obtain mild-moderate whitening of the lesion. Here again, multiple sessions at 1 to 2 week intervals are usually necessary to achieve complete closure.[102] Excessive treatment at one sitting may lead to secondary exudative detachment. For feeder vessel treatment, the afferent vessel is treated with confluent, moderately intense burns (with parameters mentioned above) until there is no spontaneous reopening. Repeat sessions are performed at 2 to 8 weekly intervals until the angioma is non-perfused.[103] Regression of retinal angioma following laser photocoagulation is shown in Figure 7.25.

YAG LASER HYALOIDOTOMY

Hemorrhage into the sub-hyaloid space overlying the macula can result in sudden and gross decrease of vision. Though the hemorrhage tends to layer over a period of time, its resolution and hence restoration of vision may

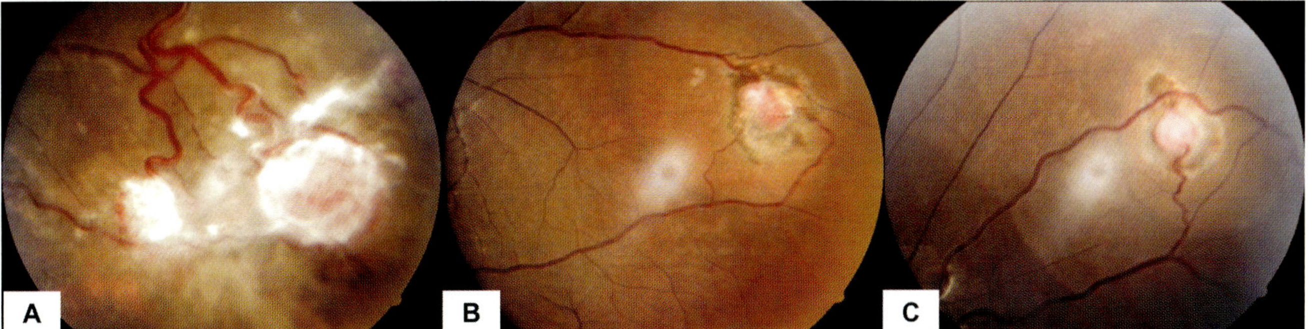

FIGURES 7.25A to C: Appearance of scarring and atrophic changes around the multiple retinal angiomas following laser in a patient with von Hippel Lindau disease.

be inordinately delayed. Apart from delayed visual recovery, premacular hemorrhage is also reported to induce late macular traction and iron toxicity.[104] Significant premacular hemorrhage is usually unilateral and may result in conditions such as diabetic retinopathy, aplastic anemia, Terson's syndrome, Valsalva retinopathy, vasculitis, ruptured retinal artery macroaneurysm, retinal vascular occlusions, etc.

Laser treatment to create a defect in the hyaloid under which the bleed is accumulated has been used to enhance resorption of premacular hemorrhage. Through the defect so created, blood escapes into the vitreous gel and is subsequently eliminated from the eye. Comparative studies have shown the procedure to be safe and effective.[105-110]

Laser is delivered through the transpupillary route using a slit lamp delivery system. Having obtained an informed consent, pupil is adequately dilated using cycloplegic-mydriatic drops. The cone angle is set at 10 degrees and laser energy is focused above the inferior extent of the hemorrhage to facilitate gravity-aided drainage of blood into the vitreous cavity. Procedure is started with an energy of 1.5 mJ using single pulse. About 5 to 6 spots may be needed to create a dehiscence and a further 8 to 10 spots of lower energy to achieve drainage of the blood.

Recommendations while deciding on the suitability of a patient with premacular hemorrhage for YAG laser hyaloidotomy include

1. Duration of hemorrhage: Premacular hemorrhage that has persisted beyond 4 weeks may be difficult to drain.

2. Size of hemorrhage: usually more than 3 disk diameters. Smaller hemorrhages may risk formation of retinal holes.

3. Absence of retinal proliferation: if present do a full scatter first. Scatter laser may not be possible if vitreous hemorrhage remains for an extended period following hyaloidotomy.

Most patients are said to recover significant vision within 4 weeks of the procedure if there is no underlying macular pathology. About 1 in 4 patients may develop non-resolving vitreous hemorrhage necessitating later vitreous surgery. Potential complications include creation of retinal hole and retinal detachment. These complications are considered infrequent when compared to the risks of undertaking vitreous surgery in these eyes. Even if the laser procedure fails it is reported not to alter the outcome of subsequent vitreous surgery. Patients with underlying choroidal/ retinal proliferation fare poorly with this procedure.

Nd: YAG VITREOLYSIS

Before considering any treatment option in patients with post surgical cystoid macular edema, it is important to ascertain its cause and nature. Angiographic cystoid macular edema alone does not warrant any treatment. In patients with clinically significant cystoid macular edema, medical, laser and surgical interventions become necessary depending on the cause and initial response to medical treatment alone. Topical non-steroidal anti-inflammatory drugs and topical or periocular cortico-steroids form the mainstay in medical management.

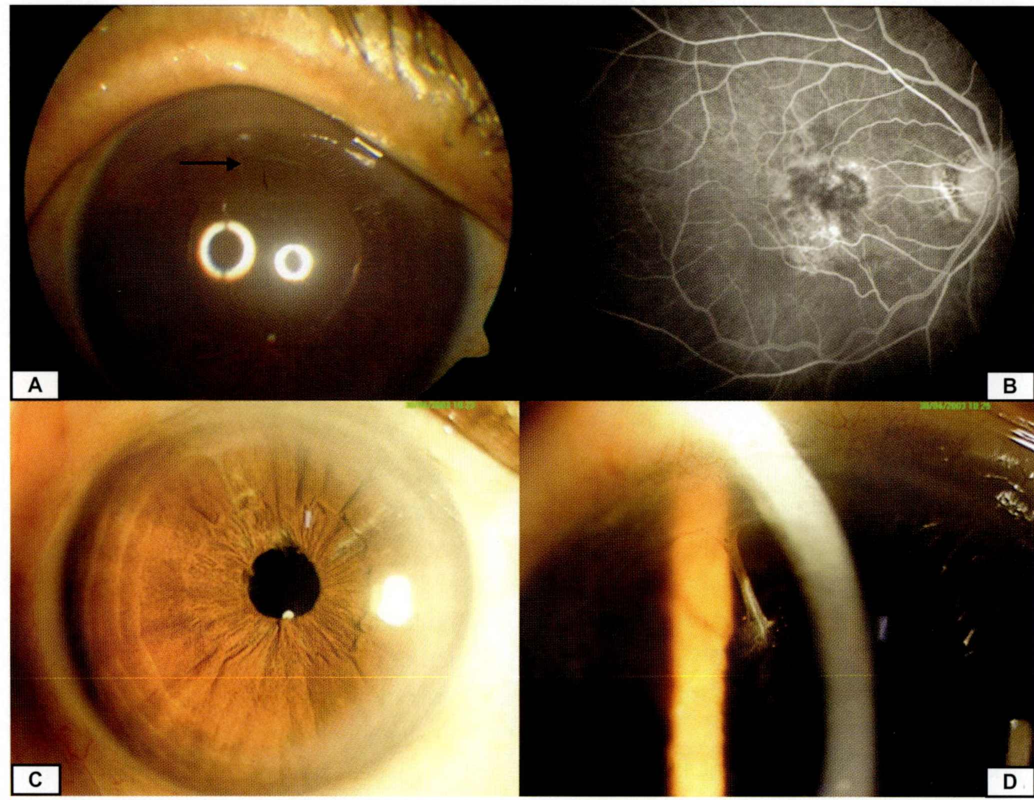

FIGURES 7.26A to D: Pre (A) and post (C, D) Nd: YAG vitreolysis photographs in a patient with post-cataract surgery cystoid macular edema (B) and vitreous incarceration into the wound. Visual acuity improved from 6/18 (20/60) to 6/12 (20/40) at the three-month follow-up.

Ketorolac tromethamine 0.5% given four times daily for three months has been found to be effective in bringing about a resolution of the macular edema. A more recent report has shown however that a dual therapy with non-steroidal anti-inflammatory drugs and topical cortico-steroids is superior to either of the drugs prescribed alone. Some authors recommend the concurrent use of oral indomethacin 25 mg thrice daily for 10 days at this stage. If no response is seen following topical therapy, one must consider injection of corticosteroids into the periocular space. The usual drugs are triamcinolone or methylprednisolone 20 mg in 0.5 ml. If no response is seen following one injection, the rationale for giving repeat injections is questionable. The next consideration should be prescription of oral corticosteroids at a dosage of 1 to 1.5 mg/kg/day, followed by a gradual taper.

When obvious aggravating factors are evident, like vitreous incarceration in the wound or intraocular lens malposition, the same should be managed early (if initial medical therapy fails or there are relapses) to prevent the edema from becoming chronic. Some authors, to manage fine vitreous strands adherent to the wound, have used YAG laser vitreolysis successfully.[111,112] This modality of treatment has the risk of producing retinal detachment and elevation of intraocular pressure.[112] In many cases, it is probably more prudent to undertake pars plana vitrectomy as vitreous adherent to the iris can also be removed.

Successful sectioning of vitreous strand going into the cataract wound in a patient with concurrent macular edema resistant to medical therapy is shown in Figure 7.26.

REFERENCES

1. Ferris FL, Fine SL, Hyman LA. Age-related macular degeneration and blindness due to neovascular maculopathy. Arch Ophthalmol 1984; 102:1640-42.

2. Bressler NM, Bressler SB, Gragoudas ES. Clinical characteristics of choroidal vascular membranes. Arch Ophthalmol 1987; 105:209-13.

3. Freund KB, Yannuzzi LA, Sorenson JA. Age-related macular degeneration and choroidal neovascularization. Am J Ophthalmol 1993; 115:786-91.

4. Singerman LJ. Growth rate of subretinal neovascularization in age-related macular degeneration. Ophthalmology 1989; 96:1422-29.

5. Klein ML, Jorizzo PA, Watzke RC. Growth features of choroidal neovascular membranes in age-related macular degeneration. Ophthalmology 1989; 96:1416-21.

6. Vander JF, Morgon CM, Shatz H. Growth rate of subretinal neovascularization in age-related macular degeneration. Ophthalmology 1989; 96:1422-29.

7. Macular photocoagulation study group: Subfoveal neovascular lesions in age-related macular degeneration: Guidelines for evaluation and treatment in the Macular photocoagulation study. Arch Ophthalmol 1991; 109:1242-57.

8. Venkatesh P, Gupta R, Verma L, Tewari HK. Evaluation of trans-scleral diode laser using diopexy probe for subfoveal choroidal neovascular membrane in age-related macular degeneration. J Clin Laser Med Surg 2004; 22:91-97.

9. Macular Photocoagulation Study Group. Laser photo-coagulation of subfoveal neovascular lesions in age-related macular degeneration: results of a randomized clinical trial. Arch Ophthalmol 1991; 109:1220-31.

10. Macular Photocoagulation Study Group. Visual outcome after laser photocoagulation for subfoveal choroidal neovascularization secondary to age-related macular degeneration: the influence of initial lesion size and initial visual acuity. Arch Ophthalmol 1994; 12:480-88.

11. Macular Photocoagulation Study Group. Laser photo-coagulation of subfoveal neovascular lesions in age-related macular degeneration. Updated findings from two clinical trials. Arch Ophthalmol 1993; 111:1200-09.

12. Macular Photocoagulation Study Group. Laser photo-coagulation for juxtafoveal choroidal neovascularization. Five year results from randomized clinical trials. Arch Ophthalmol 1994; 112:500-09.

13. Macular Photocoagulation Study Group. Argon laser photocoagulation for neovascular maculopathy. Five year results from randomized clinical trials. Arch Ophthalmol 1991; 109:1109-14.

14. Macular Photocoagulation Study Group. Laser photo-coagulation of subfoveal recurrent neovascular lesions in age-related macular degeneration. Results of a randomized clinical trial. Arch Ophthalmol 1991; 109:12320-41.

15. Yannuzzi LA. Laser photocoagulation for subretinal neovascularization. Retina 1982; 2:29-46.

16. Macular Photocoagulation Study Group. Argon laser photocoagulation for ocular histoplasmosis-results of a randomized clinical trial. Arch Ophthalmol 1983; 101:1347-57.

17. Bloom SM, Brucker AJ. Laser surgery of the posterior segment. JB Lippincott Company, Philadelphia, 1991.

18. Salvetti P, Massacesi, AL, et al. Feeder Vessel Identification: The Learning Curve. Invest Ophthalmol Vis Sci 2001; 42:1242.

19. Glaser BM, Baudo TA, Velez G, Murphy RP. Feeder vessel treatment for age-related macular degeneration with classic choroidal neovascularization. Invest Ophthalmol Vis Sci 2001; 42:1243.

20. Murphy RP, Lin SB, Glaser BM. Feeder vessel treatment for age-related macular degeneration with classic choroidal neovascularization. Invest Ophthalmol Vis Sci 2001; 42:1244.

21. Salvetti P, Massacesi, AL, et al. Feeder vessel identification: The learning curve. Invest Ophthalmol Vis Sci 2001; 42:1242.

22. Schubert HD. Topographic anatomy of the central retina and segmental choroidal circulation. In Yannuzzi LA, Flower RW, Slakter JS (Eds): Fundamentals of Indocyanine Green Angiography. St. Louis: Mosby-Year Book, 1997; p 21.

23. Apple DJ, Goldberg MF, Whinny G. Histopathology and ultra structure of the argon lesion in human retinal and choroidal vasculature. Am J Ophthalmol 1973; 75:595-609.

24. Perry DD, Reddick RL, Risco JM. Choroidal microvascular repair after argon laser photocoagulation. Am J Ophthalmol 1982; 93:787-93.

25. Perry DD, Reddick RL, Risco JM. Choroidal microvascular repair after argon laser photocoagulation: ultrastructural observations. Invest Ophthalmol Vis Sci 1984; 25:1019-26.

26. Ryan SJ. The development of an experimental model of subretinal neovascularization in diskiform macular degene-ration. Trans Am Ophthalmol Soc 1979; 77:707-45.

27. Archer DB, Gardiner TA. Experimental subretinal neovascularization. Trans Ophthalmol 1980; 100:363-368.

28. Amalric P. circulation choroidienne. C.R. symp. Int. Angiographie fluoresceinioie, Albi 1969, Karger, Basel: 1971;193-203.

29. Hayreh SS, Baines JAB. Occlusion of posterior ciliary artery. I. Effects on choroidal circulation. Br J Ophthalmol 1972; 56:719-35.

30. Hayreh SS, Baines JAB. Occlusion of posterior ciliary artery. I. Effects on choroidal circulation. Br J Ophthalmol 1972; 56:736-53.

31. Anderson DR, Davis EB. Retina and optic nerve after posterior ciliary artery occlusion: an experimental study in squirrel monkey. Arch Ophthalmol 1974; 92: 422-26.

32. Gass JDM, Blodi BA. Idiopathic juxtafoveolar retinal telangiectasis: update of classification and follow-up study. Ophthalmology 1993; 10:1536-46.

33. Casswell AG, Chaine G, Rush P, Bird AC. Paramacular telangiectasis. Trans Ophthalmol Soc UK. 1986; 105: 683-92.

34. Gass JDM, Guerry RK, Jack RL, Harris G. Choroidal osteoma. Arch Ophthalmol 1978; 96: 428-35.

35. Burke JF, Brockhurst RJ. Argon laser photocoagulation of subretinal neovascular membrane associated with osteoma of the choroid. Retina 1983; 3:304-07.

36. Grand MG, Burgess DB, Singerman LJ, Ramsey J. Choroidal osteoma: treatment of associated subretinal neovascular membranes. Retina 1984; 4:84-89.

37. Curtin BJ, Karlin DB. Axial length measurements and fundus changes in the myopic eye. Am J Ophthalmol 1971; 71: 42-53.

38. Avila MP, Weiter JJ, Jalkh AE, et al. Natural history of choroidal neovascularization in degenerative myopia. Ophthalmology 1984; 91: 1573-81.

39. Soubrane G, Coscas G. Subretinal new vessels in degenerative myopia: results of a randomized clinical trial. Invest Ophthalmol Vis Sci 1992; 33 (suppl):2564.

40. Brancato R, Pece A, Avanza P, Camesasca F. Laser treatment of macular subretinal neovascularization in pathological myopia. Fr J Ophthalmol 1989; 12: 883-86.

41. Pece A, Serini P, Avanza P, Brancato R. Recurrences after laser photocoagulation for macular subretinal neovascularization in pathologic myopia. Fr J Ophthalmol 1990; 13:24-28.

42. Pece A, Brancato R, Avanza P, et al. Laser photocoagulation of choroidal neovascularization in pathologic myopia: long term results. Int Ophthalmol 1995; 18:339-44.

43. Fuller B, Gitter KA. Traumatic choroidal rupture with late serous detachment of the macula: report of successful argon laser treatment. Arch Ophthalmol 1973; 89: 354-55.

44. Wood CM, Richardson J. Indirect choroidal ruptures: etiological factors, patterns of ocular damage, and final visual outcome. Br J Ophthalmol 1990; 74: 208-11.

45. Singerman LJ, Hatem G. Laser treatment of choroidal neovascular membranes in angioid streaks. Retina 1981; 1:75-83.

46. Geliske O, Hendrikse F, Deutman AF. A long-term follow-up of laser coagulation of neovascular membranes in angioid streaks. Am J Ophthalmol 1988; 105:299-303.

47. Lim JI, Bressler NM, Marsh MJ, et al. Laser treatment of choroidal neovascularization in patients with angioid streaks. Am J Ophthalmol 1993; 116:414-23.

48. Sickenberg M, Schmidt-Erfurth U, Miller JW, et al. A preliminary study of photodynamic therapy using verteporfin for choroidal neovascularization in pathologic myopia, ocular histoplasmosis syndrome, and angioid streaks, and idiopathic causes. Arch Ophthalmol 2000; 118:327-36.

49. Macular Photocoagulation Study Group. Krypton laser photocoagulation for idiopathic neovascular lesions. Results of a randomized clinical trial. Arch Ophthalmol 1990; 108:832-37.

50. Chan WM, Lam DS, Wong TH, et al. Photodynamic therapy with verteporfin for subfoveal idiopathic choroidal neovascularization: one-year results from a prospective case series. Ophthalmology 2003; 110:2395-2402.

51. Ho AC, Yannuzzi LA, Pisicano K, DeRosa J. The natural history of idiopathic subfoveal choroidal neovascularization. Ophthalmology 1995; 102:782-89.

52. Laatikainen L, Erkkila H. Subretinal and disk neovascularization in serpiginous choroiditis. Br J Ophthalmol 1982; 66:326-31.

53. Frank KW, Weiss H. Unusual clinical and histopathological findings in ocular sarcoidosis. Br J Ophthalmol 1983; 67:8-16.

54. Macular Photocoagulation Study Group. Krypton laser photocoagulation for neovascular lesions of ocular histoplasmosis. Results of a randomized clinical trial. Arch Ophthalmol 1987; 105:1499-1507.

55. Yannuzzi LA, Sorenson J, Spaide RF, Lipson B. Idiopathic polypoidal choroidal vasculopathy (IPCV). Retina 1990; 10:1-8.

56. Spaide RF, Yannuzzi LA, Slakter JS, et al. Indocyanine green videoangiography of idiopathic polypoidal choroidal vasculopathy. Retina 1995; 15:100-110.

57. Yannuzzi LA, Ciardella A, Spaide RF, et al. The expanding clinical spectrum of idiopathic polypoidal choroidal vasculopathy. Arch Ophthalmol 1997; 115: 478-85.

58. Zacks DN, Johnson MW. Retinal angiomatous proliferation: optical coherence tomographic confirmation of an intraretinal lesion. Arch Ophthalmol 2004; 122(6):932-33.

59. Sigelman J. Foveal drusen resorption one year after perifoveal laser photocoagulation. Ophthalmology 1991; 98: 1379-83.

60. Figueroa MS, Regueras A, Bertrand J. Laser photocoagulation to treat macular soft drusen in age-related macular degeneration. Retina 1994; 14: 391-96.

61. Ho A, Maguire M, Yoken J, et al. Laser induced drusen reduction improves visual function at 1 year. Ophthalmology 1999; 106: 1367-74.

62. Olk R, Friberg T, Stickney K, et al. Therapeutic benefits of infrared (810 nm) diode laser macular grid photocoagulation in prophylactic treatment of non-exudative age-related macular degeneration. Two-year results of a randomized pilot study. Ophthalmology 1999; 106:2082-90.

63. Gutman FA: Evaluation of a patient with central retinal vein occlusion. Ophthalmology 1983; 90: 481-83.

64. Zhao J, Sastry SM, Sperduto RD, Chew EY, Remaley NA. Arteriovenous crossing patterns in branch retinal vein occlusion: The Eye Disease Case Control Study Group. Ophthalmology 1993; 100:423-28.

65. Branch Vein Occlusion Study Group: Argon laser photocoagulation for macular edema in branch vein occlusion. Am J Ophthalmol 1984;98:271-82.

66. Branch Vein Occlusion Study Group: Argon laser scatter photocoagulation for prevention of neovascularization and vitreous hemorrhage in branch vein occlusion. Arch Ophthalmol 1986; 104:34-41.

67. The Central Vein Occlusion Study Group: Baseline and early natural history report. Arch Ophthalmol 1993; 111:1087-95.

68. The Central Vein Occlusion Study Group: Natural history and clinical management of central retinal vein occlusion. Arch Ophthalmol 1997; 115:486-91.

69. The Central Vein Occlusion Study Group: A randomized clinical trial of early panretinal photocoagulation for ischemic central vein occlusion. The CVOS Group N Report. Ophthalmology 1995; 102:1434-44.

70. The Central Vein Occlusion Study Group: Evaluation of grid pattern photocoagulation for macular edema in central vein occlusion. The CVOS Group M Report. Ophthalmology 1995; 102: 1425-33.

71. McAllister IL, Constable IJ. Laser-induced chorioretinal venous anastomosis for treatment of non-ischemic central retinal vein occlusion. Arch Ophthalmol 1995; 113:456-62.

72. Fekrat S, Goldberg MF, Finkelstein D. Laser induced chorioretinal venous anastamosis for non-ischemic central or branch retinal vein occlusion. Archives of Ophthalmol 1998; 116:43-52.

73. Leonard BC, Coupland SG, Kertes PJ, Bate R. Long-term follow-up of a modified technique for laser-induced chorioretinal venous anastomosis in non-ischemic central retinal vein occlusion. Ophthalmology 2003; 110:948-54.

74. McAllister IL, Douglas JP, Constable IJ, Yu DY. Laser-induced chorioretinal venous anastomosis for non-ischemic central retinal vein occlusion: evaluation of the complications and their risk factors. Am J Ophthalmol 1998; 126:219-29.

75. Eccarius SG, Moran MJ, Slingsby JG. Choroidal neovascular membrane after laser-induced chorioretinal anastomosis. Am J Ophthalmol 1996; 122:590-91.

76. Aktan SG, Subasi M, Akbatur H, Or M. Problems of chorioretinal venous anastomosis by laser for treatment of non-ischemic central retinal vein occlusion. Ophthalmologica 1998; 212:389-93.

77. Gilbert CM, Owens SL, Smith PD, Fine SL. Long term follow-up of central serous chorioretinopathy. Br J Ophthalmol 1984; 68:815-20.

78. Jalkh AE, Jabbour N, Avila MP, et al. I. Retinal pigment epithelial decompensation. Clinical features and natural course. Ophthalmology 1984; 91:1544-48.

79. Gass JDM, Little H. Bilateral bullous exudative retinal detachment complicating central serous chorioretinopathy during systemic corticosteroid therapy. Ophthalmology 1995; 102:737-47.

80. Robertson DM, Ilstrup D. Direct, indirect, and sham laser photocoagulation in the management of central serous chorioretinopathy. Am J Ophthalmol 1983; 95(4): 457-66.

81. Brancato R, Scialdone A, Pece A, et al. Eight-year follow-up of central serous chorioretinopathy with and without laser treatment. Graefes Arch Clin Exp Ophthalmol 1987; 225:166-68.

82. Leaver P, Williams C. Argon laser photocoagulation in the treatment of central serous retinopathy. Br J Ophthalmol 1979; 63:674-77.

83. Watzke RC, Burton TC, Woolson RF. Direct and indirect laser photocoagulation of central serous choroidopathy. Am J Ophthalmol 1979; 88:914-18.

84. Yannuzzi LA, Slakter JS, Kaufman SR, Gupta K. Laser treatment of diffuse retinal pigment epitheliopathy. Eur J Ophthalmol 1992; 2:103-14.

85. Roseman RL, Olk RJ. Grid laser photocoagulation for atypical central serous chorioretinopathy. Ophthalmic Surg. 1988; 19:786-91.

86. Jalkh AE, Jabbour N, Avila MP, et al. Retinal pigment epithelial decompensation. II: Laser treatment. Ophthalmology 1984; 91:1549-53.

87. Ricci F, Missiroli F, Cerulli L. Indocyanine green dye-enhanced micropulsed diode laser: a novel approach to subthreshold retinal pigment epithelium treatment in a case of central serous chorioretinopathy. Eur J Ophthalmol 2004; 14:74-82.

88. Piccolino CF, Eandi CM, Ventre L, et al. Photodynamic therapy for chronic central serous chorioretinopathy. Retina 2003; 23: 752-63.

89. Theodossisdias G. Evolution of congenital pit of optic disk with macular detachment in photocoagulated and nonphotocoagulated eyes. Am J Ophthalmol 1977; 83:620-31.

90. Hayreh SS. Fluids in the anterior part of the optic nerve in health and disease. Surv Ophthalmol 1978; 1-25.

91. Sobol WM, Blodi CF, Folk JC, Weingeist TA. Long-term visual outcome in patients with optic nerve pit and serous detachment of the macula. Ophthalmology 1990; 97:1539-42.

92. Schatz H, Mc Donald HR. Treatment of sensory retinal detachment associated with optic nerve pit or coloboma. Ophthalmology 1988; 85:178-86.

93. Todokoro D, Kishi S. Reattachment of retina and retinoschisis in pit-macular syndrome by surgically induced vitreous detachment and gas tamponade. Ophthalmic Surg Lasers 2000; 31:233-35.

94. Cousins SW, Flynn HW Jr, Clarkson JG. Macroaneurysms associated with retinal branch vein occlusion. Am J Ophthalmol 1990; 109:567-70.

95. Lindgren G, Sjodell L, Lindblom B. A prospective study of dense spontaneous vitreous hemorrhage. Am J Ophthalmol 1995; 119:458-65.

96. Tezel TH, Gunlap I, Tezel G. Morphometric analysis of exudative retinal arterial macroaneurysms: a geometric approach to exudates curves. Ophthalmic Res 1994; 26:332-39.

97. Rabb MF, Gagliano DA, Teske MP. Retinal artery macroaneurysms. Surv Ophthalmol 1988; 33:73-96.

98. Gass JDM. Treatment of peripheral vascular anomalies. Ophthalmology 1977; 83: 432-45.

99. Ridley ME, Shields JA, Brown GC, Tasman W. Coats' disease: evaluation of management. Ophthalmology 1982; 89:1381-87.

100. O' Hanley GP, Canny CLB. Diabetic dense premacular haemorrhage. Ophthalmology 1985; 4:507-11.

101. Hardwig P, Robertson DM. Von Hippel-Lindau disease: a familial, often lethal, multisystem phakomatoses. Ophthalmology 1984; 91:263-70.

102. Lane CM, Turner G, Gregor AJ, Bird AC. Laser treatment of retinal Angiomatosis. Eye. 1989; 3:33-38.

103. Blodi CF, Russell SR, Pulido JS, Folk JC. Direct and feeder vessel photocoagulation of retinal angioma with dye yellow laser. Ophthalmology 1990; 97: 791-97.

104. Rennie CA, Newman DK, Snead MP, Flanagan DW. Nd: YAG laser treatment for premacular subhyaloid haemorrhage. Eye 2001; 15: 519-24.

105. Adel B, Israel A, Friedman Z. Dense subhyaloid hemorrhage or sub-internal limiting membrane hemorrhage in the macula treated by Nd: YAG laser. Arch Ophthalmol 1998; 116: 1542-43.

106. Iijima H, Satoh S, Tsukahara S. Nd: YAG laser photodisruption for preretinal hemorrhage due to retinal macroaneurysm. Retina 1998; 18:430-34.

107. Gabel VP, Birngruber R, Gunther-Koszka H, et al. Nd: YAG laser photodisruption of hemorrhagic detachment of the internal limiting membrane. Am J Ophthalmol 1989; 107:33-37.

108. Tassignon MJ, Stempels N, Van Mulders L. Retrohyaloid premacular hemorrhage treated by Q-switched Nd-YAG laser. A case report. Graefes Arch Clin Exp Ophthalmol 1989; 227:440-42.

109. Ulbig MW, Mangouritsas G, Rothbacher HH, et al. Longterm results after drainage of premacular subhyaloid hemorrhage into the vitreous with a pulsed Nd: YAG Laser. Arch Ophthalmol 1998; 116:1465-69.

110. Tchah H, Rosenberg M, Larson RS, Lindstrom RL. Neodymium: YAG laser vitreolysis for treatment and prophylaxis of cystoid macular oedema. Aust N Z J Ophthalmol 1989; 17:179-83.

111. Aron-Rosa D, Greenspan DA. Neodymium: YAG laser vitreolysis. Int Ophthalmol Clin. 1985; 25:125-34.

112. Benhamou N, Glacet-Bernard A, Le Mer Y, et al. Retinal detachment following YAG laser section of vitreous strands. Apropos of 3 cases. J Fr Ophthalmol 1998; 21:495-500.

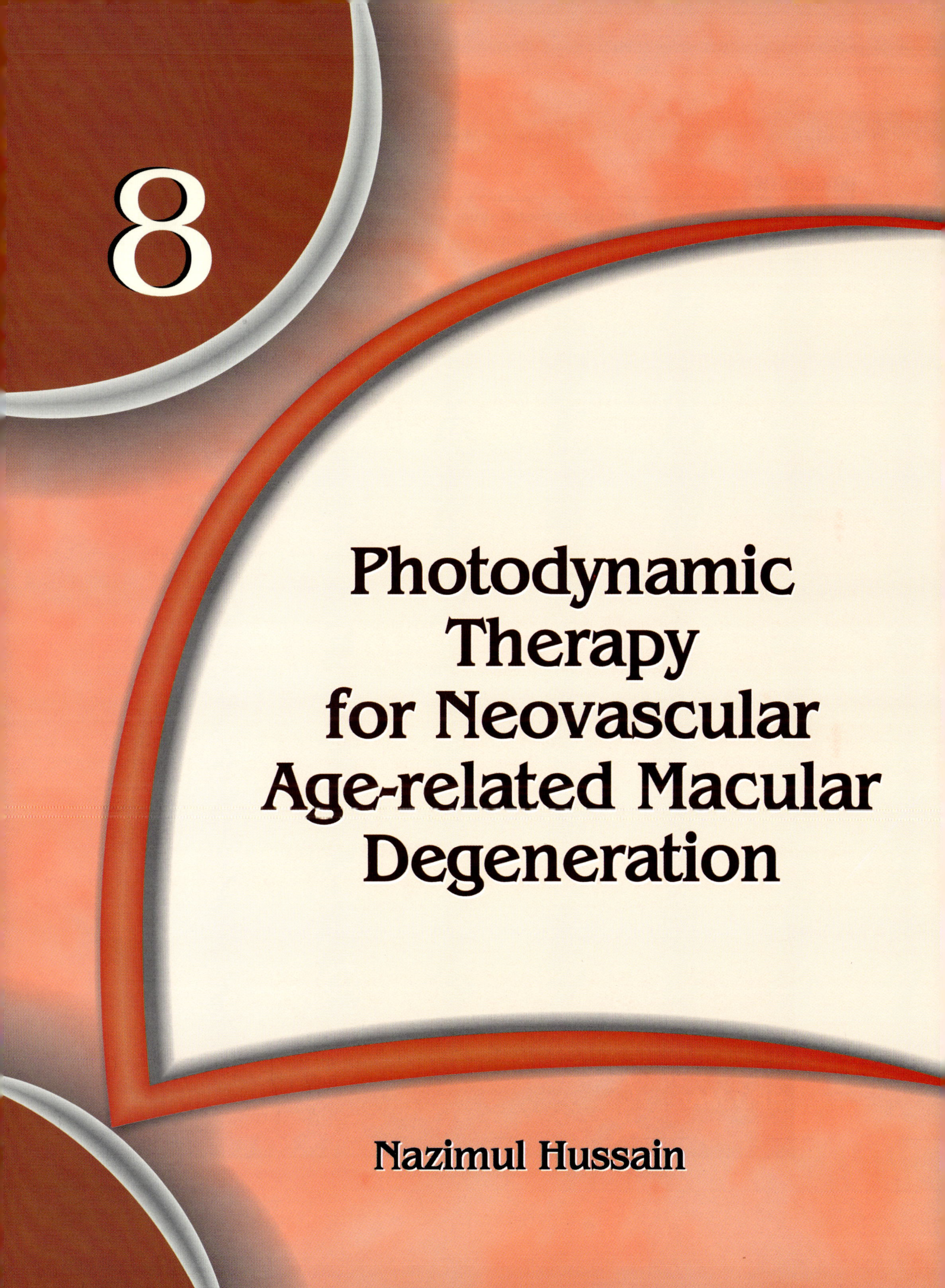

8

Photodynamic Therapy for Neovascular Age-related Macular Degeneration

Nazimul Hussain

INTRODUCTION

Verteporfin (Visudyne) is the first light activated drug approved for treatment of subfoveal choroidal neovascularization (CNV) secondary to age-related macular degeneration (AMD), pathologic myopia and other ocular conditions like ocular histoplasmosis syndrome. Until the development of photodynamic therapy with verteporfin, laser photocoagulation was the only treatment proven to be effective for CNV. This, however, was limited to juxtafoveal and extrafoveal CNV as benefit of treatment for subfoveal lesions was associated with destruction of the overlying retina and risk of immediate and irreversible loss of vision at the site of laser application. Hence, was not considered for treatment of subfoveal choroidal neovascularization. [1-33]

VERTEPORFIN

PHARMACOLOGY

The active chemical component is a benzoporphyrin derivative monoacid (BPD-MA) is a potent second generation light activated drug derived from porphyrin. It is a chlorin type molecule and exists as an equal mixture of two regioisomers (Figure 8.1), each of which consists of an enantiomeric pair that demonstrates similar pharmacologic activity *in vitro* and *in vivo*. Verteporfin has a molecular weight 718.81. It is formulated in a lipid based preparation that augments solubility in blood.

ABSORPTION

Verteporfin has a long absorption wavelength with several peaks (Figure 8.2) including a strong absorption peak

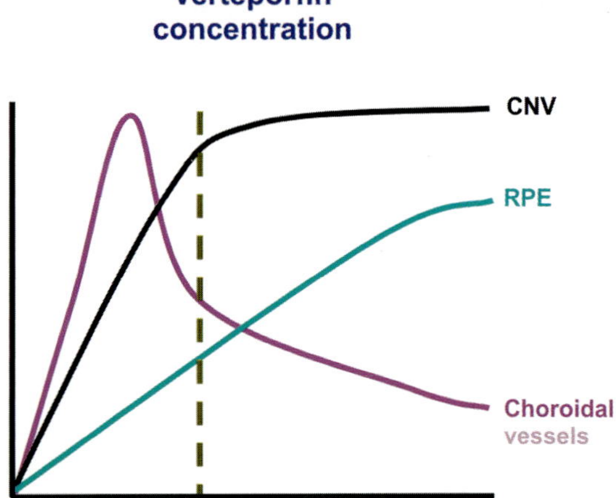

FIGURE 8.2: Verteporfin: Absorption wavelength (Novartis Ophthalmics, India)

in the 680 to 695 nm region. Verteporfin absorbs light efficiently at a wavelength of 689 nm which can penetrate a thin layer of blood or melanin. The strongest absorption peak of verteporfin is at approximately 400 nm which at the same absorption peak of oxyhemoglobin. Hence, the optimal energy absorption and suitable light source for verteporfin activation is at wavelength of 689 nm which can be achieved by using a non-thermal diode laser. The laser system has been specifically designed to deliver a high convergence parfocal beam that provides an even distribution of power over the treatment spot on the retina with low intensity at the cornea.

MECHANISM OF ACTION

There are four main stages of mechanism of action of visudyne therapy:

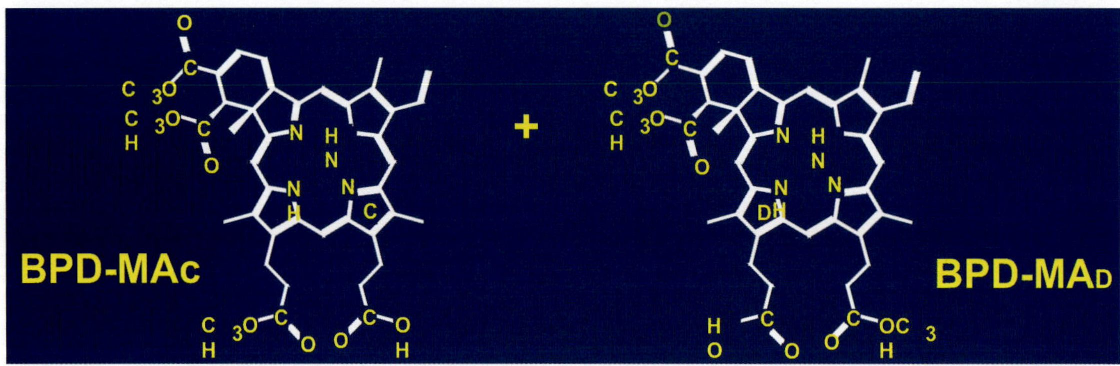

FIGURE 8.1: Verteporfin: Pharmacological structure (Novartis Ophthalmics, India)

1. *In vitro* studies have shown that lipophilic verteporfin is taken up by a process of receptor—mediated endocytosis via low density lipoprotein (LDL) receptors. Hence, after infusion, circulating verteporfin complexes with LDL.

2. LDL-verteporfin complex selectively accumulates within the new vessel. This is due to increased uptake of LDL and increased expression of LDL receptors on rapidly proliferating cells. It is then taken into the cell and binds to the intracellular or cytoplasmic components.

3. Application of non-thermal laser to the target tissue causes verteporfin to transform from a ground singlet state to an excited triplet state. From its triplet state, photochemical reactions occurs either directly via the formation of reactive free radicals (Type I mechanism) or indirectly via the transfer of its energy into ground state oxygen and highly reactive singlet oxygen (Type II mechanism; Figure 8.3). The free radical intermediates react with lipids in cellular membranes causing structural and functional cell damage. Singlet oxygen reacts directly with the cellular structures causing intermediate cell damage.

4. This reactive cellular changes cause damage to the endothelial cell lining, thereby causing red and white blood cells accumulation, platelet aggregation and fibrin clot formation. These block the lumen of the new vessels selectively while minimal damage may occur to the overlying photoreceptors and retinal pigment epithelium.

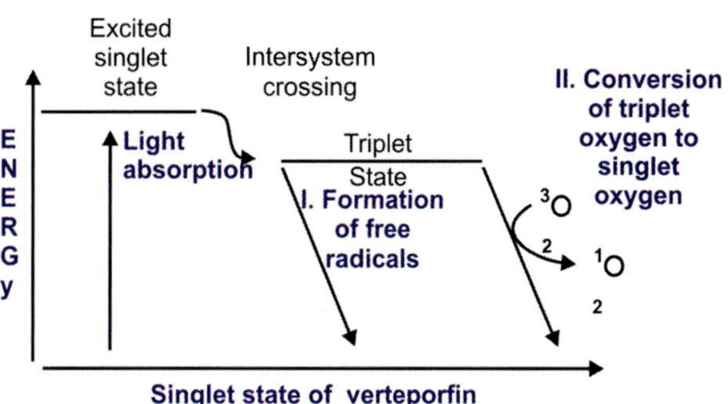

FIGURE 8.3: Photoexcitation of verteporfin

PREPARATION OF THE DRUG

Verteporfin is supplied as a lyophilized cake of 15 mg requiring reconstitution with 7 ml of sterile water. The resulting solution contains 15 mg in 7.5 ml or 2 mg/ml. After reconstitution the drug should be protected from light and used within 4 hours.

Parameters required to calculate the dosage are height and body weight. After determining the height and body weight one can use the dosage scale (Figure 8.4) to calculate the volume of drug and 5% dextrose.

After calculating the dose of visudyne and 5 % dextrose, the following steps are followed:

1. The calculated drug volume is withdrawn into a separate syringe.

2. The remaining volume of 5% dextrose is taken in a 30 ml syringe.

3. The drug volume is then injected into the 30 ml syringe to make a 30 ml of final volume to be injected.

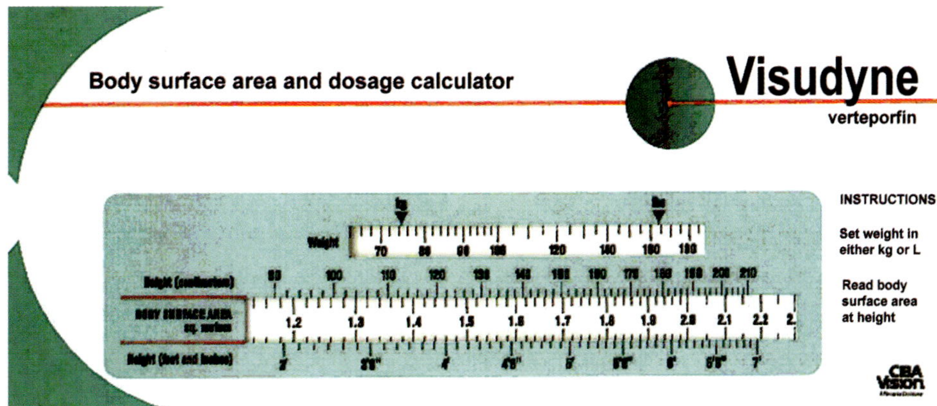

FIGURE 8.4: Dosage calculator (Novartis Ophthalmics, India)

Proper dosing is essential as under dosage can often result in inadequate treatment and over dosage can cause closure of larger retinal vessels with permanent visual loss. All the steps of reconstitution should be performed in a dimly lighted or dark room.

LASER SETTINGS

Two laser devices are currently approved for use in photodynamic therapy (PDT) with Visudyne. These are the Coherent Opal Photoactivator (Coherent, Santa Clara, USA) and Zeiss Visulas 690s laser (Zeiss Humphrey System, Dublin, USA). The laser device deliver stable power output at a wavelength of 689 nm. The light dose is 50 J/cm^2 or 600 mW/cm^2. The light energy is delivered over 83 seconds. The laser device requires the entry of spot size as well as the magnification of the fundus contact lens being used (Table 8.1).

Table 8.1: Fundus contact lens magnification

Make	Model	Magnification
Ocular Instruments, USA	Mainster Standard	1.05×
Ocular Instruments, USA	Mainster Widefield	1.50×
Volk, USA	PDT	1.50×
Volk, USA	QuadraAshperic	2.10×
Ocular Instruments, USA	3-Mirror Universal	1.08×

CALCULATION OF GREATEST LINEAR DIMENSION (GLD) AND LASER SPOT SIZE (LSD)

The spot size is determined by evaluation of fluorescein angiography using either a film based or digital angiography system. If a film based system is used then a reticule must be used taking into consideration the magnification of the camera system. Digital system is more frequently used now and this has made the calculation less cumbersome. Most of the systems are supplied with software programs. A mid-phase of fluorescein angiogram with 30° is chosen for calculation. The cursor is dragged along the lesion map and the output is read on the screen (Figure 8.5). Care must be taken to include the entire neovascular complex including pigment epithelial detachment and blocked fluorescence.

The final spot size is measured by adding 1000 microns to the GLD. A safe zone of at least 200 microns

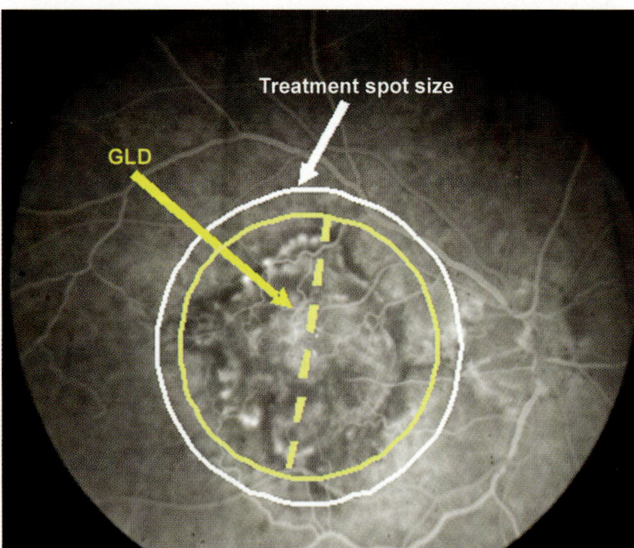

FIGURE 8.5: Shows the measured greatest linear dimension. The final spot size is measured by adding 1000 microns to the greatest linear dimension.

is recommended temporal to the margin of the optic nerve head.

TREATMENT

Photodynamic therapy is a two step procedure involving administration of Visudyne followed by activation with a non-thermal light source. The antecubital vein is preferred to reduce the complication of extravasation from smaller and more fragile veins. An infusion pump is set to deliver 3 ml of solution per minute such that 30 ml is delivered in 10 minutes. Patient is monitored carefully during infusion. Laser treatment should begin 15 minutes after the start of the infusion (5 minutes after the completion of infusion).

The spot size and the fundus lens magnification should be entered into the photoactivator. Pupil should be widely dilated and topical anesthesia instilled. The photoactivator is activated and aiming spot size beam is focused on the lesion area and foot pedal pressed to activate the drug at the area of concern. It is always a good idea to keep the fluorescein angiography image in-front at the time of treatment to identify the exact treatment site.

If extravasation occurs, infusion should be stopped immediately. If less than half (15 ml) of the dose has been administered then a better vein should be obtained.

Infusion can be restarted. If greater than 15 ml has been administered then treatment should proceed using the infused dose. Treatment can be suspended temporarily if there is excessive movement.

PRECAUTIONS

Special precautions should be taken after PDT and these needs to be explained to the patient during counseling. These are as follows:

1. Direct bright or sunlight is to be avoided for 48 hours.
2. Sunglasses have to be worn for 7 days.
3. Exposed surface needs to be protected while the patient transit from the treatment clinic to home.
4. Patient is advised to report immediately if there is any adverse events or any decrease in vision.
5. Bright halogen lights and surgical or dental operative lights have to be avoided for 7 days.

Age-related macular degeneration is the leading cause of central visual loss in adults aged more than 50 years of age. Macular Photocoagulation Study (MPS) have shown that patients treated with laser for subfoveal CNV had marginally better visual acuity than untreated eyes at 24 months. However, it was inevitably associated with rapid decline in vision followed by stabilization. The risk of immediate visual loss, irreversible damage to overlying neurosensory retina, permanent scotoma and recurrence of CNV are the drawbacks of laser treatment.

The effect of verteporfin therapy has been studied in carefully designed and controlled studies. The TAP investigations demonstrated that patients with classic subfoveal CNV due to AMD were significantly more likely to avoid at least 15 letter loss from the baseline through 2 years than the placebo group. The benefits of verteporfin therapy were found to be greatest in patients with predominantly classic CNV (lesions containing at least 50% classic CNV) at baseline regardless of lesion size. The effect on the vision of patients with predominantly classic CNV was maintained through 5 years in an open label extension study to TAP investigation.

The 48 month analysis of the open label extension of 'Treatment of Age-related Macular Degeneration with Photodynamic Therapy' (TAP) investigation indicates that in patients with predominantly classic CNV at baseline,

visual acuity remained stable between 24 and 48 months. There was very little change in visual acuity from month 24 through month 48 examinations. Forty-three percent had lost at least 15 letters from the baseline and 12.9% has lost at least 30 letters from the baseline. The mean visual acuity letter score was 50 at baseline, 41 at month 24th, 40 at month 36th and 39 at month 48th. The mean treatment rate was 3.2 in the first year, 2.2 at 2nd year and 0.4 at 4 years.

Patients treated with verteporfin for occult with no classic CNV in 'Verteporfin in Photodynamic Therapy' (VIP) trial were more likely to avoid at least 15 letters of visual acuity loss from baseline through 2 years than patients in the placebo group (p=0.032). Additionally, the greatest benefits of verteporfin therapy were found in patients with either smaller lesions (< 4 MPS disk areas) or lower levels of visual acuity (letter score < 65) with 51% had $\leq$ 15 letters loss compared to 25% of the placebo group (P< 0.001). Hence, results suggest that verteporfin therapy reduced the risk of at least 3 or 6 line visual acuity loss in occult CNV and presumed recent disease progression. Presumed recent disease was defined as the presence of blood from CNV, growth of the lesion (at least 10% increase in the greatest linear dimension of the lesion) within last 12 weeks or deterioration of best corrected visual acuity (at least 5 letters or approx. one line) within last 12 weeks. For larger lesions (> 4 MPS disk areas) or higher levels of visual acuity, 28% of patients treated with verteporfin had $\leq$ 15 letters loss compared to 48% in the placebo group. Hence, for larger lesions (> 4 MPS disk areas) therapy should be considered only if visual acuity has deteriorated to a lower level (approx. 20/50^{-1} or less). However, it does not recommend for treatment of occult with no classic CNV that > 9 MPS disk areas at presentation.

In the natural history study of minimally classic subfoveal CNV in the TAP investigation, 98 placebo treated lesions were identified as having minimally classic composition at the study entry. 40% (n=39) converted to predominantly classic CNV (21 by month 3 and 34 by month 9) irrespective of whether they were small ($\leq$ 4 MPS) at the baseline. Visual acuity benefits from verteporfin therapy was not found in the subgroup of patients with minimally classic CNV in the TAP investigation, even though treatment effect in contrast sensitivity and several secondary angiographic outcomes including reduced risk of lesion growth was observed. This may be due to undetected imbalance in the baseline lesion characteristics between the placebo and the treatment groups. It may have been possible that small ($\leq$ 4 MPS disk area) minimally classic lesions may benefit from treatment in the same way as the no classic occult small lesions as seen in the VIP trial. If conversion to classic lesion composition occurring in a setting of presumed recent disease progression, verteporfin therapy might also reduce the risk of vision loss especially if the lesion is smaller ($\leq$ 4 MPS disk area) or associated with lower level of visual acuity ($\leq$ 20/50) as observed in no classic occult lesions. It was also observed that only 20% converted to predominantly classic composition when lesion size was $\leq$ 9 MPS disk area and visual acuity $\geq$ 20/200. Hence, small minimally classic lesions if one may prefer to treat but natural history study suggest rationale to observe lesions with larger size.

The loss of contrast sensitivity is a frequent consequence of neovascular AMD and this imposes a serious impact in the quality of life and functional ability. Contrast sensitivity and visual acuity are both independent factor in the model of visual disability. It is a useful predictor of reading speed, mobility and ability to recognize visual targets such as faces or road signs. In the TAP investigation study population, patients who received verteporfin therapy lost significantly fewer letters of contrast sensitivity compared with placebo. Verteporfin treated patients lost a mean of 1.3 letters at 12 months with no further change at 24 months, whereas placebo treated patients lost a mean of 4.5 letters at 12 months and 5.2 letters at 24 months. The time-to-event analysis of the time to a loss of at least 6 or 15 letters of contrast sensitivity also showed a significant treatment benefit for patients who received verteporfin therapy. These treatment benefits were seen at the first examination at month 3 and were sustained throughout the 24 months of the study. At the month 12 examination, patients with predominantly classic lesions at baseline who were given placebo lost a mean of 5.6 letters of contrast sensitivity, where as verteporfin treated patients lost only 0.4 letters (P< 0.001). This

difference was sustained through 24 months. In the minimally classic lesion group, the difference between the placebo and verteporfin treated group was as large as seen in predominantly classic lesion group. Many vision related tasks, such as watching television or reading, depends on both contrast sensitivity and visual acuity. By reducing the risk of losing contrast sensitivity and visual acuity, verteporfin therapy may enable patients to maintain better functional abilities than they would have if they remained untreated.

As neovascular AMD affects the highly developed functions of macula. The intensity, dimension and location of central scotomas, macular fixation and reading ability vary considerably in these patients. Verteporfin therapy also influenced the scotoma size. Schmidt – Erfurth and associates [30] have shown that the mean absolute scotoma in the verteporfin group was 2.5 mm^2 at baseline and did not increase till 3rd month. It progressively increased to 6.2 mm^2 at 6 months (P<0.01) and 6.9 mm^2 at 9 months. From 12 months onwards it remained stable at 8.9 mm^2 till 18 months. Interestingly, the mean size regressed to 6.6 mm^2 at month 21 and 7.3 mm^2 at month 24 (P< 0.01 compared to month 12). In the placebo group, mean initial size (2.7 mm^2) increased to 4.82 mm^2 at month 3 and progressively increased to 11.2 mm^2 at month 6th (P< 0.01). Moderate enlargement was noted at month 12 (16.4 mm^2) and progressive growth occurred again at 21 and 24 months to 29 mm^2 and 31.5 mm^2 respectively. Hence significant larger growth occurred in the placebo group (P<0.001). Even the relative scotoma followed the similar trend in the verteporfin treated and placebo group as seen in the absolute scotoma pattern. The results for central visual field maintenance by verteporfin therapy support the TAP investigation outcomes obtained for distance visual acuity with a clear advantage for eyes receiving PDT versus placebo treatment. Continuous shrinkage of the fibrotic scar and resolution of leakage has shown that residual functional defect was only 2.5 times larger than the baseline in the verteporfin treated group while it was approximately 12 times larger than the baseline in the placebo group at the end of 24 months. Relative scotoma may reflect photoreceptor dysfunction because of intraretinal and subretinal fluid as it was located primarily in the area of intensive leakage seen angiographically. Interestingly, this was present even when leakage was absent for verteporfin therapy. Areas showing relative functional loss consistently showed dry atrophic changes at the level of retinal pigment epithelium and choriocapillaries damage. Scotometry shortly after single PDT had shown an eventual resolution of absolute scotoma and often decrease in scotoma size and intensity. This finding may imply that advanced sensory retinal damage may recover after single PDT but this advantage may be lost after repeated treatment applications. The benefit of verteporfin therapy in the reduction of central defects is significant and may further be able to be improved by optimization of treatment strategy.

The overall safety profile for verteporfin therapy was judged by the TAP and VIP study groups to be excellent, based on 3 masked, placebo controlled trials in 948 AMD patients treated and followed for 2 years. Verteporfin therapy was administered to 627 patients who received 3,334 treatment courses during 2 years. Visual disturbance events are common in the natural progression of AMD. The higher incidence of events in the verteporfin group and the temporal association with the therapy in most of these events suggests a true treatment reaction consistent with the local pharmacologic effect of verteporfin therapy. Patients in VIP and AMD trial, who had occult with no classic CNV and better visual acuity at baseline (Approx $20/50^{+1}$) reported a higher incidence of visual disturbance than the patients in TAP investigations who had classic CNV and worse visual acuity at baseline ($20/80^{-2}$). Acute severe visual acuity decrease (≥ 4 lines within 7 days of therapy) was relatively uncommon, occurring in 4.9% in VIP AMD trial and 0.7% in TAP investigations. The 5% risk of acute severe vision loss is outweighed by the net vision benefit of verteporfin therapy, which reduces the risk of moderate and severe visual loss.

Injection site reactions occurred with relatively high incidence (13.4%) in the first 12 months of TAP investigation in verteporfin treated patients. Twelve-month data showed that these events were common. Hence additional precautions were taken to avoid extravasations. These included using the largest vein possible for the injection, establishing a free flowing intravenous line before starting the verteporfin infusion and monitoring

carefully during infusion. These precautions appeared to be associated with reduced risk of subsequent injection site events, as was seen in the last half of 12 months. The incidence of photosensitivity reactions was low in verteporfin treated patients (2.4%). Most of the reaction occurred within one day of therapy. Infusion related back pain was seen in 15 patients (2.4%). Verteporfin for injection is a lipid based formulation, and it has been suggested that liposomes may activate the alternative complement pathway and the production of anaphylatoxins. This may lead to back pain phenomenon. This hypothesis was supported by a study suggesting that neutrophil margination which was quickly reversible was a possible mechanism for verteporfin related pain.

TREATMENT GUIDELINES

The algorithm for verteporfin therapy for neovascular AMD is shown in Figure 8.6.

The third round table discussion group sponsored by Novartis Ophthalmics and QLT Inc. was held in 2003 to diskuss and interpret additional data from ongoing phase 3 clinical trials and new phase II studies to consider the impact of the new data on current treatment guidelines and to agree on appropriate revisions. The guidelines were made to assists the ophthalmologists in identifying those patients where verteporfin therapy would be beneficial and follow-up pattern of these patients.

RECOMMENDATIONS[14]

1. Verteporfin therapy is recommended to treat eyes that present with a subfoveal lesion that is predominantly classic.

2. Treatment should be considered for relatively small minimally classic lesion. Also where the proportion of classic CNV is determined to be increasing and approaching 50%. If it crosses 50% treatment should be recommended.

3. Treatment should be recommended for subfoveal occult with no classic CNV and presumed recent disease progression. Presumed recent disease progression was defined as the presence of blood from the CNV, growth of the lesion (at least a 10% increase in the greatest linear dimension) within the last

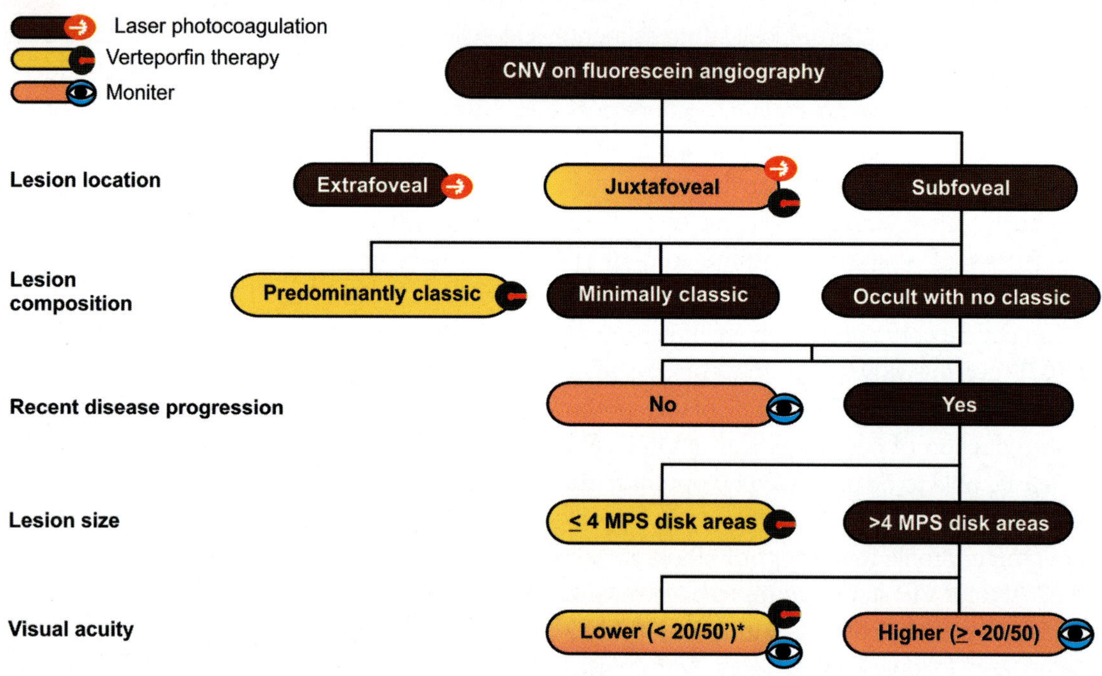

FIGURE 8.6: Algorithm for verteporfin therapy for neovascular age-related macular degeneration (Novartis Ophthalmics, India).

12 weeks or deterioration of best corrected visual acuity (at least 5 letters) within last 12 weeks. It is beneficial primarily for either smaller lesion (< 4 MPS disk area) or lower level of visual acuity (< 65 letters or ≤ 20/50). For larger lesion, therapy is considered if visual acuity is deteriorated to lower level. For lesion larger than 9 MPS disk area, therapy might be considered if associated with rapidly decreasing level of best corrected visual acuity.

4. Lesion size: Lesion size did not appear to affect the treatment benefit in predominantly classic lesion. However, above criteria is recommended for Occult with no classic and minimally classic lesions.

5. Lesion location: Verteporfin therapy is recommended for CNV that extends under the geometric centre of the foveolar avascular zone. It should also be considered for juxtafoveal lesions that are close to the fovea in which conventional laser almost certainly would extend under the foveolar avascular zone.

6. Influence of visual acuity in patient selection: At present, the lowest level of visual acuity for which verteporfin therapy should be routinely considered

is not known. It is of the opinion that it is reasonable to consider treatment, if all the criteria for therapy are met, if a patient's vision is at a level where further loss of visual acuity would be recognized as detrimental to their quality of life.

7. Criteria not influencing patient selection: The following features do not seem to affect the treatment outcome:
   - Patient age
   - Systemic arterial hypertension
   - Prior laser photocoagulation that does not extend under the center of the foveolar avascular zone
   - Treatment is also beneficial for CNV secondary to pathological myopia, angioid streaks, etc.
   - Subfoveal lesions contiguous to the optic nerve should be a contraindication to treatment. But to ensure that the optic nerve is not damaged, treatment spot should be placed at least 200 microns away from the optic nerve
   - No safety concerns have been reported for treatment of CNV in patients who have retinal vasculopathies like diabetic retinopathy or idiopathic parafoveal telangiectasis.

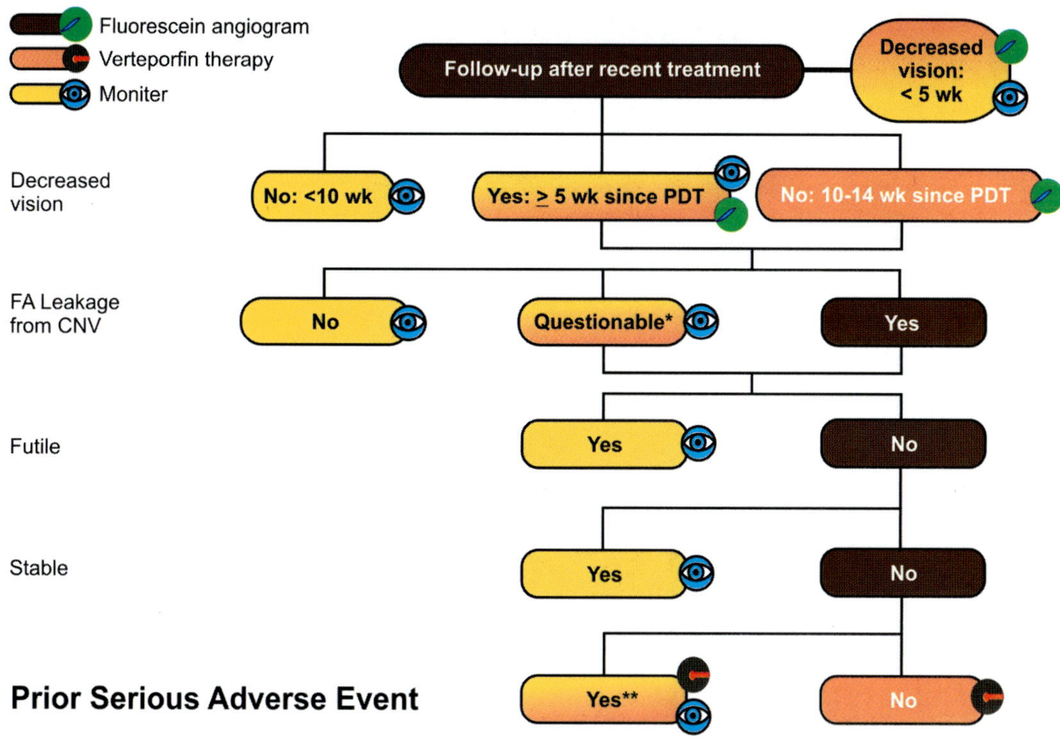

FIGURE 8.7: Algorithm for monitoring, performing fluorescein angiography and retreatment during follow-up of patients who undergo verteporfin therapy (Novartis Ophthalmics, India)

TREATMENT AND FOLLOW-UP PROCEDURES AFTER INITIAL VERTEPORFIN THERAPY

Algorithm for monitoring, performing fluorescein angiography and retreatment during follow-up of patients who undergo verteporfin therapy is shown in Figure 8.7.

The salient features are:

1. Verteporfin therapy should be initiated within 1 week of initial fluorescein angiography on which the clinical decision for treatment was based.

2. Patients should return for follow-up at least as often as every 3 months ($\pm$ 2 weeks) after initial or subsequent treatment to determine if there is any fluorescein angiography leakage from CNV.

3. If additional course of treatment is not judged to be indicated for at least 6 months then, follow-up might be scheduled at 6-month intervals and eventually at 6 to 12 months intervals. If patients notice any visual deterioration between scheduled visits, follow-up might be considered to determine whether any additional treatment is necessary.

4. Patient could receive an additional course of treatment every 3 months if there is any fluorescein angiography leakage from the CNV. Additional courses of treatment could also be considered earlier than 3 months if patient complains of vision loss, documented visual acuity loss and fluorescein angiography showing enlargement of CNV compared with fluorescein angiography performed before the most recent treatment (Figures 8.8A and B).

5. After verteporfin therapy, an extrafoveal lesion either contiguous or non-contiguous to the previously verteporfin treated lesion, conventional laser photocoagulation can be considered.

6. Patients who present with minimally classic lesion, for whom no therapy is recommended initially, should be monitored carefully so that the potential conversion to a predominantly classic lesion can be identified promptly.

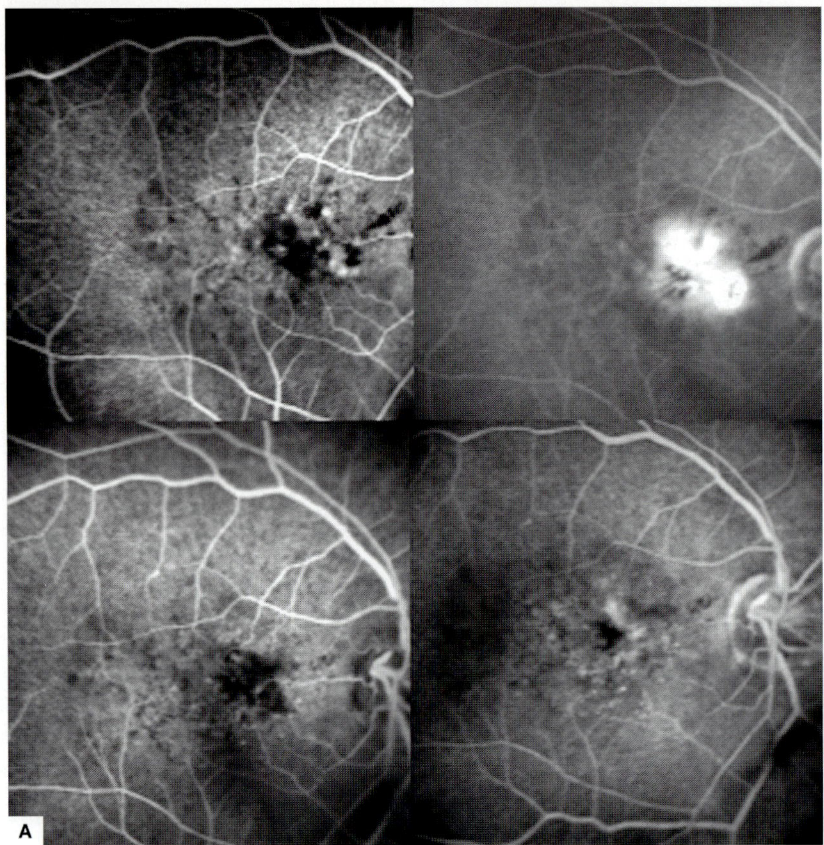

FIGURE 8.8A: Prephotodynamic therapy fluorescein angiography images of the right eye showing a predominantly classic CNV (top) with initial visual acuity of 20/125. Three months following verteporfin therapy shows still active leakage for which 2nd treatment was considered (visual acuity: 20/80).

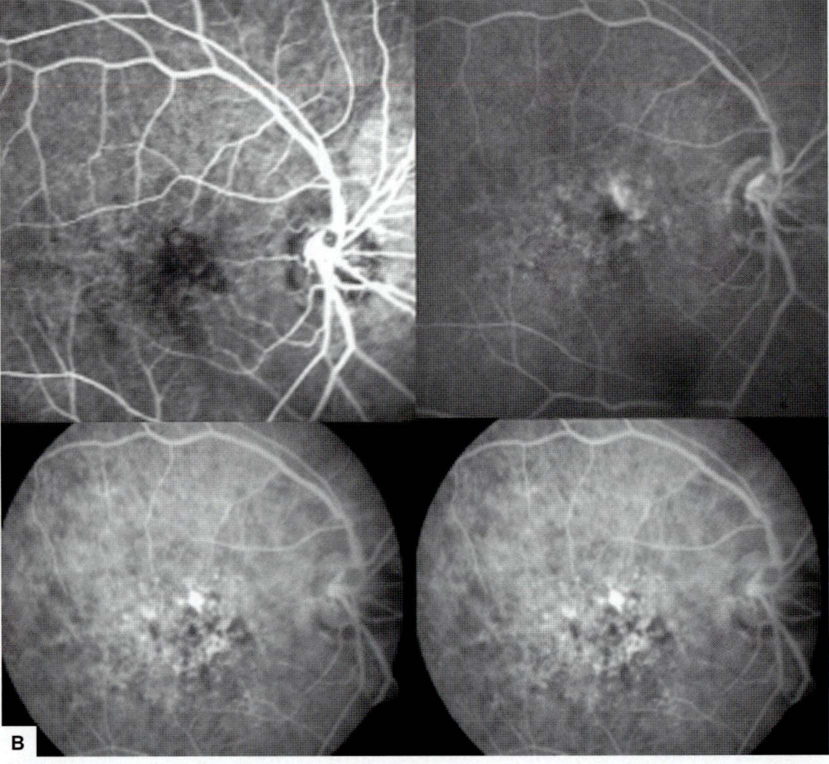

FIGURE 8.8B: Six-month follow-up fluorescein angiogram shows resolved CNV (top) and 12 months follow-up fluorescein angiogram (below) shows no active leakage. Note the retinal pigment epithelium changes in the area of treatment.

7. In patients with an occult with no classic lesion associated with both larger lesion size and better level of visual acuity, continued observation rather than cessation of follow-up is recommended. This is because some of the lesion may become predominantly classic with a lesion size and visual acuity amenable for verteporfin therapy and also some lesion may remain occult associated with progressive vision loss but still be within the visual acuity range as well as lesion size for treatment could be considered.

REFERENCES

1. Schmidt–Erfurth U, Hasan T. Mechanisms of action of photodynamic therapy with verteporfin for the treatment of age-related macular degeneration. Surv Ophthalmol 2000; 45:195-214.
2. Aveline B, Hasan T, Redmond RW. Photophysical and photosensitizing properties of benzoporphyrin derivative monoacid ring A (BPD-MA). Photochem Photobiol 1994; 59:328–35.
3. Richter AM, Yip S, Meadows H, et al. Photosensitizing potencies of the structural analogues of benzoporphyrin derivative in different biological test systems. J Clin Laser Med Surg 1996; 14:33–41.
4. Alison BA, Pritchard PH, Levy JG. Evidence for low density lipoprotein receptor mediated uptake of benzoporphyrin derivative. Br J Cancer 1994; 69:833-39.
5. Fogelman AM, Berliner JA, Van Lenten BJ, et al. Lipoprotein receptors and endothelial cells. Semin Thromb Hemost 1988; 14:206–09.
6. Schmidt–Erfurth U, Hasan T, Schomacker K, Flotte T, Birngruber R. In vivo uptake of liposomal benzoporphyrin derivative and photothrombosis in experimental corneal neovascularization. Lasers Surg Med 1995; 17:178–88.
7. Gaffney J, West D, Arnold F, et al. Differences in the uptake of modified low density lipoproteins by tissue cultured endothelial cells. J Cell Sci 1985: 79:317–25.
8. Schmidt-Erfurth U, Bauman W, Gragoudas E, et al. Photodynamic therapy of experimental choroidal melanoma using lipoprotein-delivered benzoporphyrin. Ophthalmology 1994; 101:89–99.
9. Macular Photocoagulation Study Group. Laser photocoagulation of subfoveal neovascular lesions in age-related macular degeneration: results of a randomized clinical trial. Arch Ophthalmol 1991; 109:1220–31.
10. Macular Photocoagulation Study Group. Subfoveal neovascular lesions in age-related macular degeneration: guidelines for evaluation and treatment in macular photocoagulation study. Arch Ophthalmol. 1991; 109:1242–57.
11. Treatment of Age-related Macular Degeneration with Photodynamic Therapy (TAP) study group. Verteporfin for subfoveal choroidal neovascularization in age-related macular degeneration: three year results of an open label extension of 2 randomized clinical trials – TAP report No. 5 Arch Ophthalmol 2002; 120:1307–14.
12. Treatment of Age-related macular degeneration with photodynamic therapy (TAP) study group. Verteporfin for subfoveal choroidal neovascularization in age-related macular degeneration: three year results of an open label extension of 2 randomized clinical trials. TAP report No. 7 Arch Ophthalmol 2005; 120:1283–85.
13. Verteporfin in Photodynamic Therapy (VIP) Study Group. Verteporfin therapy of subfoveal choroidal neovascularization in age-related macular degeneration: two year results of a randomized clinical trial including lesions with occult occult with no classic choroidal neovascularization – Verteporfin In Photodynamic therapy report 2. Am J Ophthalmol 2001; 131:541-60.
14. Guidelines for using Verteporfin (Visudyne) in photodynamic therapy for choroidal neovascularization due to age-related macular degeneration and other causes: Update. Verteporfin round table participants. Retina 2005; 25:119-34.
15. Verteporfin therapy of subfoveal choroidal neovascularization in age-related macular degeneration. Meta-analysis of 2 year safety results in three randomized clinical trials: Treatment of Age-related Macular Degeneration with Photodynamic Therapy and Verteporfin in Photodynamic Therapy Study Report No. 4. Retina 2004; 24:1-12.
16. Treatment of Age-related Macular Degeneration with Photodynamic Therapy (TAP) Study Group. Photodynamic therapy of subfoveal choroidal neovascularization in age-related macular degeneration with verteporfin: One year results of 2 randomized clinical trials – TAP report. Arch Ophthalmol 1999; 117:1329–45.
17. Bressler NM. Treatment of Age-related Macular Degeneration with Photodynamic Therapy (TAP) Study Group. Photodynamic therapy of subfoveal choroidal neovascularization in age-related macular degeneration with verteporfin: Two year results of 2 randomized clinical trials – TAP report 2. Arch Ophthalmol 2001; 119:198-207.
18. Cunningham CM, Kingzette M, Richards RL, et al. Activation of human complement by liposomes: A model for membrane activation of the alternate pathway. J Immunol 1979; 122:1237–42.
19. Chonn A, Cullis PR, Devine DV. The role of surface charge in the activation of the classical and alternative pathways of complement by liposomes. J Immunol 1991; 146:4234–41.
20. Devine DV, Wong K, Serrano K, et al. Liposome-complement interactions in rat serum: implications for liposome survival studies. Biochim Biophys Acta 1994; 1191:43–51.
21. Szebeni J, Wassef NM, Rudolf AS, Alving CR. Complement activation by liposome encapsulated hemoglobin in vitro: The role of endotoxin contamination. Artif Cells Blood Substit Immobil Biotechnol 1995; 23:355–63.

22. Spaide RF, Maranan L. Neutrophil margination as a possible mechanism for verteporfin infusion associated pain. Am J Ophthalmol 2003; 135:549-50.
23. Bressler SB, Pieramici DJ, Koester JM, Bressler NM. Natural history of minimally classic subfoveal choroidal neovascular lesions in the treatment of age-related macular degeneration with photodynamic therapy (TAP) investigation. Outcome potentially relevant to management – TAP Report No. 6. Arch Ophthalmol 2004; 122:325–29.
24. Verteporfin therapy of subfoveal minimally classic choroidal neovascularization in age-related macular degeneration. 2 year results of a randomized clinical trial. Visudyne in minimally classic choroidal neovascularization study group. Arch Ophthalmol 2005; 123:448–57.
25. Rubin GS, Bressler NM, The treatment of age-related macular degeneration with photodynamic therapy (TAP) study group. Effects of verteporfin therapy on contrast sensitivity. Results from the treatment of age-related macular degeneration with photodynamic therapy (TAP) investigation – TAP report No. 4. Retina 2002; 22:536-44.
26. Hakkinen L. Vision in the elderly and its use in the social environment. Scand J Soc Med (Suppl) 1984;35:5–60.
27. Leat SJ, Woodhouse JM. Reading performance with low vision aids: relationship with contrast sensitivity. Ophthalmic Physiol Opt 1993;13:9–16.
28. Maron JA, Bailey IL. Visual factors and orientation—mobility performance. Am J Optom Physiol Opt 1982; 59:413–26.
29. Evans DW, Ginsburg AP. Contrast sensitivity predicts age-related differences in highway—sign diskriminability. Hum Factors 1985; 27:637–42.
30. Schmidt-Erfurth UM, Elsner H, Terai N, et al. Effects of verteporfin on central visual field function. Ophthalmology 2004; 111:931–39.
31. Ergun E, Maar N, Radner W, et al. Scotoma size and reading speed in patients with subfoveal occult choroidal neovascularization in age-related macular degeneration. Ophthalmology 2003; 110:65–69.
32. Moller F, Bek T. Lack of correlation between visual acuity and fixation stability after photocoagulation for diabetic maculopathy. Graefes Arch Clin Exp Ophthalmol 2000; 238:566–70.
33. Bunse A, Elsner H, Laqua H, Schimdt Erfurth U. Microperimetric documentation of retinal function in photodynamic therapy of choroidal neovascularization. Klin Monastbl Augenheilkd 2000; 216:158-64.

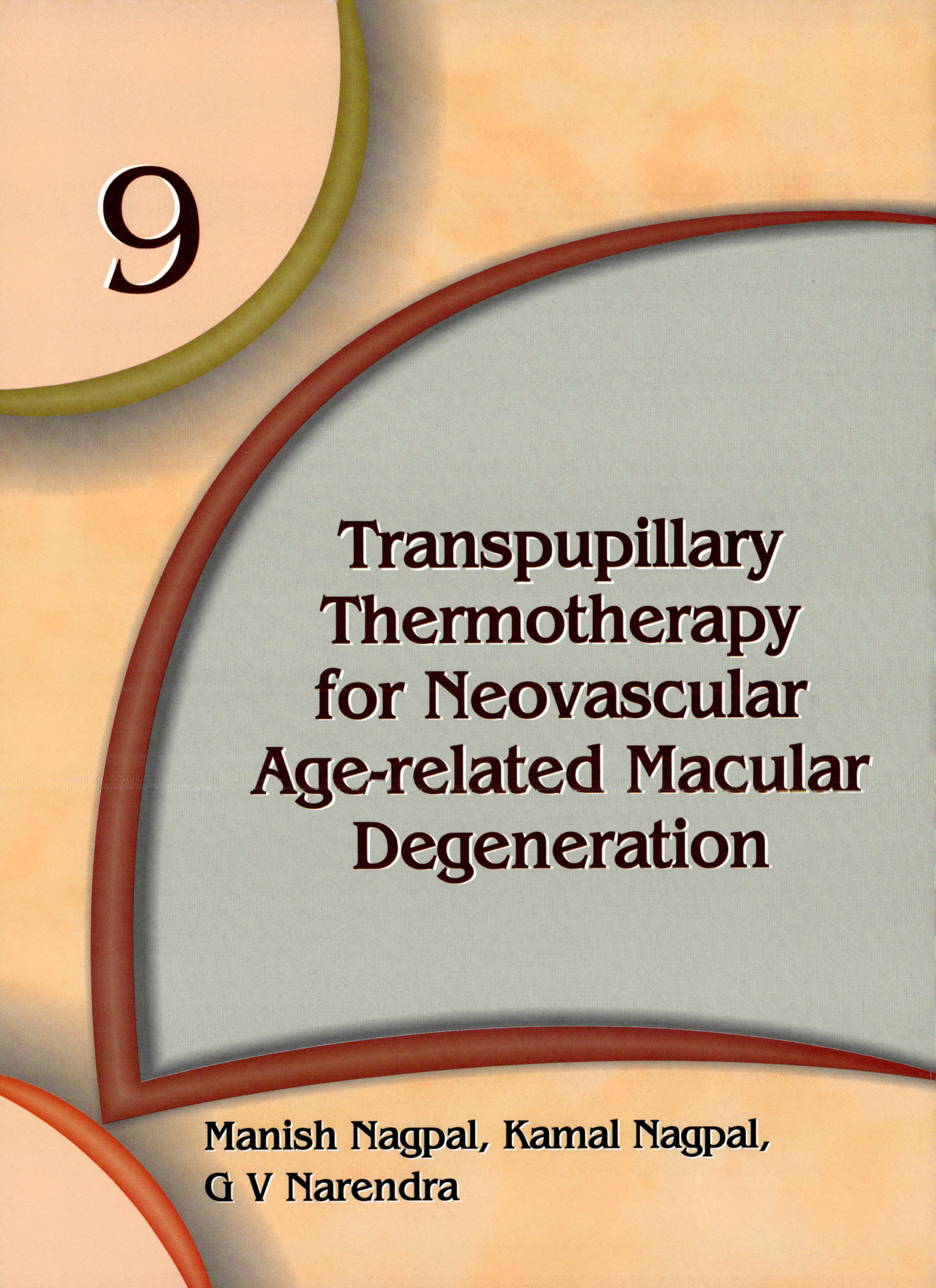

Transpupillary Thermotherapy for Neovascular Age-related Macular Degeneration

Manish Nagpal, Kamal Nagpal,
G V Narendra

INTRODUCTION

With increased life expectancy, age-related macular degeneration (AMD) has become the leading cause of irreversible visual loss among the elderly, across the globe.[1-8] Its prevalence increases sharply after the age of 65 years. Several epidemiological studies have found a 1.2 to 1.5% incidence of exudative age-related macular degeneration.[6-8] Although far less common than the non-exudative form of AMD, exudative or neovascular AMD is responsible for most cases of severe visual loss.[9]

Laser photocoagulation is the only therapy proven effective for selected patients with neovascular age related macular degeneration.[10] It has been shown to reduce the incidence of severe visual loss in patients with classic extrafoveal and juxtafoveal membranes by the Macular Photocoagulation Study (MPS) group.[11, 12] However, the MPS showed an immediate precipitous decline in central vision following laser treatment of subfoveal choroidal neovascular membrane (CNV), due to damage to the overlying neurosensory retina.[13] Also, a large proportion of the subfoveal CNV encountered clinically are occult, too large, or ill-defined. These are typically associated with poorer prognosis and do not meet the MPS guidelines for laser treatment.[14, 15] Therefore, CNV complicating AMD often remains an untreatable blinding disorder.

As a consequence, considerable effort is being directed toward developing novel treatment strategies for neovascular AMD. On one hand, laser prophylaxis to high risk drusens, in order to prevent the formation of CNV is being investigated.[16-18] On the other, the use of laser in a non-photocoagulative mode in the photodynamic therapy has been attempted.[19-22] Radiation therapy with its known antiangiogenic properties has been explored.[23-26] Pharmacological agents used for inhibition of angiogenesis such as interferon-alpha,[27] fumagillin derivatives,[28] interleukin-12,[29] thalidomide, etc. are undergoing trials for their potential beneficial role in AMD. Sub-retinal surgery with removal of subretinal blood and CNV[30-33] and the more recent macular translocation surgery[34-37] are further attempts to deal with this problem.

Lately, there have been clinical trials of the use of low irradiance, long pulse diode laser irradiation termed as "transpupillary thermotherapy" (TTT) for the management of occult and classic CNV due to AMD.[38,39] In this procedure, heat is delivered to the choroid and the retinal pigment epithelium through the pupil using a modified diode (810 nm) laser. Compared to the conventional laser photocoagulation it is found to be safer because of its greater penetrance and less absorption by xanthophyll and hemoglobin.

It was Reichel and associates[38] who demonstrated the efficacy of TTT in eyes with occult subfoveal CNV secondary to AMD. Newsom and associates[39] assessed the effectiveness of this procedure in classic and occult CNVs. They concluded that TTT is able to close CNV while maintaining visual function in patients with classic and occult CNV.

Based on encouraging initial results, we[40] conducted a study to evaluate its efficacy and to determine accurate power settings in Indian eyes. We had 99 eyes with classic and 61 eyes with occult membranes. After treatment, 80% of classic and 85% of occult membranes regressed (Figures 9.1 to 9.5). Visual improvement >/= 2 lines was seen in 29.3% and 19.6% eyes in the classic and occult group. Stabilization was noted in 39.4% and 57.4% eyes of the two groups respectively, while reduction was seen in 31.3% and 22.9% eyes with classic and occult membranes respectively. We found that Indian eyes responded to lower energy levels as compared to Caucasian eyes.

Use of TTT in ophthalmology was initiated and popularized mainly for intraocular tumors.[41-47] Reichel and associates[38] published the effectiveness of this method for the treatment of occult sub-foveal CNV. They followed 16 eyes of 15 patients for an average of 13 months following TTT. In their study, 3 eyes (19%) experienced a two or more line improvement in visual acuity, 9 eyes (56%) had stabilization of vision (no change or one line improvement) and 4 eyes (25%) showed a fall in vision by one or more lines. Recently, Newsom and associates[39] reported the use of TTT in 12 eyes with predominantly classical and 32 eyes with predominantly occult membranes and followed up these subjects for an average of 6.1 months. They showed that predominantly classic membranes were closed in 75% of eyes and

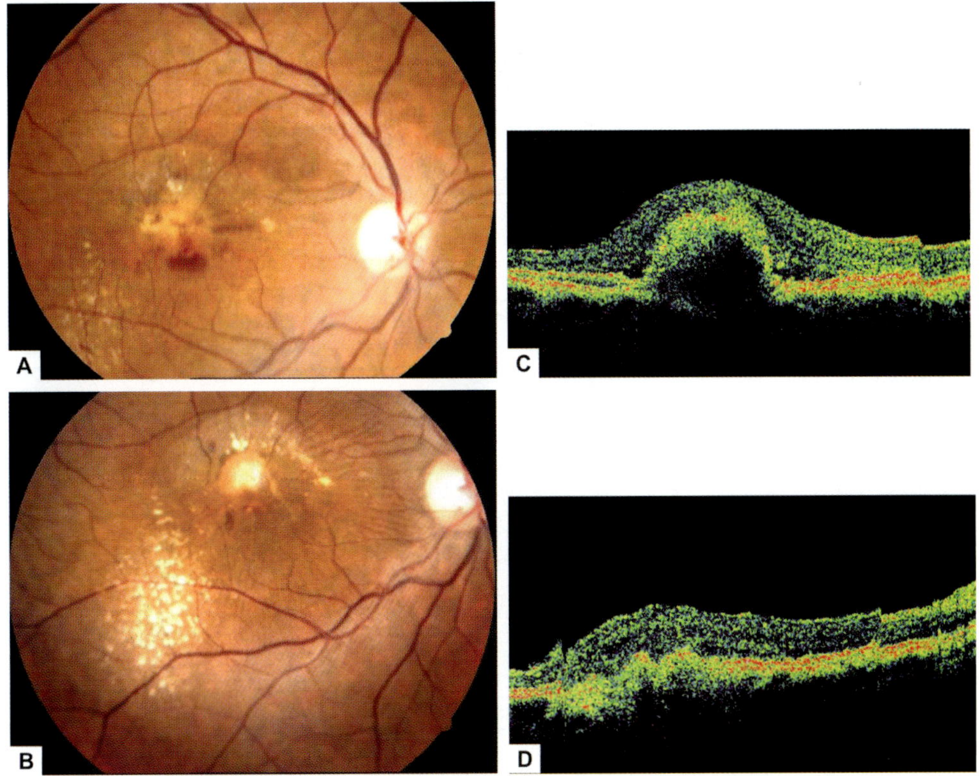

FIGURES 9.1A to D: (A, C) Pre-TTT fundus photograph and OCT. (B) Post-TTT Fundus picture reveals lessening of edema and hemorrhages. (D) Post-TTT OCT shows resolution of edema.

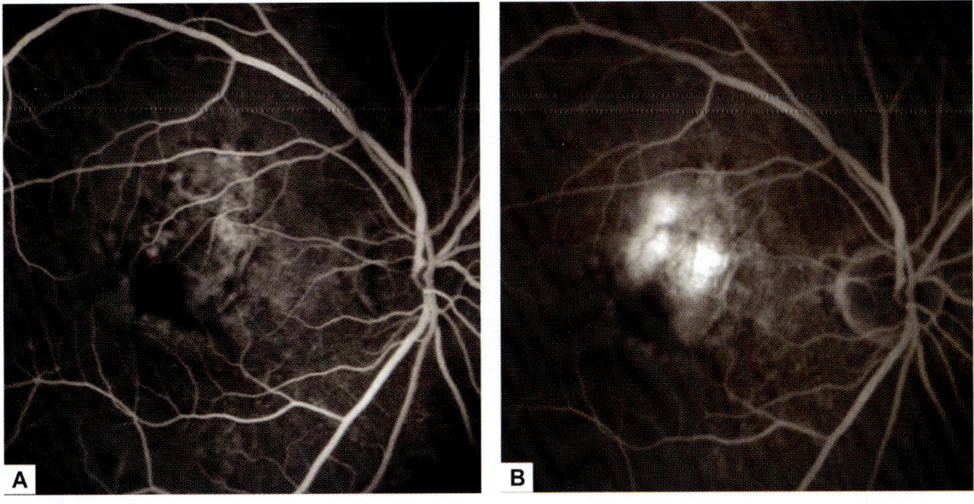

FIGURES 9.2A and B: Pre- and Post-TTT fluorescein angiograms, demonstrating lessening of leakages.

remained persistent in 25%. Predominantly occult membranes were closed in 78% of eyes and remained persistent in 12.5%. There were no recurrences in the classic membranes, while occult membranes were recurrent in 5.1%. The mean change in vision in their study group was –0.75 and –0.66. Snellen lines for the classic and occult membranes respectively. They concluded that TTT is able to close choroidal neovascular membranes, while maintaining visual function in eyes with both classic and occult disease.

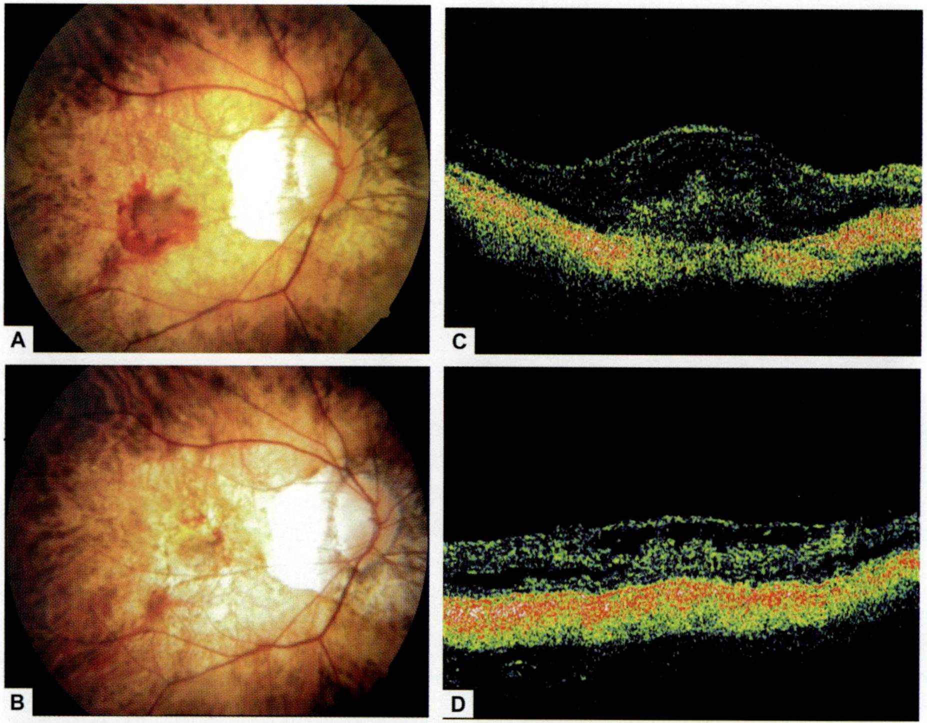

FIGURES 9.3A to D: (A, B) Pre- and Post-TTT fundus pictures. (C, D) Pre- and Post-TTT OCT contours, revealing decrease in macular thickness.

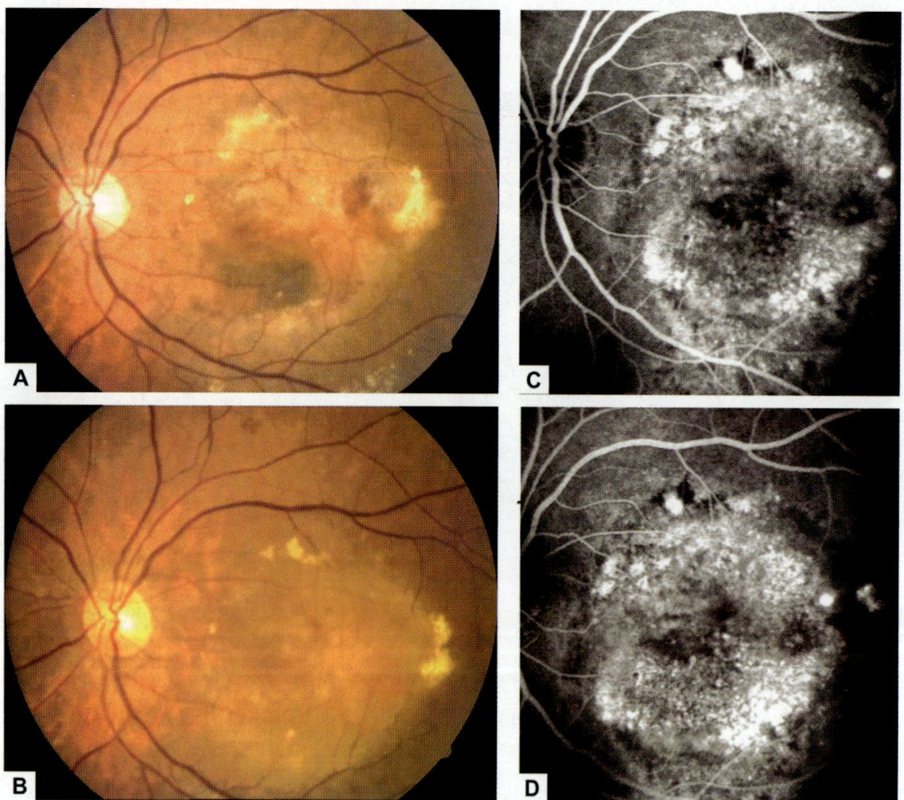

FIGURES 9.4A to D: (A, B) Pre- and Post-TTT fundus pictures. (C, D) Pre- and Post-TTT angiograms show decrease in leakage.

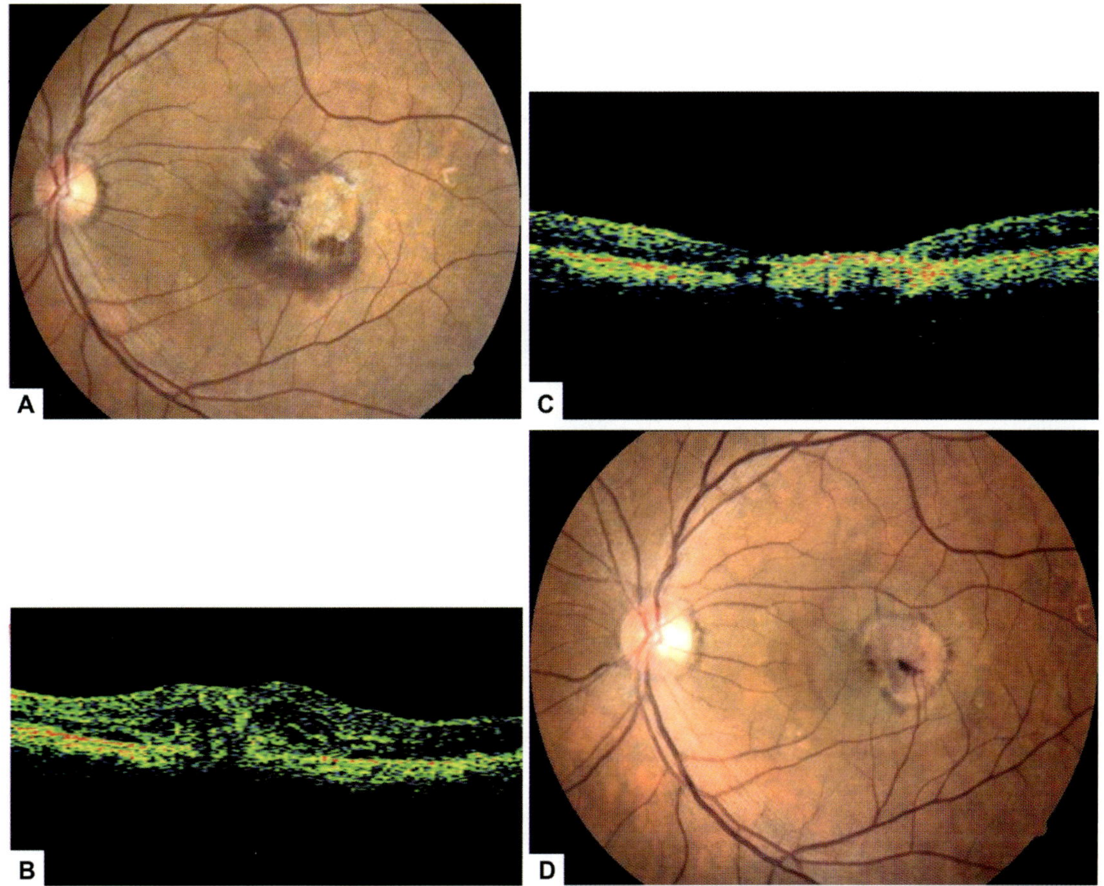

FIGURES 9.5A to D: (A,D) Pre- and Post-TTT fundus pictures. (B, C) Pre- and Post-TTT OCT pictures.

Table 9.1: Anatomical results

Number of eyes	Classic membranes	%	Occult membranes	%
Total	99		61	
Which responded to the first treatment	79	79.79%	52	85.24%
With membranes persisting after first treatment	20	20.20%	9	14.75%
Which underwent single retreatment	9	9.9%	9	14.75%
Which responded to the retreatment	4	4.4%	3	4.91%
Total anatomical success	83	83.83%	55	90.16%

Table 9.2: Visual results

	Classic membranes	%	Occult membranes	%
Visual improvement by 2 or more lines	29	29.29%	12	19.67%
Stabilization of vision (same as pre-treatment/ +/- 1 line)	39	39.39%	35	57.37%
Drop in vision by more than 1 line	31	31.31%	14	22.95%

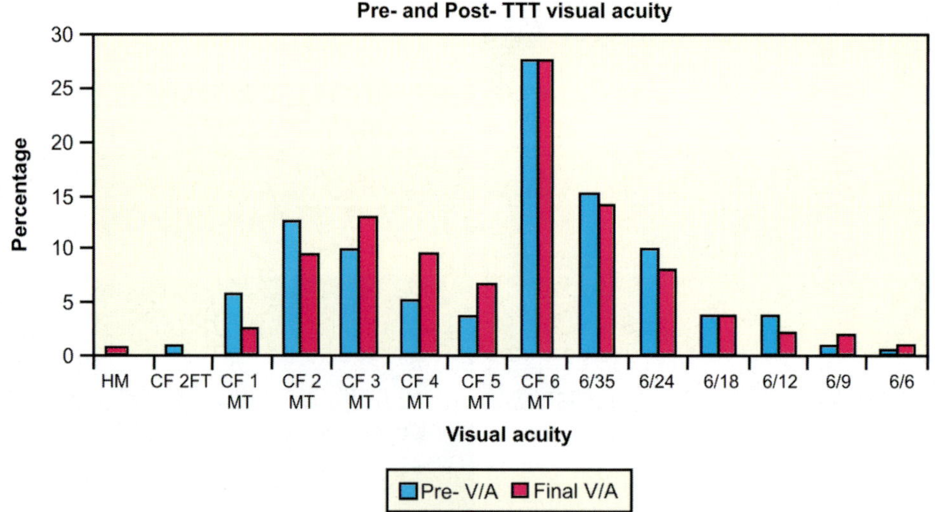

FIGURE 9.6: Pre and Post-TTT visual acuity.

Other instances, of the use of TTT for the treatment of occult and classic membranes, with promising results have also appeared in recent literature.[48-50] These results are encouraging given the grim natural history.[51,52]

A recent, unpublished data extracted for a multi-etiology TTT from our center, for a study period of 4 years from 2000 to 2004, in eyes with average period of follow up for 12 (6 months – 40 months) is as follows: The total number of eyes was 192, mean age at presentation was 59.5 years. 61% were males and 39% females. The mean duration at presentation was 8.5 months. The most common etiology was AMD –74.5% (n = 143); rest being myopia 15.6% (n=30), inflammation 5.2% (n=10), idiopathic polypoidal choroidal vasculopathy 1.6% (n=3), angioid streaks 1.6% (n=3), telangiectatic 1.6% (n=3). Most common was predominantly classic CNV, 65.1% (n=125) while the rest were occult CNV, 34.9% (n=67). Most common type was subfoveal 65.6% (n=126), followed by juxtafoveal 28.1% (n=54) and extrafoveal 6.3% (n=12). Pre-laser vision ranged from 0.001 to 1.00 (hand movement-6/6), mean 0.136(>6/60). Final post-laser vision ranged from 0.01-1.00 (counting finger 2 feet-6/6), mean 0.140 (>6/60) (Figure 9.6). Clinically, 76 eyes (39.6%) showed stabilization, 82 eyes (42.7%) showed regression and 34 eyes (17.7%) showed persistence or recurrence.

MECHANISM OF THERMOTHERAPY

Retinal absorption of optical radiation can produce photomechanical damage, photocoagulation or phototoxicity. Photomechanical retinal injuries occur when radiation from high powered military or industrial laser cause rapid chorioretinal distortion. Retinal photocoagulation occurs when radiation from lasers and other intense light sources causes thermal denaturation of chorioretinal proteins and damages other thermolabile molecular or supra molecular sub cellular components. Therapeutic retinal photocoagulation is typically performed using repetitive pulse, short pulse (<5 sec) or long pulse (>5 sec) laser sources and transpupillary transscleral or intraocular laser delivery system.

Retinal phototoxicity occurs when prolonged exposure to blue light or ultraviolet rays damage the photoreceptors by photochemical reactions. Therapeutic photochemical reactions are produced in PDT when a long pulse very low irradiance laser exposure activates a chemical photosensitizer that has been selectively absorbed in target tissues such as choroidal neovascularisation.

Transpupillary thermotherapy differs from conventional short pulse retinal photocoagulation in the sense it uses lengthy exposures and large retinal spot sizes to produce lower therapeutic retinal irradiances. It uses infrared radiation that has a deeper chorioretinal tissue penetration than visible light, decreased photoreceptor pigment bleaching, less potential Henle fiber optic transmission and negligible risk of phototoxicity which could become significant in prolonged exposures to blue or green laser sources. Hyperthermia, apoptosis and heat shock protein formation occur with long pulse which is different from the conventional short pulse laser delivery.

Melanin is the primary light absorber in retinal photocoagulation. This laser energy is converted into thermal energy and hence increases the temperature of the light absorbing tissues. The temperature rise is proportional to the retinal irradiance, i.e. laser power/area. This generated heat is conducted to the surrounding tissues, i.e. overlying neural retina, and the retina and choroid. With long exposures, heat convection because of choroidal flow moderates chorioretinal temperature rise.

Threshold laser burn is one that is barely visible and is associated with retinal pigment epithelium temperature raises from 20° for 10 seconds to 39° for 0.1 second exposure. Conventional short pulse photocoagulation is a suoprathreshold procedure associated with temperature rise as high as 40 to 60° above the normal 37°. However with long pulse TTT the maximal rise of temp is 10° C for a typical 800 mW power used in treating occult CNV, while photodynamic therapy (PDT) causes rise of nearly 2° C.

This long wavelength has low absorption in xanthophyll and is poorly absorbed by hemoglobin. These factors minimize the retinal nerve fiber layer damage and provide easy penetrance through pre and sub-retinal blood respectively. Its main site of absorption is the choroid, thereby making the treatment of choroidal lesions effective.

Henceforth, long pulse TTT has the advantage of lesser trauma to the neural tissues without losing effective action against the diseased membranes. Thus, TTT works by: thermal obliteration of vascular and retinal pigment epithelium migration, transformation and proliferation, vascular thrombosis, thermal inhibition of angiogenesis and neovascular apoptosis.

Laser power settings for retinal photocoagulation must be adjusted for fundus pigmentation and media clarity which affect absorbed retinal irradiance and thus retinal temperature rise. Similarly power absorbed is more with higher pigmentation and hence should be reduced with more pigmented fundi.

Retinal irradiance is affected by spot diameter, media and pigmentation. To produce a particular irradiance the power should be increased for any increase in diameter of the laser spot. Retinal irradiance is reduced with media opacification and hence the power must be adjusted accordingly.

PROCEDURE

Transpupillary thermotherapy is administered as sub threshold photocoagulation with no visible end point and no ophthalmoscopically apparent chorioretinal change during the treatment which results in closure of CNV and resorption of the intraretinal fluid and subretinal fluid, with little or no damage to the overlying retina.

After complete ocular examination of the patient a color photograph and angiogram of the fundus is taken to study the size and character of the CNV.

Targeting of CNVs is achieved with a diode red beam in such a way that the entire lesion is covered and it extends 100 μm beyond the borders of the lesion. Patient's fixation is monitored by observation through the slit-lamp. The beam width of either 2 mm or 3 mm is used in order to encompass the entire lesion (Figure 9.7). Before initiating the actual treatment, a pilot shot

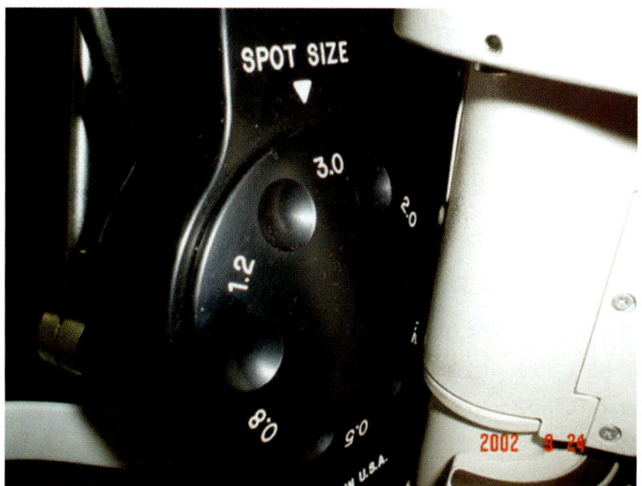

FIGURE 9.7: Adaptor for larger spot size.

is placed in each case outside the arcades and the result monitored. If whitening of the spot occurs, the power is reduced in 100 mW steps till no reaction or a faint retinal graying is seen. In our experience, a power range of 400 mW to 600 mW is adequate to produce the desired result. After this, the actual treatment is now initiated. The treatment is given for duration of 1 minute. Two adjacent 3 mm spots may be used if indicated, in order to cover larger lesions. The power of the laser is also adjusted if the spot size is reduced.

It is important to maximize and stabilize laser throughout. For that proper lenses with antireflective coating are used. The available lenses are the Goldmann's, Mainster Quadraspheric or the Volk's lenses. These have different magnifications and hence depending on that the spot diameter varies and hence should be varied. The laser beam spot size can be adjusted for different lesion sizes. For lesions larger in size than 3 mm, two strategies can be used:
- Multiple almost confluent spots
- Enlarging the aerial image through wide field lens.

It is also important to maintain an undistorted laser beam avoiding optical aberrations and astigmatic effect.

After adequate setting of the power and size the lens is apposed to the cornea and laser treatment is administered for one minute with good control of the patient. Any undue pressure over the globe should be avoided as it leads to choroidal blanching reducing the dissipation of heat. It is also important that a circular undistorted beam is obtained.

The importance of the amount of ocular pigmentation in this mode of treatment has been stressed by Auer and associates,[53] who reported choroidal atrophy in 5 of the 32 eyes that underwent TTT. These patients were originally dark haired. Similar conclusion was also drawn by others,[54] on an animal model. In our study we tried to determine the efficacy of this mode of treatment in the Indian, more pigmented eyes, which are prone to over-treatment or laser burns. Therefore as a precaution, each patient received a pilot shot outside the arcades, prior to the actual treatment. We found that these eyes responded successfully to correspondingly smaller energy levels. We used 400 mW to 600 mW for a 3 mm beam width and 300 mW for a 2 mm beam width, with high success rates. Reichel and associates[38] have used a range of 380 to 600 mW for a 2 mm beam width and from 360 to 1000 mW for a 3 mm beam width. Newsom and associates[39] recommend 500 to 700 mW energy for a 3 mm beam width and 400 to 650 mW for a 2 mm beam width.

Accurate titration of the energy attains enormous significance in this procedure, where no visible end points are desirable. This is of greater importance in the heavily pigmented Indian eyes which are more prone to foveal burns. On the other hand, under-treatment will also hamper the anatomical and functional success of the procedure. Therefore a careful balance, with precautions like pilot shots in the periphery, carefully monitoring the site of treatment and immediate abandoning of the site upon the first visible sign of a burn are mandatory. These measures will help in maximizing the benefits and reducing the complications of this procedure.

COMPLICATIONS

Several complications that have been reported in the treatment of choroidal melanoma with TTT include branch retinal artery and vein occlusion, retinal traction, retinal, choroidal and vitreous hemorrhage and retinal neovascularization.[38] The complications that have been encountered due to TTT for CNV include macular infarction and development of a classic CNV following treatment for an occult CNV.

Benner and associates[55] reported a macular infarct, diagnosed clinically and with angiography in 2.2% of their cases. They have cautioned that the presence of retinal pigment epithelial atrophy or prior laser treatment scars may contribute toward this complication. Kaga and associates[56] reported the development of a classic CNV following treatment of an occult CNV and suggested that it may be the result of cytokine release following the treatment.

McNulty and associates[57] demonstrated decreased volumetric blood flow in the retinal circulation at 24 hours post-TTT by the means of color Doppler imaging. They also showed that in the posterior ciliary arteries, which supply the choroid, there is no change at 24 hours, but at one month, there is a fall in the mean 'End Diastolic Velocity' and increase in the 'Resistive Index' in the nasal and temporal posterior ciliary arteries. Therefore, the authors suggested that TTT can cause alterations in the choroidal blood flow, perhaps by causing complete or partial occlusion of the CNV. The clinical relevance of this finding and its functional and visual implications however, are yet to be discovered.

In our study,[40] we encountered one case that developed a foveal burn despite using the similar treatment parameters, as had been used in the other eyes. Although, the treatment was stopped short at 51 seconds, she subsequently developed a scar in that area with a drop in her visual acuity.

CONCLUSION

Treatment of AMD still poses a great challenge for ophthalmologists. Newer modalities like PDT are coming up. Role of PDT in the treatment of sub-foveal classic membranes is well defined; its role in the management of occult membranes is still at an experimental stage. This is in contrast to TTT, where it is a safe and effective method of treatment for occult as well as classic CNV. Finally, PDT is an extremely expensive procedure. Thus, faced with the situation of an ever-increasing geriatric population, with increasing rates of AMD, PDT is not likely to develop into a procedure of mass treatment. This role however, can be fulfilled by TTT. Because of its easy affordability, it can be made accessible to a larger population.

REFERENCES

1. Tielsch JM. Vision problems in the US: a report on blindness and vision impairment in adults age 40 and older. In Prevent Blindness America, Schaumburg, III, 1994, Prevent Blindness.
2. Leibowitz HM, Krueger DE, Maunder LR, et al. The Framingham Eye Study monograph: an ophthalmological and epidemiological study of cataract, glaucoma, diabetic retinopathy, macular degeneration, and visual acuity in a general population of 2631 adults, 1973-1975. Surv Ophthalmol 1980;24(suppl):335-610.
3. Ganley JP, Roberts J. Eye conditions and related need for medical care among persons 1-74 years of age: United States, 1971-72, Vital Health Stat 1983;228:1-69.
4. Sommer A, Tielsch JM, Katz J, et al. Racial differences in the cause-specific prevalence of blindness in East Baltimore. N Engl J Med 1991;325:1412-17.
5. Klein R, Wang Q, Klein BE, et al. The relationship of age-related maculopathy, cataract, and glaucoma to visual acuity. Invest Ophthalmol Vis Sci 1995;36:182-91.
6. Klein R, Klein BE, Linton KL. Prevalence of age-related maculopathy: The Beaver Dam Eye Study, Ophthalmology 1992;99:933-43.
7. Mitchell P, Smith W, Attebo K, Wang JJ. Prevalence of age-related maculopathy in Australia: the Blue Mountains Eye Study. Ophthalmology 1995;102: 1450-60.
8. Vingerling JR, Dielemans I, Hoffman A, et al. The Prevalence of age-related maculopathy in Rotterdam Study, Ophthalmology 1995;102:205-20.
9. Hyman LG, Lilienfeld AM, Ferris FL, Fine SL. Senile macular degeneration: a case control study. Am J Epidemiol 1983; 118:213-27.
10. Macular Photocoagulation Study Group. Subfoveal neovascular lesion in age-related macular degeneration: guidelines for evaluation and treatment in the Macular Photocoagulation Study. Arch Ophthalmol 1991;109:1224-57.
11. Macular Photocoagulation Study Group. Argon laser photocoagulation for neovascular maculopathy: five year results from randomized clinical trials, Arch Ophthalmol 1991;109:1109-14.
12. Macular Photocoagulation Study Group. Krypton laser photocoagulation for neovascular lesion of age-related macular degeneration: results of randomized clinical trials. Arch Ophthalmol 1990;108:816-24.
13. Macular Photocoagulation Study Group. Visual outcomes after laser photocoagulation for subfoveal choroidal neovascularization secondary to age-related macular degeneration: the influence of initial lesion size and initial visual acuity. Arch Ophthalmol 1994;112:480-84.
14. Freund KB, Yannuzzi LA, Sorenson JA. Age related macular degeneration and choroidal neovascularisation. Am J Ophthalmol 1993;115:786-91.
15. Macular Photocoagulation Study Group. Laser Photocoagulation of subfoveal neovascular lesions of age-related macular degeneration: updated findings from two clinical trials. Arch Ophthalmol 1993;111:1200-09.
16. Cleadby G, Nakanishi AS, Norris JL. Prophylactic photocoagulation of the fellow eye in exudative senile maculopathy. Mod Probl Ophthalmol 1979;20:141-47.
17. Wetzig PC. Treatment of drusen-related aging macular degeneration by photocoagulation. Trans Am Ophthalmol Soc 1998;136:276-90.
18. Wetzig PC. Photocoagulation of drusen-related macular degeneration: a long-term outcome. Trans Am Ophthalmol Soc 1994;92:299-306.
19. Schmidt-Erfurth U, Hasan T, Gragoudas E, Birngruber R. Vascular targeting in photodynamic occlusion of subretinal vessels. Ophthalmology 1994;101:1953-61.

20. Miller JW, Schmidt-Erfurth U, Sickenberg M, et al. Photodynamic therapy for CNV due to age related macular degeneration with verteporfin: results of a single treatment in phase I and II study. Arch Ophthalmol 1999;117:1161-73.

21. Treatment of Age-related Macular Degeneration with Photodynamic Therapy (TAP) Study Group. Photodynamic therapy of subfoveal choroidal neo-vascularization in age related macular degeneration with verteporfin: 2 year results of 2 randomized clinical trials-TAP report # 2. Arch Ophthalmol 2001;119:198-207.

22. Verteporfin in Photodynamic Therapy (VIP) Study Group. Photodynamic therapy of subfoveal choroidal neo-vascularization in age related macular degeneration with verteporfin: 2 year results of a randomized clinical trial including lesions with occult but no classic neovascularization -VIP report # 2. Am J Ophthalmol 2001;131:541-60.

23. Hart PM, Chakravarthy U, MacKenzie G, et al. Teletherapy for subfoveal choroidal neovascularization of age-related macular degeneration: results of follow-up in a non-randomized study, Br J Ophthalmol 1996;80:1046-50.

24. Brady LW, Lahaniatis JE, Freire JE, et al. Radiation therapy for age-related 'wet-type' macular degeneration. Front Radiat Ther Oncol 2001;35:79-85.

25. Hart PM, Archer DB, Chakravarthy U. Asymmetry of disciform scarring in bilateral disease when one eye is treated with radiotherapy. Br J Ophthalmol 1995;79:562-68.

26. Spaide RF, Guyer DR, McCormick B, et al. External beam radiation therapy for choroidal neovascularization. Ophthalmology 1998;105:24-30.

27. Pharmacological Therapy for Macular Degeneration Study Group. Interferon alpha-2a is ineffective for patients with choroidal neovascularization secondary to age-related macular degeneration: results of a prospective randomized placebo-controlled clinical trial. Arch Ophthalmol 1997; 115:865-72.

28. Kusaka M, Sudo K, Fujita T, et al. Potent anti-angiogenic action of AGM-1470: comparison to the fumagillin parent. Biochem Biophys Res Commun 1991;174:1070-76.

29. Voest EE, Kenyon BM, O'Reilly MS, et al. Inhibition of angiogenesis in vivo by interleukin 12, J Natl Cancer Inst 1995;87:581-86.

30. Thomas MA, Dickinson JD, Melberg NS, et al. Visual results after surgical removal of subfoveal choroidal neovascular membranes. Ophthalmology 1994;101:1384-96.

31. Berger AS and Kaplan HJ. Clinical experience with the surgical removal of subfoveal neovascular membranes. Ophthalmology 1992;99:969-76.

32. Lambert HM, Capone A, Aaberg TM. Surgical excision of subfoveal neovascular membranes in age-related macular degeneration, Am J Ophthalmol 1992;113:257-62.

33. Thomas MA, Grand MG, Williams DF. Surgical management of subfoveal choroidal neovascularization. Ophthalmology 1992; 99:952-68.

34. Machemer R, Steinhorst UH. Retinal separation, retinotomy, and macular relocation: II. A surgical approach for age-related macular degeneration? Graefes Arch Clin Exp Ophthalmol 1993;231:635-41.

35. Nimomiya Y, Lewis JM, Hasegawa T, Tano Y. Retinotomy and Foveal Translocation for Surgical Management of Subfoveal Choroidal Neovascular Membranes. Am J Ophthalmol 1996;122:613-21.

36. Wolf S, Lappas A, Weinberger AWA, Kirchhof B. Macular translocation for surgical management of subfoveal choroidal neovascularization in patients with AMD: first results. Graefes Arch Clin Exp Ophthalmol 1999;237:51-57.

37. Toth C, Machemer R. Macular translocation: techniques and results, Vitreoretinal Update, American Academy of Ophthalmology Subspecialty Day, October,1997.

38. Reichel E, Berrocal AM, Ip MS, et al. Transpupillary thermotherapy of occult subfoveal choroidal neovascularization in patients with age-related macular degeneration. Ophthalmology. 1999;106:1908-14.

39. Newsom RSB, McAlister J, Saeed M, McHugh DA. Transpupillary thermotherapy (TTT) for the treatment of choroidal neovascularisation. Br J Ophthalmol 2001, No.2; 85:173-78.

40. Nagpal M, Nagpal K, Sharma S, et al. Transpupillary thermotherapy for treatment of choroidal neovascularization in Indian eyes. Ind J Ophthalmol 2003; 51:243-50.

41. Finger PT, Packer S, Suvitra PP, et al. Hyperthermic treatment of intraocular tumors. Arch Ophthalmol 1984;102:1477-81.

42. Kim JH, Hahn EW, Tokita N. Combination hyperthermia and radiation therapy for cutaneous malignant melanoma. Cancer 1978;41:2143-48.

43. Kim JH, Hahn EW, Tokita N, Nisce LZ. Local tumor hyperthermia in combination with radiation therapy. 1. Malignant cutaneous lesion. Cancer 1977;40:161-69.

44. Overgaard J, Overgaard M. Hyperthermia as an adjuvant to radiotherapy in the treatment of malignant melanoma. Int J Hyperthermia 1987;2:483-501.

45. Oosterhuis JA, Journee-De Korver HG, Kakebeeke-Kemme HM, Blecker JC. Transpupillary thermotherapy in choroidal melanomas. Arch Ophthalmol 1995;113:315-21.

46. Shields CL, Shields JA, DePotter P, Kheterpal S. Transpupillary thermotherapy in the management of choroidal melanoma. Ophthalmology 1996;103:1642-50.

47. Shields CL, Shields JA, DePotter P, Kheterpal S. Transpupillary thermotherapy for choroidal melanoma. Tumor control and visual results in 100 consecutive cases. Ophthalmology 1998;105:581-90.

48. Miller-Rivero NE, Kaplan HJ. Transpupillary Thermotherapy in the Treatment of Occult and Classic Choroidal Neovascularization. Invest Ophthalmol Vis Sci 2000;41:S179.

49. Petrone S, Staurenghi G, Migiliavacca L, et al. Transpupillary thermotherapy for subfoveal choroidal neovascularization in age-related macular degeneration. Invest Ophthalmol Vis Sci 2000;41:S320.

50. Kim JE, Perkins SL, Conner TB, et al. Transpupillary thermotherapy of occult subfoveal choroidal neovascularization. Invest Ophthalmol Vis Sci 2001 42:S443.

51. Bressler NM, Forst LA, Bressler SB, et al. Natural course of poorly defined choroidal neovascularization associated with macular degeneration. Arch Ophthalmol 1988;106: 1537-42.

52. Macular Photocoagulation Study Group. Recurrent choroidal neovascularization following argon laser photocoagulation for neovascular maculopathy. Arch Ophthalmol 1986;104:503-12.

53. Auer C, Tran VT, Chiou AGY, Herbort CP. Transpupillary thermotherapy (TTT) for occult subretinal neovessels: Pigmentation in adjusting diode laser power setting. Invest Ophthalmol Vis Sci 2001;42:S442.

54. Jim KH, Park TK, Yu SY, Kwak HW. Comparison of the effects of transpupillary thermotherapy (TTT) of pigmented and albino rabbit retina. Invest Ophthalmol Vis Sci 2001;42:S444.

55. Benner JD, Ahuja RM, Schwartz JC, et al. Macular infraction after transpupillary thermotherapy in the treatment of occult subfoveal choroidal neovascular membranes. Invest Ophthalmol Vis Sci 2001;42(4):S444.

56. Kaga T, Fonseca RA, Dantas MA, Spaide RF. Transient appearance of classic choroidal neovascularization after transpupillary thermotherapy for occult choroidal neovascularization. Retina 2001; 21:172-73.

57. McNulty LA, Ciulla TA, Harris A, et al. Transpupillary thermotherapy for subfoveal occult CNVM: Effect on ocular perfusion and mechanistic implications. Invest Ophthalmol Vis Sci 2001; 42:S442.

10

Vascular Endothelial Growth Factor and Anti-vascular Endothelial Growth Factor Therapy for Choroidal Neovascularization

Wai-Man Chan, Teresa T Y Lau, David T L Liu

INTRODUCTION

Vascular endothelial growth factor (VEGF) is a protein that is responsible for stimulating abnormal blood vessel growth and blood vessel leakage in diseases like diabetic retinopathy and retinal vein occlusion. Its role in the cause and progression of choroidal neovascularization (CNV) in neovascular age-related macular degeneration (neovascular AMD) has become increasingly important. By specifically blocking VEGF, there is a reduction in pathological angiogenesis.

VASCULAR ENDOTHELIAL GROWTH FACTOR

FACTORS INVOLVED IN BLOOD VESSELS ANGIOGENESIS

Angiogenesis is essential and fundamental to wound healing, tissue growth, reproduction and embryonic development. During development, new blood vessels originate from endothelial cell precursors (angioblasts) by a process called vasculogenesis or from pre-existing blood vessels by angiogenesis.[1] Both processes are mediated by paracrine growth factors. Scientific evidence are suggesting angiogenesis as the most crucial pre-requisite in harnessing a wide range of physiological as well as pathological events.[2-7] Basically, four major stages of angiogenesis have been recognized; namely, vasodilatation and hyper permeability, vessel destabilization and matrix degradation, endothelial cell proliferation and migration, lumen formation and vessel stabilization (Figure 10.1).[2] This multi-step process of remodeling helps the primitive primary plexus develop into a more differentiated secondary network via sprouting and branching of new vessels from pre-existing ones.[1] Angiogenesis is a complex biological process involving a delicate balance and interplay between a variety of molecular angiogenic (positive regulators) and angiostatic (negative regulators) factors (Table 10.1). The VEGF-A is believed to be the prime regulator of angiogenesis and takes part in all four stages of angiogenesis.[8]

HISTORICAL BACKGROUND OF VASCULAR ENDOTHELIAL GROWTH FACTOR

The first milestone in the pursuit of angiogenesis factors was engraved by Michaelson in his legendary "factor X" hypothesis in 1948. He proposed that avascular fetal retina is capable of producing a diffusible biochemical factor X to induce vascular ingrowth.[9] About two decades

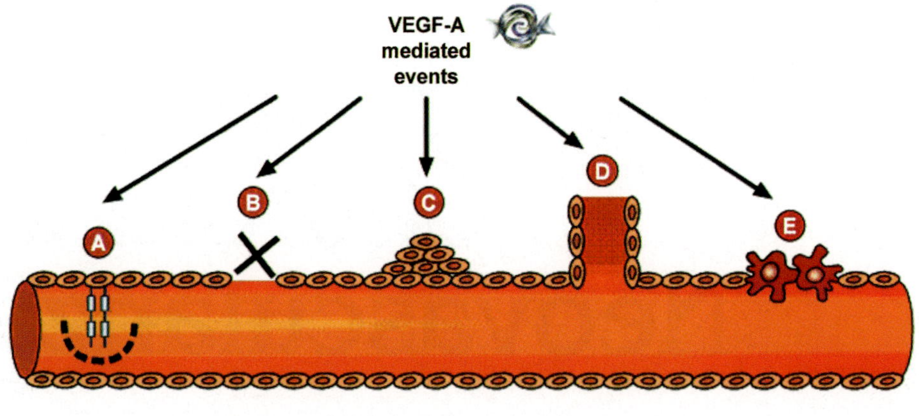

FIGURE 10.1: The role of VEGF-A in angiogenesis.

Table 10.1: Positive and negative regulators of angiogenesis

Angiogenic factors (Positive regulators)	Angiostatic factors (Negative regulators)
• Vascular endothelial growth factor (VEGF)-family	• Angiostatin
• Fibroblast growth factor (FGF)-family	• Endostatin
• Angiopoietin 1	• Angiopoietin 2
• Granulocyte colony-stimulating factor	• Pigment epithelium-derived factor (PEDF)
• Platelet-derived growth factor (PDGF)	• Thrombospondin-1
• Transforming growth factor (TGF)	• Interferon alpha (IFN-α)
• Tumor necrosis factor-alpha (TNF-α)	• Metallo-proteinase inhibitors
• Angiogenin	• Prolactin 16-kD fragment
• Insulin-like growth factor (IGF-1)	• Genistein
• Hepatocyte growth factor (HGF)	• Placental proliferin-related protein
• Interleukin-8 (IL-8)	• Platelet factor 4
• Placental growth factor (PlGF)	

later, Folkman[10] put forward a similar "tumor angiogenesis factor" hypothesis in an attempt to explain this phenomenon of tumor angiogenesis, particularly the development of metastases. First experimental verification of the hypothesis stemmed from Senger and associates[11] in their work on tumor derived factors causing increased microvascular permeability. These authors named these diffusible molecules, the vascular permeability factor. The full angiogenic potentials of this factor was later recognized from observation of their mitogenic effects on endothelial cells.[12,13] At about the same time in 1989, Leung and associates [14] successfully isolated and cloned a "new" endothelial mitogen named vascular endothelial growth factor, which was subsequently found to be identical to vascular permeability factor. Subsequently, vascular permeability factor was rechristened as VEGF.

VASCULAR ENDOTHELIAL GROWTH FACTOR FAMILY (VEGF-A, VEGF-B, VEGF-C, VEGF-D, VEGF-E AND PLGF)

The VEGF family of structurally-related growth factors has five mammalian members, namely VEGF-A, VEGF-B, VEGF-C, VEGF-D and placenta growth factor (PlGF), all encoded by separate genes. These proteins are involved in coordinating the complex physiological process of angiogenesis.

VEGF-A

VEGF-A is commonly referred to as VEGF only, is the primary driver in angiogenesis. The human VEGF-A gene has eight exons separated by seven introns.[14] Alternate exons splicing has produced six isoforms of VEGF-A with differing properties and functions.[14,15] Native VEGF-A is a homodimeric glycoprotein of 45 kDa with N-terminal signal sequence and a heparin binding domain.[16] The importance of VEGF-A in angiogenesis could be reflected from several embryonic studies.[17,18] Severe vasculature defect and embryonic fatality were evidenced after a disruption of a single allele of VEGF in mice.[17] In mice, various organs, such as brain, spinal cord, heart and kidney show VEGF-A mRNA expression whereas in the human fetus, VEGF-A mRNA is present in virtually all tissues.[26, 27] Lung, kidney and spleen have the highest production of VEGF.

Other Members

VEGF-B, VEGF-C, VEGF-D and VEGF-E (orf-virus VEGF) are other members of the VEGF family, sharing 43%, 32%, 31% and 16-27% amino acid homology respectively with VEGF-A. Expression of VEGF-B in the embryonic heart and adult cardiac and skeletal muscle suggests its role in vascularization of the musculature and development of a fully functional cardiovascular system.[21] The VEGF-B modulates VEGF activity by forming heterodimers with VEGF-A$_{165}$.[19] The VEGF-B is a weak endothelial mitogen, supported by evidence that VEGF-B deficient mice are fertile and without obvious malformation of the vascular system.[20] The VEGF-C is mainly responsible for lymphangiogenesis and maintenance of lymphatic vessels through its lymphatic endothelial receptor VEGFR-3.[22] As for VEGF-D, it is expressed in high levels in embryonic lung parenchymal tissue and is involved in lung development.[23] VEGF-E or orf-virus VEGF is a protein encoded by the orf-virus, production of which may be the effect of the genetic drift phenomenon.[24] Placenta growth factor (PlGF) increases vascular permeability, proliferation, chemotaxis and angiogenesis.[6] Its synergistic role with VEGF-A in pathological angiogenesis has also been reported.[25]

ACTIONS OF VASCULAR ENDOTHELIAL GROWTH FACTOR IN THE PROCESS OF ANGIOGENESIS

Apart from being a potent inducer of vascular permeability, VEGF is also shown to have proinflammatory and neuroprotective properties.[6,28,29]

Angiogenesis Stimulator

The first step in angiogenesis is the vasodilatation of the preexisting vessel, mediated by nitric oxide (NO).[1] The VEGF triggers vessel destabilization by degradation of the basement membrane of endothelial cells, allowing the outgrowth of endothelial cells from pre-existing vessels. Endothelial cells then reshape to invade the surrounding stroma, followed by proliferation and migration. The VEGF and angiopoietins appear to be the key mitogens responsible for these stages. The endothelial cells then migrate along a gradient of chemostatic agents through the disintegrated basement membrane. When area with reduced vessel density is reached, the endothelial cells arrange in monolayers to form tube-like structures. It is interesting to note that different isoforms of VEGF possess different vascular effects.[30] For example; $VEGF_{121}$ and $VEGF_{165}$ increase the luminal diameter while $VEGF_{189}$ reduces vessel size. The newly formed vascular tubes must be stabilized by mural cells, differentiated from nearby mesenchymal cells.

Inducer of Vascular Permeability

The VEGF is 50,000 times more potent than histamine in causing vascular permeability. It induces vessel leakage via multiple mechanisms, including fenestration, tight junction dissolution and transcellular bulk flow.[31] The increase in vascular permeability is a prerequisite and necessary step for neovascularization.[28]

Proinflammatory Effects

Inflammatory cells are known to play a role in blood retinal barrier breakdown and neovascularization formation.[32] They produce and release VEGF and VEGF receptors are also present on their cell surfaces. [32]

VEGF-A Isoforms

Via alternate splicing of the VEGF native gene, six different isoforms ($VEGF_{121}$, $VEGF_{145}$, $VEGF_{165}$, $VEGF_{183}$, $VEGF_{189}$ and $VEGF_{206}$) are isolated, with 121, 145, 165, 183, 189 and 206 amino acids respectively.[15] These isoforms differ in property and function. The $VEGF_{189}$ and $VEGF_{206}$ are mainly found on the cellular surface and extracellular matrix through their binding affinity for heparin sulfrate. The $VEGF_{121}$ and $VEGF_{165}$ are acidic polypeptides without heparin affinity and exist in unbound forms in the extracellular fluid.[33] The smallest isoform, $VEGF_{121}$, is freely soluble. The properties of native VEGF correspond closely to $VEGF_{165}$.[33] The predominant isoform, $VEGF_{165}$, possesses dual properties, either found in a freely diffusible form or in a bounded state to cell surfaces or extracellular matrix.[34] It has the optimal bioavailability and biological potency. The extracellular matrix bounded isoforms may be released in a diffusible form by plasmin cleavage at the C terminus.[33] It is interesting to note that the removal of the heparin binding domain leads to significant loss of mitogenic activity of VEGF (Figure 10.2).[35]

The $VEGF-A_{110}$ is a cleavage product of plasmin. Houck and associates [33] have shown that $VEGF_{165}$ can bind to extracellular matrix and may be released as diffusible $VEGF_{110}$ by plasmin cleavage at the C terminus. This is a measure to generate the bioactive fragment.

VASCULAR ENDOTHELIAL GROWTH FACTOR RECEPTOR DOMAIN AND ACTIONS

Three members of the VEGF Receptor (VEGFR) family have been identified so far. These three VEGFR tyrosine kinases are structurally related to the PDGF receptor family. The VEGF-A binds to two structurally related receptor tyrosine kinases: VEGFR-1 [fms-like tyrosine kinase-1 (Flt-1)] and VEGFR-2 [kinase insert domain-containing receptor or (KDR)]. Both of them possess seven

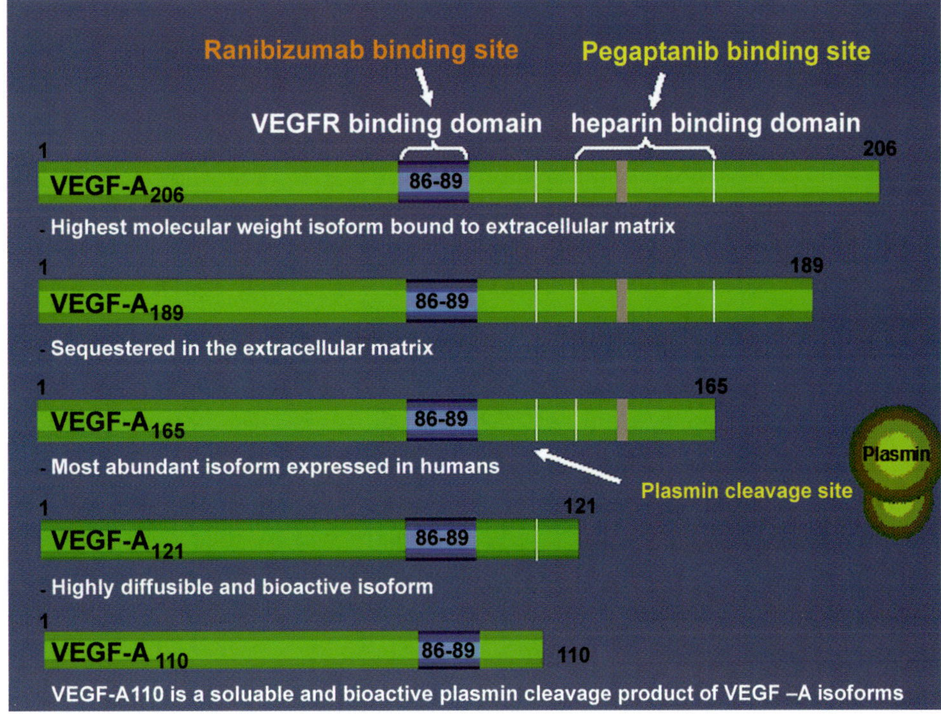

FIGURE 10.2: Different VEGF isoforms, binding domain and the VEGF- A_{110} as a cleavage product.

immunoglobulin-like domains in the extracellular domain, a single transmembrane region and a common tyrosinase kinase sequence.[36] The VEGFR-1 gene encodes two polypeptides, namely full-length membrane protein (receptor form of VEGFR-1) and a short-length soluble VEGF-binding protein (soluble form of VEGFR-1).[37] The VEGFR-1 functions as a negative regulator of VEGFR-2 and induces weak or undetectable responses on its own. The VEGFR-2 is the key receptor in mediating mitogenic, angiogenic and permeability-enhancing effects of VEGF signaling in endothelial cells. The VEGFR-3 [fms-like-tyrosine kinase (Flt-4)] also belongs to the same family of receptor tyrosine kinases but is not a receptor for VEGF-A. It binds to VEGF-C and VEGF-D in both blood vessel angiogenesis and lymphangiogenesis in wound healing and tumor angiogenesis.[38] The VEGF-C and VEGF-D also bind to VEGFR-2 but with a much lower affinity than VEGFR-3. The VEGF-B and PlGF bind with high affinity to VEGFR-1 only while VEGF-E binds specifically to VEGFR-2. Apart from receptor tyrosine kinases, there is also a group of co-receptors called neuropilins, which lack the tyrosine kinase domain of VEGF-R1 to 3. They are co-receptors for $VEGF_{165}$ that enhance VEGF-A binding to VEGFR-2. [39]

ROLE OF VASCULAR ENDOTHELIAL GROWTH FACTOR IN NORMAL PHYSIOLOGY AND ANGIOGENESIS

Embryonal Development

The VEGF-A expression could be identified in various embryonic organs including heart, kidney, spinal cord and brain. Gene targeting studies have revealed that all three VEGFRs are fundamental for embryonic vasculature development. It was noted that mice lacking VEGFR-1 expression die *in utero*.[51] Endothelial cells develop but fail to organize into normal vascular structures, which may be a reflection of the lack of normal counteracting effect from pericytes on endothelial cells in VEGFR-1 knockout mice. Similarly, knockout mice for VEGFR-2 also die *in utero*.[52] There is no vasculogenesis, hematopoietic precursors or organized blood vessels. Knockout mice for VEGFR-3 also die prematurely.[53] Vasculogenesis and angiogenesis still occur but the large blood vessels are abnormally organized.

Normal Adult

The VEGF-A has been shown to be widely involved in normal physiology and angiogenesis, for instance, in female reproductive cycle, choroid plexus epithelium in brain, glomerular epithelium in kidneys, gastrointestinal mucosa and hair follicles.[6] In ocular tissue, VEGF-A is also secreted by retinal pigment epithelial cells and VEGFR expression is found in choriocapillaris endothelium.[54] The VEGF-A secreted from the retinal pigment epithelium is postulated as a trophic factor for maintaining the integrity of the choriocapillaris endothelium.[54]

Vascular Endothelial Growth Factor in Normal Eye

Robinson and associates[55] have shown that VEGF-A, VEGFR-1 and VEGFR-2 are involved in the development of retinal vasculature. As for choroidal vasculature development, it is driven by VEGF-A secreted by the retinal pigment epithelium.[56] In adult eyes, VEGF-A mRNA is expressed in normal retina. The VEGFR-1 was reported to be expressed in microvessels in normal human retina; preferentially in pericytes.[6] This echoes VEGFR-1's auxillary function in maintaining endothelial cell differentiation and integrity. Apart from vascular tissue, all three VEGFRs were shown to be expressed in neural elements of the inner retina.[6] The VEGFR expression in neural elements indicate that VEGF also functions in non-vascular cells of the retina, with possible neurotrophic and neuroprotective effects.[6]

ROLE OF VASCULAR ENDOTHELIAL GROWTH FACTOR IN PATHOLOGICAL OCULAR DISEASES

Vascular Endothelial Growth Factor and Diabetic Retinopathy

Clinical data showed that VEGF-A may promote retinal vascular permeability by increasing vesicular transport and decreasing the occlusions between tight junctions.[57] *In vivo* studies revealed that in human non-proliferative diabetic retinopathy, there was an increased expression of VEGF-A.[58] Campochiaro and associates [59] have showed that ischemic retina may actually up-regulate VEGFR-1 receptors, leading to an increased VEGF-A sensitivity. Up-regulation of VEGFR-2 has also been implicated in the development of non-proliferative diabetic retinopathy.[60] Vascular expression of VEGFR-2 would limit the vascular permeability effect of VEGF-A, only in established diabetic retinopathy.[6] Moreover, expression of VEGFR-3 was also observed in areas of leaky retinal vessels.[61] This finding suggests the involvement of other VEGF family members, apart from VEGF-A, in the pathogenesis of diabetic retinopathy.

Vascular Endothelial Growth Factor and Choroidal Neovascularization

The role of VEGF-A in the development of choroidal neovascularization (CNV) has been established.[6] Increased VEGF-A expression was noted in surgically excised CNV, retinal pigment epithelium and vitreous of age-related macular degeneration (AMD) patients.[6] It is understood that normal retinal pigment epithelium cells secrete VEGF-A at basolateral side towards the choriocapillaris.[54] In addition, all three VEGFRs are localized on the choriocapillaris endothelium facing retinal pigment epithelium cells.[54] This paracrine relation between retinal pigment epithelium cells and choriocapillaris help maintain the viability and integrity of the choriocapillaris.[62] In AMD, this normal paracrine homeostasis may be tilted due to a thickened Bruch's membrane and much reduced hydrophilic conductivity.[63] This may cause dramatic reduction of VEGF-A reaching the choriocapillaris and atrophy of the choriocapillaris may occur.[64] As a result, outer retinal hypoxia develops and VEGF-A expression is up-regulated. Therefore, the accumulation of VEGF-A at the retinal pigment epithelium side of Bruch's membrane may incite CNV formation.[65]

ANTIVASCULAR ENDOTHELIAL GROWTH FACTOR FOR CHOROIDAL NEOVASCULARIZATION

Neovascular AMD is the leading cause of vision loss in patients over 60 years of age, particularly in western countries. Various treatments including photodynamic therapy and various laser techniques have been available to treat this condition. Recently, many new treatments have been under intense research for clinical efficacy and safety (Figure 10.3). Anti-VEGF treatment is a group of them (Table 10.2).

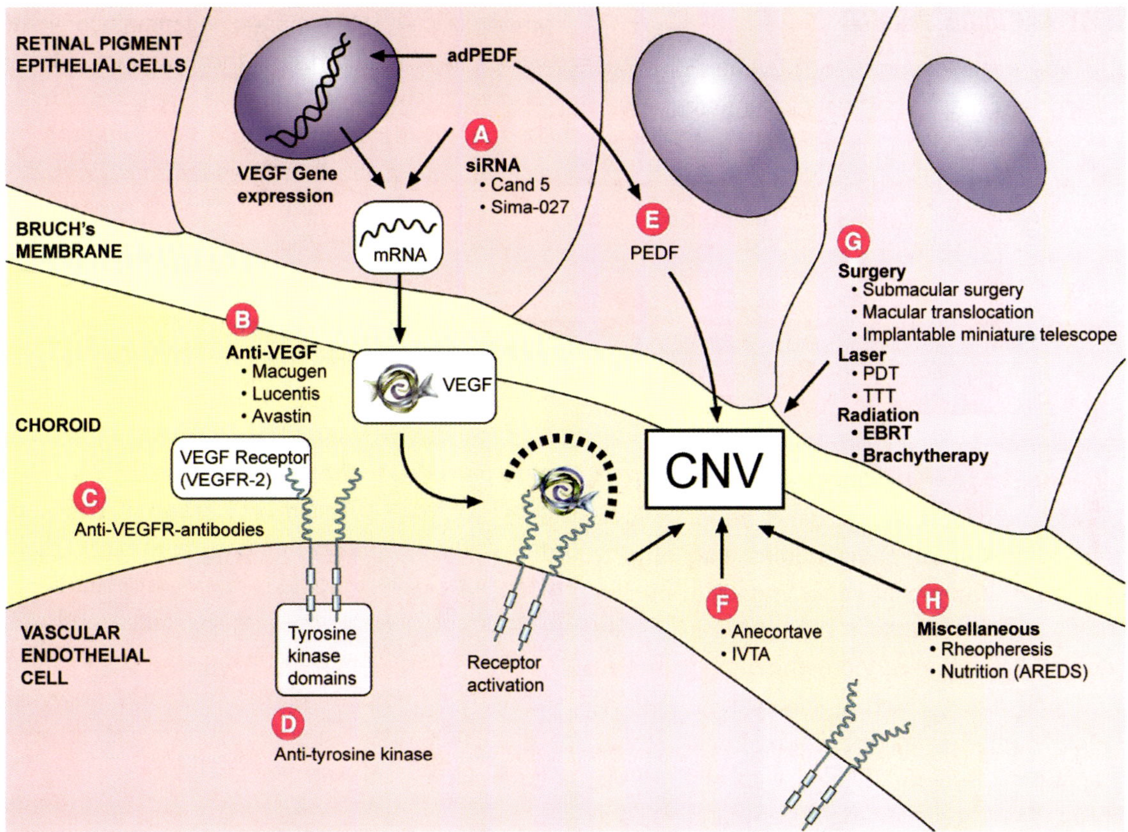

FIGURE 10.3: Treatment strategies for choroidal neovascularization.

Table 10.2: Characteristics of different anti-VEGFs

	Pegaptanib Sodium (Macugen)	Bevacizumab (Avastin)	Ranibizumab (Lucentis)
Size (MW)	50 kD	149 kD	49 kD
Nature	RNA Aptamer, VEGF antagonist	Full-length monoclonal antibody	Monoclonal antibody fragment
Mechanism of action	Binds VEGF-165 only	Binds all isoforms of VEGF	Binds all isoforms of VEGF
Recommended dosage	0.3 mg (0.9 ml)	1.25 mg (0.05 ml)	0.3 mg (0.05 ml)
Plasma half-life	10 days	20 days	10 days
Associated S/E	Hypertension, anterior chamber inflammation	Hypertension, impaired wound healing, thromboembolism, hemorrhage	Anterior and posterior inflammation
Related Clinical trials	VISION trials	SANA trials	MARINA, ANCHOR, FOCUS
FDA approval	v (for eye use)	v (for systemic use)	v (for eye use)

MACUGEN® (PEGAPTANIB SODIUM)

Pegaptanib sodium (Macugen®; Eyetech Pharmaceuticals/Pfizer) was the first anti-angiogenic therapy to be approved by US FDA for the treatment of all types of neovascular AMD in December 2004. [66,67] It is also the first aptamer to be successfully developed as a therapeutic agent for human use. [68]

Clinical Pharmacology

Pegaptanib sodium is a selective VEGF antagonist, which specifically blocks $VEGF_{165}$, [69] the VEGF-A isoform primarily responsible for pathological ocular neovascularization and vascular permeability. Pegaptanib is a RNA aptamer, a modified olionucleotide, which adopts a three-dimensional conformation that enables it to bind to extracellular VEGF. It comprises of twenty-eight nucleotides in length and terminates in a pentylamino linker, to which two 20-kilodalton monomethoxy polyethylene glycol (PEG) units are covalently attached via the two amino groups on a lysine residue. Under in vitro conditions, the aptamer binds to $VEGF_{165}$ with high affinity and specificity, thereby preventing it from binding to its cognate receptors. It was shown that pegaptanib was removed from the eye through plasma clearance and that biologically active pegaptanib could be detected in the vitreous humor of the eye for at least 28 days following a single 0.5 mg intravitreal dose. [70] No toxicities related to pegaptanib were observed following systemic and ocular administration in primate and rodent models. [71]

Clinical Trials of Pegaptanib in Neovascular AMD-VISION Trials

The safety and efficacy of pegaptanib in the treatment of CNV secondary to AMD were tested in two concurrent, prospective, randomized, double-masked, multicentric, sham controlled, pivotal trials (VISION trials - the VEGF Inhibition Study in Ocular Neovascularization). [72] In an effort to reflect the usual patient population, the trial design encompassed a broad inclusion criteria. Patients were randomized to receive pegaptanib sodium 0.3 mg, 1 mg, 3 mg by intravitreal injection or sham injection, administered every 6 weeks for 48 weeks. At week 54th, those randomized to receive pegaptanib were re-randomized (1:1) to continue pegaptanib for 48 additional weeks or to diskontinue therapy; patients originally assigned to the sham group were re-randomized to either continue in the sham group, to diskontinue sham or to receive one of the three pegaptanib doses. [73]

Efficacy and Safety of Pegaptanib after 1 Year

A total 1208 patients were randomly assigned in the two trials and 1186 of which completed 1-year follow-up. [72] Compared with 55% (164/296) of patients receiving sham injections, 70% (206/294) of patients receiving 0.3 mg of pegaptanib (p<0.001), 71% (213/300) receiving 1 mg (p<0.001) and 65% (193/296) receiving 3 mg (p=0.03) lost <15 letters of visual acuity between baseline and week 54 (primary efficacy endpoint). Higher doses were not shown to provide additional clinical benefit. Mean changes in visual acuity were −8.0 letters and −15.0 letters for patients receiving 0.3 mg and sham, respectively (p<0.0001) at week 54th. [74] There was no evidence that age, angiographic subtype, lesion size or baseline visual acuity precluded a treatment benefit. [75]

Efficacy and Safety of Pegaptanib after 2 Years

At week 54th, patients that are re-randomized to continue 0.3 mg pegaptanib demonstrated a 45% relative benefit in mean change in vision by weeks 102 as compared with those receiving usual care (p<0.01). [74] In all, 10% of patients in the pegaptanib 0.3 mg group gained at least ≥3 lines of vision after two years, compared with only 6% of patients after 1 year. The percentage of patients whose vision deteriorated to 20/200 or worse was also lower in pegaptanib-treated patients. At weeks 102, 35% of patients who received pegaptanib and 55% of patients who received usual care had visual acuities of 20/200 or worse (P<0.01). [76]

Toxicity and Possible Adverse Events

All doses of pegaptanib were well tolerated systemically. Side effects of pegaptanib were transient and mild, mostly attributable to the injection procedure. Serious ocular adverse events, such as traumatic lens injury, retinal detachments and endophthalmitis occurred with <1% of intravitreal injections. There was no evidence of either systemic toxicity or an increased risk of potential VEGF inhibition related adverse events. [73]

Conclusions

Pegaptanib was proven to reduce vision loss or stabilize vision in patients with neovascular AMD, regardless of angiographic subtype, baseline vision or lesion size. The VISION trials have convincingly shown that pegaptanib provides a statistically significant benefit to a broad spectrum of neovascular AMD patients.

AVASTIN® (BEVACIZUMAB)

Bevacizumab (Avastin Roche®, Genentech, Inc) is the FDA's approved anti-VEGF agent in the treatment of patients with metastatic colorectal cancer.[77,78] It has shown promising results, via the intravitreal route, in the treatment of neovascular ocular diseases like CNV, macular edema and proliferative diabetic retinopathy.[79-81] The use of intravitreal bevacizumab offer the advantages of using a lower dosage of drug, whilst avoiding the potential side effects associated with systemic exposure.[79]

Clinical Pharmacology

Bevacizumab is a full-length, recombinant humanized anti-VEGF monoclonal antibody that binds to all isoforms of VEGF-A, thereby inhibiting the binding of VEGF to its receptors on the surface of endothelial cells. It is derived from the same murine anti-VEGF antibody as ranibizumab. Neutralizing the biological activity of VEGF reduces vascular permeability and neovascularization, thereby, beneficial in limiting tumor growth and metastasis and in treating ocular diseases where increased vascular growth or permeability are the cause of vision loss.[7]

Clinical Trials of Bevacizumab (Systemic and Intravitreal)

In 2004, the Systemic Avastin for Neovascular AMD (SANA) study was started at the Bascom Palmer Eye Institute.[79] In this study, systemic bevacizumab was offered as salvage therapy for patients with AMD CNV, for those unsuitable for or refused photodynamic therapy (PDT). Patients received intravenous bevacizumab treatment 3 times followed by a period of close observation, with re-treatment given when there was evidence of angiographic leakage. The only significant adverse event observed was a mild elevation of blood pressure that was controlled with anti-hypertensive medication. No thromboembolic event was noted. In this study, systemic bevacizumab therapy has yielded impressive results in the treatment of neovascular AMD, with improvements in visual acuity, OCT and angiographic outcomes.

Rosenfeld and associates [79,80] have reported the use of bevacizumab systemically and intravitreal in the treatment of neovascular AMD. Intravenous administration of bevacizumab at 5 mg/kg at 2-week intervals produced a significant reduction in retinal thickening and improvement in visual acuity in a small series.[79] The intravitreal injection of 1 mg of bevacizumab was reported in a single patient with macular degeneration to cause a marked reduction in retinal thickening at 1 week after treatment, without any obvious short-term toxicity.[80] In another study by Avery and associates, [88] it was found that intravitreal bevacizumab at a dose of 1.25 mg resulted in an improvement in visual acuity from 20/200 to 20/80 in patients with neovascular AMD at 8 weeks post injection. The use of intravitreal bevacizumab offers the advantages of using a much lower dosage of drug (1/300th to 1/400th of systemic dose), whilst avoiding the rare but significant risk of thromboembolic events.[87] The results from the clinical studies on the use of bevacizumab in the treatment of CNV due to AMD and other ocular neovascular diseases have been promising. However, longer term controlled trials involving larger sample sizes are warranted to evaluate the safety and efficacy of the drug to justify its off-label use.

Toxicity and Possible Adverse Events

The bevacizumab preparation is unpreserved and contains no ingredients that are known to be toxic to the eye. Bevacizumab has been tested in rabbit eyes and no evidence of toxicity was seen by electroretinogram or visual evoked potential testing.[83,84] These findings were consistent with those by Maturi and associates, [85] whom demonstrated that no evidence of retinotoxicity noted in the short-term use of intravitreal bevacizumab in patients with neovascular AMD. When used in cancer therapy, intravenous bevacizumab at dose of 5 mg/kg every two weeks, possible adverse events observed include hypertension, impaired wound healing, hemorrhage, thromboembolic events, myocardial infarction, stroke and proteinuria.[86,87] The safety profile of intravitreal bevacizumab appeared to be more favorable. In a study by Avery and associates [88] involving 79 patients receiving intravitreal bevacizumab for the treatment of AMD CNV, no significant systemic or ocular complications were noted. This finding was consistent with that of other investigators.[89]

Conclusions

To date, the long-term intravitreal safety profile of bevacizumab remains uncertain. The theoretically longer half-life of intravitreal bevacizumab compared with ranibizumab, might increase the risk of systemic toxicity, but this risk would not be expected as high as for systemic administration, where 300 to 400 times the dose is used.[82] However, a longer half-life may also mean that less frequent administration is required. The much lower cost per dose of intravitreal bevacizumab, compared with that of pegaptanib or the anticipated cost of ranibizumab, [81] make it a promising and cost-effective treatment option for CNV for those who may not be able to afford the more expensive alternatives.

LUCENTIS® (RANIBIZUMAB)

Ranibizumab (rhuFab, Lucentis®, Genentech and Novartis Pharma AG) is another anti-VEGF agent for the treatment of neovascular ocular diseases. Preliminary results on the safety and efficacy of the drug have been promising and was in its phase III trials. [90] FDA approved its use recently.

Clinical Pharmacology

Ranibizumab is a recombinant, humanized monoclonal antibody Fab fragment designed to bind and inactivate VEGF-A, thereby inhibit vessel permeability and angiogenesis. It binds with high affinity to all VEGF-A isoforms generated by alternative mRNA splicing; namely, $VEGF_{121}$, $VEGF_{165}$ and their biologically active proteolytic cleavage product, $VEGF_{110}$.[91,92] In rodent and primate models, it has been shown to penetrate all layers of the retina after intravitreal injection—the first demonstration of retinal penetration of an anti-VEGF therapy intended for AMD.[93] This ability has been attributed to its small molecular size (48 kDa), as a full-length antibody failed to demonstrate complete retinal penetration (Table 10.3).[94] The average vitreous elimination half-life of ranibizumab in patients with 0.3 mg dose is approximately 10 days. The shorter intravitreal half-life of this antibody fragment is related to its smaller size and its significant diffusion through the retinal layers. It has been shown that Lucentis readily diffuses through the neural retina to reach the retinal pigment epithelium layer 1 hour post intravitreal injection and persists in this location for up to 7 days. Following monthly intravitreal administration of Lucentis to subjects with neovascular AMD, serum ranibizumab concentrations are found to be ~90,000-fold lower than that in vitreous levels.

Table 10.3: Different physical and pharmacologic properties between ranibizumab and bevacizumab

Features	Lucentis (Ranibizumab, antibody fragment)	Avastin (Bevacizumab, full-length antibody)
Fully penetrates all retinal layers to reach target tissue	+++	+
Rapid systemic clearance	+++	+
Low potential for immunogenicity	+++	+
Binds all VEGF-A isoforms and degradation products with high affinity	+++	+++

Systemic ranibizumab exposure is generally considered low following intravitreal administration, with plasma levels remaining below the limit of quantitation for up to 14 days post-bilateral intravitreal injections in primate models.

Preclinical Studies

Bilateral intravitreal administration of ranibizumab to cynomolgus monkeys as low as 0.25 mg/eye and as high as 2.0 mg/eye once every 2 weeks for up to 26 weeks resulted in dose-dependent effects that were limited to ocular tissues. No signs of systemic toxicity were detected. Intravitreal ranibizumab given to cynomolgus monkeys resulted in dose-dependent increases in anterior chamber flare and vitreal cell infiltrations that were greatest 48 hours after the first dose. These responses gradually diminish with subsequent injections or during recovery periods of at least 4 weeks. Perivenous retinal hemorrhage and perivascular sheathing were also observed in some animals. It was suggested that the posterior inflammation observed in animals are immune-mediated antibody responses, which has not been characteristic of the inflammatory responses seen in humans.

In non-human primates, intravitreal administration of Lucentis has been shown to penetrate the retina and reach the site of CNV with maximum retinal concentrations attained within 6 to 24 hours.[95] In another primate model of laser-induced CNV, Lucentis alone or in combination with verteporfin photodynamic therapy significantly inhibited CNV and reduced vascular leakage as seen on fluorescein angiography.[96,97] No retinotoxicity or other serious adverse effects were noted from intravitreal ranibizumab in normal primate models.[98]

Clinical Trials of Ranibizumab: Phase 1/2 studies

In Phase 1 / 2 studies in patients with primary or recurrent subfoveal neovascular AMD, intravitreal injections of Lucentis appeared to be safe and well-tolerated for treatment periods up to seven months.[99,100] Moreover, Lucentis in these studies, demonstrated encouraging signs of activity, including improvements in visual acuity, decreases in total area of leakage by fluorescein angiography and decreases in retinal thickness by optical coherence tomography over seven months of treatment. In another study, Rosenfeld *et al* reported that multiple intravitreal ranibizumab injections at escalating doses ranging from 0.3 mg to 2.0 mg were safe and well tolerated in eyes with neovascular AMD.[101] Additional trials have since been initiated to provide a more definitive evaluation of the clinical benefit of Lucentis in patients with predominantly classic or minimally classic or occult CNV.[102]

Clinical Trials of Ranibizumab- Phase 3 Studies (MARINA and ANCHOR Studies)

The clinical safety and efficacy of Lucentis have been assessed in two randomized, double-masked, sham or active controlled studies in patients with neovascular AMD. A total of 1139 patients were enrolled into the two studies. In the MARINA (Minimally Classic/ Occult Trial of the Anti-VEGF Antibody Ranibizumab in the Treatment of Neovascular AMD) study,[103] patients with minimally classic or occult with no classic CNV were randomized in a 1:1:1 ratio to sham injection or to Lucentis (0.3 mg or 0.5 mg) injected intravitreal monthly for 24 months. The ANCHOR (Anti-VEGF Antibody for the Treatment of Predominantly Classic Choroidal Neovascularization in AMD) study,[104] in contrast to the MARINA trials, involves patients with predominantly classic CNV lesions. Patients were randomized to either verteporfin PDT plus sham injection or to placebo PDT plus Lucentis (0.3 mg or 0.5 mg) monthly for 24 months.

Preliminary analysis of one-year MARINA data revealed that 95% of patients treated with Lucentis lost fewer than 15 letters at one year, compared with 62% in the control group (P<0.001). At month 12, 25% of Lucentis-treated patients in MARINA study and 36% patients in ANCHOR study gained 15 or more letters, compared with 5 and 6% of respective control patients. The differences between the Lucentis and control treatment groups in both studies were statistically significant (p<0.0001).

Toxicity and Possible Adverse Events

The ocular adverse events profiles of Lucentis in these two studies were similar to that observed in the earlier trials and there was no evidence of an increase in serious non-ocular adverse events reported. The incidences of uveitis and endophthalmitis were each <1%. [103,104]

Conclusions

Overall, patients treated with Lucentis had a significant improvement in visual acuity relative to the baseline visual acuity, whereas the control groups experienced a substantial decrease from baseline in mean visual acuity. Lucentis was shown to be superior to sham in patients with minimally classic or occult with no classic neovascular AMD. Lucentis was also demonstrated to be superior to verteporfin PDT in the treatment of patients with predominantly classic lesions.

USING OPTICAL COHERENCE TOMOGRAPHY FOR ANTI-VEGF THERAPEUTIC DECISIONS

Just as anti-VEGF is a revolution in AMD therapy, optical coherence tomography (OCT) represents a revolution in imaging. Optical coherence tomography provides clinicians with qualitative and quantitative information needed to use anti-VEGF therapy. Since OCT is fast and noninvasive, it is much more acceptable to patients than fluorescein angiography. The use of anti-VEGF therapy does not require imaging, but OCT is an ideal way to monitor our patients undergoing therapy to determine if our patients are responding favorably to treatment. [105-109] With an increasing number of treatment choices becoming available over the next few years and few studies to determine which treatments are superior, OCT will help clinicians monitor patients to determine how a patient is responding to therapy.

When treating with anti-VEGF, lesion leakage or the accumulation of fluid is the most important issue. Lesion type, size and location do not matter. If VEGF is both the angiogenic factor and the permeability factor, and if OCT can identify fluid accumulations caused by VEGF, then OCT could serve as a surrogate marker for the presence of VEGF.

Optical coherence tomography is an effective technique for identifying fluid accumulation in the retina as macular edema, under the retina as subretinal fluid and under the retinal pigment epithelium as a pigment epithelial detachment, all anatomic changes thought to be due to VEGF. It makes sense to start and stop anti-VEGF therapy based on our OCT interpretations of reversible VEGF-induced vision loss due to leakage from CNV and the presence of excess fluid in or under the macula.

Using OCT as the basis for when to inject, withhold an injection, or reinject, one can maintain the improved visual acuity and central retinal thickness outcomes in patients following their initial injections.

There are no large, randomized, controlled clinical trials using OCT to monitor any of the anti-VEGF therapies. However, two open-label non-randomized studies will use OCT imaging as the basis for when to retreat.

The PrONTO (Prospective OCT Imaging of Patients with Neovascular Age-related Macular Degeneration Treated with Intraocular Ranibizumab) study is a 2-year prospective study of 40 patients with AMD who have predominantly classic, minimally classic and occult-only CNV with central retinal thickness ≥ 300 μm by OCT imaging. Patients will receive 500 μg of Lucentis every month for 3 months. OCT imaging will be conducted on postinjection days 1, 2, 4, 7 and 14. After 3 months, patients will be reinjected only if leakage from CNV recurs as seen with OCT.

The SANA study involving Avastin is the first FDA-approved anti-VEGF therapy, but bevacizumab is only FDA-approved for the treatment of metastatic colorectal cancer. This study will include all CNV lesion types with central retinal thickness ≥ 300 μm. Patients receive 5 mg/kg Avastin every 2 weeks for two or three treatments. OCT imaging will be conducted every week for the 6 weeks, then every 2 weeks for the next 6 weeks, then every month thereafter. Patients will be reinfused with bevacizumab only if leakage from CNV recurs as detected by OCT.

OPTICAL COHERENCE TOMOGRAPHY VS FLUORESCEIN ANGIOGRAPHY

While fluorescein angiography remains the gold standard for classifying CNV in AMD, it is only a matter of time before OCT imaging overtakes fluorescein angiography as the imaging modality of choice when treating patients with CNV.

Classifying lesion type by fluorescein angiography is probably unnecessary in this new age of anti-VEGF therapy. Optical coherence tomography will be preferred by patients who prefer the fast, noninvasive testing provided by OCT when compared with fluorescein angiography.

With the increase in the number of follow-up visits and the need to make treatment decisions of whether to continue therapy, stop therapy or switch therapy, OCT imaging will prove to be an attractive alternative to fluorescein angiography.

MANAGING THE RISKS OF INTRAVITREAL INJECTION

With the introduction of anti-VEGF therapies, retinal practices are about to change. Intravitreal injection has long been an effective part of retinal practice. With continued study and care, retinal specialists will be able to safely incorporate new anti-VEGF therapy administered by intravitreal injection.

Intravitreal injection has powerful advantages, including:
- The drug is precisely introduced to the tissue where it is needed
- The blood-ocular barrier is bypassed, permitting the use of agents that would otherwise be excluded or unattainable due to systemic effects
- Immediate therapeutic intraocular concentrations soon after the injection are achieved
- Systemic toxicity is avoided.

Guidelines for Safe Injection

Until recently, there was no guideline for administering an intravitreous injection. Last year, a special panel was convened to examine how intravitreous injections could be improved. They developed preinjection, peri-injection and post-injection recommendations:[110]

The strongest recommendations of the panel:
- Exclude patients with active lid or ocular adnexal infection
- Liberally use povidone-iodine on the ocular surface, lid margins, and eye lashes

- Use lid speculum to avoid contamination of the needle with the eye lashes or eyelid margin
- Avoid extensive massage of the eyelids either pre- or postinjection (to avoid expressing meibomian glands)
- Use adequate anesthetic for each patient (topical drops and/or subconjunctival injection [single use bottles recommended)
- Use gloves for the injection procedure
- Dilate the pupil unless otherwise contraindicated; single use or fresh bottles are recommended
- Monitor/manage intraocular pressure both before and after injection Patients should be educated to know the symptoms of endophthalmitis and should be contacted within 1 week of the injection to inquire about vision loss symptoms of any complications (e.g., endophthalmitis, retinal detachment, intraocular hemorrhage, etc.).

Recommendations for which there was no clear consensus on the panel:
- Use of immediate pre- or post-injection antibiotics (little evidence to support its value as prophylaxis for endophthalmitis)
- Use of an additional 10 cc povidone-iodine as a pre-injection flush
- Use of a sterile drape
- Technique for monitoring post-injection intraocular pressure in the eye without glaucoma or underlying optic disk disease (applanation tonometry vs verifying optic disk perfusion by ophthalmoscopy).

Avoid paracentesis (prophylactic or post-injection) unless absolutely necessary.

Pre-injection Recommendations

Before injecting patients, it is important to screen them for disorders, conditions or abnormalities that may increase risks associated with intravitreal injection. A thorough risk assessment and monitoring of post-injection intraocular pressure should be perforMed Paracentesis is not the treatment of choice as softening the eye with a paracentesis before an injection adds another perfo-ration and can increase the risk of endophthalmitis. While serious allergies to povidone-iodine are rare, performing a skin-patch test in patients reporting a history of allergy is important. Any active external infections, including blepharitis, should be treated and the injection should be postponed until the infection clears. Using gloves and drapes are appropriate for the surgical field. Pre-injection antibiotics can be used at the physician's diskretion (Macugen [pegaptanib sodium injection, Eyetech/Pfizer] packaging insert requires pre-injection antibiotics; however, little data show a definite benefit). When performing a lid scrub, excessive lid manipulation should be avoided. If eye softening is desired, pressure should be applied to globe, not lids or adnexa (i.e., do not massage all of the meibomian gland material on to the ocular surface).

Peri-injection Recommendations

When performing a peri-injection, dilation is preferred for adequate visualization. Per standard practice, topical anesthetics should be applied and supplemental subconjunctival anesthetic should be considered. Prior to injection, povidone-iodine drops or wash should be applied directly to the ocular surface, lid margins and lashes. A speculum should be used to avoid any needle contact with lids and lashes. An additional drop of povidone-iodine should be administered after the speculum is in place.

The injection site should be through pars plana in the inferotemporal quadrants 3.5 mm to 4 mm from the limbus. A needle size of 27-gauge or smaller with a length of 0.5 inch to 5/8 of an inch is preferred.

The sequence of steps to intravitreal injection is: apply anesthetic, then povidone-iodine to the lids and adnexa, insert the speculum, apply a drop of povidone-iodine to the injection site and insert the needle.

Post-injection Recommendations

After intravitreal injection, antibiotics should be administered at the physician's diskretion, but not exceeding 72 hours. Intraocular pressure should be monitored routinely with intraocular lowering-lowering therapy provided when needed.

For follow-up, patients should be contacted within 1 week of the procedure and further follow-up is dictated by the patient's needs.

REFERENCES

1. Carmeliet P. Mechanisms of angiogenesis and arteriogenesis. Nat Med 2000; 6:389-95.
2. Distler JW, Hirth A, Kurowska-Stolaska M, et al. Angiogenic and angiostatic factor in the molecular control of angiogenesis. QJNM 2003; 47:149-61.
3. Ferrara N, Gerber HP, LeCounter J. The biology of VEGF and its receptors. Nature Med 2003; 9:669-76.
4. Ferrara N. VEGF and the quest for tumor angiogenesis factors. Cancer 2002; 2:795-803.
5. Schlingemann RO, van Hinsbergh VWM. Role of vascular permeability factor/vascular endothelial growth factor in eye disease. Br J Ophthalmol 1997; 81:501-12.
6. Witmer AN, Vrensen GFJM, Van Noorden CJF, et al. Vascular endothelial growth factors and angiogenesis in eye disease. Prog Ret Eye Res 2003; 22:1-29.
7. Paques M, Massin P, Gaudric A. Growth factors and diabetic retinopathy. Diabetes & Metabolism. 1997; 23:125-30.
8. Ferrara N. Vascular endothelial growth factor: molecular and biological aspects. Curr Top Microbiol Immunol 1999; 237: 1-30.
9. Michaelson IC. The mode of development of the retinal vessels and some observations of its significance in certain retinal diseases. Trans Ophthalmol Soc UK 1948; 68:137-80.
10. Folkman J. Tumor angiogenesis: role in regulation of tumor growth. Symp Soc Dev Biol 1974; 30:43-52.
11. Senger DR, Galli SJ, Dvorak AM, et al. Tumor cells secrete a vascular permeability factor that promotes accumulation of ascites fluid. Science 1983; 219:983-85.
12. Keck PJ, Hauser SD, Krivi G, et al. Vascular permeability factor, an endothelial cell mitogen related to PDGF. Science 1989; 246:1309-12.
13. Connolly DT, Heuvelman DM, Nelson R, et al. Tumor vascular permeability factor stimulates endothelial cell growth and angiogenesis. J Clin Invest 1989; 84:1470-78.
14. Leung DW, Cachianes G, Kuang WJ, et al. Vascular endothelial growth factor is a secreted angiogenic mitogen. Science 1989;246:1306-09.
15. Tischer E, Mitchell R, Hartman T, et al. The human gene for vascular endothelial growth factor. Multiple protein forms are encoded through alternative exon splicing. J Biol Chem 1991; 266:11947-54.
16. Ferrara N, Henzel WJ. Pituitary follicular cells secrete a novel heparin-binding growth factor specific for vascular endothelial cells. Biophys Res Commun 1989; 161:851-58.
17. Ferrara N, Chen H, Davis-Smyth T, et al. Vascular endothelial growth factor is essential for corpus luteum angiogenesis. Biophys Res Commun 1989; 161:851-58.
18. Gerber HP, Vu TH, Ryan AM, et al. VEGF couples hypertrophic cartilage remodeling, ossification and angiogenesis during endochondral bone formation. Nat Med 1998; 4:336-40.

19. Olofsson B, Korpelainen E, Pepper MS, et al. Vascular endothelial growth factor B (VEGF-B) binds to VEGF receptor-1 and regulates plasminogen activator activity in endothelial cells. Proc Natl Acad Sci USA 1998; 95:11709-14.

20. Bellomo D, Headrick JP, Silins GU, et al. Mice lacking the vascular endothelial growth factor-B gene (VEGF-b) have smaller hearts, dysfunctional coronary vasculature and impaired recovery from cardiac ischemia. Circ Res 2000; 86: E29-35.

21. Yancopoulos GD, Davis S, Gale NW, et al. Vascular-specific growth factors and blood vessel formation. Nature 2000; 407:242-48.

22. Kukk E, Lymboussaki A, Taira S, et al. VEGF-C receptor binding and pattern of expression with VEGFR-3 suggests a role in lymphatic vascular development. Development 1996; 122:3829-37.

23. Farnebo F, Piehl F, Lagercrantz J. Restricted expression pattern of VEGF-D in the adult and fetal mouse: high expression in the embryonic lung. Biochem Biophys Res Commun 1999; 257:891-94.

24. Meyer M, Clauss M, Lepple-Wienhues A, et al. A novel vascular endothelial growth factor encoded by Orf virus, VEGF-E, mediates angiogenesis via signaling through VEGFR-2 (KDR) but not VEGFR-1 (Flt-1) receptor tyrosine kinases. EMBO J 1999; 18:363-74.

25. Carmeliet P, Moons L, Luttun A, et al. Synergism between vascular endothelial growth factor and placental growth factor contributes to angiogenesis and plasma extravasation in pathological conditions. Nat Med 2001; 7:575-83.

26. Breier G, Albrecht U, Sterrer S, et al. Expression of vascular endothelial growth factor during embryonic angiogenesis and endothelial cell differentiation development. 1992; 114:521-32.

27. Shifren JL, Doldi N, Ferrara N, et al. In the human fetus, vascular endothelial growth factor is expressed in epithelial cells and myocytes, but not vascular endothelium: implications for mode of action. J Clin Endocrinol Metab 1994; 79:316-22.

28. Ferrara N, Houck K, Jakeman L, et al. Molecular and biological properties of the vascular endothelial growth factor family of proteins. Endocr Rev 1992; 13: 18-32.

29. Storkebaum E, Carmeliet P. VEGF: a critical player in neurodegeneration. J Clin Invest 2004; 113:14-18.

30. Hanahan D, Folkman J. Patterns and emerging mechanisms of the angiogenic switch during tumorigenesis. Cell 1996; 86:353-64.

31. Joussen AM, Murata T, Tsujikawa A, et al. Leukocyte-mediated endothelial cell injury and death in the diabetic retina. Am J Pathol 2001; 158:147-52.

32. Neufeld G, Cohen T, Gengrinovitch S, et al. Vascular endothelial growth factor (VEGF) and its receptors. FASEB J 1999; 13:9-22.

33. Houck KA, Leung DW, Rowland AM, et al. Dual regulation of vascular endothelial growth factor bioavailability by genetic and proteolytic mechanisms. J Biol Chem 1992; 267:26031-37.

34. Park JE, Keller GA, Ferrara N. The vascular endothelial growth factor (VEGF) isoforms: differential deposition into the subepithelial extracellular matrix and bioactivity of extracellular matrix-bound VEGF. Mol Biol Cell 1993; 4:1317-26.

35. Keyt BA, Berleau LT, Nguyen HV, et al. The carboxyl-terminal domain (111-165) of vascular endothelial growth factor is critical for its mitogenic potency. J Biol Chem 1996; 271:7788-95.

36. Terman BI, Carrion ME, Kovacs E, et al. Identification of a new endothelial cell growth factor receptor tyrosine kinase. Oncogene 1991; 6:1677-83.

37. Shibuya M. Structure and dual function of vascular endothelial growth factor receptor-1 (Flt-1). Int J Biochem Cell Biol 2001; 33:409-20.

38. Karkkainen MJ, Makinen T, Alitalo K. Lymphatic endothelium: a new frontier of metastasis research. Nat Cell Biol 2002; 4:E2-5.

39. Fuh G, Li B, Crowley C, et al. Requirements for binding and signaling of the kinase domain receptor for vascular endothelial growth factor. Biol Chem 1998; 273:11197-11204.

40. Waltenberger J, Claesson-Welsh L, Siegbahn A, et al. Different signal transduction properties of KDR and Flt1, two receptors for vascular endothelial growth factor. J Biol Chem 1994; 269:26988-26995.

41. Waltenberger J, Mayr U, Pentz S, et al. Functional upregulation of the vascular endothelial growth factor receptor KDR by hypoxia. Circulation 1996; 94:1647-54.

42. Gille H, Kowalski J, Li B, et al. Analysis of biological effects and signaling properties of Flt-1 (VEGFR-1) and KDR (VEGFR-2). A reassessment using novel receptor-specific vascular endothelial growth factor mutants. J Biol Chem 2001; 276: 3222-30.

43. Takagi H, King GL, Aiello LP. Identification and characterization of vascular endothelial growth factor receptor (Flt) in bovine retinal pericytes. Diabetes 1996; 45:1016-23.

44. Thakker GD, Hajjar DP, Muller WA, et al. The role of phosphatidylinositol 3-kinase in vascular endothelial growth factor signaling. J Biol Chem 1999; 274:10002-07.

45. Witmer AN, van Blijswijk BC, Dai J, et al. VEGFR-3 in adult angiogenesis. J Pathol 2001; 195:490-97.

46. Carmeliet P, Ferreira V, Breier G, et al. Abnormal blood vessel development and lethality in embryos lacking a single VEGF allele. Nature 1996; 380:435-39.

47. Ferrara N, Carver-Moore K, Chen H, et al. Heterozygous embryonic lethality induced by targeted inactivation of the VEGF gene. Nature 1996; 380:439-42.

48. Eremina V, Sood M, Haigh J, et al. Glomerular-specific alterations of VEGF-A expression lead to distinct congenital and acquired renal diseases. J Clin Invest 2003; 111:707-16.

49. Gerber HP, Vu TH, Ryan AM, et al. VEGF couples hypertrophic cartilage remodeling, ossification and

angiogenesis during endochondral bone formation. Nat Med 1999; 5:623-28.

50. Phillips HS, Hains J, Leung DW, et al. Vascular endothelial growth factor is expressed in rat corpus luteum. Endocrinology 1990; 127:965-67.

51. Fong GH, Rossant J, Gertsenstein M, et al. Role of the Flt-1 receptor tyrosine kinase in regulating the assembly of vascular endothelium. Nature 1995; 376:66-70.

52. Shalaby F, Rossant J, Yamaguchi TP, et al. Failure of blood-island formation and vasculogenesis in Flk-1-deficient mice. Nature 1995; 376:62-66.

53. Dumont DJ, Jussila L, Taipale J, et al. Cardiovascular failure in mouse embryos deficient in VEGF receptor-3. Science 1998; 282:946-49.

54. Blaauwgeers HG, Holtkamp GM, Rutten H, et al. Polarized vascular endothelial growth factor secretion by human retinal pigment epithelium and localization of vascular endothelial growth factor receptors on the inner choriocapillaris. Evidence for a trophic paracrine relation. Am J Pathol 1999; 155:421-28.

55. Robinson GS, Ju M, Shih SC, et al. Nonvascular role for VEGF: VEGFR-1, 2 activity is critical for neural retinal development. FASEB J 2001; 15:1215-17.

56. Yi X, Mai LC, Uyama M, et al. Time-course expression of vascular endothelial growth factor as related to the development of the retinochoroidal vasculature in rats. Exp Brain Res 1998; 118:155-60.

57. Kim I, Ryan AM, Rohan R, et al. Constitutive expression of VEGF, VEGFR-1, and VEGFR-2 in normal eyes. Invest Ophthalmol Vis Sci 1999; 40:2115-21.

58. Hofman P, Blaauwgeers HG, Vrensen GF, et al. Role of VEGF-A in endothelial phenotypic shift in human diabetic retinopathy and VEGF-A-induced retinopathy in monkeys. Ophthalmic Res 2001; 33:156-62.

59. Campochiaro PA. Retinal and choroidal neovascularization. J Cell Physiol 2000; 184:301-10.

60. Hammes HP, Lin J, Bretzel RG, et al. Upregulation of the vascular endothelial growth factor/vascular endothelial growth factor receptor system in experimental background diabetic retinopathy of the rat. Diabetes 1998; 47:401-06.

61. Witmer AN, Blaauwgeers HG, Weich HA, et al. Altered expression patterns of VEGF receptors in human diabetic retina and in experimental VEGF-induced retinopathy in monkey. Invest Ophthalmol Vis Sci 2002; 43:849-57.

62. Esser S, Wolburg K, Wolburg H, et al. Vascular endothelial growth factor induces endothelial fenestrations in vitro. J Cell Biol 1998;140:947-59.

63. Holz FG, Sheraidah G, Pauleikhoff D, et al. Analysis of lipid deposits extracted from human macular and peripheral Bruch's membrane. Arch Ophthalmol 1994; 112:402-06.

64. Ramrattan RS, van der Schaft TL, Mooy CM, et al. Morphometric analysis of Bruch's membrane, the choriocapillaris, and the choroids in aging. Invest Ophthalmol Vis Sci 1994; 35:2857-64.

65. Spilsbury K, Garrett KL, Shen WY, et al. Over expression of vascular endothelial growth factor (VEGF) in the retinal pigment epithelium leads to the development of choroidal neovascularization. Am J Pathol 2000; 157:135-44.

66. Eyetech Study Group. Preclinical and phase 1A clinical evaluation of an anti-VEGF pegylated aptamer (EYE001) for the treatment of exudative age-related macular degeneration. Retina 2002; 22:143-52.

67. Eyetech Study Group. Anti-vascular endothelial growth factor therapy for subfoveal choroidal neovascularization secondary to age-related macular degeneration: phase II study results. Ophthalmology 2003;110:979-86.

68. Ng EW, Shima DT, Calias P, et al. Pegaptanib, a targeted anti-VEGF aptamer for ocular vascular disease. Nat Rev Drug Diskov 2006; 5:123-32.

69. Bell C, Lynam E, Landfair DJ, et al. Oligonucleotide NX1838 inhibits VEGF 165-mediated cellular responses in vitro. In vitro Cell Dev Biol Anim 1999; 35:533-42.

70. Drolet DW, et al. Pharmacokinetics and safety of an anti-vascular endothelial growth factor aptamer (NX1838) following injection into the vitreous humor of rhesus monkeys. Pharm Res 2000; 17:1503-10.

71. Asahara T, et al. VEGF contributes to postnatal neovascularization by mobilizing bone marrow-derived endothelial progenitor cells. EMBO J 1999; 18:3964-72.

72. Gragoudas ES, Adamis AP, Cunninham ET Jr, et al. Pegaptanib for neovascular age-related macular degeneration. N Engl J Med 2004; 351:2805-16.

73. D'Amico DJ. VEGF Inhibition Study in Ocular Neovascularization (V.I.S.I.O.N.) Clinical trial group. Pegaptanib sodium for neovascular age-related macular degeneration. Two-year safety results of the two prospective, multicenter, controlled clinical trials. Ophthalmology 2006 Apr 25. Epub ahead of print.

74. The prescribing information of Macugen: http://www.macugen.com/macugen_PI.pdf (accessed on Jun 5, 2006).

75. Ng EW, Adamis AP. Targeting angiogenesis, the underlying disorder in neovascular age-related macular degeneration. Can J Ophthalmol 2005; 40:352-68.

76. Gragoudas ES. Photodynamic therapy and/or macugen update. Presented at: American Academy of Ophthalmology, October, 2005; Chicago, Illinois.

77. Hurwitz H, Fehrenbacher L, Novotny W, et al. Bevacizumab plus irinotecan, fluorouracil, and leucovorin for metastatic colorectal cancer. N Engl J Med 2004; 350:2335-42.

78. Yang JC, Haworth L, Sherry RM, et al. A randomized trial of bevacizumab, an anti-vascular endothelial growth factor antibody, for metastatic renal cancer. N Engl J Med 2003; 349:427-34.

79. Michels S, Rosenfeld PJ, Puliafito CA, et al. Systemic bevacizumab (Avastin) therapy for neovascular age-related macular degeneration twelve-week results of an uncontrolled open-label clinical study. Ophthalmology 2005; 112:1035-47.

80. Rosenfeld PJ, Moshfeghi AA, Puliafito CA. Optical coherence tomography findings after an intravitreal injection of bevacizumab (avastin) for neovascular age-related macular degeneration. Ophthalmic Surg Lasers Imaging 2005; 36:331-35.

81. Reichel E. Intravitreal bevacizumab for choroidal neovascularization and cystoid macular edema: a cost-effective treatment? Ophthalmic Surg Lasers Imaging 2005; 36:270-71.

82. Mordenti J, Cuthbertson RA, Ferrara N, et al. Comparisons of the intraocular tissue distribution, pharmacokinetics and safety of 125I-labeled full-length and Fab antibodies in rhesus monkeys following intravitreal administration. Toxicol Pathol 1999; 27:536-44.

83. Manzano RP, Peyman GA, Khan P, et al. Testing intravitreal toxicity of bevacizumab (Avastin). Retina 2006; 26:257-61.

84. Shahar J, Avery RL, Heilweil G, et al. Electrophysiologic and retinal penetration studies following intravitreal injection of bevacizumab (Avastin). Retina 2006; 26:262-69.

85. Maturi RK, Bleau LA, Wilson DL. Electrophysiologic findings after intravitreal bevacizumab (Avastin) treatment. Retina 2006; 26:270-74.

86. Van Wijngaarden P, Coster DJ, Williams KA. Inhibitors of ocular neovascularization: promises and potential problems. JAMA 2005; 293:1509-13.

87. FDA Medwatch. Barron J, Genentech. Important drug warning [letter]. Available at:http://www.fda.gov/medwatch/SAFETY/2005/Avastin_dearhcp.pdf.

88. Avery RL, Pieramici DJ, Rabena MD, et al. Intravitreal bevacizumab (avastin) for neovascular age-related macular degeneration. Ophthalmology 2006; 113:363-72.

89. Rosenfeld P. Changing strategies in the management of neovascular age-related macular degeneration. Presented at: Retina Society Meeting, September, 2005; San Diego, California.

90. Miller JW. Randomized, controlled phase III study of ranibizumab (Lucentis) for minimally classic or occult neovascular age-related macular degeneration. Paper presented at: ARCR meeting, July, 2005, Montreal, Canada.

91. Robinson CJ, Shweiki D, Itin A, et al. Hypoxia-induced expression of vascular endothelial growth factor by retinal cells is a common factor in neovascularizing ocular diseases. Lab Invest 1995; 72: 638-45.

92. Chen Y, Wiesmann C, Fuh G, et al. Selection and analysis of an optimized anti-VEGF antibody: crystal structure of an affinity-matured Fab in complex with antigen. J Mol Biol 1999; 293:865-81.

93. Gaudreault J, Webb W, Van Hoy M, et al. Pharmokinetics and retinal distribution of AMD rhufab V2 after intravitreal administration in rabbits. AAPS Pharm Sci 1999; (Suppl 1):3207.

94. Mordenti J, Cuthbertson RA, Ferrara N, et al. Comparisons of the intraocular tissue distribution, pharmacokinetics and safety of 125I-labeled full-length and Fab antibodies in rhesus monkeys following intravitreal administration. Toxicol Pathol 1999; 27:536-44.

95. Graudreault J, Fei D, Rusit J, et al. Preclinical pharmacokinetics of ranibizumab (rhuFabV2) after a single intravitreal administration. Invest Ophthalmol Vis Sci 2005; 46:726-33.

96. Krzystolik MG, Afshari MA, Adamis AP, et al. Prevention of experimental choroidal neovascularization with intravitreal anti-vascular endothelial growth factor antibody fragment. Arch Ophthalmol 2002; 120:338-46.

97. Husain D, Kim I, Gauthier D, et al. Safety and efficacy of intravitreal injection of ranibizumab in combination with verteporfin PDT on experimental choroidal neovascularization in the monkey. Arch Ophthalmol 2005; 123:509-16.

98. Kim IK, Husain D, Michaud N, et al. Effect of intravitreal injection of ranibizumab in combination with verteporfin PDT on normal primate retina and choroids. Invest Ophthalmol Vis Sci 2006; 47:357-63.

99. Heier JS. Review of Lucentis ™ (ranibizumab, rhuFab V2) phase I/II trial results: 6 month treatment of exudative AMD. Invest Ophthalmol Vis Sci 2004; 45: E-Abstract 1109.

100. Heier JS, Rosenfeld PJ, Antoszyk AN, et al. Long-term experience with Lucentis ™ (ranibizumab) in patients with neovascular age-related macular degeneration (AMD). Invest Ophthalmol Vis Sci 2005; 46: E-Abstract 1393.

101. Rosenfeld PJ, Heier JS, Hantsbarger G, et al. Tolerability and efficacy of multiple escalating doses of ranibizumab (Lucentis) for neovascular age-related macular degeneration. Ophthalmology 2006; 113:623-32.

102. Heier JS, Antoszyk AN, Pavan PR, et al. Ranibizumab for treatment of neovascular age-related macular degeneration. A Phase I/II multicenter, controlled, multidose study. Ophthalmology 2006; 113:633-42.

103. Chung CY, Kim R. A Phase III, multicenter, randomized, double-masked, sham injection-controlled study of the efficacy and safety of rhufabv2 (ranibizumab) in subjects with minimally classic or occult subfoveal neovascular age-related macular degeneration (MARINA). Study report no. CSR FVF2598g.

104. Sy JP, Schneider S, Damico L. A Phase III, multicenter, randomized, double masked, active treatment-controlled study of the efficacy and safety of rhufab v2 (ranibizumab) compared with verteporfin (Visudyne®) photodynamic therapy in subjects with predominantly classic subfoveal neovascular age-related macular degeneration (ANCHOR). Study report no. CSR FVF 2587g.

105. Hee MR, Baumal CR, Puliafito CA, et al. Optical coherence tomography of age-related macular degeneration and choroidal neovascularization. Ophthalmology 1996; 103: 1260-70.

106. Rogers AH, Martidis A, Greenberg PB, et al. Optical coherence tomography findings following photodynamic therapy of choroidal neovascularization. Am J Ophthalmol 2002; 134:566-76.

107. Ting TD, Oh M, Cox TA, et al. Decreased visual acuity associated with cystoid macular edema in neovascular age-related macular degeneration. Arch Ophthalmol 2002;120: 731-37.

108. Costa RA, Calucci D, Skaf M, et al. Optical Coherence Tomography 3: Automatic Delineation of the Outer Neural Retinal Boundary and Its Influence on Retinal Thickness Measurements. Invest Ophthalmol Vis Sci 2004;45:2399-2406.

109. Ray R, Stinnett SS, Jaffe GJ. Evaluation of image artifact produced by optical coherence tomography of retinal pathology. Am J Ophthalmol 2005; 139:18-29.

110. Aiello LP, Brucker AJ, Chang S, et al. Evolving guidelines for intravitreous injections. Retina 2004;24(5 suppl):S3-S19.

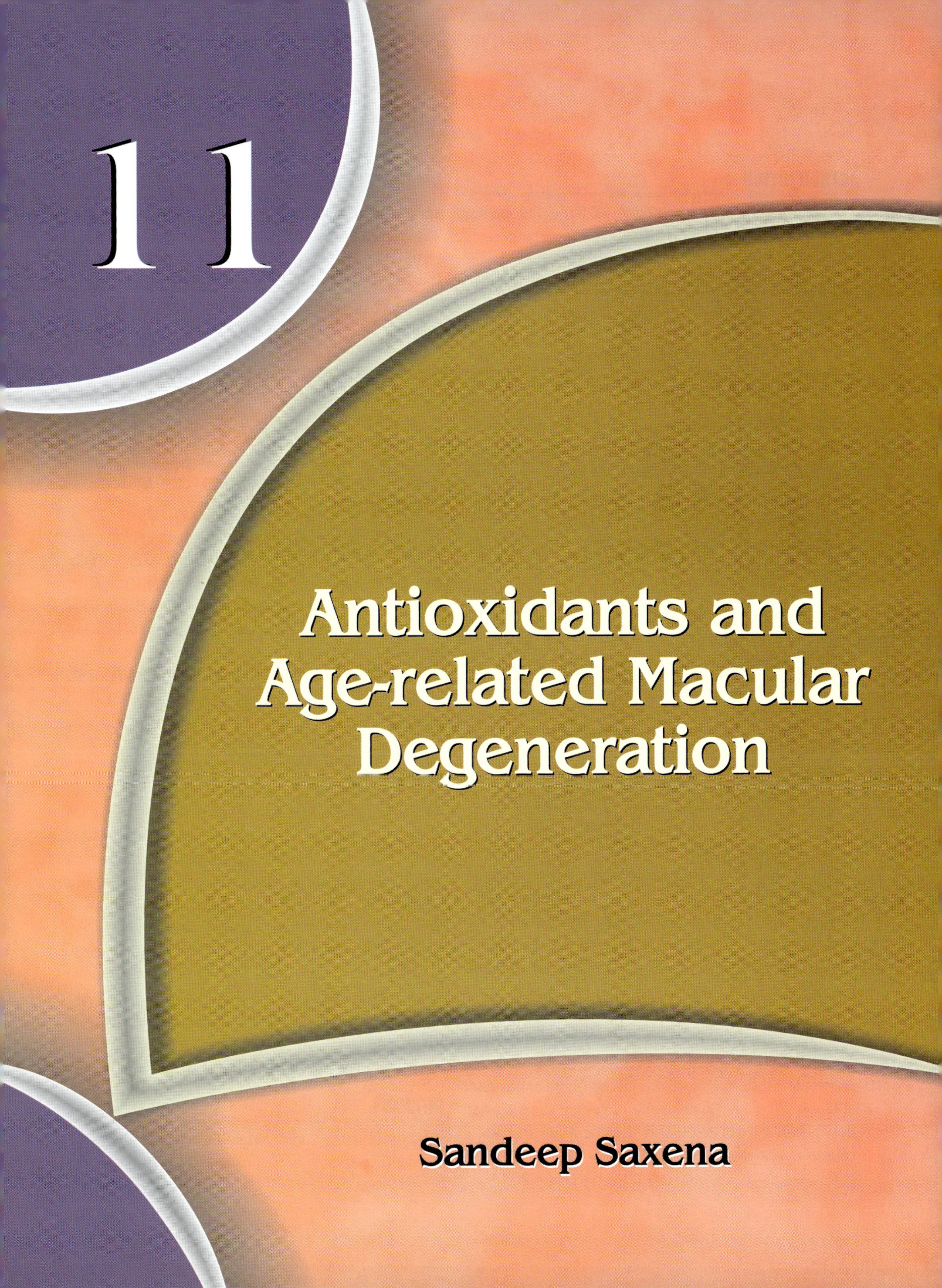

11
Antioxidants and Age-related Macular Degeneration
Sandeep Saxena

INTRODUCTION

Age-related macular degeneration (AMD) is the leading cause of irreversible vision loss in older populations. [1-4] As longevity increases, AMD is emerging as a public health issue. Age-related macular degeneration markedly compromises the quality of life among the affected elderly. In the United States, the number of people with visually impairing AMD is expected to double and reach 3 million by 2020.[5]

Despite the significance of this disease, there are no available means to prevent it and effective treatment is limited to small fraction of patients. Strategies to prevent or retard the onset of AMD are needed so that the burden of blindness and visual impairment due to this disease can be reduced.

There is increasing speculation that dietary factors, particularly antioxidants, may prevent or impede the progression of AMD. [6-13] The hypothesis that micronutrient antioxidants can protect against AMD comes from mounting evidence that oxidative stress is etiologic for AMD [14] and the observation that diets rich in fruits and vegetables and use of specific antioxidant supplements are associated with reduced risk of AMD. The theory is biologically plausible. The outer retina, rich in poly-unsaturated fatty acids, may be altered adversely by free-radical production and oxidation and, conversely may be protected by nutrients that block this oxidative damage. Antioxidants may also help maintain the integrity of the choroidal blood vessels that supply the macular region of the retina. Basic and clinical research suggests that nutritional factors may be associated with AMD. Several large observational studies and interventional trials have focused on the effects of vitamin C, vitamin E, beta-carotene, and zinc in combination or alone on the prevention of AMD.

VITAMIN C

Ascorbate is the most effective aqueous-phase antioxidant in blood. It is thought to have a protective effect against degenerative processes and degenerative disorders caused by oxidative stress.[15,16]

LIGHT DAMAGE AND VITAMIN C

In an albino rat study, in terms of pre-exposure rhodopsin levels, L-ascorbate, Na-ascorbate, and dehydroascorbate were found to protect cyclic light dark-reared rats against rod cell loss in a dose dependent manner but no such effect was found for D-ascorbate. Vitamin C supplements resulted in raised retinal ascorbate levels and were protective only if given prior to light exposure. Ascorbate supplements were also associated with preservation of rod outer segment docosahexaenoic acid suggesting that it is the antioxidant properties of vitamin C that account for its protective effect.[17]

DIETARY VITAMIN C AND AGE-RELATED MACULAR DEGENERATION

The NHANES reported that diet containing high quantity of food stuffs rich in vitamin A and C was negatively associated with AMD.[18] The Eye-Disease Case Control Study (EDCC) and the Beaver Dam Eye Study (BDES) also reported a protective effect associated with high intake of oral vitamin C, but the association was not statistically significant in these studies.[19] The Blue Mountain Eye Study (BMES) found no such protective effect for dietary ascorbate.[15]

PLASMA VITAMIN C AND AGE-RELATED MACULAR DEGENERATION

The EDCC study reported that low plasma levels of vitamin C were associated with increased risk of AMD, but high levels were not found to be protective. An anti-oxidant index comprising of plasma carotenoids, selenium, ascorbate and vitamin E were found to be inversely related to AMD.[12] The Baltimore Longitudinal Study of Aging (BLSA) reported a nonsignificant protective effect associated with the highest quintile of plasma vitamin C levels and observed a significant protective effect for an antioxidant index which included alpha-tocopherol, ascorbate, and beta-carotene.[20] These findings were however not reproduced in the POLA study.[21]

VITAMIN E

Vitamin E is the major chain-breaking antioxidant of cellular membranes, [21-23] It exists in four common forms:

alpha-tocopherol, beta-tocopherol, gamma-tocopherol and delta-tocopherol. Alpha-tocopherol is the most effective scavenger of free radicals and the most predominant tocopherol in human retina and plasma.[24,25] Selenium, a micronutrient, complements the antioxidant function of vitamin E.[15]

RETINAL LIGHT DAMAGE AND VITAMIN E

The retina contains high quantities of alpha-tocopherol in the rod outer segment ands and retinal pigment epithelium.[26,27] The concentrations are very sensitive to dietary intake of the vitamin.[28] It has been found that vitamin E content of retinal pigment epithelium is 4 to 7 times that of the neural retina and it rises with increasing age. It has also been speculated that this may be in response to increasing oxidative stress.[29]

Central neural retina closely regulates its vitamin E content, and analogies with carotenoids of macular pigment are inescapable.[30-32] Both carotenoids and alpha-tocopherol can act synergistically as free radical scavengers. Vitamin E concentration in the rhesus monkey retina-retinal pigment epithelium reaches a maximum at the fovea and at eccentricities of 1.0 mm or more and declines to a minimum at the foveal crest.[33] These minimum concentrations at the foveal crest result in an area of vulnerability accounting for the frequent occurrence of atrophic AMD at this site.

Following observations support the concept that vitamin E protects against retinal oxidative damage:[15]

- Vitamin E deficiency results in retinal degeneration, excessive retinal pigment epithelium lipofuscin, and a decrease in polyunsaturated fatty acid content of rod outer segments and the retinal pigment epithelium.[34]
- Bovine rods challenged with oxygen exhibit substantial destruction of membrane structure. This damage can be limited by high levels of endogenous vitamin E, in *in vitro* experiments.[35]
- Dark-rearing results in increased vulnerability to retinal light damage. It is associated with reduced ascorbate and vitamin E levels in the rat retina.[36,37] Some researchers, however, have failed to demonstrate that vitamin E and selenium protect against photochemical damage of the retina.[38,39]

DIETARY VITAMIN E AND AGE-RELATED MACULAR DEGENERATION

Dietary intake of vitamin E is quite difficult to estimate as its bioavailability varies considerably.[40] The BDES and the EDCC investigated the relationship between dietary intake of vitamin E and AMD. The BDES reported a significantly increased risk of large macular drusen associated with lowest versus highest quintile of past dietary intake of vitamin E.[41] The EDCC found no significant inverse association between dietary intake of vitamin E, with or without supplements and neovascular AMD.[42]

PLASMA VITAMIN E AND AGE-RELATED MACULAR DEGENERATION

The POLA study presented extensive investigation of plasma alpha-tocopherol and age-related macular degeneration.[21] Fasting blood levels of vitamin E, after multivariate adjustments showed a weak negative association with AMD. Lipid standardized plasma alpha-tocopherol had a significant inverse relationship with early and late AMD, representing a risk reduction of 82% for those in the highest quintile versus the lowest quintile. The POLA study findings are consistent with those of the BSLA and the BDES, although the statistical significance of the protective effect of serum alpha-tocopherol in the BDES was lost after adjusting for serum lipids.[43] Although the EDCC and the BMES found no significant associations between plasma levels of vitamin E and AMD, the former study did detect a significant protective effect for a serum antioxidant index which included alpha-tocopherol.[44]

VITAMIN A

Vitamin A (retinol) is essential for vision. Vitamin A must be available in the retina as a precursor of 11-*cis*-retinal for the regeneration of rhodopsin. Vitamin A exists in the following oxidation states: Retinol (an alchohol), retinal (an aldehyde) and retinoic acid (an acid). In an experiment, physiological concentrations of retinol added to liposomes composed of rod cell phospholipids were found to protect the lipids from oxidation.[45] As the chain of lipid peroxidation within the membrane is broken, a small amount of retinol may protect large concentrations of membrane lipids.

Vitamin A is also involved in the repair of cells that have been oxidatively damaged. In the retina, vitamin E is believed to protect vitamin A from oxidative degeneration.[46]

DIETARY VITAMIN A AND AGE-RELATED MACULAR DEGENERATION

The NHANES reported a 40% reduction in risk for AMD in persons who consumed food rich in vitamin A at least once per day, as compared to those who ate these food less than once per week.[15] However, this protective effect of vitamin A was not confirmed in other reports.[47,48] It is possible that the NHANES finding simply represents protective effect of dietary carotenoids, which are found in the same food.[49] The BDES also failed to detect a significant between total dietary vitamin A (provitamin A carotenoids plus retinol), or dietary retinol and early AMD, but did detect a weak inverse relationship between past consumption of provitamin A carotenoids and early AMD and a significant inverse relationship between provitamin A carotenoids and the presence of large drusen.[41]

PLASMA VITAMIN A AND AGE-RELATED MACULAR DEGENERATION

The POLA study did not detect a significant association with respect to plasma retinol and AMD.[21]

CAROTENOIDS

Carotenoids are naturally occurring pigments that are essential to photosynthetic organisms as they capture radiant energy.[50] In mammals these compounds are entirely of dietary origin. Some carotenoids can be converted to vitamin A and are therefore said to have provitamin activity. The antioxidant properties of the carotenoids are well established and include the ability to quench singlet oxygen and triplet sensitizers,[51-55] interact with free radicals[56-58] and prevent lipid peroxidation.[59-63] Carotenoids antioxidant activity is enhanced at low oxygen tension[64] and carotenoid act with other antioxidants.[65] The carotenoids appear to protect or repair alpha-tocopherol and to act synergis-

tically with vitamin C in protecting against oxidative damage.[66]

Lutein, zeaxanthin, and lycopene belong to a large class of plant pigments referred to as carotenoids. Among 25 dietary carotenoids and nine metabolites routinely found in human serum, mainly lutein, zeaxanthin, lycopene and their metabolites have been detected in ocular tissues.

An understanding of the biological sequences of limiting or supplementing with these carotenoids is only beginning to emerge. Currently, focus is on lutein, zeaxanthin, and lycopene. There is a speculation that consuming higher levels of these carotenoids lead to a higher levels in the eye and that this may confer health benefits.

LUTEIN AND ZEAXANTHIN

Primate foveas have a distinctive yellow macular pigment that is one of their recognized specializations. They were originally identified as being composed of xanthophyllic carotenoids by Wald in 1945.[67] These primary pigments were later more specifically identified as lutein and zeaxanthin by Bone and associates [68] in 1985.

Lutein and zeaxanthin are more polar than many other carotenoids, due to the presence of hydroxyl groups on the cyclic ring structure. Unlike provitamin A carotenoids (alpha and beta-carotene and cryptoxanthin), they cannot be converted to vitamin A. Their presence in tissues is due entirely to ingestion of plant sources; animal tissues do not synthesize them. However, a variety of metabolites may be found in animal sources and several exist in human blood and milk.[69]

Lutein and zeaxanthin are present in a wide variety of fruits and vegetables and impart a yellow color to the plants they are found in, such as corn. Their concentration is particularly high in leafy green vegetables such as spinach.[70] They are also present in some animal products such as egg yolk [71] due to plant products eaten by animals. Adults, on an average, consume approximately 1 to 2 mg lutein/day.[72] Level of intake varies considerably across individuals and population subgroups.[72] Currently, there is speculation that consuming higher levels of these carotenoids leads to higher levels in body tissues, particularly in the eye, and that this may confer health benefits that lower the risk of ocular diseases.

Abundance and Distribution in Blood and Tissues

Clues regarding biologic roles of lutein and zeaxanthin in health and disease may be gained with an understanding of the abundance across species.

Serum: Lutein and zeaxanthin are major serum carotenoids, along with beta-carotene, alpha-carotene and lycopene.[73] Median serum concentrations of lutein and zeaxanthin in American adults, in the Third National Health and Nutrition Examination Survey, ranged from 0.19 μmol/L in the lowest quintile to 0.79 μmol/L in the highest quintile.[72] Dietary intake of foods rich in these carotenoids has been shown to influence serum concentrations in a positive manner.[74-77] However, individual variation in serum response to intake has been observed. and may be due to factors such as varying rates of absorption and tissue uptake. Factors that influence bioavailability are described elsewhere.[78]

Tissue: Lutein and zeaxanthin have also been shown to be major carotenoids found in body tissues.[79,80] Levels of these hydroxycarotenoids vary widely across tissues. Reported concentrations of lutein and zeaxanthin are often highest in ocular tissues. In the inner retinal layer, concentrations can range from 0.1 to 1.0 pmol/mm² in tissue.[81-84] Mean concentrations in the human cataractous lens are 44.1 ng/g lens wet weight for the nuclear layer.[84] Liver lutein/zeaxanthin concentrations are often high, but vary widely from 0 to 16.2 nmol/g.[78-81] Other tissues that sometimes have relatively high levels include adrenal, adipose, pancreas, kidney and breast. [85] Levels are often reported to be lower in the lung, spleen, heart, testes, thyroid, ovary and skin. [85,86]

Macula: Macular pigment in the human retina, unlike other tissues, contains only lutein and zeaxanthin to the exclusion of other carotenoids, [87-89] and lutein/zeaxanthin concentration (1 mmol/L) is approximately 500-fold higher than the concentration in other tissues (2 μmol/ L). [90] Lutein and zeaxanthin represent a large proportion of total carotenoid in some tissues, such as adipose (44%), in which lower proportions of lycopene (39%) and beta-carotene (11%) have been reported. The proportion of these carotenoids reported in other tissues is minor. These disproportionate concentrations of lutein and zeaxanthin among tissues may indicate selective tissue uptake, possibly producing clues to their biological role. [79]

Protective Effect on Rods and Cones

There are distinctive patterns in the distribution of lutein and zeaxanthin within tissues. In the macula, the concentration of these carotenoids is the greatest in the centre and declines with increasing eccentricity.[91] An average mass per unit retinal area was reported to be 1.33 ng/mm² at the foveal centre as compared with 0.81 ng/mm² with increasing eccentricity of 1.6 to 2.5 mm.[81] Zeaxanthin is more prominent in the inner macula, averaging 60% of the total. As eccentricity increases away from the fovea, lutein becomes the dominant carotenoid. Reported ratios of lutein: zeaxanthin in the peripheral retina have been between 2:1 and 3:1. The distribution of lutein and zeaxanthin in the retina suggests a possible role for lutein in protecting the rods that are concentrated in the peripheral retina [92] and for zeaxanthin in protecting cones, which are concentrated in central retina.[81]

Metabolites of lutein and zeaxanthin have been identified in human blood and tissues;[13] however, the sources and function are largely unknown. A prevalent isomer in human retina, mesozeaxanthin, may be metabolized from dietary lutein or may be due to its ingestion because this metabolite has been identified in some foodstuff.[93]

Tissue concentrations of lutein and zeaxanthin vary widely across individuals. In the macula, a wide variability in levels of these carotenoids was observed in eyes obtained from autopsy. Median lutein/zeaxanthin concentrations in the central retina in quartile 1 vs 4 were 2.05 and 9.08 pmol/mm², respectively. In more peripheral areas of the retina, variations in concentrations also existed, and were inversely related to having a history of macular degeneration, as were levels in the central retina.[94]

The level of variation across individuals may reflect both diet and genetic factors. The premise that diet will influence lutein and zeaxanthin concentrations is supported by several investigators who have reported increases in macular pigment density with feeding of foods 6 or supplements[95] rich in these carotenoids. Genetic determination of macular pigment is supported by correlations between macular pigment density and eye color[96] and by the similarities in macular pigment density across monozygotic twins.[97] Macula pigment optical density has not been significantly correlated with differences in sex or smoking behavior.[98]

Study has shown that lutein and zeaxanthin dietary supplements raise macular pigment density and serum concentrations of these carotenoids in humans.[99]

Possible Role of Lutein and Zeaxanthin in Visual Acuity and Visibility and Macular Protection

Light must pass through the macular pigments before reaching the retinal photoreceptors. Lutein and zeaxanthin screen out significant amounts of short-wave energy. Individual variation in peak absorbance is large ranging from 0.0 to 1.5 log units.

Lutein and zeaxanthin are colored compounds, and as such, absorb visible light. Even though the structures are very similar, lutein has 10 conjugated double bonds in the molecule, whereas, zeaxanthin has 11 conjugated double bonds. As such lutein absorbs at slightly shorter wavelengths than does zeaxanthin. Both of them are effective in filtering blue light (400-475 nm), but zeaxanthin is much more effective in absorbing blue-green light at 500 nm and slightly above. [100] This ability to filter out blue light on entering the retinal tissue could, therefore, explain the presence of colored carotenoids in the macular region, but does not begin to explain why nature has selected the two xanthophylls, lutein and zeaxanthin, from more than 20 carotenoids present in the plasma. Beta-carotene, lycopene or beta-cryptoxanthin, also present in human plasma at concentrations equivalent to that of lutein and zeaxanthin,[101] would also serve as effective filters of blue light, but they have not been selected for this action. Therefore it must be some specific property of these xanthophylls that might help explain their presence in the primate retina. One such property is their disposition in biological membranes.

Dicroic properties of lutein have been studied in an attempt to explain the yellow brush or tufts, known as Haidinger brushes, observed in the macula when the eye is illuminated with polarized light. Lutein was found to be located perpendicular to the plane of the bilayer membrane.[102] Zeaxanthin resides primarily perpendicular to the plane of the membrane, whereas, beta-carotene has no preferred orientation. [103,104]

- *The acuity hypothesis:* When the emmetropic eye is in focus of middle-wave light, it will be myopic for short-wave length and slightly hyperopic for long-wave length light. [105] This effect is known as longitudinal chromatic aberration. For 460 nm light (the dominant wavelength of typical phase of daylight and peak absorption of carotenoids), the magnitude of focus error is approximately –1.2 dioptres. [106] Given optimal focus at 550 nm, much of the short wave region will be seriously out of focus. In addition of the focus problem, the wavelength dependency of the eye' focal length means that retinal image size is proportional to wavelength, i.e. the longer the wavelength the larger the retinal image. This effect is known as lateral chromatic aberration. Thus, if a disc of light is imaged on the fovea, violet-blue penumbra will result. Together, longitudinal and lateral chromatic aberrations are simply known as chromatic aberration. Max Schultze's acuity hypothesis predicts that lutein and zeaxanthin's short-wave absorption sharpen retinal images and that visual acuity is consequently improved. [107]

- *The visibility hypothesis:* In addition to blur from chromatic aberration, there is another source of optical degradation. The earth's atmosphere through which we view objects almost always contains small-suspended particles. This haze aerosol scatters short wave light more than other wavelengths and results in a bluish veiling luminance. Blue haze is a major factor that degrades visibility. Lutein and zeaxanthin may improve vision by preferentially absorbing the short-wave energy produced by the blue haze and thereby increasing both the contrast within targets and the contrast of targets with respect to their backgrounds. [107]

- *The protection hypothesis:* There have been at least two varieties of protection hypotheses advanced to account for their presence. Short-wave light is exceptionally damaging to retinal tissue.[108] The location of lutein and zeaxanthin in the inner Henle fiber layer[109] is optimal for screening vulnerable receptor outer segment from actinic short-wave light.[110] In addition to screening, they are effective quenchers of reactive oxygen species. Kirschfeld [111] first highlighted the protective role of carotenoids in eyes and photoreceptor cells. Macular pigments could also provide protection by quenching excited states of sensitizing pigments and or singlet oxygen. Macular pigments could destroy free radicals formed from exposure of light [112] whereas they may also have a direct antioxidant effect. [113] Antioxidant properties[114-118] as well as the properties associated with prooxidation have been studied. [119,120] Lutein and zeaxanthin are effective antioxidants *in vitro* and may also demonstrate this action in *ex vivo* systems, particularly those associated with evaluating their effects on low density lipoprotein oxidation. One conclusion drawn by several investigators is that if oxidation products of these carotenoids are found in a tissue such as the macula, this constitutes adequate evidence that these compounds are acting as antioxidants in that tissue.[121] However, carotenoids are not very stable compounds, and the mere presence of oxidation products cannot be considered evidence that they are acting as antioxidants, as opposed to reflecting the oxidant stress in any given tissue. [122]

The identification of oxidized by-products of lutein and zeaxanthin within the human retina is consistent with a function as retinal antioxidant. There is a large confluence of data that suggests that lutein and zeaxanthin protect the retina from light initiated oxidative damage,[123] such as experimental studies on rats,[124] quail[125] and primates.[126] Data from human has shown that the central fovea is most resistant to degenerative change. The presence of lutein and zeaxanthin in human rod outer segment membranes raises the possibility that they function as antioxidants in this cell compartment.[127]

Possible Role of Lutein and Zeaxanthin in Protection against Disease

A strong body of evidence to support a role of a nutrient or food component in the delay of chronic disease requires scientific data of a variety of different types to establish the protective role. The following important criteria may be used to establish strong evidence for a causal role of lutein and zeaxanthin in protection against chronic disease: [128]

1. *Biologic plausibility:* Evidence is required to support a known biologic mechanism by which lutein and zeaxanthin might protect against disease. Biologic plausibility is stronger with additional experimental evidence for protection demonstrated in animal models or cell culture.

2. *Consistency of relationships across human populations and study designs:* This lowers the likelihood that observations of protective relationships that are observed reflect biases associated with a particular study design, study sample or confounding factors that are unmeasured, poorly measured or unknown.

3. *Temporality:* The evidence for the hypothesized protective effect of carotenoids against the development of disease is strengthened when levels of the carotenoids in the diet or body are measured before the onset or worsening of disease. Such evidence provided by prospective studies and clinical trials, rules out the possibility that diets or body levels low in lutein or zeaxanthin area consequence of the conditions rather than an antecedent event.

4. *Strength of the relationship between level of intake and risk for disease:* Strong relationships, indicated by large odds ratio or relative risks, like consistent findings, reduce the likelihood that observations are due to unknown or unmeasured factors. Strong relative risks also indicate that the protective benefit is important.

5. *Specificity of the relationships:* Such relationship observed to lutein and zeaxanthin, rather than other aspects of diet or lifestyle that accompany the intake of foods rich in these carotenoids are challenging to demonstrate. However, such evidence can be determined systematically in large prospective studies. Randomized clinical trials can also provide evidence for a specific effect.

Role of Lutein and Zeaxanthin in Macular Degeneration

There is evidence that suggests that lutein and zeaxanthin may reduce risk for developing macular degeneration. There is also an untested possibility that they may slow progression once this condition is present. In addition, lutein may also slow degeneration of vision in patients with retinitis pigmentosa. However, only preliminary data in a very small number of eyes have been published in which lutein slowed vision loss associated with retinitis pigmentosa in one,[129] but not in another study.[130] The findings of a higher concentration of these carotenoids in rod outer segment membranes of the perifoveal retina lend support to their proposed protective role in age-related macular degeneration.[127] The chain breaking antioxidant properties of these carotenoids in peroxidative reactions of lipid membranes and quenching of free radicals seem to be of importance for inhibition of lipofuscin formation, considered an important feature in the pathogenesis of AMD.[131]

The biologic plausibility that lutein and zeaxanthin protect against the development of macular degeneration is supported by the fact that they have chemical properties that may retard the pathogenic mechanisms that are thought to promote this degenerative condition. Oxidative stress is high in eyes due to the intense light exposure and the high rate of oxidative metabolism in the retina. It is thought to contribute to age-related macular degeneration.[132] The antioxidant properties of lutein and zeaxanthin may reduce the degree to which oxidative damage promotes these diseases or may minimize the damage due to oxidative stress by limiting the degree to which oxygen penetrates membranes. However, lack of direct evidence for antioxidant protection of these carotenoids *in vivo* has also been highlighted.[133] Because these carotenoids absorb blue light, they can reduce photochemical damage that would otherwise occur in retina when exposed to light of these wavelengths,[134] it has been suggested that exposure of the retina to light can promote the development of macular degeneration.[135] Light exposure can also increase the production of free radicals in retina.[136] However, epidemiologic data to support a damaging role of light in macular degeneration is inconsistent[137] although this may reflect the difficulty in capturing actual light exposure over many years in people studied to date.

At present, there is limited data to demonstrate a role of lutein and zeaxanthin in protection against eye disease. In addition to being a relatively new field of research, there are few opportunities to investigate the biological roles of these carotenoids in macular degeneration in experimental animals such as rodents who do not have a macula. In monkeys fed diets devoid of plant pigments for several years, levels of these pigments in the macula disappear and retinal abnormalities that resemble AMD changes appear.[138] Another potential animal model with which to study the protective effects of lutein and zeaxanthin on the retina is quail. Quail retina, like the primate macula, is dominated by cone photoreceptors and concentrates lutein and zeaxanthin. Preliminary studies indicate an inverse correlation between the level of zeaxanthin in quail retina and light induced retinal cell death.[124]

Several epidemiologic studies have examined the relationship between AMD and lutein-rich foods or lutein levels in the diet or blood. A large case control study by the Eye Disease Case Control Study (EDCCS) Group compared the fasting serum samples of 615 controls to 421 patients recently diagnosed with neovascular AMD.[12] Those with lutein/zeaxanthin levels concentrations >0.67 μmol/L were 70% less likely to have AMD than those with concentrations <0.25 μmol/L. An examination of dietary intake of lutein in the year before these subjects entered the EDCCS was conducted. Among 356 cases and 520 controls, those in the highest quintile category of lutein and zeaxanthin intake (median 5757 IU) were 57% less likely to have advanced AMD than individuals in the lowest quintile category of intake (median 561 IU). Decreased odds of having AMD were observed with increasing frequency of spinach or collard greens consumption. In contrast, a retrospective study in the Beaver Dam Eye Study cohort found no significant association between lutein and zeaxanthin intake ten years prior to study enrollment and AMD. In a smaller sample of 167 case control pairs selected in the Beaver Dam cohort, no significant difference in the mean non-fasting concentrations of lutein and zeaxanthin in AMD cases and controls. However, the range of serum concentrations of lutein and zeaxanthin was not as great in this study as in the EDCCS. Subjects from the Beaver Dam cohort who were free of late stage AMD at baseline for five years and found no significant association between specific macular lesions and lutein and zeaxanthin intake either 10 years before study enrollment or at baseline. Similarly, a small case control study in the United Kingdom found no plasma differences between the mean plasma lutein concentrations of 65 patients with AMD changes and the lutein concentrations of 65 control subjects. Like the Beaver Dam cohort, most of cases had early macular changes (86%) and cases and controls had similar distribution of visual acuity. Differences in the range of lutein and zeaxanthin exposures and/or the severity of AMD examined may partly explain the inconsistent findings in these studies. The dietary intakes and blood levels of lutein and zeaxanthin were higher in the EDCCS than in the Beaver Dam population. Further, the late stage neovascular AMD was the outcome interest in the EDCCS analyses, as opposed to the earlier, more general form of AMD studied in the UK and Beaver Dam populations.[128]

The epidemiologic evidence to support the possibility that lutein and zeaxanthin have an important role in reducing the risk of cataract in humans is somewhat consistent. These carotenoids may play a role in the health of other body tissues, as well. Although these relationships are largely unexplored, there is a possibility that lutein along with other carotenoids, may protect against cancer, cardiovascular disease and other conditions that may involve the immune system.[127]

LYCOPENE

Fruits and vegetables contain several carotenoids that are routinely absorbed and metabolized by humans. [139,140] The prominent carotenoid in tomatoes is the red pigment lycopene, which is also among the major carotenoids found in human serum. [139-141] Other commonly consumed fruits that contain lycopene are pink grapefruit, papaya and apricot.[142] It has been shown that lycopene is more potent than alpha- or beta-carotene in inhibiting the cell growth of various human cancer cell lines. [143] Although lycopene has no vitamin A activity, it has been shown to possess strong antioxidant activity *in vitro*. [144] Singlet oxygen quenching capacity of lycopene, beta-carotene and tocopherols are of comparable magnitudes in plasma, when the concentration difference is taken into account, i.e. the molar singlet oxygen quenching capacity of lycopene and beta-carotene is much higher

even than that of vitamin E.[144] Lycopene has been characterized as the most efficient biological carotenoids single oxygen quencher.[145,146]

Lycopene in Ocular Tissue

2,6-cyclolycopene-1.5-diol A, which is a major oxidative metabolite of lycopene has been isolated in retina. [127] In auto-oxidation experiments, the breakdown of lycopene and beta-carotene was higher than the breakdown of lutein and zeaxanthin. The following sequence of breakdown rates was observed: lycopene > beta-carotene > zeaxanthin > lutein. The slow degradation of zeaxanthin and lutein may be suggested to explain the majority of zeaxanthin and lutein in retina. The rapid degeneration of beta-carotene and lycopene under the influence of natural sunlight and UV light is postulated to be the reason for the almost lack of those carotenoids in human retina. [147]

Lycopene and a diverse range of carotenoids have also been identified and quantified in the human ciliary body and retinal pigment epithelium/choroid. Carotenoids in human retinal pigment epithelium /choroid may provide protection by antioxidant and light-screening mechanisms. This is because retinal pigment epithelium/ choroid is subjected to comparable light exposure levels to neural retina, and carotenoids may play a role in the light-induced oxidative damage. Moreover, the retinal pigment epithelium/choroid may be an intermediate control and transfer point for lutein and zeaxanthin uptake by the neural retina from the circulating blood. [148]

DIETARY CAROTENOIDS AND AGE-RELATED MACULAR DEGENERATION

Dietary intake of carotenoids is positively related to the optical density of macular pigment for males and to their serum levels for both genders.[149] However, dietary studies should be interpreted with caution as there are many confounders. The EDCC study found that a high dietary intake of carotenoids protected against AMD.[42] Lutein and zeaxanthin were found to be most protective. The BDES study, which included a prospective arm, reported that past intake of alpha-carotene, beta-carotene and provitamin A carotenoids as well as their baseline intake was associated with significantly reduced risk of large drusen at 5 years follow-up. No such protective effect was however detected for lutein and zeaxanthin.[41] Other studies considered beta-carotene only in their investigation and did not detect a significant protective effect.[20,48] Beta-carotene is not found in human retina.[15]

SERUM CAROTENOIDS AND AGE-RELATED MACULAR DEGENERATION

Serum levels of carotenoids have the limitations that they reflect only recent nutritional intake. As macular pigment has a very slow turnover, current serum levels is of limited value. The EDCC study reported a significantly decreased risk of neovascular AMD associated with medium and high serum levels of carotenoids.[150] High levels of the individual retinal carotenoids was also found to be protective. The BDES, only reported that low levels of lycopene were associated with increased risk of AMD.[43] The BLSA and BMES measured only serum beta-carotene and failed to detect a protective effect associated with high serum levels of this carotenoid.[20,44]

ZINC

Zinc is the most abundant trace element in the human eye.[151] It plays an important role in antioxidant defenses, because it acts as a cofactor for CuZn-SOD [152] and is involved in the regulation of catalase activity.[153] Zinc induces the synthesis of metallothionein, a scavenger of hydroxyl radicals,[154] and stabilizes membrane lipids against oxidation.[155]

Despite a plausible rationale in support of the protective effect of zinc against AMD, the clinical and epidemiologic evidences are less convincing.

The EDCC and the BDES did not detect a significant relationship between serum zinc levels and the risk of AMD.[43,150] The BMES also did not find significant relationship between AMD and dietary intake of zinc.[48] In a 2-year, double-blind, randomized, placebo-controlled trial of zinc supplement with cases of neovascular AMD in one eye, although zinc supplements were associated with raised levels of this trace element at final follow-up, they were not found to affect the clinical course of the disease in a beneficial way. [156]

AGE-RELATED EYE DISEASE STUDY

According to the report from the National Eye Institute in 2002, [157] more than 1 million Americans, over 40 years of age, are blind and another 2.4 million are visually impaired. Nearly, a decade ago, the National Eye Institute initiated a multi-site clinical study called the Age-related Eye Disease Study (AREDS) [158] to examine, prospectively the effects of supplementary antioxidant vitamins and zinc on the progression of late-stage retinal and lenticular eye disease.

The AREDS was the first National Institute of Health sponsored study to be conducted with the objective to evaluate the effect of high-dose vitamins C and E, beta-carotene, and zinc supplements on AMD progression and visual acuity. This study, an 11-center double-masked clinical trial, enrolled participants in an AMD trial if they had extensive small drusen, intermediate drusen, large drusen, non central geographic atrophy, or pigment abnormalities in 1 or both eyes, or advanced AMD or vision loss due to AMD in 1 eye. At least 1 eye had best-corrected visual acuity of 20/32 or better. Participants were randomly assigned to receive daily oral tablets containing: (i) antioxidants (vitamin C, 500 mg; vitamin E, 400 IU; and beta carotene, 15 mg); (ii) zinc, 80 mg, as zinc oxide and copper, 2 mg, as cupric oxide; (iii) antioxidants plus zinc; or (iv) placebo. Main outcome measures were: (i) photographic assessment of progression to or treatment for advanced AMD and (ii) at least moderate visual acuity loss from baseline (> or =15 letters). Primary analyses used repeated-measures logistic regression with a significance level of.01, unadjusted for covariates. Serum level measurements, medical histories, and mortality rates were used for safety monitoring. Average follow-up of the 3640 enrolled study participants, aged 55 to 80 years, was 6.3 years, with 2.4% lost to follow-up. Comparison with placebo demonstrated a statistically significant odds reduction for the development of advanced AMD with antioxidants plus zinc (odds ratio [OR], 0.72; 99% confidence interval [CI], 0.52-0.98). The odds ratios for zinc alone and antioxidants alone are 0.75 (99% CI, 0.55-1.03) and 0.80 (99% CI, 0.59-1.09), respectively. Participants with extensive small drusen, non-extensive intermediate size drusen, or pigment abnormalities had only a 1.3% 5-year probability of progression to advanced AMD. Odds reduction estimates increased when these 1063 participants were excluded (antioxidants plus zinc: OR, 0.66; 99% CI, 0.47-0.91; zinc: OR, 0.71; 99% CI, 0.52-0.99; antioxidants: OR, 0.76; 99% CI, 0.55-1.05). Zinc and antioxidants plus zinc significantly reduced the odds of developing advanced AMD in this higher-risk group. The only statistically significant reduction in rates of at least moderate visual acuity loss occurred in persons assigned to receive antioxidants plus zinc (OR, 0.73; 99% CI, 0.54-0.99). No statistically significant serious adverse effect was associated with any of the formulations. Following are the conclusions of this study: Persons older than 55 years should have dilated eye examinations to determine their risk of developing advanced AMD. Those with extensive intermediate size drusen, at least 1 large druse, non central geographic atrophy in 1 or both eyes, or advanced AMD or vision loss due to AMD in 1 eye, and without contraindications such as smoking, should consider taking a supplement of antioxidants plus zinc such as that used in this study.

SUMMARY

INTERVENTIONAL TRIALS

1. Newsome and associates[159] reported the first randomized, double-masked, placebo-controlled trial (n = 151 for a follow-up of 12 to 24 months) to show a salutary effect of an oral zinc supplement (100 mg zinc sulphate twice a day) on AMD progression.
2. Stur and associates,[156] in a randomized, double-masked, placebo-controlled trial (n = 112 for a 2-year follow-up) using the same dose of oral zinc supplement (200 mg zinc sulphate daily), found no effect on the occurrence of AMD in the unaffected eye of patients (mean age, 71.5 years) with exudative AMD in the other eye.
3. The Age-related Eye Disease Study (AREDS)[158] was designed to investigate the role of high-dose vitamin C (500 mg), vitamin E (400 IU ≈ 273 mg), beta-carotene (15 mg), and zinc (80 mg of zinc as zinc oxide) on both AMD and cataract. For AREDS, 4757 subjects (age, 55-80 years; mean age, 69 years) were recruited from 11 retinal specialty clinics between 1992 and 1998. Participants were grouped into 4 main categories according to AMD stage. Those who were in category 1 (no signs of AMD; n = 1117) were not included in the AMD trial analyses and did not receive zinc supplementation. Those who were in categories 2-4 (small drusen, intermediate drusen, and advanced AMD in 1 eye; n = 3640) were randomly assigned to 1 of 4 arms: a. Antioxidants; b. Zinc; c. Antioxidants plus zinc; or d. Placebo. The results showed that the combination of zinc plus antioxidants or zinc alone offers modest benefit with respect to progression from extensive intermediate drusen, large drusen, or noncentral geographic atrophy to advanced AMD over a mean follow-up time of 6.3 years. The effect was not seen with antioxidants alone. There was no statistically significant effect of delay in progression of early AMD, but this lack of effect could be due in part to the relatively short duration of the trial.
4. The Alpha Tocopherol Beta Carotene (ATBC) trial[160] (n = 29,133 for 5-8 years of follow-up) was originally designed to investigate the effect of vitamin E (alpha-tocopherol; 50 mg/d) and beta-carotene (20 mg/d) in the prevention of lung cancer. Ophthalmologic examinations on a random sample of 941 smoking males aged ≥ 65 years at the end of this trial indicated that long-term alpha-tocopherol or beta-carotene supplementation does not affect the occurrence of early AMD.[17] The small number (n = 12) of more advanced AMD (neovascular or geographic atrophy) precluded the possibility of evaluating the treatment effect for advanced AMD.
5. The AMD branch of the Vitamin E, Cataract, and Age-related Maculopathy Trial (VECAT) randomized 1193 subjects (age, 55-80 years) into 2 groups (vitamin E 500 IU daily and placebo) and followed them for 4 years to investigate the effect of vitamin E on the prevention of early AMD.[161] The study concluded that daily vitamin E supplement use does not alter rates of development or progression of early AMD.

OBSERVATIONAL STUDIES

1. Dietary Ancillary Study of the Eye Disease Case-Control Study (n = 356 cases vs 520 controls),[43]

found that a higher dietary intake of carotenoids was associated with a lower risk for AMD. Among the specific carotenoids, lutein and zeaxanthin were most strongly associated with a reduced risk for AMD. Consistent with these observations, several food items rich in carotenoids, such as spinach or collard greens, were also found to be inversely associated with AMD. The intake of preformed vitamin A (retinol), vitamin E, or total vitamin C consumption was not associated with a statistically significant reduced risk for AMD, although a possibly lower risk for AMD was suggested among those with higher intake of vitamin C, particularly from foods.

2. The Beaver Dam Eye Study (BDES) is a population-based cohort study (n = 4926; aged 43-84 years at baseline 1988-1990) in Beaver Dam, Wisconsin. As part of the nutrition study in the BDES, a sample of 1586 persons was used to evaluate the associations between antioxidants and zinc and the 5-year (1993-1995) incidence of early AMD. [42] A food-frequency questionnaire was administered at baseline to collect dietary information for that time period and a period of time 10 years earlier (1978-1980). Side-by-side comparisons of baseline vs follow-up fundus photographs were conducted to identify eyes that showed progression of signs of age-related maculopathy. Modest inverse associations were observed between intakes of provitamin A carotenoids and dietary vitamin E and the incidence of large drusen, and between zinc (diet plus supplements) and the incidence of pigment abnormalities. No significant inverse associations were found between antioxidants or zinc intake and the incidence of overall early maculopathy. The authors implied that associations between specific antioxidants and the incidence of distinct macular lesions may be biologically important. Because there was no adjustment for multiple comparisons that resulted from the high numbers of nutrients and analyses examined, it is possible that some findings which appear as statistically significant may be seen by chance alone.

3. In the Physicians' Health Study I (PHS I) cohort (n = 21,120 male), during an average of 12.5 person-years of follow-up, users of vitamin E supplements who did not have a diagnosis of AMD at baseline (1982) had a possible, but non-significant, 13% reduced risk of AMD, and users of multivitamins had a possible, but non significant, 10% reduced risk compared with nonusers. [162] Also in PHS I, users of vitamin C supplements had only a 3% reduced risk. The authors concluded that large reductions in the risk of AMD are unlikely among persons who self-select for supplemental use of antioxidant vitamin C or E or multivitamins. Because the exceptionally low incidence may imply that a substantial number of cases in that cohort were unidentified, under-ascertainment or differential ascertainment of the disease may have biased the results. Furthermore, the low prevalence of cigarette smoking and exclusion of subjects with a history of cardiovascular diseases from the PHS I cohort may also partially explain the negative findings and limit its generalizability to other cohorts.

4. In a large prospective follow-up study of the Nurses' Health Study (NHS; n = 66,572) and the Health Professionals Follow-up Study (HPFS; n = 37,636), Cho and associates,[163] did not find a significant protective effect of moderate zinc intake (either from food, supplements, or combined) on the occurrence of AMD. The median total zinc intake was 25.5 mg/d for women in the NHS and 40.1 mg/d for men in the HPFS. Because few people used zinc supplements (especially at high dose), it was impossible to evaluate the effectiveness of high-dose zinc in the prevention of AMD. Furthermore, because of the small number of late-stage AMD cases in both cohorts, they did not have enough power to detect modest effects of zinc on the prevention of late-stage AMD.

5. In another follow-up study of the same cohorts (NHS, n = 77,562; HPFS, n = 40,866), Cho and associates[164] found that participants (women, men, or combined) who consumed 3 or more servings per day of fruits had significantly reduced risk of neovascular AMD compared with those who consumed less than 1.5 servings per day. They did not find significant associations between intakes of vegetables, antioxidant vitamins (including vitamin A, C, E, and multivitamins), or carotenoids (including alpha-carotene, beta-carotene, beta-cryptoxanthin,

lycopene, and lutein/zeaxanthin) with either early or neovascular AMD. However, as indicated above, the small number of late AMD lesions in both cohorts may have limited their ability to detect modest associations.

6. In a 5-year follow-up study of the Blue Mountains Eye Study (BMES) in Australia, Flood and colleagues[165] did not find associations or trends to suggest possible associations between the occurrence of early AMD and baseline intake of alpha-carotene, beta-carotene, beta-cryptoxanthin, lutein and zeaxanthin, lycopene, retinol, vitamin A, and zinc. Their finding of a harmful effect of vitamin C intake in this study was attributed to chance, because previous studies reported a potential beneficial association between vitamin C and AMD. The authors suggested that consumption of usual levels of antioxidants from diet or from supplements may have no influence on the course of AMD and implied the need for much higher levels of antioxidants than usual intakes for any protection to manifest.

7. Rotterdam Study, a population-based prospective study, indicated that antioxidants as present in normal daily foods significantly reduced the risk of developing AMD, especially with intake of vitamin E and zinc. An above-median intake of all 4 nutrients, including beta-carotene (median − 3.6 mg), vitamin C (median = 114 mg), vitamin E (median = 13 IU), and zinc (median = 9.6 mg), was associated with a 35% reduced risk of AMD at a mean follow-up of 8.0 years in persons older than 55 years.[166] This result was independent of supplement use. The results imply that dietary intake of much lower levels of the micronutrients that were used in the AREDS formulation can substantially reduce the risk of developing AMD.

FOCUS ON LUTEIN AND ZEAXANTHIN

These macular pigments are entirely of dietary origin. Their higher dietary intake is related to lower risk for AMD. Bioavailability is one of the important issues in this inconsistency. There is considerable interindividual variability with respect to absorption of carotenoids, and,

recently, obesity,[167] another risk factor for AMD, has been proposed to interact with lutein-zeaxanthin to affect the risk for AMD.[168] Currently, there is no published clinical trial indicating whether or not lutein-zeaxanthin supplements prevent or delay the progression of AMD in humans. However, an ongoing study, AREDS II, which aims to increase our understanding of the role of nutrients used in the AREDS formulation as well as potential contributions of lutein-zeaxanthin in the development of AMD,[169] will provide valuable information.

RECOMMENDATIONS

The available evidence indicates a protective role for antioxidants with respect to diminished risk for onset or progression of AMD. There is increasing evidence that certain types of dietary fat and carbohydrate, which have already been related to the risk of diabetes and cardiovascular diseases,[170,171] affect the risk of AMD.[172,173]

In terms of lifestyle, recommendation for patients who smoke is to quit smoking. In terms of diet, persons at high risk of AMD, such as those with early or intermediate signs of AMD (large drusen and pigment abnormalities) or those with a family history of AMD, should be advised to consume more foods containing antioxidants. Such a diet, in addition to possibly slowing AMD, has the added advantage of reducing the risk for major systemic diseases. Foods high in antioxidants include:

- Whole grains (vitamin E, zinc)
- Spinach (beta-carotene, lutein-zeaxanthin)
- Citrus fruits (vitamin C)
- Broccoli (vitamin C, lutein-zeaxanthin)
- Green peppers (vitamin C)
- Nuts (vitamin E) and
- Dairy products (zinc).

A multivitamin can be recommended as well, especially for those with inadequate or irregular diets. Patients with signs of intermediate disease or advanced AMD in 1 eye may be advised to take the AREDS-type supplements.

REFERENCES

1. National Advisory Eye Council, Report of the Retinal and Choroidal Diseases Panel. Vision research- A National Plan:

1983-1987, Bethesda, Md: US Dept of Health and Human Services; 1984. National Institute of Health Publication 83-2471.

2. Klein R, Klein B, Linton KLP. Prevalence of age-related maculopathy: the Beaver Dam Study. Ophthalmology 1992;99:933-43.

3. Tomany SC, Wang JJ, Van Leeuwen R, et al. Risk factors for incident age-related macular degeneration: pooled findings from 3 continents. Ophthalmology 2004;111:1280-87.

4. Seddon J, Chen C. Epidemiology of age-related macular degeneration. In Ryan SJ (Ed); Retina, Vol. Two. Medical Retina, 4th ed. St. Louis: Mo: CV Mosby; 2005.

5. Friedman DS, O'Colmain BJ, Munoz B, et al. Prevalence of age-related macular degeneration in the United States. Arch Ophthalmol 2004;122:564-72.

6. Organisciak DT, Wang HM, Li Z, Li ZY, Tso MOM. The protective effect of ascorbate in retinal light damage of rats. Invest Ophthalmol Vis Sci 1985;26:1580-88.

7. Tso MOM, Woodford BJ, Lam KW. Distribution of ascorbate in normal primate retina after photic injury: a biochemical, morphological correlated study. Curr Eye Res 1984;3:181-91.

8. Katz ML, Parker KR, Handelman GJ, Bramel TL, Dratz EA. Effects of antioxidant nutrient deficiency on the retina and retinal pigment epithelium of albino rats: a light and electron microscopic study. Exp Eye Res 1982;34:339-69.

9. Hayes KC. Retinal degeneration in monkeys induced by deficiencies of vitamin E or A. Invest Ophthalmol Vis Sci 1974;13:499-510.

10. Young RW. Solar radiation and advanced-age-related macular degeneration. Surv Ophthalmol 1988;32:252-69.

11. Goldberg J, Flowerdew G, Smith E, Brody JA, Tso MOM. Factors associated with age-related macular degeneration: an analysis of data from the First National Health and Nutrition Examination Survey. Am J Epidemiol 1988;128:700-10.

12. The Eye Disease Case-Control Study Group. Antioxidant status and neovascular age-related macular degeneration. Arch Ophthalmol 1993;111:104-09.

13. Blumenkranz MS, Russell SR, Robey MG, Blumenkranz RK, Penneys N. Risk factors in age-related maculopathy complicated by choroidal neovascularization. Ophthalmology 1986;96:552-58.

14. Winkler BS, Boulton ME, Gottsch JD, Sternberg P. Oxidative damage and age-related macular degeneration. Mol Vis 1999;5:32.

15. Beatty S, Koh H, Henson D. The role of oxidative stress in the pathogenesis of age-related macular degeneration. Surv Ophthalmol 2000;45:115-34.

16. Harman D. The aging process. Proc Natl Acad Sci USA. 1981;78:7124-28.

17. Organisiack DT, Wang HM, Li ZY, et al. The protective effect of ascorbate in retinal light damage of rats. Invest Ophthalmol Vis Sci 1985;26:1580-88.

18. Goldberg J, Flowerdew G, Smith E, et al. Factors associated with age-related macular degeneration. An analysis of data from the first national health and nutrition examination survey. Am J Epidemiol 1988;128:700-10.

19. The Eye Disease Case-Control Study Group. Antioxidant status and neovascular age-related macular degeneration. Arch Ophthalmol 1993;111:104-09.

20. West S, Vitale S, Hallfrisch J, et al. Are antioxidants or supplements protective for age-related macular degeneration? Arch Ophthalmol 1994;112:222-27.

21. Delcourt C, Cristol JP, Tessier F, et al. Factors associated with age-related macular degeneration and antioxidant status in POLA study. POLA study group. Pathologies Oculaires Liees a l'Age. Arch Ophthalmol 1999;117:1384-90.

22. Chow CK. Vitamin E and oxidative stress. Free Rad Biol Med 1991;11:215-32.

23. Packer L. Interactions among antioxidants in health and disease:vitamin E and redox cycle. Proc Soc Exp Biol Med 1992;2000:271-76.

24. Packer L, Landvik S. Vitamin E in biological systems. Adv Exp Med Biol 1990;264:93-103.

25. Alvarez RA, Liou GL, Fong SL, et al. Levels of alpha-and gamma-tocopherol in human eyes: evaluation of the possible IRBP in intraocular alpha- tocopherol transport. Am J Clin Nutr 1987;46:481-87.

26. Handelman GJ, Machlin LJ, Fitch K, et al. Oral alpha-tocopherol supplements decrease plasma gamma-tocopherol levels in humans. J Nutr 1985;115:807-13.

27. Friedrichson T, Kalbach HL, Buck P, van Kuijk FJ. Vitamin E in macular and peripheral tissues of the human eye. Curr Eye Res 1995;14:693-701.

28. Hunt DF, Organisciak DT, Wang HM, et al. Alpha-tocopherol in the developing rat retina: a high pressure liquid chromatographic analysis. Curr Eye Res 1984;3:1281-88.

29. Stephens RJ, Negi DS, Short SM, et al. Vitamin E distribution in ocular tissues following long-term dietary depletion and supplementation as determined by micro dissection and gas chromatography-mass spectrophotometry. Exp Eye Res 1988;47:237-45.

30. Organisciak DT, Berman ER, Wang HM, Feeney-Burns L. Vitamin E in human neural retina and retinal pigment epithelium: effect of age. Curr Eye Res 1987;6:1051-55.

31. Handelman GJ, Snodderly DM, Krinsky NI, et al. Biological control of primate macular pigment. Biochemical and densitometric studies. Invest Ophthalmol Vis Sci 1991;32:257-67.

32. Snodderly DM, Auran JD, Delori FC. The macular pigment II. Spatial distribution in primate retinas. Invest Ophthalmol Vis Sci 1984;25:674-85.

33. Snodderly DM, Handelman GJ, Adler AJ. Distribution of individual macular pigment carotenoids in central retina of macaque and squirrel monkeys. Invest Ophthalmol Vis Sci 1991;32:268-79.

34. Crabtree DV, Adler AJ, Snodderly DM. Radial distribution of tocopherols in rhesus monkey retina and retinal pigment epithelium-choroid. Invest Ophthalmol Vis Sci 1996;37:61-76.

35. Hayes KC. Retinal degeneration in monkeys induced by deficiencies of vitamin E and A. Invest Ophthalmol Vis Sci 1978;13:499-510.

36. Farnsworth CC, Dratz EA. Oxidative damage of retinal rod outer segment membranes and the role of vitamin E. Biochim Biophys Acta 1976;443;556-70.

37. Birch DG, Jacobs GH. Light-induced damage to photopic and scotopic mechanisms in the rat depends on rearing conditions. Exp Neurol 1980;68:269-83.

38. Feeney-Burns L, Gao CL, Tidwell M. Lysosomal enzyme cytochemistry of human RPE, Bruchs membrane and drusen. Invest Ophthalmol Vis Sci 1987;28:1138-47.

39. Katz ML, Eldred GE. Failure of vitamin E to protect the retina against damage resulting from bright cyclic light exposure. Invest Ophthalmol Vis Sci 1989;30:3090-99.

40. Stone WL, Katz ML, Lurie M, et al. Effects of dietary depletion and supplementation as determined by microdissection and gas chromatography-mass spectrometry. Exp Eye Res. 1988;47:237-245.

41. Acuff RV, Thedford SS, Hidiroglou NN, et al. Relative bioavailability of RRR- and all-rac-alpha-tocopheryl acetate in humans: studies using deuterated compounds. Am J Clin Nutr 1994;60:397-402.

42. VandenLangdenberg GM, Mares-Perlman JA, Klein R, et al. Associations between antioxidant and zinc intake and the 5-year incidence of early age- related maculopathy in the Beaver Dam Eye Study. Am J Epidemiol 1998;148:204-14.

43. Seddon JM, Ajani UA, Sperduto RA, et al. Dietary carotenoids, vitamins A, C, and E, and advanced age-related macular degeneration. Eye Disease Case-control Study Group. JAMA 1994;272:1413-20.

44. Mares-Perlman JA, Brady WE, Klein R, et al. Serum antioxidants and age- related macular degeneration in a population-based case-control study. Arch Ophthalmol 1995;113:1518-23.

45. Smith W, Mitchell P, Rochester C. Serum beta carotene, alpha tocopherol, and age-related maculopathy: the Blue Mountains Eye Study. Am J Ophthalmol 1997;124:838-40.

46. Keys SA, Zimmerman WF. Antioxidant activity of retinol, glutathione, and taurine in bovine photoreceptor cell membranes. Exp Eye Res 1999;68:693-02.

47. Robison WG, Kuwabara T, Bieri JG. The roles of vitamin E and unsaturated fatty acids in the visual process. Retina 1982;2:263-81.

48. Blumenkranz MS, Russell SR, Robey MG, et al. Risk factors in age-related maculopathy complicated by choroidal neovascularization. Ophthalmology 1986;93:552-58.

49. Smith W, Mitchell P, Webb K, et al. Dietary antioxidants and age-related maculopathy: the Blue Mountains Eye Study. Ophthalmology 1999;106:761-77.

50. Sommerburg O, Keunen JE, Bird AC, et al. Fruits and vegetables that are sources of lutein and zeaxanthin: the macular pigment in human eyes. Br J Ophthalmol 1998; 82:907-10.

51. Krinsky NI. The protective function of carotenoid pigments. In Giese AL (Ed): Photophysiology, New York, Academic Press, 1968; pp 123-95.

52. Conn PF, Schalch W, Truscott TG. The singlet oxygen and carotenoid interaction. J Photochem Photobiol B. 1991; 11:41-47.

53. Foote CS, Denny RW. Chemistry of singlet oxygen. VII Quenching by beta-carotene. J Am Chem Soc 1968; 90: 6233-35.

54. Krinsky NI, Deneke SM. Interaction of oxygen and oxy-radicals with carotenoids. J Natl Cancer Inst 1982;69:205-10.

55. Oliveros E, Braun AM, Aminian-Saghafi T, et al. Quenching of singlet oxygen by carotenoid derivatives: kinetic analysis by near infra-red luminescence. New J Chem 1994;18:535-39.

56. Tinkler JH, Bohm F, Schalch W, Trusscott TG. Dietary carotenoids protect human cells from damage. J Photochem Photobiol B 1994;26:283-85.

57. Bohm F, Tinkler JH, Truscott TG. Carotenoids protect against cell membrane damage by the nitrogen dioxide radical. Nat Med 1995;1:98-99.

58. Burton GW, Ingold KU. Beta-carotene: an unusual type of lipid antioxidant. Science 1984;224:569-73.

59. Hill TJ, Land EJ, McGarvey DJ, et al. interactions between carotenoids and the CCI302 radical. J Am Chem Soc 1995; 8322-26.

60. Anderson SM, Krinsky NI. Protective action of carotenoid pigments against photodynamic damage to liposomes. Photochem Photobiol 1973;18:403-08.

61. Lim BP, Nagao A, Terao J, et al. Antioxidant activity of xanthophylls on peroxyl radical-mediated phospholipids peroxidation. Biochim Biophys Acta 1992;1126:178-84.

62. Packer L. Antioxidant action of carotenoids in vitro and in vivo and protection against oxidation of human low-density lipoproteins. Ann NY Acad Sci 1993;691:48-60.

63. Vile GF, Winterbourn CC. Inhibition of adriamycin-promoted microsomal lipid peroxidation by beta-carotene, alpha-tocopherol and retinol at high and low oxygen partial pressures. FEBS Lett 1988;238:353-56.

64. Zhang LX, Cooney RV, Bertrams JS. Carotenoids enhance gap junctional communication and inhibit lipid peroxidation in C3H/10T1/2 cells: relationship to their cancer chemo-preventive action. Carcinogenesis 1991;12:2109-14.

65. Jorgensen K, Skibsted LH. Carotenoid scavenging of radicals. Effect of carotenoid structure and oxygen partial pressure on antioxidative activity. Z Lebensm Unters Forsch 1993;196:423-29.

66. Edge R, McGarvey DJ, Truscott TG. The carotenoids as antioxidants-a review. J Photochem Photobiol B 1997; 41: 189-200.

67. Wald G. Human vision and spectrum. Nature 1945;101: 653-58.

68. Bone RA, Landrum JT, Tarsis SL. Preliminary identification of the human macular pigment. Vis Res 1985;25:1531-39.

69. Khachik F, Bernstein P, Garland DL. Identification of lutein and zeaxanthin oxidation products in human and monkey retinas. Invest Ophthalmol Vis Sci 1997;38:1802-11.

70. Mangels AR, Holden JM, Beecher GR, et al. Carotenoid content of fruits and vegetables: an evaluation of analytic data. J Am Diet Assoc 1993;93:284-96.

71. Bailey CA, Chen BH. Chromatographic analyses of xanthophylls in egg yolks from laying hens fed turf Bermuda grass (Cynodon dactylon) meal. J Food Sci 1989;54:584-86.

72. Mares-Perlman JA, Fisher A, Klein R, et al. Lutein and zeaxanthin in the diet and serum and their relation to age-related maculopathy in the Third National Health and Nutrition Examination Survey. Am J Epidemiol 2001; 153: 424-32.

73. Parker RS. Carotenoids in human blood and tissues. J Nutr 1989;119:101-04.

74. Hammond BR, Johnson EJ, Russell EJ, et al. Dietary modification of human macular pigment density. Invest Ophthalmol Vis Sci 1997;38:1795-1801.

75. Landrum JT, Bone RA, Joa H, et al. Sprague KE. A one-year study of the macular pigment: the effect of 140 days of a lutein supplement. Exp Eye Res 1997;64:57-62.

76. Johnson EJ, Hammond RB, Yeum KJ, et al. Relation among serum and tissue concentrations of lutein and zeaxanthin and macular pigment density. Am J Clin Nutr 2000;71:1555-62.

77. Bone RA, Landrum JT, Dixon Z, et al. Lutein and zeaxanthin in the eyes, serum and diet of human subjects. Exp Eye Res 2000;71:239-45.

78. Zaripheh S, Erdman JW. Factors that influence the bioavailability of xanthophylls. J Nutr 2002;132:531S-534S.

79. Kaplan LR, Lau JM, Stein EA. Carotenoid composition, concentrations and relationships in various human organs. Clin Physiol Biochem 1990;8:1-10.

80. Schmitz HH, Poor CL, Wellman RB, Erdman JW. Concentrations of selected carotenoids and vitamin A in human liver, kidney and lung tissue. J Nutr 1991;121: 1613-21.

81. Bone RA, Landrum JT, Fernandez L, Tarsis SL. Analysis of macular pigment by HPLC: retinal distribution and age study. Invest Ophthalmol Vis Sci 1988;29:843-49.

82. Handelman GJ, Dratz EA, Reay CC, van Kuijk JG. Carotenoids in the human macula and whole retina. Invest Ophthalmol Vis Sci 1988;29:850-55.

83. Bone RA, Landrum JT, Friedes LM, et al. Distribution of lutein and zeaxanthin stereoisomers in the human retina. Exp Eye Res 1997;64:211-18.

84. Yeum KJ, Shang F, Schalch W, et al. Fat-soluble nutrient concentrations in different layers of human cataractous lens. Curr Eye Res 1999;19:503-05.

85. Zhang S, Tang G, Russell RM, et al. Measurements of retinoids and carotenoids in breast adipose tissue and a comparison of concentrations in breast cancer cases and control subjects. Am J Clin Nutr 1997;66:626-32.

86. Wingerath T, Sies H, Stahl W. Xanthophyll esters in human skin. Arch Biochem Biophys 1998;355:271-74.

87. Snodderly DM, Handelman GJ, Adler AJ. Distribution of individual macular pigment carotenoids in central retina of macaque and squirrel monkeys. Invest Ophthalmol Vis Sci 1991;32:268-79.

88. Handelman GJ, Snodderly DM, Krinsky NI, Russell MD. Biological control of primate macular pigment. Biochemical and densitometric studies. Invest Ophthalmol Vis Sci 1991;32:257-67.

89. Bone RA, Landrum JT, Hime GW, et al. Stereochemistry of the macular carotenoids. Invest Ophthalmol Vis Sci 1993;34:2033-40.

90. Schmitz HH, Poor CL, Gugger ET, Erdman JW. Analysis of carotenoids in human and animal tissues. Methods Enzymol 1993;214:102-16.

91. Bone RA, Landrum JT. Distribution of macular pigment components, zeaxanthin and lutein in human retina. Methods Enzymol 1992;213:360-67.

92. Sommerburg O, Siems GW, Hurst SJ, et al. Lutein and zeaxanthin are associated with photoreceptors in the human retina. Curr Eye Res 1999;19:491-95.

93. Maoka T, Arai A, Shimizu M, Matsuno T. The first isolation of enantiometric and mesozeaxanthin in nature. Comp Biochem Physiol 1986;83:121-24.

94. Bone RA, Landrum JT, Mayne ST, et al.. Macular pigment in donor eyes with and without AMD: a case-control study. Invest Ophthalmol Vis Sci 2001;42:235-40.

95. Berendschot TJM, Goldbohm AR, Klopping WA, et al. Influence of lutein supplementation on macular pigment, assessed with two objective techniques. Invest Ophthalmol Vis Sci 2000;41:3322-26.

96. Hammond BR, Jr, Curran-Celentano J, Judd S. Sex differences in macular pigment optical density: relation to plasma carotenoid concentrations and dietary patterns. Vis Res 1996;36:2001-12.

97. Hammond BR, Fuld K, Curran-Celentano J. Macular pigment density in monozygotic twins. Invest Ophthalmol Vis Sci 1995;36:2531-41.

98. Curran-Celentano J, Hammond BR, Ciulla TA, et al.. Relation between dietary intake, serum concentrations and retinal concentrations of lutein and zeaxanthin in adults in a Mid West population. Am J Clin Nutr. 2001;74:796-802.

99. Bone RA, Landrum JT, Guerra LH, Ruiz CA. Lutein and zeaxanthin dietary supplements raise macular pigment density and serum concentrations of these carotenoids in humans. J Nutr 2003;133:992-98.

100. Landrum JT, Bone RA. Lutein, zeaxanthin and the macular pigment. Arch Biochem Biophys 2001;385:28-40.

101. Krinsky NI, Russell MD, Handelman GJ, Snodderly DM. Structural and geometrical isomers of carotenoids in human plasma. J Nutr 1990;120:1654-61.

102. Bone RA, Landrum JT. Macular pigment in Henle fibre membranes: a model for Haidenger's brushes. Vis Res 1984;24:103-08.

103. Gabrielska J, Gruszecki WI. Zeaxanthin (dihydroxy-beta-carotene) but not beta carotene rigidifies lipid membranes: a ^{1}H-NMR study of carotenoids-egg phosphatidylcholine liposomes. Biochem Biophys Acta 1996;1285:167-74.

104. Sujak A, Gabrielska J, Grudzinski W, et al. Lutein and zeaxanthin as protectors of lipid membranes against oxidative damage: the structural aspects. Arch Biochem Biophys 1999;371:301-07.

105. Gilmartin B, Hogan RE. The magnitude of longitudinal chromatic aberration of the human eye between 458 and 633 nm. Vis Res 1985;25:1747-53.

106. Howarth PA, Bradley A. The longitudinal chromatic aberration of the human eye and its correction. Vis Res 1986;26:361-66.

107. Wooten BR, Hammond BR. Macular pigment: influences on visual acuity and visibility. Prog Retinal Eye Res 2002; 21:225-40.

108. Ham WT, Ruffolo JJ, Mueller HA, et al. Histologic analysis of photochemical lesions produced in rhesus retina by short wavelength light. Invest Ophthalmol Vis Sci 1978;17:1029-35.

109. Snodderly DM, Auran JD, Delori FC. The macular pigment.II. Spatial distribution in primate retinas. Invest Ophthalmol Vis Sci 1984;25:674-85.

110. Junghans A, Sies H, Stahl W. Macular pigment lutein and zeaxanthin as blue light filters studied in liposomes. Arch Biochem Biophys 2001;391:160-64.

111. Kirschfeld K. Carotenoid pigments: their possible role in protecting against photooxidation in eyes and photoreceptor cells. Proc R Soc Lond 1982;B216:71-85.

112. Haegerstrom-Portnoy G. Short-wave length-sensitive-cone sensitivity loss with aging: a protective role for macular pigment? J Opt Soc Am 1988;A5:2140-44.

113. Weiter JJ, Delori F, Dorey CK. Central sparing of annular macular degeneration. Am J Ophthalmol 1988;106:286-92.

114. Krinsky NI. Carotenoid protection against oxidation. Pure Appl Chem 1979;51:649-60.

115. Krinsky NI. Antioxidant functions of carotenoids. Free Rad Biol Med 1989;7:617-35.

116. Palozza P, Krinsky NI. Antioxidant effects of carotenoids in vitro and in vivo: an overview. Methods Enzymol 1992; 213:403-20.

117. Krinsky NI. The antioxidant and biological properties of the carotenoids. Ann N Y Acad Sci 1998;854:443-47.

118. Krinsky NI. Carotenoids as antioxidants. Nutrition. 2001;17:815-17.

119. Palozza P. Prooxidant actions of carotenoids in biologic systems. Nutr Rev 1998;56:257-65.

120. Young AJ, Lowe GM. Antioxidant and prooxidant properties of carotenoids. Arch Biochem Biophys 2001;385:20-27.

121. Bernstein PS, Khachik F, Carvalho LS, Muir GJ, Zhao DY, Katz NB. Identification and quantification of carotenoids and their metabolites in the tissues of the human eye. Exp Eye Res 2001;72:215-23.

122. Jandacek RJ. The canary in the cell: a sentinel role for beta-carotene. J Nutr 2000;130:648-51.

123. Beatty S, Murray IJ, Henson DB, et al. Macular pigment and risk of age-related macular degeneration in subjects from the North European population. Invest Ophthalmol Vis Sci 2001;42:4390-4446.

124. Li Z, Tso MOM. A research of Lycium barbarum in rescue of retina from photic injury in rats. Chin J Ocular Fundus Diseases 1995;11:31-33.

125. Dorey CK, Toyoda Y, Thomson L, et al. Light-induced photoreceptor apoptosis is correlated with dietary and retinal levels of 3R, 3R-zeaxanthin. Invest Ophthalmol Vis Sci 1997;38:S38.

126. Neuringer M, Klein ML, Snodderly DM. Effects of carotenoids depletion and N-3 fatty acid status on macular defects in Rhesus monkeys. Invest Ophthalmol Vis Sci 1999;40:S164.

127. Rapp LM, Maple SS, Choi JH. Lutein and zeaxanthin concentrations in rod outer segment membranes from perifovea and peripheral human retina. Invest Ophthalmol Vis Sci 2000;41:1200-09.

128. Mares-Perlman JA, Millen AE, Ficek TL, Hankinson SE. The body of evidence to support a protective role for lutein and zeaxanthin in delaying chronic disease. Overview. J Nutr 2002;132:518S-524S.

129. Dagnelie G, Zorge IS, McDonald TM. Lutein improves visual function in some patients with retinal degeneration: a pilot study via internet. Optometry 2000;71:147-64.

130. Aleman TS, Duncan JL, Bieber ML, et al. Macular pigment and lutein supplementation in retinitis pigmentosa and usher syndrome. Invest Ophthalmol Vis Sci 2001;42:1873-81.

131. Sundelin SP, Nilsson SEG. Lipofuscin formation in retinal pigment epithelial cells is reduced by antioxidants. Free Rad Biol Med 2001;31:217-25.

132. Mares-Perlman JA, Klein R. Diet and age-related macular degeneration. In: Taylor A (ed). Nutritional and environmental influences on the eye. Boca Raton, CRC Press, 1999, pp 5-24.

133. Krinsky NI. Possible biological mechanisms for a protective role of xanthophylls. J Nutr 2002;132:540S-542S.

134. Sliney DH, Mueller HA, Ham WT. Retinal sensitivity to damage from short wave length light. Nature (London) 1976; 260:153-55.

135. Borges J, Li Z, Tso MOM. Effects of repeated public exposures on the monkey macula. Arch Ophthalmol 1990; 108:727-33.

136. Dayhaw-Barker P. Ocular photosensitization. Photochem Photobiol 1986;46:1051-55.

137. McCarty C, Taylor HR. Light and risk for age-related eye diseases. In Taylor A (Ed): Nutritional and environmental influences on the eye. Boca Raton, CRC Press, 1999; pp 135-160.

138. Malinow MR, Feeney-Burns L, Peterson LH, et al. Diet-related macular anomalies in monkeys. Invest Ophthalmol Vis Sci 1980;19:857-63.

139. Khachik F, Beecher GR, Goli MB, Lusby WR. Separation, identification and quantification of carotenoids in fruits, vegetables and human plasma by high performance liquid chromatography. Pure Appl Chem 1991;63:71-80.

140. Khachik F, Beecher GR, Goli MB, Lusby WR. Separation and quantification of carotenoids in foods. In Packer L (Ed): Methods in Enzymology. New York, Academic Press, 1992; pp 347-359.

141. Khachik F, Goli MB, Beecher GR, et al. The effect of food preparation on qualitative and quantitative distribution of major carotenoids constituents of tomatoes and several green vegetables. J Agric Food Chem 1998;46:4885-90.

142. Khachik F, Beecher GR, Lusby WR. Separation, identification and quantification of the major carotenoids in extracts of apricots, peaches, cantaloupe and pink grape fruit by liquid chromatography. J Agric Food Chem 1989;37:1465-73.

143. Levy J, Bosin E, Feldman B, et al. Lycopene is a more potent inhibitor of human cancer cell proliferation than either alpha or beta carotene. Nutr Cancer 1995;24:257-66.

144. DiMascio P, Kaiser S, Sies H. Lycopene as the most efficient biological carotenoids singlet oxygen quencher. Arch Biochem Biophys 1989;274:532-38.

145. Kennedy TA, Lieber DC. Peroxyl radical oxidation of beta-carotene: formation of beta-carotene epoxides. Chem Res Toxicol 1991:4:290-95.

146. Kennedy TA, Lieber DC. Peroxyl radical scavenging by beta-carotene in lipid bilayers. J Biol Chem 1992;267:4658-63.

147. Siems WG, Sommerburg O, van Kuijk FJGM. Lycopene and beta-carotene decompose more rapidly than lutein and zeaxanthin upon exposure to various pro-oxidants in vitro. Biofactors 1999;10:105-13.

148. Khachik F, Carvalho L, Bernstein PS, et al. Chemistry, distribution and metabolism of tomato carotenoids and their impact on human health. Exp Biol Med 2002:227:845-51.

149. Hammond BR Jr, Curran-Celetano J, Judd S, et al. Sex differences in macular pigment optical density: relation to plasma carotenoid concentrations and dietary patterns. Vision Res 1996;36:2001-12.

150. The Eye Disease Case-Control Study Group. Risk factors for age-related macular degeneration. Arch Ophthalmol 1992; 111:104-09.

151. Karcioglu ZA. Zinc in the eye. Surv Ophthalmol 1982;27:114-22.

152. Marklund SL, Westman NG, Lundgren E, et al. Copper and zinc-containing superoxide dismutase, manganese-containing superoxide dismutase, catalase, and glutathione peroxide in normal and neoplastic human cell lines and normal human tissues. Cancer Res 1982;42:1955-61.

153. Tate DJ Jr, Miceli MV, Newsome DA. Zinc induces catalase expression in cultured fetal human retinal pigment epithelium cells. Curr Eye Res 1997;16:1017-23.

154. Sato M, Bremner I. Oxygen free radicals and metallothionein. Free Rad Biol Med 1993;14:325-27.

155. Thomas JP, Bachowski GJ, Girotti AW. Inhibition of cell membrane lipid peroxidation by cadmium- and zinc-metallothioneins. Biochim Biophys Acta 1986;884:448-61.

156. Stur M, Tittl M, Reitner A, et al. Oral zinc and the second eye in age-related macular degeneration. Invest Ophthalmol Vis Sci 1996;37:1225-35.

157. National Eye Institute. Vision problems in the U.S. – prevalence of adult vision impairment and age-related eye diseases in America, 4th ed. Schaumberg, IL, Prevent Blindness America, 2002.

158. Age-related Eye Disease Study Research Group. A randomized, placebo-controlled, clinical trial of high-dose supplementation with vitamin C and E, beta-carotene, and zinc for age-related macular degeneration and vision loss. AREDS Report No. 8. Arch Ophthalmol 2001;119:1417-36.

159. Newsome DA, Swartz M, Leone NC, Elston RC, Miller E. Oral zinc in macular degeneration. Arch Ophthalmol 1988;106:192-98.

160. The Alpha-Tocopherol BCCPSG. The effect of vitamin E and beta carotene on the incidence of lung cancer and other cancers in male smokers. N Engl J Med 1994;330:1029-35.

161. Taylor HR, Tikellis G, Robman LD, McCarty CA, McNeil JJ. Vitamin E supplementation and macular degeneration: randomized controlled trial. BMJ 2002;325:11.

162. Christen WG, Ajani UA, Glynn RJ, et al. Prospective cohort study of antioxidant vitamin supplement use and the risk of age-related maculopathy. Am. J Epidemiol 1999; 149: 476-84.

163. Cho E, Stampfer MJ, Seddon JM, et al. Prospective study of zinc intake and the risk of age-related macular degeneration. Ann Epidemiol 2001;11:328-36.

164. Cho E, Seddon JM, Rosner B, Willett WC, Hankinson SE. Prospective study of intake of fruits, vegetables, vitamins, and carotenoids and risk of age-related maculopathy. Arch Ophthalmol 2004;122:883-92.

165. Flood V, Smith W, Wang JJ, Manzi F, Webb K, Mitchell P. Dietary antioxidant intake and incidence of early age-related maculopathy: the Blue Mountains Eye Study. Ophthalmology 2002; 109:2272-78.

166. van Leeuwen R, Boekhoorn S, Vingerling JR, et al. Dietary intake of antioxidants and risk of age-related macular degeneration. JAMA 2005;294:3101-07.

167. Seddon JM, Cote J, Davis N, Rosner B. Progression of age-related macular degeneration: association with body mass index, waist circumference, and waist-hip ratio. Arch Ophthalmol 2003;121:785-92.

168. Johnson EJ. Obesity, lutein metabolism, and age-related macular degeneration: a web of connections. Nutr Rev 2005; 63:9-15.

169. Chew EY, Clemons T. Vitamin E and the age-related eye disease study supplementation for age-related macular degeneration. Arch Ophthalmol 2005;123:395-96.

170. Hu FB, Willett WC. Optimal diets for prevention of coronary heart disease. JAMA 2002;288:2569-78.

171. Schulze MB, Hu FB. Primary prevention of diabetes: what can be done and how much can be prevented? Annu Rev Public Health 2005;26:445-67.

172. Seddon JM, Cote J, Rosner B. Progression of age-related macular degeneration: association with dietary fat, transunsaturated fat, nuts, and fish intake. Arch Ophthalmol 2003;121:1728-37.

173. Chiu CJ, Hubbard LD, Armstrong J, et al. Dietary glycemic index and carbohydrate in relation to early age-related macular degeneration. Am J Clin Nutr. 2006;83:880-86.

12

Intravitreal Triamcinolone Acetonide in Macular Diseases

Carsten H Meyer, Robert F Degenring

INTRODUCTION

Angiogenesis is frequently accompanied by inflammation, and infiltration in biologic tissue.[1-6] The accumulation of inflammatory cells increases with expression of vascular endothelial growth factor (VEGF). To limit the inflammatory and angiogenic reaction, numerous drugs are currently evaluated. The antiangiogenic effect of steroids was first diskovered by Shubik and associates,[7] who observed that systemically applied methylprednisolone inhibited tumor-induced angiogenesis. Corticosteroids have several well-established antiangiogenic, antifibrotic and antipermeability properties and belong to the first line treatment regime of ocular inflammatory disease.

Corticosteroids effect the vascular cascade by inhibiting the expression of VEGF,[8-13] thus inhibiting extracellular matrix metalloproteinases turnover, reducing basic fibroblast growth factor-induced migration, down-regulating intercellular adhesion molecule (ICAM)-1 expression and decreasing major histocompatibility complex-II antigen expression.[14,15] Steroids have also an indirect angiostatic affect of inhibiting inflammatory cells, e.g. leukocytes, monocytes or macrophages, which may release cytokines or additional proangiogenic growth factors.[16]

The anti-inflammatory effect of steroids is larger than its angiostatic effect. This anti-inflammatory effect correlates in the expression of cell surface markers,[17,18] secretion of proinflammatory and angiogenic cytokines and the stabilization of cell membranes or tight junctions.[14,15,19-22] Steroids suppress the accumulation of inflammatory cells[23] and diminish the synthesis of inflammatory mediators such as prostaglandins and leukotrienes.[24] These anti-inflammatory effects may change the blood-ocular barrier function in the eye.[25,26]

While natural glucocorticoids (cortisone or hydrocortisone) contain strong mineralocorticoid properties; synthetic analogs like dexamethasone, prednisone or triamcinolone acetonide contain mainly anti-inflammatory properties. Triamcinolone has been used as an intravitreal antiangiogenesis drug in animal models. Intravitreal triamcinolone acetonide (IVTA) can significantly reduce retinal neovascularization and fibrosis in rabbit (Figure 12.1).[27-30]

Recently, its therapeutical potential has expanded to the posterior segment in humans to treat edematous, proliferative and neovascular diseases.[31] Intravitreal triamcinolone acetonide has increasingly been applied in pilot studies for the treatment of vascular age-related macular degeneration (AMD), diabetic retinopathy and diabetic maculopathy.

RATIONALE FOR INTRAVITREAL DRUG DELIVERY

Systemic steroid application can achieve sufficient drug delivery at the posterior segment of the eye; however long-term administration may cause elevated blood glucose, Cushing's disease or elevated blood pressure.

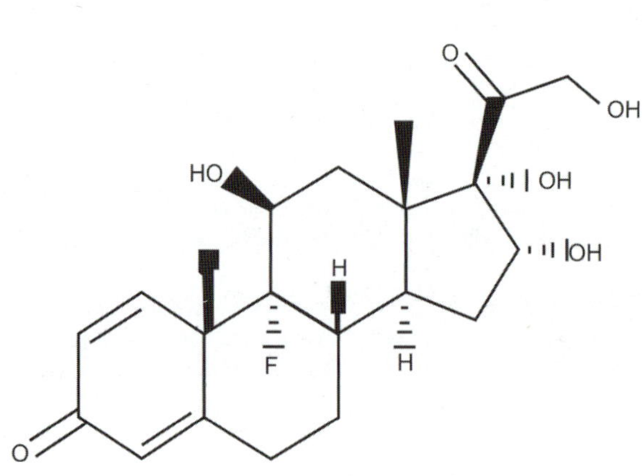

Formula: $C_{24}H_{31}FO_6$; M_r = 434,51

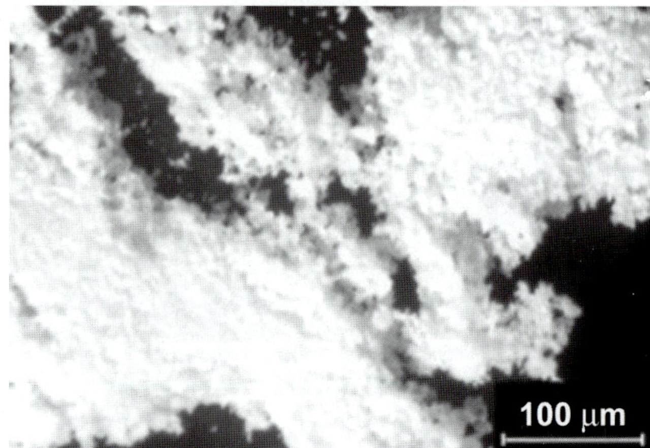

Particle size 2-50 µm

FIGURE 12.1: Triamcinolone acetonide.

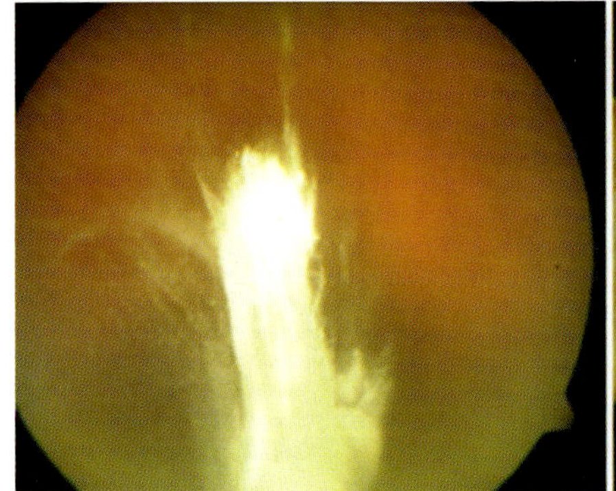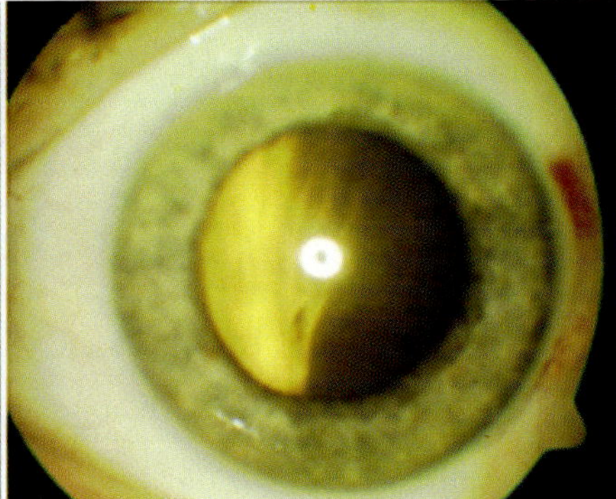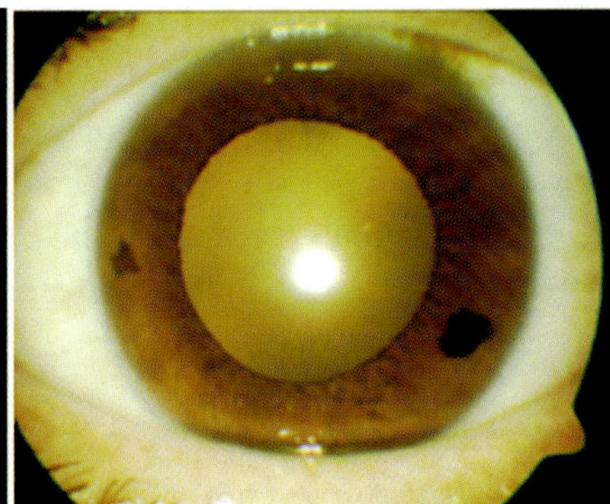

FIGURE 12.2: Intravitreal triamcinolone acetonide.

However, the disadvantage of topical application is that the ointment may not penetrate deep enough, limiting the therapeutic effect. To overcome this limitation, Machemer, Hida, Tano and McCuen suggested applying corticosteroids intravitreally in order to achieve locally therapeutic levels with prolonged concentrations.[27-29,32-36]

PHARMACOKINETICS OF INTRAVITREAL TRIAMCINOLONE ACETONIDE

After IVTA the drug attaches to the collagen net of the vitreous[37] and persists in the vitreous cavity for months;[38-40] its elimination depends on the status of the vitreous as well as the applied drug dosage. Beer and associates[41] calculated after a single 4 mg IVTA, a mean half-life elimination of 3.2 days in vitrectomized eyes compared with 18.6 days in non-vitrectomized eyes (Figure 12.2).

TRIAMCINOLONE IN NEOVASCULAR AGE-RELATED MACULAR DEGENERATION

Multiple angiogenic growth factors contribute to choroidal neovascularization in AMD, including VEGF and pigment epithelium-derived factor (PEDF). The VEGF is a major stimulus for CNV-development and its expression in surgically excised CNV from human eyes. The PEDF inhibits the migration of endothelial cells and the development of experimental retinal and choroidal neovascularization.[42-50]

Clinical Findings

Several case-studies on vascular AMD reported promising results. Penfold and associates[51] employed intravitreal triamcinolone on exudative AMD-patients and diskovered reduced visual loss and stabilized CNV with less leakage on fluorescein angiogram. This clinical study was subsequently confirmed by other studies.[52-56] Ranson and associates[57] demonstrated that intravitreal triamcinolone stabilized recurrent CNV in patients after laser treatments.[57] Another study involving 13 AMD-patients with occult or predominantly occult CNV treated with IVTA 25 mg and observed an increased visual improvement from 0.17 to 0.32 (approximately 20/125 to 20/63; Snellen's charts) after one injection. Similar increases in visual acuity from 0.17 to a mean maximum of 0.32 (approximately 20/125) were reported by Jonas et al[58] after the first injection in another study of 13 eyes with occult or predominantly occult CNV due to AMD who received IVTA 25 mg. A second additional injection improved the VA from 0.15 to 0.23 (approximately 20/125 to 20/80), compared to unchanged vision in all placebo group.

Importantly, the only large-scale ($n = 151$), randomized, controlled, double-masked study of IVTA 4 mg determined that although IVTA significantly reduced the growth of vascular lesions in eyes with classic CNV, there was no significant reduced risk of developing severe vision loss between IVTA and the placebo.[59] Although IVTA was generally well tolerated, there was an increased incidence of mild or moderate elevation of intraocular pressure and significant progression of cataracts.

The current evidence suggests that IVTA should not be used as a monotherapy for vascular AMD. In the authors' opinion, the benefits of IVTA-monotherapy do not outweigh the possible risk of developing increased intraocular pressure, cataract formation or endophthalmitis. Novel treatments approaches including anti-VEGF inhibitors or corticosteroids in combination with photodynamic therapy has the potential to not only stabilize visual acuity but also to increase visual acuity in patients vascular AMD.

Triamcinolone with Photodynamic Therapy in Neovascular Age-related Macular Degeneration

A. The combination of IVTA with photodynamic therapy (PDT) is based on the pathogenesis of AMD and its response to PDT.[60-65] Photodynamic therapy causes a short-term antiangiogenic effect on neovascular vessels. Both, chronic AMD as well as PDT generate free radicals, leading to an upregulation of growth factors, e.g. VEGF (Figure 10.3). [48,66-70]

The combination of PDT with triamcinolone may further benefit the therapy for several reasons:

B. Photodynamic therapy has been shown to induce a rapid inflammatory response including infiltration of leukocytes and increased expression of cytokines. First, there is collateral damage to the adjacent choriocapillaris and retinal pigment epithelium and increase in edema and local VEGF-production.[71,72]

C. Inflammatory cells are commonly seen in histopathological examination of CNV specimens.[45,46,49] Choroidal neovascular have other constituents, such as inflammatory cells and other signs of inflammation,[73] which may not be affected short-term and are unlikely to be affected over a longer period by conventional PDT.

D. Tomographic evaluations by OCT has shown an increase in edema following verteporfin therapy.[74-79]

E. Re-growth of the neovascularization occurs with resumption of vascular leakage.[57,80,81] These patients require retreatment to restrain the leakage from the new vessels in an attempt to limit visual loss.

Intravitreal triamcinolone acetonide has been used in pilot studies to treat neovascular AMD. Penfold and associates[51] and Challa and associates[52] published case series and Danis and associates[53,82] reported a small randomized trial reporting improvement in treated

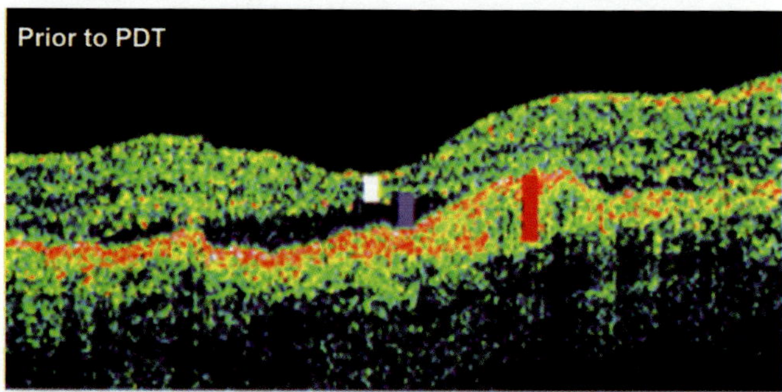

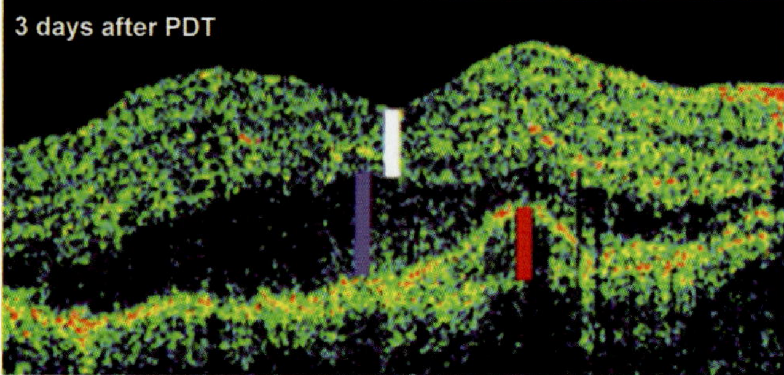

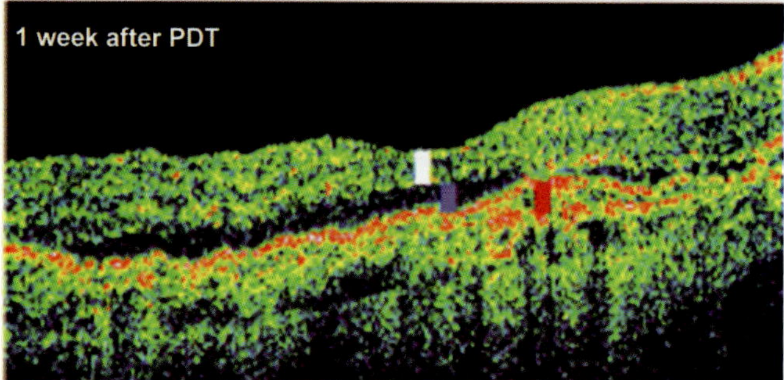

FIGURE 12.3: OCT prior to photodynamic therapy: The white bar indicates the thickness of the retina, the blue bar the subretinal fluid accumulation and the red bar the elevation of the fibrovascular pigment epithelial detachment. Three days after photodynamic therapy the subretinal fluid increased significantly, while the retinal thickness and the occult choroidal neovascularization remained clinically unchanged. One week after photodynamic therapy is the subretinal fluid reduced and the choroidal neovascularization starts to shrink, while the retinal contour and thickness becomes normalized.

patients relative to controls. A randomized clinical trial of a single dose of 4 mg intravitreal triamcinolone demonstrated a smaller growth of the lesion at 3 months in treated patients but no significant difference in visual acuity at 1 year.

Augustin and Schmidt-Erfurth[83-85] described outcomes from a prospective, open-label, non-comparative, single-center study involving 199 patients. Purified triamcinolone acetonide was administered intravitreally 16 hours after PDT, at a dose of 25 mg (n = 184). The group had a mean follow-up of 65 weeks. The 199 eyes in the series had a mean visual acuity of 20/125 (range, 20/32 to hand motion) and a mean lesion size of 3,425 μm. Lesions of any composition were eligible for treatment. The lesions were subfoveal in 80.4% of the 199 eyes, juxtafoveal in 10.1%, and extrafoveal in 9.5%. The mean number of treatments necessary for complete regression was 1.32. Compared with the baseline value, visual acuity at last visit for all eyes had improved by a mean of 1.1 lines, and the effect was even more evident when measured with laser interferometry (mean +1.26 lines). In subgroup analyses, visual acuity improved in all lesion composition groups and in lesions larger and smaller than 2,600 μm. However, at this time of follow-up, the changes compared with baseline were statistically significant only in eyes with subfoveal lesions and lesions >2,600 μm. This means that the results are not driven by the juxta- and extrafoveal lesions. Analysis of mean number of lines changed showed nearly 60% of eyes had increased visual acuity (>1 line and up to 7 lines) and >70% showed improvement or real stabilization with loss of less than 1 line. In 20% of eyes, VA decreased by 1 to 3 lines and only 8% of eyes lost more than 3 lines of visual acuity. A side-to-side comparison of these results with other studies clearly shows that this combination approach leads to a response rate of >90%.

Anti-inflammatory agents such as triamcinolone acetonide with the addition of PDT may therefore minimize visual disturbances occurring as a result of localized edema. Combination treatment [61-64] of neovascular AMD using PDT plus IVTA appears to improve visual outcomes and reduce the number of re-treatments necessary to achieve lesion regression when compared with standard PDT alone and can therefore counteract both AMD-related and PDT-induced inflammatory reactions, in addition to any direct effects on CNV. Preventing inflammation or edema may minimize or prevent vision disturbances.

The introduction of an adjunctive antiangiogenic therapy to PDT may enhance the therapeutic effect of intravitreal steroids. Intravitreal triamcinolone acetonide seems to reduce the growth of CNV and the need for PDT-retreatment. However, intravitreal steroids are associated with raised intraocular pressure, which may persist for months, thus requiring filtration as well as cataract surgery. These secondary effects would not be expected from PDT using verteporfin alone.

Intravitreal triamcinolone persists in the vitreous cavity, extending the duration of treatment against the neovascular complex. [32, 40] There are possible side effects from both PDT, IVTA as well as many potential interactions as well. The stabilization of visual acuity observed after treatment with verteporfin therapy correlates with a significant reduction in CNV growth and progressive resolution of leakage.[65] However, recanalization of the neovascular complex can occur after initial closure following PDT. [80] Patients may therefore require additional treatment with PDT, although the number of treatments required has been shown to decrease over time.

DIABETIC RETINOPATHY

In diabetic retinopathy, exists a link between inflammation and VEGF.[86] Increasing evidence suggests that VEGF may cause inflammation by inducing ICAM-1 expression and leukocyte adhesion.[86, 87] When ICAM-1 bioactivity is blocked, VEGF induced blood-retinal barrier breakdown is suppressed; and similarly, when VEGF-bioactivity is blocked, ICAM-1 upregulation, leukocyte adhesion, and blood-retinal-barrier breakdown are all reduced. Studies with animals[33] and humans have evaluated the hypothesis that inflammation is a possible cause for diabetic retinopathy.[88]

Increasing evidence suggests that microvascular changes may partially result from inflammation. In experimental diabetes, leukocytes migrate and adhere to the retinal vasculature,[18] appearing to bind to the endothelial cell layer via cellular adhesion molecules such as intercellular adhesion molecule-1 (ICAM-1) on the vasculature and α2-integrins on the leukocytes. Other molecules, such as vascular cell adhesion molecule-1 and α 4 β1-integrin (VLA-4, a leukocyte ligand for vascular cell adhesion molecule-1, fibronectin, and osteopontin) may also be involved.[88] Leukocyte migration into the neural retina is associated with the breakdown of the blood-retinal barrier, premature endothelial cell death, and capillary ischemia, all of which occur before any funduscopic changes. [18] The relation between leukocytes and these changes is obvious when diabetic rats are treated with cellular adhesion inhibitors (anti-ICAM-1 or α2-integrin antibodies) that reduce leukocyte adhesion and prevent blood-retinal barrier breakdown and endothelial cell injury. Mice deficient in the ICAM-1 or α2-integrin gene exhibit no retinal vascular change after 11 months of experimental diabetes. [27, 87]

Acellular capillaries and retinal hemorrhages have been prevented in diabetic dogs with the use of long-term aspirin therapy and anti-inflammatory agents have suppressed blood-retinal barrier breakdown in rat. [88]

Angiostatic steroids, such as 2-zethoxyestradiol (an endogenous metabolite of estrogen), have shown promise in preventing tumor neovascularization in experimental models. Intravitreal steroid injections potently inhibit preretinal neovascularization in pig and rat models, [73, 82] whereas in a rat retinopathy of prematurity model, anecortave acetate inhibits retinal neovascularization, in part by the induction of (PAI)-1 mRNA, a plasminogen activator inhibitor. [88] In patients who underwent pars plana vitrectomy for treatment of PDR, an intravitreal injection of 15 to 20 mg of crystalline triamcinolone acetonide resulted in regression of pre-existing rubeosis in 12 of 29 patients, [89] and an intravitreal injection of 20 mg triamcinolone acetonide led to regression of rubeosis in proliferative glaucoma caused by proliferative diabetic retinopathy or ischemic central vein occlusion.

DIABETIC MACULAR EDEMA

Macular edema is the most common cause of visual loss among diabetics. The incidence of diabetic macular edema over a 10-year period is 13.9 to 25%. [90] The pathogenesis of diabetic macular edema is the result of an increase in retinal vascular permeability factors, such as interleukin 6, VEGF and leakage of intravascular fluid from microaneurysms and abnormal retinal capillaries into the intraretinal and subretinal space from a general blood retinal barrier breakdown. [91,92] Machemer and associates [28] proposed the use of intravitreal cortisone to locally inhibit intraocular inflammation, cell proliferation and neovascularization. Although cortisone mainly suppresses the intraocular inflammation locally,

it also inhibits the expression of vascular growth factors, and contributes to the integrity of the blood retinal barrier. [27,33]

For diabetic macular edema, an intravitreal injection of triamcinolone acetonide is thought to decrease vascular permeability during inflammation (Figure 12.4). [93-95] In one prospective series of 26 eyes (in 20 patients) that received a single 25 mg intravitreal injection, visual acuity improved significantly ($P < 0.001$) from 0.12 ± 0.08 at baseline to a maximum of 0.19 ± 0.14 during mean follow-up of 6.64 ± 6.10 months. However, there was no significant change in a matched, but not randomized, control group of 16 patients who underwent macular grid laser photocoagulation. Predictably, about 35% of treated patients experienced elevated intraocular pressure which was controlled with topical medication only. [95] In another study of 16 eyes with clinically significant macular edema that failed to respond to laser photocoagulation treatments, an intravitreal injection of triamcinolone resulted in mean improvement in visual acuity of 2.4, 2.4, and 1.3 Snellen lines at 1, 3, and 6 months follow-up intervals, respectively. The central macular thickness, measured by OCT, decreased by 55, 57.5, and 38%, respectively, over these same intervals from an initial pretreatment mean of 540.3 μm. Reinjection was performed in three of eight eyes after 6 months due to the recurrence of macular edema; which is commonly encountered, even at higher triamcinolone acetonide dosages. [95] Long-term safety and efficacy of repeated intravitreal injections is uncertain, but encouraging results promote the need for developing long-term sustained release devices for corticosteroid therapy.

RETINAL VEIN OCCLUSION

Cystoid macular edema (CME) is the major cause for decreased visual acuity in patients following branch or central retinal vein occlusion.

Central Retinal Vein Occlusion

While neovascular complications of central retinal vein occlusion (CRVO) can be treated with panretinal laser photocoagulation, macular laser photocoagulation can reduce angiographic evidence of macular edema.

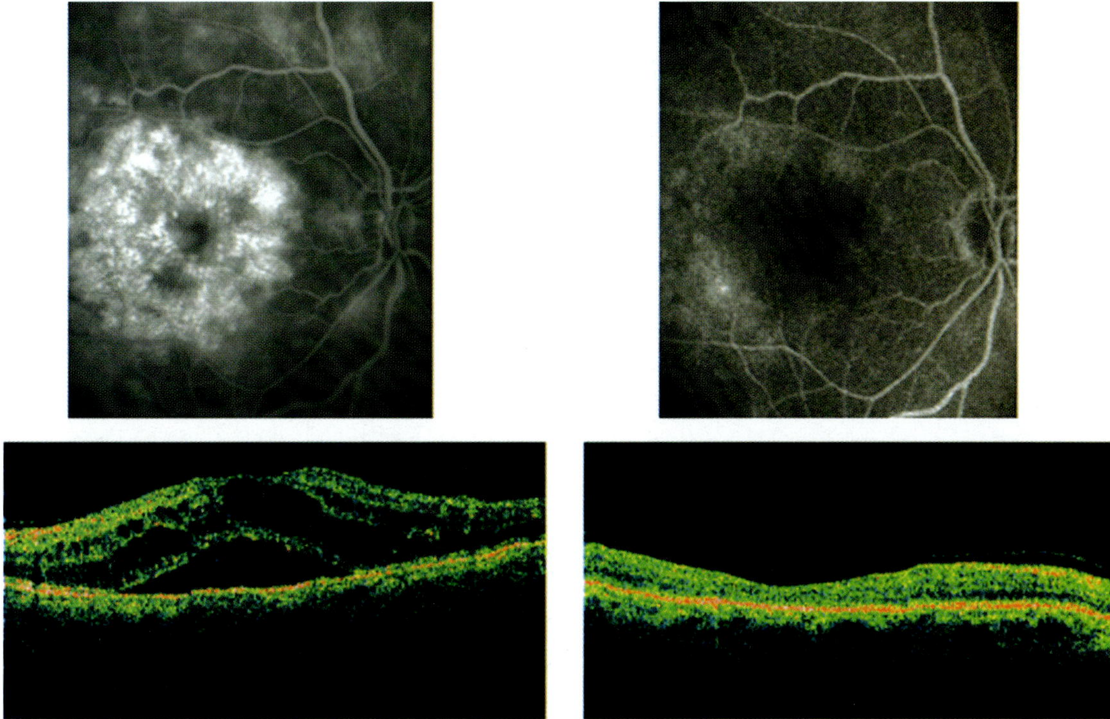

FIGURE 12.4: Fifty-year-old patient visual acuity prior to intravitreal triamcinolone acetonide with visual acuity 0.2 and 0.4, 6 weeks later.

However, macular laser photocoagulation is not capable of improving macular function.[96] No other treatments proven effective in terms of visual acuity are available either.

After promising case reports,[97, 98] a number of recent studies have investigated the effect of IVTA on CME and visual acuity after CRVO.[99-105] All studies reported a clear morphological improvement in terms of a reduction of retinal thickness or resolution of CME, and a corresponding functional improvement by increased visual acuity (Figures 12.5A to C). In the only randomized clinical trial to date, Ramezani and associates[104] demonstrated a therapeutic effect of IVTA in 13 eyes after acute CRVO less than 2 months old. The effect was greatest at months first and second after the injection and decreased to month 4th. In a prospective comparative non-randomized trial of 33 eyes Jonas and assocaites[101] found a significantly improved visual acuity in the treatment group for up to three months after IVTA. Visual acuity in the control group deteriorated during follow-up. Within the treatment group the visual acuity increase was higher in the non-ischemic subgroup than in eyes with ischemic CRVO. A better outcome in eyes with non-

ischemic CRVO compared to eyes with ischemic CRVO was also reported by Ip and associates.[100] In another non-randomized trial, 60% of eyes treated with IVTA due to non-ischemic CRVO had a final visual acuity of 20/40 or better versus only 20% in the observation group. Forty percent of the untreated patients had a final visual acuity worse than 20/200, while none of the treated patients did.[99] Most studies found a positive effect of IVTA for three or four months, which may last up to 6 months, but was not sustained at 1 year.[102,105] Re-injections are frequently necessary.

Branch Retinal Vein Occlusion

In contrast to laser treatment of CME following CRVO, macular laser photocoagulation has been shown to be effective with regard to the reduction of macular edema and improving VA after branch retinal vein occlusion.[106] Macular laser photocoagulation still is the standard therapy for CME after branch retinal vein occlusion (BRVO).

As with CRVO, early case reports have demonstrated an efficacy of IVTA after BRVO (Figures 12.6A and B).[107]

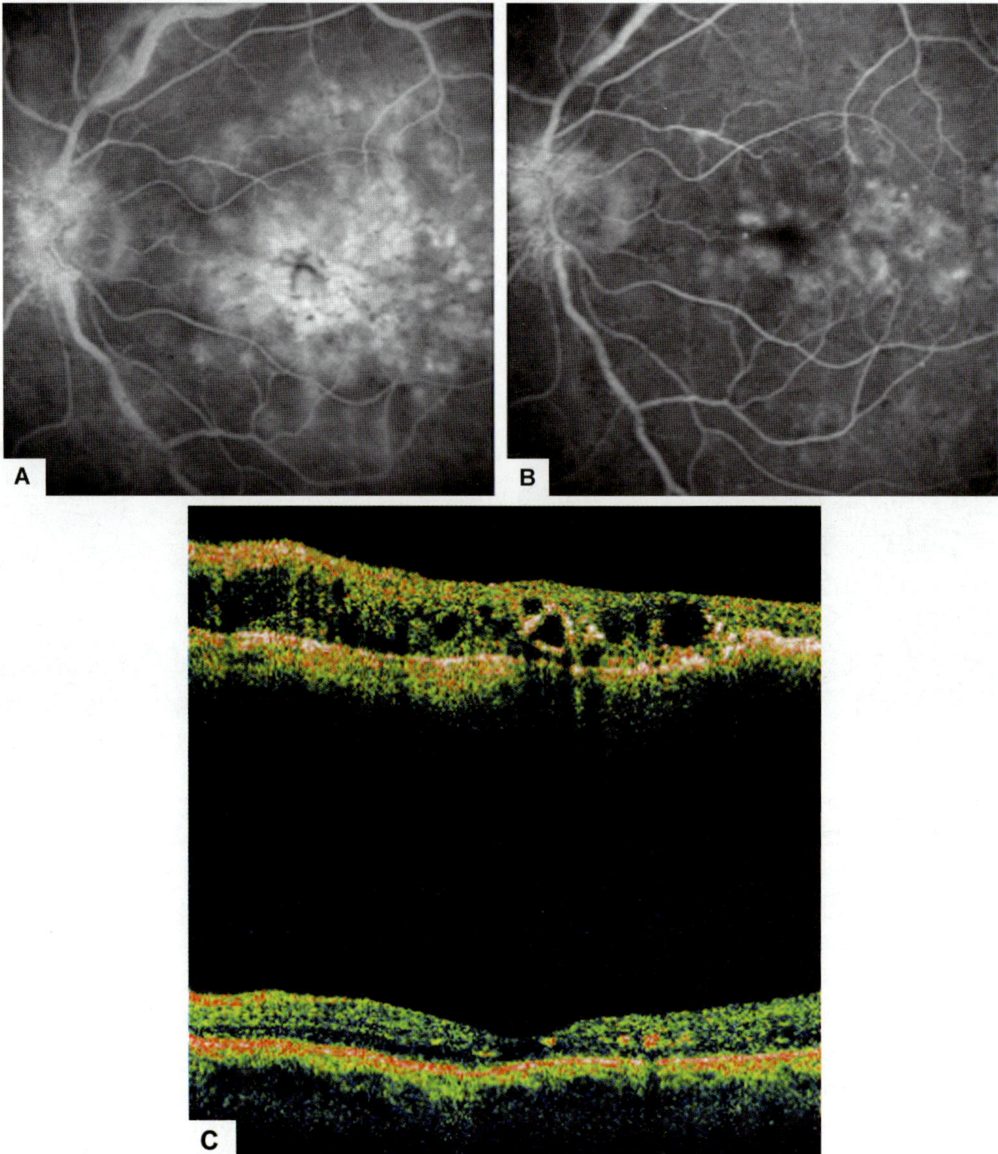

FIGURES 12.5A to C: (A) Cystoid macular edema due to central retinal vein occlusion due to CRVO. VA 20/50. (B) Reduced extravasation 5 weeks after intravitreal triamcinolone acetonide. Visual acuity increased to 20/40. (C) Pre- and post-treatment OCT showing resolution of macular edema.

Recently published investigations consistently reported a significant VA increase after IVTA. In a comparative non-randomized study 15 eyes treated with IVTA primarily achieved better results than 19 control eyes treated with macular laser photocogulation for BRVO for up to 6 months. [108] On the other hand, IVTA may still be effective after macular laser photocoagulation failed to improve macular edema after BRVO.[109] Jonas and associates[110] compared a IVTA study group with a non-randomized control group. The gain in visual acuity was significantly higher in the study group than in the control group one and two months after IVTA. While treated eyes without macular ischemia improved significantly, there was no significant change in treated eyes with macular ischemia.

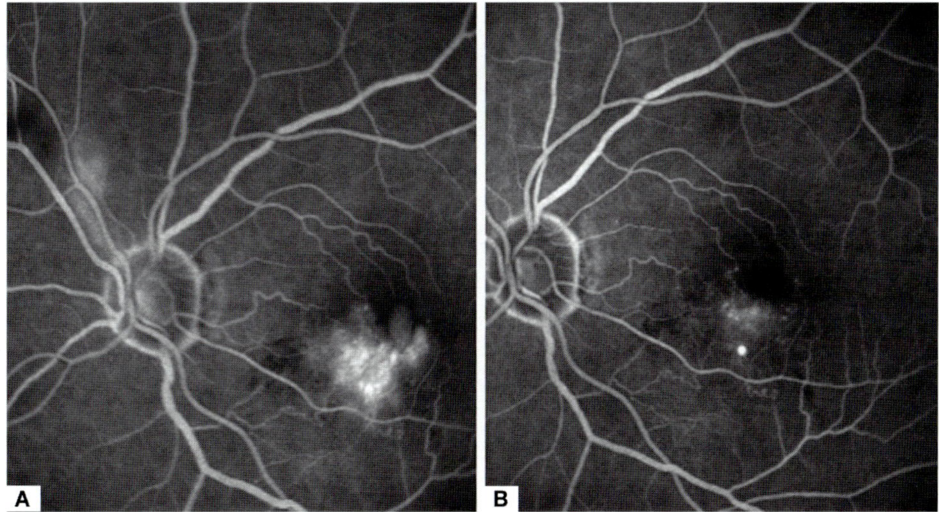

FIGURES 12.6A and B: (A) Cystoid macular edema due to branch retinal vein occlusion. Visual acuity was 20/100. (B) Reduced cystoid macular edema 5 weeks after intravitreal triamcinolone acetonide. Visual acuity increased to 20/40.

Chen and associates [111,112] reported an anatomic and visual acuity improvement after IVTA also for long standing BRVO associated with macular ischemia, but this effect was also temporarily. As with CRVO, re-injections are frequently necessary.

OTHER INDICATIONS

Intravitreal triamcinolone acetonide has been used as a treatment trial in nearly all kinds of macular edema. Most publications on the subject were case reports or case series studies.

Pseudophakic macular edema may occur even after uncomplicated cataract (and other types of intraocular) surgery. It often resolves spontaneously, but some cases are persistent. In small case series studies of three to eight eyes a clear functional and anatomic benefit IVTA has been reported.[113-115] However, as in other indications, the regression of CME was temporary and re-injections had to be performed (Figures 12.7A to C).

Young and associates[116] reported a resolution of CME secondary to uveitis in 6 cases resistant to other steroid delivery routes in 6 patients. The treatment effect lasted for up to 6 months. In a similar study, Antcliff and associates[117] demonstrated complete anatomic and to some extent functional success in long term refractory inflammatory CME. In a case report of a single patient who refused systemic immunosuppression for chronic posterior uveitis, she was managed over a period of three years with IVTA. She developed cataract and increased intraocular pressure, but maintained good vision. In a publication on IVTA for refractory CME in Behcet's disease 7 of 10 eyes showed improvement of visual acuity after three months, but in 5 eyes CME recurred and IVTA had to be repeated.[118]

Intravitreal triamcinolone acetonide has also been applied for treatment of juxtafoveal telangiectasia. In two treated eyes macular morphology and visual acuity improved, but no treatment effect was seen in a third eye.[119, 120] One eye that received IVTA after prior focal laser photocoagulation exhibited extensive resolution of CME which however was not accompanied by functional improvement.[121]

COMPLICATIONS OF INTRAVITREAL TRIAMCINOLONE ACETONIDE

Complications after IVTA can be categorized into two groups: drug-related complications (e.g. intraocular pressure increase, cataract induction/progression, toxic effects) and procedure-related complications (infectious endophthalmitis, vitreoretinal complications and others).

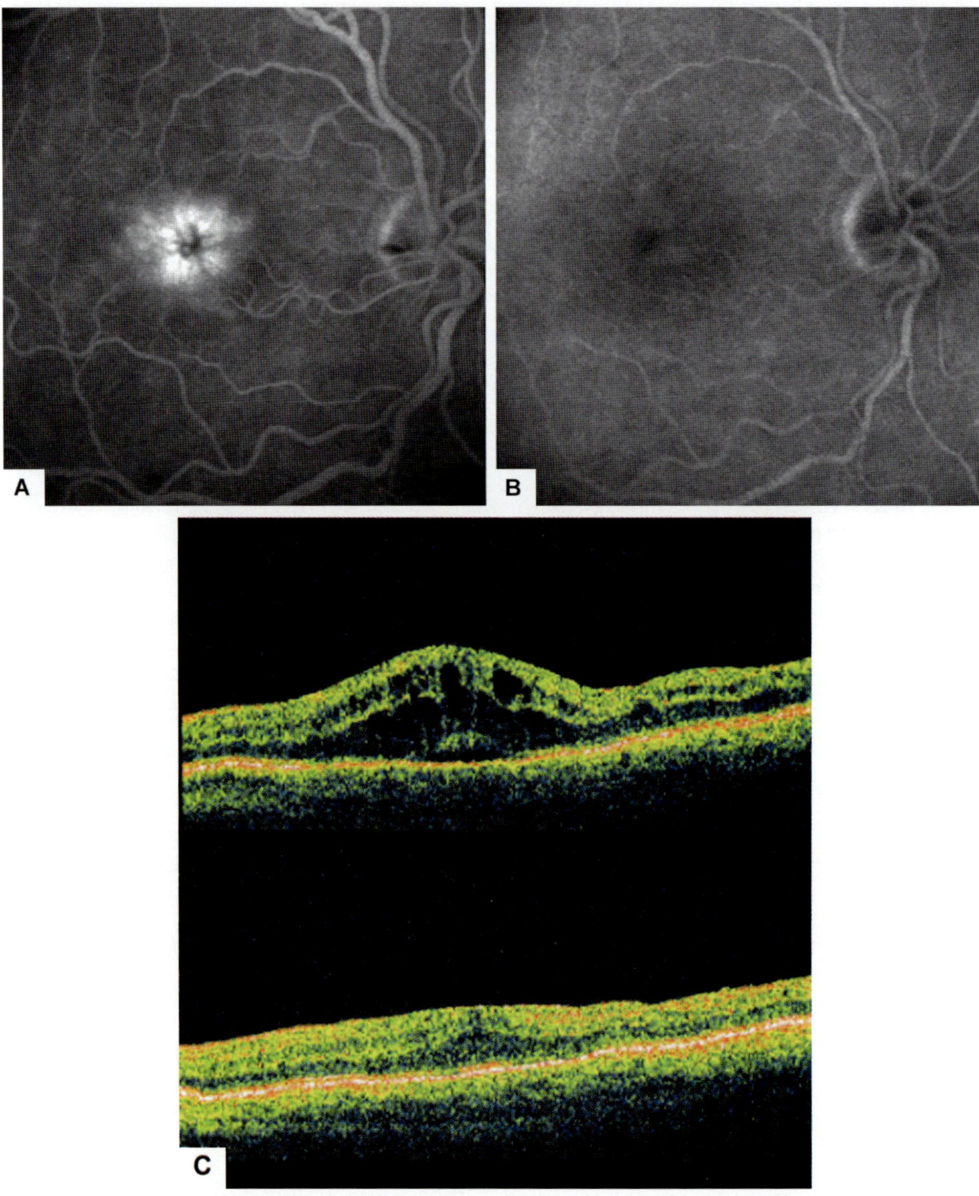

FIGURES 12.7A to C: (A) Pseudophakic cystoid macular edema. Visual acuity was 20/100. (B) Psudophakic cystoid macular edema 5 weeks after intravitreal triamcinolone acetonide. Visual acuity improved to 20/32. (C) Pre- and post-treatment OCT.

SECONDARY STEROID-INDUCED OCULAR HYPERTENSION OR OPEN-ANGLE GLAUCOMA

An increase of the intraocular pressure is a well known phenomenon after prolonged use of steroid eyedrops or periocular injections. Consequently, secondary steroid-induced ocular hypertension (or open-angle glaucoma, if damage to optic nerve head occurs) can frequently be found after IVTA. After IVTA of 25 mg an intraocular pressure increase to more than 21 mm Hg occurs in 41.2% and an intraocular pressure increase to values exceeding 35 mm Hg in 5.5%. [122] Usually, intraocular pressure can be lowered sufficiently by standard topical anti-glaucoma medication. In about 1% of the eyes, however, filtering surgery may become necessary. The intraocular pressure increase after IVTA can start as early as one week after IVTA and is manifest 1 to 2 months after IVTA in most eyes that are *steroid responders*. In some eyes, however, the intraocular pressure may rise even more than 3 months after IVTA, even if they were vitrectomized previously, and some eyes may need filtering surgery even 8 months after IVTA with triamcinolone crystals still being visible in the inferior vitreous cortex. [39, 122] After applying a dosage of 25 mg IVTA the intraocular pressure usually returns to preinjection values after 7 to 9 months without further medication.

While younger age of the patient is a positive risk factor for steroid-induced intraocular pressure elevation, this does not apply for presence of diabetes mellitus, reason for IVTA, refraction, and, interestingly, to the best knowledge so far, pre-existing open-angle glaucoma. [122]

The overall incidence of steroid induced intraocular pressure increase after IVTA is about 40%. Analyzing a number of studies, there does not seem to be a marked difference of the intraocular pressure reaction after different dosages of 4.25 mg IVTA. [122-126]

CATARACT INDUCTION OR PROGRESSION

Like intraocular pressure elevation, cataract formation is a well known complication after prolonged steroid use irrespective of the administration route. A number of studies confirmed cataract formation also after IVTA.[127-130] In the elderly phakic population, IVTA may lead to cataract surgery in 15 to 20% after 1 year. Another study reported a clinically significant opacification of the crystalline lens in up to 50% of the phakic eyes. [131] This may not be a major problem, as cataract surgery can be performed after IVTA without a markedly elevated risk of intra- or postoperative complications, [130, 132] and many of the injected eyes of elderly patients have pre-existing incipient or provect cataract anyway.

Recent studies found posterior subcapsular cataract development to be associated with a secondary intraocular pressure increase after IVTA, and posterior subcapsular cataract development to be more frequent after single IVTA injections. After multiple injections all-layer cataracts were more prevalent. [127, 128] Damage to the crystalline lens as a procedure-related complication

is possible when injecting into the vitreous cavity, however this complication has not been reported yet in the context of IVTA. Inadvertent lens damage can be avoided with an adequate injection technique.

TOXIC EFFECTS

Toxic effects are a major concern in the use of intravitreal medication. Intravitreal steroids have been shown to be adequately safe in a number of animal and human studies.[35,38,129,133-138] In the case of direct contact of triamcinolone crystals to the retina or the optic nerve head no damage was clinically detectable (unpublished data).[139, 140] However, there is experimental evidence of a retinal pigment epithelium-cytotoxicity after direct physical contact to triamcinolone in vitro.[141] Furthermore, the vehicle of commercially available triamcinolone solutions may show intraocular toxicity.[34,142,143] These facts, as well as conclusions drawn from observations with sterile endophthalmitis, suggest that a removal of the vehicle before injecting into the eye seems to be advisable. However, the direct use of the commercial solution is widely accepted as well.

ENDOPHTHALMITIS

It is essential to distinguish between 3 different types of endophthalmitis after IVTA.

Infectious endophthalmitis is the most devastating, potentially blinding complication after IVTA. The frequency of infectious endophthalmitis in large IVTA studies ranged between 0.0% in a series of 1135 injections and 0.87% in a series of 992 IVTA.[144-146] It has been speculated that intraocular immunosuppression due to IVTA may contribute to the relatively high risk of endophthalmitis in some studies as compared to other intraocular surgery, e.g. standard cataract surgery. In conclusion, these studies suggest that the risk of an infectious endophthalmitis may be low (<1:1000) if the injection is performed under sterile conditions using a povidone iodine disinfection, lid drape, and lid speculum. An interesting and clinically important observation is that eyes presenting with infectious endophthalmitis after IVTA often exhibit much less pain than eyes with endophthalmitis after other intraocular surgery.

Non-infectious or sterile endophthalmitis has been reported in up to 6.7% after IVTA. [147-149] Symptoms were blurred vision, hypopyon, pain, vitritis and others within 2 days after IVTA. In some of the patients the inflammatory response resolved without specific treatment under close observation, in other patients, vitrectomy was performed to treat presumed infectious endophthalmitis, but cultures were negative and the eyes recovered rapidly. Mean time to presentation of symptoms was 1.5 days.[149] The reason for sterile endophthalmitis has not been clearly identified yet. However, it is likely that one or more of the additives and preservatives (esp. benzyl alcohol) of the commercial triamcinolone preparations may be the causative agent of this inflammatory reaction. [143] Another reason for this assumption is that sterile endophthalmitis has been described in studies that used an unpurified triamcinolone suspension only, and it has not been described in studies including a great number of eyes using purified triamcinolone with the solvent agent removed. [144] Presumed non-infectious endophthalmitis may not be clearly distinguished from infectious endophthalmitis in all cases.

Pseudoendophthalmitis is characterized by an accumulation of white triamcinolone crystals in the inferior anterior chamber angle forming a pseudohypopyon.[150,151] This may be the case if triamcinolone crystals are washed from the vitreous cavity into the anterior chamber through a defect of the separating diaphragm built by lens, capsule and zonules. It might be a diagnostic problem to differentiate between a painless hypopyon and a pseudohypopyon, but on high magnification of the slit lamp the crystalline structure of triamcinolone can be recognized in many cases of pseudohypopyons. Triamcinolone crystals in the anterior chamber usually resolve spontaneously and no reports on chamber angle or endothelial damage due to pseudohypopyons have been published yet. In pilot studies intracameral steroids have been applied to treat endothelial immune reactions after penetrating keratoplasty. [152]

RHEGMATOGENOUS RETINAL DETACHMENT—INTRAOCULAR HEMORRHAGE

As the IVTA is carried out in the posterior segment of the eye, de-arranging the vitreous body, possibly exerting tractional forces upon the vitreous base, and occasionally leading to vitreous incarceration into the injection site due to reflux of intraocular fluid, one might expect, that rhegmatogenous retinal detachment may a frequent complication after IVTA. Fortunately this is not the case. In most studies no postoperative rhegmatogenous retinal detachments have been reported (Figure 12.8).[129, 153] This is consistent with our own experience of more than 2500 injections. Intraocular hemorrhages following IVTA have only been reported anecdotally. The risk of intraocular bleeding may be elevated in cases with present intraocular (especially iris or retina) neovascularization in the short phase of ocular hypotony if a paracentesis is performed.

VITREOUS PROLAPSE/INTRAOCULAR LENS DECENTRATION

In eyes with compromised compartments, e.g. due to zonulolysis, a sulcus fixated IOL with open posterior capsule, aphakia and others, a vitreous prolapse into the anterior chamber with or without incarceration into a paracentesis may occur. A sulcus IOL may dislocate. In a series of more than 600 injections of 25 mg IVTA (0.2 ml, paracentesis performed to reduce the intraocular pressure) this complication occurred in about 0.5%, and was treated with anterior vitrectomy.[154] The reason for this finding is the rapid increase of volume in the posterior segment of the eye during injection.

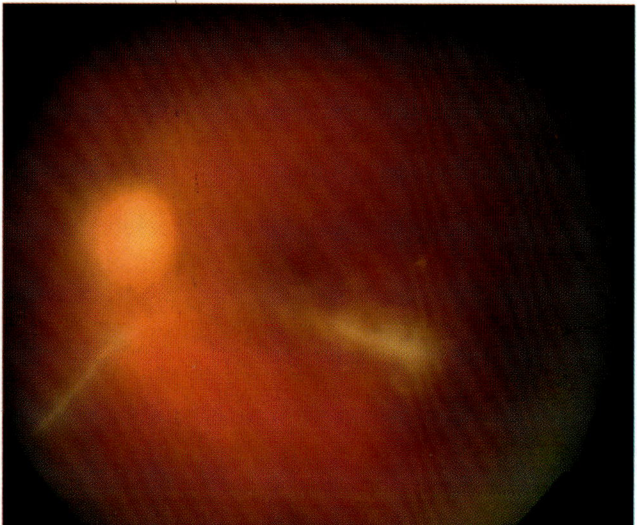

FIGURE 12.8: Intraocular hemorrhage following intravitreal triamcinolone acetonide injection.

POSTINJECTIONAL INTRAOCULAR PRESSURE INCREASE / CENTRAL RETINAL ARTERY OCCLUSION

The rapid and marked intraocular pressure increase during injection may also lead to functional central retinal artery occlusion, which can be perceived by the patient as a darkening or loss of light perception immediately after the injection. While a paracentesis does not have to be performed routinely with an injection volume of up to 0.1 ml, it has to be performed using 0.2 ml.[124] In any case of intravitreal injection, light perception must be checked immediately after the injection, and the surgeon has to assure that the intraocular pressure is not dangerously high before finishing the surgical procedure.

Intravitreal triamcinolone acetonide has a significant profile of adverse reactions and side effects. Using adequate techniques and follow-up, the risk is tolerable and most complications can be well managed without damage to the eye.

CONCLUSIONS

Intravitreal corticosteroids have been used as an adjunctive therapy for proliferative retinopathy, choroidal neovascularization, uveitic and pseudophakic macular edema, idiopathic juxtafoveal telangiectasia, and others. The safety and efficacy of IVTA has been well studied in animal models and clinical studies. These studies showed that IVTA does not have a toxic effect on intraocular tissue however; it can be toxic to the retinal Müller cells, outer plexiform and nuclear layers when administered in higher doses.

At present, laser photocoagulation is recommended for selected eyes with juxtafoveal and extrafoveal CNV due to AMD, while PDT has been proven effective for patients with subfoveal lesions composed of predominantly classic CNV (regardless of lesion size), and has demonstrated efficacy in treating small minimally classic or occult with no classic lesions with evidence of recent progression. While triamcinolone acetonide appeared promising in pilot studies, currently available evidence suggests that it cannot be recommended as a monotherapy for CNV due to AMD in the absence of evidence that it is safe and effective in large-scale clinical trials. The potential to reduce inflammation and edema and

prevent re-growth of CNV by combining PDT and IVTA is an interesting concept and there have been promising results in early pilot studies. Future studies are warranted to determine the balance between the potential benefits of administering triamcinolone acetonide to patients receiving PDT and the possible possibly risks of an increase in intraocular pressure and progression of cataract.

REFERENCES

1. Aiello LP, Pierce EA, Foley ED, et al. Suppression of retinal neovascularization in vivo by inhibition of vascular endothelial growth factor VEGF using soluble VEGF-receptor chimeric proteins. Proc Natl Acad Sci USA 1995; 92:10457-61.
2. Gross J, Azizkhan RG, Biswas C, et al. Inhibition of tumor growth, vascularization, and collagenolysis in the rabbit cornea by medroxyprogesterone. Proc Natl Acad Sci USA 1981;78:1176-80.
3. Ingber DE, Madri JA, Folkman J. A possible mechanism for inhibition of angiogenesis by angiostatic steroids: induction of capillary basement membrane dissolution. Endocrinology 1986;119:1768-75.
4. Michaelson IC. The mode of development of the vascular system of the retina with some observations on its significance for certain retinal disease. Trans Ophthalmol Soc UK 1948;68:137-80.
5. Miller J, Adamis AP, Shima DT, et al. Vascular endothelial growth factor (vascular permeability factor) is temporally and spatially correlated with ocular angiogenesis in a primate model. Am J Pathol 1994; 145:574-84.
6. Wise GN. Retinal neovascularization. Trans Am Ophthalmol Soc 1956;54:729-826.
7. Shubik P, Feldman R, Garcia II, Warren BA. Vascularization induced in the cheek pouch of the Syrian hamster by tumor and nontumor substances. J Natl Cancer Inst 1976; 57: 769-74.
8. Fischer S, Renz D, Schaper W, Karliczek GF. In vitro effects of dexamethasone on hypoxia-induced hyperpermeability and expression of vascular endothelial growth factor. Eur J Pharmacol 2001; 411:231-43.
9. Folkman J, Ingber DE. Angiostatic steroids. Method of diskovery and mechanism of action. Ann Surg 1987; 206:374-83.
10. Gao H, Qiao X, Gao R, et al. Intravitreal triamcinolone does not alter basal vascular endothelial growth factor mRNA expression in rat retina. Vision Res 2004; 44:349-56.
11. Nauck M, Karakiulakis G, Perruchoud AP, et al. Corticosteroids inhibit the expression of the vascular endothelial growth factor gene in human vascular smooth muscle cells. Eur J Pharmacol 1998; 341:309-15.
12. Sears JE, Hoppe G. Triamcinolone acetonide destabilizes VEGF mRNA in Müller cells under continuous cobalt stimulation. Invest Ophthalmol Vis Sci 2005; 46:4336-41.

13. Wang YS, Friedrichs U, Eichler W, et al. Inhibitory effects of triamcinolone acetonide on bFGF-induced migration and tube formation in choroidal microvascular endothelial cells. Graefes Arch Clin Exp Ophthalmol 2002; 240:42-48.

14. Penfold PL, Wen L, Madigan MC, et al. Triamcinolone acetonide modulates permeability and intercellular adhesion molecule-1 (ICAM-1) expression of the ECV304 cell line: implications for macular degeneration. Clin Exp Immunol 2000;121:458-65.

15. Penfold PL, Wong JG, Gyory J, Billson FA. Effects of triamcinolone acetonide on microglial morphology and quantitative expression of MHC-II in exudative age-related macular degeneration. Clin Experiment Ophthalmol 2001; 29:188-92.

16. Kaiser PK. Steroids for choroidal neovascularization. Am J Ophthalmol 2005; 539:533-35.

17. Gollnick SO, Evans SS, Baumann H, et al. Role of cytokines in photodynamic therapy-induced local and systemic inflammation. Br J Cancer 2003; 88:1772-79.

18. Joussen AM, Murata T, Tsujikawa A, et al. Leukocyte-mediated endothelial cell injury and death in the diabetic retina. Am J Pathol 2001; 158:147-52.

19. Brooks HL Jr, Caballero S Jr, Newell CK, et al. Vitreous levels of vascular endothelial growth factor and stromal-derived factor 1 in patients with diabetic retinopathy and cystoid macular edema before and after intraocular injection of triamcinolone. Arch Ophthalmol 2004; 122:1801-07.

20. Itakura H, Akiyama H, Hagimura N, et al. Triamcinolone acetonide suppresses interleukin-1 beta-mediated increase in vascular endothelial growth factor expression in cultured rat Muller cells. Graefes Arch Clin Exp Ophthalmol 2005; 28:1-6.

21. Meyer RF, Smolin G, Hall JM, Okumoto M. Effect of local corticosteroids on antibody-forming cells in the eye and draining lymph nodes. Invest Ophthalmol 1975; 14:138-44.

22. Penfold PL, Wen L, Madigan MC, et al. Modulation of permeability and adhesion molecule expression by human choroidal endothelial cells. Invest Ophthalmol Vis Sci 2002; 43:3125-30.

23. Bhattacherjee P, Williams RN, Eakins KE. A comparison of the ocular anti-inflammatory activity of steroidal and nonsteroidal compounds in the rat. Invest Ophthalmol Vis Sci 1983; 24:1143-46.

24. Umland SP, Nahrebne DK, Razac S, et al. The inhibitory effects of topically active glucocorticoids on IL-4, IL-5, and interferon gamma production by cultured primary CD4+ T cells. J Allergy Clin Immunol 1997; 100:511-19.

25. Augustin AJ, Dick HB, Koch F, Schmidt-Erfurth U. Correlation of blood-glucose control with oxidative metabolites in plasma and vitreous body of diabetic patients. Eur J Ophthalmol 2002; 12:94-101.

26. Edelman JL, Lutz D, Castro MR. Corticosteroids inhibit VEGF-induced vascular leakage in a rabbit model of blood-retinal and blood-aqueous barrier breakdown. Exp Eye Res 2005; 80:249-58.

27. Antoszyk AN, Gottlieb JL, Machemer R, Hatchell DL. The effects of intravitreal triamcinolone acetonide on experimental preretinal neovascularization. Graefe's Arch Clin Exp Ophthalmol 1993; 231:34-40.

28. Machemer R, Sugita G, Tano Y. Treatment of intraocular proliferations with intravitreal steroids. Trans Am Ophthalmol Soc 1979; 77:171-80.

29. Tano Y, Chandler D, Machemer R. Treatment of intraocular proliferation with intravitreal injection of triamcinolone acetonide. Am J Ophthalmol 1980; 90:810-16.

30. Wilson CA, Berkowitz BA, Sato Y, et al. Treatment with intravitreal steroid reduces blood retinal barrier breakdown due to retinal photocoagulation. Arch Ophthalmol 1992; 110:1155-59.

31. Jonas JB, Kreissig I, Degenring RF. Intravitreal triamcinolone acetonide for treatment of intraocular proliferative, exudative, and neovascular diseases. Prog Retin Eye Res 2005; 24:587-611.

32. Degenring RF, Jonas JB. Serum levels of triamcinolone acetonide after intravitreal injection. Am J Ophthalmol 2004; 137:1142-43.

33. Chandler DB, Hida T, Sheta S, et al. Improvement in efficacy of corticosteroid therapy in an animal model of proliferative vitreoretinopathy by pretreatment. Graefes Arch Clin Exp Ophthalmol 1987; 225:259-65.

34. Hida T, Chandler D, Arena JE, Machemer R. Experimental and clinical observations of the intraocular toxicity of commercial corticosteroid preparations. Am J Ophthalmol 1986 15; 101:190-95.

35. McCuen BW 2nd, Bessler NM, Tano Y, et al. The lack of toxicity of intravitreally administered triamcinolone acetonide. Am J Ophthalmol 1981; 91:785-88.

36. Schindler RH, Chandler D, Thresher R, Machemer R. The clearance of intravitreal triamcinolone acetonide. Am J Ophthalmol 1982; 93:415-17.

37. Doi N, Uemura A, Nakao K, Sakamoto T. Vitreomacular adhesion and the defect in posterior vitreous cortex visualized by triamcinolone-assisted vitrectomy. Retina 2005; 25:742-45.

38. Kivilcim M, Peyman GA, El-Dessouky ES, et al. Retinal toxicity of triamcinolone acetonide in silicone-filled eyes. Ophthalmic Surg Lasers 2000; 31:474-78.

39. Meyer CH, Mennel S, Schmidt JC. Intravitreal triamcinolone acetonide may increase the intraocular pressure even in vitrectomized eyes after more than 3 months. Am J Ophthalmol 2005; 140:766-67.

40. Scholes GN, O'Brien WJ, Abrams GW, Kubicek MF. Clearance of triamcinolone from vitreous. Arch Ophthalmol 1985; 103:1567-69.

41. Beer PM, Bakri SJ, Singh RJ, et al. Intraocular concentration and pharmacokinetics of triamcinolone acetonide after a single intravitreal injection. Ophthalmology 2003; 110: 681- 86.

42. Dawson DW, Volpert OV, Gillis P, et al. Pigment epithelium derived factor: a potent inhibitor of angiogenesis. Science 1999; 285:245-48.

43. Ishibashi T, Hata Y, Yoshikawa H, et al. Expression of vascular endothelial growth factor in experimental choroidal neovascularization. Graefe's Arch Clin Exp Ophthalmol 1997; 235:159-67.

44. Kvanta A, Algvere PV, Berglin L, Seregard S. Subfoveal fibrovascular membranes in age-related macular degeneration express vascular endothelial growth factor. Invest Ophthalmol Vis Sci 1996; 37:1929-34.

45. Lopez PF, Grossniklaus HE, Lambert HM, et al. Pathologic features of surgically excised subretinal neovascular membranes in age-related macular degeneration. Am J Ophthalmol 1991; 112:647-56.

46. Lopez PF, Sippy BD, Lambert HM, et al. Transdifferentiated retinal pigment epithelial cells are immunoreactive for vascular endothelial growth factor in surgically excised age-related macular degeneration-related choroidal neovascular membranes. Invest Ophthalmol Vis Sci 1996; 37:855-68.

47. Mori K, Duh E, Gehlbach P, et al. Pigment epithelium-derived factor inhibits retinal and choroidal neovascularization. J Cell Physiol 2001; 188:253-63.

48. Schmidt-Erfurth U, Schlotzer-Schrehard U, Cursiefen C, et al. Influence of photodynamic therapy on expression of vascular endothelial growth factor (VEGF), VEGF receptor 3, and pigment epithelium-derived factor. Invest Ophthalmol Vis Sci 2003; 44:4473-80.

49. Seregard S, Algvere PV, Berglin L. Immunohistochemical characterization of surgically removed subfoveal fibrovascular membranes. Graefe's Arch Clin Exp Ophthalmol 1994; 232:325-29.

50. Spilsbury K, Garrett KL, Shen WY, et al. Over expression of vascular endothelial growth factor (VEGF) in the retinal pigment epithelium leads to the development of choroidal neovascularization. Am J Pathol 2000; 157:135-44.

51. Penfold PL, Gyory JF, Hunyor AB, Billson FA. Exudative macular degeneration and intravitreal triamcinolone. A pilot study. Aust N Z J Ophthalmol 1995;23:293 98.

52. Challa JK, Gillies MC, Penfold PL, et al. Exudative macular degeneration and intravitreal triamcinolone: 18 month follow up. Aust New Zealand J Ophthalmol 1998; 26:277-81.

53. Danis RP, Ciulla TA, Pratt LM, Anliker W. Intravitreal triamcinolone acetonide in exudative age-related macular degeneration. Retina 2000; 20:244-50.

54. Degenring RF, Jonas JB. Photodynamic therapy in combination with intravitreal triamcinolone for myopic choroidal neovascularization. Acta Ophthalmol Scand. 2005; 83:621.

55. Jonas JB, Akkoyun I, Budde WM, et al. Intravitreal reinjection of triamcinolone for exudative age-related macular degeneration. Arch Ophthalmol 2004; 122:218-22.

56. Jonas JB, Kreissig I, Hugger P, et al. Intravitreal triamcinolone acetonide for exudative age related macular degeneration. Br J Ophthalmol 2003; 87:462-68.

57. Ranson NT, Danis RP, Ciulla TA, Pratt L. Intravitreal triamcinolone in subfoveal recurrence of choroidal neovascularization after laser treatment in macular degeneration. Br J Ophthalmol 2002; 86:527-29.

58. Jonas JB, Degenring RF, Kreissig I, et al. Exudative age-related macular degeneration treated by intravitreal triamcinolone acetonide. A prospective comparative nonrandomized study. Eye 2005;19:163-70.

59. Gillies MC, Simpson JM, Luo W, et al. A randomized clinical trial of a single dose of intravitreal triamcinolone acetonide for neovascular age-related macular degeneration: one-year results. Arch Ophthalmol 2003; 121:667-73.

60. Meyer CH, Lapolice DJ, Fekrat S. Functional changes after photodynamic therapy with verteporfin. Am J Ophthalmol 2005; 139:214-15.

61. Spaide RF, Sorenson J, Maranan L. Combined photodynamic therapy with verteporfin and intravitreal triamcinolone acetonide for choroidal neovascularization. Ophthalmology 2003; 110:1517-25.

62. Spaide RF, Sorenson J, Maranan L. Combined photodynamic therapy and intravitreal triamcinolone for nonsubfoveal choroidal neovascularization. Retina 2005;25: 685-90.

63. Spaide RF, Sorenson J, Maranan L. Photodynamic therapy with verteporfin combined with intravitreal injection of triamcinolone acetonide for choroidal neovascularization. Ophthalmology 2005; 112:301-04.

64. Spaide RF. Rationale for Combination Therapies for Choroidal Neovascularization. Am J Ophthalmol 2006; 141:149-56.

65. Treatment of Age-Related Macular Degeneration with Photodynamic Therapy (TAP) Study Group. Verteporfin therapy of subfoveal choroidal neovascularization in patients with age-related macular degeneration: additional information regarding baseline lesion composition's impact on vision outcomes - TAP report No. 3. Arch Ophthalmol 2002; 120:1443-54.

66. Krebs I, Binder S, Stolba U. A new treatment regimen in combined intravitreal injection of triamcinolone acetonide and photodynamic therapy. Graefes Arch Clin Exp Ophthalmol 2005; 6·1-5

67. Kroll P, Meyer CH. Which AMD-patient benefits from which therapy best? A comparison of different treatment approaches for vascular age-related macular degeneration [editorial]. Br J Ophthalmol 2006; 90:128-30.

68. Nicolo M, Ghiglione D, Lai S, et al. Occult with no classic choroidal neovascularization secondary to age-related macular degeneration treated by intravitreal triamcinolone and photodynamic therapy with verteporfin. Retina 2006; 26:58-64.

69. Rechtman E, Danis RP, Pratt LM, Harris A. Intravitreal triamcinolone with photodynamic therapy for subfoveal choroidal neovascularization in age related macular degeneration. Br J Ophthalmol 2004; 88:344-47.

70. Smithen LM, Spaide RF. Photodynamic therapy and intravitreal triamcinolone for a subretinal neovascularization in bilateral idiopathic juxtafoveal telangiectasis. Am J Ophthalmol 2004;138:884-86.

71. Gelisken F, Lafaut BA, Inhoffen W, et al. Clinicopathological findings of choroidal neovascularization following verteporfin photodynamic therapy. Br J Ophthalmol 2004; 88:207-11.

72. Grisanti S, Tatar O, Canbek S, et al. Immunohistopathologic evaluation of choroidal neovascular membranes following verteporfin-photodynamic therapy. Am J Ophthalmol 2004; 137:914-23.

73. Ciulla TA, Criswell MH, Danis RP, Hill TE. Intravitreal triamcinolone acetonide inhibits choroidal neovascularization in a laser-treated rat model. Arch Ophthalmol 2001;119:399-404.

74. Mennel S, Liu F, Meyer CH. Optical coherence tomography in photodynamic therapy. Br J Ophthalmol 2005; 89:928-29.

75. Mennel S, Meyer CH, Eggarter F, Peter S. Transient serous retinal detachment in classic and occult choroidal neovascularization after photodynamic therapy. Am J Ophthalmol 2005; 140:758-60.

76. Mennel S, Meyer CH, Schmidt JC, Rodrigues EB. Dreidimensionale Optische Kohärenz Tomographie (3D-OCT) zur Verlaufskontrolle von Makulaödemen nach intravitrealer Triamcinolon Applikation. Spektrum Augenheilkd. 2004;18: 48-54.

77. Mennel S, Meyer CH. Transient visual disturbance after photodynamic therapy. Am J Ophthalmol 2005; 139:748-49.

78. Mennel S, Peter S, Meyer CH, Thumann G. Effect of photodynamic therapy on the function of the outer blood-retinal barrier in an in vitro model. Graefes Arch Clin Exp Ophthalmol 2006; 19:1-7.

79. Mennel S, Rodrigues EB, Meyer CH, Schmidt JC. Macular edema induced by photodynamic therapy in age-related macular degeneration. Ocular Pharmacology and Therapeutics 2004; pp. 247-54.

80. Schmidt-Erfurth U, Michels S, Barbazetto I, Laqua H. Photodynamic effects on choroidal neovascularization and physiological choroid. Invest Ophthalmol Vis Sci 2002; 43:830-41.

81. Schmidt-Erfurth U. Advances in photodynamic therapy and antiangiogenic combination strategies. Acta Ophthalmol Scand 2004; 82:357.

82. Danis RP, Bingaman DP, Yang Y, Ladd B. Inhibition of preretinal and optic nerve head neovascularization in pigs by intravitreal triamcinolone acetonide. Ophthalmology 1996;103:2099-2104.

83. Schmidt-Erfurth U, Michels S, Augustin A. Perspectives on verteporfin therapy combined with intravitreal corticosteroids. Arch Ophthalmol 2006;124:561-63.

84. Augustin AJ, Schmidt-Erfurth U. Verteporfin and intravitreal triamcinolone acetonide combination therapy for occult choroidal neovascularization in age-related macular degeneration. Am J Ophthalmol 2006: 141:638-45.

85. Augustin AJ, Schmidt-Erfurth U. Verteporfin therapy combined with intravitreal triamcinolone in all types of choroidal neovascularization due to age-related macular degeneration. Ophthalmology. 2006; 113:14-22.

86. Adamis AP. Is diabetic retinopathy an inflammatory disease? Br J Ophthalmol 2002; 86:363-65.

87. Lu M, Perez LV, Ma N, et al. VEGF increases retinal vascular ICAM-1 expressionin vivo. Invest Ophthalmol Vis Sci 1999; 40:1808-12.

88. Joussen AM, Poulaki V, Mitsiades N, et al. Nonsteroidal anti-inflammatory drugs prevent early diabetic retinopathy via TNF-alpha suppression. FASEB J 2002; 16: 438-40.

89. Jonas JB, Hayler JK, Sofker A, Panda-Jonas S. Intravitreal injection of crystalline cortisone as adjunctive treatment of proliferative diabetic retinopathy. Am J Ophthalmol 2001; 131:468-71.

90. Congdon N, O'Colmain B, Klaver CC, et al, Eye Diseases Prevalence Research Group. Causes and prevalence of visual impairment among adults in the United States. Arch Ophthalmol 2004;122:477-85.

91. Jonas JB, Kreissig I, Kamppeter B, Degenring RF. Intravitreal triamcinolone acetonide for the treatment of intraocular edematous and neovascular diseases. Ophthalmologe 2004; 101:113-20.

92. Jonas JB. Intravitreal triamcinolone acetonide for treatment of intraocular oedematous and neovascular diseases. Acta Ophthalmol Scand 2005; 83:645-63.

93. Bonini-Filho MA, Jorge R, Barbosa JC, et al. Intravitreal injection versus sub-Tenon's infusion of triamcinolone acetonide for refractory diabetic macular edema: a randomized clinical trial. Invest Ophthalmol Vis Sci 2005; 46:3845-49.

94. Cardillo JA, Melo LA Jr, Costa RA, et al. Comparison of intravitreal versus posterior sub-Tenon's capsule injection of triamcinolone acetonide for diffuse diabetic macular edema. Ophthalmology 2005; 112:1557-63.

95. Jonas JB, Kreissig I, Sofker A, Degenring RF. Intravitreal injection of triamcinolone for diffuse diabetic macular edema. Arch Ophthalmol 2003; 121:57-61.

96. The Central Vein Occlusion Study Group. Evaluation of grid pattern photocoagulation for macular edema in central vein occlusion. The Central Vein Occlusion Study Group M report. Ophthalmology 1995; 102:1425-33.

97. Greenberg PB, Martidis A, Rogers AH, et al. Intravitreal triamcinolone acetonide for macular oedema due to central retinal vein occlusion. Br J Ophthalmol 2002; 86:247-48.

98. Jonas JB, Kreissig I, Degenring RF. Intravitreal triamcinolone acetonide as treatment of macular edema in central retinal vein occlusion. Graefes Arch Clin Exp Ophthalmol 2002; 240:782-83.

99. Bashshur ZF, Ma'luf RN, Allam S, et al. Intravitreal triamcinolone for the management of macular edema due to nonischemic central retinal vein occlusion. Arch Ophthalmol 2004; 122:1137-40.

100. Ip MS, Gottlieb JL, Kahana A, et al. Intravitreal triamcinolone for the treatment of macular edema associated with central retinal vein occlusion. Arch Ophthalmol 2004;122:1131-36.

101. Jonas JB, Akkoyun I, Kamppeter B, et al. Intravitreal triamcinolone acetonide for treatment of central retinal vein occlusion. Eur J Ophthalmol 2005;15:751-58.

102. Krepler K, Ergun E, Sacu S, et al. Intravitreal triamcinolone acetonide in patients with macular oedema due to central

retinal vein occlusion. Acta Ophthalmol Scand 2005; 83:71-75.

103. Park CH, Jaffe GJ, Fekrat S. Intravitreal triamcinolone acetonide in eyes with cystoid macular edema associated with central retinal vein occlusion. Am J Ophthalmol 2003; 136:419-25.

104. Ramezani A, Entezari M, Moradian S, et al. Intravitreal triamcinolone for acute central retinal vein occlusion; a randomized clinical trial. Graefes Arch Clin Exp Ophthalmol (In press).

105. Williamson TH, O'Donnell A. Intravitreal triamcinolone acetonide for cystoid macular edema in nonischemic central retinal vein occlusion. Am J Ophthalmol 2005; 139:860-66.

106. The Branch Vein Occlusion Study Group. Argon laser photocoagulation for macular edema in branch vein occlusion. The Branch Vein Occlusion Study Group. Am J Ophthalmol 1984; 98:271-82.

107. Degenring RF, Kamppeter B, Kreissig I, Jonas JB. Morphological and functional changes after intravitreal triamcinolone acetonide for retinal vein occlusion. Acta Ophthalmol Scand 2003; 81:399-401.

108. Ozkiris A, Evereklioglu C, Erkilic K, Ilhan O. The efficacy of intravitreal triamcinolone acetonide on macular edema in branch retinal vein occlusion. Eur J Ophthalmol 2005; 15:96-101.

109. Ozkiris A, Evereklioglu C, Erkilic K, Dogan H. Intravitreal triamcinolone acetonide for treatment of persistent macular oedema in branch retinal vein occlusion. Eye 2006; 20:13-17.

110. Jonas JB, Akkoyun I, Kamppeter B, et al. Branch retinal vein occlusion treated by intravitreal triamcinolone acetonide. Eye 2005; 19:65-71.

111. Chen SD, Lochhead J, Patel CK, Frith P. Intravitreal triamcinolone acetonide for ischaemic macular oedema caused by branch retinal vein occlusion. Br J Ophthalmol 2004; 88:154-55.

112. Chen SD, Sundaram V, Lochhead J, Patel CK. Intravitreal triamcinolone for the treatment of ischemic macular edema associated with branch retinal vein occlusion. Am J Ophthalmol 2006; 141:876-83.

113. Benhamou N, Massin P, Haouchine B, et al. Intravitreal triamcinolone for refractory pseudophakic macular edema. Am J Ophthalmol 2003; 135:246-49.

114. Conway MD, Canakis C, Livir-Rallatos C, Peyman GA. Intravitreal triamcinolone acetonide for refractory chronic pseudophakic cystoid macular edema. J Cataract Refract Surg 2003; 29:27-33.

115. Jonas JB, Kreissig I, Degenring RF. Intravitreal triamcinolone acetonide for pseudophakic cystoid macular edema. Am J Ophthalmol 2003; 136:384-86.

116. Young S, Larkin G, Branley M, Lightman S. Safety and efficacy of intravitreal triamcinolone for cystoid macular oedema in uveitis. Clin Experiment Ophthalmol 2001; 29:2-6.

117. Antcliff RJ, Spalton DJ, Stanford MR, et al. Intravitreal triamcinolone for uveitic cystoid macular edema: an optical coherence tomography study. Ophthalmology 2001;108:765-72.

118. Karacorlu M, Mudun B, Ozdemir H, et al. Intravitreal triamcinolone acetonide for the treatment of cystoid macular edema secondary to Behcet disease. Am J Ophthalmol 2004; 138:289-91.

119. Alldredge CD, Garretson BR. Intravitreal triamcinolone for the treatment of idiopathic juxtafoveal telangiectasis. Retina 2003; 23:113-16.

120. Martinez JA. Intravitreal triamcinolone acetonide for bilateral acquired parafoveal telangiectasis. Arch Ophthalmol 2003; 121:1658-59

121. Li KK, Goh TY, Parsons H, et al. Use of intravitreal triamcinolone acetonide injection in unilateral idiopathic juxtafoveal telangiectasis. Clin Experiment Ophthalmol 2005; 33:542-44

122. Jonas JB, Degenring RF, Kreissig I, et al. Intraocular pressure elevation after intravitreal triamcinolone acetonide injection. Ophthalmology. 2005;112:593-98.

123. Bakri SJ, Beer PM. The effect of intravitreal triamcinolone acetonide on intraocular pressure. Ophthalmic Surg Lasers Imaging 2003; 34:386-90.

124. Dwinger MC, Pieper-Bodeewes I, Eter N, Holz FG. Variations in intraocular pressure (IOP) and necessity for paracentesis following intravitreal triamcinolone injection. Klin Monatsbl Augenheilkd 2005; 222:638-42.

125. Smithen LM, Ober MD, Maranan L, Spaide RF. Intravitreal triamcinolone acetonide and intraocular pressure. Am J Ophthalmol 2004; 138:740-43.

126. Wingate RJ, Beaumont PE. Intravitreal triamcinolone and elevated intraocular pressure. Aust N Z J Ophthalmol 1999; 27:431-32.

127. Cekic O, Chang S, Tseng JJ, et al. Cataract progression after intravitreal triamcinolone injection. Am J Ophthalmol 2005; 139:993-98.

128. Gillies MC, Kuzniarz M, Craig J, et al. Intravitreal triamcinolone-induced elevated intraocular pressure is associated with the development of posterior subcapsular cataract. Ophthalmology 2005; 112:139-43.

129. Gillies MC, Simpson JM, Billson FA, et al. Safety of an intravitreal injection of triamcinolone: results from a randomized clinical trial. Arch Ophthalmol 2004;122:336-40.

130. Jonas JB, Degenring R, Vossmerbauemer U, Kamppeter B. Frequency of cataract surgery after intravitreal injection of high-dosage triamcinolone acetonide. Eur J Ophthalmol 2005; 15:462-64.

131. Thompson JT. Cataract formation and other complications of intravitreal triamcinolone for macular edema. Am J Ophthalmol 2006; 141:629-37.

132. Jonas JB, Kreissig I, Degenring RF. Cataract surgery after intravitreal injection of triamcinolone acetonide. Eye 2004; 18:361-64.

133. Dierks D, Lei B, Zhang K, Hainsworth DP. Electroretinographic effects of an intravitreal injection of triamcinolone in rabbit retina. Arch Ophthalmol 2005; 123:1563-69.

134. Jaffe GJ, Yang CH, Guo H, et al. Safety and pharmacokinetics of an intraocular fluocinolone acetonide sustained delivery device. Invest Ophthalmol Vis Sci 2000; 41:3569-75.

135. Jonas JB, Degenring R, Kreissig I, Akkoyun I. Safety of intravitreal high-dose reinjections of triamcinolone acetonide. Am J Ophthalmol 2004; 138:1054-55.

136. Kwak HW, D'Amico DJ. Evaluation of the retinal toxicity and pharmacokinetics of dexamethasone after intravitreal injection. Arch Ophthalmol 1992; 110:259-66.

137. Nabih M, Peyman GA, Tawakol ME, Naguib K. Toxicity of high-dose intravitreal dexamethasone. Int Ophthalmol 1991;15:233-35.

138. Soto-Pedre E. Purification of triamcinolone acetonide suspension for intravitreal injection. Br J Ophthalmol 2006; 90:123-24.

139. Enaida H, Sakamoto T, Ueno A, et al. Submacular deposition of triamcinolone acetonide after triamcinolone-assisted vitrectomy. Am J Ophthalmol 2003; 135:243-46.

140. Sakamoto T, Koga H, Noda Y, Ishibashi T. Optic disk cup filled with triamcinolone. Retina 2002; 22:516-18.

141. Szurman P, Kaczmarek R, Spitzer MS, et al. Differential toxic effect of dissolved triamcinolone and its crystalline deposits on cultured human retinal pigment epithelium (ARPE19) cells. Exp Eye Res; in press.

142. Kai W, Yanrong J, Xiaoxin L. Vehicle of triamcinolone acetonide is associated with retinal toxicity and transient increase of lens density. Graefes Arch Clin Exp Ophthalmol 2006; 2:1-8.

143. Morrison VL, Koh HJ, Cheng L, et al. Intravitreal toxicity of the kenalog vehicle (benzyl alcohol) in rabbits. Retina 2006; 26:339-44.

144. Jonas JB, Kreissig I, Spandau UH, Harder B. Infectious and noninfectious endophthalmitis after intravitreal high-dosage triamcinolone acetonide. Am J Ophthalmol 2006; 141:579-80.

145. Moshfeghi DM, Kaiser PK, Scott IU, et al. Acute endophthalmitis following intravitreal triamcinolone acetonide injection. Am J Ophthalmol 2003; 136:791-96.

146. Westfall AC, Osborn A, Kuhl D, et al. Acute endophthalmitis incidence: intravitreal triamcinolone. Arch Ophthalmol 2005; 123:1075-77.

147. Nelson ML, Tennant MT, Sivalingam A, et al. Infectious and presumed noninfectious endophthalmitis after intravitreal triamcinolone acetonide injection. Retina 2003; 23:686-91.

148. Roth DB, Chieh J, Spirn MJ, et al. Noninfectious endophthalmitis associated with intravitreal triamcinolone injection. Arch Ophthalmol 2003; 121:1279-82.

149. Moshfeghi DM, Kaiser PK, Bakri SJ, et al. Presumed sterile endophthalmitis following intravitreal triamcinolone acetonide injection. Ophthalmic Surg Lasers Imaging 2005; 36:24-29.

150. Chen SD, Lochhead J, McDonald B, Patel CK. Pseudohypopyon after intravitreal triamcinolone injection for the treatment of pseudophakic cystoid macular oedema. Br J Ophthalmol 2004; 88:843-44.

151. Jonas JB, Hayler JK, Panda-Jonas S. Intravitreal injection of crystalline cortisone as adjunctive treatment of proliferative vitreoretinopathy. Br J Ophthalmol 2000; 84:1064-67.

152. Reinhard T, Sundmacher R. Adjunctive intracameral application of corticosteroids in patients with endothelial immune reactions after penetrating keratoplasty: a pilot study. Transpl Int 2002; 15:81-88.

153. Jonas JB, Kreissig I, Degenring RF. Retinal complications of intravitreal injections of triamcinolone acetonide. Graefes Arch Clin Exp Ophthalmol 2004; 242:184-85.

154. Degenring RF, Sauder G. Vitreous prolapse and IOL dislocation during intravitreal injection of triamcinolone acetonide. Graefes Arch Clin Exp Ophthalmol 2005; 20:1-2.

13

Surgeries for Epiretinal Membrane, Vitreomacular Traction Syndrome, Idiopathic Macular Hole, Choroidal Neovascularization, Diabetic Macular Edema and Myopic Foveoschisis

Sandeep Saxena, Masahito Ohji,
Nancy M Holekamp, Matthew A Thomas

INTRODUCTION

Modern vitreous surgery through the pars plana is now one of the most effective tools for treating posterior segment disease. Macular pucker, vitreomacular traction syndrome, macular hole, subfoveal choroidal neovascular membrane, and submacular hematoma comprise the spectrum of macular disease. Innovative and exciting developments in the field of macular surgery offer promise to patients with these conditions that were previously thought to be incurable.

EPIRETINAL MEMBRANES

Epiretinal membranes are fine, nonvascular fibrotic membranes on the surface of the retina. They can cause a wrinkling or a puckering effect on the retinal surface, interfering with its function. These membranes can occur as a primary idiopathic disorder (Figure 13.1), as a limited form of proliferative vitreoretinopathy after successful retinal reattachment surgery (Figures 13.2A and B), or as an associated finding in numerous other ocular disorders.[1] Machemer first described the surgical removal of epiretinal membranes using pars plana vitrectomy.[2] Surgical intervention has proved to be beneficial to patients who experience significant visual loss related to epiretinal membranes.

In idiopathic epiretinal membranes, Roth and Foos[3] proposed that glial cells of retinal origin proliferate through

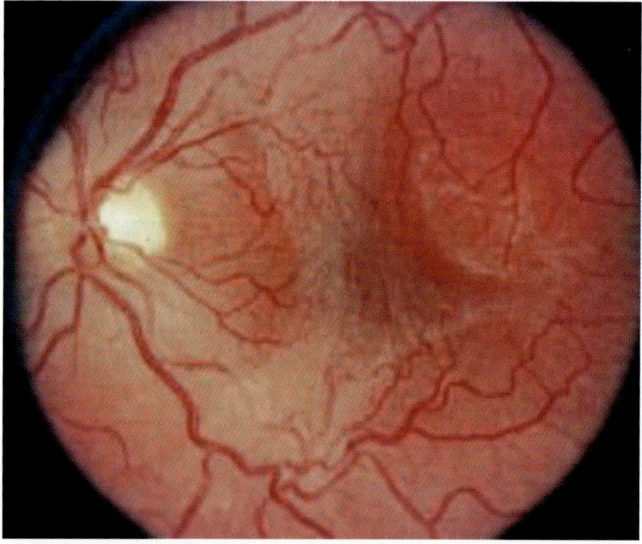

FIGURE 13.1: Idiopathic macular pucker.

defects in the internal limiting membrane. Bellhorn and associates[4] demonstrated that glial cells from the neurosensory retina migrating through breaks in the inner lamina were responsible for producing epiretinal membranes. These breaks were usually associated with posterior vitreous separation.[5] Vitreous detachment might contribute to the development of these membranes through several mechanisms. Vitreous detachment can lead to retinal breaks, liberating retinal pigment epithelial cells into the vitreous cavity, which can subsequently attach to the posterior retina and proliferate. Disruption

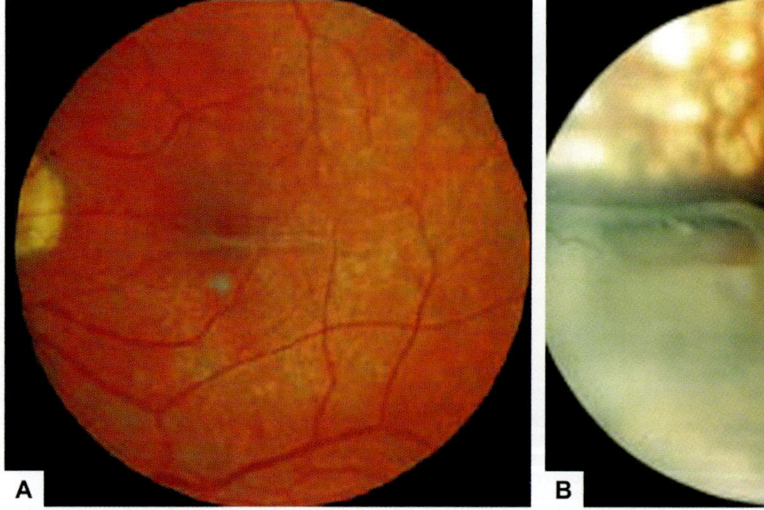
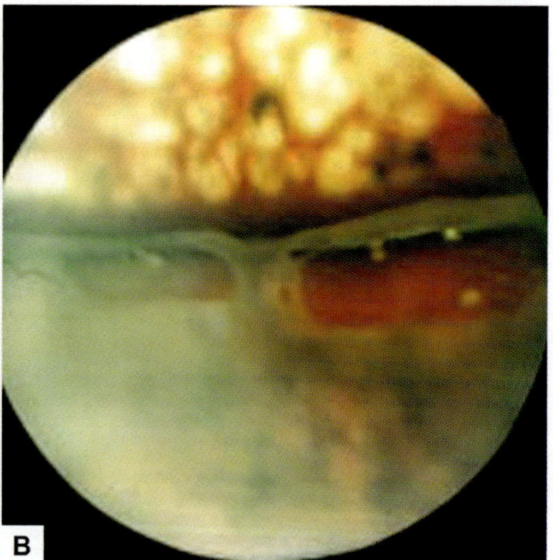

FIGURES 13.2A and B: (A) Macular pucker as a limited form of proliferative vitreoretinopathy.
(B) Open break on inferior buckle following successful retinal reattachment surgery.

of the internal limiting membrane at the time of posterior vitreous detachment could allow fibrous astrocytes access to the retinal surface to proliferate and create an extracellular matrix.[4,5] Vitreous hemorrhage, inflammation, or both at the time of vitreous detachment might stimulate cellular proliferation. In cases of epiretinal membrane formation before the vitreous detaches, glial cells may grow into the vitreous cavity. As the epiretinal membrane extends over the retina, a layer of vitreous is trapped against the inner limiting lamina. This relationship between the membrane and vitreous explains one mechanism by which spontaneous separation of epiretinal membranes could occur with subsequent vitreous separation.[6] Other cell types that contribute to epiretinal membrane formation include fibrocytes, myofibroblasts, macrophages, inflammatory cells, hyalocytes, retinal pigment epithelial cells, and vascular endothelial cells.[7-10] Significant amounts of collagen are present in all surgically removed membranes.[11] Once formed, both idiopathic and secondary epiretinal membranes behave similarly. After an initial period of growth and contraction, epiretinal membranes are morphologically and visually stable in approximately 90% of patients.

CLINICAL FEATURES

Visual symptoms from epiretinal membranes manifest as a continuum from no symptoms to severe visual dysfunction and are usually related to the severity of the membrane. In fact the majority of patients with idiopathic epiretinal membranes are asymptomatic.[12] When minimally symptomatic, patients usually complain of mild metamorphopsia, and visual acuity remains 20/40 or better indicating that only the inner retinal surface is involved. In eyes with marked distortion of the retina patients may have severe metamorphopsia and visual acuity of less than 20/200.[13-18] Less commonly, central photopsia, macropsia, or diplopia is noted.[19-23] The level of vision may also be related to preexisting retinal detachment.[18] In fact, vision is usually reduced further in eyes with epiretinal membranes that occur after retinal detachment.[24] Mechanisms for these symptoms include tissue covering or distorting macula, vascular leakage with cystoid macular edema, low-lying traction macular detachment, and obstructed axoplasmic flow.[25,26]

The clinical characteristics vary according to the degree of the membrane. Gass[19] has proposed a classification scheme for epiretinal membranes. Translucent membranes unassociated with retinal distortion are grade 0 (cellophane maculopathy). Membranes that cause irregular wrinkling of the inner retina are grade 1 (crinkled cellophane maculopathy). Opaque membranes that cause obscuration of the underlying vessels and marked full-thickness retinal distortion are grade 2 (macular pucker).

An asymptomatic patient may have a glinting, irregular light reflex caused by a subtle epiretinal membrane. These "cellophane membranes" usually do not have a distinct edge.

If the translucent membrane is more apparent, it can appear to cover the entire macula and even extend anteriorly beyond the vascular arcades. The full extent of an epiretinal membrane is best appreciated at the time of surgery, and sometimes idiopathic membranes can be stripped out past the equator.[12] When internal membrane "contraction" or "shrinkage" is observed, there is an associated tractional effect on the entire inner retina, which produces fine retinal striae radiating from the center of the membrane, and tortuosity of retinal vessels (Figure 13.3). However, the membrane can extend beyond the area of retinal striae. In more severe and visually debilitating epiretinal membranes, vascular tortuosity with tethering and straightening of vessels occurs distal to the center of membrane contraction[12] (Figure 13.4). If the membrane is centered distal to the macula, foveal ectopia can occur that causes complaints of diplopia. Occasionally, the epiretinal membrane lifts the sensory fovea off the retinal pigment epithelium in a subtle, shallow, tabletop manner. Cystoid macular edema may be present (Figures 13.5A and B). Pigmentation may also be present in the membrane. This may be caused by the presence of retinal pigment epithelial cells and occurs mainly in eyes with peripheral retinal breaks or a history of prior retinal detachment.[27-30] Studies have shown an especially high incidence (75 to 93%) of posterior vitreous detachment in eyes with idiopathic epiretinal membranes.[3,8,13-17,31-34] Partial or complete posterior vitreous detachment were also noted intraoperatively in 90% of eyes undergoing vitrectomy for idiopathic epiretinal membranes.[32]

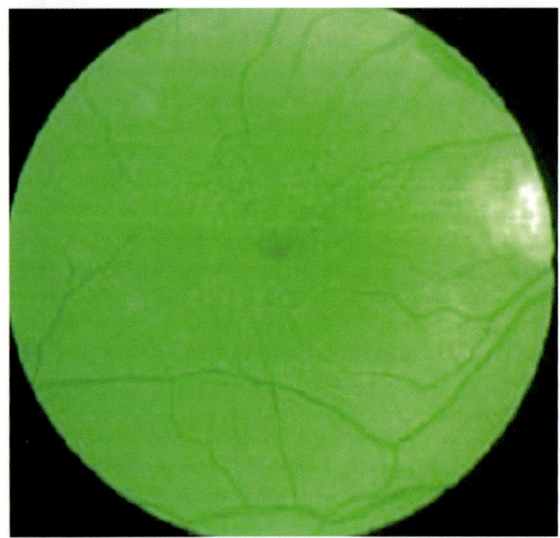

FIGURE 13.3: Red-free photograph demonstrates fine retinal striae radiating from center of membrane.

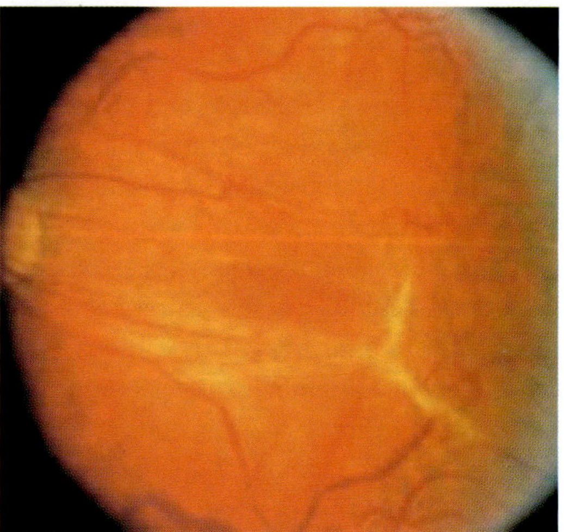

FIGURE 13.4: Tethering and straightening of retinal vessels occurs distal to the center of membrane contraction.

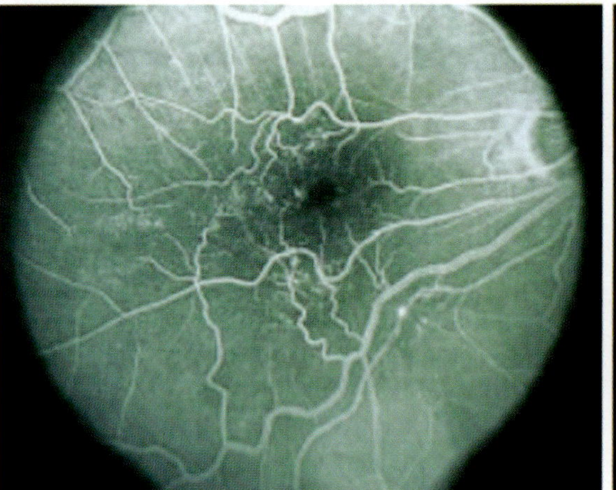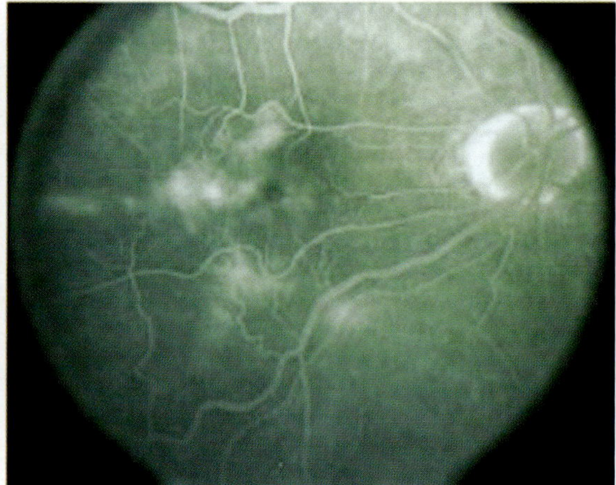

FIGURE 13.5A and B: (A) Retinal vascular tortuosity and capillary incompetence are seen in the early arteriovenous phase of fluorescein angiography. (B) Late frames of the angiogram demonstrate cystoid macular edema.

NATURAL HISTORY

The prevalence of epiretinal membranes varies with the underlying condition.[1] The majority of patients with symptomatic idiopathic epiretinal membranes are older than 50 years. Bilateral involvement occurs in 10 to 20% of cases.[14,16,34,35] Clinically significant epiretinal membranes affecting the macula occur in 4 to 8% of eyes after otherwise successful surgery for retinal detachment.[36-38] The prevalence of epiretinal membrane increases by 71.4% during the first 6 months after uneventful extracapsular cataract extraction with posterior chamber intraocular lens implantation. Thereafter, the prevalence remains about the same. Newly formed epiretinal membranes are probably induced by the uneventful surgery. Although new-onset membranes usually do not preclude good visual acuity, they can cause metamorphopsia postoperatively.[39] Most epiretinal membranes are stable after an initial period of growth and contraction.[21] Sidd and associates[15] in a study of 72 eyes with epiretinal membranes affecting the macula, found no change in the appearance of the membrane and the retina when reexamined an average of 31 months later. Seventy-three percent of the eyes maintained similar visual acuity during follow-up interval, and only rarely did vision improve or worsen markedly. Wiznia [16] found visual loss of 2 or more Snellen lines, in 6 (12%) of 47 eyes, during a follow-up interval averaging 38 months. Occasionally, spontaneous separation of epiretinal membrane from the retinal surface can result in improvement in visual acuity. [8,21,40-44] Such a phenomenon has been observed in eyes with idiopathic membranes,[21,40] membranes after retinal detachment[43] retinal vascular disorders,[44] and previous anterior segment surgery.[40] The observation of spontaneous separation of epiretinal membranes stimulated thinking that vitreous surgery might be used to peel these membranes from the retinal surface in selected cases.[2]

SURGICAL CASE SELECTION

No absolute criteria exist for recommending vitrectomy for epiretinal membrane. Indications depend mainly on the visual needs of each patient.[45,46] No form of treatment is known for mild epiretinal membranes.[1] The optimal time for removal of epiretinal tissue is probably 6 to 8 weeks after the eye becomes symptomatic.[1] Rapid progression is most common in cases with macular pucker after retinal detachment surgery. The epiretinal membrane is mature after 6 to 8 weeks and usually can be removed completely. In idiopathic cases, membrane growth is generally slow and surgery is recommended when the patient has substantial impairment of vision or severe metamorphopsia. The postoperative visual acuity may improve if the membrane has been present for a few months; however, the potential for improvement is reduced if the membrane has been present for an especially prolonged time. [25,47,48] Other preoperative prognostic factors regarding final visual acuity include preoperative vision and the presence of cystoid macular edema. Eyes with preoperative visual acuity of 20/70 or better have an improved postoperative visual acuity after vitrectomy for macular pucker. However, such eyes have been found to improve significantly fewer lines overall compared with those eyes with visual acuity of 20/80 or worse. [48,49] Therefore, unless the patient is seriously hampered by symptoms of metamorphopsia, vitrectomy for macular pucker is often not advocated unless the visual acuity is in the range of 20/70 or worse.[1,25,48] The

presence of preoperative retinal vascular leakage and cystoid macular edema has been found to correlate with less visual improvement postoperatively. [47-50] However, Margherio and associates [51] did not find any association between preoperative cystoid macular edema and lower postoperative vision. Removal of epiretinal membrane is usually associated with a later reduction in vascular leakage and retinal edema. [19,52,53]

SURGICAL TECHNIQUE

A conventional vitrectomy technique is used in the management of macular pucker. A complete posterior vitreous detachment is nearly always present. Sometimes the vitreous is not separated from the retina in young patients and in eyes with membranes associated with inflammatory conditions. The entire central vitreous gel is removed in aphakic and pseudophakic eyes. The anterior portion of central vitreous gel is spared in phakic eyes to decrease the possibility of trauma to the lens.[51] Previously operated eyes with relatively high scleral buckles must be approached cautiously to avoid tearing the retina protruding over the buckle.[49,51] The most accessible edge of the epiretinal membrane is engaged with a vitreoretinal pic. This is followed by a slight to-and-fro motion with gentle elevation (Figure 13.6). If there is no pre-existing elevation of the edge, the pic is

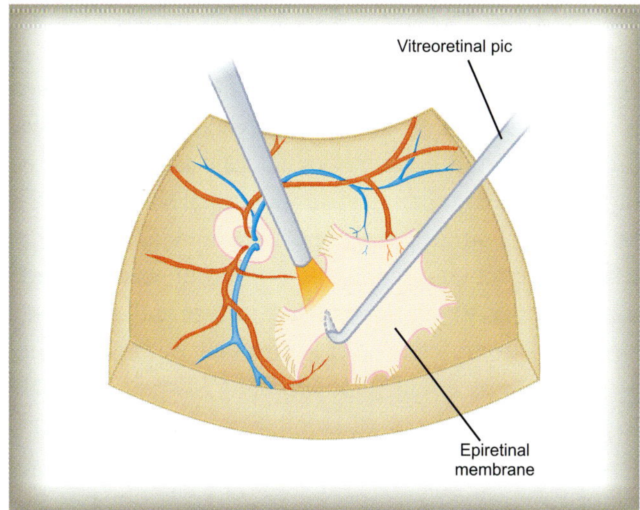

FIGURE 13.6: The most accessible edge of the epiretinal membrane is engaged with a vitreoretinal pic

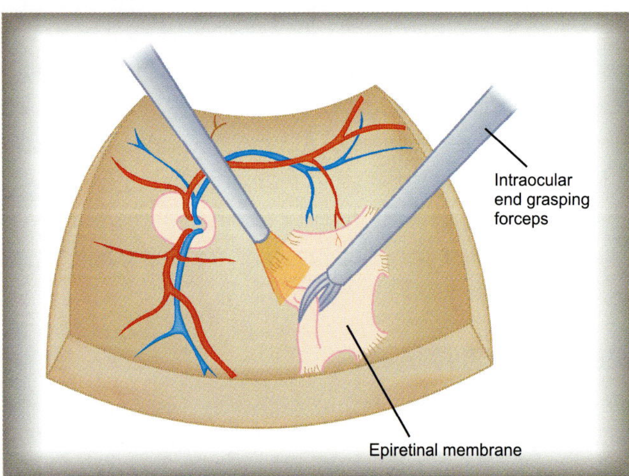

FIGURE 13.7: Epiretinal membrane is grasped with an intraocular forceps

used to apply centripetal traction on the membrane near its margin, until the edge becomes elevated.[1] Often radiating striae, present in the inner retina central to the margin of the membrane, aid in the identification of the edge. A barbed microvitreoretinal blade is often used to create a plane between the epiretinal membrane and internal limiting membrane. After the edge is identified and dissection started, a vitreoretinal pic is used to avoid fragmentation of the membrane. After a portion of the membrane has been separated from the retina, it is grasped with an intraocular forceps (Figure 13.7). The membrane is usually removed as a single piece, although it may be necessary to engage it sequentially to tease it from the retinal surface. If an abnormally firm area of attachment to the retina is encountered, the membrane is amputated with an intraocular scissors or a vitrectomy probe. Once the epiretinal membrane is removed, the underlying retina may have an abnormal sheen, and the inner retinal surface may appear wrinkled. Prominent whitening probably represents obstruction of retrograde axoplasmic flow in the inner retinal surface and disappears in 48 to 72 hours after surgery.[52] This change is important to recognize to avoid misinterpreting it intraoperatively as an additional layer of membrane. Petechial hemorrhages commonly occur along the inner retinal surface as the membrane is removed,[52] and denote that separation occurs at the level of the internal limiting membrane. Such minimal bleeding is usually self-limited,

but may require temporarily increased intraocular pressure by elevation of the infusion bottle. Finally, at the close of each vitrectomy the retina must be carefully inspected by indirect ophthalmoscopy with peripheral scleral depression to rule out iatrogenic peripheral retinal breaks at the time of surgery.

Trypan Blue-assisted Epiretinal Membrane Removal

Trypan blue concentration of 0.06% is obtained by further dilution of a commercially available 0.15% trypan blue solution (DORC, Dutch Ophthalmic Research Center, Zuidland, The Netherlands) with balanced salt solution (BSS Plus, Alcon Laboratories, Fort Worth, Texas, U.S.A). Then, 0.5 ml of a 0.06% trypan blue solution is dropped over the macula after fluid-air exchange or under continuous infusion over the posterior pole under direct visualization. After 1 minute the dye is removed. Visible epiretinal membrane is removed using an end-gripping forceps. If the retinal surface still has a glistening aspect without slight whitening as a sign of removed internal limiting membrane, the internal limiting membrane is incised and then peeled off using the end-gripping forceps.

Indocyanine Green-assisted Epiretinal Membrane Removal

Twenty-five milligrams of indocyanine green dye is reconstituted with 1.0 ml of sterile water. After the indocyanine green was completely dissolved, 4.0 ml of balanced salt solution is added to the solution to attain a final indocyanine green concentration of 0.5%. Then 0.6 to 0.8 ml of indocyanine green solution is instilled directly over the posterior pole using a 27-gauge blunt needle. The indocyanine green was left in the vitreous cavity for three minutes with scleral plugs in place. After removal of the indocyanine green with active suction, the internal limiting membrane is stained except in those areas where the epiretinal membrane is adherent to the internal limiting membrane. The staining is more intense in the posterior pole. The indocyanine green - stained internal limiting membrane is cut and peeled off in a circular fashion. As a result, the internal limiting membrane is removed together with the epiretinal membrane.

COMPLICATIONS

Retinal breaks occur peripherally in 4 to 6% of eyes[26,32,48,54,56] and near the macula in fewer than 1%.[14,29,35,37] Retinal detachment is reported to occur in 3 to 6% of cases.[26,45,47,51] It appears to be more common in patients with macular pucker after prior retinal detachment (7%)[53] than in those with idiopathic epiretinal membranes (1%).[2] The incidence of postoperative nuclear sclerosis of the crystalline lens is reported to range from 12 to 68%.[32,45-49,51,56] The rate of recurrent epiretinal membrane causing reduction in the best postoperative vision has been reported to range from 0 to 5%.[11,25,26,47,51,57] Recurrent membranes occur in both idiopathic epiretinal membrane (5%)[58] and macular pucker after retinal detachment (2.5%).[54] Intraoperative hemorrhage and retinal tears and postoperative progressive nuclear sclerosis, retinal tears causing detachments, macular edema and retinal pigmentary epitheliopathy have been reported.[59] Kim and associates[60] reported a case of visual field defect caused by damage of the nerve fiber layer associated with an internal limiting lamina defect after uneventful epiretinal membrane peeling. A nasal step and mild inferior arcuate scotoma developed without any associated glaucoma. Adhesion between epiretinal membrane and retinal tissue in the area of the internal limiting lamina defect may result in damage of the nerve fiber layer and visual field defect. Uemura and associates[61] reported visual field defects postoperatively, in four of seven eyes (57%) with indocyanine green-assisted internal limiting membrane peeling. None of the eyes without indocyanine green -assisted internal limiting membrane peeling had a visual field defect. They suggested that peripheral visual field defects might occur after vitrectomy with indocyanine green-assisted internal limiting membrane peeling.

The teratogenic and carcinogenic potential of trypan blue is well known.[62,63] In the animal studies, it was administered via intraperitoneal injection in dosages varying between 100 mg/kg and 300 mg/kg. However, for cataract surgery, trypan blue is injected locally at a dose of approximately 0.005 mg/kg. Peroperative use of trypan blue at a concentration of 0.1% in anterior chamber surgery for the vital staining of corneal endo-thelium did not produce ocular complication after an 8-year follow-up.[64] Trypan blue is also used to facilitate capsulorhexis during phacoemulsification procedures in the absence of a red fundus reflex.[65] No signs of toxicity were detected with light and electron microscopy after continuous exposure of 0.06% trypan blue to the retina for 1 month in an *in vivo* rabbit model.[66] Recently, trypan blue was also used successfully to stain epiretinal membranes during surgery for proliferative vitreoretinopathy.[67] No adverse reactions were observed up to 3 months after surgery

RESULTS

In patients who underwent surgery for idiopathic epiretinal membranes, postoperative vision improved at least two Snellen lines in 78 to 87% of eyes.[2,52,55,61] In the series of de Bustros and associates,[54] vision was unchanged in 9% and worse in 4% of the eyes. In patients who underwent surgery for macular pucker after prior retinal tear or retinal detachment, vision improved at least two Snellen lines in 63 to 100% of eyes.[3,31] In a series of 119 eyes reported by Clarkson and associates,[31] 104 eyes (88%) had visual improvement, 8 eyes (7%) had no change in vision, and 7 eyes (5%) had loss of vision. No difference was seen in the rate of improvement based on whether or not the macula had been damaged by the prior detachment, but the level of final visual acuity was substantially better if the macula had not been detached.[1] Less frequently, vision returns to normal after surgical removal of epiretinal membrane. Margherio and associates,[51] in their series of 184 eyes with idiopathic epiretinal membranes, reported final visual acuity of 20/30 or better in 14% of eyes and 20/50 or better in 44% of eyes. In the series of de Bustros and associates,[54] only 2% of eyes achieved final visual acuity of 20/20, and 22% had final visual acuity of 20/40 or better. Fifteen (28%) of 51 eyes obtained final visual acuity of 20/40 or better if the macula was not detached previously, whereas 9 (16%) of 52 eyes achieved a similar level of visual acuity if the macula was involved by prior detachment. McDonald and associates,[45] in their series of 33 eyes, reported a mean preoperative visual acuity of 20/100 and a mean postoperative visual acuity of 20/50. Pesin and associates [46] reported the largest series of 270 eyes treated with pars plana vitrectomy and membrane peeling. Visual improvement of two or more lines was achieved in 58% of eyes at 3 to 5 years. In addition to visual changes, metamorphopsia is frequently reduced postoperatively. This cannot be quantitated easily.

Trypan blue (0.06%) stained both internal limiting membrane and epiretinal membrane and might be a useful tool in vitreoretinal surgery. Trypan blue might be especially applicable in cases in which the borders of the epiretinal membrane are difficult to define. [68-71] However, according to Rodrigues and associates[72] and Meyer and associates[73] trypan blue stains the epiretinal membrane but not the internal limiting membrane. Staining of internal limiting membrane during macular pucker surgery may not have deleterious effects.[74,75] Indocyanine green-assisted surgery for macular pucker might have an adverse effect on functional outcome.[76] Indocyanine green helps in distinguishing posterior vitreous from internal limiting membrane. [77,78] Negative indocyanine green staining of epiretinal membrane has also been reported. Internal limiting membrane is stained except in those areas where the epiretinal membrane is adherent to the internal limiting membrane.[79]

The development or progression of postoperative nuclear sclerosis is the most common complication of successful vitrectomy in elderly patients.[80,81] Saito and associates[80] treated idiopathic epiretinal membrane with non-vitrectomizing vitreous surgery in an attempt to prevent postoperative nuclear sclerosis. Neither intravitreal infusion nor vitrectomy of any kind was performed during the procedure. There was no difference in the rate of development or progression of nuclear sclerosis or the degree of myopic shift between operated and control eyes during the postoperative follow-up period of 9 months. Simultaneous cataract surgery and vitrectomy for idiopathic epiretinal membrane removal results in visual improvement in the majority of patients.[82] The characteristics of epiretinal membrane in young patients are quite different in many cases from those in adults in terms of thickness and adherence. Removal of epiretinal membrane in young patients is feasible and safe although the membrane may focally adhere strongly to retinal vessels. Visual acuity is usually improves significantly after surgery, but recurrences are more frequent than in adults.[83] After surgery for idiopathic epiretinal membranes combined with pseudohole, visual outcome is good, and pseudohole has no adverse prognostic value. Pseudohole disappears inconstantly after surgery, but its persistence does not preclude good postoperative visual recovery.[84]

ROLE OF OPTICAL COHERENCE TOMOGRAPHY

Optical coherence tomograms were correlates with visual acuity, slit-lamp biomicroscopy, fluorescein angiography, and fundus photography. Based on optical coherence tomography, the epiretinal membrane was clearly separated from the retina with focal points of attachment or globally adherent (no observed separation). Optical coherence tomography was able to provide a structural assessment of the macula that was useful in the preoperative and postoperative evaluation of epiretinal membrane surgery. Quantitative measurements and the assessment of membrane adherence with optical coherence tomography may be useful in characterizing the surgical prognosis of eyes with an epiretinal membrane.[85] Epiretinal membranes may be partially separated from the macula, with tractional focal point(s) of attachment to the macular region or totally adherent to the macular region. The membranes were barely visible by optical coherence tomography or not visible in few cases. Intraoperatively, the surgeon was guided in the peeling procedures. A significant correlation was found between visual acuity and macular thickness before surgery and at the end of the postoperative follow-up. Optical coherence tomography images provide very useful information for the surgical indication, intraoperative management and postoperative outcome of patients.[86] Macular thickness decreases after epiretinal membrane surgery, but the macular profile rarely returns to normal.[87] There was a significant difference in the pattern of membrane attachment to the retina in idiopathic epiretinal membranes with those of secondary epiretinal membranes. [88] Secondary epiretinal membranes are more likely to be characterized by focal retinal adhesion than are primary epiretinal membranes. Primary epiretinal membranes tend to be globally adherent.

VITREOMACULAR TRACTION SYNDROME

Vitreomacular traction syndrome has been described as a distinct clinical entity.[1] This syndrome comprises a broad spectrum of easily missed clinical findings, ranging from total peripheral vitreous separation with residual foveal attachment to multiple areas of subtle traction retinal detachment caused by persistent, focal, posterior, and peripheral vitreous attachment.[8,18,20,89-94] The vitreomacular traction syndrome may represent a subset of idiopathic macular pucker (one without complete posterior vitreous detachment) and it may very well represent a premacular hole condition (albeit with low risk).[95] Because it has features that distinguish it from these entities, it deserves separate recognition.[96] The hallmark of vitreomacular traction syndrome is persistent anterior to posterior traction on the macula via a directly observable, persistent vitreoretinal attachment. The vitreous attachment margin can be observed because it is separated peripherally. This allows sharp contrast between the linear profiles formed by the vitreous and optically clear post-vitreous fluid. The attachment most commonly includes a one- to six-disk area zone centered on the fovea. It is usually contiguous with the optic nerve head, yielding a horizontally oriented oval or hourglass configuration of the margins. The zone of vitreous attachment also includes premacular tissue that mimics a macular pucker. The cystic macular changes stain with fluorescein and the extent of premacular tissue approximates the zone of persistent vitreous attachment.[95]

The pathogenesis of vitreomacular traction syndrome is unknown. Two possible sequences may occur. Firstly, completion of subsequent vitreous separation may be prevented by epiretinal cellular proliferation. Secondly, an incomplete vitreous separation may lead to epiretinal membrane proliferation. The latter sequence seems more likely, because the visual loss tends to be progressive and the macular tissue has been observed in some cases to increase in size and extent with further follow-up.[95] At the time of age-related vitreous syneresis and posterior vitreous detachment, the vitreous remains attached to the posterior pole. Some individuals have an unusually strong attachment between the posterior vitreous cortex, macula, and peripapillary retina.[97-100] Vitreous cortex remnants have been found at the fovea after spontaneous vitreous detachment, which possibly indicates some degree of vitreoretinal adhesion that may not have been lysed during posterior vitreous separation.[101] This supports the concept that during posterior vitreous detachment the cortical vitreous can remain attached to the posterior pole and cause traction on the macula. The occurrence of macular pucker after vitreous separation in the vitreomacular traction syndrome can result from traction-induced stimulation of proliferative cells or it may be caused by proliferation of hyalocytes stranded within persistent vitreous surface strands.[8] Transmission electron microscopy of removed epimacular tissue specimens has shown glial and contractile elements.[99] Reese and associates[102] demonstrated the cystic histopathologic macular changes associated with vitreomacular traction syndrome. Another histopathologic study reported a case of macular macrocystic changes in association with persistent vitreoretinal adhesion.[103]

CLINICAL FEATURES

The age, symptoms, and clinical appearance of patients with vitreomacular traction syndrome are similar to those with idiopathic macular pucker. The symptoms include decreased vision, metamorphopsia, and monocular diplopia. The visual symptoms may worsen gradually because persistent traction causes retinal vascular incompetence, leakage, and cystic degeneration. Alternatively, spontaneous release of the traction can occur, resulting in visual improvement. Reported cases of spontaneous peeling of an epiretinal membrane[41,43,104,105] may actually be cases in which the vitreous detachment progressed to completion and pulled the epiretinal tissue along with it. Contact lens examination of the posterior pole may show subtle areas of traction retinal detachment, cystic macular changes, retinal striae, a thickened posterior hyaloid face, an epiretinal membrane, and tractional changes on the optic nerve head. Persistent posterior vitreous attachment is best seen at the posterior margin of the vitreous attachment. The characteristic area of residual posterior vitreous attachment and remacular tissue often involves a horizontally oriented, dumbbell-shaped area that encircles the macula and optic nerve head. Peripapillary vitreous traction appears as a ring of fibrous adherence lying on the optic nerve surface, the "fleshy doughnut" sign. [106] McDonald and associates [106] categorized eyes anatomically as having either "classic" vitreomacular syndrome (eyes with 360° midperipheral vitreous detachment) or "variable" vitreomacular traction syndrome (eyes with a variety of midperipheral areas of vitreous separation). There is a variable amount of fibrous proliferation ranging from a diffuse cellophane-like macular appearance in mild cases to more discrete, heavy fibrous bands in more severe cases. [95] Although rare, persistent vitreomacular traction can lead to low-traction retinal detachment. Two reported cases of idiopathic traction retinal detachment without posterior vitreous detachment may represent such a case of severe vitreomacular traction syndrome. [107] Although the retina can be surgically attached in these cases, visual improvement may be limited by chronic detachment, premacular fibrosis, cystoid macular edema, or macular schisis.[108] Cystic changes in the macula are seen more frequently than in idiopathic macular pucker. Fluorescein leakage has been observed more frequently than for idiopathic macular pucker [17,89] (Figure 13.8). However, many cases may not show leakage. [90] An association with

vitreous cells and a higher prevalence in phakic patients has been noted.[8,90]

NATURAL HISTORY

Jaffe [8,90] reported visual acuity that ranged from 20/25 to 20/70 in patients with the vitreomacular traction syndrome. The series of Smiddy and associates [89] represented patients who underwent surgery and thus their reported preoperative visual acuities were worse, ranging from 20/40 to 20/300. Two of the 16 fellow eyes had macular abnormalities, including epiretinal membrane and lamellar macular hole. Jaffe [90] reported spontaneous release of the vitreoretinal adhesion, with moderate improvement in vision and symptoms in 5 of 10 patients usually within 2 weeks, although it occurred in one patient 5 months after presentation. Hikichi and associates [109] reported the natural history of vitreoretinal traction syndrome in 53 consecutive symptomatic eyes. Of the 81% of eyes with cystoid macular changes at the initial diagnostic examination, 67% had cystoid changes that persisted during the median follow-up period of 60 months. In 64% of all eyes, visual acuity at the time of final examination decreased two Snellen lines or more from the initial measurement, and complete posterior vitreous detachment developed in 11% of eyes. The number of eyes with resolved cystoid changes or stable visual acuity was significantly higher when complete vitreomacular separation occurred.

SURGICAL CASE SELECTION

Correctly diagnosing the vitreomacular traction syndrome allows the surgeon to inform the patient of prognosis and therapy. Idiopathic macular pucker can mimic vitreomacular traction syndrome because epiretinal membrane formation is common and vitreous insertion into the retinal surface may be difficult to observe. The relation of the vitreous to the retina, even in cases with epimacular proliferation, is the predominant feature that separates idiopathic macular pucker from vitreomacular traction syndrome.[95] In true epiretinal membranes, posterior vitreous separation is almost always present.[110] Another diagnostic difficulty lies in differentiating vitreomacular traction syndrome from impending macular

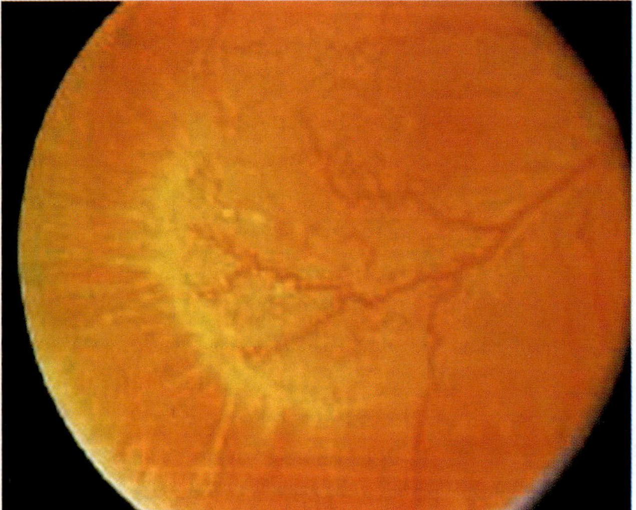

FIGURE 13.8: The margin of persistent vitreous attachment in the inferotemporal macula is easily seen.

hole.[92,111] The main distinguishing feature is observation of direct vitreomacular traction. Visual acuity is typically better in stage I macular hole than it is in vitreomacular traction syndrome, although patients with mild cases of vitreomacular traction syndrome may have good vision. Central serous chorioretinopathy and cystoid macular edema can also mimic vitreomacular traction syndrome. The distinguishing features between these clinical entities can usually be best observed with contact lens and biomicroscopy.

SURGICAL TECHNIQUE

A standard three-port vitrectomy is performed to remove anterior to posterior vitreous traction. In cases with formed vitreous membranes, the posterior hyaloid is identified and elevated in an "en bloc" fashion using a vitreoretinal pic or a bent needle. Subsequently, the posterior hyaloid is removed along with any contiguous preretinal tissue. Special care is taken to avoid direct macular trauma. Frequently, it is impossible to determine the vitreoretinal relationship preoperatively. The vitreoretinal relationship can be determined intraoperatively using oblique intraocular illumination, noting the effect of gentle tractional forces on the macula. During surgery, Margherio and associates[91] divided the elements of vitreomacular traction into three types. Type 1 vitreomacular traction (noted in 73% of eyes) consists of tangential traction alone. Type 2 vitreomacular traction syndrome (noted in 19% of the eyes) is of anteroposterior variety. Type 3 (noted in 8% of eyes) is a combination of types 1 and 2. This classification has not been widely advocated, however.

COMPLICATIONS

Complications of vitreous surgery for vitreomacular traction syndrome include accelerated nuclear sclerosis,[91,106] epiretinal membrane formation,[106] retinal breaks,[106] retinal detachment, and macular holes.[91]

RESULTS

Smiddy and associates[89] reported improvement in Snellen visual acuity by two lines or more in 10 of 16 eyes. The final visual acuity was 20/70 or better in 9 of 16 eyes.

McDonald and associates[106] reported improvement in vision of two or more lines in 75% of eyes, with 40% obtaining 20/50 visual acuity or better. Melberg and associates[108] reported their experience with vitrectomy for vitreomacular traction syndrome with macular detachment. In seven of nine eyes (78%), the macula was attached after surgery. Visual acuity improved in four eyes and became worse in one eye.

IDIOPATHIC MACULAR HOLE

Recent advances in the pathogenesis, classification, and surgical intervention of idiopathic macular holes have generated a renewed interest in this entity. Better indicators of visual outcome as well as refinements in the surgical technique have led to improvements in the success of macular hole surgery.

Clinical characterization and theories on the pathogenesis of macular hole have continued to evolve.[112] Although originally thought to be the result of trauma,[113] it is now recognized that most macular holes occur in the absence of antecedent injury and are referred to as idiopathic. Theories for the pathogenesis of idiopathic macular holes have included progressive thinning of the foveal tissue[114] and prehole cyst formation.[115,116] The primary pathogenic role of the vitreous was suggested by studies that indicated a low relative risk for macular hole formation in eyes with complete posterior vitreous detachment.[114,115,117] Gass[92] and Gass and Johnson[111] proposed a theory whereby shrinkage of adherent cortical vitreous and subsequent tangential vitreous traction first cause a circumscribed foveolar detachment (stage I) followed by early retinal dehiscence (stage II), then enlargement of the macular hole with vitreofoveal separation (stage III) and finally complete posterior vitreous detachment (stage IV). Guyer and Green[118] proposed three mechanisms of tangential traction on the macula, including fluid movements and counter currents, cellular remodeling of cortical vitreous, and contraction of a cellular membrane on the inner surface of the tapered cortical vitreous. Gass[92] emphasized the difficulty in distinguishing posterior vitreous detachment from a zone of posterior vitreous liquefaction and attached posterior cortical vitreous over the macula. He also emphasized that unless the posterior cortical vitreous contains the vitreous condensation ring (Weiss' ring) over the optic nerve, an operculum, or a pseudo-operculum, the diagnosis of posterior vitreous detachment is uncertain. Smiddy and associates [119] discovered the presence of a thin transparent structure adherent to the retina during vitrectomy for prevention of macular holes and provided a correlate to Gass' hypothesis. Results of histopathologic examination of the excised tissue confirmed its vitreous nature.[120] Kishi and Shimizu [121] described a posterior precortical vitreous pocket in older patients with a layer of cortical vitreous over the macula. Kishi and associates[122] proposed tractional elevation of Henle's fiber layer with intraretinal cyst formation as the initial feature

of macular hole development. Gordon and associates[123] reported five cases of full-thickness macular hole formation in eyes with a pre-existing, complete, posterior vitreous detachment and concluded that in these instances, some mechanism other than tangential traction by prefoveal vitreous cortex was responsible.

CLINICAL FEATURES

Idiopathic macular holes occur most frequently in the sixth decade of life. Table 13.1 summarizes the biomicroscopic findings of various stages of macular hole.[124] According to Gass,[124] stage IA and IB lesions represent focal foveal detachments secondary to vitreous traction. A 100 to 200 μm diameter yellow spot is the earliest

Table 13.1: Biomicroscopic classification of idiopathic macular hole

Stages	Biomicroscopic findings	Anatomic interpretation
IA (impending hole)	Central yellow spot Loss of foveolar depression No vitreofoveolar separation	Early serous detachment of foveolar retina
IB (impending or occult hole)	Yellow ring with bridging interface Loss of foveolar depression No vitreofoveolar separation	For small ring, serous foveolar detachment with lateral displacement of xanthophyll; for larger ring, central occult foveolar hole with centrifugal displacement of foveolar retina and xanthophyll, with bridging contracted prefoveolar vitreous cortex
II	Eccentric oval, crescent, or horseshoe retinal defect inside edge of yellow ring Central round retinal defect Rim of elevated retina — with prefoveolar opacity — without prefoveolar opacity	Hole (tear) in contracted prefoveolar vitreous bridging round retinal hole, no loss of foveolar retina Hole with pseudo-operculum[a], rim of retinal detachment Hole, no posterior vitreous detachment from optic disk and macula
III	Central round ≥400 µm diameter retinal defect No Weiss' ring, Rim of elevated retina — with prefoveolar opacity — without prefoveolar opacity	Hole with pseudo-operculum, no posterior vitreous detachment Hole with no posterior vitreous detachment from optic disk and macula
IV	Central round retinal defect, rim of elevated retina, Weiss' ring — with prefoveolar opacity[b] — without prefoveolar opacity	Hole with pseudo-operculum and posterior vitreous detachment from optic disk and macula Hole and posterior vitreous detachment from optic disk and macula

[a] Pseudo-operculum contains no retinal receptors.
[b] Prefoveolar opacity usually found near temporal border of Weiss' ring.
Source: Modified from Gass JDM. Reappraisal of biomicroscopic classification of stages of development of a macular hole. Am J Ophthalmol 1995;119:752-9.

change observed. With progression, a 200 to 350 μm yellowish ring develops. Fine radiating striae are often seen surrounding the yellow ring. The vision is in the range of 20/25 to 20/70. Within several weeks to months, a full-thickness dehiscence develops. This dehiscence often starts eccentrically, and then opens in a "can-opener" fashion to form a crescentic retinal defect, then a horseshoe-shaped hole, and finally a round hole with an operculum. In some cases, the dehiscence starts centrally, with gradual enlargement of the hole, and no operculum develops. A ring of retinal detachment usually surrounds the hole. As the hole enlarges, the vision generally decreases and within several months it progresses to a fully developed hole that measures approximately 500 μm in diameter. When present, the operculum is suspended over the hole by the detached vitreous cortex. With time, round yellow deposits on the central retinal pigment epithelium, epiretinal membranes that cause contracture of the internal limiting membrane, depigmentation of the pigment epithelium under the cuff of retinal elevation, and a pigmentary demarcation ring defining the outer margin of the retinal detachment may be observed. Vision is usually in the range of 20/70 to 20/400. Posterior vitreous separation from the macula and disk develops in a small percentage of cases. Eyes with idiopathic macular hole lose vision secondary to tissue dehiscence, cystic changes, and retinal cuff elevation with photoreceptor degeneration. Clinical observations have led to the impression that the macular hole and cuff enlarge secondary to persistent tangential traction from the vitreous, tangential traction from epiretinal membranes, and the development of large cystic spaces within the surrounding cuff.[125]

NATURAL HISTORY

The natural history of idiopathic macular hole is well established. Idiopathic macular holes usually lead to a decrease in visual acuity in the range of 20/100 to 20/400.[111,114,115,126-130] Histopathologic studies[131,132] have shown variable photoreceptor degeneration around the hole suggesting the inability to support good vision. However, characterization of visual status using scanning laser ophthalmoscope indicates that good visual function may persist at the edge of the hole. Aaberg[127] noted vision of 20/100 to 20/400 in 80% of 73 eyes, with nearly half at a level of 20/200. McDonnell and associates[115] observed vision of 20/100 to 20/400 in most of their 17 eyes. Morgan and Schatz[114] reported vision of 20/100 to 20/400 in 60% of 132 eyes and 20/80 or better vision in 30%. Yuzawa and associates[133] observed that the incidence of apparent disappearance of idiopathic full-thickness macular holes was low. Improvement in visual acuity was greater in those cases in which macular holes disappeared in a relatively short period of time. Kakehashi and associates[134] found that foveal detachment and macular break resolution seem to result from the release or weakening of vitreous traction on the fovea. Reattachment of the fovea preserves fair to good visual acuity. Hikichi and associates[135] noted progression of stage II lesions to stage III and IV in 67% and 29% of eyes, respectively. They concluded that even though vitreomacular separation can improve the prognosis of a macular hole, stage II lesions usually will develop an enlarged hole and decreased visual acuity. Fisher and associates[136] suggested that fellow eyes in patients with unilateral idiopathic macular holes have a relatively favorable natural history and that kinetic ultrasound examination can help determine which of these fellow eyes is at highest risk of full-thickness macular hole developing. Akiba and associates[137] found that 10 (37%) of 27 eyes that had an impending macular hole without vitreous separation from the fovea progressed to a fully developed macular hole. Akiba and associates[138] also reported that 14 fellow eyes (37%) of 38 eyes with stage I macular hole or unilateral full-thickness macular hole went on to development of full-thickness macular hole. Guyer[139] reported that only 2 of 19 (10.5%) of the premacular hole lesions in their series progressed to macular hole formation. A resolved flat, reddish lesion was observed in 15 of 19 (79%) of their patients. Kokame and associates[140] found that eyes with stage I macular holes with best corrected visual acuity between 20/50 and 20/80 had a 66% risk of progression to full-thickness macular hole, whereas eyes with best corrected visual acuity between 20/25 and 20/40 had a 30% risk of progression to full-thickness macular hole. The Vitrectomy for Macular Hole Study Group [141] has recently reported the baseline characteristics, natural history, and risk factors for progression in eyes with stage II macular holes. Forty-one eyes (37 patients) were analyzed; 19 eyes were randomized to observation (vs. surgery). Mean Snellen visual acuity was 20/66 at baseline. Centric stage II holes usually had a small break (201 μm average diameter) with a dark yellow ring and without significant retinal elevation. Eccentric stage II holes had a high maximum/minimum diameter ratio and an incomplete cuff of subretinal fluid or yellow ring. Posterior vitreous detachment prevalence was 32% (8/25) and 0% (0/16) in the centric and eccentric hole groups, respectively. Progression rate to stage III or IV was 74%. Progression rate to stage III was 100% in eyes with pericentral hyperfluorescence and 55% in eyes without pericentral hyperfluorescence. Enlargement occurred in 100% of eccentric holes and 60% of centric holes. This group concluded that eccentric and centric holes might have a different pathogenesis. In addition to purely tangential traction, some component of obliquely oriented anteroposterior vitreous traction component may be important for pathogenesis of senile macular holes, particularly stage II eccentric macular holes. Epiretinal membranes are common in eyes with full-thickness idiopathic macular holes. Although epiretinal membrane prevalence increases with severity and size of the macular hole, the presence of epiretinal membrane are not closely correlated with visual acuity. These factors may be important in considering the removal of epiretinal membrane during vitrectomy for macular hole.[142]

Macular hole reopening is reported to occur in 9.5% of cases. The cause of reopening might have been any anatomic stress such as epiretinal membrane formation or macular edema. However, in most of the reopened cases, no definite cause is evident.[143]

Stage I macular holes can initially be observed. However, excellent visual and surgical results can be obtained in stage I holes with poor vision, or with acute progression to full-thickness holes.[144]

SURGICAL CASE SELECTION

Many conditions that mimic macular holes have a favorable natural course and require different surgical maneuvers or are not amenable to surgical intervention. Premacular hole lesions are often misdiagnosed [145,146] and many conditions can masquerade as full-thickness macular holes. [147] An epiretinal membrane with a pseudohole can be confused with a macular hole. The pseudohole usually allows better vision than does the macular hole. In addition, the pseudohole does not have a halo of fluid, an operculum, or yellow deposits at the level of retinal pigment epithelium. A foveal detachment due to central serous retinopathy can be mistaken for a stage Ia macular hole. Both appear as a yellow spot; however, fluorescein angiography can distinguish these two entities. Central serous retinopathy occurs in young to middle-aged men, whereas idiopathic macular holes usually affect elderly women. Cystoid macular edema can also mimic the yellow spot of a stage I lesion. Fluorescein angiography and a history of cataract extraction can be useful in differentiating between these two conditions. The early yellow lesion of solar retinopathy can also appear similar to a stage I lesion. A central drusen or retinal pigment epithelium depigmentation with a small amount of subretinal fluid and a central fibrocellular epiretinal membrane with a macular detachment have been described as mimicking an impending macular hole. The vitreomacular traction syndrome can mimic an impending macular hole. Vitreous traction on the macula due to an incomplete vitreous detachment is responsible for this lesion. These disorders can be distinguished by examination of the vitreous.

A full-thickness macular hole is most accurately diagnosed clinically using a fundus contact lens and slit lamp biomicroscopy. Supplemental tests that can assist in or allow for more accurate diagnosis include Amsler grid testing,[148] testing for a Watzke-Allen sign,[149] and fluorescein angiography. Amsler grid testing is sensitive in detecting any form of macular abnormality, but is not specific enough to be useful in establishing a diagnosis of macular hole, and preoperative testing has not been standardized. [150] The Watzke-Allen test and to a greater degree the laser-aiming beam test further improve the accuracy of diagnosis of full thickness macular holes. The major advantage of these tests is that they are simple to perform, can be done in the office, and are easily accessible.[150] Watzke-Allen sign testing in all patients with clinically defined macular holes shows a break or thinning of the slit beam. Thinning of the beam is seen in both macular hole and pseudomacular hole cases. Therefore, thinning is not as specific as a total break in the slit beam in full-thickness macular hole. The laser-aiming beam test may yield similar diagnostic information, allowing the clinician to test focal areas of the retina for a scotoma. A 50 μ spot laser-aiming beam can be hidden in the macular lesion in all patients with clinically defined full-thickness macular hole. This contrasts with the finding in pseudohole eyes, which could detect the 50 μ spot. In addition, the inability to detect a 200 or 500 μ spot size is noted only by patients with macular holes. Thus, the absolute scotoma detected by the laser beam test is sensitive and specific for full-thickness macular holes. Other ancillary tests, such as focal electroretinography,[151] scanning laser ophthalmoscopy,[152-154] confocal laser tomographic analysis systems,[155] monochromatic photography,[156] and laser biomicroscopy,[157,158] have been applied to the study of macular holes with some success. These modalities are not available or feasible for many clinical practices, however. Echographic features of idiopathic macular hole correlate reasonably accurately with clinical features.[159,160] A pseudo-operculum is a focal condensation of the vitreous cortex suspended on detached invisible posterior hyaloid membrane, in front of either intact foveolar retina or full thickness macular hole.[161] It is demonstrable ultrasonographically.[161] Its presence in front of intact foveolar retina indicates evidence of vitreofoveal separation and low risk of developing a macular hole. Optical coherence tomography has been found effective in distinguishing full-thickness macular holes from partial thickness holes, macular holes, and cysts. It has been successful in staging macular holes and providing a quantitative measure of hole diameter and the amount of surrounding macular edema. It can also detect small separations of the posterior hyaloid from the retina.[162] Careful patient selection is critical to a successful outcome. The ideal candidate would be a patient with bilateral holes of relatively recent onset, with vision in the better eye less than or equal to 20/100. Patients with unilateral symptomatic holes with recently reduced vision to 20/70 or worse are also good candidates.[163] As reported anatomic success rates for macular surgery increase, a method of accurately predicting postoperative visual acuity has increased clinical utility. Both laser interferometer and potential acuity meter have been found to be modestly accurate. Laser interferometer was found to be more accurate in predicting a visual acuity of 20/50 or better.[164]

Long-term follow-up of unoperated macular holes demonstrates progression in hole size and stage, vision loss which generally stabilizes at the 20/200 to 20/400 level, a redistribution and reduced number of yellow nodular opacities at the level of the retinal pigment epithelium, and the development of retinal pigment epithelial atrophy surrounding the macular hole, resulting in a "bull's eye" macular appearance.[165]

MANAGEMENT

Limited visual improvement in eyes with laser photocoagulation, in an effort to flatten the localized detachment around the hole, has been reported.[166,167] This type of treatment could damage potentially viable photoreceptors at the margins of the macular hole. The new understanding of the pathogenesis of this disorder led to the hypothesis that vision might stabilize or improve if it were possible to relieve the traction, reduce the cystic changes, and reattach the cuff of detached retina surrounding the hole. The surgical objectives for repair of macular holes include relief of all tangential traction and retinal tamponade. Identification and removal of the cortical vitreous or posterior hyaloid and removal of fine epiretinal membranes around the hole relieve tangential traction. Tamponade is provided by total gas-fluid exchange with SF_6 or C_3F_8 and strict face-down positioning for at least one week.[168] Most eyes with macular hole have uniform intraoperative vitreous findings.[169] A zone of collapsed vitreous fibers usually lies anterior to a posteriorly optically clear cavity. In most instances, the vitreous cortex or posterior hyaloid is invisible and remains attached to the underlying internal limiting membrane of the retina. In some cases, the presence of a focally detached vitreous is suggested by an operculum floating above the macular hole.

After surgical removal of the central vitreous, it is necessary to develop and/or complete a posterior vitreous detachment. Using active aspiration (150-250 mm Hg), a silicone-tipped suction cannula is gently swept over the retinal surface near the major arcades or the optic nerve. The area immediately around the hole is avoided. The silicone tip is noted to flex once the cortical vitreous is engaged (Figure 13.9). This has been termed the "fish-strike sign" [170] or "divining rod sign." Once engaged, a posterior vitreous detachment can be created by continuous suction with anterior posterior-tangential traction while the tip is moved over the retinal surface (Figure 13.10). The dissection is carried from the area of initial detachment to adjacent attached areas in an attempt to complete the detachment from the posterior retina to the equatorial zone. Vitrectomy probe with "cutter off" can also be used. The cutter's large port engages the vitreous more firmly and is more efficient in peeling the cortex from the optic nerve. Once the posterior cortical vitreous is engaged near the optic nerve, it can be peeled from the nerve with continued suction and traction. It is common to create small disk and retinal hemorrhages during this process. Once the vitreous separates from the optic nerve it will usually separate easily to the posterior vitreous base with further gentle traction. Once the posterior hyaloidal dissection has been initiated, the vitreous cortex becomes visible as a thickened

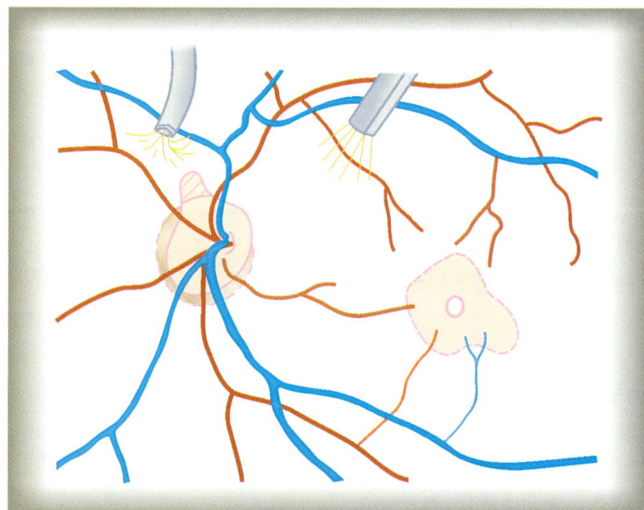

FIGURE 13.10: With continuous suction and anterior-posterior-tangential traction, a posterior vitreous detachment can be created.

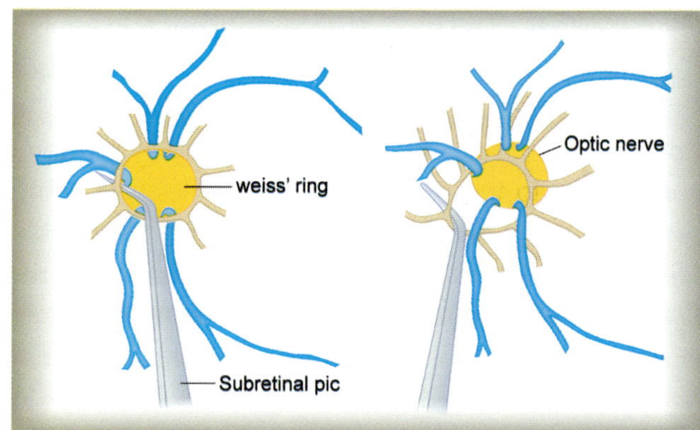

FIGURE 13.11: A 36-gauge subretinal pic is used to engage the posterior hyaloid near the optic nerve and pull off the Weiss' ring.

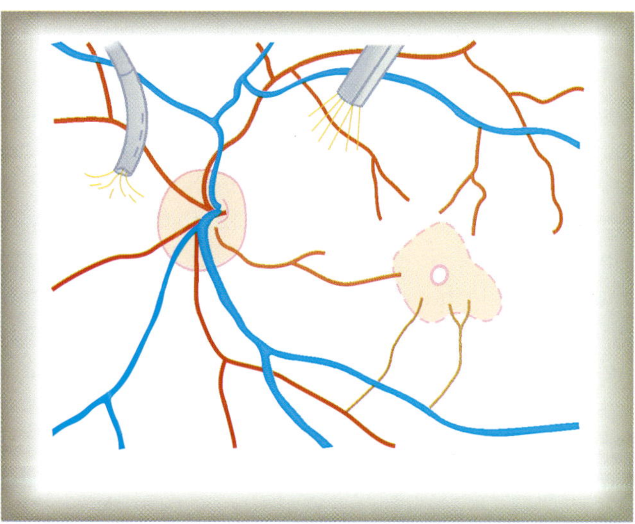

FIGURE 13.9: A silicone-tipped cannula flexes once the cortical vitreous is engaged.

transluscent sheet, especially the oblique illumination. Occasionally, the disk attachments are so firm that tissue forceps, or pic manipulation is required to complete the posterior vitreous detachment in these areas. A 36-gauge subretinal pic can be useful in engaging the posterior hyaloid near the optic nerve and then pulling off Weiss's ring (Figure 13.11). Frequently, an operculum is detected as a glial fragment attached to the vitreous cortex. Frequently, an operculum or pseudo-operculum can be detected as a luteal-colored fragment attached to the vitreous cortex. A ring of condensed vitreous (Weiss' ring) is observed over the disk corresponding to previous vitreopapillary attachment. If the vitreous cortex is not removed it will become apparent during the completion of the air-fluid exchange as a gelatinous substance on the retinal surface.

Ryan and associates [171] described the use of intravitreal autologous blood to identify posterior cortical vitreous. We believe that this procedure is not necessary for the identification of posterior cortical vitreous. Once the vitreous is completely detached, vitrectomy is completed. If residual vitreous cortex is present, it becomes apparent during completion of the air-fluid exchange as a gelatinous substance on the surface of the retina. Fifty percent of operated eyes have some degree of epiretinal membrane proliferation. [172] These epiretinal membranes, unlike typical epiretinal membranes, tend to be finer and more friable, and at times are densely adherent to the retina. The epiretinal membranes may be present surrounding the hole or can involve only a few clock hours. A microbarbed myringotomy blade is used to create an edge in the epiretinal membrane, which is grasped with tissue forceps and stripped. One disk area around the macular hole is checked and liberated from epiretinal membranes to ensure the relief of traction. During this maneuver, it is common to create small hemorrhages around the hole. Damage to the inner retina is avoided, an early sign of which may be the development of fluffy whitish areas. Prolonged intense illumination from the light pipe near the macula is avoided to prevent phototoxicity. A total air-fluid exchange is performed and effort is made to dehydrate the vitreous cavity. The shallow fluid in the base of the optic disk cup is aspirated repeatedly, with a soft-tipped cannula, until fluid no longer collects. A non-expansive concentration of long-acting gas is exchanged for air. Postoperatively, strict prone positioning is prescribed. At the 1-week visit if the edges of the macular hole are flattened and imperceptible with flattening of the cuff of retinal detachment, anatomic success is assured. However, if the edges are still visible and the cuff elevated, anatomic failure is probable.

INTERNAL LIMITING MEMBRANE PEELING

Rationale for internal limiting membrane peeling is as follows:

- Relaxation of tangential traction of internal limiting membrane itself
- Removal of possible cause of persistent fine retinal fold
- Removal of epiretinal proliferation
- Removal of diffusion barrier
- Differences between internal limiting membrane and retina.

SURGICAL TECHNIQUE

Internal Limiting Membrane Peeling

The first step is puncturing the internal limiting membrane with a sharp-tipped and barbed microvitreoretinal blade in the superior macula about half disk diameter away from the macular hole. Once the internal limiting membrane is punctured, the microvitreoretinal blade is drawn gently across the surface of the retina for a short distance until a small opening is created. There is typically a white "fluffy" appearance to this opening and occasionally a fleck of hemorrhage. A pic is advanced and wiggled slightly from side to side in an effort to engage only the internal limiting membrane and not the nerve fiber layer. Once a proper dissection plane is established, effort is made to tunnel beneath the internal limiting membrane in a counter-clockwise direction, creating a pocket to work in. An intermittent slight lifting motion is used to peel the internal limiting membrane off the nerve fiber layer ahead of the instrument tip. The internal limiting membrane is often not visible over the instrument tip, but a slight movement of the retina in the direction of the pic indicates that it has been engaged. Once the internal limiting membrane is elevated this extent, it can be grasped with an internal limiting membrane or end-gripping forceps and peeled around the macular hole.

Indocyanine Green-assisted Internal Limiting Membrane Peeling

Indocyanine green dye is prepared as follows:

a. 25 mg of indocyanine green dye is diluted with 0.5 ml of distilled water. Then 4.5 ml of balanced salt solution (BSS) is added to make 0.5% solution.

b. 25 mg of dry indocyanine green substance is first dissolved with 5 ml sterile distilled water. One milliliter of this solution was then diluted with 9 ml of BSS plus. Indocyanine green with a concentration of 0.05%

is then applied to stain the internal limiting membrane. 0.2 to 0.5 ml of diluted indocyanine green is placed/sprayed over the retina under normal infusion. The dye is washed out immediately. After removal of the indocyanine green, internal limiting membrane peeling is performed.

Internal limiting membrane peeling can be done as follows:

1. *Directly grasping the internal limiting membrane* by forceps.
2. *Creating a tear/rent in internal limiting membrane* by:
   i. Barbed microvitreoretinal blade or bent 28-gauge needle.
   ii. Tano's diamond-dusted membrane scraper: It is a useful tool for membrane separation during vitreous surgery. A diamond-dusted silicone cannula is fashioned from flexible silicone tubing with a beveled tip and coated with diamond fragments. It has been found to be particularly useful for removing residual vitreous cortex and epiretinal membranes from around the hole. It is also effective in removing "immature membranes" in proliferative vitreoretinopathy. The diamond-dusted silicone cannula is a useful tool for removing thin epiretinal membranes and vitreous cortex that may be difficult or nearly impossible to remove safely using other techniques.
   iii. Silicone brush.
   iv. Suction with a back-flush needle.
3. *Completion of internal limiting membrane peeling:* The unstained, underlying retina is readily apparent in contrast to the green-stained internal limiting membrane. Subsequently, the flap of internal limiting membrane is easily grasped and peeled with a diamond dusted intraocular forceps. Continuous curvilinear maculorhexis is performed. The contrast enables the surgeon to monitor precisely the extent and the completeness of the internal limiting membrane peeling. Subtle frills of internal limiting membrane are not left at the edge of macular hole. The bare area free of internal limiting membrane is intended to be one disk diameter surrounding the macular hole. Persisting autofluorescence of the macular area or the optic nerve is observed up to 3 months after surgery.

Infracyanine Green-assisted Internal Limiting Membrane Peeling

To prepare the infracyanine green solution (SERB, Paris, France), a 25 mg vial of infracyanine green is dissolved in 5 ml of glucose 5% solution to obtain final infracyanine green concentration of 0.5% with an osmolarity of 309 mosm/kg. After closure of the infusion line, 0.2 ml of this solution is instilled directly into the posterior vitreous cavity over the macula using a blunt cannula. After 2 minutes, the infusion line is reopened and the excess of dye was removed from the vitreous cavity using a backflush cannula. The internal limiting membrane that had been in contact with the dye is stained green diffusely.

Trypan Blue-assisted Internal Limiting Membrane Peeling

A 0.5 to 1 ml of trypan blue 0.06% (Visionblue, DORC International, The Netherlands) is injected under continuous infusion over the posterior pole under direct visualization, staining the internal limiting membrane. Alternatively, after fluid-air exchange, the dye is placed over the macula under air sufflation. Air fluid-exchange is done to aspirate the dye. A 20-gauge bent microvitreoretinal blade is then used to incise the membrane, and diamond dusted intraocular forceps are used to remove it in a circumferential manner 360 degrees around the macular hole.

Triamcinolone-assisted Vitrectomy

The preservative of triamcinolone acetonide is removed with a filter and rinsed with balanced salt solution. The triamcinolone acetonide particles (40 mg) are then resuspended in 2 ml of balanced salt solution. Following core vitrectomy, triamcinolone acetonide suspension is injected over the posterior pole. The posterior hyaloid is clearly observed. Separation of the hyaloid from the optic nerve head and posterior retina is then performed. Next, a subtotal vitrectomy was performed. The triamcinolone acetonide suspension is injected again over the posterior pole, and excess triamcinolone acetonide is aspirated with a backflush needle. Numerous particles of triamcinolone acetonide are observed as white specks on the posterior retina. The internal limiting membrane is then grasped with an intraocular forceps and peeled in a circumferential manner around the macular hole. The peeled area was clearly observed as an area lacking the white specks left by the triamcinolone acetonide. Several particles of triamcinolone acetonide are observed on the peeled internal limiting membrane. Triamcinolone acetonide tends to stick to the residual vitreous cortex on the internal limiting membrane or to the internal limiting membrane itself. The peeled area of the membrane is clearly confirmed by the lack of white specks left elsewhere by the triamcinolone acetonide. The internal limiting membrane can be easily peeled in a circumferential manner as using indocyanine green. A small amount of triamcinolone acetonide often deposits in the macular hole, however. Local toxicity of triamcinolone acetonide to the neural retina and retinal pigment epithelium is unknown.

Perfluorocarbon liquid-assisted Internal Limiting Membrane Peeling in Macular Hole Associated with Detachment

Stripping the internal limiting membrane is supposed to be beneficial in attaching the retina in retinal detachment because of macular hole. However, it is difficult to lift up and strip the internal limiting membrane over extensively detached retinas because such retinas are very mobile. To evade this difficulty, flattened the detached retina can be flattened with perfluorocarbon liquid and peeling of internal limiting membrane is done in the presence of perfluorocarbon liquid. The internal limiting membrane flap is easily turned up and enlarged with the posterior counter traction by perfluorocarbon liquid.

In another technique, the subretinal fluid is drained with the vitreous probe held over the macular hole and operating in the aspirating mode (200 mm Hg). Once the macular hole has flattened, the infusion is stopped, and perfluoro-n-octane is injected slowly as a single large bubble over the posterior pole. Following the injection and gradual retinal attachment, indocyanine green (0.5%, 270 mosm) is instilled (approximately 2 ml of the solution) over the macula at the retina–perfluoro-n-octane interface. The infusion is reopened following indocyanine

green injection, and the intravitreal dye is washed out. The dye between the perfluoro-n-octane bubble and the retina is then flushed with an injection of balanced salt solution at the perfluoro-n-octane–retina interface using a soft-tip needle attached to a syringe. The internal limiting membrane is stained green and became clearly visible under the perfluoro-n-octane. The dye also stained the retinal pigment epithelium within the hole. Passage of the dye into the subretinal space does not occur. The internal limiting membrane is removed using standard micro end-gripping forceps.

Tamponade

Gas: A non-expansive concentration of long-acting gas (C_3F_8) is exchanged for air. Postoperatively, 24-hour a day strict prone positioning for 5 to 7 days is prescribed. Face down positioning increases the buoyancy effect of gas bubble, which may augment the surface tension effects of intraocular gas tamponade, which in turn may enhance the anatomic closure of macular holes.

Silicone oil: Silicone oil eliminates the need for face-down positioning allows immediate return of normal functioning and unrestricted air travel and possibly eliminates visual field defects. It requires a second procedure to remove it after 2 to 3 months, and is possibly not as effective as gas tamponade. The rate of hole closure is significantly lower than for C_3F_8 gas. Silicone oil may be considered if: the patient is either unable or unwilling to maintain face-down position postoperatively, early return to normal activity is necessary, patient is monocular and postoperative air travel is required.

RESULTS

Impending Macular Holes

Several studies have suggested that vitrectomy may be beneficial for patients with an impending macular hole. Smiddy and associates [119] reported arrest of progression of macular hole in 80% of eyes with premacular hole lesions. Improved vision was noted in 41% of these eyes. Jost and associates [173] reported arrest in progression of stage I macular hole in 90% of eyes at risk for formation of full thickness macular hole. Improvement in vision, with 58% attaining a visual acuity of 20/25 or better, was reported. Four eyes were noted to have stage II macular holes at the time of vitrectomy. Two of these four eyes did not show progressive macular hole formation and had 20/25 visual acuity. Margherio and associates [127] reported a series of 106 consecutive symptomatic eyes considered to be at high risk of idiopathic macular hole formation that underwent vitrectomy with membrane peeling. Two eyes were found to have small microholes involving the fovea. Postoperatively, in both cases full-thickness holes continued to evolve, with further deterioration in visual acuity. A prospective, multicentric trial was undertaken to study the role of vitreous surgery in impending macular holes. [174,175] The study was conducted on patients with full-thickness macular holes in their first eye (stages III and IV) and signs and symptoms of stage I macular holes in their fellow eye (study eye). Patients were randomized to surgery or observation. A full-thickness macular hole developed in 37% of the surgery group and in 40% of the observed group. Because of low recruitment the study was terminated before enough cases were enrolled to achieve statistical significance. [176]

Stage II Macular Holes

Chambers and associates [177] reported a consecutive series treated with pars plana vitrectomy in which surgical manipulation of the prefoveal layer of cortical vitreous

was avoided for stage I and stage II macular holes. The tangential and anteroposterior traction was relieved remote to the macula. No significant improvement in vision occurred in eyes with stage II macular holes, but visual acuity improved in 87% of the patients with stage I holes. Ruby and associates [178] reported the results for the treatment of stage II macular holes: 61% of the eyes had a visual acuity of 20/50 or better while only 18% had a visual acuity of 20/200 or worse. Seventy-five percent of the eyes showed a stable appearance of a very small hole, a decrease in the hole size, or a resolution of the full-thickness defect (Figures 13.12A and B). Compared with observation alone, surgical intervention in stage 2 macular holes results in a significantly lower incidence of hole enlargement and appears to be associated with better outcome in some measures of visual acuity.[179]

Stages III and IV Macular Holes

Kelly and Wendel [169] reported the results of a pilot study for the treatment of stages III and IV full-thickness macular holes. Although 58% of their patients showed anatomic flattening of the macula and 73% of these improved by two or more Snellen lines of visual acuity, only 25% of all these patients had a visual acuity of 20/50 or better postoperatively, and 50% had 20/200 or worse. Subsequent follow-up study [180] on 152 consecutive eyes

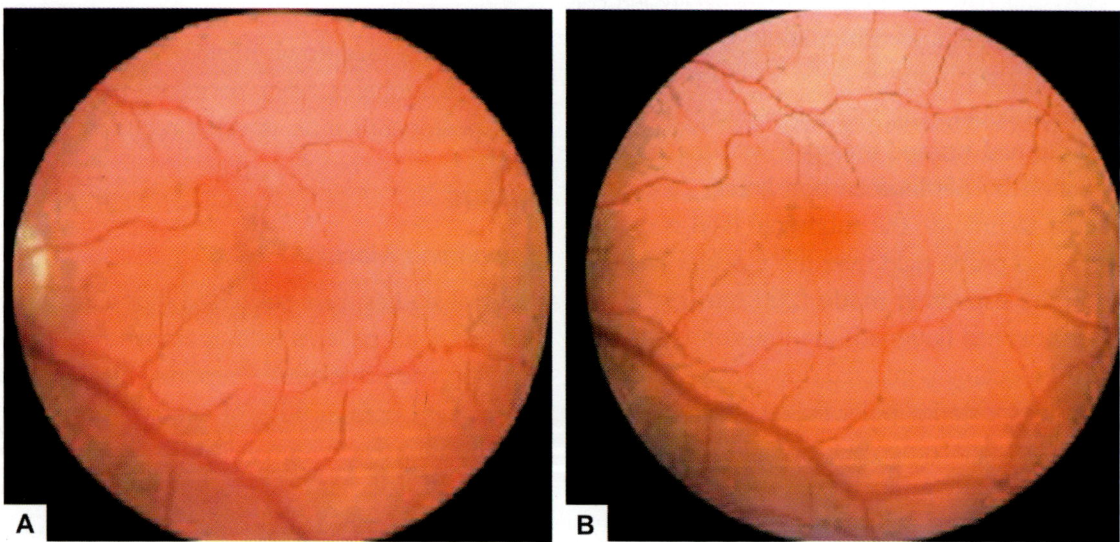

FIGURES 13.12A and B: (A) Preoperative stage II macular hole. Watzke-Allen sign is present. (B) Postoperative fundus photograph shows closed macular hole. Visual acuity is 20/25-1. Watzke-Allen sign is absent.

showed an improved anatomic success of 73%, but the percentage of patients with excellent central visual acuity has remained relatively low, at 26%, with visual acuity of 20/40 or better. Ryan and Gilbert[181] reported the surgical treatment of recent-onset full-thickness idiopathic macular holes. In the early group (symptoms <6 months), 56% of the patients gained at least three lines of vision. Anatomic success rate was seen with one operation in 75% and with two operations in 87.5%. Stage II holes had a final anatomic success rate of 94.4%. In the late group (symptoms >6 months), closure of the hole with one operation was seen in 60% (Figures 13.13A and B). Glaser and associates[182] used transforming growth factor alpha 2 (TGF alpha 2) as a pharmacologic adjuvant in surgery on macular holes. In the subset of patients given the highest dose of TGF alpha 2 (1330 ng), 91% improved two or more Snellen lines, but only 45% had visual acuity of 20/50 or better. In a subsequent study, Lansing and associates[183] reported a 96% anatomic success rate with 48% of the patients having visual acuity of 20/40 or better. Preliminary anatomic results of a multicentric, prospective study demonstrated that a single application of TGF alpha 2 had a statistically significant beneficial effect on resolution of the subretinal cuff surrounding a macular hole when used in conjunction with standardized vitrectomy for full-thickness macular holes.[184] Thompson and associates[185] reported that a

longer duration intraocular gas tamponade from 16% C_3F_8 gives a much higher rate of successful closure of macular holes and improved visual acuity using vitrectomy and TGF alpha 2 than does air. Subsequently, a large, prospective randomized study sponsored by the pharmaceutical company that manufactures TGF alpha 2, found TGF alpha 2 to be no more efficacious in closing macular holes than placebo. Liggett and associates[186] have proposed the use of human autologous serum for treatment of full-thickness macular holes. In a small pilot study, all of the 11 eyes had resolution of the surrounding subretinal fluid and flattening of the macular hole, and showed improvement of at least two lines or more in visual acuity. A larger randomized, controlled trial has not been done. The recovery of 20/20 visual acuity, the disappearance of focal hyperfluorescence corresponding with the macular hole angiographically, and the disappearance of absolute central scotomas observed in some patients after macular hole surgery suggest that centripetal movement of paracentral retinal receptors and their xanthophyll can occur after retinal reattachment.[187,188] There does appear to be an inverse relationship between duration of symptoms and both anatomic success and visual improvement. Holes of shorter duration have better anatomic and visual results following surgery compared with long-standing holes. Visual results routinely lag 6 weeks behind anatomic success, with about

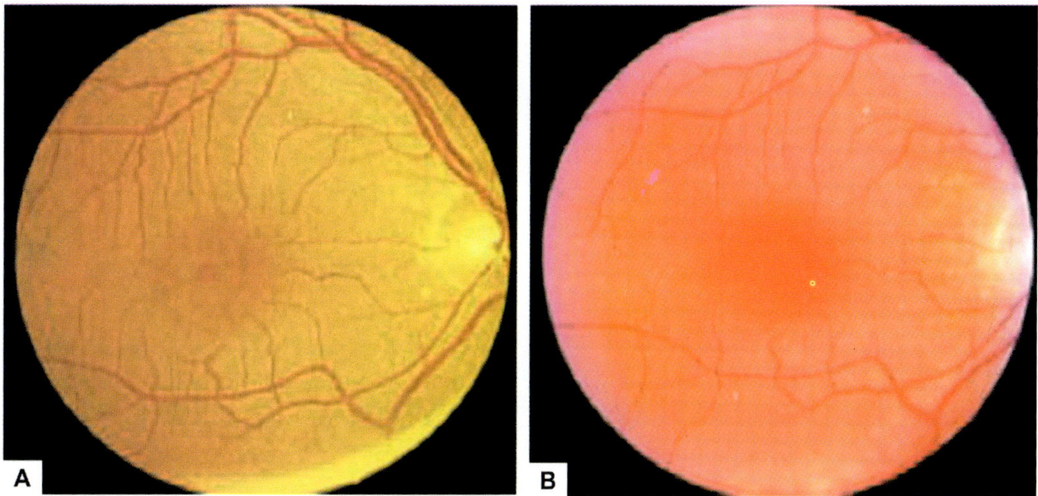

FIGURES 13.13A and B: (A) Preoperative stage III macular hole. Visual acuity is 20/200. (B) Postoperative stage III macular hole. Visual acuity is 20/40.

75% of the anatomically successful eyes improving by two lines or more of visual acuity. The release of macular traction creates the necessary environment for gas tamponade to reattach the cuff surrounding the macular hole in most cases. The role of chorioretinal and epiretinal proliferation in reattachment is unclear. The etiology of anatomic failure is uncertain. Patient noncompliance in postoperative prone positioning and subsequent inadequate tamponade, production of traction by residual epiretinal membranes, intrinsic retinal changes that cause stiffness, and prevention of retinal reattachment possibly plays a role. Experience with reoperation has been limited. If failure is believed to be secondary to residual epiretinal membranes, reoperation has been successful. If noncompliance with postoperative prone positioning is thought to be the cause of failure, newly motivated patients can be given a second chance. Macular holes can reopen after initial surgical repair. Those cells that can lead to the closure of an idiopathic macular hole can also contribute to its recurrence if the reparative process goes awry. [189] Krypton laser photocoagulation and fluid gas exchange for recurrent macular hole have been reported.[190]

Macular holes of > or = 2 years' duration may be more difficult to close successfully than are more recent macular holes, and the visual improvement appears to be less favorable. Many eyes with chronic macular holes gain substantial visual acuity, so vitreous surgery can be considered in selected eyes with chronic macular holes based on visual needs.[191] Although vitrectomy is a risk factor for nuclear sclerosis progression, the duration of vitrectomy does not increase the risk.[192]

Patients with chronic systemic illness such as arthritis may be unable to carry out this postoperative regime. Thus there has been a need for alternative techniques that would eliminate such a regime. In patients who underwent macular hole surgery using silicone oil without any postoperative posturing, the anatomical results have been reported to be similar in 80% cases in keeping with those reported in other studies using gas tamponade. However, the visual results are disappointing and less rewarding than those obtained after successful surgery using gas tamponade.[193]

Visual acuity in patients after anatomically successful macular hole surgery continues to improve even beyond 1 year after surgery. Although substantial improvement occurs soon after cataract extraction, further improvement in visual acuity continues for 2 years thereafter.[194] The retinal pigment epithelium alterations and retinal detachments are common after macular hole surgery and result in significantly reduced postoperative visual acuity.[195]

According to Tornambe and associates [196] successful macular hole closure is possible without face-down positioning. This technique may be an alternative for patients with macular holes in pseudophakic eyes that are unable to assume face-down posturing. Combining cataract surgery with this technique for macular hole repair is reasonable for phakic patients who cannot maintain prone positioning. Major disadvantages of combined surgery include the morbidity of the second procedure and removal of a visually insignificant cataract. This approach should be considered for those patients unable to tolerate face-down positioning.

After macular hole surgery, anatomically unsuccessful closure of the hole correlates with small enlargements in the diameter of the macular hole and its surrounding subretinal fluid cuff, and with a slight decrease in visual acuity. Macular hole closure after repeat surgery improves visual acuity outcome in the majority of retreated eyes.[197]

COMPLICATIONS

The most common complication of a vitrectomy for impending macular hole and a full-thickness macular hole is the occurrence or progression of nuclear sclerotic cataracts. Of the patients treated for macular holes, 20 to 33% require cataract extraction postoperatively [169] Nuclear sclerotic cataracts progress substantially after macular hole surgery with a long-acting intraocular gas tamponade.[198]

Park and associates[199] noted posterior segment complications in 23% of their cases. These included peripheral retinal breaks (3%), rhegmatogenous retinal detachment from a peripheral retinal break (14%), enlargement of the hole (2%), and late reopening of the hole (2%), retinal pigment epithelium loss under the hole

(1%), photic toxicity (1%), and endophthalmitis (1%). Iatrogenic retinal breaks tend to be in the inferior and temporal retina, which establishes the need for greater intraoperative surveillance in these areas. [200] Peripheral retinal tears may develop during stripping of cortical vitreous. The free edge of the macular hole is mobile and susceptible to incarceration during aspiration maneuvers, which can lead to tearing and enlargement of the hole.[169] During membrane stripping or fluid aspiration care must be taken to avoid excessive traction and inadvertent damage to the edge of the macular hole and inner retina. Retinal pigment epitheliopathy after macular hole surgery may portend a guarded visual prognosis in affected patients undergoing successful macular hole repair (Figure 13.14). This may be the result of individual patient sensitivities to manipulation, direct trauma, or prolonged exposure to the endoilluminator.[169] Poliner and Tornambe [201] hypothesized that combination of prolonged intraocular gas contact and light exposure exceeding threshold for an already compromised macula appear to be responsible for this pigmentary pattern. According to Charles, [202] retinal pigment epithelium changes seem more likely to be secondary to trauma to the retinal pigment epithelium and photoreceptors and occur secondary to precipitous suction removal of thick subretinal fluid through macular holes. Duker [203] hypothesized that the persistence of subretinal fluid may be as important as individual susceptibility or overall light exposure for the development of this epitheliopathy. Late reopening can complicate initially successful macular hole surgery and may occur in at least 4.8% of initially successful operations. Reopening has been documented to occur at between 2 and 22 months, and it has been hypothesized that the growth of an epiretinal membrane plays a part in at least some of the eyes. Repeat vitrectomy with gas injection can result in re-closure of the hole and improvement in vision.[204] Kokame[205] reported late recurrence of macular hole in an eye with impending macular hole, which initially resolved after surgical intervention. The mechanism of late recurrence may be similar in impending and full-thickness macular holes. [205] Smiddy [206] also noted macular hole development after surgical peeling of epiretinal membrane over the macula.

Thus macular holes can develop in certain situations in which the posterior cortical vitreous has been removed from the macula, either surgically or by natural posterior vitreous detachment.[206]

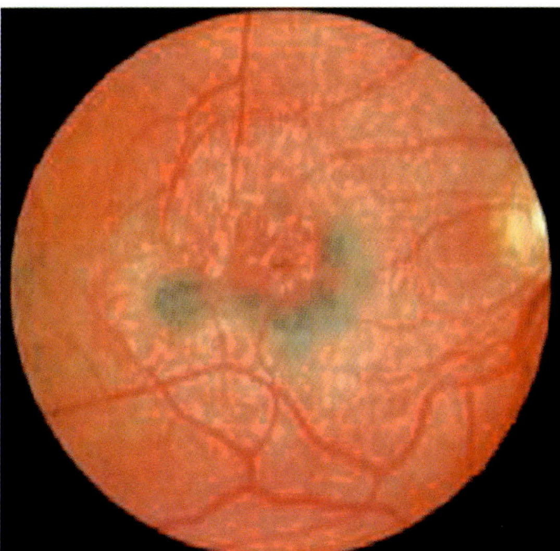

FIGURE 13.14: Retinal pigment epitheliopathy following vitrectomy and gas-fluid exchange for stage IV macular hole. Although the hole is closed, the patient sees a ring scotoma, and visual acuity is 20/150.

Holekamp and associates [207] reported ulnar neuropathy as a complication of macular hole surgery.

A significant temporal field defect may occur in patients after otherwise uncomplicated surgery for macular holes. The cause is unclear; however, reduction in nerve fiber layer thickness from the superior and nasal peripapillary area suggests that acute surgical release of the posterior hyaloid and the use of long-acting intraocular gas may in certain patients result in visual field defects. The most common visual field defect is dense and wedge-shaped and involves the temporal visual field. Although unclear, the etiology may involve trauma to the peripapillary retinal vasculature or nerve fiber layer during elevation of the posterior hyaloid or during aspiration at the time of air-fluid exchange, followed by compression and occlusion of the retinal peripapillary vessels during gas tamponade.[208-211] Visual field defects can occur following vitrectomy and gas-fluid exchange for macular hole. Two categories of scotomas have been observed: peripheral and relative arcuate. The cause of peripheral visual field loss is unclear. Increased intraocular pressure may be the cause of relative arcuate scotomas.[212] Peripheral visual field defects after macular hole surgery can be a complication of very low incidence. A rather low-pressure set during air-fluid exchange as well as special aspects of the surgical technique may be responsible for this low incidence of peripheral visual field defects.[213] Small, mostly asymptomatic, paracentral scotomata as a complication after vitrectomy for idiopathic macular hole have not been reported in the literature so far. Whether they are caused by trauma to the nerve fibers during surgery or other factors remain unknown.[214] Fundus changes become apparent after surgery, and they are progressive. Therefore, it is important to examine eyes with visual field defects for a follow-up period of several years.[215] The location of the visual field defect correlated with the location of the infusion cannula. The incidence of this visual field defect was influenced strongly by the infusion air pressure. The visual field defect may be caused by the mechanical damage of air infusion.[216] Dehydration injury of the nerve fiber layer during the fluid-air exchange should be considered as a possible cause of visual field defect after pars plana vitrectomy for macular hole.[217] Passing air used for fluid-air exchange through water seems to prevent visual field defects after vitrectomy for macular hole surgery. Visual field defects that occur after room air is used may result from desiccation of the retina by room air.[218]

Some eyes develop increased intraocular pressure after vitreous surgery for macular hole, and the increase occurs most frequently between two days and two weeks postoperatively.[219]

Internal Limiting Membrane Peeling Complications

Intravitreal indocyanine green-assisted internal limiting membrane peeling improves anatomic success in macular hole surgery, but it may potentially lead to unfavorable visual acuity outcome and peripheral visual field loss. Fundus fluorescence is observed after indocyanine green.[220-238] Smiddy and associates [239]did not find internal limiting membrane peeling essential in macular hole surgery.

Retina exposed to indocyanine green concentrations used in human vitreoretinal surgery had greater retinal pigment epithelial atrophy and outer retinal degeneration than control eyes undergoing the same surgery without indocyanine green. Eyes filled with infusion fluid during indocyanine green injection had less damage to the retinal pigment epithelium and outer retina than did air-filled eyes receiving indocyanine green. Potential damage to the neurosensory retina is associated with the intra-operative administration of the indocyanine green solution. Whether toxic effects of the dye itself cause this, mechanical trauma to the retina or other mechanisms remains unknown. It has also been suggested that intravitreal application of indocyanine green may cause retinal damage by altering the cleavage plane to the innermost retinal layers. That may result in less improvement of visual acuity and unexpected visual field defects. The underlying mechanisms of action remain unclear.[240-248]

Macular hole surgery with peeling of the internal limiting membrane without the use of adjuvants or internal limiting membrane staining leads to good functional long-term results. Paracentral scotomata remain subclinical in most cases and may be due to a mechanical trauma of the nerve fiber layer. Anatomical changes of the macula following vitrectomy with removal of the internal limiting membrane are infrequent. However, paracentral scotomata observed in our series might be caused by a trauma to the nerve fibers during internal limiting membrane peeling.[249,250] Altered uptake of infrared diode laser by retina after intravitreal indocyanine green dye and internal limiting membrane peeling has been reported.[251] Indocyanine green and intense light exposure in retinal pigment epithelium cells causes photosensitizing toxicity that is reduced when sodium in the solvent is eliminated and replaced with other cations. Eliminating sodium from the solvent reduces indocyanine green uptake into retinal pigment epithelium and its associated photosensitizing toxicity. This reconstitution method of indocyanine green may be helpful for safer intravitreal indocyanine green use in macular hole surgery.[252]

Dilutions of indocyanine green as recommended in the literature may alter the structure of the retina to some degree. Possible factors responsible for this inadvertent action may include:

1. Concentration,
2. Osmolarity, pH
3. Time of tissue contact, and
4. Mechanical factors from more forceful traction during peeling.[253]

The use of silicone oil in macular hole surgery with internal limiting membrane peeling may complicate the postoperative outcome. Internal limiting membrane defects may facilitate the entry of silicone oil into the retina, leading to accumulation of oil vacuoles.[254] Infracyanine green-assisted removal of the retinal internal limiting membrane appears to induce a high incidence of anatomical closure, with good visual outcome.[255]

MISCELLANEOUS

Combining cataract surgery with vitrectomy surgery may prevent a later second operation for post-vitrectomy cataract formation.[256] Biometry after macular hole surgery should be corrected by subtracting the depth of the foveolar crater (0.5 mm, the estimated depth of the foveolar crater) from the measured axial length.[257] C_3F_8 gas has proved to be a more effective tamponade than silicone oil with respect to achieving initial closure of macular holes. Eyes receiving an oil tamponade required significantly more reoperations to achieve a similar rate of hole closure compared with eyes undergoing a gas tamponade. Final visual acuity was better for gas-operated eyes than for silicone-operated eyes.[258]

Perfluorohexyloctane merits further evaluation for ocular endotamponade in patients with persisting macular holes.[259]

ROLE OF OPTICAL COHERENCE TOMOGRAPHY

Optical coherence tomography plays an important role in the diagnosis and management of macular hole. According to Tornambe[260] optical coherence tomography images and a simple model suggest macular hole formation may be due to a defect in the inner retina with secondary vitreous fluid accumulation into the middle and outer retinal tissue. Idiopathic macular holes have one of two patterns early after surgical closure, simple closure or a bridge formation. Visual improvement starts after the fovea assumes a normal configuration. The bridge formation appears to reflect an early phase and fragile condition in the anatomic closure of macular holes.[261] A small macular hole appears to be closed by 3 days after vitrectomy with gas tamponade. Although we cannot generalize to all sizes of macular hole, our findings suggest that small macular holes are closed much earlier than reported and that the duration of maintaining a prone position can be shortened.[262] There is a close correlation between the stage of the macular hole and the degree of posterior vitreous detachment. This close correlation suggests that progression of idiopathic macular hole is related to enlargement of the posterior vitreous detachment. [263] Ullrich and associates [264] assessed macular holes according to the classification by Gass with optical coherence tomography before pars plana vitrectomy. Macular hole diameters were determined at the level of the retinal pigment epithelium (base diameter) and at the minimal extent of the hole (minimum diameter). Calculated hole form factor (HFF) was correlated with the postoperative anatomical success rate and best corrected visual acuity. The duration of symptoms was correlated with base and minimum diameter of the macular hole. In eyes without anatomical closure of the macular hole after one surgical approach the base diameter and the minimum diameter were significantly larger than in cases with immediate post surgical closure. There was a significant negative correlation between both the base and the minimum diameter of the hole and the postoperative visual function. In all patients with HFF >0.9 the macular hole was closed following one surgical procedure, whereas in eyes with HFF <0.5 anatomical success rate was 67%. Better postoperative visual outcome correlated with higher HFF. Preoperative measurement of macular hole size with optical coherence tomography can provide a prognostic factor for postoperative visual outcome and anatomical success rate of macular hole surgery. The duration of symptoms did not correlate with the diameters measured. Base and minimum diameters especially seem to be of predictive value in macular hole surgery. Visual outcome after anatomic closure of macular holes by vitrectomy is closely related to the structure of the center of the fovea postoperatively.[265]

The repaired macular holes were classified by the optical coherence tomography images by Uemoto and associates[266] as being of "good shape" (nearly normal foveal contour) or "poor shape" (abnormal foveal contour with flat fovea and steep edge or with a thick retina without a foveal pit). Internal limiting membrane peeling may provide better anatomical success and recovery of the macular shape, but the postoperative visual acuity and improvement of visual acuity were not related to the morphological results.

Optical coherence tomography findings of postoperative macular hole closure status correlate well with the clinical findings. Careful clinical examination alone may be adequate in determining the surgical anatomical end points in the majority of patients after macular hole surgery.[267]

The postoperative closure of idiopathic macular holes following vitreous surgery was related to the preoperative macular hole diameter determined by optical coherence tomography, with lesions smaller than 400 microns demonstrating higher success rates. A trend toward greater visual acuity improvement was demonstrated for idiopathic macular holes smaller than 400 microns. Late reopening was only seen in macular holes that were 400 microns or larger measured by optical coherence tomography. Preoperative analysis and measurement of idiopathic macular holes with optical coherence tomography may help delineate postoperative expectations for successful anatomical closure of the macular hole, visual acuity, and long-term closure.[268]

Vitrectomy surgery for impending macular hole based on optical coherence tomography has also been suggested.[269] It is possible to repair macular holes by using optical coherence tomography to guide the dissection of the vitreous from the macular hole followed by limited vitrectomy. By using a less invasive approach, it may be possible to repair macular holes in less operative time and with fewer complications. A microspatula knife is used to dissect the connection between the vitreous and the retina previously delineated by optical coherence tomography. The posterior vitreous was not stripped from the retinal surface. Limited vitrectomy over the hole was performed to create a space for a gas bubble.[270]

SUBMACULAR SURGERY

In the last several years, a surge of interest has been seen in submacular surgery. Candidates for this surgery consist primarily of individuals with subfoveal choroidal neovascularization and those with submacular hemorrhage.

SUBFOVEAL CHOROIDAL NEOVASCULARIZATION

Choroidal neovascularization is a principal cause of loss of central visual function in adults. Choroidal neovascular membranes disrupt normal macular anatomy (including the critical photoreceptor-retinal pigment epithelial interface); leak serum or formed blood elements, or both; and lead to irreversible loss of overlying photoreceptors.[271] When fibrovascular membranes grow beneath the center of the foveal avascular zone, the visual prognosis is generally poor. Choroidal neovascular membranes are most frequently caused by age-related macular degeneration and presumed ocular histoplasmosis syndrome, although neovascularization may be observed as a complication of other ocular conditions.[272-286]

NATURAL HISTORY

The visual prognosis is related to the underlying etiology of the subfoveal choroidal neovascular membrane. Bressler and associates [287] found that 70% of eyes with subfoveal membranes secondary to age-related macular degeneration had visual acuities of 20/200 or worse within 2 years. The Macular Photocoagulation Study Group [288] reported 3- and 4-year visual outcomes in eyes followed in two randomized clinical trials of laser photocoagulation for subfoveal choroidal neovascular membrane secondary to age-related macular degeneration. Four years after enrollment in the subfoveal new choroidal neovascularization study, 39 (47%) of 83 untreated eyes and 17 (22%) of 77 laser-treated eyes had lost six or more lines of visual acuity from baseline levels. At the 3-year examination in the subfoveal recurrent choroidal neovascularization study, 21 (36%) of 58 untreated eyes and 6 (12%) of the treated eyes had lost six or more lines of visual acuity from baseline levels. Eyes with presumed ocular histoplasmosis syndrome do better; as many as 14% may retain visual acuity of 20/40 despite subfoveal vessels. [289,290] However, 90% of eyes with visual acuity of 20/200 or less still will have severely reduced visual acuity after 3 years. Only 7% of membranes in eyes with choroidal neovascular membrane secondary to presumed ocular histoplasmosis syndrome undergo spontaneous involution with improvement in visual acuity.[291] Fibrovascular membranes, regardless of etiology, usually continue to grow without treatment. Vander and associates[292] documented an average growth rate of 9 μm a day in eyes with neovascular membranes in age-related macular degeneration. Enlarging membranes beneath the fovea often lead to disciform scars with poor visual function.

MANAGEMENT

The objective in treating choroidal neovascular membrane is to destroy the abnormal neovascular tissue and limit its damaging effects. Over the last 20 years, laser photocoagulation has been shown to be effective in the management of extrafoveal and juxtafoveal membranes of various etiologies. [293-300] The Macular Photocoagulation Study Group [301-303] and other investigators. [304,305] have demonstrated a marginal benefit of laser treatment compared with observation in certain eyes with age-related macular degeneration even when the neovascular tissue lies beneath the center of the fovea. One of the principal limitations of laser photocoagulation is the concomitant damage to overlying neurosensory retina.[306] This is particularly harmful when the membrane is under the center of the fovea because central vision is almost always significantly reduced after treatment. [307] Surgical removal is an alternative means of eradicating subfoveal choroidal neovascular membrane with potentially less damage to neurosensory retina and, in some cases, better visual function.

In 1988, de Juan and Machemer[308] reported four cases of submacular scar removal using modern vitrectomy techniques. Following vitrectomy, a large circumferential retinotomy was made on the temporal side of the macula, allowing direct access to and dissection of the submacular tissue. Because of a high incidence of proliferative vitreoretinopathy and retinal detachment, as well as discouraging visual results, this technique was not widely employed. Blinder and associates [309] proposed a similar technique creating large-flap retinotomies (between 200 and 260 degrees), modified by the preoperative administration of barrier photocoagulation treatment. Understanding the importance of subfoveal retinal pigment epithelium integrity following subfoveal scar removal, they combined their technique with transposition retinal pigment epithelial flaps and homologous retinal pigment epithelial grafts with limited success.[310] In 1991, Thomas and Kaplan[311] reported a different approach to subfoveal neovascular membrane removal in presumed ocular histoplasmosis syndrome. The technique emphasized making a small retinotomy away from the center of the fovea; through this incision, the subfoveal neovascular complex was accessed and removed from the eye. A small retinotomy does not require laser photocoagulation at the conclusion of the procedure, thus preventing thermal damage to juxtafoveal retina, retinal pigment epithelium, and choriocapillaris.[312] The surgical technique has now become established.[313-320] Emphasis has been placed on the design and development of smaller-gauge instruments to facilitate subretinal tissue manipulation while minimizing retinal pigment epithelial and photoreceptor trauma. However, the principal limitations of the surgical technique arise from the concomitant damage to adjacent ocular structures associated with the choroidal neovascular membrane, especially in age-related macular degeneration. Thus case selection is of critical importance. [321]

CASE SELECTION

As with any new technique, the determination of appropriate case selection awaits the outcome of a randomized, prospective clinical trial that is currently under way. With our experience of the past 6 years, it appears that choroidal neovascular membranes anterior to the retinal pigment epithelium seem to have the best surgical prognosis, as preservation of the retinal pigment epithelium is a critical factor in the subsequent recovery of central visual function. If the goal of surgery is regaining central foveal function, then surgical removal of a subfoveal, choroidal neovascular membrane is advised if it appears to lie anterior to the retinal pigment epithelium. Contact lens examination of the macula combined with color-stereo views and stereoscopic fluorescein angiography helps in determining the membrane's location.

The following clinical findings may suggest that the neovascular complex lies anterior to the retinal pigment epithelium:

1. A well-defined edge with an abrupt transition to underlying retinal pigment epithelium.
2. An anterior location apparent on stereoscopic viewing,
3. A thin layer of subretinal blood outlining the edges of a neovascular complex and the subjacent retinal pigment epithelium.
4. A pigmented border (which corresponds to the rim of hypofluorescence occasionally seen angiographically) outlining the location of the membrane (Figures 13.15A and B). Some lesions that are indeed anterior to retinal pigment epithelium may lack a sharp border perhaps because of their recent onset. Additionally, fibrin may obscure the border with underlying retinal pigment epithelium.

Angiographic findings suggestive of an anterior location of the membrane include the following:

1. A distinct boundary between the hyperfluorescence of the membrane and background choroidal fluorescence.
2. A rim of blocked fluorescence between the two.
3. Compact angiographic appearance.
4. Homogenous hyperfluorescence.
5. Clearly visible lacy vascular pattern.
6. Anterior location apparent on stereoangiogram viewing and
7. Absence of late staining surrounding tissues (indicative of occult or sub-retinal pigment epithelium neovascularization) (Figures 13.16A to C). Membranes posterior to the retinal pigment epithelium tend to have clinical and angiographic findings that are the opposite of those for anterior membranes.

INSTRUMENTATION

Thomas and associates[322] have developed instruments that greatly facilitate subretinal removal of choroidal neovascular membranes and hematomas. Subsequently, Thomas and Ibanez[323] have developed a newer generation of subretinal instruments.

Angled Subretinal Pic

The angled pic, having a 20-gauge shaft, a 130-degree bend, and a flattened tip tapering to 0.305 mm (36-gauge) has been developed. The blade is used to perforate neurosensory retina to create the initial retinotomy, to push against and disconnect the neovascular complex and to dissect gently under the neovascular complex.

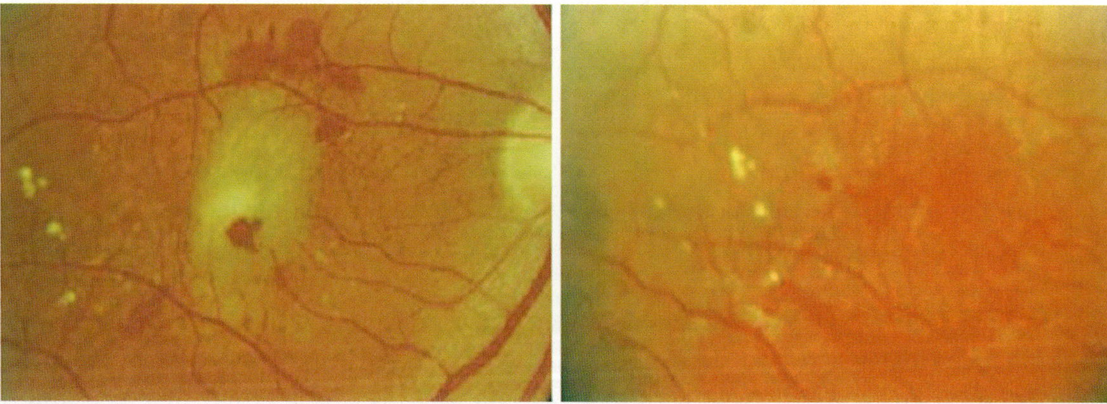

FIGURES 13.15A and B: (A) This compact subfoveal neovascular membrane appears to lie anterior to the retinal pigment epithelium, has a slightly pigmented border, and is partially outlined by a thin layer of subretinal blood. (B) A one-day postoperative photograph confirms that the membrane was anterior to retinal pigment epithelium and could be safely removed without damaging underlying structures.

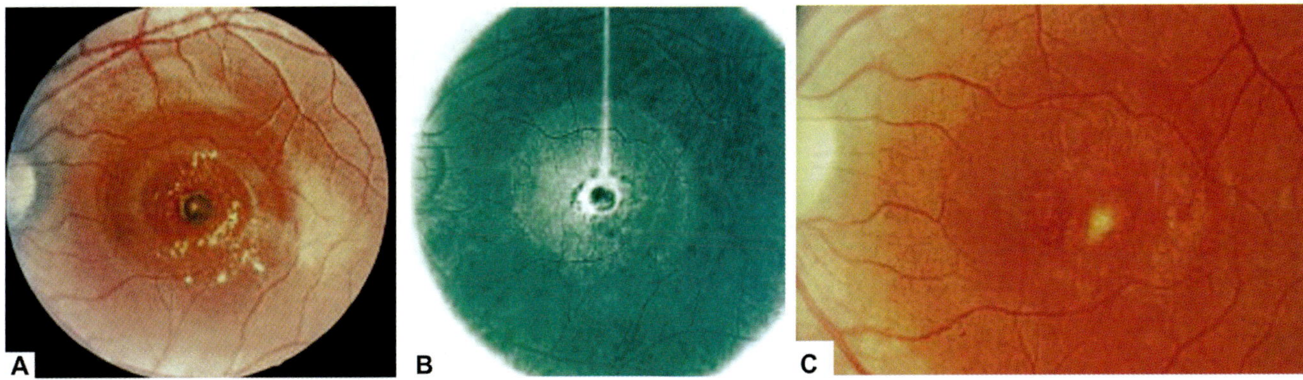

FIGURES 13.16A to C: (A) Compact, hyperpigmented subfoveal neovascular membrane with preoperative visual acuity of 20/200. (B) The angiographic appearance is favorable for surgical removal. (C) The membrane is completely removed without disturbing underlying retinal pigment epithelium except for the focus of hypopigmentation at the ingrowth site. Visual acuity is 20/20.1.

Subretinal Infusion Cannula

The 20-gauge needle tapers to 33-gauge proximal to the 130-degree angle. The angled, slightly beveled 33-gauge tip measures 3.2 mm in length.

A syringe filled with balanced salt solution is connected via a short piece of intravenous tubing to the hand piece and allows gentle infusion into the subfoveal space as opposed to refluxing into the vitreous cavity. Rarely (if retinotomies are large), subretinal fluid can be aspirated through a 30- or 33-gauge straight cannula. The smaller caliber tip can facilitate aspiration of subretinal fluid with less risk of engaging neurosensory retina around the edges of a small retinotomy.

Subretinal Forceps

In many cases the trunk of vascular ingrowth from the choroid firmly tethers the subretinal membrane. In most cases, it is necessary to grasp this stalk to disconnect it. A 20-gauge, positive-action, horizontal forceps, with an angle of 130 degrees, narrow opposing blades (0.61 mm width of closed tips), and a tip length of 2.4 mm, has been designed. These forceps can be used to effectively pass behind the loosened membrane, grasp the stalk, and extract the membrane through the retinotomy. The current 20-gauge, horizontal subretinal forceps have been designed with blades that are slightly thinner yet grasp more firmly than earlier forceps. The superior grasping force is achieved by having the tips close first, so that the intrinsic spring of the metal tips gives additional force as the blades are pressed together. These have a 130-degree angle from the shaft and a length of 3.2 mm from the bend. Vertical action forceps are only occasionally useful in special situations. These narrow subretinal forceps have a fixed lower blade and an active anterior blade. When fully opened, the tips are separated by 1 mm. Peyman and Kwang [324] have designed a subretinal forceps consisting of a 25-gauge curved shaft housing a retractable, three-pronged tip resembling a rake in the open position. They believe this rake tip may be helpful in disconnecting choroidal neovascular membrane from surrounding retinal pigment epithelium especially in age-related macular degeneration. In our experience, the neovascular complex usually breaks free from the surrounding, more normal subretinal tissue when traction is exerted on the main complex.

Subretinal Scissors

Horizontal subretinal scissors having a blade length of approximately 3 mm angled at 130-degree from the shaft have been developed. These scissors may be used to separate a laser scar from its overlying neurosensory retinal adhesion or to section recurrent membranes from their adjacent laser scars. Vertical subretinal scissors having a blade length of approximately 3 mm angled at 130-degree from the shaft have been developed. Rarely, one encounters a neovascular complex in which it is helpful to section the membrane into two pieces before extracting the tissue from the subretinal space.

SURGICAL TECHNIQUE

Current surgical technique is most effective in those cases in which the membrane lies predominantly anterior to the retinal pigment epithelium and thus can be removed without extracting large areas of retinal pigment epithelium.

Sclerotomy Site

A standard three-port pars plana vitrectomy is performed. The placement of sclerotomies is critical. The surgeon should study the angiogram and decide preoperatively where the retinotomy is to be placed to avoid damaging major vessels and to provide adequate access to the subretinal membrane. These factors usually dictate that the retinotomy be created in a straight temporal location and thus the superotemporal sclerotomy should be made near the horizontal meridian. If a sewn-on ring system is used to hold a corneal contact lens, it is sometimes advantageous to rotate the fixation flanges superotemporally and inferonasally from the horizontal to allow a nearly horizontal placement of the temporal port. Occasionally, these horizontal sclerotomy sites bleed more than they do when placed more superiorly, but this has not proved to be a significant complication.

Removal of Posterior Hyaloid

Although there are no data to support the importance of removing the posterior hyaloid, its removal is attempted in every case, as described earlier.

Retinotomy

The placement of retinotomy takes into account: (i) the exact location and extent of the membrane under the fovea, (ii) the presence of presumed adhesions between the neurosensory retina and underlying tissue (previous photocoagulation scars and/or evidence of pigment migration into neurosensory retina or retinochoroidal vascular anastomoses), (iii) the dimensions of the subretinal instruments (specifically, the length of the angled instrument tips that determines how far away from the fovea the retinotomy can be made and still allow the tips to reach the membrane), and (iv) the topographic anatomy of the neurosensory retina and nerve fiber layer.

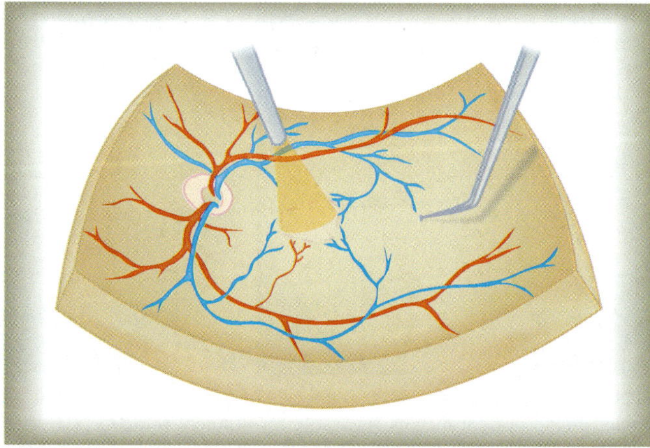

FIGURE 13.17: For a right-handed surgeon in a right eye, a straight temporal retinotomy is often best.

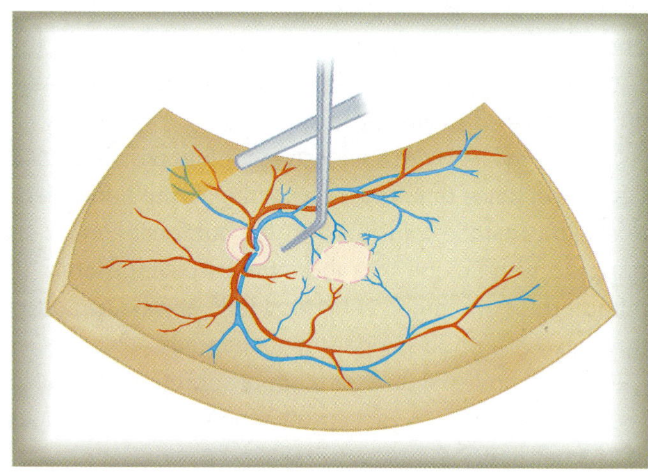

FIGURE 13.18: For a right-handed surgeon in a left eye a retinotomy can be created superonasal to the fovea without significant damage to the papillomacular bundle.

In most cases, these factors dictate a straight temporal or slightly superotemporal location for the retinotomy (Figure 13.17). However, a retinotomy can be created superonasal to the fovea (Figure 13.18). With 33- and 36-gauge instruments, the retinotomies are small enough that no significant damage to the papillomacular bundle occurs. Besides being in the most advantageous location, the retinotomy should be as small as possible. Initially, the retinal surface was lightly diathermized and then the microvitreoretinal blade was used to tease open a small hole. Currently, a 120-degree angled, sharply pointed 36-gauge subretinal pic is used to pierce undiathermized neurosensory retina. While intraocular pressure is raised, the tip can be pushed through neurosensory retina to achieve a very tiny retinotomy. As the pic is obliquely advanced through the neurosensory retina, transient blanching of the choriocapillaris may be seen. Rarely, the local retinal pigment epithelium underlying the retinotomy site may be scraped as the pic enters the subretinal space but this can be avoided by gently lifting the pic as the retina is perforated. A small hemorrhage can occur as retinal capillaries are cut, but this always responds to the increased intraocular pressure and is limited. Greve and associates [325] described a technique of retinotomy in non-diathermized retina. The direction of retinotomy is parallel to the nerve fiber layer. By incising the retina parallel to the nerve fiber layer, the directional forces on the surface of the retina created by the nerve fiber layer's inherent plasticity pull the walls of the retinotomy together, creating a self-sealing retinotomy.

Creation or Enhancement of Neurosensory Detachment

After retinotomy, an angled 33-gauge infusion cannula is introduced beneath the retina and the balanced salt solution is infused to elevate the neurosensory retina (Figure 13.19). This is accomplished by gently pushing on the plunger of a syringe that is connected to the hub of the needle by a short piece of tubing. To avoid trapping air bubbles within the tip, balanced salt solution is gently infused as the instrument is entered into the eye and before the subretinal space is entered. Slow infusion is very important, as this step can lead to the development of a retinal break, especially in areas of strong chorioretinal adhesions. Excessive infusion pressure can tear the retina. A neurosensory detachment can also be created or enhanced by injecting balanced salt solution using a controlled infusion pump.[326] As the fluid enters the subretinal space, attention is directed to edges of the laser scars or adhesions to the underlying membrane, or both.

Removal of Neovascular Membrane

The subretinal membrane is dislodged from the underlying retinal pigment epithelium and the overlying neurosensory retina with the aid of a pointed, 36-gauge subretinal pic (Figure 13.20). The sharp end of the pic is very helpful in engaging the edges of the neovascular complex, and facilitating its separation from the underlying retinal pigment epithelium. The pic is moved in a pivoting or rotating manner to avoid stretching or enlarging the retinotomy. In most cases, the neovascular complex dislodges easily from the underlying subfoveal retinal pigment epithelium but remains attached to the edge of a laser scar or to the stalk of choroidal vascular ingrowth. Occasionally, horizontal subretinal scissors are necessary to cut firm adhesions. If the retina is not mobilized over the entire photocoagulation scar, separation is achieved at least far enough into the scar to allow manipulation and extraction of the membrane

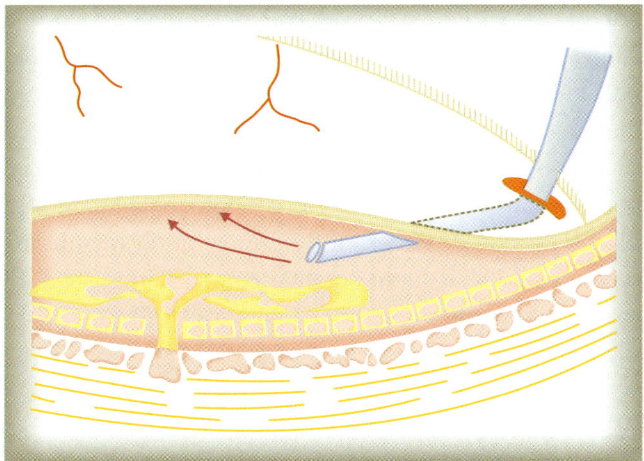

FIGURE 13.19: A gentle infusion of balanced salt solution through a 33-gauge cannula creates a small neurosensory retinal detachment.

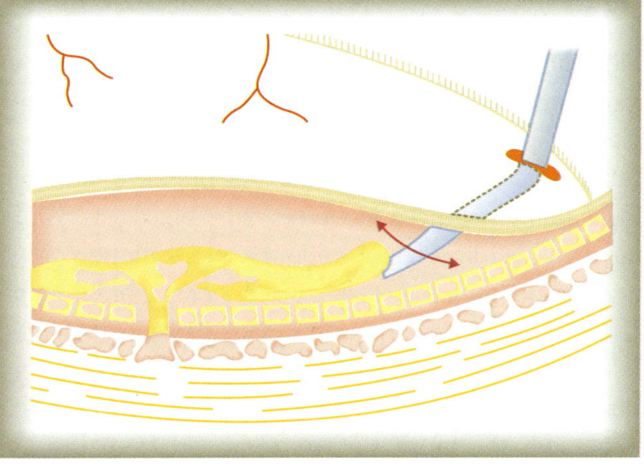

FIGURE 13.20: The neovascular tissue is dislodged from underlying retinal pigment epithelium with the aid of a pointed, 36-gauge subretinal pic.

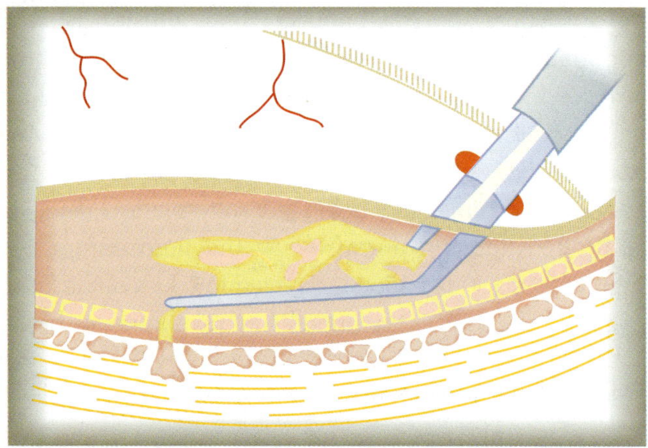

FIGURE 13.21: Horizontal subretinal forceps are used to firmly grasp the neovascular tissue and slowly remove it from the subretinal space.

without tearing adjacent retina. Trauma to foveal photoreceptors from either the pic or scissors is avoided. A positive-action horizontal forceps is introduced (closed) through the retinotomy, which has usually enlarged during the subretinal manipulation. The opened blades are placed around the stalk or the adhesion, with the membrane in front of the blades. Gentle traction with the blades held closed breaks the connection (Figure 13.21). If traction on the retina is seen, the membrane is released and further separation of the complex from neurosensory retina is accomplished. If excessive tugging and displacement of retinal pigment epithelium are seen, consideration is given to using the subretinal scissors to cut the stalk rather than breaking it with the forceps. When the vascular connection from the choroid is about to be severed, the intraocular pressure is raised to approximately 80 mm Hg. Minimal hemorrhage is often encountered when the membrane is removed. The intraocular pressure is elevated for at least one minute and any evidence of rebleeding is observed while the pressure is slowly lowered. When these measures fail, hemostasis can be achieved by subretinal endophotocoagulation. Most membranes are easily grasped with horizontal subretinal forceps. Vertical action forceps may be needed to extract relatively thin disks of neovascularization that have been disconnected from the choroid. Once hemostasis is achieved, the membrane is removed from the eye through the sclerotomy. Dividing a large membrane with intraocular forceps or a vitrector is preferable to enlarging

the sclerotomy. Scleral plugs are placed and the retina is inspected with indirect ophthalmoscopy and scleral depression to verify that no peripheral tears have occurred.

A complete air-fluid exchange is performed. Standard extrusion needles or silicone-tipped needles are used to aspirate over the optic nerve. The angled 33-gauge cannula can be used to aspirate subretinal fluid at the retinotomy. This generally everts the edges of the retinotomy, allowing for better closure. If the retinotomy is small and the surgeon desires a small gas tamponade, balanced salt solution is gently reinfused over the optic nerve after the vitreous cavity has been dry for a few minutes. The eye is almost completely filled with fluid and the patient is asked to be face down postoperatively. In early cases, endolaser photocoagulation of the retinotomy was done. Smaller gauged instrumentation allows for the creation and preservation of a small retinotomy that does not require laser photocoagulation. This prevents thermal damage to neurosensory retina, retinal pigment epithelium, and choriocapillaris, thus preserving extrafoveal retinal function and decreasing the size of a postoperative scotoma.

COMPLICATIONS

Two changes in the milieu that occur in the setting of choroidal neovascular membrane have a practical impact on surgical technique and visual prognosis: cystoid macular edema and fibrin- or photocoagulation-related retinal adhesion to choroidal neovascular membrane.[327] Cystoid changes render the fovea vulnerable to iatrogenic macular hole during fluid-assisted separation of the retina from the subjacent neovascular complex. Incomplete separation of the overlying retina from underlying choroidal neovascular membrane or prior photocoagulation scar places the fovea at risk of avulsion during membrane removal.[327] Other intraoperative complications are subretinal hemorrhage, retinal tear, and retinal detachment.[328,329]

POSTOPERATIVE MANAGEMENT

Patients are examined at 24 hours and at 1 week after surgery for signs of infection, retinal detachment, or elevated intraocular pressure. Three weeks after surgery, the view is usually adequate to clinically detect the presence or absence of subfoveal retinal pigment epithelium. Occasionally, residual subretinal blood will obscure the underlying tissues for a longer period of time. Within the first month, angiography is repeated to evaluate for recurrence of neovascularization. Not uncommonly, the site of the original choroidal ingrowth stalk demonstrates recurrent neovascularization. Often this site is not subfoveal and therefore slit lamp laser photocoagulation can be employed to ablate the recurrence. Since the membranes can recur in more than one third of cases within 6 months, close follow-up is essential.

ADJUNCTS TO SURGERY

Subretinal Endophotocoagulation

Transretinal laser photocoagulation invariably damages the underlying retinal pigment epithelium and the overlying neurosensory retina, thus minimizing the prospect for visual function in the treated site.[330,331] Selected delivery of laser energy within the subretinal space could theoretically allow for the obliteration of a subretinal choroidal neovascular complex and reduce damage to the overlying photoreceptor layer. Subretinal endophotocoagulation in rabbits has shown that low- to moderate-intensity burns (<1.0 W) preserve the overlying retina, and high-laser energy powers (>1.0 W) will cause coagulative necrosis of the outer retinal layers.[332] Thomas and Ibanez[333] developed a subretinal laser delivery system as an adjunct to the surgical excision of subfoveal choroidal neovascular membranes. A 31-gauge subretinal endolaser probe is used; it takes advantage of the difference in the index of refraction between silica and balanced salt solution to produce a down and forward laser beam. Strong unrelenting adhesions to previous laser or inflammatory chorioretinal scars occasionally preclude safe excision of a neovascular complex. When this situation is encountered, the firm adhesion or stalk of neovascular ingrowth can be cut with subretinal scissors and photocoagulated (outside the fovea) with the subretinal endolaser probe, minimizing damage to subfoveal retinal pigment epithelium, choriocapillaris, and the overlying neurosensory retina. In other instances, a small, subfoveal neovascular complex anterior to the retinal pigment epithelium is found intraoperatively to have a larger subretinal pigment epithelium component, the excision of which can lead to the development of a large retinal pigment epithelium tear. In these cases, the anterior component of the neovascular complex can be reflected and photocoagulated in an extrafoveal location. Finally, subretinal endophotocoagulation also allows for the obliteration of a bleeding subretinal stump that has failed to respond to elevated intraocular pressure.

Pharmacologic Therapy

Given the limitations of photocoagulation and surgical intervention, many investigators have searched for drugs to control choroidal neovascularization. Interferon (INF) alfa-2a initially attracted widespread attention, but results have been discouraging. It is an endogenous glycoprotein with antiproliferative, immunoregulatory, antiviral, and antiangiogenic properties,[334-339] and has been reported to be beneficial in the treatment of subretinal neovascularization.[340,341] The early experience reported by Thomas and Ibanez[342] was disappointing. In a prospective study, patients with recurrent subfoveal neovascularization following surgical excision and patients with subfoveal choroidal neovascularization without previous surgical excision received INF alfa-2a in a dose of 3.0 to 6.0 million units/m^2 body surface area every other night for an average of 12 weeks. Use of INF alfa-2a did not improve visual acuity or fluorescein angiographic appearance of subfoveal neovascular membranes in 90% of cases and was associated with significant side effects, including fever, alopecia, leukopenia, thrombocytopenia, elevated liver enzymes, and suicidal tendencies.

Chan and associates[343] reported an efficacy and toxicity study on the treatment of choroidal, neovascular membranes by INF alfa-2a. The regression of choroidal neovascularization was minimal. Toxic effects that interfered with patients' performance status were associated with the treatment. It is possible that higher doses may achieve a therapeutic response. In the future, better drug delivery systems may allow for the selective intraocular administration of high doses of INF alfa-2a, thus bypassing its toxicity. Unfortunately, a multinational, randomized, prospective study has revealed no treatment benefit. [344] Other antineovascular agents that are being evaluated include thalidomide and peptide inhibitors of integrin molecules.

Tissue Plasminogen Activator

Tissue plasminogen activator (t-PA) is a fibrinolytic agent[345] that activates plasminogen specifically in the presence of fibrin and whose activity is enhanced in the presence of fibrin.[346] Tissue plasminogen activator has been used as an adjunct to the surgical removal of subfoveal, choroidal neovascular membranes by Thomas and associates.[347] At a concentration of 6ug/0.1 ml, t-PA was injected into the subretinal space and 30 to 40 minutes were allowed to elapse for fibrin breakdown to occur. The t-PA dissolved the fibrin rim surrounding recent subfoveal membranes but was less effective on more mature lesions. These authors proposed that enzymatic dissolution of the fibrin rim resulted in less shearing of surrounding photoreceptors and retinal pigment epithelium when more recent subretinal neovascular membranes were grasped and removed. In contrast, with older membranes, the pseudopod-like strands of mature organized fibrin were more adherent and more manipulation was required for membrane removal. No increased bleeding occurred in these patients when the membranes were removed. Although t-PA may be a useful intraoperative tool, in our experience, gentle mechanical pressure against the edge of the neovascular complex usually "peels up" the fibrin rim without disturbing retinal pigment epithelium (unless the complex has grown beneath the retinal pigment epithelium).

Liquid Perfluorocarbons

Perfluoro-*N*-octane has been used to assist in the evacuation of subretinal hemorrhage and fluid, and to facilitate endophotocoagulation of the retinotomy site.[348] Perfluoro-*N*-octane was injected after membrane removal to reattach the retina and tamponade bleeding. An air-fluid exchange with removal of the perfluoro-*N*-octane was performed before sclerotomy closure. Simple air-fluid exchange appears to achieve the same ends.

RESULTS

Thomas and Kaplan[311] treated two patients with presumed ocular histoplasmosis subfoveal neovascular membranes and progressive visual acuity loss to 20/400. Visual acuity returned to 20/20 with 7 months follow-up in one patient and to 20/40 with 3 months follow-up in the other patient. Lambert and associates [348] reported the results of surgical excision of 10 consecutive, subfoveal choroidal neovascular membranes in patients with age-related macular degeneration. Six of these patients showed mixed visual improvement at 1 month and 3 month follow-up. Thomas and associates [328] reported surgical management of subfoveal choroidal neovascular membrane in 33 eyes with age-related macular degeneration, 20 eyes with presumed ocular histoplasmosis syndrome, and 5 eyes with miscellaneous etiologies. Five eyes also received subfoveal retinal pigment epithelial patches. With limited follow-up, significant improvement in vision (defined as 2 Snellen lines) was achieved in 7 of 22 eyes with age-related macular degeneration choroidal neovascular membrane removal, 0 of 4 eyes with age-related macular degeneration choroidal neovascular membrane removal and retinal pigment epithelial patches, and 1 of 7 eyes with age-related macular degeneration choroidal neovascular membrane disconnection. Significant improvement was achieved in 6 of 16 eyes with presumed ocular histoplasmosis syndrome choroidal membrane removal and 0 of 4 eyes with presumed ocular histoplasmosis syndrome choroidal neovascular membrane disconnection. In 5 eyes with miscellaneous choroidal neovascular membrane, 2 improved. Choroidal neovascular membrane recurred in 29%. Berger and Kaplan [349] reported their series of 15 patients with presumed ocular histoplasmosis syndrome and 19 patients with age-related macular degeneration followed for an average of 4 months postoperatively. Snellen visual acuity improved by two lines or more in 8 of 15 (53%) cases of presumed ocular histoplasmosis syndrome. Fourteen of 19 (74%) cases of age-related macular degeneration showed either slight improvement or stabilization of vision.

Thomas and associates[329] updated their surgical experience and explored possible correlations between preoperative characteristics and final postoperative visual acuity in 67 eyes with presumed ocular histoplasmosis syndrome, 41 eyes with age-related macular degeneration, 10 eyes with myopia, 9 eyes with multifocal choroiditis, 8 eyes with idiopathic choroidal neovascular membrane, 4 eyes with angioid streaks, and 8 eyes with miscellaneous etiologies for choroidal neovascularization. In eyes with presumed ocular histoplasmosis syndrome, mean follow-up was 10.5 months. Visual acuity was stable or improved in 56 (83%) eyes and was 20/40 or greater in 21 (31%) eyes. Mean interval to best visual acuity was 3 months. In eyes with age-related macular degeneration, mean follow-up was 15 months. Visual acuity was improved in only 5 (12%) eyes and was 20/40 or greater in only 2 (5%) eyes. The interval to best visual acuity was 5 months. Recurrence rates of 37% (presumed ocular histoplasmosis syndrome) and 27% (age-related macular degeneration) had no statistically significant effect on final visual outcome. Patients with focal disorders of the retinal pigment epithelium-Bruch's membrane complex appear to have a better surgical outcome than do those with diffuse disease. Adelberg and associates,[326] in their retrospective analysis of surgical removal of choroidal neovascular membrane in myopia, angioid streaks, and other disorders, found visual acuity to be stable in 10 of 17 (59%) eyes, improved by two or more Snellen lines in 6 (35%) eyes, and decreased in 1 (6%) eye. Postoperative visual acuity of better than 20/80 was achieved in only a minority of eyes. Ormerod and associates [350] reported long-term outcomes after the surgical removal of advanced neovascular membranes in age-related macular degeneration. The mean choroidal neovascular membrane size was 7 disk diameters. Surgically induced mean retinal pigment epithelium defect was 14 standard disk areas in size. Eight of 10 patients improved one to two lines of Snellen visual acuity postoperatively. A 2-year recurrence rate of 40% was observed. Connor and associates [351] surgically removed extrafoveal fibrotic choroidal neovascular membrane in a patient with age-related macular degeneration. Visual acuity improved from 20/200 to 20/25. Melberg and associates [352] reported their experience with recurrent neovascularization after subfoveal surgery in 120 patients with presumed ocular histoplasmosis syndrome. In 42%

of all eyes, recurrence developed in an average time of 4.4 months. Recurrent choroidal neovascular membrane location was subfoveal in 66% of eyes. Surgical excision of subfoveal neovascular membranes may result in recovery of excellent visual acuity in patients with presumed ocular histoplasmosis syndrome but not in patients with age-related macular degeneration. Gass[353] offered a rational explanation for these reported visual outcomes. He provided histopathologic evidence from autopsy eyes to propose a classification scheme. In type 1 choroidal neovascularization, as typically seen in individuals older than 50 years with age-related macular degeneration, the new vessels that arise in the choroid usually grow within the subpigment epithelial space and not in the subneurosensory retinal space. In type 2 choroidal neovascularization, typically seen in younger individuals with presumed ocular histoplasmosis syndrome, the new vessels are partly engulfed by a monolayer of proliferating retinal pigment epithelium and lie anterior to normal retinal pigment epithelium in the subneurosensory retinal space. Surgical excision of presumed ocular histoplasmosis syndrome membrane permits retention of intact normal retinal pigment epithelium, reapproximation of the retinal receptors, and native pigment epithelium and may be associated with remarkable return of visual acuity. [353]

SELECTED CASES

Case 1

An 82-year-old man had developed a fibrotic disciform scar in the left eye 3 years before presentation. Choroidal neovascularization developed in the right eye for which he underwent photocoagulation. Recurrent neovascular tissue arose predominantly superior to the fovea, and best corrected visual acuity dropped to 20/300. Given the clinical appearance of the lesion (well defined borders with blood apparently outlining a cleavage plane between the recurrent membrane and underlying retinal pigment epithelium), the referring retinal specialist believed that surgical removal of the complex might be preferable to additional laser (Figures 13.22A and B). Indeed during surgery, the membrane peeled up from underlying retinal pigment epithelium and came out in one piece with the

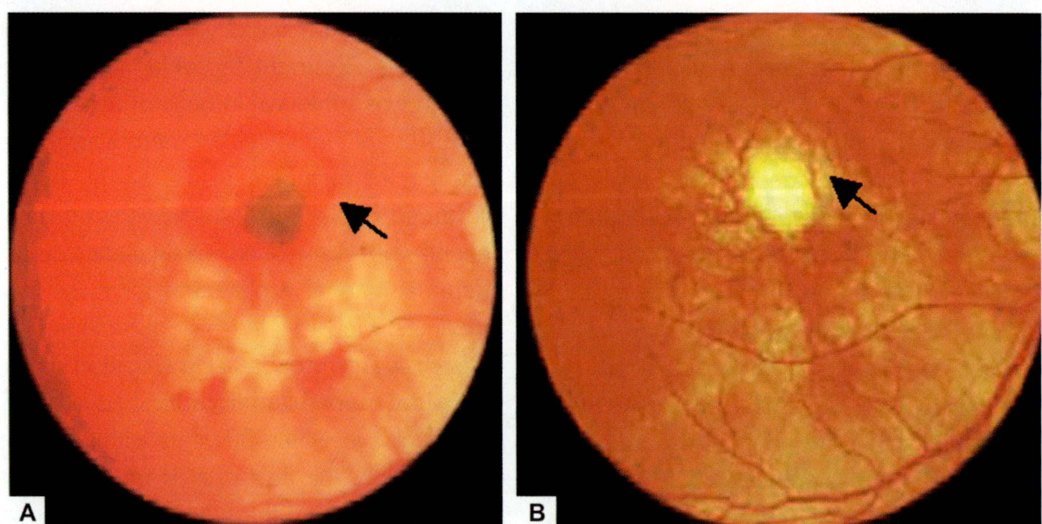

FIGURES 13.22 A and B: (A) Fundus appearance of a neovascular membrane. Note the blood, which appears to outline a clear border between the neovascular complex and underlying tissue. (B) Postoperative clinical appearance.The atrophic white spot is the site of laser scar removal. The retinal pigment epithelium appears thinned where the membrane previously lay, but the tissue appears intact.

prior laser scar. Within 3 months, visual acuity had improved to 20/40.

Case 2

A 57-year-old man presented with some drusen and pigment disturbance in both eyes, and an occult choroidal neovascular process was juxtafoveal in location in the right eye. He underwent laser photocoagulation; however, a subfoveal recurrence developed.

Best corrected visual acuity was 20/400 before surgery (Figures 13.23A and B). During the vitrectomy, the recurrent neovascular complex could be reflected from the underlying foveal retinal pigment epithelium, and the entire complex was removed. Postoperatively, a hyperpig-

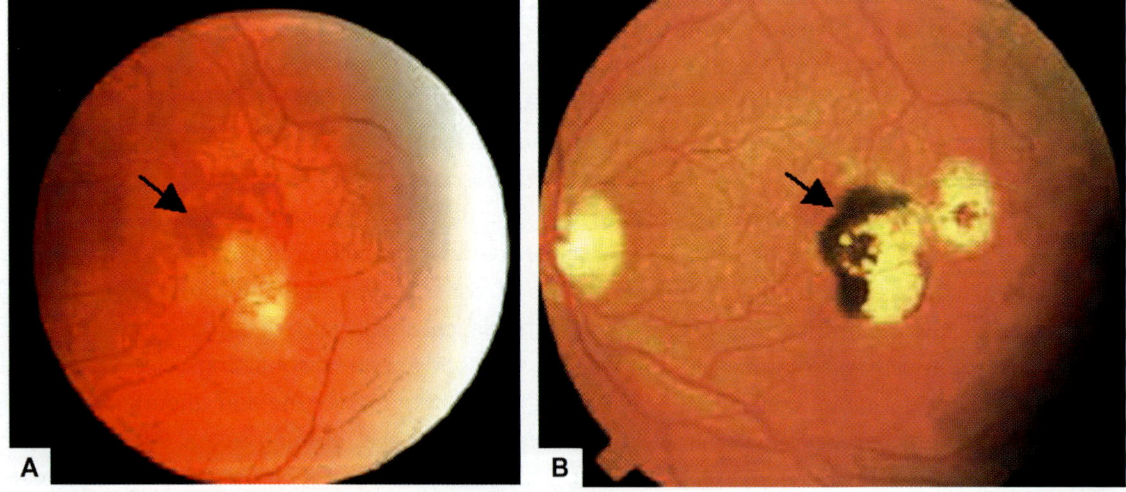

FIGURES 13.23A and B: (A) Preoperative appearance of recurrent subfoveal choroidal neovascularization (following laser). Best corrected visual acuity was 20/400). (B)Four years after surgery, the subfoveolar retinal pigment epithelium has become densely pigmented, but vision remains 20/20. The atrophic scar temporal in the macula is the site of the retinotomy, which was lasered to create a chorioretinal adhesion. It is now understood that laser treatment of retinotomies is almost never required.

mented reaction in the central retinal pigment epithelium developed with a dark black appearance. Visual acuity improved to 20/20 and has remained at this level with 4-year follow-up.

SUBMACULAR SURGERY TRIAL

The safety and possible efficacy of submacular surgery have been questioned.[354,355] It is appropriate to proceed with a randomized, controlled, prospective multicenter clinical trial to further evaluate subfoveal surgery. A pilot study for the submacular surgery trial has evaluated surgery in four categories.[356]

Group 1 includes eyes with age-related macular degeneration and subfoveal choroidal neovascular membranes in which the benefit of laser photocoagulation was minimal. Randomization is between surgery and observation. Group 2 includes eyes with age-related macular degeneration and recurrent subfoveal choroidal neovascular membranes that are deemed eligible for photocoagulation according to the Foveal Photocoagulation Study. Randomization is between surgery and laser photocoagulation. Group 3 includes eyes with age-related macular degeneration in which submacular hemorrhage comprises more than 50% of the macular lesion. Randomization is between surgery and observation. Group 4 includes eyes with presumed ocular histoplasmosis syndrome and idiopathic subfoveal choroidal neovascularization. Randomization is between surgery and observation. It is hoped that National Institute of Health funding will allow these pilot studies to expand into large multicentric studies. By carefully following the prospective protocol established in the submacular surgery trial data will be collected that will help define the appropriate role of submacular surgery in the management of patients with these difficult problems.

SUBMACULAR HEMORRHAGE

Blood beneath the neurosensory retina almost always originates from the choroidal circulation. Trauma to choroidal vessels can produce hemorrhage: from blunt or penetrating trauma, from inadvertent surgical trauma with a deep suture during scleral buckling or from drainage of subretinal fluid either internally or externally.[357,358] In the absence of trauma, hemorrhage can occur secondary to choroidal neovascularization.[359,360] Small hemorrhages frequently accompany the ingrowth of vessels from the choroid through Bruch's membrane. Extensive hemorrhages are believed to occur as a result of rupture of large choroidal vessels that extend into fibrovascular complexes. Vessels in fibrovascular scars have been observed to have arterial and venous characteristics and are continuous with choroidal arteries and veins, respectively.[361] Leakage of blood or serous fluid from the neovascular tissue leads to detachment of the retinal pigment epithelium and produces pressure on the artery and vein as they enter the fibrovascular scar. This pressure reportedly leads to necrosis of the artery and, when it ruptures, massive hemorrhage occurs with accumulation of blood under the retinal pigment epithelium, under neurosensory retina, and in some cases in the vitreous cavity.[362]

MECHANISM OF RETINAL INJURY

Subretinal blood is toxic to the outer retina and has been documented to cause irreversible photoreceptor damage.[363,364] Laboratory animal studies have shown that the degree of retinal destruction is correlated with the duration of contact of the retina with hemorrhage. These animal studies show that damage can occur as early as 1 hour,[365] with moderate to severe outer retinal destruction at 3 to 7 days and full-thickness retinal degeneration by day.[14,363,366,367] Subretinal blood clots form a mechanical barrier between the retina and the retinal pigment epithelium. This can inhibit metabolic exchange between retina and retinal pigment epithelium.[363] Retinal toxicity can result from iron liberated from hemoglobin that is released from degenerating erythrocytes.[364] Glatt and Machemer[363] showed that subretinal blood clot adherence and retraction caused tractional forces on the photoreceptors, which led to outer retinal damage. The role of fibrin in causing retinal damage associated with subretinal hemorrhage was better defined by Toth and associates.[365] They suggested that a fibrinolytic agent be used to dissolve the fibrin meshwork, thereby preventing the shearing effect on the photoreceptors. Benner and associates [368] demonstrated that t-PA could be safely used in the subretinal space at concentrations of 2.5 to 200.0 mg/liter. Higher doses caused severe, irreversible toxic effects to the photoreceptor- retinal pigment epithelium complex. The toxic effects of t-PA were attributable to the carrier vehicle. Coll and associates [369] reported the effect of intravitreal t-PA on experimental subretinal hemorrhage. Intravitreal t-PA 1 day after subretinal injection of blood in rabbits facilitated more rapid lysis of clotted blood; however, retinal damage was not prevented.

Hemorrhage is a frequent concomitant finding in age-related macular degeneration-associated maculopathy because of the intrinsic fragility of the vessels present in choroidal neovascularization. Subretinal blood either beneath the neurosensory retina or beneath the retinal pigment epithelium can have profound impact on the visual prognosis.

Blood presents a significant impediment to visualization of the pathologic process. Thus one objective in the management of hemorrhagic age-related macular degeneration is improving visualization to allow therapy. Subretinal blood (particularly thick blood) has long been considered toxic to photoreceptors and thus harmful to vision.

Lincoff and associates [370] determined the cellular mechanism that allows subretinal hemorrhage to cloud the vitreous. Thick subretinal hemorrhage causes necrosis of the overlying retina. Fragments of the erythrocytes infiltrate the retina and cross an intact internal limiting membrane to cloud the vitreous. Rapid necrosis of the retina occurs over thick subretinal hemorrhage and indicates the need for early displacement of the hemorrhage from the macula if function is to be preserved and breakthrough prevented.

Ito and associates [371] found that methemoglobin induced peroxidation of retinal unsaturated phospholipids directly and by releasing iron.

Terasaki and associates [372] evaluated changes in preoperative and postoperative macular electroretinograms in 5 eyes undergoing surgical drainage of macular subretinal hemorrhage using rt-PA. In all eyes, preoperative electroretinographic response was remarkably reduced or not recordable. Postoperative visual acuity improved, and electroretinographic response recovered to about one half the amplitude of the fellow eye in every eye with a normal fellow eye. A nearly non-recordable preoperative response on macular electroretinogram indicates severe dysfunction of the photoreceptors caused by the submacular hemorrhage. A postoperative recovered macular electroretinogram suggests that photoreceptor function is at least partially reversible with surgical intervention.

NATURAL HISTORY

The visual outcome of subretinal hemorrhage varies depending on the extent, location, and thickness of the hemorrhage. [373] Gillies and Lahav [374] reported three patients with age-related macular degeneration, myopia, and trauma with neither thick nor large subretinal hemorrhages. Their initial visual acuities of counting fingers (2 eyes) and 20/400 improved to 20/40 in 6 months, 20/25 in 3 months, and 20/67 in 6 months, respectively. Fekrat and associates [375] reviewed the natural history of 41 eyes with submacular hemorrhages and found a trend toward declining visual acuity over time. The median overall change between the initial and 3-year visual acuities was a loss of four lines. Eyes with larger and thicker hemorrhages had poorer visual acuity outcomes.

Subretinal hemorrhage associated with neovascular age-related macular degeneration generally carries a poor visual prognosis. In most reviews, macular lesions in which >/= 50% of the surface area is blood are defined as hemorrhagic. Avery and associates reported a mean loss of 3.5 lines of acuity during 36 months of follow-up of such eyes. Forty-four percent had lost 6 or more lines of acuity over the 3 years of follow-up. [376] Thick blood elevating retina, size of hemorrhage, and size of the entire lesion correlated with worse visual outcome in this series. Earlier, Bennett and associates [377] reviewed the cases of 29 patients with large subfoveal hemorrhages followed for an average of 3 years. Thicker hemorrhages had poorer final visual acuity than did thinner hemorrhages. Eyes with age-related macular degeneration had a worse final visual acuity than did non-age-related macular degeneration eyes. Eyes with choroidal rupture fared better than other eyes. The presence of age-related macular degeneration, rather than the thickness of the hemorrhage, was the factor most predictive of poor outcome as had also been seen in a previous series by Bennett and associates.[377] A larger series by Scupola and associates[378] found a similar grim visual outcome. Visual acuity in eyes with thick hemorrhage fell from 20/500 on presentation to 20/2000 with mean follow-up of 24 months. Subretinal hemorrhage (even thick clots) without choroidal neovascularization may clear with some improvement in acuity without intervention. The visual prognosis in these non- age-related macular degeneration eyes is significantly better than in hemorrhagic age-related macular degeneration.[379]

MANAGEMENT

In 1983, Dellaporta[380] described passing an endo-diathermy needle through retina, choroid, and sclera in a patient with a 10-week history of massive, posterior pole subretinal hemorrhage and a visual acuity of 3/200. The cauterized hole in the retina allowed the blood to spill into the vitreous cavity and vision returned to 20/25. Hanscom and Diddie[381] first used modern vitrectomy techniques, internal retinotomy, endodrainage of blood, and air-fluid exchange in the management of submacular hemorrhage. de Juan and Machemer[308] used vitrectomy and a combination of drainage and irrigation of subretinal clot and disciform scar removal. Early surgical intervention to avoid toxicity from subretinal hemorrhage was stressed by Slusher.[382]

CASE SELECTION

Multiple preoperative, intraoperative, and postoperative factors have an impact on the visual result following surgery for submacular hemorrhage. Preoperative factors, including the baseline health of the neurosensory retina and submacular retinal pigment epithelium, the presence of choroidal neovascularization, disciform scarring, or previous foveal photocoagulation will determine the postoperative visual potential. The health status of the retinal pigment epithelium and neurosensory retina can also influence the tolerance of these tissues to the noxious effects of subretinal blood. Eyes with age-related macular degeneration may have more extensive and diffuse photoreceptor/retinal pigment epithelium dysfunction and less metabolic reserve than eyes without age-related macular degeneration (i.e. eyes with choroidal neovascular membranes due to presumed ocular histoplasmosis syndrome, macroaneurysm, or idiopathic causes). This may partially explain why eyes without age-related macular degeneration are more likely to have visual improvement following surgery than are eyes with age-related macular degeneration. The duration of submacular hemorrhage may also be an important factor. Progressive photoreceptor destruction has been observed to occur for up to 14 days following introduction of experimental subretinal hemorrhage. Postoperative visual function may also be affected by photoreceptor and/or retinal pigment epithelium trauma induced by surgical manipulations in the subretinal space as well as intraoperative and postoperative complications. In the absence of results from clinical trials, case selection remains unclear. The Randomized, Prospective Submacular Surgery Trial is comparing surgical removal of large submacular hemorrhage secondary to age-related macular degeneration. No randomization trials have been proposed for hematomas of other etiologies. Hence, at the present time only impressions regarding case selection can be offered. Relatively thin hemorrhages unassociated with choroidal neovascularization often do well with observation. Thick hemorrhage without known choroidal neovascularization may be appropriate for removal. Thick hemorrhages with probable choroidal neovascularization remain controversial. Recent-onset hemorrhages probably have a better surgical result than do older hemorrhages and may be appropriate for t-PA use (Figures 13.24A and B).

Observation

Given the poor natural history of hemorrhagic age-related macular degeneration, observation is of limited appeal in cases with thick subretinal hemorrhage. In cases with thin blood, watchful waiting may be reasonable. As a thin hemorrhage clears, indocyanine green imaging may become feasible and reveal treatable pathology.

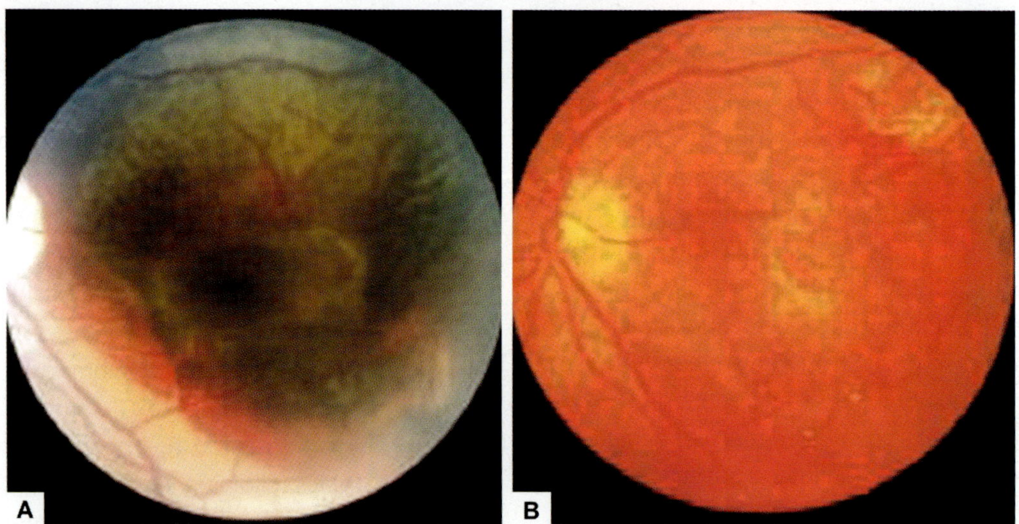

FIGURES 13.24A and B: (A) The thickness of submacular hemorrhage is better appreciated on higher magnification. (B) Three months postoperatively, the macula is free of subretinal hemorrhage. The causative neovascular membrane was superotemporal. Visual acuity returned to 20/70.

Thermal Laser and Photodynamic Therapy

Thin hemorrhages may be absorbed and subsequently allow more informative angiography. It may be reasonable to treat some hemorrhagic cases involving thin blood with thermal laser, especially if indocyanine green hot spots are identified. In a review of 30 cases, Kramer and associates[383] found that 2/3rd of the eyes had treatable lesions (hot spots or plaques) when imaged with indocyanine green, while only 1 in 6 had treatable lesions based on fluorescein angiography. Occasionally, it is appropriate to treat visible choroidal neovascular membrane with photodynamic therapy. As the hemorrhage clears, additional angiography may show the need for more laser.

Vitrectomy with Mechanical Clot Extraction, without Tissue Plasminogen Activator (t-PA)

Given the poor prognosis of hemorrhagic age-related macular degeneration with thick blood, many investigators have explored vitrectomy to remove the clot and associated choroidal neovascularization. Visual acuity has been almost universally poor (20/200) or worse, and a high rate of complications including retinal detachment with proliferative vitreoretinopathy have been common. Mechanical extraction of blood clot is also being evaluated in submacular surgery trials. Mechanical removal of the choroidal neovascular membrane/clot may be appropriate in select cases.

Vitrectomy with Clot Removal Following Subretinal Tissue Plasminogen Activator Injection

Tissue plasminogen activator is an endogenous serine protease with a molecular weight of 70,000. t-PA forms a complex with fibrin to activate plasminogen to plasmin, which in turn lyses fibrin into soluble degradation products, thus achieving clot lysis.[384]

t-PA has a theoretical appeal in managing subretinal hemorrhage: facilitation of liquefaction of thick clots to allow extrafoveal displacement and modulation of the fibrin-neurosensory retinal interaction that may cause shearing of photoreceptors.[385]

It is hypothesized that dealing with liquefied blood may be less traumatic to neurosensory retina than mechanical clot removal.

Surgical technique: Pars plana vitrectomy with posterior hyaloid removal is followed by subretinal injection of t-PA (10-12 micrograms per 0.1 ml). Twenty to 40 minutes pass with t-PA bathing the clot before active irrigation is done through the same or adjacent retinotomy to flush out the dissolved blood. Some blood always remains; the goal is to remove most of the thick, large clots. Some surgeons advocate grasping and removing the causative neovascular complex, if visible, whereas others intentionally leave it in place.

Pneumatic Displacement with or without Tissue Plasminogen Activator

Heriot pioneered the management of subretinal hemorrhage with intravitreal t-PA and gas injection without vitrectomy in 1997.

Surgical technique: The injection procedure was performed with the patient under retrobulbar anesthesia. Fifty micrograms of commercial recombinant tissue plasminogen activator (rt-PA) solution in a volume of 50 microliters, is drawn in a tuberculin syringe and injected slowly into the midvitreous cavity through a 30-gauge needle. After an aqueous tap to reduce intraocular pressure, 0.5 ml of 100% sulfur hexafluoride gas is injected into the vitreous cavity. Both injections are administered via the pars plana in the superotemporal quadrant, 3 mm posterior to the limbus in pseudophakic patients and 3.5 mm posterior to the limbus in phakic patients. Patients were then instructed to maintain prone positioning for 72 hours. Whenever blood displacement from under the fovea was not complete, prone positioning was continued for an additional 24 to 48 hours.

Krepler and associates [386] assessed the efficacy and safety of intravitreal injection of rt-PA (25 micrograms) and 0.5 ml sulfur hexafluoride gas for displacement of subretinal hemorrhages in age-related macular degeneration. Displacement of subretinal blood was successful within the first week after surgery in 10 of 11 patients. This was accompanied by visual improvement in eight patients. Hattenbach and associates [387] investigated the efficacy and safety of treating 43 eyes with submacular hemorrhages secondary to age-related macular degeneration with 50 micrograms intravitreous rt-PA and 0.5 ml sulfur hexafluoride gas. Final visual acuity was improved two or more lines in 13 eyes (30%), stable in 26 (61%), and two or more lines worse in 4 eyes (9%). Duration of hemorrhage <or=14 days was associated with a better gain of lines of vision. Overall, complete displacement of blood from under the fovea was achieved in 35 eyes (81%). Handwerger and associates [388] reviewed 14 eyes

who received low-dose intravitreal t-PA (18-50 micrograms) and expansile gas (0.3-0.4 ml of perfluoropropane) for thrombolysis and displacement of submacular hemorrhage. After the procedure, patients maintained face-down positioning for 1 to 3 days. Submacular blood was completely displaced from the fovea in 10 (71%) of the 14 patients and partially displaced in 3 (21%). Early (<2 months) postoperative visual acuity improved by 2 or more lines in 8 patients (57%). Schulze and Hesse [389] assessed factors predicting final visual outcome after displacement of subretinal hemorrhage by intravitreally injected t-PA and gas in patients suffering from age-related macular degeneration. The best visual outcome after t-PA and gas injection can be expected in patients with preoperative acuity of less than 0.1 caused by a small submacular hemorrhage. In the presence of large submacular hemorrhage (diameter >5 mm) an increase in visual acuity after therapy is unlikely. Hesse and associates [390] quantified the effect of intravitreally injected t-PA and an expanding gas on freshly formed submacular hemorrhage. Patients were treated with an intravitreal injection of 50 micrograms t-PA, and 24 hours later, with an expanding gas. A significant shift of the geometric center toward the inferior retinal periphery out of the macula was found after gas injection. Enlargement of subretinal hemorrhage in a gravity-dependent manner indicates submacular liquefaction of the clot after t-PA treatment. An intravitreal injection of gas 24 hours later can significantly displace the submacular hemorrhage inferiorly. Hassan and associates [391] investigated the efficacy and safety of treating thick submacular hemorrhages with intravitreous t-PA and pneumatic displacement in 15 eyes with acute (<3 weeks) thick subretinal hemorrhage involving the center of the macula in eyes with pre-existing good visual acuity. Hemorrhages were secondary to age-related macular degeneration in 13 eyes and macroaneurysm and trauma in 1 eye each. Patients received intravitreous injection of commercial t-PA solution (25-100 micrograms in 0.1-0.2 ml) and expansile gas (0.3-0.4 ml of perfluoropropane or sulfur hexafluoride) for thrombolysis and displacement of submacular hemorrhage. The procedure resulted in complete displacement of thick submacular hemorrhage out of the foveal area in all the eyes. Final visual acuity improved by 2 lines or greater in 10 (67%) of 15 eyes and measured 20/80 or better in 6 (40%) of 15 eyes. Complications included breakthrough vitreous hemorrhage in three eyes and endophthalmitis in one eye. Ohji and associates [392] assessed the efficacy and complications of intravitreal injection of perfluoropropane gas for displacement of subretinal hemorrhage, without the use of t-PA. Pure perfluoropropane gas (0.4-0.5 ml) was injected into the vitreous cavity in 4 eyes with age-related macular degeneration and one eye with ruptured retinal arterial macroaneurysm. The patients were instructed to maintain a prone position. Final visual acuity improved in all cases, ranging from 20/15 to 20/220. Gas injected into the vitreous cavity can displace subretinal hemorrhage without the use of tissue plasminogen activator in some cases. Visual acuity after gas injection may be improved, making this treatment an alternative to evacuation of subretinal hemorrhage with vitrectomy. These results are similar to those seen in vitrectomy, but complications are significantly reduced. The most frequent complication is breakthrough hemorrhage. Controversy remains regarding the potential retinal toxicity of intravitreal t-PA. To minimize risks, most surgeons commonly use a concentration of 50 micrograms per 0.1 ml or less for intravitreal injection. Subretinal recombinant tissue plasminogen activator injection has also been used along with pneumatic displacement of thick submacular hemorrhage in age-related macular degeneration.[393]

Vitrectomy, Subretinal Injection of t-PA and Fluid-gas Exchange

A hybrid approach with the goals of maximizing clot lysis while minimizing the risk of trauma to the retina and retinal pigment epithelium can be taken.

Surgical technique: Following pars plana vitrectomy and posterior hyaloid removal, a bent 36-gauge needle is used to inject 25 or 50 micrograms of t-PA per 0.1 ml directly into the clot. Complete fluid-air exchange is performed and the eye is left with a full fill of either 20% SF6 gas or air. Postoperatively, face down positioning is advised. Haupert and associates [394] described this procedure for displacement of large, thick submacular hemorrhage in patients with age-related macular degeneration. With surgery, subretinal hemorrhage was displaced from the fovea in all 11 cases. Final postoperative visual acuity ranged from 20/70 to light perception, with improvement in eight (73%) cases. This technique displaces submacular hemorrhage from the fovea and can improve vision in patients with age-related macular degeneration.

Other Techniques

Tissue plasminogen activator has been used as an adjunct in the surgical removal of submacular hemorrhage. It is usually used intraoperatively, but may not provide enough time for effective fibrinolysis, especially for a large hemorrhage. Chaudhry and associates [395] conducted a study to evaluate the efficiency and safety of preoperative use of t-PA for large submacular hemorrhages. Five eyes with large submacular hemorrhage secondary to age-related macular degeneration underwent subretinal injection of t-PA 24 hours before surgery. All hemorrhages were less than seven days old and at least 3 mm thick. Four of the five eyes (80%) showed improved visual acuity after surgery and 3/5 (60%) attained visual acuity of 20/200 or better. Kamei and associates [396] used t-PA and perfluorocarbon liquid in surgical removal of submacular hemorrhage, in 22 eyes, which underwent pars plana vitrectomy. The hemorrhages were liquefied with tissue plasminogen activator, squeezed into the vitreous cavity with perfluorocarbon liquid, and then evacuated. Efficacy of the procedure was judged by the best postoperative corrected visual acuity, which was 20/100 or better in 16 eyes (73%). Submacular hemorrhage recurred in four (18%) eyes, epiretinal membrane formed in three (14%) eyes, and retinal detachment occurred in three (14%) eyes. Best-corrected final visual acuity was improved postoperatively in 18 (82%) of the 22 eyes, unchanged in three (14%) eyes, and decreased in one (5%) eye, final visual acuity was 20/200 or better in 15 eyes (68%) and limited in other eyes by subretinal hemorrhage of greater than 30 days' duration or subfoveal neovascularization. Use of tissue plasminogen activator and perfluorocarbon liquid in surgical removal of submacular hemorrhage may improve the outcome of surgery by reducing surgically induced retinal damage. Jonas and

Jager [397] reported on the use of perfluorohexyloctane as a heavy liquid to temporarily tamponade the fovea for the prevention of recurrent massive subfoveal hemorrhage in 7 patients with exudative age-related macular degeneration. The patients underwent pars plana vitrectomy, drainage of the subretinal blood, and foveal endotamponade with perfluorohexyloctane. The perfluorohexyloctane was removed after 98 days (range 22-118 days) after the primary surgery in a second pars plana intervention. In six patients (85.7%) the subretinal hemorrhage removed during the first pars plana vitrectomy did not recur after removal of perfluorohexyloctane. In the seventh, however, a subretinal hemorrhage re-developed five days after release of perfluorohexyloctane. Perfluorohexyloctane may be a useful additional tool for preventing the recurrence of subfoveal re-bleeding in exudative age-related macular degeneration. Matsuo and associates [398] described a new surgical strategy, planned two-step vitrectomy, for a large and thick submacular hemorrhage involving 3 or more quadrants of the fundus. In a first-step vitrectomy, a retinotomy was made in the posterior pole, after any vitreous hemorrhage had been removed. Following fluid-gas exchange with no laser photocoagulation around the retinotomy, patients took a facedown position for a few days to a week to facilitate subretinal hemorrhage movement to the vitreous cavity and anterior chamber. In a second-step surgery, the hemorrhage in the vitreous cavity and anterior chamber was washed out. The remaining subretinal hemorrhage was aspirated, and the retina was reattached with fluid-gas exchange and laser photocoagulation around the retinotomy. The planned two-step vitrectomy is a safer and more effective procedure for removing a large quantity of subretinal hemorrhage in a shorter period of surgical time, compared with hemorrhage removal in a single vitrectomy.

SPECIAL CONSIDERATIONS

Patients with neovascular age-related macular degeneration who are chronically anticoagulated (on warfarin) have a higher risk of this devastating complication. Tilanus and associates, [399] in their retrospective study of age-related macular degeneration cases complicated by massive subretinal and vitreous hemorrhage found no difference between the hemorrhagic cases and controls but they did find that the massive hemorrhage patients were 12 times more likely than controls to use warfarin.

Subretinal Hemorrhage in other Clinical Conditions

Large submacular hemorrhages may occur after photodynamic therapy with verteporfin in age-related macular degeneration patients with subfoveal choroidal; neovascular membrane. Even in the absence of acute severe visual acuity decrease, submacular hemorrhage after verteporfin therapy can be associated with severe vision loss and preclude determining if additional therapy should be given.[400-403] Submacular hemorrhage may also be associated with laser *in situ* keratomileusis and central serous retinopathy. Central serous retinopathy may also be complicated by massive subretinal hemorrhage.[402,403] Shiraga and associates [404] reported the visual outcome of surgical treatment of submacular hemorrhage associated with idiopathic polypoidal choroidal vasculopathy in 8 eyes treated with pars plana vitrectomy and tissue plasminogen activator-assisted removal of subretinal blood or intravitreal 100% sulfur hexafluoride gas injection without t-PA. Postoperatively, laser treatment was performed for active polypoidal lesions outside the foveal avascular zone in four eyes. The best-corrected visual acuity improved (by 3 or more lines) or stabilized in seven of the eight eyes. Four eyes had a final best-corrected visual acuity of 20/40 or better, and three eyes had a final best-corrected visual acuity of 20/50 to 20/200. Surgical intervention may be of benefit in eyes with submacular hemorrhage associated with idiopathic polypoidal choroidal vasculopathy. Morse and associates[405] described the clinical features of 49 patients with advanced proliferative diabetic retinopathy who underwent vitrectomy and were found to have subretinal hemorrhages. In general, removal of subretinal hemorrhages was not necessary to achieve macular anatomic attachment, and most patients experienced improved visual function after surgery. Diabetic subretinal hemorrhages may indicate a retinal break, and, therefore, careful ophthalmic inspection should be performed in these patients. Chen and associates[406] evaluated the efficacy of rt-PA and SF6 in displacing submacular hemorrhage in patients who had scleral buckling procedures complicated by the development of submacular hemorrhage. Sequential intravitreal injections of 50 microgram rt-PA in 0.1 ml and 0.4 cc SF$_6$ were performed in eight patients. Submacular hemorrhage was totally or partially displaced extramacular in all patients on the day after rt-PA and SF6 injection. Vitreous hemorrhage was present in all patients. The retina was attached in all patients and no recurrent retinal detachment was noted. Visual acuity was improved at 6 months after treatment in all seven of the patients with macula-off retinal detachments compared to the preoperative visual acuity. Use of intravitreal air bubble for displacing submacular hemorrhage during scleral buckling surgery has also been reported. [407] Humayun and associates [408] reported intraoperative pharmacologic lysis of recent submacular hemorrhage with rt-PA followed by surgical drainage of the unclotted blood in patients with retinal arterial macroaneurysms in nine eyes. All nine eyes had improved final corrected visual acuity after surgery, and eight eyes (89%) attained a corrected visual acuity of 20/60 or better. Sudden severe vitreous hemorrhage may be an immediate complication after intravitreal injection of tissue plasminogen activator and gas for treatment of submacular hemorrhage associated with retinal arterial macroaneurysm.[409]

COMPLICATIONS

Substantial postoperative complications have been seen following surgical removal of subretinal hemorrhage. Postoperative retinal detachment, proliferative vitreoretinopathy, recurrent subretinal hemorrhage, subretinal fibrosis, cataract, and optic atrophy have been reported.

RESULTS

Hanscom and Diddie[381] reported evacuation of subretinal hemorrhage of 1 week's duration from two patients (age-related macular degeneration and a ruptured macroaneurysm). Visual acuity improved from counting fingers and hand motions to 20/400 by 3 months and 20/80 at 1 month, respectively. De Juan and Machemer [308] obtained improved, though limited, visual acuity in three of four patients with exudative age-related macular degeneration and large submacular hemorrhage. These patients had subretinal hemorrhage for a greater than 1 week duration. Wade and associates [359] evacuated subretinal hemorrhage greater than five disk diameters in 14 patients. Five patients had massive subretinal hemorrhages associated with age-related macular degeneration. The other nine patients had hemorrhagic retinal detachments, scleral buckling complications that led to subretinal hemorrhage, traumatic retinal detachments, and sickle cell disease. All five age-related macular degeneration eyes had preoperative visual acuities of 20/200 or worse and postoperative visual acuities of 5/200 or less. Three other eyes had improved visual acuity postoperatively. Age-related macular degeneration was associated with guarded recovery of visual acuity. Vander and associates [410] reported 11 patients, of whom 4 (36%) showed improved visual acuity after evacuation of the subretinal blood. However, retinal detachments with proliferative vitreoretinopathy developed postoperatively in 36% of patients and cataracts occurred postoperatively in another 36%. Because of the high rate of postoperative complications, the authors did not recommend evacuation of such large subretinal hemorrhages. Peyman and associates [411] reported t-PA-assisted removal of subretinal hemorrhage. One (33%) of three eyes had improved visual acuity and the other two eyes were stabilized. In the series of Lewis, [412] only eyes with recently documented good vision before the hemorrhage in the affected eye underwent surgery. Twenty (83%) of these 24 eyes showed an improvement in visual acuity. Eight eyes (33%) had postoperative visual acuity of 20/200 or better. In the series of Lim and associates, [413] 5 (28%) of 18 eyes showed an improved visual acuity of two lines or more. The use of perfluoro-*N*-octane showed a trend toward better postoperative visual acuity outcomes. The perfluoro-*N*-octane served to tamponade the retinotomy site and keep the t-PA in the subretinal space during the waiting period. The subsequent use of perfluoro-*N*-octane to express blood from the subretinal space may limit the manipulation required and thus spare the underlying retinal pigment epithelium and the overlying retina from mechanical trauma and cellular loss. Ibanez and associates, [414] in their 47 cases of submacular hemorrhage removal, noted that age-related macular degeneration eyes had a poor prognosis overall with or without use of t-PA. Recently, Kamei and associates [415] reported surgical removal of submacular hemorrhage using t-PA and perfluorocarbon liquid. Best postoperative corrected final visual acuity was 20/100 or better in 16 (73%) of the 22 eyes. Despite the significant interest in the surgical removal of submacular hemorrhages, the visual outcomes in all reported series have been disappointing. However, the natural history of these eyes is often poor. Thus, a trial comparing surgery to observation appears to be warranted. The submacular surgery trial includes large age-related macular degeneration-associated hemorrhages in such a randomized comparison. The submacular surgery trial currently is investigating the benefit of surgically evacuating massive submacular hemorrhage versus observing these eyes. [416] In addition the recognition that preserving the retinal pigment epithelium is related to better visual acuity outcomes will aid in selecting those cases with subretinal hemorrhage without associated subretinal pigment epithelial hemorrhage. [413]

VITRECTOMY FOR DIABETIC MACULAR EDEMA

Macular edema is a major cause of visual loss in a number of ocular disorders, including diabetes, retinal vein occlusion, postoperative edema (Irvine–Gass), uveitis, vitreomacular traction syndrome, and retinitis pigmentosa. The reasons discussed for the development of persistent macular edema are diverse. Breakdown of the blood–retinal barrier and vitreoretinal traction are probably the most relevant factors. [417,418] Treatment of persistent macular edema remains a major challenge. Best analyzed is the clinical course of the macular edema in diabetes. The ETDRS study demonstrated that early photocoagulation of a clinically significant macular edema in diabetic patients reduces the visual loss by half in a subgroup of eyes with mild to moderate non-proliferative diabetic retinopathy. [419] Nevertheless, in about 50% of the patients laser photocoagulation fails to improve the functional and anatomical outcome. [420] For macular edema due to other underlying conditions, potential treatment approaches are even more limited. Central retinal vein occlusion leads to a poor visual outcome in

most cases, especially in ischemic types or in eyes with persistent macular edema. The central vein occlusion study group reported a visual acuity of 20/100 or less after 3 years in 58% of the patients and an improvement by 2 lines or more in only 20% of cases. Treatment with laser photocoagulation or isovolemic hemodilution has no significant impact on the visual outcome of eyes with central retinal vein occlusion and macular edema. [421] Similar limited success is reported for treatment of persistent macular edema in patients with uveitis. In 21-52% of patients with uveitis a clinically significant macular edema with decrease of the visual acuity is found. [422] Long-term examinations demonstrate a persistent reduction in visual acuity in 74% of the patients despite anti-inflammatory treatment with topical non-steroidal anti-inflammatory drugs, steroids and systemic anti-inflammatory and immunosuppressive agents. Similarly, topical and systemic treatment with carbonic anhydrase inhibitors failed to reduce the macular edema. [423]

CLINICAL CHARACTERISTICS

Diffuse diabetic macular edema is macular thickening due to diffuse leakage from a generally dilated macular retinal capillary bed in eyes with diabetic retinopathy. Sometimes it is further classified based on the presence of macular cysts. It is often bilateral. Hard exudates may be variable, from none to extensive. Attached posterior hyaloid often may be present and appears as thickened and taut. Fluorescein angiography reveals diffuse leakage from retinal capillaries and possibly from the choriocapillaris across the retinal pigment epithelium. There may be associated shallow (10 microns or greater) macular detachment detectable by optical coherence tomography. Associated systemic factors may include cardiovascular or renal fluid retention, and systemic hypertension.

RATIONALE

In recent years it has become evident that the vitreous must play a role in various aspects of diabetic retinopathy. The exact role of the vitreous is, however, in many aspects still ill defined. There are structural changes of the vitreous, as for instance vitreous liquefaction and posterior vitreous detachment, which are associated with the occurrence and earlier onset of diabetic retinopathy. Further there are angiogenic and angioinhibitory factors in the vitreous which influence neovascularization by means of endothelial cell proliferation. Photocoagulation of the retina can cause structural changes (posterior vitreal detachment) and histological changes (increased hyalocytes activity), which can protect against the progression of proliferative diabetic retinopathy. The role of vitrectomy in protecting against proliferative diabetic retinopathy is generally related to the removal of the vitreal scaffold. But vitrectomy can also induce changes in the oxygenation of the eye. If complete detachment of the posterior vitreous can be achieved it might be possible to further slow the progression of diabetic retinopathy. It is possible that in the future, manipulation of the vitreous by means of enzymes and lasers can play a role in the treatment and prevention of diabetic retinopathy.[424]

The physiologic mechanism of photocoagulation can be seen in the following steps. The physical light energy is absorbed in the melanin of the retinal pigment epithelium. The adjacent photoreceptors are destroyed and are replaced by a glial scar and the oxygen consumption of the outer retina is reduced. Oxygen that normally diffuses from the choriocapillaris into the retina can now diffuse through the laser scars in the photoreceptor layer without being consumed in the mitochondria of the photoreceptors. This oxygen flux reaches the inner retina to relieve inner retinal hypoxia and raise the oxygen tension. As a result, the retinal arteries constrict and the blood flow decreases. Hypoxia relief reduces production of growth factors such as vascular endothelial growth factor and neovascularization is reduced or stopped. Vasoconstriction increases arteriolar resistance, decreases hydrostatic pressure in capillaries and venules and reduces edema formation according to Starling's law. Vitrectomy also improves retinal oxygenation by allowing oxygen and other nutrients to be transported in water currents in the vitreous cavity from well oxygenated to ischemic areas of the retina. Vitrectomy and retinal photocoagulation both improve retinal oxygenation and both reduce diabetic macular edema and retinal neovascularization.[425]

Vitreous surgery may improve perifoveal microcirculation in the eyes of diabetic patients with cystoid macular edema and resolve the macular edema. Improvement of perifoveal microcirculation may be an important factor affecting visual outcome.[426] In addition, the removal of the vitreous might have a beneficial effect due to a potential accumulation of growth factors and inflammatory cytokines in the vitreous gel. Leukocyte-mediated endothelial cell damage and apoptosis in experimental diabetes have been demonstrated to increase the vascular permeability.[427] Also, vitreous levels of Angiotensin II and vascular endothelial growth factor have been reported to be elevated in diabetic macular edema patients irrespective of the status of posterior vitreous detachment. Angiotensin II and vascular endothelial growth factor may be induced in the eyes and be related to the pathogenesis.[428] In another study, altered vitreous levels of interleukin-6 and vascular endothelial growth factor have been related to diabetic macular edema.[429] Ikeda and associates[430] investigated the pathogenesis of honeycombed cystoid macular edema in patients with diabetes and demonstrated a strong correlation between an attached posterior hyaloid membrane and the presence of honeycombed cystoid macular edema. They suggested that retinal traction by the posterior hyaloid membrane is involved in the pathogenesis of honeycombed cystoid changes in diabetic patients. In order to further improve fluid diffusion from the retinal tissue, a removal of the remaining barrier between the vitreous cavity and the retina might be a promising approach. The internal limiting membrane is thought to be formed by the footplates of the Müller cells. However, there is controversy as to whether the internal limiting membrane can be considered a real basement membrane.[431] Peeling of the internal limiting membrane has been performed previously to reduce vitreoretinal traction and in combination with the removal of macular epiretinal membranes. How internal limiting membrane peeling reduces diabetic macular edema is unclear; however, it is likely that the peeling can only increase diffusion of fluid from the retinal tissue by eliminating the barrier function of the internal limiting membrane, a pseudomembrane formed by the endplates of Müller-cells, which is thought to act as a diffusion barrier between the retina and the vitreous. The blood-retinal barrier as evidenced by fluorescein angiography, in contrast, seems to be unaffected. Blood-retinal barrier breakdown as seen in persistent macular edema is the result of several pathophysiological alterations which have been investigated clinically and experimentally, including increased passive permeability, structural defects of junction molecules, and increased expression of permeability factors.[432-436] It is much more likely that internal limiting membrane peeling merely reduces the diffusion barrier towards the vitreous and thus is more efficient in patients with preexisting interface alterations. With respect to the inflammation-mediated fluid accumulation, intravitreal application of triamcinolone in combination with internal limiting membrane peeling could be a promising approach. A reduction in the inflammatory response most likely plays a role. However, there is currently no broad-based clinical investigation analyzing the long-term effect of these treatment approaches on persistent macular edema and its interaction with internal limiting membrane peeling.

SURGICAL TECHNIQUE

The surgical technique includes pars plana vitrectomy that utilizes the standard three port incisions. After core vitrectomy, the remaining cortical vitreous is aspirated with a flexible tipped cannula or a vitreous cutter to create posterior hyaloid detachment. After confirming the presence of a sheet-like posterior hyaloid membrane, including Weiss's ring, the remaining vitreous, up to vitreous base is removed.

Intraocular injection of triamcinolone acetonide during a vitrectomy visualizes the transparent vitreous and that this method helps surgeons to obtain complete separation of the posterior vitreous from the retina. A triamcinolone acetate aqueous suspension is left standing for 30 minutes, and the vehicle of triamcinolone acetonide is discarded. The remaining triamcinolone (40 mg) suspension is mixed with 2.5 ml of balanced salt solution. Next, 0.5 to 1.0 ml of triamcinolone suspension is injected with a 27-gauge needle into the midvitreous cavity. The triamcinolone granules are trapped in the gel structure of the residual vitreous cortex. After this procedure, residual vitreous cortex is typically seen on the retina as either a diffuse membrane or small islands. Residual posterior vitreous cortex could not be visualized without using the triamcinolone acetonide suspension.

Posterior hyaloidal separation can also be achieved using triamcinolone acetonide. A core vitrectomy was performed and 0.5-1.0 ml of triamcinolone suspension was injected with a 23-gauge needle into the midvitreous cavity. The triamcinolone granules were trapped in the gel structure of the vitreous. Then, posterior cortical vitreous appears as a white gel and a break of posterior hyaloid cortex appears on the temporal retinal vein. Next, the edge of the hyaloid cortex break is held by the gentle aspiration of the vitrectomy probe. The separation of the posterior hyaloid from the retina can be easily started from this edge by gentle cutting and mild aspiration (less than 50 mm Hg). During this procedure, the posterior hyaloid is clearly seen as a white colored vitreous. Even after this procedure, the residual vitreous cortex was sometimes left on the retina as islands. The thin layer of vitreous cortex that is visualized with triamcinolone acetonide is removed, using Tano's diamond dusted membrane eraser or brush back-flush needle.

The internal limiting membrane is stained with 0.125% of indocyanine green dye under balanced salt solution. The dye is removed immediately after injection to minimize possible complication. Internal limiting membrane is removed using an asymmetric forceps or other microforceps.

In order to visualize the peripheral vitreous, a triamcinolone suspension is sprayed onto the peripheral vitreous, so that the peripheral vitreous appears as a white gel. Peripheral vitreous is removed as much as possible. Removal of peripheral vitreous after internal limiting membrane peeling can decrease the postoperative concentration of indocyanine green dye in the vitreous cavity, reducing its possible toxicity. Thereafter, an attempt is made to wash out the residual triamcinolone granules from the eye. The vitreous with triamcinolone is removed with a vitrectomy probe. Although small amounts of triamcinolone granules (<1 mg) are usually left on the inferior retina, they disappear within 2 weeks after pars plana vitrectomy.

Results of surgery are shown in Figures 13.25A to D.

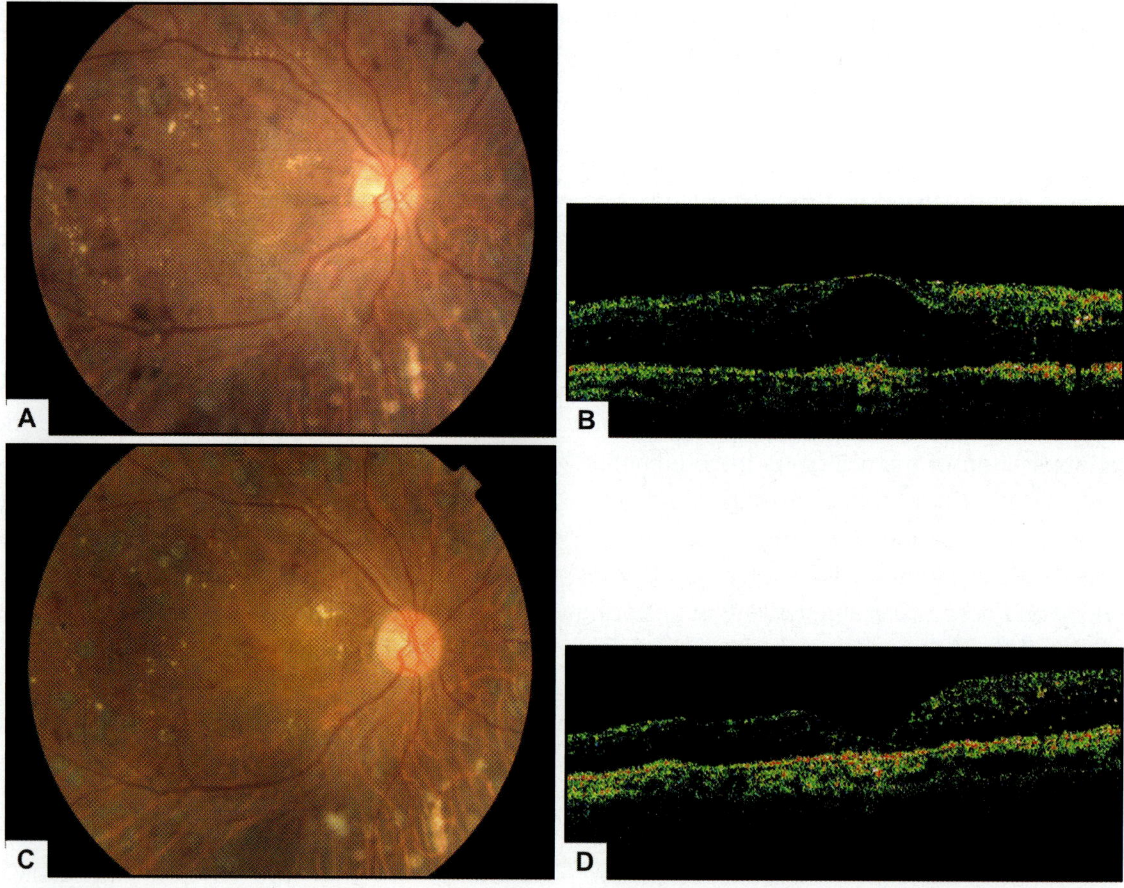

FIGURE 13.25A to D: (A) A 69-year-old female with cystoid macular edema due to diabetic retinopathy. Fundus examination revealed taut posterior vitreous membrane. Visual acuity was 20/250 preoperatively. (B) Optical coherent tomography disclosed marked cystoid macular edema. (C) Macular edema was resolved following vitrectomy combined with internal limiting membrane removal. (D) Optical coherent tomography showed reduction of macular edema and recovery of foveal depression.

RESULTS

Vitrectomy for Diffuse Diabetic Macular Edema with Taut Posterior Hyaloid

Lewis and associates [437] performed pars plana vitrectomy with separation of the posterior hyaloid in 10 eyes with diabetic macular edema and traction associated with a thickened and taut premacular posterior hyaloid. Nine of the 10 eyes had previous macular photocoagulation. Preoperative fluorescein angiography showed a deep and diffuse pattern of leakage in the macula. Postoperatively, vision improved in nine eyes. The macular traction and edema resolved in eight eyes and decreased in two. Complications included a vitreous hemorrhage, a rhegmatogenous retinal detachment, cataract formation, and a mild epimacular membrane, each occurring in one eye. They conclude that vitreous surgery can improve the visual prognosis of some eyes with diabetic macular traction and edema associated with a thickened and taut posterior hyaloid.

Harbour and associates [438] also found that vitrectomy effectively improved visual acuity in some eyes with diabetic macular edema associated with traction from a thickened and taut posterior hyaloid membrane. Despite careful preoperative examination with a fundus contact lens, however, in some patients it might be difficult to assess how the posterior hyaloid membrane contributes to the macular edema. In selected patients, early surgical intervention may be associated with better visual outcome.

Pendergast and associates [439] also found that in eyes with persistent diffuse diabetic macular edema with a taut premacular posterior hyaloid face unresponsive to laser therapy, vitrectomy with removal of the posterior hyaloid appeared to be beneficial in some cases. They observed that careful selection of eyes with favorable preoperative clinical characteristics might improve surgical outcomes.

Mechanism for improvement could be release of vitreous traction that created or exacerbated diabetic macular edema, as well as flattening of a shallow macular detachment if present.

Vitrectomy for Diffuse Diabetic Macular Edema Without Taut Posterior Hyaloid

La Heij and associates [440] found that in eyes with diabetic macular edema without evident macular traction from a thickened vitreous membrane, vitrectomy resulted in the resolution of macular edema, with an improvement in visual acuity in the majority of cases. Eyes without preoperative macular photocoagulation had a significantly higher percentage visual improvement than eyes without preoperative macular laser treatment.

In another study, Yamamoto and associates [441] observed that vitrectomy with removal of epimacular membrane was generally an effective procedure in reducing diabetic macular edema, and the outcome did not depend on the presence absence of posterior vitreous detachment and epimacular membrane. In a non-randomized clinical trial by Otani and Kishi,[442] eyes that underwent surgery were compared with untreated fellow eyes to assess the efficacy of vitrectomy for diabetic macular edema. In eyes with diabetic macular edema that underwent surgery, the foveal thickness significantly decreased after vitrectomy. It was concluded that vitrectomy might be effective for treating diabetic macular edema. Ikeda and associates[443,444] also reported improvement after vitrectomy in eyes with attached or detached posterior hyaloid. Tachi and Ogino[445] also reported that after vitrectomy and posterior vitreous detachment, macular edema resolved, and diffuse fluorescein leakage disappeared in 35 of 36 eyes examined at the 12th month. Visual acuity improved significantly. According to Saika and associates,[446] surgical detachment of the posterior vitreous combined with gas or air tamponade led to morphologically reduced macular edema and improved visual acuity. Mechanism for improvement could be the elimination of fluid containing a chemical mediator in a premacular liquefied pocket and the exchange of this fluid for fresh aqueous fluid.

Vitrectomy with Internal Limiting Membrane Peeling

Gandorfer and associates [447] found that vitrectomy including removal of the internal limiting membrane led to expedited resolution of diffuse diabetic macular edema and improvement of visual acuity without subsequent epiretinal membrane formation. Complete release of tractional forces and inhibition of reproliferation of fibrous astrocytes seemed to be prudent in the eyes of patients with diabetes and advanced vitreoretinal interface disease of the macula. Stefaniotou and associates [448] also reported better results with internal limiting membrane peeling. In eyes with diffuse diabetic macular edema vitrectomy seems to be effective, but additional internal limiting membrane peeling presented better results. Pars-plana vitrectomy with internal limiting membrane peeling reduced macular edema in most cases. In contrast, visual acuity improved significantly in lesser number of the treated eyes only. The discrepancy between anatomical and functional results of internal limiting membrane removal in chronic diabetic macular edema may be caused by structural changes of the macula due to long-standing edema. Radetzsky and associates [449] evaluated the efficacy of internal limiting membrane peeling in persistent macular edema. This retrospective review analyzed a series of 23 eyes from 23 patients with persistent macular edema. The main diagnoses were uveitis (anterior, intermediate, posterior and panuveitis) (n=9), central retinal vein occlusion (n=4), diabetic retinopathy (n=5), vitreoretinal traction syndrome (n=2), and Irvine-Gass syndrome (n=3). Nine eyes had undergone phacoemulsification previously and two eyes had been subjected to combined phacoemulsification and internal limiting membrane peeling. The eyes were tamponaded with gas (3), silicone oil (5) or air (11). In four cases no endotamponade was used. Improvement in visual acuity of 2 lines or more was regarded as significant. Visual acuity improved after 3 months in 9 of the 23 patients. After 6 months and at the follow-up, a significant improvement was found in 6/21 and 7/21 patients. This improvement was predominantly seen in patients with uveitis (5/9), or diabetic maculopathy (3/5). One patient with Irvine-Gass syndrome showed a significant reduction, one with vitreoretinal traction an improvement in visual acuity. The group of patients with central retinal vein occlusion showed no significant change during the follow-up. The choice of endotamponade did not alter the visual acuity outcome. Different patient groups responded differently to internal limiting membrane peeling. Although overall significant visual acuity improvement was observed in only one third of all cases 12 months after internal limiting membrane peeling for persistent macular edema, patients with uveitis and non-proliferative diabetic maculopathy demonstrated a benefit. The lack of long-term improvement in the majority of cases is in accordance with the hypothesis that internal limiting membrane peeling may reduce the intraretinal edema, but does not affect the underlying mechanism causing macular edema. So far, only diabetics have shown improvement (still unproven) from internal limiting membrane peeling, and this study provides no justification for extending the treatment to macular edema of other causes.

Triamcinolone-assisted Vitrectomy

Sakamoto and associates [450] determined the effect of a triamcinolone-assisted pars plana vitrectomy on the visibility of hyaloid during surgery and the postoperative clinical outcome. The vitreous body was clearly seen by means of triamcinolone during surgery, which greatly helped in performing a posterior hyaloid resection safely and thoroughly. Diabetic macular edema eyes which received triamcinolone-assisted pars plana vitrectomy showed significantly less breakdown of the blood-ocular barrier than those with routine pars plana vitrectomy. Triamcinolone improved the visibility of the hyaloid and the safety of the surgical procedures during pars plana vitrectomy and also inhibited the postoperative break-down of the blood-ocular barrier.

Sonoda and associates [451] visualized the residual vitreous cortex on the retinal surface after surgical posterior vitreous separation during a pars plana vitrectomy. Diabetic eyes more often demonstrated the diffuse type of residual vitreous cortex, even after surgical posterior vitreous separation.

Vitrectomy for Removal of Submacular Hard Exudates

Yang [452] analyzed the surgical results of eyes with massive hard exudates secondary to diabetic macular edema treated with combined pars plana vitrectomy, posterior hyaloid removal, focal endolaser treatment, and panretinal photocoagulation and concluded that combined surgery may offer an opportunity for improvement of vision and reduction of massive macular exudates in patients with severe diabetic macular edema.

Takagi and associates [453] reported a new surgical approach for removing massive foveal hard exudates in diabetic macular edema and determined the expression of vascular endothelial growth factor in the excised specimens. Pars plana vitrectomy for removal of massive foveal exudates was performed. Postoperative best-corrected visual acuity improved by two or more lines of Snellen equivalent. They concluded that surgical removal of foveal hard exudates might be effective in low-vision patients with diabetic maculopathy. Vascular endothelial growth factor might play a role in the formation and persistence of foveal hard exudates in diabetic macular edema. However, according to Takaya and associates,[454] visual improvement could not be obtained for a long period after removing submacular hard exudates in most of the patients. They suggested that diabetic maculopathy should be treated before massive exudate deposits appear in the macula.

Effect of Preoperative Factors on Vitrectomy

Kojima and associates[455] determined the effect of preoperative factors on the foveal thickness following vitrectomy for diabetic macular edema. Preoperative low HbA(1c) and postoperative pseudophakia were independently associated with the decrease in foveal thickness. The greater reduction in foveal thickness in eyes with an intraocular lens probably resulted from a relatively larger amount of vitreous being removed during the vitrectomy. Because the decrease in foveal thickness may be related to the preoperative glycemic control and the amount of vitreous, these factors should be considered in the planning for vitrectomy.

Effect on Focal Macular Electroretinogram after Vitrectomy

Terasaki and associates [456] evaluated the changes in the focal macular electroretinogram and foveal retinal thickness after vitrectomy for diabetic macular edema. A disparity in the time course and degree of recovery of the foveal thickness and macular retinal function was found in eyes after vitrectomy. Part of the functional recovery could be attributed to decreased retinal thickness and the absorption of the subretinal fluid.

Role of Plasmin in Vitrectomy

Williams and associates [457] in a pilot study assessed the use of autologous plasmin enzyme as an adjunct to vitreous surgery in eyes with macular tractional retinal detachment, and refractory macular edema. All autologous plasmin enzyme-treated eyes achieved spontaneous or easy removal of the posterior hyaloid including one eye that had vitreoschisis over areas of detached retina. All eyes treated with autologous plasmin enzyme had resolution of intraretinal edema.

COMPLICATIONS

Yamamoto and associates [458] determined the complications, in 65 eyes, after pars plana vitrectomy for diabetic macular edema. The intraoperative and postoperative complications included peripheral retinal tear in 3 (4.6%) eyes, postoperative rhegmatogenous retinal detachment in 1 (1.5%) eyes, neovascular glaucoma in 3 (5%) eyes, recurrent vitreous hemorrhage in 1 (1.5%) eyes, hard exudates in the center of the macula in 3 of 56 (4.6%) eyes, postoperative epiretinal membrane formation in 9 (13.8%) eyes, and a lamellar macular hole in 1 (1.5%) eyes. In another study, Yang [452] also reported intraoperative and postoperative complications included angle closure glaucoma), persistent vitreous hemorrhage, choroidal detachment, intravitreal fibrin formation, epiretinal membrane formation, and neovascular glaucoma. Formation of macular hole after peeling of internal limiting membrane has also been reported.[459]

ROLE OF OPTICAL COHERENCE TOMOGRAPHY

Giovannini and associates [460] assessed the role of optical coherence tomography in the evaluation and follow-up after vitrectomy for diabetic macular edema: optical coherence tomography revealed two patterns of edema. The first group (15 eyes) was characterized by widespread thickening of the neurosensory retina with an increased nonhomogeneous reflectivity of the inner retinal layers; cystoid-like spaces of absent or reduced reflectivity in the neurosensory retina were also present. In the second group (3 eyes), a cystoid macular edema with a dome-shaped foveal profile because of a markedly increased retinal thickness in the foveal region was observed. The disappearance of the physiologic foveal profile was always seen. Biomicroscopy revealed an increased reflex of the inner limiting membrane in the first group and minimal alterations in the second one. The restoration of the normal foveal profile and the reduction of the retinal thickness on the optical coherence tomography were evident in all cases one month after surgery. Optical coherence tomography appears to be a useful tool in the diagnosis and management of diabetic macular edema and in the monitoring of the morphological changes after vitrectomy. Otani and Kishi [461] demonstrated the intraretinal changes of macular edema and the process of edema absorption after vitrectomy, by optical coherence tomography. During the process of macular edema absorption, intraretinal fluid appeared to move into the subretinal space in some cases. Best-corrected visual acuity improvement was greater in eyes with less preoperative increase in thickness of neurosensory retina.

Yamamoto and associates [441] observed that the foveal retinal thickness does not decrease linearly but fluctuated: The mean postoperative retinal thickness decreased significantly 7 days after surgery, then remained unchanged for approximately 1 month, and thereafter gradually decreased until 4 months. Because the postoperative reduction in retinal thickness is not complete until 4 months, the assessment of vitrectomy on foveal thickness should not be made until this time. Massin and associates [462] reported the use of optical coherence tomography for evaluation of diffuse diabetic macular edema before and after vitrectomy. They observed that vitrectomy was beneficial in eyes with diffuse macular edema combined with vitreomacular traction but not in eyes without traction. Optical coherence tomography allowed diagnosis of subtle vitreomacular traction and provided precise preoperative and postoperative assessments of macular thickness.

Presently, multicenter, randomized, masked, controlled trial comparing eyes receiving Retisert (0.5 mg fluocinolone acetonide) implant, and eyes receiving a Retisert in conjunction with vitrectomy, to control eyes receiving placebo implant in conjunction with vitrectomy is underway. Diabetic Macular Edema Vitrectomy Study is another prospective, randomized clinical trial evaluating the role of vitrectomy with internal limiting membrane peeling versus standard therapy (grid laser photocoagulation) for diffuse diabetic macular edema.

MACULAR TRANSLOCATION

Macular translocation is a new approach in the management of subfoveal disease. Macular translocation can be defined as any surgery that has a primary goal of relocating the central neurosensory retina or fovea intraoperatively or postoperatively specifically for the management of macular disease.

RATIONALE

In the early, potentially reversible stages of neovascular age-related macular degeneration, visual deterioration may be secondary to such factors as subretinal fluid and hemorrhage in the fovea. In the later likely irreversible stages of the disease, fibrovascular proliferation causes permanent damage of the photoreceptors.[463] Therefore, by moving the neurosensory retina in an eye with recent-onset subfoveal lesion to a new location with presumably healthier retinal pigment epithelium and choriocapillaris away from the lesion, the fovea may be able to recover or maintain its visual function. In addition, moving the fovea away from such subfoveal lesions as choroidal neovascularization may permit the removal of the choroidal neovascularization or its destruction by laser photocoagulation.

INDICATIONS

Currently, the most common subfoveal lesion treated with this surgery is choroidal neovascularization related to age-related macular degeneration, ocular histoplasmosis syndrome, or pathologic myopia. Other potentially suitable lesions include retinal pigment epithelium defects created after removal of subfoveal choroidal neovascularization that is located in the subretinal pigment epithelial space (type 1 choroidal neovascularization), such as that commonly found in age-related macular degeneration.

Some surgeons have combined surgical removal of choroidal neovascularization with macular translocation so that the fovea can be relocated to an area outside the retinal pigment epithelium defect associated with choroidal neovascularization removal.[464-470] Others have used macular translocation to manage this complication at a subsequent operation.[471]

TERMINOLOGY

Various forms of macular translocation have been described by names such as retinal relocation, retinal translocation,[464,470,472-475] and foveal translocation.[465-467,476,477] Because the surgery is primarily employed for the management of macular disorders and the foveal displacement may be in the superior, inferior, or nasal direction, the term macular translocation appears to be a good term to describe the entire spectrum of procedures.

Macular translocation with punctate retinotomy has also been called limited macular translocation, because the surgery is less extensive than macular translocation with large or 360-degree retinotomy and achieves a smaller postoperative foveal displacement compared with these techniques.[472,473,478,479] Macular translocation with 360-degree retinotomy achieves a greater postoperative foveal displacement, and some have called it full macular translocation.[463]

CLASSIFICATION

Several different techniques currently in use may be classified according to the size of the retinotomy/retinotomies used.

The retinotomy may be a focal, tiny, punctate perforation in the retina made by a 39-gauge or 41-gauge retinal hydrodissection cannula (that is, macular translocation with punctate retinotomy, also called limited macular translocation) or a larger curvilinear "incision" of the retina that may be either 360-degrees around the periphery of the retina (that is, macular translocation with 360-degree or complete circumferential retinotomy, also called full macular translocation or large but less than 360-degree (that is, macular translocation with large or "partial"/incomplete circumferential retinotomy).[464-467,474,480-484] Macular translocation with punctate retinotomy may be performed with[470-473,483-485,487] or without[487] a chorioscleral shortening procedure.

The chorioscleral shortening may be effected by either chorioscleral infolding (also known as scleral imbrication or scleral inpouching)[466,467,473,475,478,479,485,488,489] or chorioscleral outfolding (also known as scleral outpouching.[486,488]

Macular translocation techniques using transscleral retinal hydrodissection to detach the retina and not requiring any retinotomy have also been described [464,472-475] and, may be grouped together with macular translocation with punctate retinotomy.

SURGICAL PRINCIPLES

To displace the neurosensory retina relative to the underlying retinal pigment epithelium, choroid, sclera, and subfoveal lesion, a physical separation of the neurosensory retina from the underlying layers is necessary. Hence, all forms of macular translocation involve planned retinal detachment and subsequent retinal reattachment. Macular translocation with large or 360-degree retinotomy requires retinopexy and internal tamponade with silicone oil or long-acting gas, whereas macular translocation with punctate or no retinotomy only requires temporary air tamponade.

MECHANISMS FOR FOVEAL DISPLACEMENT

The different forms of macular translocation allow foveal displacement by one or more of the following mechanisms.

Disinsertion of Retina from its Anterior Attachment

The retina, even when "totally detached," is attached at the ora serrata and the optic disk. By freeing the retina from its anterior attachment, macular translocation with large or 360-degree retinotomy allows the retina or macula to pivot around the optic disk and be displaced after retinal reattachment.[464,465,470]

Redundancy of Retina Relative to Underlying Eyewall

In macular translocation with punctate retinotomy, chorioscleral shortening by either chorioscleral infolding or chorioscleral outfolding is usually necessary to cause redundancy of the retina relative to the eyewall (sclera, choroid, and retinal pigment epithelium). This relative redundancy allows the retina to be displaced, sometimes with a retinal fold in the inferior periphery after an inferior macular translocation Unlike chorioscleral infolding, chorioscleral outfolding reduces the internal surface area of the eyewall without requiring the retina to "drape" the infolded eyewall. Thus, the extent of postoperative foveal displacement may be greater with this technique. Use of chorioscleral outfolding with scleral clips achieved a greater postoperative foveal displacement than chorioscleral infolding in porcine eyes.[488] Successful macular translocation in humans with both chorioscleral infolding and with sutured chorioscleral circumferential or radial outfolding has also been demonstrated.[486] However, in those patients, the postoperative foveal displacement was not increased by the sutured chorioscleral outfolding techniques.

Stretching of Retina

It is possible to achieve effective macular translocation without large or 360-degree retinotomy and without scleral shortening.[487] It is likely that in such a case, redundancy of the retina is created by stretching the retina during subretinal injection of balanced salt solution. The postoperative upright head positioning allows the buoyancy of an air bubble to support the superior retina while the effect of gravity stretches the redundant retina downward.

PATTERN OF POSTOPERATIVE RETINAL DISPLACEMENT

The fovea may be displaced superiorly, inferiorly, or even nasally after macular translocation. Inferior macular translocation denotes inferior movement of the neurosensory macula relative to the underlying tissues, and superior macular translocation implies macular displacement in the opposite direction. Nasal macular translocation moves the fovea toward the optic disk. Because of the attachment of the papillomacular bundle at the optic disk, meaningful temporal macular translocation is not likely possible. The pattern in which various points on the retina are displaced differs in the different types of macular translocation. Also, different points on the same retina may have different amounts of displacement.

EFFECTIVE MACULAR TRANSLOCATION

Anatomically successful macular translocation may be described as "effective" and this may be defined as successful intraoperative or postoperative relocation of the fovea overlying a subfoveal lesion to an area outside the border of the lesion, that is, a previously subfoveal lesion becomes either juxtafoveal (1 to 199 m from the foveal center) or extrafoveal (200 m or more from the foveal center) after the surgery. This anatomic success is dependent on two major considerations.

   i. Minimum desired translocation is related to the size, shape, and eccentricity of the subfoveal lesion.

   ii. Postoperative foveal displacement is dependent on such factors as achieving the desired planned retinal detachment and the surgical technique used.

MINIMUM DESIRED MACULAR TRANSLOCATION

The size of the subfoveal lesion is a factor in determining the postoperative anatomic relationship of the foveal center to the lesion. Some investigators have retported the size of the lesion in terms of area [469,482] or diameter,[466] or shown fundus photographs of the lesions,[464-468,473,476,481,485] and others have given no indication of the size of the lesions in their series.[470] In general, small subfoveal lesions are more likely to become juxtafoveal or extrafoveal after macular translocation compared with larger lesions, assuming the lesions are the same shape and similarly centered on the foveal center. However, subfoveal lesions not uncommonly are centered eccentrically relative to the fovea. A lesion that is eccentrically centered superiorly relative to the fovea

is more likely to become juxtafoveal or extrafoveal after an inferior macular translocation compared with another lesion that is eccentrically centered downward relative to the fovea, assuming that the net postoperative foveal displacement is identical in both cases.

The key dimension to consider when planning macular translocation is not simply the size, shape, or eccentricity of the lesion but the distance between the foveal center and a point either on the inferior or superior border of the lesion. This distance is the minimum desired translocation.

The temporal edge of the optic disk rather than the center of the disk is taken as the pivoting point of the fovea, because the papillomacular bundle enters the optic disk from temporally close to this point. This is therefore the point on which the papillomacular bundle would pivot when the fovea is relocated after macula translocation. (The pivot of the entire macular is an arcuate line of attachment at the temporal margin of the disk). Subfoveal lesions of the same size but different eccentricities may have different minimum desired translocations), whereas subfoveal lesions of different sizes may have the same minimum desired translocation. Such lesions as parafoveal laser scar should be taken into consideration when determining the minimum desired translocation. For nasal macular translocation, the minimum desired translocation is the distance between the foveal center and the nasal border of the lesion.

Although the minimum desired translocation is the smallest postoperative foveal displacement in which macular translocation may be considered effective, the preferred translocation distance is usually larger than this distance so that the foveal center becomes relocated a reasonable distance away from the subfoveal lesion. It may seem ideal to displace the foveal center as far away from the subfoveal lesion as possible, but this is not necessarily always the case. This is in part because large postoperative foveal displacement is associated with severe, and sometimes intractable, postoperative diplopia and/or cyclotropia that may require corrective muscle surgery.[477] In addition, because the macula differs from extramacular areas in having the greatest density of retinal pigment epithelium melanin pigmentation[490] and a lobular choroidal angioarchitecture that allows for extremely fast circulation,[491] whether extramacular retinal pigment epithelium and choroid can support foveal function as well as those in the macula is unknown.

ESTIMATION OF POSTOPERATIVE FOVEAL DISPLACEMENT

A simple technique can be used to estimate the amount of postoperative foveal displacement without resorting to sophisticated imaging equipment. This is done by first measuring on the preoperative fluorescein angiogram the distance from a predetermined retinal landmark (such as a retinal vascular bifurcation) located superior to the subfoveal lesion to a specific point along the inferior edge of the lesion ("choroidal" landmark) The two points are chosen such that a line joining the two points is close to and roughly parallel to the "path" of the foveal displacement. A similar measurement using the same landmarks is performed on the postoperative angiogram. The absolute difference between these two measurements estimates the amount of foveal displacement. If the time difference between the preoperative and postoperative angiograms is within 2 weeks, the size and characteristics of the choroidal neovascularization on the postoperative angiogram tend not to change significantly. A more precise method to measure the postoperative foveal displacement is to superimpose a digitized postoperative angiogram over the preoperative angiogram using a computer software program.[486] The median postoperative foveal displacement normally achieved can be derived by analyzing data collected either retrospectively or prospectively in a series of consecutive cases operated by the surgeon. This information, when considered together with the minimum desired translocation of a particular eye, gives some useful idea of the likelihood of effective macular translocation. If the minimum desired translocation in an eye is equal to the median postoperative foveal displacement normally achieved, barring any complication, the eye has an approximately 50% chance of achieving effective macular translocation after the surgery. If the minimum desired translocation is less than the median postoperative foveal displacement, the eye has a greater than 50% chance of achieving effective macular translocation and vice versa. If the macular translocation is combined with choroidal

neovascularization removal, this rule may not apply if the area of the retinal pigment epithelium defect accompanying the choroidal neovascularization removal differs greatly from the original area of the choroidal neovascularization.

It is also possible to consider the minimum desired translocation in terms of the angle subtended at the temporal edge of the optic disk by the foveal center and a point on the inferior or superior edge of the subfoveal lesion depending on whether the macular translocation is inferior or superior. However, this method cannot be applied to nasal macular translocation.

Macular translocation surgery is still under development, and although the Committee on Ophthalmic Procedures Assessment Retinal Panel of the American Academy of Ophthalmology did not find strong evidence to answer the question of whether macular translocation is effective in treating visual loss from age-related macular degeneration,[492] preliminary results in some case series have been encouraging for both neovascular age-related macular degeneration and myopic neovascular maculopathy. [465-467,470,473,476,479,487]

LIMITED MACULAR TRANSLOCATION

de Juan and associates described the limited translocation technique. This technique is based on the concept of creating neurosensory retinal redundancy by shortening sclera/retinal pigment epithelium relative to neurosensory retina. This technique eliminates the need for large retinotomies and associated complications. Indications and case selection for limited macular translocation are shown in Table 13.2.

SURGICAL PROCEDURE

Pars plana vitrectomy is followed by removal of posterior hyaloid. A 41-gauge cannula is used to create detachment of temporal retina by means of self-sealing retinotomies. Scleral imbrication is created using in-pouching technique with scleral sutures or outpouching technique using clips. Fluid-air exchange is done and upright positioning is recommended for 24 to 36 hours. Postoperative laser photocoagulation to choroidal neovascular membrane is performed.

Results of surgery are shown in Figures 13.26 to 13.28.

Table 13.2: Limited macular translocation: Indications and case selection

A. Subfoveal CNV secondary to age-related macular dege neration
1. Poor prognosis for visual improvement or stabilization following current standard care treatments mandates the need to find better options.
2. Ideal case has fellow eye with disciform process.
3. Small lesion, center of fovea to inferior edge of choroidal neovascular membrane, 1.0 mm (minimum translocation distance).
4. Recent loss of vision, reversible neurosensory changes:
   a. Symptoms < 3 months.
   b. Recent lesions (previous non-foveal treatment).
   c. Presenting vision >20/400.
5. Scanning laser ophthalmoscope findings:
   a. Stable central fixation has highest predictive value for good visual outcome (>20/200).
   b. Eccentric fixation has highest negative predictive value for good visual outcome.
B. Pathological myopia, ocular histoplasmosis, angioid streaks, multifocal choroiditis, and idiopathic causes:
1. Natural history of subfoveal choroidal neovascular membrane may be better than age-related macular degeneration.
2. Selection of patient similar to above parameters.

Surgical Technique of Macular Translocation with 360-degree Retinotomy

Crystalline lens removal is necessary to ensure visibility and maneuverability in the peripheral fundus in phakic eyes. Phacoemulsification and intraocular lens implantation are performed at the beginning of the surgery.

Core vitrectomy is performed via a standard three-port pars plana approach. The surgeon must either confirm or create a posterior vitreous detachment, since adherent vitreous may cause postoperative retinal detachment or proliferative vitreoretinopathy. However, it is often difficult to detect residual vitreous cortex intraoperatively by simple observation alone. Intravitreal injection of triamcinolone dramatically facilitates visibility of the vitreous cortex.[493] After creation of the posterior vitreous detachment, peripheral vitrectomy is performed with scleral indentation. Removal of the peripheral vitreous is crucial for macular translocation with 360-degree retinotomy to facilitate maneuvering of the retina during surgery and to prevent postoperative proliferative vitreoretinopathy.

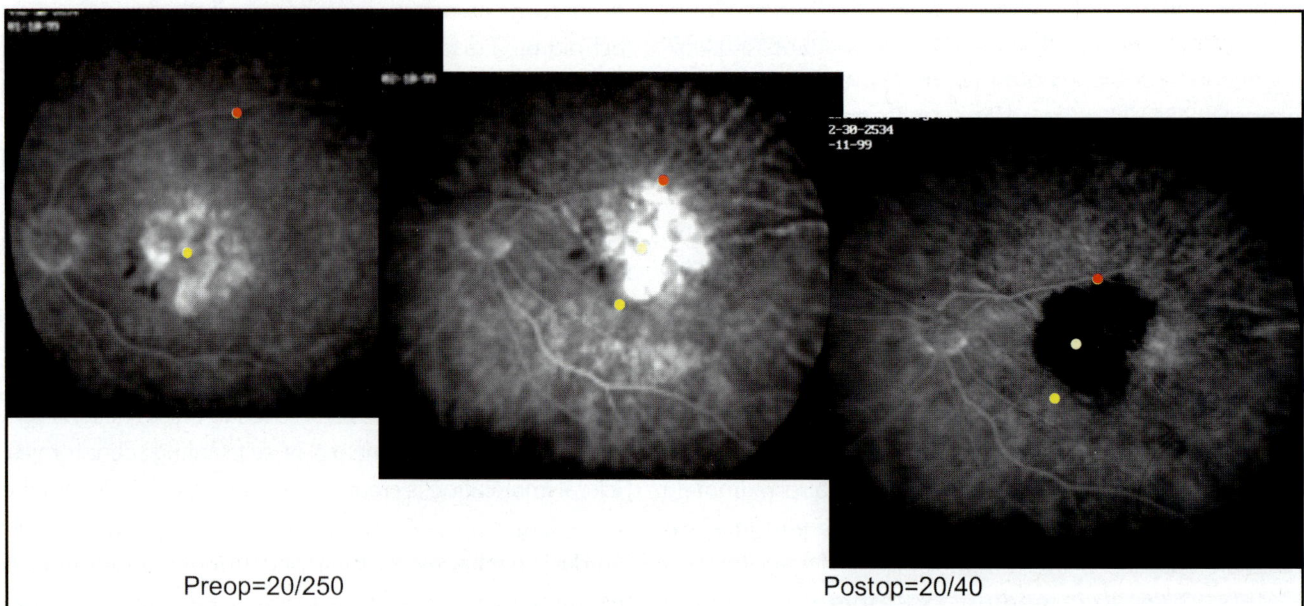

FIGURE 13.26: Limited macular translocation: Age-related macular degeneration with large subfoveal choroidal neovascular membrane. (Corresponding retinal landmarks are marked with color dots for comparison in pre- and postoperative figures).

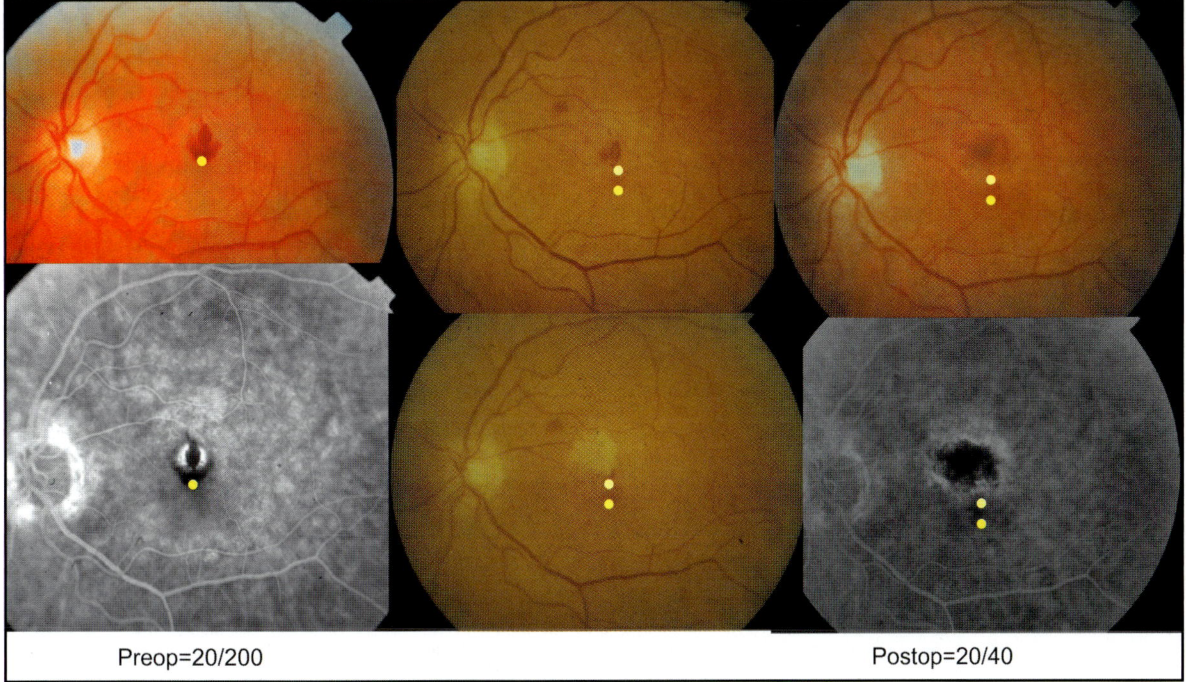

FIGURE 13.27: Limited macular translocation: Age-related macular degeneration with large juxtafoveal choroidal neovascular membrane with hemorrhagic edge extending subfoveally. (Corresponding retinal landmarks are marked with color dots for comparison in pre- and postoperative figures).

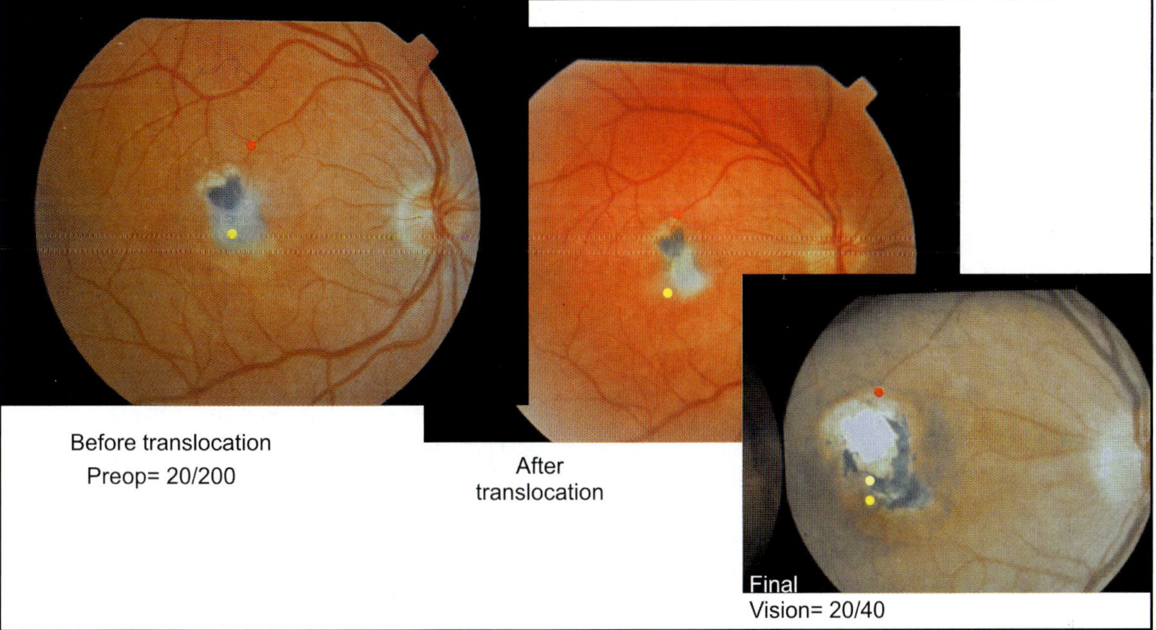

FIGURE 13.28: Limited macular translocation: A 21-year old punctate inner choroidopathy patient who initially had argon laser for juxtafoveal membrane, then subfoveal recurrence for which photodynamic therapy was performed and limited macular translocation and removal of choroidal neovascular membrane was done for persistent subfoveal choroidal neovascular membrane (Corresponding retinal landmarks are marked with color dots for comparison in pre- and postoperative figures).

The retinal detachment may be created with either trans-scleral or transretinal infusion of balanced saline solution into the subretinal space; the latter technique is often performed. A 39- or 41-gauge polyimide flexible needle may be used for the transretinal infusion. Balanced salt solution is infused into the subretinal space with the needle.[494] A 20-gauge silicone-tipped needle might be used to complete the total retinal detachment.[495] Intraocular pressure should be kept lower to facilitate enlargement of the retinal detachment. Fluid-air exchange might be necessary to complete the total retinal detachment at the posterior pole.

A circumferential 360-degree retinotomy should be created using a vitreous cutter or scissors as peripherally as possible to preserve functioning retina, minimize exposed retinal pigment epithelium, and prevent hemorrhage. The retina is then flipped, and the choroidal neovascular membrane and/or subretinal hemorrhage is removed under direct visualization using forceps.

The retina at the posterior pole is unfolded and flattened using liquid perfluorocarbon, followed by rotation of the retina. The retina is then gently rotated clockwise or counterclockwise around the axis of the optic nerve head using a soft-tipped cannula.[496] After the retina is translocated to the appropriate position, additional perfluorocarbon liquid is injected to achieve complete retinal reattachment. Photocoagulation is applied to the peripheral retina and intentional retinal breaks made with a 39-gauge needle. Finally, perfluorocarbon is directly exchanged with silicone oil.

Silicone oil is usually removed 2 to 3 months late. Extraocular muscle surgery is performed if the patient complains of a tilted image or diplopia, but it could be performed simultaneously with translocation surgery.[470]

Results of surgery are shown in Figures 13.29 to 13.31.

VISUAL OUTCOMES

Ohji and Tano[470] have performed macular translocation with 360-degree retinotomy in 36 eyes with choroidal neovascular membrane due to age-related macular degeneration. The fovea was translocated between 1,250 μm and 5,870 μm (mean, 3,340 μm). The visual acuity improved by two lines or more in seven eyes (19%) and was maintained within two lines in 19 eyes (53%). Several reports on visual outcomes after total macular translocation in eyes with age-related macular degeneration

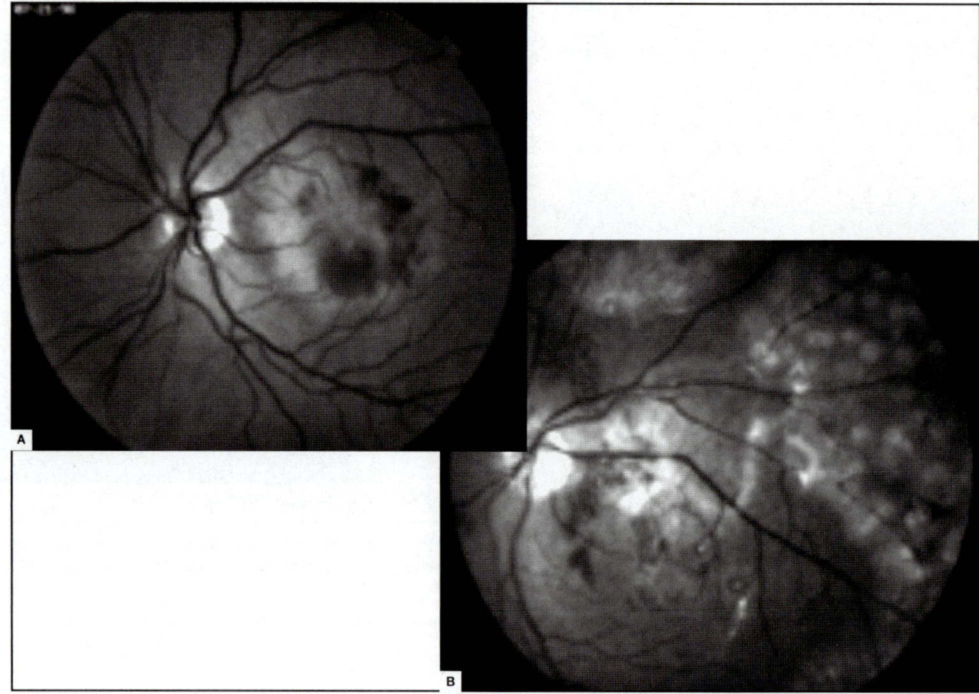

FIGURE 13.29: Macular translocation with 360-degree retinotomy: (A) Preoperative, (B) Postoperative.

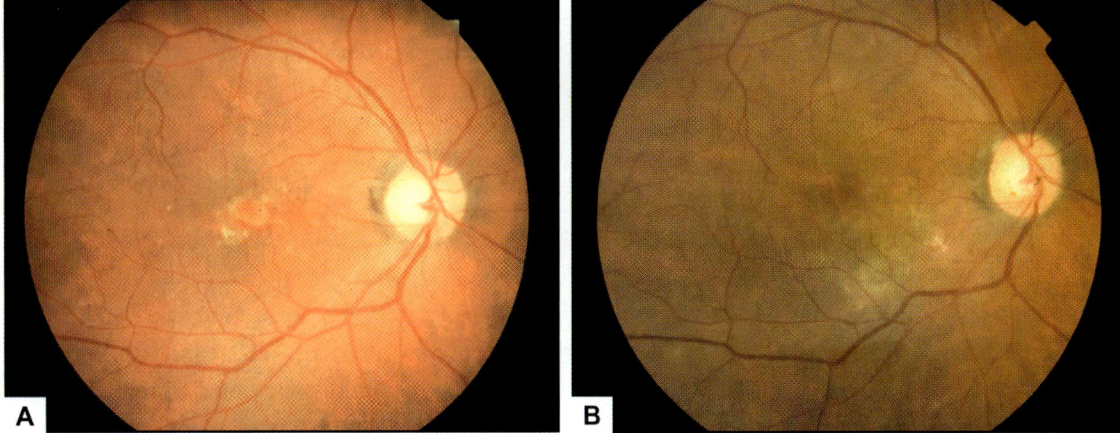

FIGURES 13.30A and B: (A) Macular translocation with 360-degree retinotomy: A 67-year-old male with subfoveal choroidal neovascular membrane due to age-related macular degeneration with visual acuity was 20/160 preoperatively. (B) Macular translocation with 360-degree retinotomy: The retina was rotated upward by 25 degrees followed by counter-rotation of the eyeball. Visual acuity improved to 20/25.

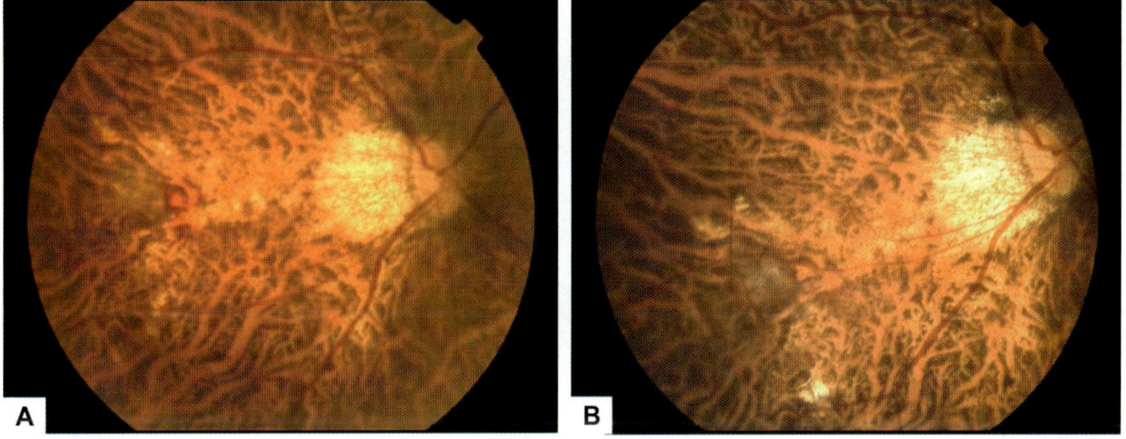

FIGURES 13.31A and B: (A) Macular translocation with 360 degree retinotomy: A 45-year-old male with subfoveal choroidal neovascular membrane due pathological myopia. Visual acuity was 20/200 preoperatively. (B) Macular translocation with 360-degree retinotomy: The retina was rotated by 18-degree followed by counter-rotation of the eyeball. Visual acuity improved to 20/15 and has been maintained until the last visit, 3 years postoperatively.

have been published. A meta analysis of the reports revealed that visual acuity improved in 39% of eyes and was maintained in another 39%.[470, 497-504] Macular translocation might achieve better visual outcomes than other treatments.[505]

Near vision might even be more important than far vision. Improved near vision might be achieved in more eyes than improved far vision. Eckardt and associates[470] reported that near vision of 0.4 or better was achieved in 18 eyes of 30 eyes (60%), and Lai and associates[506] also reported good reading ability, which is very important for performing activities of daily living. Reading ability

is another important measurement to evaluate improvement in daily activities. Critical print size that is a factor reflecting reading ability improves after macular translocation. The improvement of the critical print size correlates with subjective visual improvement.[507]

A wide peripheral visual field is also important in addition to improved visual acuity. Restriction of the peripheral visual fields is of great concern in total macular translocation because a 360-degree retinotomy must be created at the peripheral retina. The peripheral visual field measured with the V/4 isopter in Goldmann perimetry postoperatively constricted 78 to 90% of the preoperative visual field.[508] A circumferential retinotomy should be performed as peripherally as possible.[507]

The electroretinogram could be reduced after macular translocation surgery because a total retinal detachment must be created during surgery. The amplitude of the full-field electroretinogram decreased and the implicit time lengthened postoperatively, presumably due to creation of a total retinal detachment.[508] The focal electroretinogram improved in most cases after macular translocation surgery likely because of improved macular function.[509]

Electro-oculogram was performed to measure changes after 360-degree retinotomy and macular translocation for subfoveal choroidal neovascular membrane in patients with age-related macular degeneration. The mean dark trough decreased significantly by 64% postoperatively.[510] A significant correlation between the reduction of the dark trough and the visual acuity was also found. Surgical trauma reduces the dark trough.

Postoperative diplopia is another serious complication that develops in about 10% of cases, because the fovea is rotated substantially. Diplopia diminished spontaneously in some cases without additional treatment and decreased dramatically in most cases after extraocular surgery.[511] Binocular function such as stereopsis or motor fusion is difficult to achieve.[512] Peripheral fusion could also be achieved in some cases.[513]

COMPLICATIONS

Various postoperative complications can develop because macular translocation surgery involves many procedures. Retinal detachment and diplopia are the most important of the complications. Postoperative retinal detachment reportedly develops in 20 to 40% of cases. Although improvements in surgical techniques and surgical instruments reduced the incidence of retinal detachment, postoperative retinal detachment including proliferative vitreoretinopathy is still the most serious complication.[514]

MYOPIC FOVEOSCHISIS

Myopic foveoschisis is common in high myopia. Vitrectomy with vitreous cortex removal, internal limiting membrane peeling, and gas tamponade could be useful to treat myopic foveoschisis in highly myopic eyes.

Tractional force of the epiretinal membrane may cause myopic foveoschisis. Optical coherence tomography has provided more information and indicated that different subtypes of myopic foveoschisis may have processes specific to their development. For instance, local posterior vitreous detachment at the posterior retina as well as a preretinal strand between the edge of the macular hole and the posterior vitreous surface often are observed in myopic foveoschisis in which a macular hole develops. This indicates that a macular hole associated with myopic foveoschisis may develop as the result of posterior vitreous detachment, which generates anteroposterior traction and consequent retinal tearing at the fovea. Another possible mechanism is retinal vascular traction on the retina.

Collagen fiber and cellular component are suggested to play an important role in developing myopic foveoschisis. Internal limiting membrane peeling may be essential for vitrectomy for myopic foveoschisis.[515]

SURGICAL TECHNIQUE

Surgery is performed under local anesthesia in most cases.

Phacoemulsification is performed at the beginning of the surgery, followed by intraocular lens implantation. Core vitrectomy is performed with a standard 3-port vitrectomy system. Vitreous cortex is visualized with injection of triamcinolone acetonide. Visualization of vitreous cortex allows surgeons to confirm residual vitreous cortex. Although so-called posterior vitreous detachment is found in many cases, thin layer of vitreous cortex remains attached to the posterior retina in most cases. The thin layer of vitreous cortex that is visualized with triamcinolone acetonide is removed, using Tano's diamond dusted membrane eraser or brush back-flush needle. Internal limiting membrane is stained with 0.125% of indocyanine green dye under balanced salt solution. The dye is removed immediately after injection to minimize possible complication. Internal limiting membrane is removed using an asymmetric forceps or other microforceps. Peripheral vitreous is removed as much as possible. Removal of peripheral vitreous after internal limiting membrane peeling can decrease the postoperative concentration of indocyanine green dye in the vitreous cavity, reducing its possible toxicity. Fluid-air exchange followed by injection of 20% sulfur hexafluoride.

RESULTS

Ikuno and associates[516] performed vitrectomy including vitreous cortex removal, internal limiting membrane peeling, and gas tamponade in 6 eyes. Patients were followed for at least 6 months. The foveal detachment resolved completely in five eyes and partially in one eye. Best-corrected visual acuity improved more than two lines in all eyes (100%) 6 months postoperatively. Scanning laser ophthalmoscope microperimetry showed smaller scotoma compared with preoperatively and stabilized fixation. On the other hand, according to Kwok and associates[517] vitrectomy without internal limiting membrane peeling followed by gas tamponade appeared to result in favorable visual and anatomical outcomes for treating myopic foveoschisis in highly myopic eyes. The results are comparable with studies in which internal limiting membrane removal was performed.

Retinal microfolds are common in eyes with myopic foveoschisis after vitrectomy with internal limiting membrane peeling, and they seem to be generated as the result of insufficient flexibility of the sclerotic retinal arteriole during axial length elongation in highly myopic eyes. OCT-ophthalmoscope examination confirmed the location of the microfold coincided exactly with that of retinal arteriole. The presence of microfolds was not significantly related to the postoperative visual acuity. This finding suggests that the inward tractional force on the

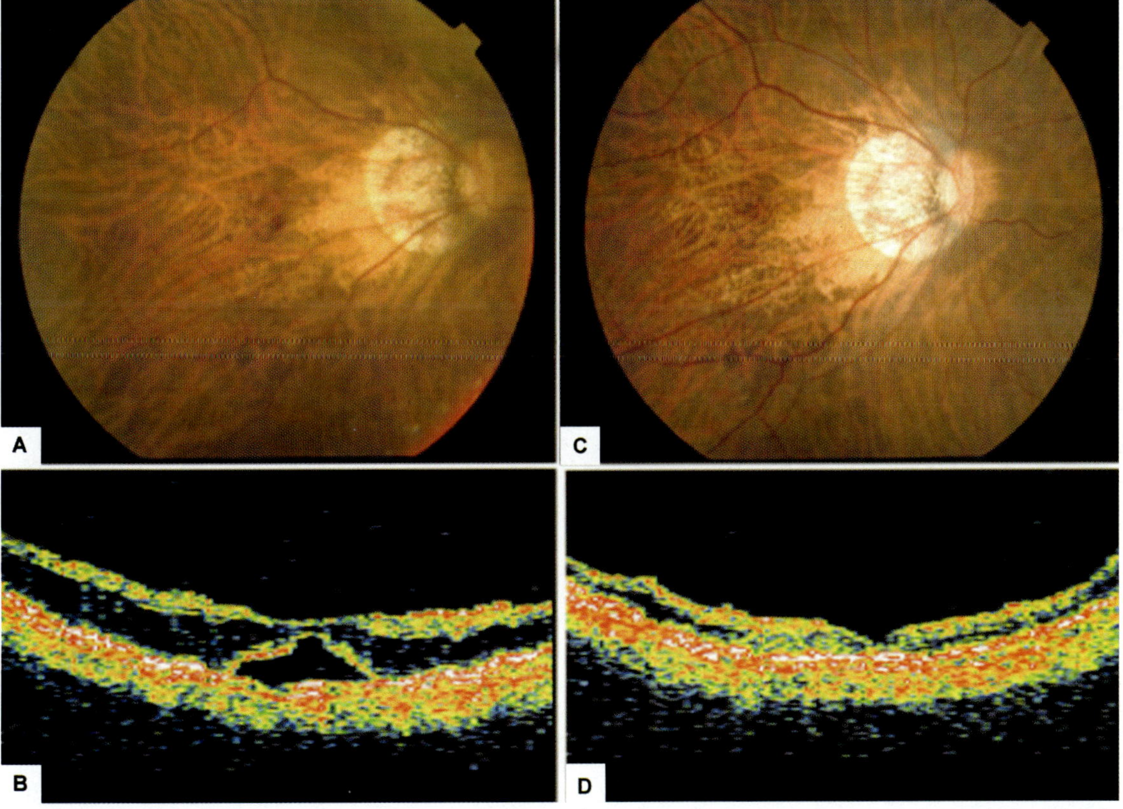

FIGURE 13.32: Preoperative fundus appearance of patients who underwent vitrectomy for myopic foveoschisis. (A) Color fundus photograph shows almost normal fundus, except for myopic atrophy. (B) However, OCT shows apparent foveal detachment and retinoschisis. Fundus appearance, 6 months after surgery. (C) The color fundus image has not changed from preoperatively. (D) However, the OCT image shows complete resolution of the foveal detachment and consequent visual improvement (Prof Yasuo Tano MD, Japan).

retina along the arteriole may be closely related to the pathogenesis of vitreoretinal diseases specific to high myopia, including myopic foveoschisis or paravascular microhole formation.[518]

The incidence of retinal microfolds is 2.9%, and thus they are not uncommon in highly myopic eyes without vitrectomy. The coincident appearance of the folds and vessels suggests that inflexibility of the retinal vessels and retinal stretching attributable to ocular elongation may cause the microfolds. The presence of these microfolds indicates that inward retinal vascular traction could be common in highly myopic eyes.[519]

Reoperation including complete vitreous cortex removal and internal limiting membrane peeling could be beneficial for patients with persistent myopic foveoschisis after primary surgery, indicating that vitreous cortex removal and internal limiting membrane peeling are critical in treating myopic foveoschisis.[520]

Vitrectomy for macular holes associated with myopic foveoschisis may be performed. Although significant visual improvement occurs in less than 50% of cases, vitrectomy can be beneficial for some cases.[521]

Results of surgery are shown in Figures 13.32A to D.

ROLE OF OPTICAL COHERENCE TOMOGRAPHY

After surgery, OCT typically shows that foveal detachment gradually resolves over time. Foveal detachment completely resolves soon after surgery in some cases; however, other cases can take longer than 6 months to resolve, probably depending on the viscosity of the subretinal or intraretinal fluid. Although there is a risk of macular hole formation even after surgery, 80% to 90% of patients have improved visual acuity. The surgery usually results in stabilization of the fixation point in scanning laser ophthalmoscope microperimetry, indicating that retinal function has improved.

REFERENCES

1. Sjaarda RN, Michels RG. Macular pucker. In Ryan SJ (Ed): Retina (2nd edn) vol. 3. St. Louis: Mosby, 1994;2301-11.
2. Machemer R. Die chirurgische entfernung von epiretinalen makulamembranen (macular puckers). Klin Monatsbl Augenheilkd 1978;173:36-42.
3. Roth AM, Foos RY. Surface wrinkling retinopathy in eyes enucleated at autopsy. Trans Am Acad Ophthalmol Otolaryngol 1971;75:1047-59.
4. Bellhorn MB, Friedman AH, Wise GN, Henkind P. Ultrastructure and clinicopathologic correlation of idiopathic preretinal macular fibrosis. Am J Ophthalmol 1975;79:366-73.
5. Foos RY. Vitreoretinal juncture—simple epiretinal membranes. Graefe's Arch Clin Exp Ophthalmol 1974;189:231-50.
6. Wise GN. Macular changes after venous obstruction. Arch Ophthalmol 1957;58:544-57.
7. Green WR, Kenyon KR, Michels RG, et al. Ultrastructure of epiretinal membranes causing macular pucker after retinal re-attachment surgery. Trans Ophthalmol Soc UK 1979; 99: 63-77.
8. Jaffe NS. Macular retinopathy after separation of vitreoretinal adherence. Arch Ophthalmol 1967;78:585-91.
9. Kenyon KR, Michels RG. Ultrastructure of epiretinal membrane removed by pars plana vitreoretinal surgery. Am J Ophthalmol 1977;83:815-23.
10. Machemer R, van Horn DL, Aaberg TM. Pigment epithelial proliferation in human retinal detachment with massive periretinal proliferation. Am J Ophthalmol 1978;85:181-191.
11. Trese M, Chandler DB, Machemer R. Macular pucker. II. Ultrastructure. Graefe's Arch Clin Exp Ophthalmol 1983;221:16-26.
12. McDonald HR, Schatz H, Johnson RN. Introduction to epiretinal membranes. In Ryan SJ (Ed): Retina, (2nd edn); vol. 3. St. Louis: Mosby, 1994;1819-25.
13. Pearlstone AD. The incidence of idiopathic preretinal macular gliosis. Ann Ophthalmol 1985;17:378-80.
14. Scudder MJ, Eifrig DE. Spontaneous surface wrinkling retinopathy. Ann Ophthalmol 1975;7:333-41.
15. Sidd RJ, Fine SL, Owens SL, Patz A. Idiopathic preretinal gliosis. Am J Ophthalmol 1982;94:44-8.
16. Wiznia RA. Natural history of idiopathic preretinal macular fibrosis. Ann Ophthalmol 1982;14:876-8.
17. Hirokawa H, Jalkh AE, Takahashi M, et al. Role of vitreous in idiopathic premacular fibrosis. Am J Ophthalmol 1986;101:166-9.
18. Wise GN. Congenital preretinal macular fibrosis. Am J Ophthalmol 1975;79:363-5.
19. Gass JDM. Stereoscopic atlas of macular diseases. St. Louis: Mosby-Year Book, 1987:694-712.
20. McDonald HR, Aaberg TM. Idiopathic epiretinal membranes. Semin Ophthalmol 1986;1:189-95.
21. Schatz H. Essential fluorescein angiography: a compendium of 100 classic cases. San Francisco: Pacific Medical Press, 1982.
22. Wise GN. Preretinal macular fibrosis (an analysis of 90 cases). Trans Ophthalmol Soc UK 1972;92:131-40.
23. Wise GN. Congenital preretinal macular fibrosis. Am J Ophthalmol 1975;79:363-5.
24. Tanenbaum HL, Schepens CL, Elzeneiny I, Freeman HM. Macular pucker following retinal detachment surgery. Arch Ophthalmol 1970;83:286-93.

25. Michels RG. A clinical and histopathologic study of epiretinal membranes affecting the macula and removed by vitreous surgery. Trans Am Acad Ophthalmol Soc 1982;80:580-656.

26. Michels RG. Vitrectomy for macular pucker. Ophthalmology 1984;91:1384-8.

27. Cherfan GM, Smiddy WE, Michels RG, et al. Clinicopathologic correlation of pigmented epiretinal membranes. Am J Ophthalmol 1988;106:536.

28. Dellaporta A. Macular pucker and peripheral retinal lesions. Trans Am Ophthalmol Soc 1973;71:329-40.

29. Laqua H. Pigmented macular pucker. Am J Ophthalmol 1978;86:56-8.

30. Robertson DM, Buettner H. Pigmented preretinal membranes. Am J Ophthalmol 1977;83:824-29.

31. Clarkson JG, Green WR, Massof D. A histopathologic review of 168 cases of preretinal membrane. Am J Ophthalmol 1977;84:1-17.

32. de Bustros S, Thompson JT, Michels RG, et al. Vitrectomy for idiopathic epiretinal membranes causing macular pucker. Br J Trans Am Ophthalmol Soc 1973;71:329-40.

33. Foos RY. Surface wrinkling retinopathy. In Freeman HM, Hirose T, Schepens CL (Eds): Vitreous Surgery and Advances in Fundus Diagnosis and Treatment. New York: Appleton-Century-Crofts, 1977.

34. Spitznas M, Leuenberger R. Die primare epiretinale Gliose. Kiln Montsbl Augenheilkd 1977;171:410-20.

35. Wilson DJ, Green WR. Histopathologic study of the effect of retinal detachment surgery on 49 eyes obtained postmortem. Am J Ophthalmol 1987;103:167-79.

36. Hagler WS, Aturaliya U. Macular puckers after retinal detachment surgery. Br J Ophthalmol 1971;55:451-7.

37. Lobes LA, Jr, Burton TC. The incidence of macular pucker after retinal detachment pucker. Am J Ophthalmol 1978; 85:72-7.

38. Francois-Cedilla J, Verbraeken H. Relationship between the drainage of the subretinal fluid in retinal detachment surgery and the appearance of macular pucker. Ophthalmologica 1979;179:111-4.

39. Jahn CE, Minich V, Moldaschel S, et al. Epiretinal membranes after extracapsular cataract surgery. J Cataract Refract Surg 2001;27:753-60.

40. Allen AW Jr, Gass JDM. Contraction of a perifoveal epiretinal membrane simulating a macular hole. Am J Ophthalmol 1976;82:684-91.

41. Gass JDM. Photocoagulation of macular lesions. Trans Am Acad Ophthalmol Otolaryngol 1971;75:580-608.

42. Messner KH. Spontaneous separation of preretinal macular fibrosis. Am J Ophthalmol 1977;83:9-11.

43. Schwartz A. In Dellaporta A (Ed): Discussion; Macular Pucker and Preretinal Lesions. Trans Am Ophthalmol Soc 1973; 71:329-40.

44. Sumers KD, Jampol LM, Goldberg FM, Huamonte FU. Spontaneous separation of epiretinal membranes. Arch Ophthalmol 1980;98:318-20.

45. McDonald HR, Verre WP, Aaberg TM. Surgical management of idiopathic epiretinal membranes. Ophthalmology 1986; 93:978-83.

46. Pesin SR, Bovino JA. Macular pucker. In Bovino JA (Ed): Macular Surgery. Norwalk, CT: Appleton and Lange 1994:1-10.

47. Poliner LS, Olk RJ, Grand MG, et al. The surgical management of premacular fibroplasia. Arch Ophthalmol 1988; 106:761-64.

48. Rice TA, de Bustros S, Michels RG, et al. Prognostic factors in vitrectomy for epiretinal membranes of the macula. Ophthalmology 1986;93:602-10.

49. Pesin SR, Olk RJ, Grand MG, et al. Vitrectomy for premacular fibroplasia. Prognostic factors, long term follow-up, and time course of visual improvement. Ophthalmology 1991; 98:1109-14.

50. Rowen RL, Glaser BM. Retinal pigment epithelial cell release: a chemoattractant for astrocytes. Arch Ophthalmol 1985;103:704-7.

51. Margherio RR, Cox MS Jr, Trese MT, et al. Removal of epimacular membranes. Ophthalmology 1985;92:1075-83.

52. Michels RG. Vitreous surgery for macular pucker. Am J Ophthalmol 1981;92:628-39.

53. Shea M. The surgical management of macular pucker in rhegmatogenous retinal detachment. Ophthalmology 1980;87:70-4.

54. de Bustros S, Rice TA, Michels RG, et al. Vitrectomy for macular pucker after treatment of retinal tears or retinal detachment. Arch Ophthalmol 1988;106:758-60.

55. Michels RG, Gilbert HD. Surgical management of macular pucker after retinal reattachment. Am J Ophthalmol 1979;88:925-29.

56. de Bustros S, Thompson JT, Michels RG, et al. Nuclear sclerosis after vitrectomy for idiopathic epiretinal membranes. Am J Ophthalmol 1988;105:160-4.

57. Charles S. Vitreous Microsurgery, 2nd edn. Baltimore: Williams and Wilkins, 1987.

58. Mittelman D, Green WR, Michels RG, de la Cruz Z. Clinicopathologic correlation of an eye after surgical removal of an epiretinal membrane. Retina 1989;9:143-7.

59. Donati G, Kapetanios AD, Pournaras CJ. Complications of surgery for epiretinal membranes. Graefe's Arch Clin Exp Ophthalmol 1998;236:739-46.

60. Kim CY, Lee JH, Lee SJ, et al. Visual field defect caused by nerve fiber layer damage associated with an internal limiting lamina defect after uneventful epiretinal membrane surgery. Am J Ophthalmol 2002;133:569-71.

61. Uemura A, Kanda S, Sakamoto Y, Kita H. Visual field defects after uneventful vitrectomy for epiretinal membrane with indocyanine green-assisted internal limiting membrane peeling. Am J Ophthalmol 2003;136:252-7.

62. Chung KT. The significance of azo-reduction in the mutagenesis and carcinogenesis of azo dyes. Mutat Res 1983;114:269-81.

63. Schmidt KL, Milner K, Hilburn PJ, Schmidt WA. Ultrastructure of trypan blue induced ocular defects: I. Retina and lens. Teratology 198;28:131-44.

64. Norn MS. Per operative trypan blue vital staining of corneal endothelium: eight years' follow up. Acta Ophthalmol 1980;58:550-5.

65. Melles GR, de Waard PW, Pameyer JH, Beekhuis HW. Trypan blue capsule staining to visualize the capsulorhexis in cataract surgery. J Cataract Refract Surg 2000;25:7-9.

66. Veckeneer M, van Overdam K, Monzer J, et al. Ocular toxicity study of trypan blue injected into the vitreous cavity of rabbit eyes. Graefe's Arch Clin Exp Ophthalmol 2001;239:698-704.

67. Feron E, M. Veckeneer M, Parys-Van Ginderdeuren R, et al. Trypan blue staining of epiretinal membranes in proliferative vitreoretinopathy. Arch Ophthalmol 2002; 120:141-4.

68. Teba FA, Mohr A, Eckardt C, et al. Trypan blue staining in vitreoretinal surgery. Ophthalmology 2003;110:2409-2412.

69. Haritoglou C, Eibl K, Schaumberger M, et al. Functional outcome after trypan blue-assisted vitrectomy for macular pucker: a prospective, randomized, comparative trial. Am J Ophthalmol 2004;138:1-5.

70. Perrier M, Sebag M. Epiretinal membrane surgery assisted by trypan blue. Am J Ophthalmol 2003;135:909-11.

71. Li K, Wong D, Hiscott P, et al. Trypan blue staining of internal limiting membrane and epiretinal membrane during vitrectomy: visual results and histopathological findings. Br J Ophthalmol 2003;87:216-9.

72. Rodrigues EB, Meyer CH, Schmidt JC, Kroll P. Trypan blue stains the epiretinal membrane but not the internal limiting membrane. Br J Ophthalmol 2003;87:1431-72.

73. Meyer CH, Rodrigues EB, Kroll P. Trypan blue has a high affinity to cellular structures such as epiretinal membrane. Am J Ophthalmol 2004;137:207-8.

74. Hasegawa T, Emi K, Ikeda T, et al. Long-term prognosis of internal limiting membrane peeling for idiopathic epiretinal membrane. Nippon Ganka Gakkai Zasshi 2004;108:150-6

75. Park DW, Dugel PU, Garda J, et al. Macular pucker removal with and without internal limiting membrane peeling: pilot study. Ophthalmology 2003;110:62-4.

76. Haritoglou C, Gandorfer A, Gass CA, et al. The effect of indocyanine green on functional outcome of macular pucker surgery. Am J Ophthalmol 2003;135:328-37.

77. Eshita T, Ishida S, Shinoda K, Kitamura S, Inoue M, Oguchi Y, Yamazaki Indocyanine green can distinguish posterior vitreous cortex from internal limiting membrane during vitrectomy with removal of epiretinal membrane. Retina 2002;22:104-6.

78. Eshita T, Inoue M, Kazuto Y, Shinoda K, Ishida S. Indocyanine green can distinguish posterior vitreous cortex from internal limiting membrane during vitrectomy with removal of epiretinal membrane. Retina 2003;23:427.

79. Foster RE, Petersen MR, Da Mata AP, et al. Negative indocyanine green staining of epiretinal membranes. Retina 2002;22:106-8.

80. Saito Y, Lewis JM, Park I, et al. Nonvitrectomizing vitreous surgery: a strategy to prevent postoperative nuclear sclerosis. Ophthalmology 1999;106:1541-5.

81. Sawa M, Saito Y, Hayashi A, et al. Assessment of nuclear sclerosis after nonvitrectomizing vitreous surgery. Am J Ophthalmol 2001;132:356-62.

82. Alexandrakis G, Chaudhry NA, Flynn HW Jr, Murray TG. Combined cataract surgery, intraocular lens insertion, and vitrectomy in eyes with idiopathic epiretinal membrane. Ophthalmic Surg Lasers 1999;30:327-28.

83. Benhamou N, Massin P, Spolaore R, et al. Surgical management of epiretinal membrane in young patients. Am J Ophthalmol 2002;133: 358-64.

84. Massin P, Paques M, Masri H, et al. Visual outcome of surgery for epiretinal membranes with macular pseudoholes. Ophthalmology 1999;106:580-5.

85. Wilkins JR, Puliafito CA, Hee MR, et al. Characterization of epiretinal membranes using optical coherence tomography. Ophthalmology 1996;103:2142-51.

86. Azzolini C, Patelli F, Codenotti M, et al. Optical coherence tomography in idiopathic epiretinal macular membrane surgery. Eur J Ophthalmol 1999; 9:206-11.

87. Massin P, Allouch C, Haouchine B, et al. Optical coherence tomography of idiopathic macular epiretinal membranes before and after surgery. Am J Ophthalmol 2000;130:732-39.

88. Mori K, Gehlbach PL, Sano A, et al. Comparison of epiretinal membranes of differing pathogenesis using optical coherence tomography. Retina 2004;24:57-62.

89. Smiddy WE, Michels RG, Glaser BM, de Bustros S. Vitrectomy for macular traction caused by incomplete vitreous separation. Arch Ophthalmol 1988;106:624-8.

90. Jaffe NS. Vitreous traction at the posterior pole of the fundus due to alterations in the vitreous posterior. Trans Am Acad Ophthalmol Otolaryngol 1967;71:642-2.

91. Margherio RR, Trese MT, Margherio AR, Cartright K. Surgical management of vitreomacular traction syndromes. Ophthalmology 1989;96: 1437-45.

92. Gass JDM. Idiopathic senile macular hole: its early stages and pathogenesis. Arch Ophthalmol 1988;106:629-39.

93. Michels RG. A clinical and histopathologic study of epiretinal membranes affecting the macula and removal by vitreous surgery. Trans Am Ophthalmol Soc 1982;80:580-56.

94. Carter JB, Michels RG, Glaser BM, de Bustros S. Iatrogenic retinal breaks complicating pars plana vitrectomy. Ophthalmology 1990;97:848-54.

95. Smiddy WE. Vitreomacular traction syndrome. In Bovino JA, (Ed): Macular Surgery. Norwalk, CT: Appleton and Lange 1994:11-26.

96. Smiddy WE, Michels RG, Green WR. Morphology, pathology, and surgery for idiopathic macular disorders. Retina 1990;10:288-96.

97. Sebag J. Age-related differences in the human vitreoretinal interface. Arch Ophthalmol 1991;109:966-71.

98. Foos RY, Wheeler NC. Vitreoretinal juncture. Synchysis senilis and posterior vitreous detachment. Ophthalmology 1982; 89:1502-12.

99. Smiddy WE, Green WR, Michels RG, de la Cruz Z. Ultrastructural studies of vitreomacular traction syndrome. Am J Ophthalmol 1989;107:177-85.

100. Sebag J. Anatomy and pathology of the vitreo-retinal interface. Eye 1992;6:541-52.

101. Kishi S, Demaria C, Shimizu K. Vitreous cortex remnants at the fovea after spontaneous vitreous detachment. Int Ophthalmol 1986;9:253-60.

102. Reese AB, Jones IR, Cooper WC. Vitreomacular traction syndrome confirmed histologically. Am J Ophthalmol 1970;60:975-7.

103. Tolentino FI, Schepens CL. Edema of the posterior pole after cataract extraction. Arch Ophthalmol 1965;74:781-6.

104. Byer NE. Spontaneous disappearance of early postoperative preretinal traction. Arch Ophthalmol 1973;90:133-5.

105. Greven GM, Slusher MM, Weaver RG. Epiretinal membrane release and posterior vitreous detachment. Ophthalmology 1988;95:902-5.

106. McDonald HR, Johnson RN, Schatz HA. Surgical results in the vitreomacular traction syndrome. Ophthalmology 1994;101:1397-1403.

107. Thomas EL, Michels RG, Rice TA, et al. Idiopathic progressive unilateral vitreous fibrosis and secondary traction retinal detachment. Retina 1982;2:134-44.

108. Melberg NS, Williams DA, Balles MW, et al. Vitrectomy for vitreomacular traction syndrome with macular detachment. Retina 1995;15:192-7.

109. Hikichi T, Yoshida A, Trempe CL. Course of vitreomacular traction syndrome. Am J Ophthalmol 1995;119:55-61.

110. Smiddy WE, Maguire AM, Green WR, et al. Idiopathic epiretinal membranes. Ultrastructural characteristics in clinical pathologic correlation. Ophthalmology 1989;96:811-21.

111. Gass JDM, Johnson RN. Idiopathic macular holes. Observations, stages of formation, and implication for surgical intervention. Ophthalmology 1988;95:912-24.

112. Madreperala SA, McCuen BW II, Hickinbotham D, Green WR. Clinicopathologic correlation of surgically removed macular hole opercula. Am J Ophthalmol 1995;120:197-207.

113. Lister W. Holes in the retina and their clinical significance. Br J Ophthalmol 1924;8:1-20.

114. Morgan CM, Schatz H. Idiopathic macular holes. Am J Ophthalmol 1985;99:437-44.

115. McDonnell PJ, Fine SL, Hillis AI. Clinical features of idiopathic macular cysts and holes. Am J Ophthalmol 1982;93:777-86.

116. Kornzweig AL, Feldstein M. Studies of the eye in old age, II. Hole in the macula: a clinical-pathologic study. Am J Ophthalmol 1950;33:243-7.

117. Trempe CL, Weiter JJ, Furukawa H. Fellow eyes in cases of macular hole: biomicroscopic study of the vitreous. Arch Ophthalmol 1986;104:93-5.

118. Guyer DR, Green WR. Idiopathic macular holes and precursor lesions. In Franklin RM (Ed): Proceedings of the Symposium on Retina and Vitreous, New Orleans Academy of Ophthalmology, New Orleans. New York: Kugler, 1993:135-62.

119. Smiddy WE, Michels RG, Glaser BM, de Bustros S. Vitrectomy for impending macular holes. Am J Ophthalmol 1988;105:371-6.

120. Campochiaro PA, Van Neil E, Vinores SA. Immunocytochemical labeling of cells in cortical vitreous from patients with premacular hole lesions. Arch Ophthalmol 1992;110:371-7.

121. Kishi S, Shimizu K. Posterior precortical vitreous pocket. Arch Ophthalmol 1990;108:979-82.

122. Kishi S, Kamei Y, Shimizu K. Traction elevation of Henle's fiber layer in idiopathic macular holes. Am J Ophthalmol 1995;120:486-96.

123. Gordon LW, Glaser BM, Darmakusuma Ie, et al. Full-thickness macular hole formation in eyes with a pre-existing complete posterior vitreous detachment. Ophthalmology 1995;102:1702-5.

124. Gass JDM. Reappraisal of biomicroscopic classification of stages of development of a macular hole. Am J Ophthalmol 1995;119:752-9.

125. Smith RG, Hardman-Lea SJ, Galloway NR. Visual performance in idiopathic macular holes. Eye 1990;4:190.

126. Yaoeda H. Clinical observation on macular hole. Nippon Ganka Gakkai Zasshi 1967;71:1723-36.

127. Margherio RR, Schepens CL. Macular breaks. I. Diagnosis, etiology, and observations. Am J Ophthalmol 1972;74:219-32.

128. Aaberg TM, Blair CJ, Gass JDM. Macular holes. Am J Ophthalmol 1970;69:555-62.

129. James M, Feman SS. Macular holes. Graefe's Arch Clin Exp Ophthalmol 1980;215:59-63.

130. Bidwell AE, Jampol LM, Goldberg MF. Macular holes and excellent visual acuity: case report. Arch Ophthalmol 1988;106:1350.

131. Frangieh GT, Green WR, Engel HM. A histopathologic study of macular cysts and holes. Retina 1981;1:311-36.

132. Guyer DR, Green WR, de Bustros S, Fine SL. Histopathologic features of idiopathic macular holes and cysts. Ophthalmology 1990;97:1045-51.

133. Yuzawa M, Watanabe A, Takahashi Y, Matsui M. Observations of idiopathic full-thickness macular holes. Arch Ophthalmol 1994;112: 1051-56.

134. Kakehashi A, Schepens CL, Akiba J, et al. Spontaneous resolution of foveal detachments and macular breaks. Am J Ophthalmol 1995;120:767-75.

135. Hikichi T, Yoshida A, Akiba J, et al. Prognosis of stage II macular holes. Am J Ophthalmol 1995;119:571-5.

136. Fisher YL, Slakter JS, Yannuzzi LA, Guyer DR. A prospective natural history study and kinetic ultrasound evaluation of idiopathic macular holes. Ophthalmology 1994;101:5-11.

137. Akiba J, Yoshida A, Trempe CL. Risk of developing a macular hole. Arch Ophthalmol 1990;108:1088-90.

138. Akiba J, Kakehashi A, Arzabe CW, Trempe CL. Fellow eyes in idiopathic macular hole cases. Ophthalmic Surg 1992;23:594-7.

139. Guyer DR, de Bustros S, Diener-West M, Fine SL. The natural history of idiopathic macular holes and cysts. Arch Ophthalmol 1992;110:1264-8.

140. Kokame GT, de Bustros S. The Vitrectomy for Prevention of Macular Hole Study Group. Visual acuity as a prognostic indicator in stage I macular holes. Am J Ophthalmol 1995;119:112-4.

141. Kim JW, Freeman WR, El-Haig W, et al. The Vitrectomy for Macular Hole Study Group. Baseline characteristics, natural history, and risk factors to progression in eyes with stage II macular holes. Results from a prospective randomized clinical trial. Ophthalmology 1995;102:1818-29.

142. Cheng L, Freeman WR, Ozerdem U, et al. Prevalence, correlates, and natural history of epiretinal membranes surrounding idiopathic macular holes. Vitrectomy for Macular Hole Study Group. Ophthalmology 2000; 107:853-9.

143. Paques M, Massin P, Blain P, et al. Long-term incidence of reopening of macular holes. Ophthalmology 2000;107:760-5.

144. Kokame GT. Management options for early stages of acutely symptomatic macular holes. Am J Ophthalmol 2002; 133(2):276-8.

145. Gass JDM, Joondeph BC. Observations concerning patients with suspected impending macular holes. Am J Ophthalmol 1990;109:638-46.

146. Fish RH, Anand R, Izbrand DJ. Macular pseudoholes: clinical features and accuracy of diagnosis. Ophthalmology 1992;99:1665-70.

147. Smiddy WE, Gass JDM. Masquerades of macular holes. Ophthalmic Surg 1995;26:16-24.

148. Amsler M. Quantitative and qualitative vision. Trans Ophthalmol Soc UK 1949;69:397.

149. Watzke RC, Allen L. Subjective slitlamp beam sign for macular disease. Am J Ophthalmol 1969;68:449-53.

150. Martinez J, Smiddy WE, Kim J, Gass JDM. Differentiating macular holes from macular pseudoholes. Am J Ophthalmol 1994;117:762-7.

151. Birch DG, Jost BF, Fish GE. The focal electroretinogram in fellow eyes of patients with idiopathic macular holes. Arch Ophthalmol 1988;106: 1558-63.

152. Sjaarda RN, Frank DA, Glaser BM, et al. Resolution of an absolute scotoma and improvement of relative scotoma after successful macular surgery. Am J Ophthalmol 1993;116:129-39.

153. Acosta F, Lashkari K, Reynaud X, et al. Characterization of functional changes in macular holes and cysts. Ophthalmology 1991;98:1820-3.

154. Weinberger D, Stiebel H, Gaton H, et al. Three-dimensional measurements of idiopathic macular holes using a scanning laser tomograph. Ophthalmology 1995;102:1445-49.

155. Bartsch DU, Intaglietta M, Bille JF, et al. Confocal laser tomographic analysis of the retina in eyes with macular hole formation and other focal macular diseases. Am J Ophthalmol 1989;108:277-87.

156. Oritz RG, Lopez PF, Lambert HM, et al. Examination of macular vitreoretinal interface disorders with monochromatic photography. Am J Ophthalmol 1992;113:243-47.

157. Ogura Y, Shahidi M, Mori MT, et al. Improved visualization of macular hole lesions with laser biomicroscopy. Arch Ophthalmol 1991;109:957-61.

158. Kiryu J, Ogura Y, Shahidi M, et al. Enhanced visualization of vitreoretinal interface by laser biomicroscopy. Ophthalmology 1993;100: 1040-3.

159. Dugel PU, Smiddy WE, Byrne SF, et al. Macular hole syndrome: echographic findings with clinical correlation. Ophthalmology 1994;101:815-21.

160. Kokame GT. Clinical correlation of ultrasonographic findings in macular holes. Am J Ophthalmol 1995;119:441-51.

161. Van Newkirk MR, Gass JDM, Callanan D, et al. Follow-up and ultrasonographic examination of patients with macular pseudo-operculum. Am J Ophthalmol 1994; 117: 13-8.

162. Hee MR, Puliafito CA, Wong C, et al. Optical coherence tomography of macular holes. Ophthalmology 1995; 102:748-56.

163. Sjaarda R. Macular hole. Int Ophthalmol Clin 1995;35:105-22.

164. Smiddy WE, Thomley M, Knighton RW, Feuer WJ. Use of the potential acuity meter and laser interferometer to predict visual acuity after macular hole surgery. Retina 1994;14:305-9.

165. Casuso LA, Scott IU, Flynn HW Jr, et al. Long-term follow-up of unoperated macular holes. Ophthalmology 2001; 108:1150-5.

166. Schocket SS, Lakhanpal V, Xiaoping M, et al. Laser treatment of macular holes. Ophthalmology 1988;95:574-82.

167. Makabe R. Kryptonlaserkoagulation bei idiopathischem makulaloch. Klin Monatsbl Augenheilkd 1990;196:202-4.

168. Melberg NS, Meredith TA. Success with macular hole surgery. Ophthalmology 1996;103:200-1.

169. Kelly NE, Wendel RT. Vitreous surgery for idiopathic macular holes: results of a pilot study. Arch Ophthalmol 1991; 109: 654-9.

170. Mein CE, Flynn HW Jr. Recognition and removal of the posterior cortical vitreous during vitreoretinal surgery for impending macular holes. Am J Ophthalmol 1991;111:611-3.

171. Ryan EA, Lee S, Chern S. Use of intravitreal autologous blood to identify posterior cortical vitreous in macular hole surgery. Arch Ophthalmol 1995;113:822-3.

172. Wendel RT, Patel AC. Full-thickness macular hole. In Bovino JA (Ed): Macular Surgery. Norwalk, CT: Appleton and Lange, 1994:49-60.

173. Jost BF, Hutton WL, Fullet DG, et al. Vitrectomy in eyes at risk for macular hole formation. Ophthalmology 1990;97:843-7.

174. de Bustros S. Early stages of macular holes: to treat or not to treat. Arch Ophthalmol 1990;108:979-82.

175. de Bustros S. Vitrectomy for prevention of macular hole study. Arch Ophthalmol 1991;109:1057.

176. de Bustros S. The Vitrectomy for Prevention of Macular Holes Study Group. Vitrectomy for prevention of macular holes: results of a randomized clinical trial. Ophthalmology 1994;101:1055-60.

177. Chambers RB, Davidorf FH, Gresak P, Stief WC. Modified vitrectomy for impending macular holes. Ophthalmic Surg 1991;22:730-4.

178. Ruby AJ, Williams DF, Grand MG, et al. Pars plana vitrectomy for treatment of stage II macular holes. Arch Ophthalmol 1994;112:359-64.

179. Kim JW, Freeman WR, Azen SP, et al. Prospective randomized trial of vitrectomy or observation for stage 2 macular holes. Vitrectomy for Macular Hole Study Group. Am J Ophthalmol 1996;121:605-14.

180. Wendel RT, Patel AC, Kelly NE, et al. Vitreous surgery for macular holes. Ophthalmology 1993;100:1671-6.

181. Ryan EH, Gilbert HD. Results of surgical treatment of recent-onset full-thickness idiopathic macular holes. Arch Ophthalmol 1994;112:1545-53.

182. Glaser BM, Michels RG, Kupperman BD, et al. Transforming growth factor-beta 2 for the treatment of full-thickness macular holes. Ophthalmology 1992;99:1162-73.

183. Lansing MB, Glaser BM, Liss H, et al. The effects of pars plana vitrectomy and transforming growth factor beta 2 without epiretinal membrane peeling on full thickness macular holes. Ophthalmology 1993;100:868-72.

184. Smiddy WE, Glaser BM, Thompson JT, et al. Transforming growth factor beta-2 significantly enhances the ability to flatten the rim of subretinal fluid surrounding macular holes. Preliminary anatomic results of a multicenter prospective randomized study. Retina 1993;13:296-301.

185. Thompson JT, Glaser BM, Sjaarda RN, et al. Effects of intraocular bubble duration in the treatment of macular holes by vitrectomy and transforming growth factor beta-2. Ophthalmology 1994,101.1195-1200.

186. Liggett PE, Skolik S, Horio B, et al. Human autologous serum for the treatment of full-thickness macular holes: a preliminary study. Ophthalmology 1995;102:1071-6.

187. Funata M, Wendel RT, de la Cruz Z, Green WR. Clinicopathologic study of bilateral macular holes treated with pars plana vitrectomy and gas tamponade. Retina 1992;12:289-98.

188. Madreperla SA, Geiger GL, Funata M, et al. Clinicopathologic correlation of a macular hole treated by cortical vitreous peeling and gas tamponade. Ophthalmology 1994;101:682-6.

189. Fekrat S, Wendel RT, de la Cruz Z, Green WR. Clinicopathologic correlation of an epiretinal membrane associated with a recurrent macular hole. Retina 1995;15:53-7.

190. Del Priore LV, Kaplan HJ, Bonham RD. Laser photocoagulation and fluid-gas exchange for recurrent macular hole. Retina 1994;14:381-2.

191. Thompson JT, Sjaarda RN, Lansing MB. The results of vitreous surgery for chronic macular holes. Retina 1997;17:493-501.

192. Cheng L, Azen SP, El-Bradey MH, et al. Duration of vitrectomy and postoperative cataract in the vitrectomy for macular hole study. Am J Ophthalmol 2001;132:881-7.

193. Karia N, Laidlaw A, West J, et al. Macular hole surgery using silicone oil tamponade. Br J Ophthalmol 2001; 85: 1320-3.

194. Leonard RE 2nd, Smiddy WE, Flynn HW Jr, Feuer W. Long-term visual outcomes in patients with successful macular hole surgery. Ophthalmology 1997;104:1648-52.

195. Banker AS, Freeman WR, Kim JW, et al. Vision-threatening complications of surgery for full-thickness macular holes. Vitrectomy for Macular Hole Study Group. Ophthalmology 1997;104:1442-52.

196. Tornambe PE, Poliner LS, Grote K. Macular hole surgery without face-down positioning: a pilot study. Retina 1997;17:179-85.

197. Leonard RE 2nd, Smiddy WE, Flynn HW Jr. Visual acuity and macular hole size after unsuccessful macular hole closure. Am J Ophthalmol 1997;123:84-9.

198. Thompson JT, Glaser BM, Sjaarda RN, Murphy RP. Progression of nuclear sclerosis and long-term visual results of vitrectomy with transforming growth factor beta-2 for macular holes. Am J Ophthalmol 1995;119:48-54.

199. Park SS, Marcus D, Duker JS, et al. Posterior segment complications after vitrectomy for macular hole. Ophthalmology 1995;102:775-81.

200. Sjaarda RN, Glaser BM, Thompson JT, et al. Distribution of iatrogenic retinal breaks in macular hole surgery. Ophthalmology 1995;102:1387-92.

201. Poliner LS, Tornambe PE. Retinal pigment epitheliopathy after macular hole surgery. Ophthalmology 1992;99:1671-77.

202. Charles S. Retinal pigment epithelium abnormalities after macular hole surgery. Retina 1993;13:176. Letter.

203. Duker JS. Retinal pigment epitheliopathy after macular hole surgery. Ophthalmology 1993;100:1604-5. Letter.

204. Duker JS, Wendel RT, Patel AC, Puliafito CA. Late reopening of macular holes following initial successful vitreous surgery. Ophthalmology 1994;101:1373-8.

205. Kokame GT. Recurrence of macular holes. Ophthalmology 1995;102:172-3. Letter.

206. Smiddy WE. Atypical presentations of macular holes. Arch Ophthalmol 1993;111:626-31.

207. Holekamp NM, Meredith TA, Landers MB, et al. Ulnar neuropathy as a complication of macular hole surgery. Arch Ophthalmol 1999;117:1607-10.

208. Hutton WL, Fuller DG, Snyder WB, Fellman RL, Swanson WH. Visual field defects after macular hole surgery: a new finding. Ophthalmology 1996;103:2152-8.

209. Boldt HC, Munden PM, Folk JC, Mehaffey MG. Visual field defects after macular hole surgery. Am J Ophthalmol 1996;122:371-81.

210. Pendergast SD, McCuen BW 2nd. Visual field loss after macular hole surgery. Ophthalmology 1996;103:1069-77.

211. Ezra E, Arden GB, Riordan-Eva P, et al. Visual field loss following vitrectomy for stage 2 and 3 macular holes. Br J Ophthalmol 1996;80:519-25.

212. Paques M, Massin P, Santiago PY, et al. Visual field loss after vitrectomy for full-thickness macular holes. Am J Ophthalmol 1997;124:88-94.

213. Gass CA, Haritoglou C, Messmer EM, et al. Peripheral visual field defects after macular hole surgery: a complication with decreasing incidence. Br J Ophthalmol 2001;85:549-51.

214. Haritoglou C, Ehrt O, Gass CA, et al. Paracentral scotomata: a new finding after vitrectomy for idiopathic macular hole. Br J Ophthalmol 2001;85:231-3.

215. Yonemura N, Hirata A, Hasumura T, Negi A. Fundus changes corresponding to visual field defects after vitrectomy for macular hole. Ophthalmology 2001;108:1638-43.

216. Hirata A, Yonemura N, Hasumura T, et al. Effect of infusion air pressure on visual field defects after macular hole surgery. Am J Ophthalmol 2000;130:611-6.

217. Welch JC. Dehydration injury as a possible cause of visual field defect after pars plana vitrectomy for macular hole. Am J Ophthalmol 1997;124:698-9.

218. Ohji M, Nao-I N, Saito Y, et al. Prevention of visual field defect after macular hole surgery by passing air used for fluid-air exchange through water. Am J Ophthalmol 1999;127:62-66.

219. Thompson JT, Sjaarda RN, Glaser BM, Murphy RP. Increased intraocular pressure after macular hole surgery. Am J Ophthalmol 1996;121:615-22.

220. Spaide RF. Persistent intraocular indocyanine green staining after macular hole surgery. Retina 2002;22:637-9.

221. Ando F, Sasano K, Ohba N, et al. Anatomic and visual outcomes after indocyanine green-assisted peeling of the retinal internal limiting membrane in idiopathic macular hole surgery. Am J Ophthalmol 2004;137:609-14.

222. Weinberger AW, Schlossmacher B, Dahlke C, et al. Fundus fluorescence after indocyanine green. Ophthalmology 2004; 111:849-50

223. Ciardella AP, Schiff W, Barile G, et al. Persistent indocyanine green fluorescence after vitrectomy for macular hole. Am J Ophthalmol 2003;136:174-7.

224. Ashikari M, Ozeki H, Tomida K, et al. Retention of dye after indocyanine green-assisted internal limiting membrane peeling. Am J Ophthalmol 2003;136:172-4.

225. Stec LA, Ross RD, Williams GA, et al. Vitrectomy for chronic macular holes. Retina 2002;24:341-7.

226. Oz O, Fudemberg SJ, Cakir B, et al. Predictors of success in macular hole surgery with emphasis on the internal limiting membrane (ILM) and ILM peeling. Ophthalmic Surg Lasers Imaging 2004;35:207-14.

227. Rezende FA, Kapusta MA. Internal limiting membrane: ultrastructural relationships, with clinical implications for macular hole healing. Can J Ophthalmol 2004;39:251-9.

228. Schmidt JC, Rodrigues EB, Meyer CH, et al. A modified technique to stain the internal limiting membrane with indocyanine green. Ophthalmologica 2004;218:176-9.

229. Ben Simon GJ, Desatnik H, Alhalel A, et al. Retrospective analysis of vitrectomy with and without internal limiting membrane peeling for stage 3 and 4 macular hole. Ophthalmic Surg Lasers Imaging 2004;35:109-15.

230. Sheidow TG, Blinder KJ, Holekamp N, et al. Outcome results in macular hole surgery: an evaluation of internal limiting membrane peeling with and without indocyanine green. Ophthalmology 2003;110:1697-1701.

231. Kwok AK, Lai TY, Man-Chan W, Woo DC. Indocyanine green assisted retinal internal limiting membrane removal in stage 3 or 4 macular hole surgery. Br J Ophthalmol 2003;87:71-4.

232. Da Mata AP, Burk SE, Riemann CD, et al. Indocyanine green-assisted peeling of the retinal internal limiting membrane during vitrectomy surgery for macular hole repair. Ophthalmology 2001;108:1187-92.

233. Gandorfer A, Messmer EM, Ulbig MW, Kampik A. Indocyanine green selectively stains the internal limiting membrane. Am J Ophthalmol 2001;131:387-8.

234. Mester V, Kuhn F. Internal limiting membrane removal in the management of full-thickness macular holes. Am J Ophthalmol 2000;129:769-77.

235. Kadonosono K, Itoh N, Uchio E, et al. Staining of internal limiting membrane in macular hole surgery. Arch Ophthalmol 2000;118:1116-8.

236. Park DW, Sipperley JO, Sneed SR, et al. Macular hole surgery with internal-limiting membrane peeling and intravitreous air. Ophthalmology 1999;106:1392-7.

237. Eckardt C, Eckardt U, Groos S, et al. Removal of the internal limiting membrane in macular holes: clinical and morphological findings. Ophthalmology 1997;94:545-51.

238. Smiddy WE, Feuer W, Cordahi G. Internal limiting membrane peeling in macular hole surgery. Ophthalmology 2001;108:1471-6.

239. Schechter RJ. Retinal pigment epithelial changes after macular hole surgery with indocyanine green-assisted internal limiting membrane peeling. Am J Ophthalmol 2002;134:151.

240. Ho JD, Chen HC, Chen SN, Tsai RJ. Reduction of indocyanine green-associated photosensitizing toxicity in retinal pigment epithelium by sodium elimination. Arch Ophthalmol 2004;122:871-8.

241. Czajka MP, McCuen BW 2nd, Cummings TJ, et al. Effects of indocyanine green on the retina and retinal pigment epithelium in a porcine model of retinal hole. Retina 2004;24:275-82.

242. Ho JD, Tsai RJ, Chen SN, Chen HC. Cytotoxicity of indocyanine green on retinal pigment epithelium: implications for macular hole surgery. Arch Ophthalmol 2003;121:1423-9.

243. Maia M, Haller JA, Pieramici DJ, et al. Retinal pigment epithelial abnormalities after internal limiting membrane peeling guided by indocyanine green staining. Retina 2004;24:157-60.

244. Rivett K, Kruger L, Radloff S. Membrane peeling in macular hole repair: Does it make a difference? Graefe's Arch Clin Exp Ophthalmol 2004;242:393-6.

245. Engelbrecht NE, Freeman J, Sternberg P Jr, et al. Retinal pigment epithelial changes after macular hole surgery with indocyanine green-assisted internal limiting membrane peeling. Am J Ophthalmol 2002;133:89-94.

246. Gass CA, Haritoglou C, Schaumberger M, Kampik A. Functional outcome of macular hole surgery with and without indocyanine green-assisted peeling of the internal limiting membrane. Graefe's Arch Clin Exp Ophthalmol 2003;241:716-20.

247. Hirata A, Inomata Y, Kawaji T, Tanihara H. Persistent subretinal indocyanine green induces retinal pigment epithelium atrophy. Am J Ophthalmol 2003;136:353-5.

248. Haritoglou C, Gandorfer A, Gass CA, et al. Indocyanine green-assisted peeling of the internal limiting membrane in macular hole surgery affects visual outcome: a clinicopathologic correlation. Am J Ophthalmol 2002;134: 836-41.

249. Haritoglou C, Gass CA, Schaumberger M, et al. Long-term follow-up after macular hole surgery with internal limiting membrane peeling. Am J Ophthalmol 2002;134:661-6.

250. Haritoglou C, Gass CA, Schaumberger M, et al. Macular changes after peeling of the internal limiting membrane in macular hole surgery. Am J Ophthalmol 2001;132:363-8.

251. Blem RI, Huynh PD, Thall EH. Altered uptake of infrared diode laser by retina after intravitreal indocyanine green dye and internal limiting membrane peeling. Am J Ophthalmol 2002;134:285-6.

252. Ho JD, Tsai RJ, Chen SN, Chen HC. Removal of sodium from the solvent reduces retinal pigment epithelium toxicity caused by indocyanine green: implications for macular hole surgery. Br J Ophthalmol 2004;88:556-9.

253. Gandorfer A, Haritoglou C, Gass CA, et al. Indocyanine green-assisted peeling of the internal limiting membrane may cause retinal damage. Am J Ophthalmol 2001;132:431-3.

254. Chung J, Spaide R. Intraretinal silicone oil vacuoles after macular hole surgery with internal limiting membrane peeling. Am J Ophthalmol 2003;136:766-7.

255. Van De Moere A, Stalmans P. Anatomical and visual outcome of macular hole surgery with infracyanine green-assisted peeling of the internal limiting membrane, endodrainage, and silicone oil tamponade. Am J Ophthalmol 2003; 136:879-87.

256. Lahey JM, Francis RR, Fong DS, et al. Combining phacoemulsification with vitrectomy for treatment of macular holes. Br J Ophthalmol 2002;86:876-8.

257. Cohen D. Intraocular lens power calculation after macular hole surgery. J Cataract Refract Surg 2002;28:1485-6.

258. Lai JC, Stinnett SS, McCuen BW. Comparison of silicone oil versus gas tamponade in the treatment of idiopathic full-thickness macular hole. Ophthalmology 2003;110: 1170-4.

259. Jonas JB, Jager M. Perfluorohexyloctane endotamponade for treatment of persisting macular hole. Eur J Ophthalmol 2003;13:103-4.

260. Tornambe PE. Macular hole genesis: the hydration theory. Retina 2003;23:421-4.

261. Takahashi H, Kishi S. Tomographic features of early macular hole closure after vitreous surgery. Am J Ophthalmol 2000;130:192-6.

262. Sato H, Kawasaki R, Yamashita H. Observation of idiopathic full-thickness macular hole closure in early postoperative period as evaluated by optical coherence tomography. Am J Ophthalmol 2003;136:185-7.

263. Ito Y, Terasaki H, Suzuki T, et al. Mapping posterior vitreous detachment by optical coherence tomography in eyes with idiopathic macular hole. Am J Ophthalmol 2003;135: 351-5.

264. Ullrich S, Haritoglou C, Gass C, et al. Macular hole size as a prognostic factor in macular hole surgery. Br J Ophthalmol 2002;86:390-3.

265. Mikajiri K, Okada AA, Ohji M, et al. Analysis of vitrectomy for idiopathic macular hole by optical coherence tomography. Am J Ophthalmol 1999;128:655-7.

266. Uemoto R, Yamamoto S, Aoki T, et al. Macular configuration determined by optical coherence tomography after idiopathic macular hole surgery with or without internal limiting membrane peeling. Br J Ophthalmol 2002;86:1240-2.

267. Kwok AK, Lai TY, Yip WW. Correlation of clinical and optical coherence tomography findings in postoperative macular hole closure status. Ophthalmic Surg Lasers Imaging 2003;34:25-32.

268. Ip MS, Baker BJ, Duker JS, et al. Anatomical outcomes of surgery for idiopathic macular hole as determined by optical coherence tomography. Arch Ophthalmol 2002; 120:29-35.

269. Fujii GY, De Juan E, Bressler NM. Vitrectomy surgery for impending macular hole based on optical coherence tomography. Retina 2001;21:389-92.

270. Spaide RF. Macular hole repair with minimal vitrectomy. Retina 2002;22:183-6.

271. Gass JDM. Pathogenesis of disciform detachment of the neuroepithelium. III. Senile disciform macular degeneration. Am J Ophthalmol 1967;63:617-44.

272. Lopez PF, Grossniklaus HE, Lambert HM, et al. Pathologic features of surgically excised subretinal neovascular membranes in age-related macular degeneration. Am J Ophthalmol 1991;112:647-56.

273. Grossniklaus HE, Martinez JA, Brown VB, et al. Immunohistochemical and histochemical properties of surgically excised subretinal neovascular membranes in age-related macular degeneration. Am J Ophthalmol 1992; 114:464-72.

274. Hotchkiss ML, Fine SL. Pathologic myopia and choroidal neovascularization. Am J Ophthalmol 1981;91:177-183.

275. Hampton GR, Kohen D, Bird AC. Visual prognosis of disciform degeneration in myopia. Ophthalmology 1983; 90:923-6.

276. Avila MP, Weiter JJ, Jalkh AE, et al. Natural history of choroidal neovascularization in degenerative myopia. Ophthalmology 1984;91:1573-81.

277. Singerman LJ, Hatem G. Laser treatment of choroidal neovascular membranes in angioid streaks. Retina 1981;1:75-83.

278. Clarkson JG, Altman RD. Angioid streaks. Surv Ophthalmol 1982;26:235-46.

279. Lim JI, Bressler NM, Marsh MJ, Bressler SB. Laser treatment of choroidal neovascularization in patients with angioid streaks. Am J Ophthalmol 1993;116:414-23.

280. Klein R, Lewis RA, Myers SM, Myers FL. Subretinal neovascularization associated with fundus flavimaculatus. Arch Ophthalmol 1978;96:2054-7.

281. Miller SA, Bresnick GH, Chandra SR. Choroidal neovascular membrane in Best's vitelliform macular dystrophy. Am J Ophthalmol 1976;82:252-5.

282. Callanan D, Gass JDM. Multifocal choroiditis and choroidal neovascularization associated with the multiple evanescent dot syndrome and acute idiopathic blind spot enlargement syndrome. Ophthalmology 1992;99:1678-85.

283. Morgan CM, Schatz H. Recurrent multifocal choroiditis. Ophthalmology 1986;93:1138-47.

284. Beebe WE, Kirkland C, Price J. A subretinal neovascular membrane as a complication of endogenous *Candida endophthalmitis*. Ann Ophthalmol 1987;19:207-9.

285. Wysynski RE, Grossniklaus HE, Frank KE. Indirect choroidal rupture secondary to blunt ocular trauma: a review of eight eyes. Retina 1988;8:237-43.

286. Ruby AJ, Jampol LM, Goldberg MF, et al. Choroidal neovascularization associated with choroidal hemangiomas. Arch Ophthalmol 1992;110:658-61.

287. Bressler SB, Bressler NM, Fine SL, et al. Natural course of choroidal neovascular membranes within the foveal avascular zone in senile macular degeneration. Am J Ophthalmol 1982;93:157-63.

288. Macular Photocoagulation Study Group. Laser photocoagulation of subfoveal neovascular lesions of age-related macular degeneration. Updated findings from two clinical trials. Arch Ophthalmol 1993;111:1200-09.

289. Olk RJ, Burgess DB, McCormick PA. Subfoveal and juxtafoveal subretinal neovascularization in the presumed ocular histoplasmosis syndrome: visual prognosis. Ophthalmology 1984;91:1592-1602.

290. Kleiner RC, Ratner CM, Enger C, Fine SL. Subfoveal neovascularization in the ocular histoplasmosis syndrome: a natural history study. Retina 1988;8:225-9.

291. Campochiaro PA, Morgan KM, Conway BP, Stathos J. Spontaneous involution of subfoveal neovascularization. Am J Ophthalmol 1990;109:668-75.

292. Vander JF, Morgan CM, Schatz H. Growth rate of subretinal neovascularization in age related macular degeneration. Ophthalmology 1989;96:1422-9.

293. Macular Photocoagulation Study Group. Argon laser photocoagulation for senile macular degeneration: results of a randomized clinical trial. Arch Ophthalmol 1982;100:912-8.

294. Macular Photocoagulation Study Group. Krypton laser photocoagulation for neovascular lesions of age-related macular degeneration: results of randomized clinical trial. Arch Ophthalmol 1990;108:816-24.

295. Macular Photocoagulation Study Group. Argon laser photocoagulation for neovascular maculopathy: three-year results from randomized clinical trials. Arch Ophthalmol 1986;104:694-701.

296. Macular Photocoagulation Study Group. Argon laser photocoagulation for ocular histoplasmosis: results of a randomized clinical trial. Arch Ophthalmol 1983;101:1347-57.

297. Macular Photocoagulation Study Group. Argon laser photocoagulation for neovascular maculopathy: five year results from randomized clinical trials. Arch Ophthalmol 1991;109:1109-14.

298. Macular Photocoagulation Study Group. Recurrent choroidal neovascularization after argon laser photocoagulation for neovascular vasculopathy. Arch Ophthalmol 1986;104:503-12.

299. Macular Photocoagulation Study Group. Persistent and recurrent neovascularization after krypton laser photocoagulation for neovascular lesions of age-related macular degeneration. Arch Ophthalmol 1990;108:825-31.

300. Macular Photocoagulation Study Group. Persistent and recurrent neovascularization after krypton laser photocoagulation for neovascular lesions of ocular histoplasmosis. Arch Ophthalmol 1989;107:344-52.

301. Macular Photocoagulation Study Group. Laser photocoagulation of subfoveal neovascular lesions in age-related macular degeneration: results of a randomized clinical trial. Arch Ophthalmol 1991;109:1220-31.

302. Macular Photocoagulation Study Group. Laser photocoagulation of subfoveal recurrent neovascular lesions in age-related macular degeneration: results of a randomized clinical trial. Arch Ophthalmol 1991;109:1232-41.

303. Macular Photocoagulation Study Group. Subfoveal neovascular lesions in age-related macular degeneration: guidelines for evaluation and treatment in the Macular Photocoagulation Study. Arch Ophthalmol 1991;109:1242-57.

304. Sorensen JA, Yannuzzi LA, Shakin JL. Recurrent subretinal neovascularization. Ophthalmology 1985;92:1059-74.

305. Coscas G, Soubrane G, Ramahefasolo C, Fardeau C. Perifoveal laser treatment for subfoveal choroidal new vessels in age-related macular degeneration: results of a randomized clinical trial. Arch Ophthalmol 1991;109:1258-65.

306. Green WR. Clinicopathologic studies of treated choroidal neovascular membranes: a review and report of two cases. Retina 1991;11:328-56.

307. Fine SL, Wood WJ, Isernhagen RD. Laser treatment for subfoveal neovascular membranes in ocular histoplasmosis syndrome: results of a pilot randomized clinical trial. Arch Ophthalmol 1993;111:19-20.

308. de Juan E Jr, Machemer R. Vitreous surgery for hemorrhagic and fibrous complications of age-related macular degeneration. Am J Ophthalmol 1988;105:25-9.

309. Blinder KJ, Peyman GA, Paris CL, Gremillion CM Jr. Submacular scar excision in age-related macular degeneration. Int Ophthalmol 1991;15:215-22.

310. Peyman GA, Blinder KJ, Paris CL, et al. A technique for retinal pigment epithelium transplantation for age related macular degeneration secondary to extensive subfoveal scarring. Ophthalmic Surg 1991;22:102-8.

311. Thomas MA, Kaplan HJ. Surgical removal of subfoveal neovascularization in the presumed ocular histoplasmosis syndrome. Am J Ophthalmol 1991;111:1-7.

312. Dickinson JD, Aguilar HE, Thomas MA. Retinotomies in subfoveal surgery: neither laser nor long acting gas tamponade is required. Presented at American Academy of Ophthalmology meeting, 1994.

313. Thomas MA. The use of vitreoretinal surgical techniques in subfoveal choroidal neovascularization. Curr Opin Ophthalmol 1992;3:349-56.

314. Thomas MA, Williams DF, Grand MG. Surgical removal of submacular hemorrhage and subfoveal choroidal neovascular membranes. Int Ophthalmol Clin 1992;32:173-88.

315. Ibanez HE, Thomas MA. Surgical approach to subfoveal neovascularization and submacular hemorrhage. Semin Ophthalmol 1994;9:56-64.

316. Ibanez HE, Thomas MA. Surgical excision of subfoveal choroidal neovascularization. Ophthalmol Clin North 1994; 7:51-7.

317. Thomas MA, Ibanez HE. Surgical excision of subfoveal neovascular membranes and subretinal strands. In Tasman W, Jaeger EA, (Eds): Duane's Clinical Ophthalmology. Philadelphia: Lippincott, 1994:1-10.

318. Thomas MA. Surgical removal of subfoveal choroidal neovascular membranes. In Ryan SJ, (Ed): Retina. 2nd edn; vol. 3. St. Louis: Mosby, 1994:2385-93.

319. Thomas MA. Surgical removal of subfoveal choroidal neovascular membranes. In Lewis H, Ryan SJ, (Eds): Medical and Surgical Retina: Advances, Controversies, and Management. St. Louis: Mosby, 1994:63-81.

320. Thomas MA. Vitrectomy surgery for subfoveal choroidal neovascularization and submacular hemorrhage. In Bovino JA, (Ed): Macular Surgery. Norwalk, Appleton and Lange, 1994;135-64.

321. Bressler NM. Submacular surgery. Are randomized trials necessary? Arch Ophthalmol 1995;113:1557-60.

322. Thomas MA, Lee CA, Pesin S, Lowe M. New instruments for submacular surgery. Am J Ophthalmol 1991;12:733-4.

323. Thomas MA, Ibanez HE. Instruments for submacular surgery. Retina 1994;14:84-7.

324. Peyman GA, Kwang KJ. A new subretinal forceps. Retina 1995;15:87-8.

325. Greve MDJ, Peyman GA, Millsap CM. Direction and location of retinotomy for removal of subretinal neovascular membranes. Ophthalmic Surg 1995;26:330-3.

326. Adelberg DA, Del Priore LV, Kaplan HJ. Surgery for subfoveal membranes in myopia, angioid streaks, and other disorders. Retina 1995;15:198-05.

327. Capone A Jr. Submacular surgical procedures. Int Ophthalmol Clin 1995;35:83-93.

328. Thomas MA, Grand MG, Williams DF, et al. Surgical management of subfoveal choroidal neovascularization. Ophthalmology 1992;99:952-96.

329. Thomas MA, Dickenson JD, Melberg NS, et al. Visual results after surgical removal of subfoveal choroidal neovascular membranes. Ophthalmology 1994;101:1384-96.

330. Smiddy WE, Fine SL, Green WR, et al. Clinicopathologic correlation of krypton red, argon blue-green, and argon green photocoagulation in the human fundus. Retina 1984;4:15-21.

331. Thomas EL, Apple DJ, Swartz M, et al. Histopathologic and ultrastructure of krypton and argon laser lesions in human retina-choroid. Retina 1984;4:22-39.

332. Eldrini AA, Ogden TE, Ryan SJ. Subretinal endophotocoagulation: a model of subretinal neovascularization in the rabbit. Retina 1991;11: 244-9.

333. Thomas MA, Ibanez HE. Subretinal endophotocoagulation in the treatment of choroidal neovascularization. Am J Ophthalmol 1993;116: 279-85.

334. Baron S, Tyring SK, Fleischmann WR Jr, et al. The interferons: mechanisms of action and clinical applications. JAMA 1991;266:1375-83.

335. Spiegel RJ. Clinical overview of alpha interferon: studies and future directions. Cancer 1987;59:626.

336. Volberding PA, Mitsuyasu RT, Golando JP, Spiegel RJ. Treatment of Kaposi's sarcoma with interferon alfa-2b (Intron A). Cancer 1987;59 (suppl 3): 620.

337. de Wit R, Schattenkerk JK, Boucher CA, et al. Clinical and virological effects of high-dosage recombinant interferon-alpha in disseminated AIDS-related Kaposi's sarcoma. Lancet 1988;2:1214.

338. Brouty-Boye D, Zetter BR. Inhibition of cell motility by interferon. Science 1980;208:516-518.

339. White CW, Wolf SJ, Korones DN, et al. Treatment of childhood angiomatous disease with recombinant interferon alpha-2a. J Pediatr 1991;118:59-66.

340. Fung WE. Interferon alpha-2a for treatment of age-related macular degeneration. Am J Ophthalmol 1991;112:349-50.

341. Spiegel RJ. Dosage and toxicity. Alpha interferon: dosage, toxicity and antibody formation. In Silver HKB, (Ed): Interferons in Cancer Treatment: Biologic Activity and Clinical Toxicity of Interferons, Clinical Response to Systemic Interferons, Alternate Routes of Administration. Missiaugo, Ontario: MES Medical Education Services, 1986:17-27.

342. Thomas MA, Ibanez HE. Interferon alpha-2a in the treatment of subfoveal choroidal neovascularization. Am J Ophthalmol 1993;115:563-8.

343. Chan CK, Kempin SJ, Noble SK, Palmer GA. The treatment of choroidal neovascular membranes by alpha interferon. Ophthalmology 1994;101:289-300.

344. Pharmacological Therapy for Macular Degeneration Study Group. Interferon alfa-2a is ineffective for patients with choroidal neovascularization secondary to age-related macular degeneration. Arch Ophthalmol 1997;115:865-872.

345. Collen D, Stassen JM, Marafino BJ, et al. Biological properties of human tissue-type plasminogen activator obtained by expression of recombinant DNA in mammalian cells. J Pharmacol Exp Ther 1984;231:146-52.

346. Tiefenbaum AJ, Robison AK, Kurnik PB, et al. Clinical pharmacology in patients with evolving myocardial infarction of tissue-type plasminogen activator produced by recombinant DNA technology. Circulation 1985;71:110-6.

347. Thomas JW, Lopez PF, Lambert HM. Tissue plasminogen activator in the surgical excision of subfoveal choroidal neovascular membranes. Ophthalmic Surg 1995;26:374-6.

348. Lambert HM, Capone A Jr, Aaberg TM, et al. Surgical excision of subfoveal neovascular membranes in age-related macular degeneration. Am J Ophthalmol 1993;115:563-8.

349. Berger AS, Kaplan HJ. Clinical experience with the surgical removal of subfoveal choroidal neovascular membranes: short-term post-operative results. Ophthalmology 1992;99:969-76.

350. Ormerod LD, Puklin JE, Frank RN. Long-term outcomes after the surgical removal of advanced subfoveal neovascular membranes in age-related macular degeneration. Ophthalmology 1994;101:1201-10.

351. Connor TB, Wolf MD, Arrindel EL, Mieler WF. Surgical removal of an extra foveal fibrotic choroidal neovascular membrane with foveal serous detachment in age-related macular degeneration. Retina 1994;14:125-9.

352. Melberg NS, Thomas MA, Dickinson JD, Valluri S. Managing recurrent neovascularization after subfoveal surgery in presumed ocular histoplasmosis syndrome. Ophthalmology 1996;103:1064-7.

353. Gass JDM. Biomicroscopic and histopathologic considerations regarding the feasibility of surgical excision of subfoveal neovascular membranes. Am J Ophthalmol 1994;118:285-98.

354. Russell SR, Crapotta JA, Zerbolio DJ. Surgical removal of subfoveal neovascularization. Ophthalmology 1993;100:795-6. Letter.

355. Schachat AP. Should we recommend vitreous surgery for patients with choroidal neovascularization? Arch Ophthalmol 1994;112:459-61. Editorial.

356. Submacular Surgery Trials. Manual of Procedure, September 1995. Baltimore: Johns Hopkins, 1995.

357. Bennett SR, Folk JC, Blodi CF, Klugman M. Factors prognostic of visual outcome in patients with subretinal hemorrhages. Am J Ophthalmol 1990;109:33-7.

358. Wade EC, Flynn HW, Olsen KR, et al. Subretinal hemorrhage management by pars plana vitrectomy and internal drainage. Arch Ophthalmol 1990;108:973-8.

359. Lewis H. Management of submacular hemorrhage. In Lewis H, Ryan SJ, (Eds): Medical and Surgical Retina: Advances, Controversies, and Management. St. Louis: Mosby, 1994:54-62.

360. Campochiaro PA, Morgan KM, Conway BP, Stathos J. Spontaneous involution of subfoveal neovascularization. Am J Ophthalmol 1990;109:668-75.

361. Williams DF, Thomas MA. Vitrectomy for removal of submacular hemorrhage. In Ryan SJ, (Ed): Retina. 2nd edn; vol. 3. St. Louis: Mosby, 1994;2557-9.

362. El Baba F, Jarrett WH, Harbin TS, et al. Massive hemorrhage complicating age-related macular degeneration. Ophthalmology 1986;93:1581-92.

363. Glatt H, Machemer R. Experimental subretinal hemorrhage in rabbits. Am J Ophthalmol 1982;94:762-63.

364. Koshibu A. Ultrastructural studies on absorption of experimentally produced subretinal hemorrhage: III. Absorption of erythrocyte breakdown products and retinal hemosiderosis at the late stage. Nippon Ganka Gakkai Zasshi 1979;83:386-400.

365. Toth CA, Morse LS, Hjelmeland LM, Landers MB. Fibrin directs early retinal damage after experimental subretinal hemorrhage. Arch Ophthalmol 1991;109:1731-4.

366. Lewis H, Resnick SC, Flannery JG, Straasma BR. Tissue plasminogen activator treatment of experimental subretinal hemorrhage. Am J Ophthalmol 1991;111:197-204.

367. Johnson MW, Olsen KR, Hernandez E. Tissue plasminogen activator treatment of experimental subretinal hemorrhage. Retina 1991;11:250-8.

368. Benner JD, Morse LS, Toth CA, et al. Evaluation of a commercial recombinant tissue-type plasminogen activator preparation of the subretinal space of the cat. Arch Ophthalmol 1991;109:723-9.

369. Coll GE, Sparrow JR, Marinovic A, Chang S. Effects of intravitreal tissue plasminogen activator on experimental subretinal hemorrhage. Retina 1995;319-26.

370. Lincoff H, Madjarov B, Lincoff N, et al. Pathogenesis of the vitreous cloud emanating from subretinal hemorrhage. Arch Ophthalmol 2003;121:91-6.

371. Ito T, Nakano M, Yamamoto Y, et al. Hemoglobin-induced lipid peroxidation in the retina: a possible mechanism for macular degeneration. Arch Biochem Biophys 1995;316:864-72.

372. Terasaki H, Miyake Y, Kondo M, Tanikawa A. Focal macular electroretinogram before and after drainage of macular subretinal hemorrhage. Am J Ophthalmol 1997;123:207-11.

373. Lim JI. Subretinal hemorrhage. Int Ophthalmol Clin 1995;35:95-104.

374. Gillies A, Lahav M. Absorption of retinal and subretinal hemorrhages. Ann Ophthalmol 1983;15:1068-74.

375. Fekrat S, Avery RL, MacCumber M, Bressler NM. Natural history of subretinal hemorrhage in age-related macular degeneration (AMD). Invest Ophthalmol Vis Sci 1993;34(suppl):1133.

376. Avery RL, Fekrat S, Hawkins BS, Bressler NM. Natural history of subfoveal hemorrhage in age-related macular degeneration. Retina 1996;16:183-9.

377. Bennett SR, Folk JC, Blodi CF, Klugman M. Factors prognostic of visual outcome in patients with sub-retinal hemorrhage. Am J Ophthalmol 1990;109:33-7.

378. Scupola A, Coscas G, Soubrane G, Balestrazzi E. Natural history of macular degeneration. Ophthalmologica 1999;213:97-102.

379. Berrocal MH, Lewis ML, Flynn HW Jr. Variations in the clinical course of submacular hemorrhage. Am J Ophthalmol 1996;122:486-93.

380. Dellaporta A. Retinal damage from subretinal hemorrhage. Am J Ophthalmol 1983;95:568-70.

381. Hanscom TA, Diddie KR. Early surgical drainage of macular subretinal hemorrhage. Arch Ophthalmol 1987;105:1722-23.

382. Slusher MM. Evacuation of submacular hemorrhage: technique and timing. In Morris R, (Ed): Vitreoretinal surgery and technology. vol. 1. Thorofare: Slack, 1989:238.

383. Kramer M, Mimouni K, Priel E, et al. Comparison of fluorescein angiography and indocyanine angiography for imaging of choroidal neovascularization in hemorrhagic age-related macular degeneration. Am J Ophthalmol 2000; 129:495-500.

384. Hochman MA, Seery CM, Zarbin MA. Pathophysiology and management of subretinal hemorrhage. Surv Ophthalmol 1997;42:195-13.

385. Toth CA, Morse LS, Hjelmeland LM, Landers MB. Fibrin directs early retinal damage after experimental subretinal hemorrhage. Arch Ophthalmol 1999;109:723-9.

386. Krepler K, Kruger A, Tittl M, et al. Intravitreal injection of tissue plasminogen activator and gas in subretinal hemorrhage caused by age-related macular degeneration. Retina 2000;20:251-6.

387. Hattenbach LO, Klais C, Koch FH, Gumbel HO. Intravitreous injection of tissue plasminogen activator and gas in the treatment of submacular hemorrhage under various conditions. Ophthalmology 2001;108:1485-92.

388. Handwerger BA, Blodi BA, Chandra SR, et al. Treatment of submacular hemorrhage with low-dose intravitreal tissue plasminogen activator injection and pneumatic displacement. Arch Ophthalmol 2001;119:28-32.

389. Schulze SD, Hesse L. Tissue plasminogen activator plus gas injection in patients with subretinal hemorrhage caused by age-related macular degeneration: predictive variables for visual outcome. Graefe's Arch Clin Exp Ophthalmol 2002; 240:717-20.

390. Hesse L, Schroeder B, Heller G, Kroll P. Quantitative effect of intravitreally injected tissue plasminogen activator and gas on subretinal hemorrhage. Retina 2000;20:500 5.

391. Hassan AS, Johnson MW, Schneiderman TE, et al. Management of submacular hemorrhage with intravitreous tissue plasminogen activator injection and pneumatic displacement. Ophthalmology 1999;106:1900-6.

392. Ohji M, Saito Y, Hayashi A, et al. Pneumatic displacement of subretinal hemorrhage without tissue plasminogen activator. Arch Ophthalmol 1998;116:1326-32.

393. Olivier S, Chow DR, Packo KH, et al. Subretinal recombinant tissue plasminogen activator injection and pneumatic displacement of thick submacular hemorrhage in age-related macular degeneration. Ophthalmology 2004; 111:1201-8.

394. Haupert CL, McCuen BW. 2nd, Jaffe GJ, et al. Pars plana vitrectomy, subretinal injection of tissue plasminogen activator, and fluid-gas exchange for displacement of thick submacular hemorrhage in age-related macular degeneration. Am J Ophthalmol 2001;131:208-15.

395. Chaudhry NA, Mieler WF, Han DP, et al. Preoperative use of tissue plasminogen activator for large submacular hemorrhage. Ophthalmic Surg Lasers 1999;30:176-80.

396. Kamei M, Tano Y, Maeno T, et al. Surgical removal of submacular hemorrhage using tissue plasminogen activator and perfluorocarbon liquid. Am J Ophthalmol 1996; 121: 267-75.

397. Jonas JB, Jager M. Perfluorohexyloctane endotamponade for treatment of subfoveal hemorrhage. Eur J Ophthalmol 2002;12:534-6.

398. Matsuo T, Shiraga F, Takasu I. Planned two-step vitrectomy for extremely large and thick subretinal hematoma. Acta Ophthalmol Scand 2001;79:533-7.

399. Tilanus MA, Vaandrager W, Cuypers MH, et al. Relationship between anticoagulant medication and massive intraocular hemorrhage in age-related macular degeneration. Graefe's Arch Clin Exp Ophthalmol 2000;238:482-5.

400. Do DV, Bressler NM, Bressler SB. Large submacular hemorrhages after verteporfin therapy. Am J Ophthalmol 2004;137:558-60.

401. Axer-Siegel R, Ehrlich R, Rosenblatt I, et al. Bilateral macular hemorrhage after laser *in situ* keratomileusis. Graefe's Arch Clin Exp Ophthalmol 1999;237:611-3.

402. Kwok AK, Lai TY, Cheng AC, Lam DS. Central serous chorioretinopathy complicated by massive bilateral subretinal haemorrhage. Br J Ophthalmol 2000;84:936-7.

403. Kwok AK, Lai TY, Cheng AC, Lam DS. Massive subretinal haemorrhage associated with central serous chorioretinopathy. Eye 2001;15:121-3.

404. Shiraga F, Matsuo T, Yokoe S, et al. Surgical treatment of submacular hemorrhage associated with idiopathic polypoidal choroidal vasculopathy. Am J Ophthalmol 1999;128:147-54.

405. Morse LS, Chapman CB, Eliott D, et al. Subretinal hemorrhages in proliferative diabetic retinopathy. Retina 1997;17:87-93.

406. Chen SN, Ho CL, Kuo YH, Ho JD. Intravitreous tissue plasminogen activator injection and pneumatic displacement in the management of submacular hemorrhage complicating scleral buckling procedures. Retina 2001;21:460-3.

407. Sarrafizadeh R, Williams GA. Submacular hemorrhage during scleral buckling surgery treated with an intravitreal air bubble. Retina 2000;20:415-7.

408. Humayun M, Lewis H, Flynn HW Jr, et al. Management of submacular hemorrhage associated with retinal arterial macroaneurysms. Am J Ophthalmol 1998;126:358-61.

409. Kokame GT. Vitreous hemorrhage after intravitreal tissue plasminogen activator (t-PA) and pneumatic displacement of submacular hemorrhage. Am J Ophthalmol 2000;129: 546-7.

410. Vander JF, Federman JL, Greven CL, et al. Surgical removal of massive subretinal hemorrhage associated with age-related macular degeneration. Ophthalmology 1991;98:23-7.

411. Peyman GA, Nelson NC Jr, Alturki W, et al. Tissue plasminogen activating factor assisted removal of subretinal hemorrhage. Ophthalmic Surg 1991;22:575-82.

412. Lewis H. Intraoperative fibrinolysis of submacular hemorrhage with tissue plasminogen activator and surgical drainage. Am J Ophthalmol 1994;118:559-68.

413. Lim JI, Drews-Botsch C, Sternberg P Jr, et al. Submacular hemorrhage removal. Ophthalmology 1995;102:1393-9.

414. Ibanez HE, Williams DA, Thomas MA, et al. Surgical management of submacular hemorrhage: a series of 47 consecutive cases. Arch Ophthalmol 1995;113:62-9.

415. Kamei M, Tano Y, Maeno T, et al. Surgical removal of submacular hemorrhage using tissue plasminogen activator and perfluorocarbon liquid. Am J Ophthalmol 1996;121:267-75.

416. Capone A Jr, Sternberg P Jr. Advances in submacular surgery. Am J Ophthalmol 1994;118:659-63.

417. Sander B, Larsen M, Engler C, et al. Diabetic macular oedema: a comparison of vitreous fluorometry, angiography, and retinopathy. Br J Ophthalmol 2002;86:316-20.

418. Vinores SA, Derevjanik NL, Mahlow J, et al. Electron microscopic evidence for the mechanism of blood-retinal barrier breakdown in diabetic rabbits: comparison with magnetic resonance imaging. Pathol Res Pract 1998;194:497-505.

419. Early Treatment Diabetic Retinopathy Study Group. Early Treatment Diabetic Retinopathy Study Report number 1. Photocoagulation for diabetic macular edema. Arch Ophthalmol 1985;103:1796-1806.

420. Kremser BG, Kunze C, Troger J, et al. Grid pattern photocoagulation for diabetic macular edema: long term visual results. Ophthalmologica 1996;210:160-2.

421. The Central Vein Occlusion Study Group. Evaluation of grid pattern photocoagulation for macular edema in central vein occlusion. Ophthalmology 1995;102:1425-33.

422. Zimmerman PL. Pars planitis and other intermediate uveitis. In Yanoff M, Duker JS (Eds): Ophthalmology. St. Louis: Mosby 1999;10.1-10.6.

423. Dugel PU, Rao NA, Ozler S, et al. Pars plana vitrectomy for intraocular inflammation-related cystoid macular edema unresponsive to corticosteroids. Ophthalmology 1992;99:1535-41.

424. Hendrikse F, Yeo KT. Role of the vitreous body in diabetic retinopathy. Klin Monatsbl Augenheilkd 1993;203:319-23.

425. Stefansson E. The therapeutic effects of retinal laser treatment and vitrectomy: a theory based on oxygen and vascular physiology. Acta Ophthalmol Scand 2001;79:435-40.

426. Kadonosono K, Itoh N, Ohno S. Perifoveal microcirculation before and after vitrectomy for diabetic cystoid macular edema. Am J Ophthalmol 2000;130:740-4.

427. Joussen AM, Poulaki V, Qin W, et al. Retinal vascular endothelial growth factor induces intercellular adhesion molecule-1 and endothelial nitric oxide synthase expression and initiates early diabetic retinal leukocyte adhesion *in vivo*. Am J Pathol 2002;160:501-9.

428. Funatsu H, Yamashita H, Ikeda T, et al. Relation of diabetic macular edema to cytokines and posterior vitreous detachment. Am J Ophthalmol 2003;135:321-7.

429. Funatsu H, Yamashita H, Ikeda T, et al. Vitreous levels of interleukin-6 and vascular endothelial growth factor are related to diabetic macular edema. Ophthalmology 2003;110:1690-6.

430. Ikeda T, Sato K, Katano T, Hayashi Y. Attached posterior hyaloid membrane and the pathogenesis of honeycombed cystoid macular edema in patients with diabetes. Am J Ophthalmol 1999;127:478-9.

431. Nishihara H. Studies on the ultrastructure of the inner limiting membrane of the retina-distribution of anionic sites in the inner limiting membrane of the retina. Acta Soc Ophthalmol Jpn 1991;95:951-8.

432. Barber AJ, Antonetti DA, Gardner TW. Altered expression of retinal occludin and glial fibrillary acidic protein in experimental diabetes. Invest Ophthalmol Vis Sci 2000;41:3561-8.

433. De Vries C, Escobedo JA, Ueno H, et al. The fms-like tyrosine kinase, a receptor for vascular endothelial growth factor. Science 1992;255:989-91.

434. Sander B, Larsen M, Engler C, et al. Diabetic macular oedema: a comparison of vitreous fluorometry, angiography, and retinopathy. Br J Ophthalmol 2002;86:316-20.

435. Tolentino MJ, Miller JW, Gragoudas ES, et al. Intravitreous injections of vascular endothelial growth factor produce retinal ischemia and microangiopathy in an adult primate. Ophthalmology 1996;103:1820-8.

436. Vinores SA, Derevjanik NL, Mahlow J, et al. Electron microscopic evidence for the mechanism of blood-retinal barrier breakdown in diabetic rabbits: comparison with magnetic resonance imaging. Pathol Res Pract 1998;194:497-505.

437. Lewis H, Abrams GW, Blumenkranz MS, Campo RV. Vitrectomy for diabetic macular traction and edema associated with posterior hyaloidal traction. Ophthalmology 1992;99:753-9.

438. Harbour JW, Smiddy WE, Flynn HW Jr, Rubsamen PE. Vitrectomy for diabetic macular edema associated with a thickened and taut posterior hyaloid membrane. Am J Ophthalmol 1996;121:405-13.

439. Pendergast SD, Hassan TS, Williams GA, et al. Vitrectomy for diffuse diabetic macular edema associated with a taut premacular posterior hyaloid. Am J Ophthalmol 2000;130:178-86.

440. La Heij EC, Hendrikse F, Kessels AG, Derhaag PJ. Vitrectomy results in diabetic macular oedema without evident vitreomacular traction. Graefe's Arch Clin Exp Ophthalmol 2001;239:264-70.

441. Yamamoto T, Akabane N, Takeuchi S. Vitrectomy for diabetic macular edema: the role of posterior vitreous detachment and epimacular membrane. Am J Ophthalmol 2001;132:369-77.

442. Otani T, Kishi S. A controlled study of vitrectomy for diabetic macular edema. Am J Ophthalmol 2002;134:214-9.

443. Ikeda T, Sato K, Katano T, Hayashi Y. Vitrectomy for cystoid macular oedema with attached posterior hyaloid membrane in patients with diabetes. Br J Ophthalmol 1999;83:12-4.

444. Ikeda T, Sato K, Katano T, Hayashi Y. Improved visual acuity following pars plana vitrectomy for diabetic cystoid macular

edema and detached posterior hyaloid. Retina 2000;20:220-2.

445. Tachi N, Ogino N. Vitrectomy for diffuse macular edema in cases of diabetic retinopathy. Am J Ophthalmol 1996;122:258-60.

446. Saika S, Tanaka T, et al. Surgical posterior vitreous detachment combined with gas/air tamponade for treating macular edema associated with branch retinal vein occlusion: retinal tomography and visual outcome. Graefe's Arch Clin Exp Ophthalmol 2001;239:729-32.

447. Gandorfer A, Messmer EM, Ulbig MW, Kampik A. Resolution of diabetic macular edema after surgical removal of the posterior hyaloid and the inner limiting membrane. Retina 2000;20:126-33.

448. Stefaniotou M, Aspiotis M, Kalogeropoulos C, et al. Vitrectomy results for diffuse diabetic macular edema with and without inner limiting membrane removal. Eur J Ophthalmol 2004 ;14:137-43.

449. Radetzky S, Walter P, Fauser S, et al. Visual outcome of patients with macular edema after pars plana vitrectomy and indocyanine green-assisted peeling of the internal limiting membrane. Graefe's Arch Clin Exp Ophthalmol 2004;242:273-8.

450. Sakamoto T, Miyazaki M, Hisatomi T, et al. Triamcinolone-assisted pars plana vitrectomy improves the surgical procedures and decreases the postoperative blood-ocular barrier breakdown. Graefe's Arch Clin Exp Ophthalmol 2002;240:423-9.

451. Sonoda KH, Sakamoto T, Enaida H, et al. Residual vitreous cortex after surgical posterior vitreous separation visualized by intravitreous triamcinolone acetonide. Ophthalmology 2004;111:226-30.

452. Yang CM. Surgical treatment for severe diabetic macular edema with massive hard exudates. Retina 2000;20:121-5.

453. Takagi H, Otani A, Kiryu J, Ogura Y. New surgical approach for removing massive foveal hard exudates in diabetic macular edema. Ophthalmology 1999;106:249-56.

454. Takaya K, Suzuki Y, Mizutani H, et al. Long-term results of vitrectomy for removal of submacular hard exudates in patients with diabetic maculopathy. Retina 2004;24:23-9.

455. Kojima T, Terasaki H, Nomura H, et al. Vitrectomy for diabetic macular edema: effect of glycemic control [HbA(1c)], renal function (creatinine) and other local factors. Ophthalmic Res 2003;35:192-8.

456. Terasaki H, Kojima T, Niwa H, et al. Changes in focal macular electroretinograms and foveal thickness after vitrectomy for diabetic macular edema. Invest Ophthalmol Vis Sci 2003;44:4465-72.

457. Williams JG, Trese MT, Williams GA, Hartzer MK. Autologous plasmin enzyme in the surgical management of diabetic retinopathy. Ophthalmology 2001;108:1902-5.

458. Yamamoto T, Hitani K, Tsukahara I, et al. Early postoperative retinal thickness changes and complications after vitrectomy for diabetic macular edema. Am J Ophthalmol 2003;135:14-9.

459. Yoon KC, Seo MS. Macular hole after peeling of the internal limiting membrane in diabetic macular edema. Ophthalmic Surg Lasers Imaging 2003;34:478-9.

460. Giovannini A, Amato G, Mariotti C, Scassellati-Sforzolini B. Optical coherence tomography findings in diabetic macular edema before and after vitrectomy. Ophthalmic Surg Lasers 2000;31:187-91.

461. Otani T, Kishi S. Tomographic assessment of vitreous surgery for diabetic macular edema. Am J Ophthalmol 2000;129:487-94.

462. Massin P, Duguid G, Erginay A, et al. Optical coherence tomography for evaluating diabetic macular edema before and after vitrectomy. Am J Ophthalmol 2003;135:169-77.

463. Green WR, Enger C. Age-related macular degeneration histopathologic studies. The 1992 Lorenz E Zimmerman lecture. Ophthalmology 1993;100:1519-35.

464. Machemer R, Steinhorst UH. Retinal separation, retinotomy, and macular relocation II: a surgical approach for age-related macular degeneration. Graefe's Arch Clin Exp Ophthalmol 1993;231:635-41.

465. Ninomiya Y, Lewis JM, Hasegawa T, Tano Y. Retinotomy and foveal translocation for surgical management of subfoveal choroidal neovascular membranes. Am J Ophthalmol 1996;122:613-21.

466. Ohji M, Fujikado T, Saito Y, et al. Foveal translocation: a comparison of two techniques. Sem Ophthalmol 1988;13:52-61.

467. Fujikado T, Ohji M, Hayashi A, et al. Anatomic and functional recovery of the fovea after foveal translocation surgery without large retinotomy and simultaneous excision of a neovascular membrane. Am J Ophthalmol 1998;126:839-42.

468. Wolf S, Lappas A, Weinberger AWA, Kirchof B. Macular translocation for surgical management of subfoveal choroidal neovascularizations in patients with AMD: first results. Graefe's Arch Clin Exp Ophthalmol 1999;237:51-7.

469. Lewis H, Kaiser PK, Lewis S, Estafanous M. Macular translocation for subfoveal choroidal neovascularization in age-related macular degeneration: a prospective study. Am J Ophthalmol 1999;128:135-40.

470. Eckardt C, Eckardt U, Conrad HG. Macular rotation with and without counter-rotation of the globe in patients with age-related macular degeneration. Graefe's Arch Clin Exp Ophthalmol 1999;237:313-25.

471. Fujii GY, de Juan E, Thomas MA, et al. Limited macular translocation for the management of subfoveal retinal pigment epithelial loss following submacular surgery. Am J Ophthalmol (in press).

472. Imai K, Loewenstein A, de Juan E, Translocation of the retina for management of subfoveal choroidal neovascularization I: experimental studies in the rabbit eye. Am J Ophthalmol 1998;125:627-34.

473. de Juan E, Loewenstein A, Bressler NM, Alexander J. Translocation of the retina for management of subfoveal choroidal neovascularization II: a preliminary report in humans. Am J Ophthalmol 1998;125:635-46.

474. Machemer R, Steinhorst UH. Retinal separation, retinotomy, and macular relocation I: experimental studies in the rabbit eye. Graefe's Arch Clin Exp Ophthalmol 1993;231:629-34.

475. Imai K, de Juan E. Experimental surgical macular relocation by scleral shortening. ARVO abstracts. Invest Ophthalmol Vis Sci 1996;37 (suppl) S116.

476. Fujikado T, Ohji M, Saito Y, et al. Visual function after foveal translocation with scleral shortening in patients with myopic neovascular maculopathy. Am J Ophthalmol 1998;125:647-56.

477. Cekic O, Ohji M, Hayashi A, et al. Foveal translocation surgery in age-related macular degeneration. Lancet 1999;354:340.

478. Ng EW, Fujii GY, Au Eong KG, et al. Limited macular translocation for recurrent subfoveal choroidal neovascularization. ARVO abstracts. Invest Ophthalmol Vis Sci 2000;41 (suppl) S540.

479. Pieramici DJ, de Juan E, Fujii GY, et al. Limited inferior macular translocation for the treatment of subfoveal choroidal neovascularization secondary to age-related macular degeneration. Am J Ophthalmol 2000;130:419-28.

480. Toth CA. Full macular translocation surgery for AMD. 15th Biennial Eye Research Seminar, Los Angeles, California, September 26 to 29, 1999;30-1.

481. Seaber JH, Machemer R. Adaptation to monocular torsion after macular translocation. Graefe's Arch Clin Exp Ophthalmol 1997;235:76-81.

482. Akduman L, Karavellas MP, MacDonald CJ, et al. Macular translocation with retinotomy and retinal rotation for exudative age-related macular degeneration. Retina 1999;19:418-23.

483. Toth CA, Machemer R. Macular translocation. In Berger JW, Fine SL and Maguire MG (Eds): Age-related Macular Degeneration. Philadelphia: Mosby 1999;353-62.

484. Roider J, Hermann W, Kobuch K, et al. Ca++/Mg+ free solutions as an adjunct during 360-degree macular translocation surgery in AMD—clinical and experimental findings. ARVO abstracts. Invest Ophthalmol Vis Sci 2000;41 (suppl) S540.

485. Harlan JB, de Juan E, Bressler NM. Retinal translocation with unplanned translocation of the retinal pigment epithelium. The Wilmer Retina Update 1999;5:3-8.

486. Meyer CH, Benner JD, Winter KP, et al. Distance of movement with three different macular translocation techniques in humans (scleral outpouching, scleral imbrication, 360 retinotomy). ARVO abstracts. Invest Ophthalmol Vis Sci 2000;41 (suppl) S540.

487. de Juan E, Vander JF. Effective macular translocation without scleral imbrication. Am J Ophthalmol 1999;128:380-2.

488. Kamei M, Roth DB, Lewis H. Macular translocation using scleral clips to create an outpouching radial fold of the sclera, choroid and retinal pigment epithelium. ARVO abstracts. Invest Ophthalmol Vis Sci 2000;41 (suppl) S540.

489. Phillips SJ, Fujii GY, Pieramici DJ, et al. Persistent and recurrent neovascularization after successful macular translocation for subfoveal choroidal neovascularization of age-related macular degeneration. ARVO abstracts. Invest Ophthalmol Vis Sci 2000;41 suppl:S541.

490. Tso MOM, Friedman E. The retinal pigment epithelium I: comparative histology. Arch Ophthalmol 1967;78:641-9.

491. Yoneya S, Tso MOM. Angioarchitecture of the human choroid. Arch Ophthalmol 1987; 105:681-7.

492. American Academy of Ophthalmology. Macular translocation. Ophthalmology 2000;107:1015-8.

493. Peyman GA, Cheema R, Conway MD, Fang T. Triamcinolone acetonide as an aid to visualization of the vitreous and the posterior hyaloid during pars plana vitrectomy. Retina 2000;20:554-5.

494. Loewenstein A, Rader RS, Shelley TH, de Juan E. A flexible infusion micro-cannula for subretinal surgery. Ophthalmic Surg Lasers 1997;28:774-5.

495. Kubota A, Harino S, Ohji M, Tano Y. Modified technique to create a retinal detachment during macular translocation surgery. Am J Ophthalmol 2003;135:105-6.

496. Ohji M, Tano Y, Scheller GD, Chang S. New soft-tipped instruments for foveal translocation surgery with 360-degree retinotomy. Arch Ophthalmol 2000;118:1422-4.

497. Ohji M, Fujikado T, Kusaka S, et al. Comparison of three techniques of foveal translocation in patients with subfoveal choroidal neovascularization due to age-related macular degeneration. Am J Ophthalmol 2001;132:888-96.

498. Wolf S, Lappas A, Weinberger AWA, Kirchhof B. Macular translocation for surgical management of subfoveal choroidal neovascularization in patients with AMD: first results. Graefe's Arch Clin Exp Ophthalmol 1999;237:51-7.

499. Okita K, Ogino N, Saitou Y, et al. Macular translocation with 360-degree retinotomy for age-related macular degeneration. Atarashii Ganka (Journal of the Eye) 2001;18:1217-20.

500. Toth CA, Freedman SF. Macular translocation with 360-degree peripheral retinectomy impact of technique and surgical experience on visual outcomes. Retina 2001;21:293-303.

501. Terasaki H, Miyake Y, Suzuki T, et al. Change in full-field ERGs after macular translocation surgery with 360° retinotomy. Invest Ophthalmol Vis Sci 2002;43:452-7.

502. Aisenbrey S, Lafaut BA, Szurman P, et al. Macular translocation with 360 degrees retinotomy for exudative age-related macular degeneration. Arch Ophthalmol 2002;120:451-9.

503. Pertile G, Claes C. Macular translocation with 360 degree retinotomy for management of age-related macular degeneration with subfoveal choroidal neovascularization. Am J Ophthalmol 2002;134:560-5.

504. Abdel-Meguid A, Lappas A, Hartmann K, et al. One year follow up of macular translocation with 360 degree retinotomy in patients with age related macular degeneration. Br J Ophthalmol 2003;87:615-21.

505. Tano Y. Edward Jackson Memorial Lecture Pathologic myopia-Where are we now? Am J Ophthalmol 2002; 134:645-60.

506. Lai JC, Lapolice DJ, Stinnett SS, et al. Visual outcomes following macular translocation with 360 degrees peripheral retinectomy. Arch Ophthalmol 2002;120:1317-24.

507. Fujikado T, Asonuma S, Ohji M, et al. Reading ability after macular translocation surgery with 360-degree retinotomy. Am J Ophthalmol 2002;134:849-56.

508. Kubota A, Ohji M, Kusaka S, et al. Evaluation of the peripheral visual field after foveal translocation. Am J Ophthalmol 2001;132:581-4.

509. Luke C, Aisenbrey S, Luke M, et al. Electrophysiological changes after 360 degrees retinotomy and macular translocation for subfoveal choroidal neovascularization in age related macular degeneration. Br J Ophthalmol 2001; 85:928-32.

510. Terasaki H, Ishikawa K, Niwa Y, et al. Changes in focal macular ERGs after macular translocation surgery with 360 degrees retinotomy. Invest Ophthalmol Vis Sci 2004;45:567-73.

511. Luke C, Alteheld N, Aisenbrey S, et al. Electro-oculographic findings after 360 degrees retinotomy and macular translocation for subfoveal choroidal neovascularization in age-related macular degeneration. Graefe's Arch Clin Exp Ophthalmol 2003;241:710-5.

512. Freedman SF, Holgado S, Enyedi LB, Toth CA. Management of ocular torsion and diplopia after macular translocation for age-related macular degeneration: prospective clinical study. Am J Ophthalmol 2003;136: 640-8.

513. Freedman SF, Rojas M, Toth CA. Strabismus surgery for large-angle cyclotorsion after macular translocation surgery. J AAPOS 2002;6:154-62.

514. Sato M, Terasaki H, Ogino N, et al. Strabological findings after macular translocation surgery with 360 degrees retinotomy. Invest Ophthalmol Vis Sci 2003;44:1939-44.

515. Bando H, Ikuno Y, Choi JS, et al. Ultrastructure of internal limiting membrane in myopic foveoschisis. Am J Ophthalmol 2005;139:197-9.

516. Ikuno Y, Sayanagi K, Ohji M, et al. Vitrectomy and internal limiting membrane peeling for myopic foveoschisis. Am J Ophthalmol 2004;137:719-24.

517. Kwok AK, Lai TY, Yip WW. Vitrectomy and gas tamponade without internal limiting membrane peeling for myopic foveoschisis. Br J Ophthalmol 2005;89:1180-3.

518. Ikuno Y, Gomi F, Tano Y. Potent retinal arteriolar traction as a possible cause of myopic foveoschisis. Am J Ophthalmol 2005;139:462-7.

519. Sayanagi K, Ikuno Y, Gomi F, Tano Y. Retinal vascular microfolds in highly myopic eyes. Am J Ophthalmol 2005; 139:658-63.

520. Sayanagi K, Ikuno Y, Tano Y. Reoperation for persistent myopic foveoschisis after primary vitrectomy. Am J Ophthalmol 2006;14:414-7.

521. Ikuno Y, Tano Y. Vitrectomy for macular holes associated with myopic foveoschisis. Am J Ophthalmol 2006;141: 774-6.

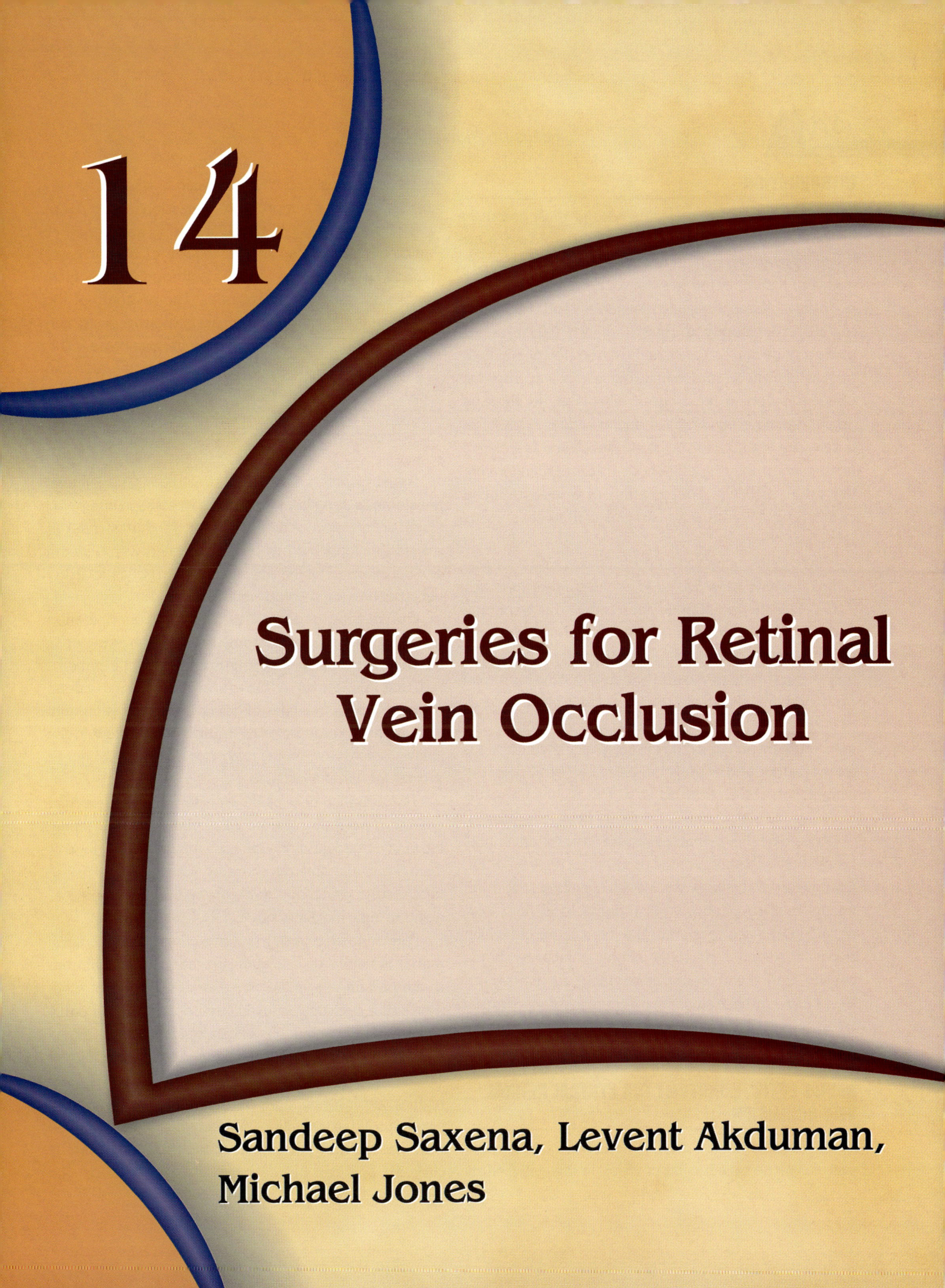

14

Surgeries for Retinal Vein Occlusion

Sandeep Saxena, Levent Akduman, Michael Jones

INTRODUCTION

Retinal vein occlusions are the second most common vision threatening retinal vascular disorders. Our therapeutic armamentarium for functional improvement was very limited in the past for all types of retinal vein occlusions. Also pathogenic mechanism and risk factors are not completely understood yet. Argon-laser-photocoagulation can prevent the development and treat neovascularization successfully, but is unable to improve visual function in most cases. Thrombolytic therapy applied systemically is limited due to serious side effects but may be helpful when injected intraocularly. Isovolemic hemodilution may be efficacious in central retinal vein occlusion (CRVO). The creation of a laser-induced chorioretinal venous anastomosis showed serious complications.

Since 1999, numerous reports on successful surgical techniques have been published. A new surgical approach in CRVO is the radial optic neurotomy. This technique was primarily performed under the hypothesis of decompression of the central vein by cutting the scleral ring. Meanwhile there is some evidence that the formation of chorioretinal shunts may be the decisive factor in cases of successfully performed radial optic neurotomy. Due to inconsistent and rare data this surgical procedure needs further evaluation. Another surgical option is the cannulation of the occluded vein. This technique seems to be feasible but the clinical results still have to be proved.

It could be shown that the dissection of the adventitial sheath with separation of the artery from the vein at the arteriovenous crossing where branch retinal vein occlusion occurs may re-establish the retinal blood flow with reduction of macular edema. But it is still unclear which step of the surgery (vitrectomy, internal limiting membrane peeling, and sheathotomy) is causative for the results. Despite several uncertainties and open questions, surgical techniques are likely to overcome the desolate therapeutic situation for retinal vein occlusion of the past.[1]

RADIAL OPTIC NEUROTOMY FOR CENTRAL RETINAL VEIN OCCLUSION

Central retinal vein occlusion is the second most common vascular cause of reduction of vision in the eye. Central retinal vein occlusion can be associated with severe irreversible visual loss with improvement of vision in only 20%.[2]

The pathogenesis of CRVO is poorly understood.[3,4] Pathological evidence suggests the site of obstruction is situated at the lamina cribrosa, although histological samples of early CRVO are rare.[5] The anatomy of the normal central retinal vein appears to show a constriction of the vein as it passes through the lamina cribrosa.[6] This may predispose the vein to occlusion, thereby reducing its retinal blood flow.[7] Secondary ischemia of the retina occurs from the stasis of blood flow in the capillaries caused by back pressure from the occluded venous system.

As yet there is no established treatment. Chorioretinal anastomosis using laser has been successful in improving vision in the non-ischemic variant of the disorder in selected patients but has been associated with frequent complications.[8] This therapy is not used in ischemic CRVO because of a high complication rate.

Opremcak and associates[9] described an operation involving pars plana vitrectomy and incision of the optic nerve on the nasal side (neurotomy) in 11 patients resulting in improvement in vision in eight eyes with an average gain of five lines of Snellen acuity. It is thought that the neurotomy helps to improve blood flow in the central retinal vein by relieving pressure on the vein as it exits the lamina cribrosa.[10]

Theoretically, pars plana vitrectomy and intraocular gas injection may increase oxygenation to the retina. However, removal of the vitreous may allow angiogenic factors into the anterior chamber increasing the risk of neovascular glaucoma; therefore, panretinal photocoagulation may be required.[11]

Pars plana vitrectomy may have beneficial effects upon retinal ischemia by allowing circulation in the vitreous cavity of fluid oxygenated by unaffected retina or other sites in the eye such as the ciliary body. This may partly explain the advantageous effects of early vitrectomy on diabetic retinopathy. Using the principles of Fick's diffusion equation it has been speculated that the insertion of a high molecular weight gas into the vitreous cavity might also improve oxygenation. At least 95% of ocular blood flow passes through ciliary circulation primarily the choroid. This can be regarded as a source of oxygen divided from the vitreous cavity by a semi permeable membrane—that is, the retina. The perfluoropropane gas draws oxygen and other small molecular weight gases through the retina into the vitreous cavity in an active equilibrium. Hopefully the oxygen can be utilized by the ischemic retinal tissues. Gradually the perfluoropropane gas is lost over a period of 2 months. Theoretically, this may reduce neovascular complications over the crucial early period of the CRVO natural history.[12]

Many CRVO patients gradually develop capillary non-perfusion up to 3 months after onset with iris neovascularization usually occurring in the first 6 months. Iris neovascularization occurs in 45 to 80% of patients with ischemic CRVO.[10] There was a risk that pars plana vitrectomy would allow release of angiogenic factors into the anterior chamber causing severe neovascular glaucoma. Hence pan retinal photocoagulation may be beneficial. The number of burns given is much less than the dosage applied in the CRVO study. This strategy was successful in reversing the neovascularization.[11]

The mechanism of action of the neurotomy is uncertain. The intention is to decompress the central retinal vein in the nerve. However, eyes with neurotomy have evidence of the formation of blood vessels in the neurotomy site. Perhaps these represent a chorioretinal anastomosis aiding venous drainage from the retina. However, one will need to examine the effect of pars plana vitrectomy in these patients before they attribute changes to the neurotomy.[11]

SURGICAL TECHNIQUE

Rationale behind this surgical technique is to decompress the vein near the lamina cribrosa. A special neurotomy knife has been designed to incise the scleral ring nasally. After a routine 3-port pars plana vitrectomy, the knife is inserted radial to the ring and the scleral fibers are cut. Thus the injury to the nerve fibers is minimized and the papillomacular bundle is avoided. Reports of successful results have varied. Improvement is indicated by disappearance of hemorrhages and edema rapidly (Figure 14.1A and B).

Most of the studies on radial optic neurotomy have not defined the depth of the incision. Complications following a deeper incision have been described. Wrede and associates [13] performed a histological study to evaluate the required depth for radial optic neurotomy. Serial sections of the area of the optic nerve head were performed in 19 eye bank eyes. The distance between the inner surface of the optic disk and the outer limit of the cribriform plate was measured. Ten additional eye bank eyes underwent 2 mm deep experimental radial optic neurotomy using the Spaide CRVO Knife (DORC, Netherlands). The cutting depth was assessed histologically by serial cuts. The distance between the inner surface

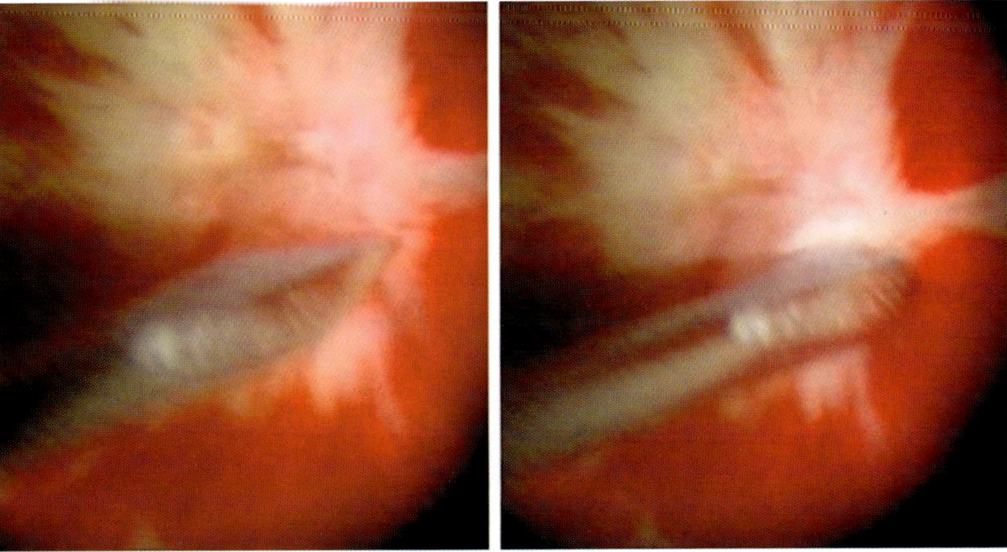

FIGURES 14.1A and B: Radial optic neurotomy (Manish Nagpal, MS, India)

of the disk and the outer limit of the cribriform plate measured 1.35+/–0.3 mm (shrinkage-revised value: 1.45 mm). The experimental radial optic neurotomy showed cutting depths of 1.53+/–0.3 mm (shrinkage-revised value: 1.65 mm). Based on normal eyes, a cutting depth of 1.45 mm is sufficient to cut through the cribriform plate. This might change during central retinal vein occlusion because possible papillary edema due to central retinal vein occlusion has to be considered. Even under controlled experimental conditions radial optic neurotomy leads to great variation in incision depths. The development of a knife with a fixed penetration depth would be helpful.

PATHOANATOMY

Radial optic neurotomy remains a controversial method of treatment for central retinal vein occlusion. Histopathologic changes in the porcine eye without retinal vein occlusion after radial optic neurotomy have been studied. Radial optic neurotomy was performed in 14 normal eyes of 12 Yorkshire Cross pigs. One radial stab incision at the edge of the nasal optic nerve head was made using a 20-gauge microvitreoretinal blade (Visitec) while the intraocular pressure was elevated. Surgery was concluded when hemostasis was achieved. Weekly ophthalmoscopic examinations were performed. Group 1 eyes (4 eyes of 2 pigs) were enucleated at the end of surgery. Group 2 eyes (4 eyes of 4 pigs) were enucleated 1 week postoperatively, and group 3 eyes (4 eyes of 4 pigs) were enucleated 3 weeks postoperatively. In group 4 (2 eyes of 2 pigs), animals underwent vitrectomy and radial optic neurotomy, and eyes were enucleated 3 weeks postoperatively. Ophthalmoscopic examination demonstrated engorged blood vessels at the radial optic neurotomy site up to 3 weeks after surgery with minimal or no hemorrhage. Histological examination of the optic nerve demonstrated foci of hemorrhage, interstitial edema, reactive gliosis, and rare inflammatory cells. At 3 weeks, there was complete axonal nerve fiber loss distal to the neurotomy site. After radial optic neurotomy, marked gliosis and complete axonal nerve fiber loss occur at the neurotomy site. Although bleeding was rare intraoperatively in this porcine model, hemorrhage and interstitial edema were present within the optic nerve at the neurotomy site histologically.[14] Another study demonstrated the fundus and histopathological changes in the normal miniature pig eye after radial optic neurotomy. The retina radial to the site of radial optic neurotomy darkened gradually with the increasing curvature of the major retinal arteries. The filling time intervals from the retinal artery to the retinal vein were prolonged. At the incision site, there was a loss of nerve fibers, which were subsequently replaced by collagenous tissue. No anastomotic vessels formed by the end of the study. Postoperatively, the retinal circulation seemed somewhat sluggish compared with that seen preoperatively. Segmental retinal nerve atrophy eventually formed. The study postulated that the procedure itself may not be the sole factor for the formation of shunt vessels.[15]

Histopathologic evidence demonstrated displaced fragments of Bruch's membrane surrounded by retinal tissue at the nasal side of the papilla. A discrete scar was noted at this site that reached the cribriform plate without involving the adjacent sclera or the retinal vessels. The optic nerve showed advanced atrophy with a small temporal sector of viable nerve fibers. Histopathologic findings after radial optic neurotomy do not provide evidence for the postulated mechanism of action.[16]

RESULTS

Radial optic neurotomy is designed to release proposed pressure within the scleral canal. Opremcak and associates[9] performed pars plana vitrectomy with radial optic neurotomy on 11 consecutive patients with severe, hemorrhagic CRVO with visual acuities of 20/400 or less. There were no complications noted with this procedure. All patients had clinical improvement as determined by fundus examination, photography, and fluorescein angiography. Postoperative visual acuities were equal or improved in 82% of patients. Eight of the patients (73%) had rapid improvement of visual acuity with an average gain of five lines of vision. Surgical decompression of CRVO via radial optic neurotomy was found to be technically feasible and initially safe procedure that is associated with rapid reperfusion of the retina.

Opremcak and associates[17] subsequently performed pars plana vitrectomy with RON was performed on 117 consecutive patients with CRVO and severe loss of vision (defined as 20/200 or worse). No serious complications noted with this procedure. Anatomical and clinical improvement as determined by fundus examination, fundus photography, and fluorescein angiography was found in 95% of patients. Snellen visual acuity improved by an average of 2.5 lines in 71% of patients. Two or more lines were gained in 53% of patients, and > or = 4 lines were gained in 25%. Anterior segment neovascularization was found in 6% of patients with CRVO.

Opremcak and associates[18] performed radial optic neurotomy with simultaneous, adjunctive intraoperative triamcinolone in patients with CRVO to ascertain any anatomic or visual benefit of this combined approach on 63 consecutive patients with CRVO and visual acuity of 20/200 or worse. At the end of the case, 4 mg of triamcinolone was injected into the vitreous cavity. Clinical improvement as determined by fundus examination, photography, and fluorescein angiography was noted in 93% of patients. Snellen visual acuity improved by an average of three lines in 68% of all patients. Two or more lines were gained in 44% of patients and four or more lines were gained in 20% of patients. Anterior segment neovascularization developed in 7% of patients. Persistent cystoid macular edema was noted in 17%. These outcomes were similar to patients undergoing radial optic neurotomy alone without triamcinolone. Elevated intraocular pressure was noted in 25% of patients and one patient developed endophthalmitis. Clinical resolution of the CRVO and improved visual function noted in combined procedure paralleled outcomes following radial optic neurotomy alone. Radial optic neurotomy with triamcinolone was associated with a higher incidence of elevated intraocular pressure and endophthalmitis.

Williamson and associates[19] treated eight eyes with ischemic CRVO with pars plana vitrectomy, mild panretinal photocoagulation, and intraocular perfluoropropane gas injection. Radial optic neurotomy was performed in four eyes. No patients suffered from neovascular glaucoma. Visual recovery was seen in patients with and without neurotomy. Fundus photography demonstrated reduced engorgement of retinal veins in two of the patients with neurotomy and one with vitrectomy alone. Optical coherence tomography demonstrated macular edema in three patients with neurotomy and all patients with vitrectomy alone. Segmental visual field loss was seen in one patient with neurotomy suggesting damage to the optic nerve head. Pars plana vitrectomy was found to be safe in ischemic CRVO. Combined with mild pan retinal photocoagulation and intraocular gas injection the risk of neovascular glaucoma was low. Neurotomy can be added to try to improve the chances of recovery of central vision but may cause additional peripheral visual field loss.

Weizer and associates[20] reviewed initial experience with radial optic neurotomy as treatment for retinal vein occlusion. Mean preoperative visual acuity was 4/200. Preoperatively, the vein occlusion was perfused in one (20%), nonperfused in one (20%), and indeterminate in three (60%). Mean postoperative visual acuity was 20/400 at last follow-up. Four patients (80%) had improvement in visual acuity and one (20%) worsened. Two patients (40%) improved to 20/80 postoperatively. In four cases (80%), disk congestion improved and intraretinal hemorrhage reabsorbed more quickly than would be expected without treatment. Time to the venous phase of fluorescein angiography improved slightly in three cases (60%) postoperatively. Perfusion status as determined by fluorescein angiography was not significantly altered postoperatively. One patient (20%) had resolution of macular edema postoperatively as shown by volumetric optical coherence tomography. One patient developed choroidovitreal neovascularization and one developed iris neovascularization postoperatively, both of which responded to panretinal photocoagulation. Le Rouic and associates[21] reported the results of radial optic neurotomy in 10 eyes. Mean visual acuity on an ETDRS chart increased from 30+/–12 points preoperatively to 42+/–15 points at the 3-month visit, and mean macular thickness decreased from 580+/–150 micro m to 361+/–52 microns. Mean visual acuity of the five patients followed-up for 6 months was 52.8+/

–20 points. No visual loss was observed. None of the patients underwent laser photocoagulation or has presented with neovascularization. Optociliary veins developed in three eyes and a retinochoroidal anastomosis within the disk incision was observed in two eyes. Their preliminary results were encouraging when compared to the reported natural progression of severe central retinal vein occlusion. A bypass of the site of occlusion is a possible mechanism for radial optic neurotomy.

Furino and associates[22] evaluated the efficacy of radial optic neurotomy, internal limiting membrane peeling, and intravitreal triamcinolone acetonide for central retinal vein occlusion in eight eyes. After 5 months, best-corrected visual acuity significantly improved, intraocular pressure was well controlled, and fluorescein angiography showed perfused state and reduction of the number of retinal hemorrhages in all eyes. Optical coherence tomography revealed significant reduction of macular thickness. Bleeding in the neurotomy site occurred in 3 cases.

Zambarkakji and associates[23] observed an improvement in visual acuity score and a corresponding reduction in foveal thickness and macular volume following radial optic neurotomy, but macular edema persisted in 60% of patients. Nagpal and associates[24] found radial optic neurotomy to be better than the natural course in eyes with CRVO, with vision < 6/60. Martinez-Jardon and associates[25] did not find improvement in visual function (by multifocal ERG) or visual acuity although macular thickness did improve after radial optic neurotomy. This technique may be associated with potential risks. Randomized studies are needed to corroborate these results. Lerche and Richard[26] found radial optic neurotomy to be a safe and feasible procedure. The results indicated the potential to improve visual acuity while typical complications due to surgery or vein occlusion did not occur during the first three months. Patelli and associates[27] reported that optical coherence tomography demonstrated resolution of the macular edema in all the treated eyes, however, this resolution was not always accompanied with an improvement in visual acuity.

Garcia-Arumi and associates[28] evaluated the incidence of chorioretinal anastomosis after radial optic neurotomy and to determine its effect on visual acuity and foveal thickness in 14 patients with central retinal vein occlusion. Eight patients (57.1%) gained 1 or more lines of visual acuity while the visual acuity of 6 patients (42.9%) improved by 2 or more lines (mean visual acuity, 20/80) (mean visual acuity gain, 3 lines). The decrease in macular thickness was statistically significant (median, 282 microns). Retinochoroidal shunts developed in 6 eyes (42.9%) at the site of the radial optic neurotomy. Improvement in visual acuity and a decrease in foveal thickness were observed on optical coherence tomography. Improvement may occur because of optic nerve decompression, vitrectomy, and by inducing new chorioretinal shunts that drain retinal circulation to the choroid and accelerate resolution of retinal edema.

Spaide and associates[29] evaluated six patients who had undergone radial optic neurotomy for central retinal vein occlusion for the presence of retinal choroidal collateral circulation and to correlate these collaterals with changes in macular thickness during follow-up. The mean time from onset of the central retinal vein occlusion to the radial optic neurotomy was 2.3 months. One patient had no collateral vessels, three patients had significant collaterals, and two patients had moderate-caliber collaterals. The mean central macular thickness preoperatively was 1,021 microns and the mean central macular thickness postoperatively was 733 microns. The change in macular thickness was highly correlated with the degree of development of collaterals from the retinal to the choroidal circulation. Although all patients had a radial optic neurotomy a significant determinant in reduction of macular edema was the presence of retinal-choroidal collateral circulation. This suggests that there may be additional mechanisms, other than simple release of alleged pressure in the scleral canal, for any observed effects from radial optic neurotomy.

Nomoto and associates[30] evaluated the effects of radial optic neurotomy on retinal circulation in 15 eyes with CRVO by indocyanine green (ICG) videoangiography and a computer-assisted image analysis. Within 72 hours before the surgery and at 3 months after the surgery, ICG videoangiography was performed with a scanning laser ophthalmoscope, and the images were transferred to a computer. Two measurement points were selected, one on a main retinal artery close to the optic disk and the other on the corresponding retinal vein. At each point, fluorescence intensities were serially measured, and dye dilution curves were obtained. Retinal circulation times (DeltaT(50)) before and after the surgery were calculated. Mean preoperative DeltaT(50) was 6.46 +/–1.36 seconds, and mean postoperative DeltaT(50) was 6.80 +/–2.50 seconds. In 8 of 15 eyes, T(50) decreased by 6.8% to 29.6% after the surgery. In the seven eyes that developed chorioretinal anastomosis at the site of RON, DeltaT(50) decreased after the surgery. In contrast, DeltaT(50) decreased postoperatively in only one of the eight eyes without chorioretinal anastomosis. Best-corrected visual acuity improved significantly after the surgery in the group of eyes with improvement in DeltaT(50), but not in the group of eyes without improvement in DeltaT(50). Some degree of retinal circulation improvement occurred in approximately half of these eyes, which appears to be correlated with the development of chorioretinal anastomosis.

Horio and associates[31] calculated retinal blood flow from dye dilution curves of videofluorescein angiograms in seven eyes which underwent radial optic neurotomy. At 1 week after surgery, the retinal blood flow was significantly reduced. At 6 months after surgery, the retinal blood flow was not significantly different from the preoperative retinal blood flow, although chorioretinal anastomoses were found in all seven eyes. The foveal thickness was significantly decreased. The postoperative visual acuity was better than the preoperative visual acuity by two or more lines in three out of seven eyes, and was worse in two eyes. Neither radial optic neurotomy nor chorioretinal anastomoses improved the retinal blood flow but macular edema was improved. These findings suggested that removal of the vitreous could reduce macular edema as in diabetic macular edema. However, the possibility that the changes represent the natural course of this disease could not be excluded.

Horio and associates[32] in another study demonstrated that a further reduction of retinal blood flow can occur after radial optic neurotomy, and blood flow in the chorioretinal anastomoses may be insufficient to prevent the event.

Chalam and Shah [33] found that radial optic neurotomy resulted in rapid improvement in visual acuity, central fixation, and macular scotoma as measured by a liquid crystal display microperimeter.

Mennel and associates[34] performed radial optic neurotomy in combined cilioretinal artery and central retinal vein occlusion.

Result of radial optic optic neurotomy is shown in Figures 14.2 and 14.3.

COMPLICATIONS

Patients undergoing radial optic neurotomy should be closely observed to minimize the risk of complication. Chorioretinal neovascularization through the radial cut of the optic disk after radial optic neurotomy may occur.[35,36] Choroidovitreal neovascularization may also occur.[20]

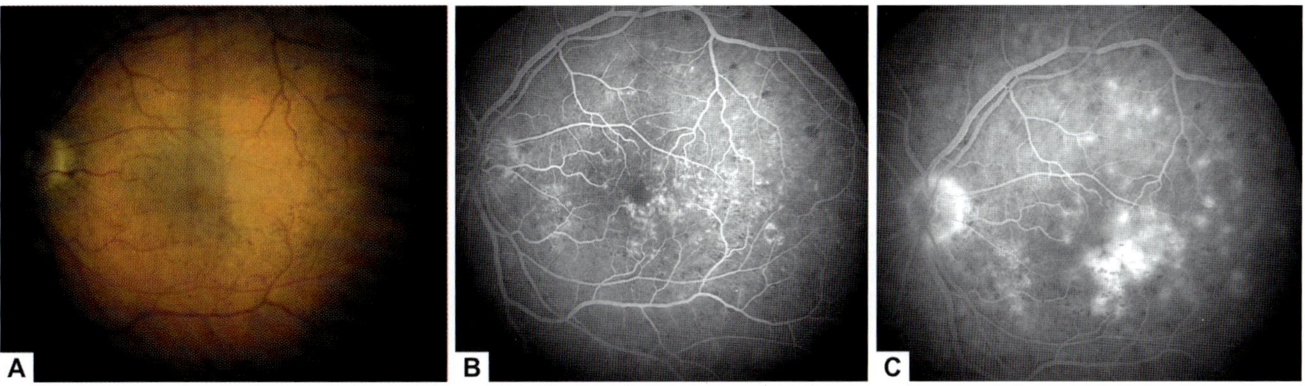

FIGURES 14.2A to C: Radial optic neurotomy: Pre-treatment

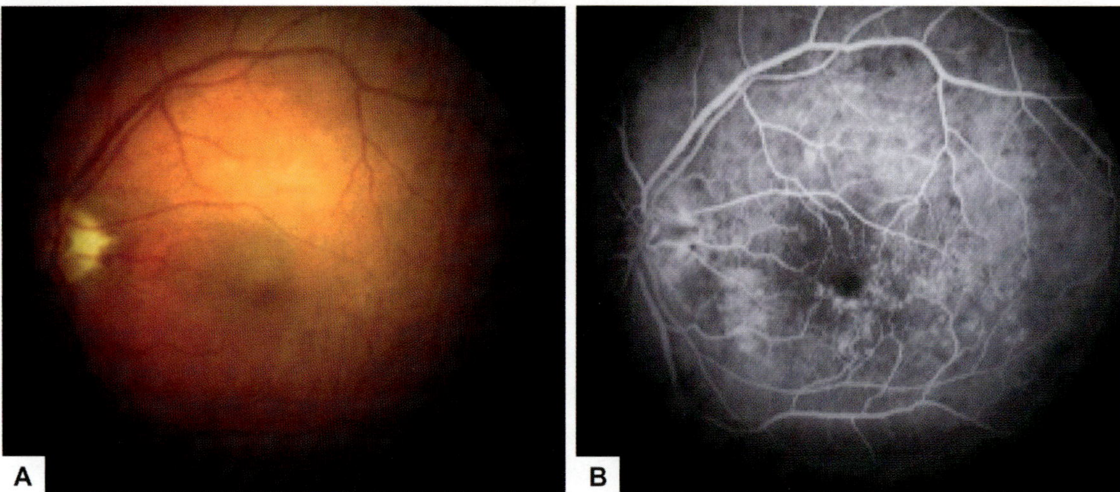

FIGURES 14.3A and B: Radial optic neurotomy: Post-treatment

Incising the optic nerve to create the neurotomy has risks. Bleeding may occur from the neurotomy site.[22,37,38] Peroperative bleed from the incision can be easily controlled by elevation of the intraocular pressure which indicates damage to the vasculature around the optic nerve. Infusion of liquid perfluoro-carbon seems to be effective to arrest arterial bleeding from the radial optic neurotomy site.[38] Central retinal artery occlusion has also been reported after radial optic neurotomy.[39]

Peripapillary retinal detachment may also follow radial optic neurotomy.[40] While performing vitrectomy for CRVO, the induction of posterior vitreous detachment may deroof a foveal cyst in the highly edematous macula to form a macular hole. A small macular hole, however, may close spontaneously without further intervention.[41]

Visual field loss after radial optic neurotomy for the treatment of CRVO is a frequent complication.[42-44] Postoperatively, sectoral visual field loss arising from the optic head has been found by Goldmann perimetry, and a thin nerve fiber bundle defect has also been noted. Microperimetry demonstrated an absolute nerve fiber bundle defect arising from the radial cut at the optic disk. A postoperative defect in the temporal visual field consistent with the incision to the optic disk has also been reported in another study. However, this visual field defect appears to be well tolerated by most patients.[44] The etiology of this visual loss appears to be a combination of mechanical trauma to the nerve fiber layers and ischemia of the optic disk circulation.[42]

SHEATHOTOMY FOR BRANCH RETINAL VEIN OCCLUSION

Branch retinal vein occlusion (BRVO) is a significant cause of visual loss attributed to retinal vascular disease and is second only to diabetic retinopathy. Branch retinal vein occlusion nearly always occurs at an arteriovenous crossing because of compression of the vein by the artery, resulting in hemodynamic abnormalities in the vein, including thrombus formation, reversal of flow toward the artery, and arteriovenous collateral formation. Relatively little information is available on the natural history of BRVO; most of what exists is derived from clinical trials, including the Branch Vein Occlusion Study. Current treatment options focus on treating sequelae of the occluded venous branch, such as macular edema, retinal neovascularization, vitreous hemorrhage, and traction retinal detachment.

Mechanical narrowing of the venous lumen at these intersections is thought to play a pathoetiologic role in BRVO. A novel therapeutic approach is decompression of the arteriovenous crossing, which has had promising initial results including restoration of vision and reversal of hemodynamic abnormalities. A prospective, controlled, clinical trial is being organized to determine the role of arteriovenous sheathotomy in the treatment of BRVO.[45]

SURGICAL TECHNIQUE

3 port pars plana vitrectomy is done including induction of posterior vitreous detachment if need be. Sheathotomy knife is used to incise the common adventitious sheath between the artery and the vein at the crossing involved in the occlusive process (Figure 14.4). The site of occlusion is identified from the clinical picture and the fluorescein angiography. Peeling of the internal limiting membrane and intravitreal triamcinolone are optional steps in the surgical procedure.

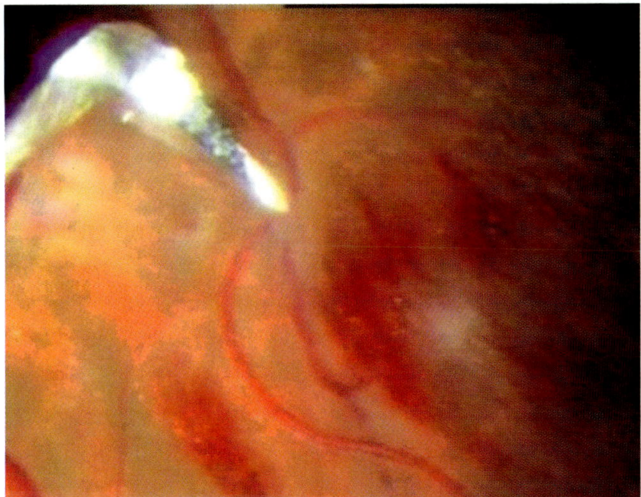

FIGURE 14.4: Sheathotomy at arteriovenous crossing (Manish Nagpal, MS, India)

RESULTS

Opremcak and Bruce[46] performed surgical decompression of BRVO via arteriovenous crossing sheathotomy in 15 patients with decreased visual acuity due to macular hemorrhage, edema, and ischemia. Reperfusion of the retina was achieved by surgically separating the overlying retinal arteriole from the venule via vitrectomy and adventitial sheathotomy techniques. All patients showed clinical improvement. Postoperative visual acuities were equal or improved in 80% of patients. Ten of the 15 subjects (67%) had improved visual acuity with an average gain of four lines of vision. Surgical decompression of BRVO via sheathotomy is a technically feasible procedure that can result in rapid reperfusion of the retina.

Shah and associates[47] reported on five eyes with best-corrected visual acuity of less than 20/200 secondary to branch retinal vein occlusion that underwent pars plana vitrectomy and arteriovenous adventitial sheathotomy and were followed postoperatively for a mean of 6.5 years. In four of five eyes, the best-corrected visual acuity improved to 20/30 to 20/70. In the remaining eye, visual acuity remained at finger counting secondary to macular ischemia. Arteriovenous adventitial sheathotomy may be beneficial for select patients with poor vision secondary to branch retinal vein occlusion.

Mason and associates[48] evaluated the efficacy and safety of arteriovenous sheathotomy surgery to decompress branch retinal vein occlusion. Twenty eyes underwent vitrectomy and surgical decompression by means of arteriovenous sheathotomy were compared with 20 control eyes (10 observation and 10 laser treated). The mean preoperative visual acuity was 20/250 in the surgical group and 20/180 in the control group. The mean 14-month visual acuity was 20/63 in the surgical group and 20/125 in the control group. Seventy-five percent of the surgical group halved their visual angle compared with 40% of the control group. Average lines of visual acuity gained were 4.55 in the surgical group and 1.55 in the control group. They concluded that surgical arteriovenous sheathotomy to decompress BRVO resulted in significantly better visual outcomes than a matched control group of observation and laser-treated eyes.

In a clinical trial by Lerche and Richard,[49] 12 patients with ischemic BRVO underwent surgical decompression. Arteriovenous sheathotomy was performed 0.5 to 6 months after retinal vein occlusion. Follow up-time was 3 months. After sheathotomy, visual acuity increased significantly from log MAR 0.74 (decimal 0.18) to 0.56 (0.32) in EDTRS charts. Surgical or early complications did not occur during the 3-month control period. Improvement of retinal blood flow during angiography was demonstrated in 75% of the patients. In 50% of the patients all non-perfusion areas had disappeared. For patients with retinal vein occlusion, sheathotomy was found to be a safe and feasible.

Martinez-Soroa and associates[50] initial results have also been encouraging, not only regarding visual acuity improvement, but also because of a decreased risk of neovascularization.

Horio and Hroguchi[51] determined the effect of arteriovenous sheathotomy on retinal blood flow. Seven eyes of 7 patients with BRVO underwent sheathotomy and were followed for more than 6 months. At 1 week postoperatively, the retinal blood flow in the affected vessels was significantly improved from 14.1 +– 5.7 to 27.3 +/– 11.3 pixel (2)/sec (P < 0.01), and the foveal thickness was significantly reduced from 536 +/– 84 to 366 +/– 134 microns. However, the retinal blood flow was reduced again to 11.7 +/– 7.7 pixel (2)/sec at 1 month postoperatively, and the foveal thickness was increased to 424 +/– 184 microns. Arteriovenous sheathotomy led to a transient improvement of the retinal blood flow and was effective in reducing macular edema. It is not clear whether the transient effect of sheathotomy affects the long-term visual acuity and macular edema.

Yamaji and associates[52] quantitatively evaluated the effects of arteriovenous crossing sheathotomy on retinal circulation in 18 consecutive 18 eyes. Changes in retinal circulation after the surgery were evaluated by fluorescein videoangiography with a scanning laser ophthalmoscope and by image analysis using dye dilution technique. At a venule distal to the responsible arteriovenous crossing site and a normal venule, the circulation time (T50) from the beginning of filling to 50% filling of the peak intensity was calculated. The time difference (DeltaT50) between T50 at the point on the affected venule and that at the point on the normal venule, which represents the filling delay at the venule distal to the arteriovenous crossing site, was compared between before and early after the surgery. The preoperative DeltaT50 was 1.36 +/–1.15 seconds (mean +/– SD), and the postoperative DeltaT50 was 0.72 +/– 0.77 seconds. In 11 of the 18 eyes, DeltaT50 decreased by 20% or more after the surgery. In the other 7 eyes, DeltaT50 was unchanged or slightly increased after the surgery. Although a randomized controlled study is needed to confirm the effectiveness of sheathotomy on visual function, this technique could be effective for improving the delay in perfusion in the affected venule.

Kube and associates[53] assessed retinal hemodynamics, arteriovenous passage time of the affected and unaffected branches, at first and at maximal venous filling. Changes in the foveal avascular zone were calculated to determine foveal structural changes. Sheathotomy lead to a significant decrease of arteriovenous passage time

and may ameliorate retinal perfusion in the affected branch.

Recent onset BRVO, responsible for a visual acuity of 20/40 or less has been estimated to be good candidates for this procedure. Le Rouic and associates [54] reported on the results of the prospective evaluation of three eyes (in three patients) with recent onset BRVO which underwent surgical decompression. Initial visual acuity was 20/80, 20/80, and 20/200. After 11, 10, and 9 months follow-up, visual acuity was 20/80, 20/200, and 20/200. In two eyes, an increase of the area of retinal non-perfusion was treated with peripheral laser photocoagulation. No cataract, retinal tears or retinal detachment were observed. Although feasible, sheathotomy did not lead to a significant visual improvement in their patients. They concluded that dissection of the arteriovenous crossing could have induced vascular trauma. Furthermore, vitrectomy with posterior hyaloid detachment alone could be of benefit in the treatment of branched retinal vein occlusions.

Charbonnel and associates[55] analyzed 13 eyes. An improvement in visual acuity of two ETDRS lines or more was observed in nine eyes (69%). The mean gain was 1.9 ETDRS lines. The absence of previous posterior vitreous detachment (PVD), poor initial visual acuity and the presence of retinal ischemia were correlated to the improvement in vision. Eyes with initial posterior vitreous detachment had a mean loss postoperatively of 5.7 lines, but eyes without posterior vitreous detachment experienced a gain of 4.2 lines. Macular edema decreased significantly (preoperative thickness: 714 microns, postoperative thickness: 353 microns, whereas the aspect of the vein at the crossing and the non-perfused area remained unchanged. They concluded that vitrectomy with sheathotomy seems to be of benefit in the management of BRVO, particularly in eyes with no previous posterior vitreous detachment, and the main postoperative feature was the decrease in macular edema. The surgical detachment of posterior hyaloid could be as important (or more) as the sheathotomy itself.

Fujimoto and associates [56] examined the efficacy of arteriovenous adventitial sheathotomy. Eighty-three patients (83 eyes) who had macular edema in BRVO for 26 weeks or less underwent pars plana vitrectomy and internal limiting membrane The eighty-three eyes were divided into 38 eyes with sheathotomy (sheathotomy group) and 45 eyes without sheathotomy (non-sheathotomy group). The mean absorption period for macular edema was 3.4 months in the sheathotomy group and 4.2 months in the non-sheathotomy group, and the mean difference between pre- and postoperative visual acuity at one year was 0.37 and 0.28, respectively. There was no significant difference between the two groups. There was no significant factor related to the absorption period for macular edema, but the difference between preoperative visual acuity and postoperative visual acuity at one year was significant. They concluded that sheathotomy may have no additional effect on the absorption of macular or the improvement of visual acuity after vitrectomy.

Cahill and associates[57] in a retrospective review categorized eyes as having resolution (group 1), reduction (group 2), or persistence (group 3) of cystoid macular edema. Of the 27 eyes identified, eight (29.6%) had resolution, 14 (51.8%) had reduction, and five (18.6%) had persistence of cystoid macular edema. Median preoperative visual acuity was similar in all groups. Overall median follow up was 12.0 months. Eyes in group 1 had significantly better median postoperative visual acuity than eyes in groups 2 and 3 (0.6, 1.0, and 2.0 respectively). A higher percentage of group 1 eyes had evidence of postoperative retinal perfusion (83.0% v 21.43% and 40.0%). Complete resolution of cystoid macular edema after sheathotomy occurred in one third of patients, and postoperative vision improved significantly in this group. However, in the majority of cases, despite an improvement in cystoid macular edema, there was no improvement in vision after sheathotomy.

Yamamoto and associates[58] compared the results of vitrectomy with or without arteriovenous crossing sheathotomy. Twenty eyes underwent sheathotomy (AS group), and 16 eyes underwent posterior vitreous detachment (PVD group). The mean postoperative best-corrected visual acuities were significantly better in both the AS and the PVD group. Foveal thickness decreased significantly 1 month after surgery in both groups and continued to decrease up to 12 months. Postoperative

fluorescein angiography showed reperfusion of the occluded vein in 10 eyes in the AS group and 2 eyes in the PVD group, and formation of shunt vessels at the arteriovenous crossing site or around the macular region in all of the other eyes of both groups. Both arteriovenous sheathotomy and simple posterior vitreous detachment significantly reduced macular edema associated with BRVO. However, there was no significant difference in the improvement of macular function following either procedure. Postoperative improvement of retinal circulation by either reperfusion of the occluded vein or collateral vessel formation was found. This accounted for functional and morphologic improvements.

Garcia-Arumi and associates[59] reported the surgical recanalization of the occluded vein using a bimanual technique and recombinant tissue plasminogen activator (tPA) and its effect on final visual acuity. Arteriovenous sheathotomy was performed, using a bimanual technique, followed by fluid-air exchange and injection of 25 mg of recombinant tPA over the area of the occluded vein. Intraoperative sectioning of the common arteriovenous sheath was achieved in all 40 patients. Thrombus release was observed in 11 cases (27.5%) and was correlated with early surgery and better final visual recovery. Optical coherence tomography showed macular thickness that decreased by greater than 40% in 31 patients (77.5%) compared with preoperatively, and correlated to postoperative visual acuity (P < 0.001). The mean visual acuity increased from 20/100 to 20/40, with 70% of patients gaining three or more lines of visual acuity. They concluded that surgical venous decompression and injection of recombinant tPA may effectively manage macular edema secondary to BRVO, thus improving anatomic and visual outcome. Early surgical intervention may obtain maximum final visual recovery.

Internal limiting membrane peeling has recently given interesting results in the management of macular edema in diabetic patients, even in the absence of vitreomacular tractions. Becquet and associates[60] performed internal limiting membrane peeling associated with arteriovenous crossing sheathotomy on six eyes and internal limiting membrane peeling alone on six eyes. At 6 months, postoperative visual acuity was improved in all patients (mean VA=20/40; range, 20/125-20/20), with an average gain of three lines of vision (or 14 ETDRS points). On automated field testing, the mean corrected defect improved from 3.4+/–0.9dB to 2.3+/–0.9dB. On OCT, mean foveal thickness decreased from 419+/–57 micro m to 233+/–10 microns. No difference was noted between simple vitrectomy with internal limiting membrane peeling and arteriovenous crossing sheathotomy in terms of visual acuity, visual field, or foveal thickness improvement. Their findings suggest that internal limiting membrane removal for macular edema may improve the functional prognosis in patients with branch retinal vein occlusion. Adventitial sheathotomy did not yield further functional benefits in these cases. Asensio and associates[61] also reported that therapeutical effect of sheathotomy in treatment of macular non ischemic macular edema secondary to branch retinal vein occlusion, and the additional performance of internal limiting membrane maculorhexis may improve visual prognosis.

Lakhanpal and associates[62] evaluated a new technique of 25-gauge transvitreal limited arteriovenous-crossing manipulation without vitrectomy (LAM), for the treatment of BRVO complicated by macular hemorrhage and/or macular edema recalcitrant to grid laser photo-coagulation. Twelve eyes of 12 patients underwent LAM for BRVO using the 25-gauge nitinol flexible-extendable blunt pick. Restoration of blood flow was noted in all patients and was based on intraoperative reestablishment of a red column of erythrocytes through the previously closed vessel. Mean visual acuity improved from 20/200 (logarithm of the minimal angle of resolution [LogMAR] +/– SD, 1.00 +/– 0.32) preoperatively to 20/70 (LogMAR +/– SD, 0.56 +/– 0.28) (P = 0.0003) at the final visit. Eleven (92%) of 12 eyes had >or=2 lines of visual improvement. Five eyes (45%) had final visual acuity of 20/50 or better. Mean macular thickness +/– SD improved from 401.0 +/– 73.2 to 178.7 +/– 19.6 microns at the final visit. No statistically significant difference was noted in cataract progression or intraocular pressure. All patients were observed for at least 12 weeks. LAM may achieve outcomes comparable with those of arteriovenous adventitial sheathotomy for complicated BRVO.

Fujii and associates[63] found that optical coherence tomography can detect an early positive effect of sheathotomy surgery on macular edema, and scanning laser ophthalmoscope can document associated improvement in fixation stability.

Two cases of uncommon branch retinal vein occlusion (BRVO) with vein overlying artery at occlusion site that can be found in less than 1% who underwent retinal venule sheathotomy without separation of retinal vessel for decompression of BRVO have been reported. [64] Both patients had macular hemorrhage, edema, and area of macular capillary nonperfusion. The retinal venules were dissected around the crossing site without separation of retinal vessels. Intraoperative dilation, pulsation and restoration of downstream blood flow of the involved venules were observed. In the first patient, at 1 day, 2 weeks, and 6 weeks postoperatively, visual acuity improved to 20/120, 20/30, and 20/20, respectively, and remained unchanged at 12 months postoperatively. In the second patient, visual acuity improved to 20/80 on the first day postoperatively and improved to 20/60 at 1 week follow up and continuously improved to nearly normal at 2 months postoperatively then patient lost contact. Postoperative fundus fluorescein angiogram showed dilated and improved perfusion with decreased macular edema in both cases. Optical coherence tomography confirmed remarkable reduction of retinal thickness (from 874 microns preoperatively to 420 microns at 1 week postoperatively) in the second patient. Retinal venule sheathotomy without separation of retinal vessel for decompression of BRVO with venule overlying arteriole at occlusion site could be effective for improving visual acuity and decreased macular edema.

Result of sheathotomy for branch retinal vein occlusion is shown in Figures 14.5 and 14.6.

COMPLICATIONS

Perforation of retinal vein may occur during sheatho-tomy.[65] Retinal detachment may also occur after surgery.

Retinal vein occlusions remain as the second commonest sight threatening vascular disorder. Despite its frequency treatments are unsatisfactory and include several that have not been tested by large, well designed,

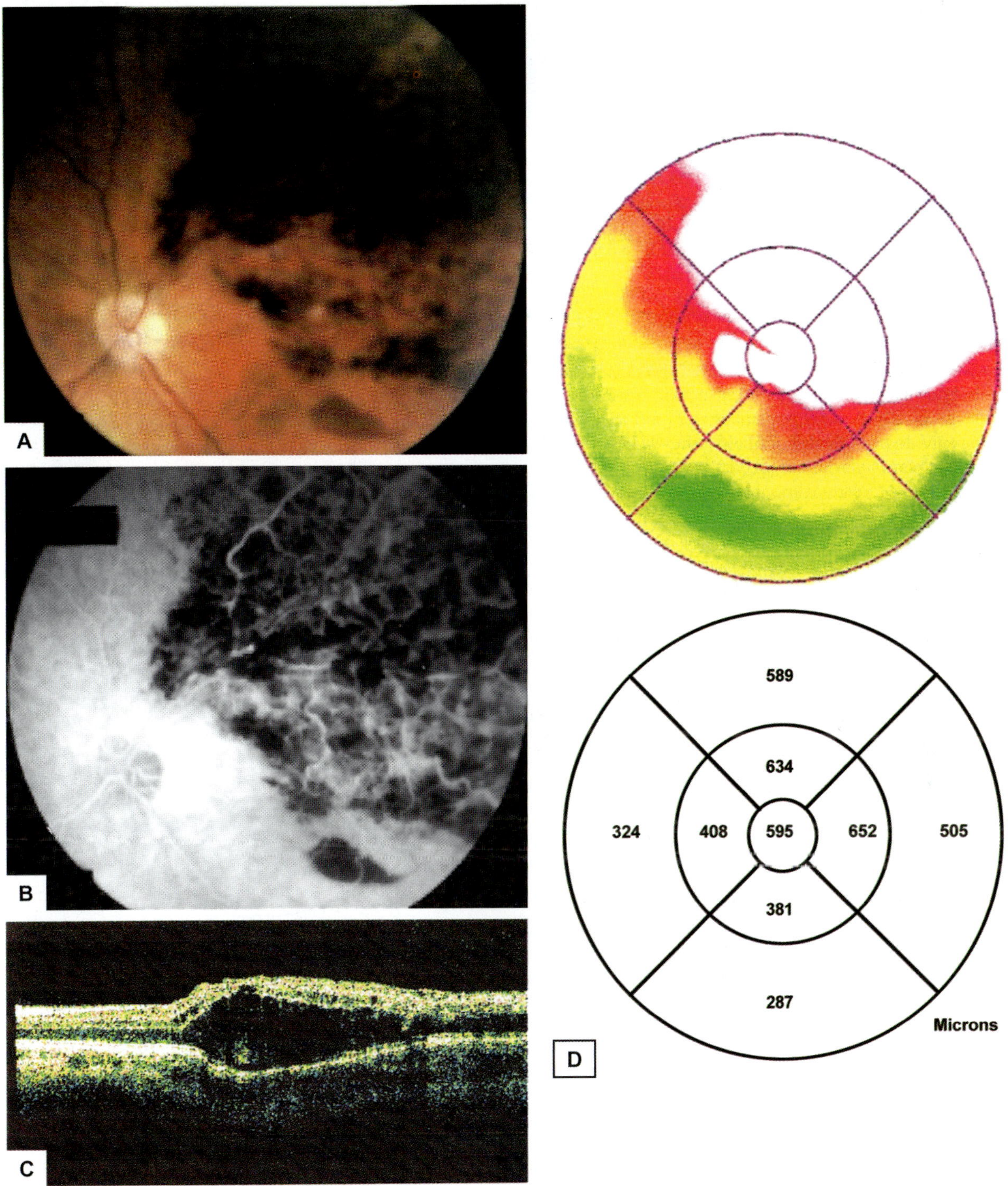

FIGURES 14.5A to D: Sheathotomy: Pre-treatment

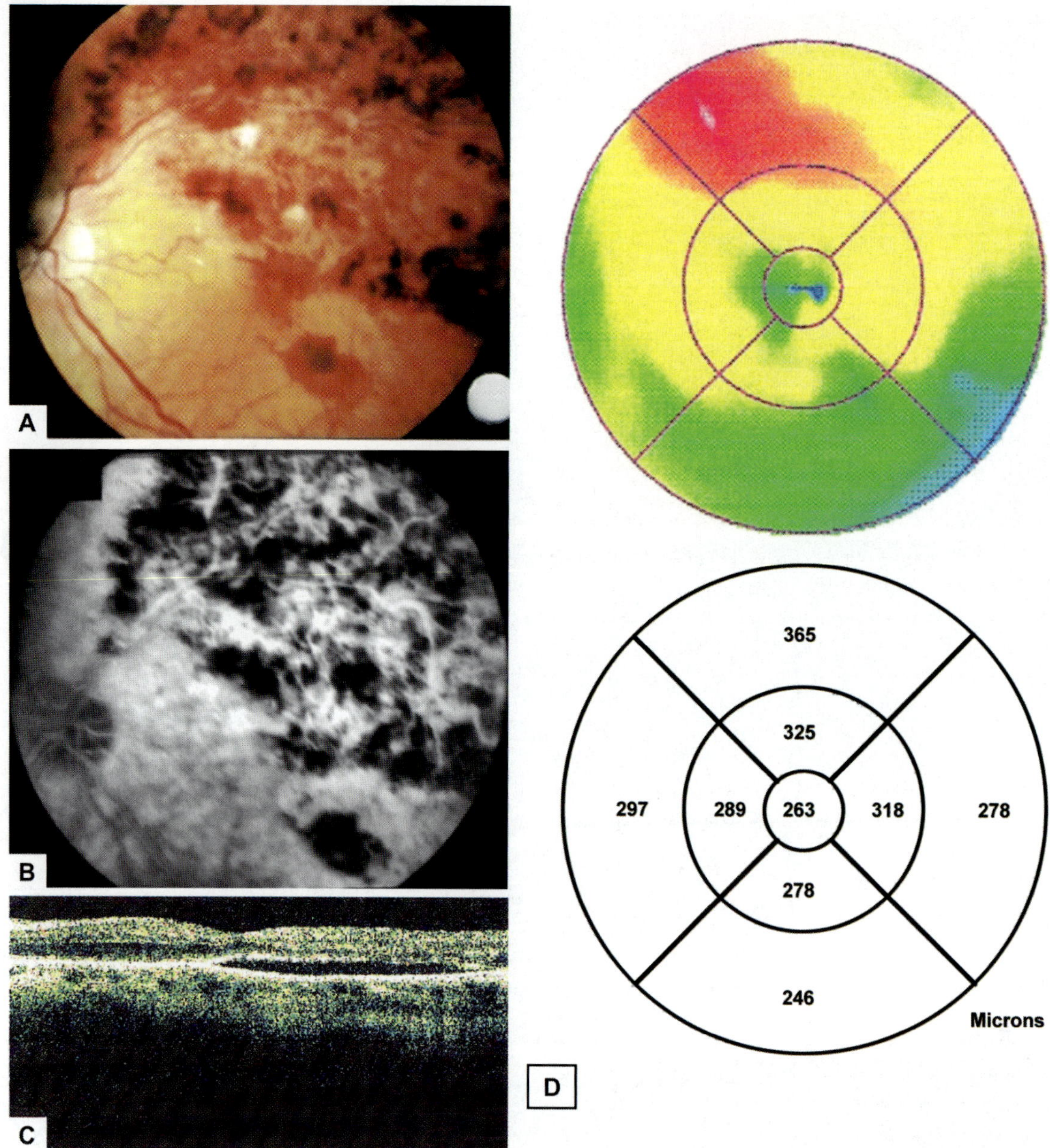

FIGURES 14.6A to D: Sheathotomy: Post-treatment

prospective, randomized controlled trials. There is also the lack of long term follow up in many of the available small uncontrolled studies, and the timings of interventions are haphazard. Isovolemic hemodilution is of limited benefit and should be avoided in patients with concurrent cardiovascular, renal, or pulmonary morbidity. Evidence to date does not support any therapeutic benefit from radial optic neurotomy, optic nerve decompression, or arteriovenous crossing sheathotomy on its own. Vitrectomy combined with intravenous thrombolysis may offer promise for CRVO. Similarly, vitrectomy combined with arteriovenous sheathotomy intravenous tissue plasminogen activator may offer benefits for BRVO. Retinal vein occlusions occur at significantly high frequency to allow future prospective randomized controlled studies to be conducted to evaluate the role of different therapeutic modalities singly or in combination.[66]

REFERENCES

1. Mester U. Surgical approach to retinal vein occlusion. Klin Monatsbl Augenheilkd. 2005; 222:299-308.
2. The Central Vein Occlusion Study Group. Natural history and clinical management of central retinal vein occlusion. Arch Ophthalmol 1997; 115:486-91.
3. Van Heuven WA, Hayreh MS, Hayreh SS. Pathogenesis of 'central retinal vein occlusion'. Bibl Anat 1977:1-5.
4. Hayreh SS, van Heuven WA, Hayreh MS. Experimental retinal vascular occlusion. I. Pathogenesis of central retinal vein occlusion. Arch Ophthalmol. 1978; 96:311-23.
5. Green WR, Chan CC, Hutchins GM, et al. Central retinal vein occlusion: a prospective histopathologic study of 29 eyes in 28 cases. Trans Am Ophthalmol Soc 1981; 79:371–422.
6. Taylor AW, Sehu W, Williamson TH, et al. Morphometric assessment of the central retinal artery and vein in the optic nerve head. Can J Ophthalmol 1993; 28:320-24.
7. Williamson TH, Baxter GM. Central retinal vein occlusion, an investigation by color Doppler imaging. Blood velocity characteristics and prediction of iris neovascularization. Ophthalmology 1994; 101:1362-72.
8. McAllister IL, Douglas JP, Constable IJ, et al. Laser-induced chorioretinal venous anastomosis for nonischemic central retinal vein occlusion: evaluation of the complications and their risk factors. Am J Ophthalmol 1998; 126:219-29.
9. Opremcak EM, Bruce RA, Lomeo MD, et al. Radial optic neurotomy for central retinal vein occlusion: a retrospective pilot study of 11 consecutive cases. Retina 2001; 21:408-15.
10. Williamson TH. Central retinal vein occlusion: what's the story? Br J Ophthalmol 1997; 81:698-704.
11. Singh Hayreh S, Opremcak EM, Bruce RA, et al. Radial optic neurotomy for central retinal vein obstruction. Retina 2002, 22.374-77.
12. Central Vein Occlusion Study Group. Central vein occlusion study of photocoagulation therapy. Baseline findings. Online J Curr Clin Trials 1993;Doc No 95:6021.
13. Wrede J, Varadi G, Volcker HE, Dithmar S. Radial optic neurotomy for central retinal vein occlusion—how deep should it be? Ophthalmologe. 2005 Nov 22; [Epub ahead of print]
14. Czajka MP, Cummings TJ, McCuen BW 2nd, et al. Radial optic neurotomy in the porcine eye without retinal vein occlusion. Arch Ophthalmol 2004; 122:1185-89.
15. Tao Y, Jiang YR, Li XX, et al. Fundus and histopathological study of radial optic neurotomy in the normal miniature pig eye. Arch Ophthalmol 2005; 123:1097-1101.
16. Vogel A, Holz FG, Loeffler KU. Histopathologic findings after radial optic neurotomy in central retinal vein occlusion. Am J Ophthalmol 2006; 141:203-5.
17. Opremcak EM, Rehmar AJ, Ridenour CD, Kurz DE. Radial optic neurotomy for central retinal vein occlusion: 117 consecutive cases. Retina 2006; 26:297-305.
18. Opremcak EM, Rehmar AJ, Ridenour CD, et al. Radial optic neurotomy with adjunctive intraocular triamcinolone for central retinal vein occlusion: 63 consecutive cases. Retina 2006; 26:306-13.
19. Williamson TH, Poon W, Whitefield L, et al. A pilot study of pars plana vitrectomy, intraocular gas, and radial neurotomy in ischemic central retinal vein occlusion. Br J Ophthalmol 2003; 87:1126-29.
20. Weizer JS, Stinnett SS, Fekrat S. Radial optic neurotomy as treatment for central retinal vein occlusion. Am J Ophthalmol 2003; 136:814-19.
21. Le Rouic JF, Becquet F, Zanlonghi X, et al. Radial optic neurotomy for severe central retinal vein occlusion: preliminary results. J Fr Ophtalmol 2003; 26:577-85.
22. Furino C, Ferrari TM, Boscia F, et al. Combined radial optic neurotomy, internal limiting membrane peeling, and intravitreal triamcinolone acetonide for central retinal vein occlusion. Ophthalmic Surg Lasers Imaging 2005; 36:422-5.
23. Zambarakji HJ, Ghazi-Nouri S, Schadt M, et al. Vitrectomy and radial optic neurotomy for central retinal vein occlusion: effects on visual acuity and macular anatomy. Graefes Arch Clin Exp Ophthalmol 2005; 243:397-405.
24. Nagpal M, Nagpal K, Bhatt C, Nagpal PN. Role of early radial optic neurotomy in central retinal vein occlusion. Indian J Ophthalmol 2005; 53:115-20.
25. Martinez-Jardon CS, Meza-de Regil A, Dalma-Weiszhausz J, et al. Radial optic neurotomy for ischaemic central vein occlusion. Br J Ophthalmol 2005; 89:558-61.
26. Lerche RC, Richard G. Radial optic neurotomy in ischemic central retinal vein occlusion. Klin Monatsbl Augenheilkd 2005; 222:134-41.
27. Patelli F, Radice P, Zumbo G, et al. Optical coherence tomography evaluation of macular edema after radial optic neurotomy in patients affected by central retinal vein occlusion. Semin Ophthalmol 2004;19:21-24.
28. Garcia-Arumi J, Boixadera A, Martinez-Castillo V, et al. Chorioretinal anastomosis after radial optic neurotomy for central retinal vein occlusion. Arch Ophthalmol 2003; 121:1385-91.
29. Spaide RF, Klancnik JM Jr, Gross NE. Retinal choroidal collateral circulation after radial optic neurotomy correlated with the lessening of macular edema. Retina 2004; 24:356-9.
30. Nomoto H, Shiraga F, Yamaji H, et al. Evaluation of radial optic neurotomy for central retinal vein occlusion by indocyanine green videoangiography and image analysis. Am J Ophthalmol 2004; 138:612-9.
31. Horio N, Horiguchi M. Retinal blood flow and macular edema after radial optic neurotomy for central retinal vein occlusion. Am J Ophthalmol 2006; 141:31-4.
32. Horio N, Horiguchi M. Central retinal vein occlusion with further reduction of retinal blood flow one year after radial optic neurotomy. Am J Ophthalmol 2005; 139:926-7.
33. Chalam KV, Shah VA. Resolution of macular scotoma after radial optic neurotomy in central retinal vein occlusion. Ophthalmic Surg Lasers Imaging 2006; 37:72-5.

34. Mennel S, Droutsas K, Meyer CH, et al. Radial optic neurotomy in combined cilioretinal artery and central retinal vein occlusion. Br J Ophthalmol 2005; 89:642-3.

35. Schneider U, Inhoffen W, Grisanti S, et al. Chorioretinal neovascularization after radial optic neurotomy for central retinal vein occlusion. Ophthalmic Surg Lasers Imaging 2005; 36:508-11.

36. Bakri SJ, Beer PM. Choroidal neovascularization after radial optic neurotomy for central retinal vein occlusion. Retina 2004; 24:610-11.

37. Gauntt CD, Williamson TH, Sanders MD. Relationship of the distal optic nerve sheath to the circle of Zinn. Graefes Arch Clin Exp Ophthalmol 1999; 237:642-7.

38. Takaya K, Suzuki Y, Nakazawa M. Massive hemorrhagic retinal detachment during radial optic neurotomy. Graefes Arch Clin Exp Ophthalmol 2006; 244:265-7.

39. Yamamoto S, Takatsuna Y, Sato E, Mizunoya S. Central retinal artery occlusion after radial optic neurotomy in a patient with central retinal vein occlusion. Am J Ophthalmol 2005; 139:206-7.

40. Samuel MA, Desai UR, Gandolfo CB. Peripapillary retinal detachment after radial optic neurotomy for central retinal vein occlusion. Retina 2003; 23:580-3.

41. Shukla D, Rajendran A, Kim R. Macular hole formation and spontaneous closure after vitrectomy for central retinal vein occlusion. Graefes Arch Clin Exp Ophthalmol 2006 Mar 8; [Epub ahead of print].

42. Schneider U, Inhoffen W, Grisanti S, Bartz-Schmidt KU. Characteristics of visual field defects by scanning laser ophthalmoscope microperimetry after radial optic neurotomy for central retinal vein occlusion. Retina 2005; 25:704-12.

43. Feltgen N, Herrmann J, Hansen L. Visual field defect after radial optic neurotomy. Ophthalmologe 2005; 102:802-4.

44. Tsujikawa A, Hangai M, Kikuchi M, et al. Visual field defect after radial optic neurotomy for central retinal vein occlusion. Jpn J Ophthalmol 2006;50:158-60.

45. Cahill MT, Fekrat S. Arteriovenous sheathotomy for branch retinal vein occlusion. Ophthalmol Clin North Am 2002; 15:417-23.

46. Opremcak EM, Bruce RA. Surgical decompression of branch retinal vein occlusion via arteriovenous crossing sheathotomy: a prospective review of 15 cases. Retina 1999; 19:1-5.

47. Shah GK, Sharma S, Fineman MS, et al. Arteriovenous adventitial sheathotomy for the treatment of macular edema associated with branch retinal vein occlusion. Am J Ophthalmol 2000; 129:104-6.

48. Mason J 3rd, Feist R, White M Jr, et al. Sheathotomy to decompress branch retinal vein occlusion: a matched control study. Ophthalmology 2004; 111:540-5.

49. Lerche RC, Richard G. Arteriovenous sheathotomy in venous thrombosis. Klin Monatsbl Augenheilkd 2004; 221:479-84.

50. Martinez-Soroa I, Ruiz Miguel M, Ostolaza JI, et al. Surgical arteriovenous decompression (sheathotomy) in branch retinal vein occlusion: retrospective study. Arch Soc Esp Oftalmol 2003;78:603-8.

51. Horio N, Horiguchi M. Effect of arteriovenous sheathotomy on retinal blood flow and macular edema in patients with branch retinal vein occlusion. Am J Ophthalmol 2005; 139:739-40.

52. Yamaji H, Shiraga F, Tsuchida Y, et al. Evaluation of arteriovenous crossing sheathotomy for branch retinal vein occlusion by fluorescein videoangiography and image analysis. Am J Ophthalmol 2004; 137:834-41.

53. Kube T, Feltgen N, Pache M, et al. Angiographic findings in arteriovenous dissection (sheathotomy) for decompression of branch retinal vein occlusion. Graefes Arch Clin Exp Ophthalmol 2005; 243:334-8.

54. Le Rouic JF, Bejjani RA, Rumen F, et al. Adventitial sheathotomy for decompression of recent onset branch retinal vein occlusion. Graefes Arch Clin Exp Ophthalmol 2001; 239:747-51.

55. Charbonnel J, Glacet-Bernard A, Korobelnik JF, et al. Management of branch retinal vein occlusion with vitrectomy and arteriovenous adventitial sheathotomy, the possible role of surgical posterior vitreous detachment. Graefes Arch Clin Exp Ophthalmol 2004; 242:223-8.

56. Fujimoto R, Ogino N, Kumagai K, et al. The efficacy of arteriovenous adventitial sheathotomy for macular edema in branch retinal vein occlusion. Nippon Ganka Gakkai Zasshi 2004;108:144-9.

57. Cahill MT, Kaiser PK, Sears JE, Fekrat S. The effect of arteriovenous sheathotomy on cystoid macular oedema secondary to branch retinal vein occlusion. Br J Ophthalmol 2003; 87:1329-32.

58. Yamamoto S, Saito W, Yagi F, et al. Vitrectomy with or without arteriovenous adventitial sheathotomy for macular edema associated with branch retinal vein occlusion. Am J Ophthalmol 2004; 138:907-14.

59. Garcia-Arumi J, Martinez-Castillo V, Boixadera A, et al. Management of macular edema in branch retinal vein occlusion with sheathotomy and recombinant tissue plasminogen activator. Retina 2004; 24:530-40.

60. Becquet F, Le Rouic JF, Zanlonghi X, et al. Efficiency of surgical treatment for chronic macular edema due to branch retinal vein occlusion. J Fr Ophthalmol 2003; 26:570-76.

61. Asensio Sanchez VM, Rodriguez Bravo I, Botella Oltra G. Adventitial sheathotomy in branch retinal vein occlusion with non ischemic macular edema. Arch Soc Esp Oftalmol 2004; 79:347-52.

62. Lakhanpal RR, Javaheri M, Ruiz-Garcia H, et al. Transvitreal limited arteriovenous-crossing manipulation without vitrectomy for complicated branch retinal vein occlusion using 25-gauge instrumentation. Retina 2005; 25:272-80.

63. Fujii GY, de Juan E Jr, Humayun MS. Improvements after sheathotomy for branch retinal vein occlusion documented

by optical coherence tomography and scanning laser ophthalmoscope. Ophthalmic Surg Lasers Imaging 2003; 34:49-52.

64. Rodanant N, Thoongsuwan S. Sheathotomy without separation of venule overlying arteriole at occlusion site in uncommon branch retinal vein occlusion. J Med Assoc Thai 2005; 88(Suppl)9:S143-50.

65. Dieguez Millan JM, Suner Capo M, Olea Vallejo JL. Intraoperative rupture of the vein in an arteriovenous crossing sheathotomy. Arch Soc Esp Oftalmol 2002; 77: 575-8.

66. Shahid H, Hossain P, Amoaku WM. The management of retinal vein occlusion: is interventional ophthalmology the way forward? Br J Ophthalmol 2006; 90:627-39.

15

Step by Step Macular and Allied Surgeries

Sandeep Saxena

INTRODUCTION

Macular diseases are an important cause of visual disability. Epiretinal membrane, macular hole, vitreomacular traction syndrome, subfoveal choroidal neovascular membrane, submacular hemorrhage, diabetic macular edema, myopic foveoschisis, and optic disk pit with macular schisis are some of the treatable disorders.

Modern vitreous surgery through the pars plana is one of the most effective tools for treating such diseases. Innovative developments in the field of macular surgery offer promise to patients with these conditions. Modern vitreoretinal instrumentation, viewing systems and newer techniques such as use of triamcinolone acetonide, during surgery, have revolutionized macular surgery. Surgeries for retinal vein occlusion also seem to relieve macular involvement.

In this chapter, step by step macular and allied surgeries are shown.

POSTERIOR HYALOID REMOVAL

Step by step surgery for removal of posterior hyaloid using triamcinolone acetonide is shown in Figure 15.1.

EPIRETINAL MEMBRANE

- Step by step surgery for removal of epiretinal membrane is shown in Figure 15.2.
- Step by step surgery for removal of epiretinal membrane using triamcinolone acetonide is shown in Figure 15.3.

MACULAR HOLE

- Step by step macular hole surgery using trypan blue dye for epiretinal membrane staining and indocyanine green dye for internal limiting membrane staining is shown in Figure 15.4.
- Step by step macular hole surgery using triamcinolone acetonide is shown in Figure 15.5.

DIABETIC MACULAR EDEMA

Step by step surgery for diabetic macular edema using indocyanine green dye for internal limiting membrane peeling is shown in Figure 15.6.

MYOPIC FOVEOSCHISIS

Step by step surgery for myopic foveoschisis using indocyanine green dye for internal limiting membrane peeling is shown in Figure 15.7.

SURGERIES FOR RETINAL VEIN OCCLUSION

RADIAL OPTIC NEUROTOMY

Step by step radial optic neurotomy surgery for central retinal vein occlusion is shown in Figure 15.8.

ARTERIOVENOUS SHEATHOTOMY

Step by step arteriovenous sheathotomy surgery for branch retinal vein occlusion is shown in Figure 15.9.

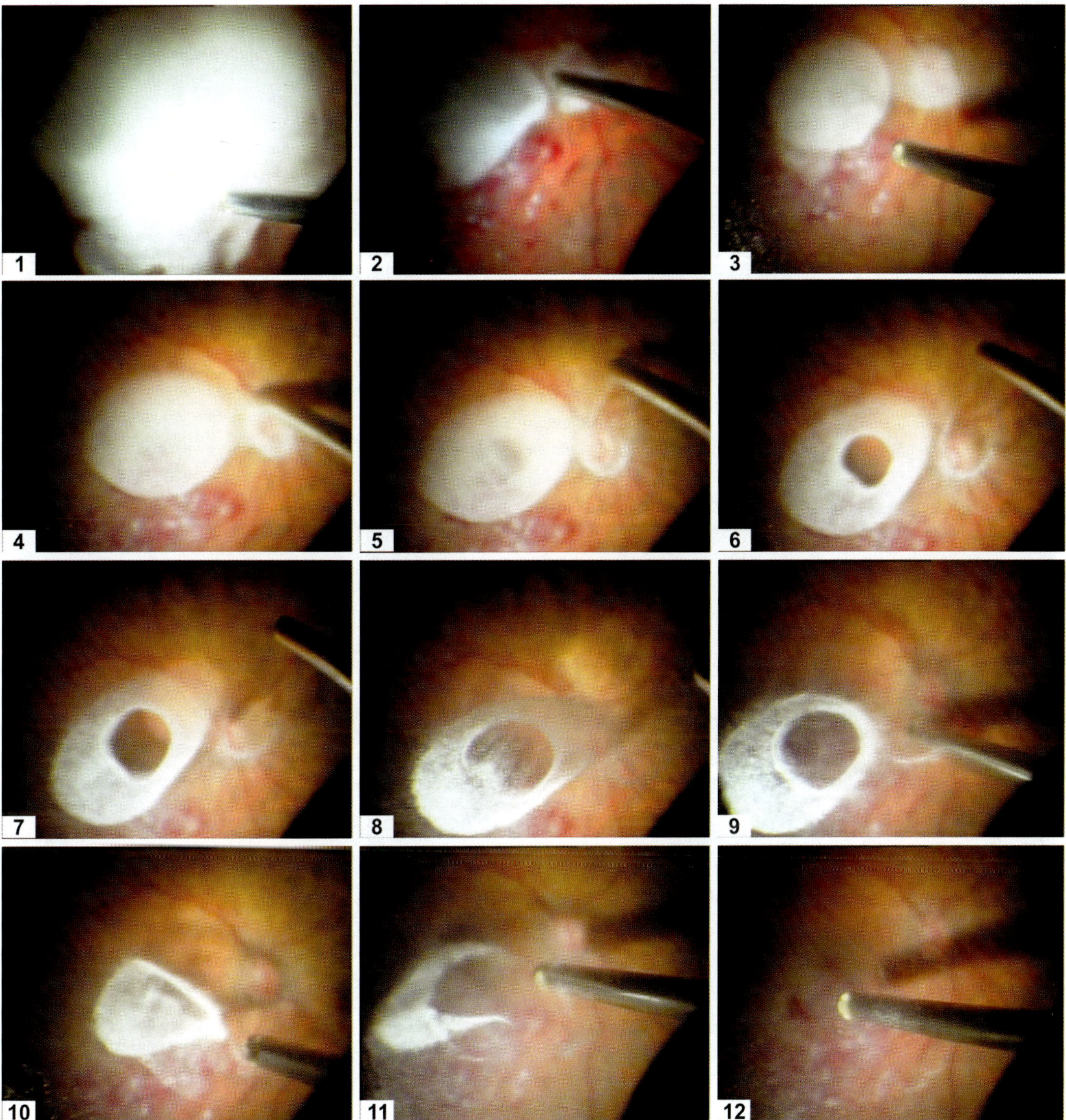

FIGURE 15.1: Posterior hyaloid removal using triamcinolone acetonide (Manish Nagpal MS, India).

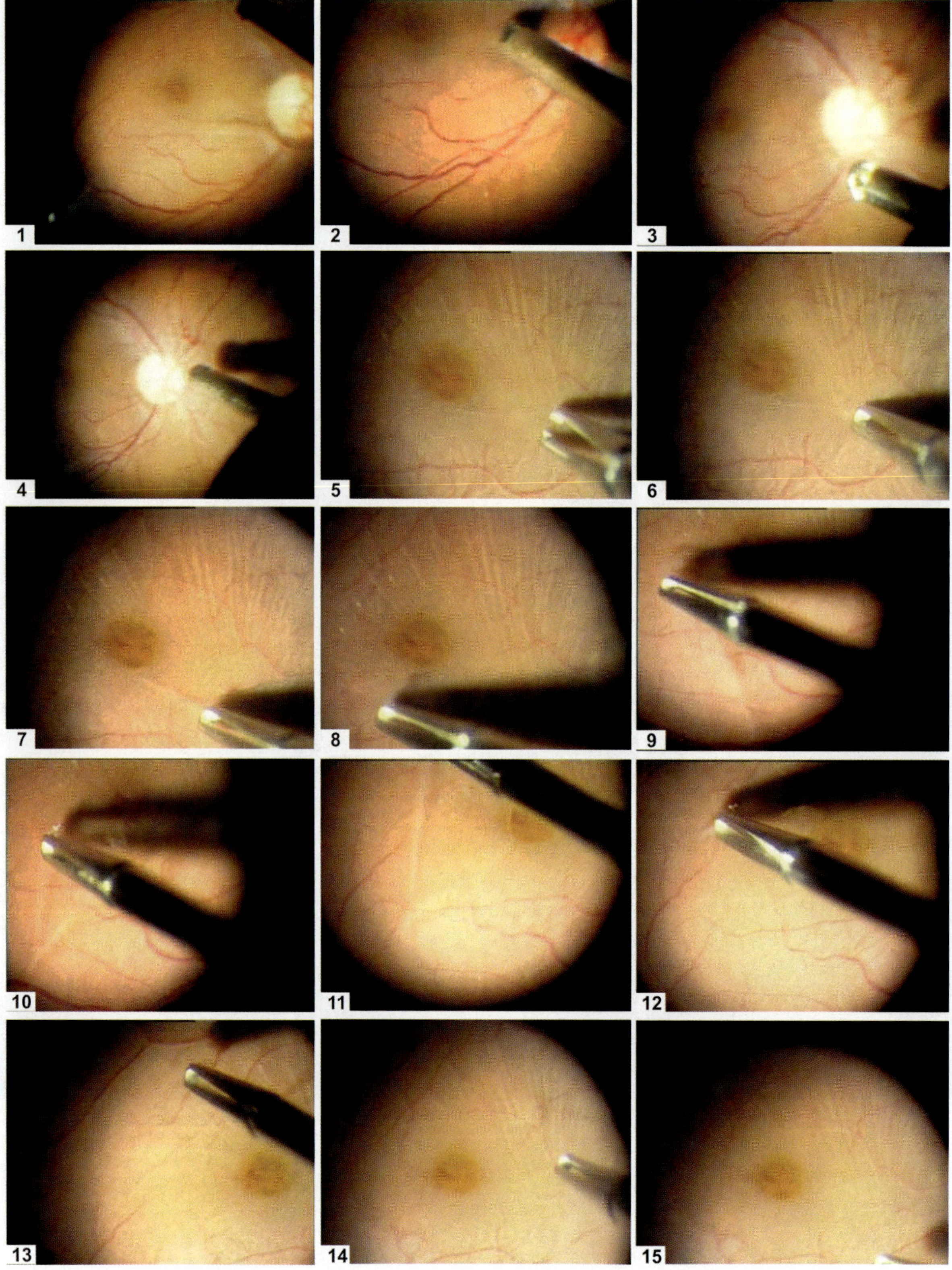

FIGURE 15.2: Epiretinal membrane removal (Manish Nagpal, MS, India).

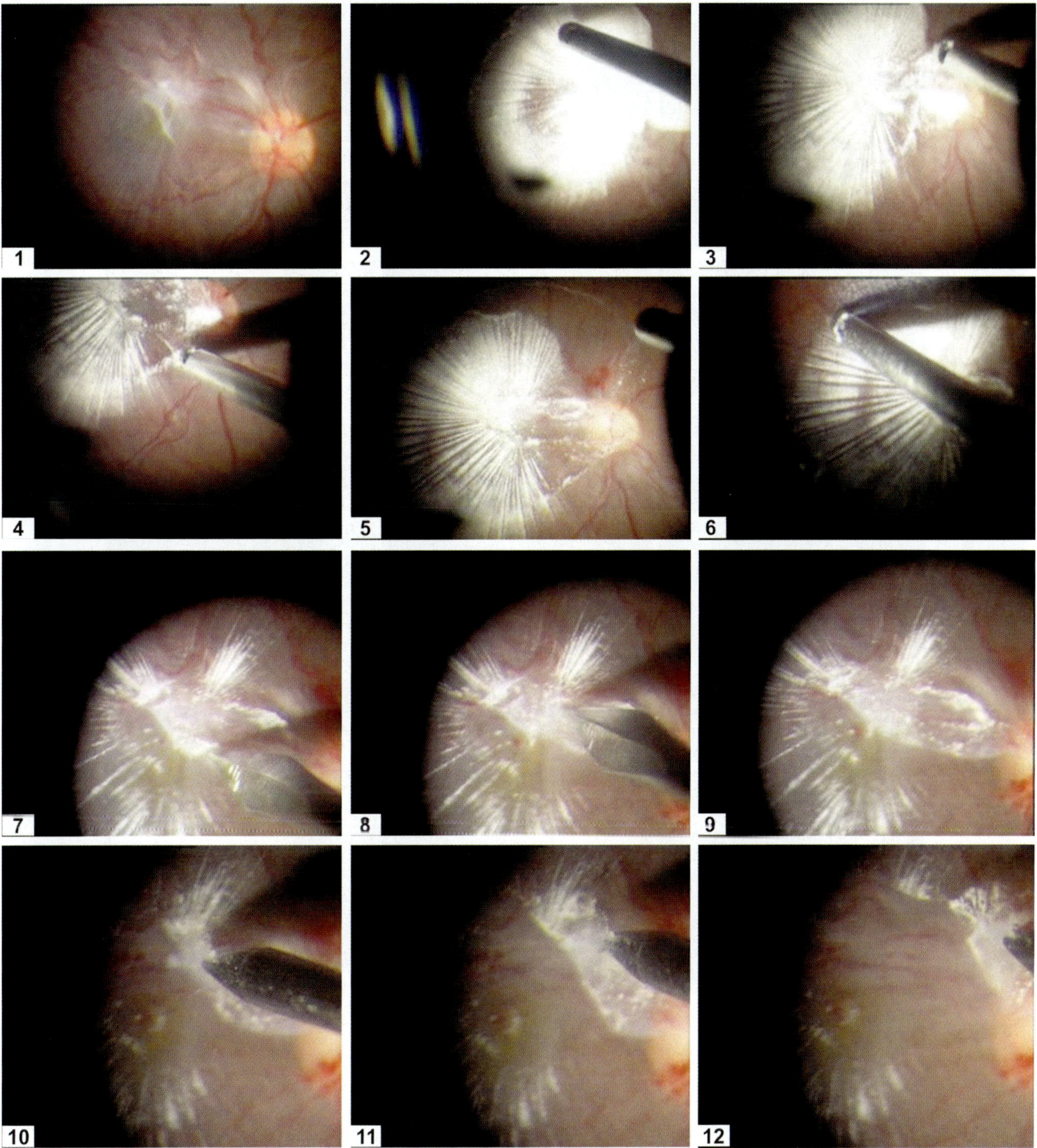

FIGURE 15.3: Epiretinal membrane removal using triamcinolone acetonide (Manish Nagpal, MS, India).

Focus on Macular Diseases

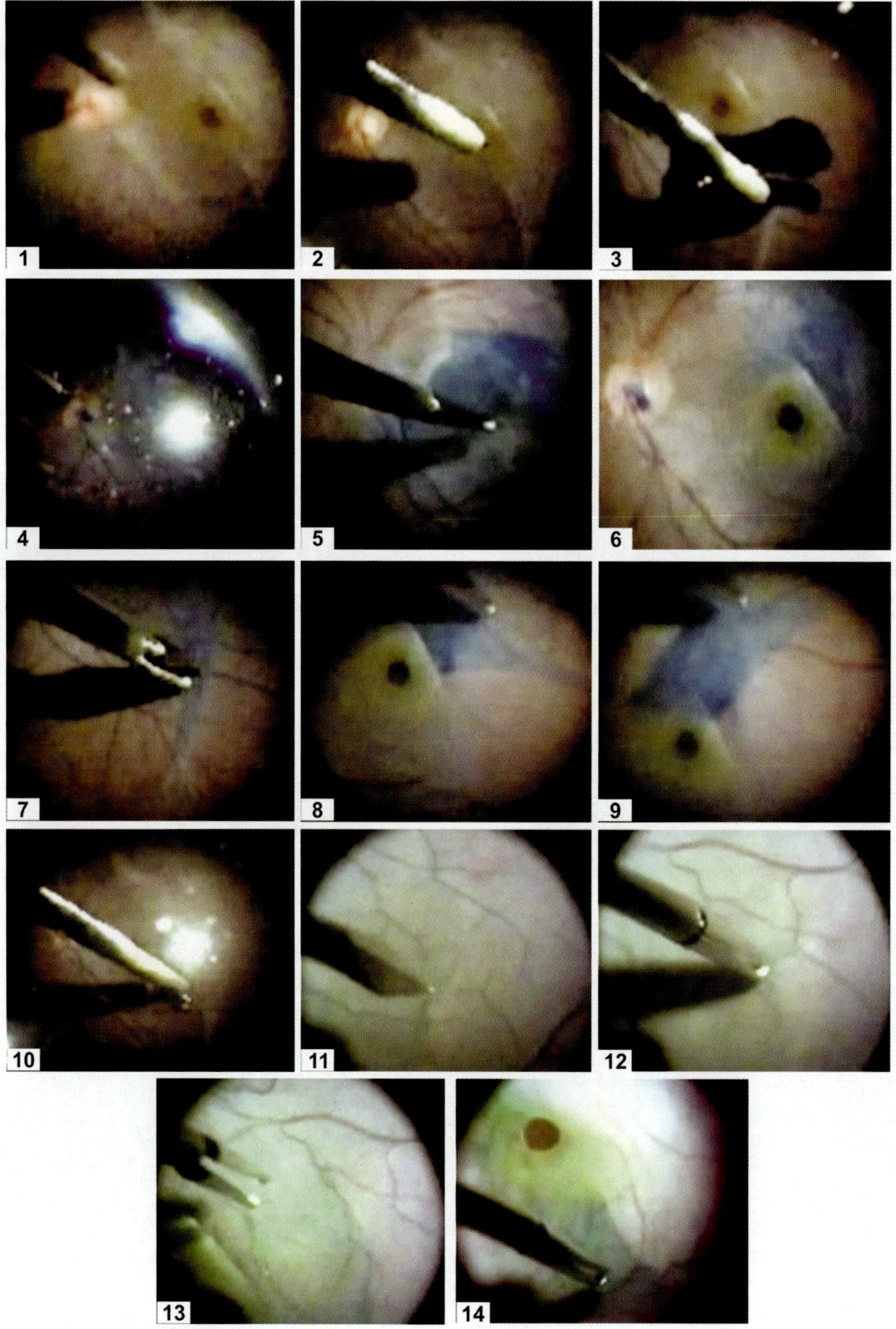

FIGURE 15.4: Step by step macular hole surgery using trypan blue dye for epiretinal membrane staining and indocyanine green dye for internal limiting membrane staining (Nazimul Hussain, MS, India).

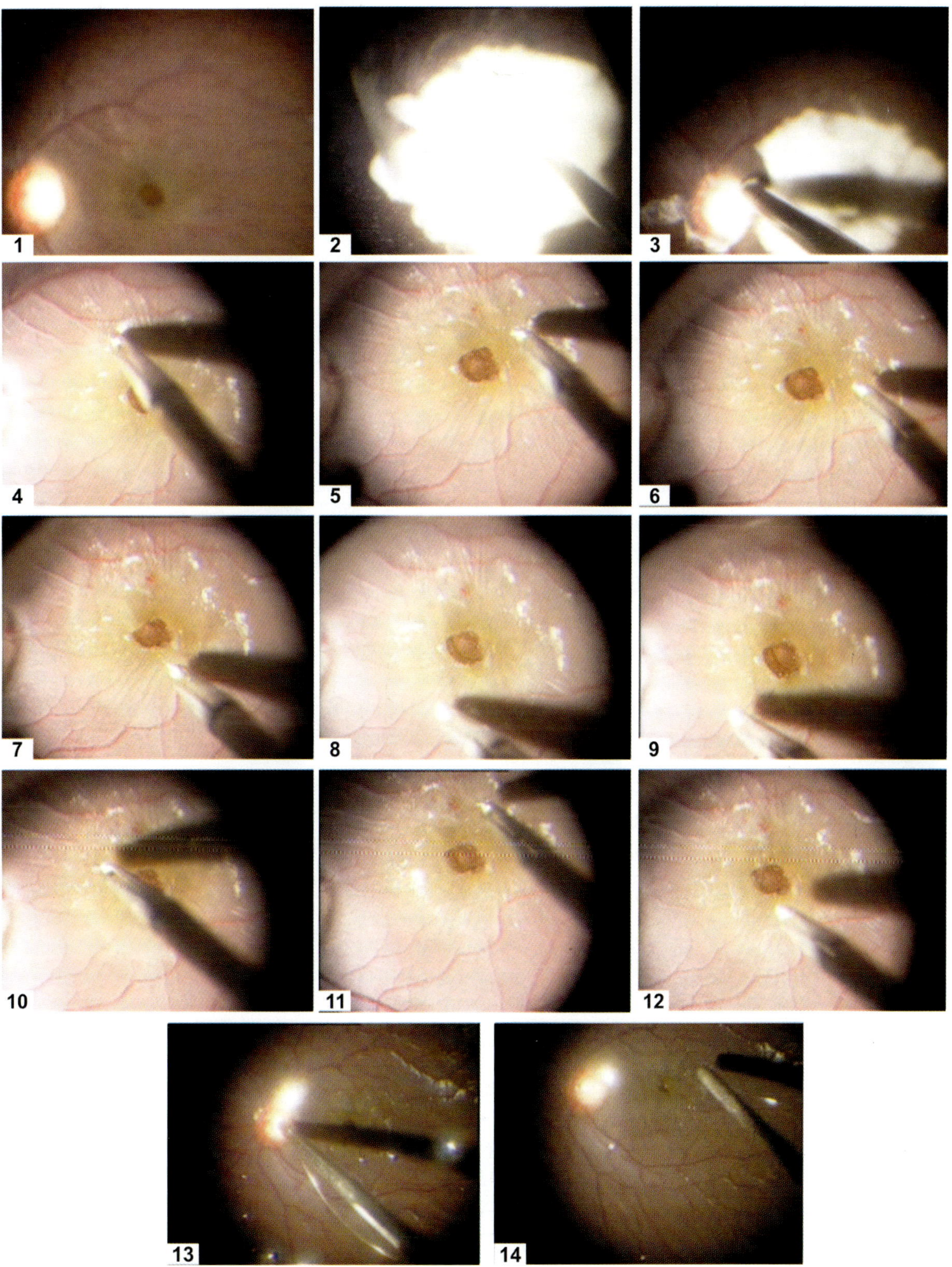

FIGURE 15.5: Macular hole surgery using triamcinolone acetonide
(Manish Nagpal, MS, India).

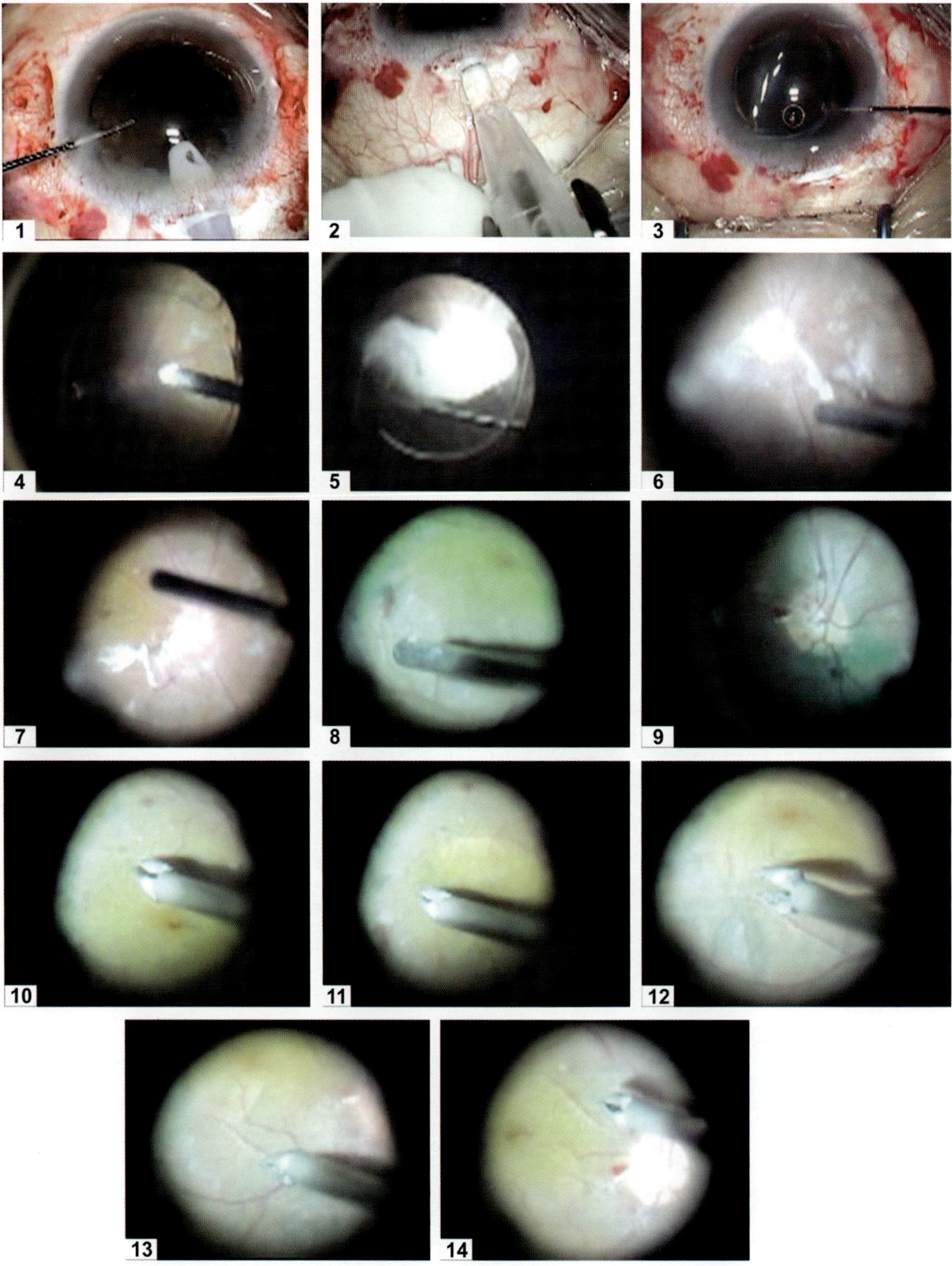

FIGURE 15.6: Surgery for diabetic macular edema using indocyanine green dye for internal limiting membrane peeling (Prof Masahito Ohji MD, Japan).

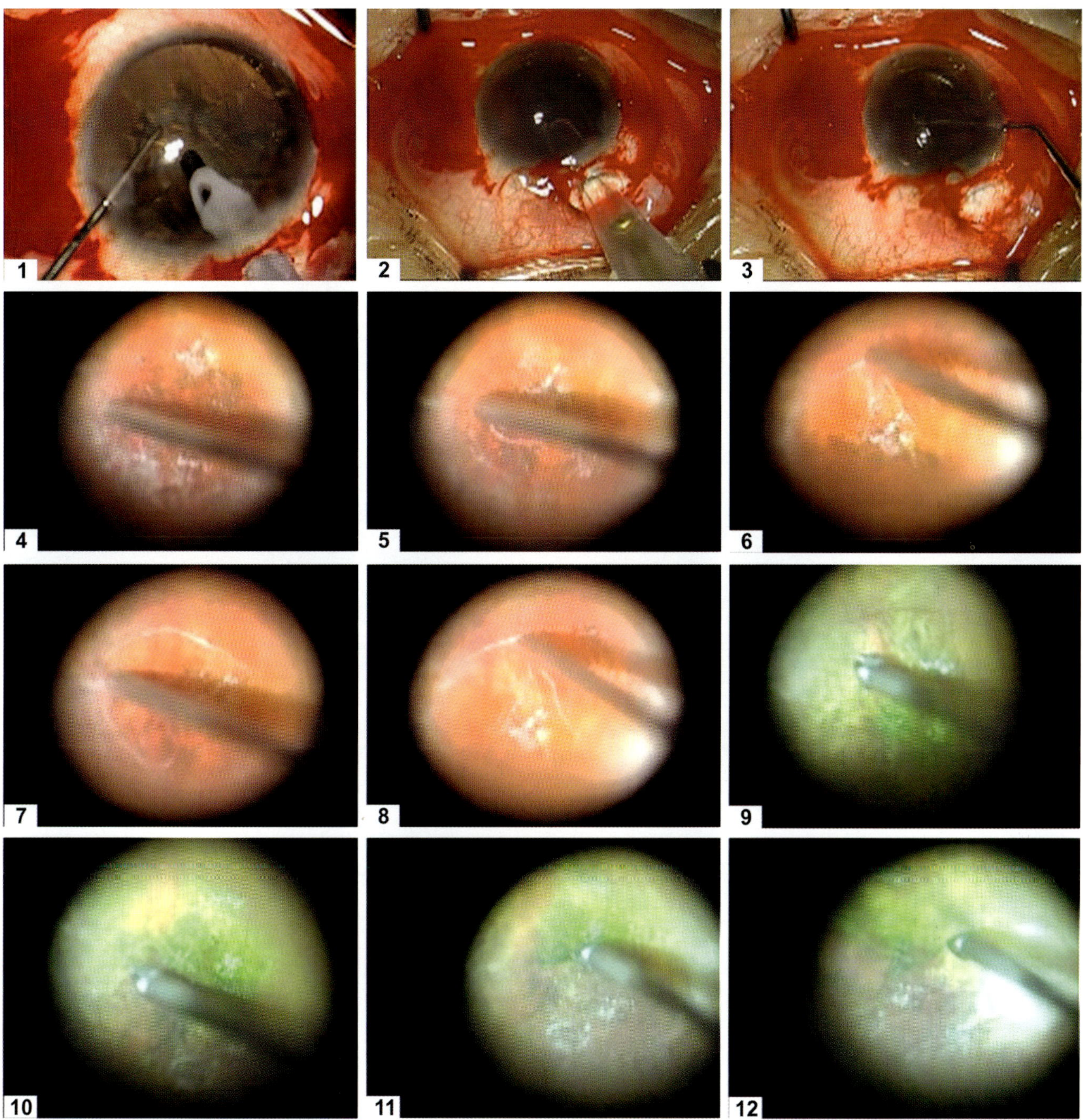

FIGURE 15.7: Surgery for myopic foveoschisis using indocyanine green dye for internal limiting membrane peeling (Prof Masahito Ohji MD, Japan).

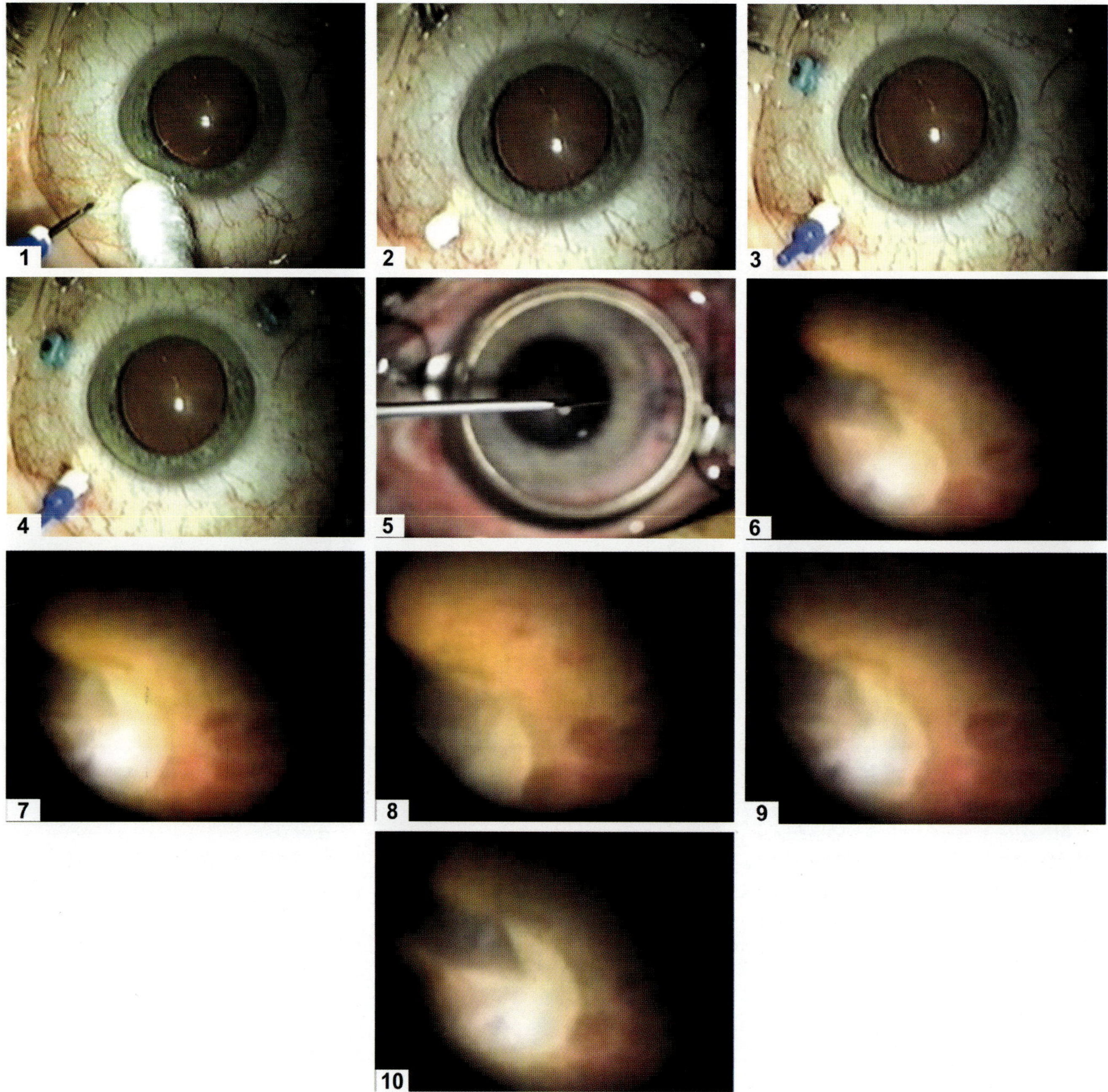

FIGURE 15.8: Radial optic neurotomy surgery for central retinal vein occlusion (Levent Akduman MD, USA).

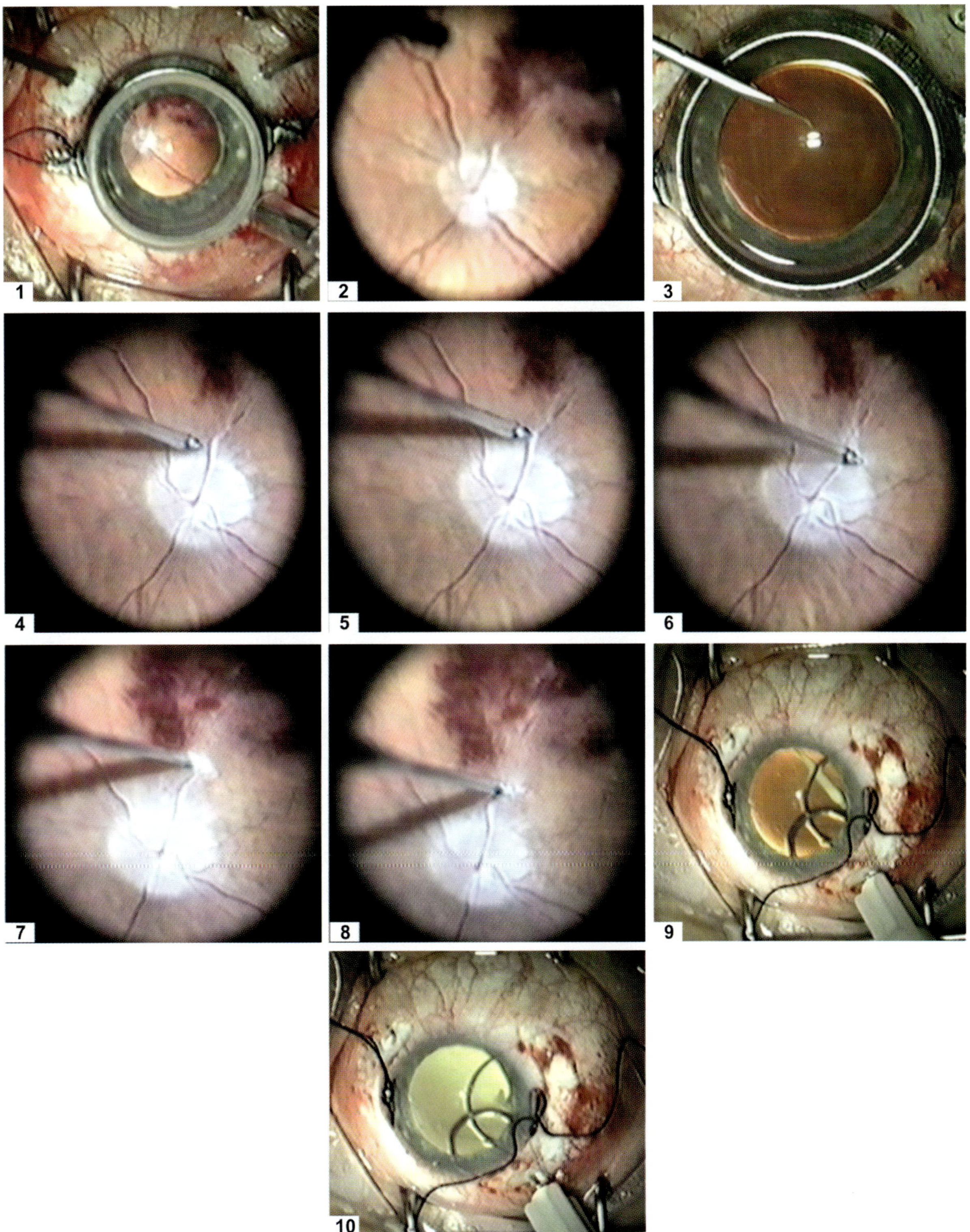

FIGURE 15.9: Arteriovenous sheathotomy for branch retinal vein occlusion (Levent Akduman MD, USA).

16

Macular Involvement in Posterior Uveitis

Jyotirmay Biswas, S Sudharshan

INTRODUCTION

Posterior uveitis is one of the vision threatening diseases, especially when the macula is involved. Several posterior uveitic entities involve the macula, which can either be infectious or non-infectious. In addition, many of these conditions develop choroidal neovascular membrane, especially in the healed stage. Common posterior uveitic entities are presented.

CAUSES/DIFFERENTIAL DIAGNOSIS

1. Infective causes
   a. Toxoplasmosis
   b. Toxocariasis
   c. Tuberculosis
   d. Herpetic
2. Non-infective causes
   a. Acute posterior multifocal placoid pigment epitheliopathy
   b. Multiple evanescent white dot syndrome
   c. Macular geographic helicoid peripapillary choroidopathy
   d. Multifocal choroiditis
   e. Punctate inner choroidopathy
   f. Birdshot choroidopathy
   g. Presumed ocular histoplasmosis syndrome
   h. Sub retinal fibrosis and uveitis syndrome
   i. Harada's disease
   j. Sympathetic ophthalmia
   k. Retina pigment epithelitis (Krill's disease)
   l. Sarcoidosis.

INFECTIONS

TOXOPLASMOSIS

Toxoplasmosis is caused by the obligate intracellular protozoan *Toxoplasma gondii*. Although it affects humans and animals, the feline species is the only definitive host.[1] It is the most common cause of posterior uveitis in the immunocompetent patients. Prevalence is higher in tropical countries than in arid or cold areas.[2]

Cats are the definitive host of *T gondii*, but many other animals and humans serve as intermediate hosts. Humans can be infected with *T gondii* by ingesting either material contaminated with infectious oocysts or tissue cysts contained in raw or undercooked meat from another intermediate host. Outbreak of ocular toxoplasmosis due to possible municipal water contamination has been reported recently.[3] It can also be transmitted by transplantation of infected organs, through blood transfusion, and through laboratory accidents.[2] Transplacental transmission of *T gondii* is the only form of human-to-human transmission of toxoplasmosis. Infection of the fetus occurs in 40% of the cases when the mother is infected during pregnancy.[2]

Most cases of toxoplasmosis in the immunocompetent host are subclinical or benign. Congenital toxoplasmosis, the more severe form, is most commonly acquired during the last trimester of pregnancy and the infants are usually asymptomatic.[1] Infection during the first three months is more severe and can lead to death and spontaneous abortion[1]. Although it has a self limiting course in immunocompetent patients, it can recur and lead to irreversible visual loss should ocular structures critical to good vision (the macula and the optic nerve) be involved.[2] Acquired toxoplasmosis in immunocompetent hosts is asymptomatic in 70 to 90% of the cases.[2] In the immunocompromised host, toxoplasmosis poses unique diagnostic and therapeutic challenges.

Clinical Features

Toxoplasmic retinochoroiditis is unilateral in 72 to 83% of the cases.[2] Ocular infection may be the only manifestation of congenital toxoplasmosis; 10% of the patients have ocular lesions without clear evidence of disease in other organs.[1, 2] Ocular toxoplasmosis occurs from activation of cysts deposited in or near the retina. Focal necrotizing retinitis is the characteristic lesion. Peripheral retinochoroidal scars are the most common ocular finding occurring in 82% of the patients.

However, *Toxoplasma* has a strong predilection for the posterior pole, particularly the macular region,[1] this location occurring in more than 50% of the cases.[2] Typical congenital toxoplasmic retinochoroiditis presents as a macular cicatricial lesion, consisting in radial deposition of pigment around a central necrotic zone (Figure 16.1). It affects primarily the retina, with secondary involvement of the choroid and the vitreous. Anterior uveitis is a

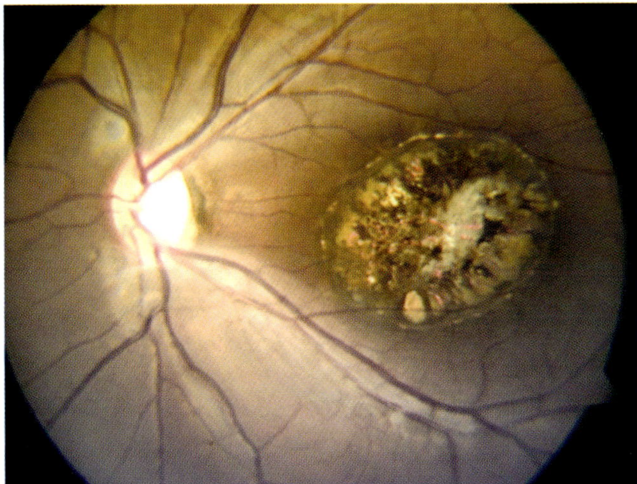

FIGURE 16.1: Typical deep punched out congenital *Toxoplasma* retinochoroiditis scar.

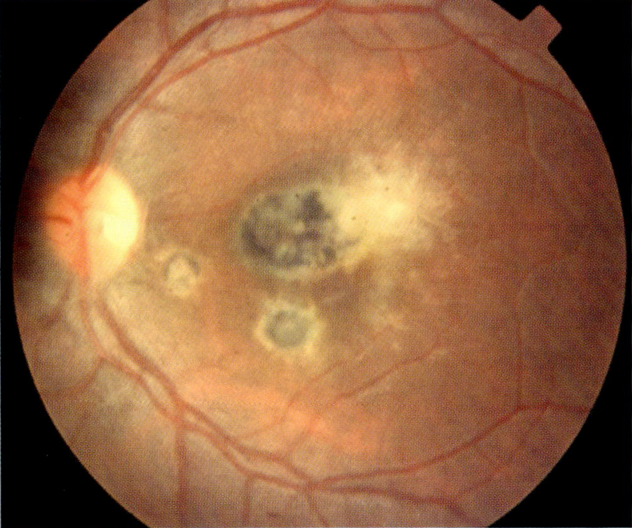

FIGURE 16.2A: Active retinochoroiditis at the edge of an old toxoplasmic scar.

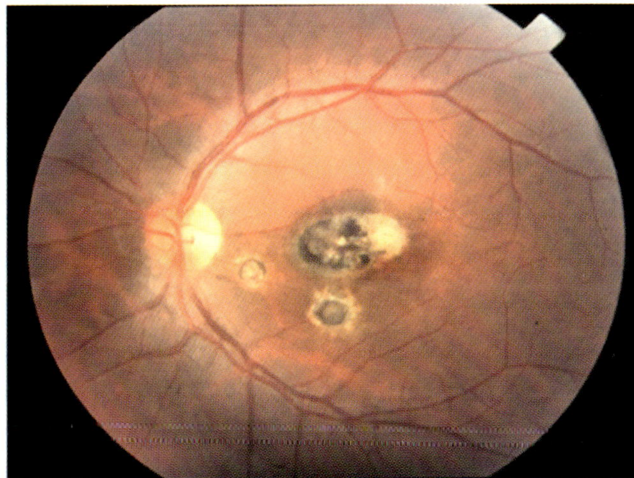

FIGURE 16.2B: Healed choroiditis at the edge of an old toxoplasmic scar.

complication of the retinochoroiditis, and the presence of the parasite in the anterior segment has been demonstrated in immunocompromised patients.[2]

Recurrent lesions frequently develop at the borders of the old *Toxoplasma* scars (Figures 16.2A and B), so called satellite lesions. Classically, the initial lesion starts in the superficial retina gradually involving the full thickness retina, adjacent choroid, vitreous and even sclera. A yellowish white or grey exudative lesion is seen with ill defined borders because of surrounding area of retinal edema. The size of the lesion varies from a fraction of the disk to about two quadrants of the retina. Adjacent choroiditis, retinal vasculitis, hemorrhage and vitritis may be seen. An active lesion accompanied by a severe vitreous inflammatory reaction will have the classic "headlight in the fog" appearance (Figures 16.3A and B). Healed scar typically has well defined borders with central retinochoroidal atrophy and peripheral pigment epithelial hyperplasia.

Toxoplasma presenting as serous macular detachment has been reported.[4] Other uncommon presentations include punctate outer retinal toxoplasmosis, retinal vasculitis and anterior uveitis. The patient may also present with complications, most common of all being secondary glaucoma.[1] Others include cataract, vitreous hemorrhage, retinal detachment, choroidal neovascular membrane (Figure 16.4), cystoid macular edema, vascular occlusions and optic atrophy.

Neuroretinitis: It typically consists of active lesions localized to the juxtapapillary region, aggressively involving the retina and optic nerve.[5] It presents with papillitis with disk hemorrhages, venous engorgement and overlying vitritis. Later, a juxtapapillary retinochoroiditis and macular star develop. *Toxoplasma* neuroretinitis is an ophthalmic emergency and requires prompt treatment[1] (Figures 16.5A and B).

Diagnosis

Diagnosis of ocular *Toxoplasma* is based mainly on clinical findings. Serological studies are helpful in suspected cases

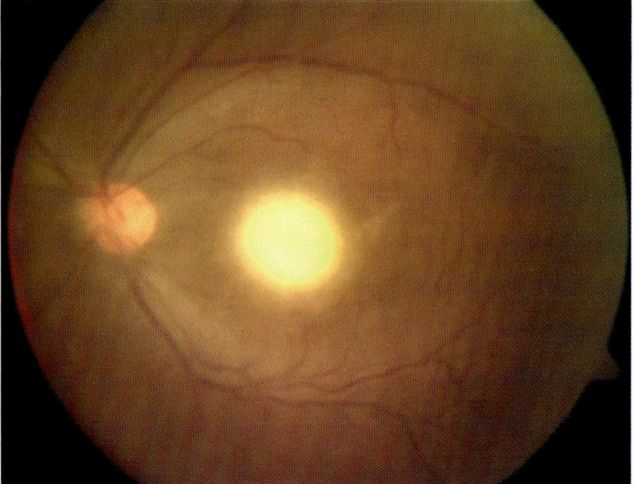

FIGURE 16.3A: Classic "headlight in the fog" appearance.

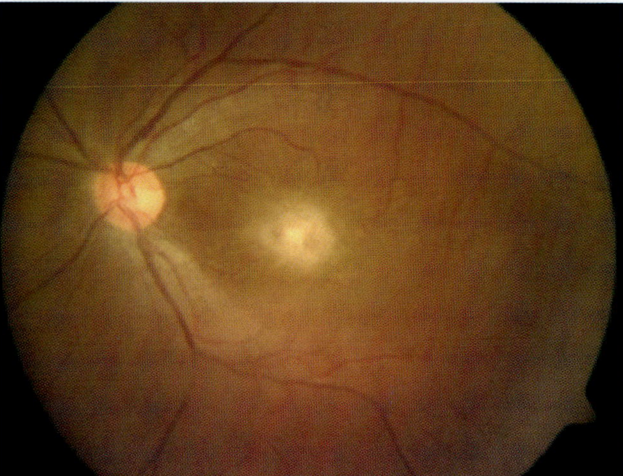

FIGURE 16.3B: Resolving *Toxoplasma* retinochoroidal lesion one-month after therapy.

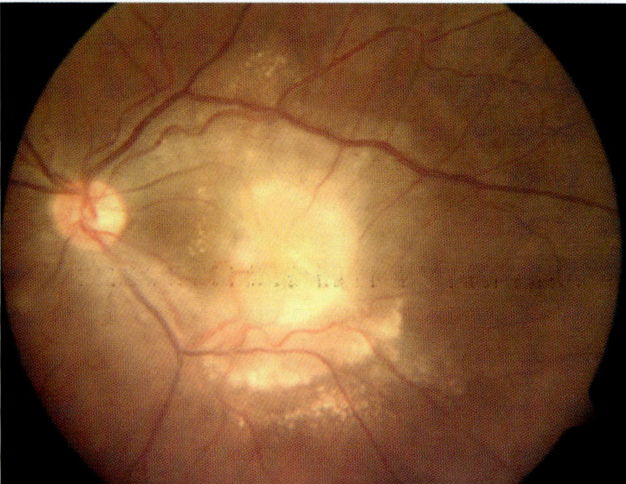

FIGURE 16.4: Post-*Toxoplasma* retinochoroiditis choroidal neovascular membrane.

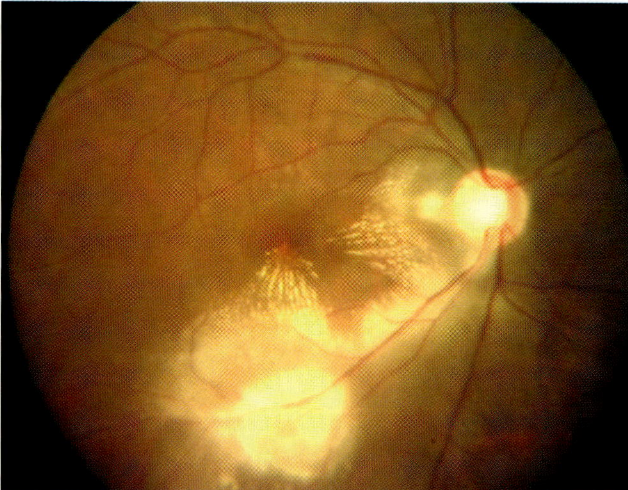

FIGURE 16.5A: Active *Toxoplasma* neuroretinitis: pre-treatment.

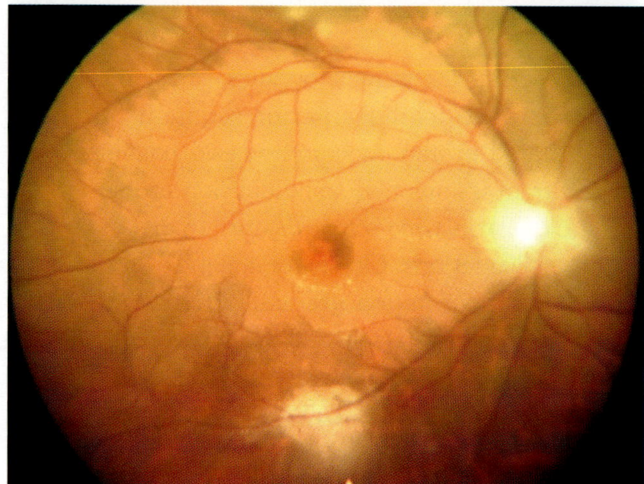

FIGURE 16.5B: Resolved *Toxoplasma* neuroretinitis: post-treatment.

or the ones with atypical presentation. However, high titers of positive *Toxoplasma* in the normal human population complicate the results of serology. Antibody detection and characterization, when associated with clinical findings, help in differentiating between recently acquired and chronic infections.[2] There are several serological tests for detection of *Toxoplasma* specific antibodies, which include the Sabin- Feldman dye test (Gold standard), complement fixation test, hemagglutination test, immunofluorescence antibody test, enzyme-linked immunosorbent assay (ELISA), immunoblotting and immunosorbent agglutination assay (ISAGA).[1] Polymerase chain reaction (PCR) is an important tool in making the diagnosis of ocular toxoplasmosis especially in cases of equivocal serology. Polymerase chain reaction and Goldman Witmer (GW) co-efficient analysis have been compared by various groups and both are found to be equally important.[6,7] In case of diagnostic dilemma, aqueous or vitreous samples may be evaluated for the presence of *Toxoplasma* DNA sequences, using this technique, with high degree of specificity and sensitivity. Antibodies titers are measured in aqueous humor and serum and Witmer-Goldman coefficient is calculated. Analysis of IgG, IgM and IgA increases the sensitivity of aqueous humor study.[1,6,7] Viral necrotizing retinopathy closely mimics *Toxoplasma* infection in immunocompromised as well as in immunocompetent individuals.[8] Polymerase chain reaction has shown to be particularly helpful in immunocompromised patients.

In newborns, the 'TORCH' infections are the major source of infection. They include toxoplasmosis, rubella, cytomegalovirus, herpes simplex virus infections and others including congenital syphilis. Other ocular entities that may be confused with toxoplasmosis include macular coloboma, primary hyperplastic primary vitreous, and retinoblastoma.

Fundus fluorescein angiography and indocyanine green angiography may be helpful in confirming the activity of the lesion and to detect complications.[9] Optical coherence tomography (OCT) is especially helpful in detecting complications such as epiretinal membrane, vitreoretinal traction, cystoid macular edema and choroidal neovascularization[2].

Treatment

Despite recent advances, an ideal combination that destroys the tissue cysts and prevents recurrence has not been found.[1, 10-12] Current therapies are targeted mainly at the active disease. A combination of the following drugs are used:

Pyrimethamine—(loading dose: 100 mg (1st day), 75 mg 2nd day, 50 mg—3rd day and followed by 25 mg once daily and

Sulfadiazine—4 G daily divided in every 6 hours)—for 4 to 6 weeks, is effective against acute toxoplasmosis in immunocompetent adults. These two drugs work synergistically against the tachyzoite form of *T. gondii*.

Other drugs used in various combinations include: Clindamycin[12] (150-450 mg/dose every 6-8 hours—maximum dose: 1.8 gm/day), Trimethoprim + sulphamethoxazol –160 mg/800 mg – one tablet twice daily.

Spiramycin—2 gm/ day in two divided doses.

Azithromycin—loading dose 1 G - 1st day, followed by 500 mg once daily for 3 weeks, Atovaquone[11]—750 mg every 6 hours for 4 to 6 weeks.

Oral corticosteroids must be initiated at least 24 hours after starting anti parasitic drugs and they must be discontinued at least 10 days before stopping specific drugs.[2]

Common combination regimens include:
1. Pyrimethamine, sulfadiazine, folinic acid and prednisolone.
2. Pyrimethamine, sulfadiazine, clindamycin, folinic acid and prednisolone.
3. Pyrimethamine, clindamycin/azithromycin, folinic acid and prednisolone.

Topical steroids and mydriatics can be used in cases with anterior uveitis based on severity. A newer fluoroquinolone, trovafloxacin has got a potent activity against *Toxoplasma* and seems to be a promising agent. Therapy for immunocompromised patients uses the same regimens for longer durations till resolution. After complete resolution of lesions, long term prophylaxis is continued in these patients till CD4 counts rises above 200 cells/ml for 6 or more months and then discontinued.[2]

Therapy regimens used during pregnancy:
1. First trimester—Spiramycin and sulfadiazine.
2. Second trimester (>14 weeks)—Spiramycin, sulfadiazine, pyrimethamine and folinic acid.
3. Third trimester—Spiramycin, pyrimethamine and folinic acid.

Treatment of the mother reduces the likelihood of congenital transmission.

Standard regimen for newborns is pyrimethamine, sulfadiazine and folinic acid.

Surgical treatment such as pars plana vitrectomy may be tried to remove vitreous opacities or to relieve the persistent vitreoretinal traction. Toxoplasmic choroidal neovascular membrane has been treated with Verteporfin photodynamic therapy with good results.[13]

In cases where optic nerve or macula is spared from the active disease, prognosis remains good. In some cases, however, macular scars, secondary glaucoma, choroidal neovascular membrane, retinal detachment cause a profound visual loss.

TOXOCARIASIS

Toxocariasis is an infection caused by the accidental ingestion of larvae of the dog roundworm *Toxocara canis* or the cat roundworm *Toxocara cati*. The soil of parks and playgrounds is commonly contaminated with the eggs of *T canis,* and infection may cause human disease in the liver, lung, muscle, eye, and brain.

Dogs or cats act as an intermediate host while the humans acquire the infection by eating contaminated soil containing toxocara larvae, or by ingesting contaminated meat. Children who have pica and are in close contact with puppies are particularly vulnerable. In the human intestine the second stage larvae migrate through the intestinal wall and enter the blood stream via the portal circulation, finally traveling to the small vessels of the end organs where they encyst. Once in the tissue, the larvae are encysted by the focal granulomatous reaction, where they can remain alive for months or even years. The granulomas are found in the brain, liver, lung and eye. The humans are an end host for the parasite as it cannot migrate back to the intestines and complete its lifecycle.

Clinical Features

Clinically, human infestation can take three different forms. The two classical expressions are visceral larva migrans and ocular toxocariasis. The third clinical manifestation has been called the covert toxocariasis.[1]

Various clinical manifestations according to the decreasing preference of the parasite are:
1. Granuloma in the peripheral retina and vitreous.
2. Posterior pole granuloma.
3. Chronic endophthalmitis.
4. Optic nerve involvement.
5. Anterior segment involvement.

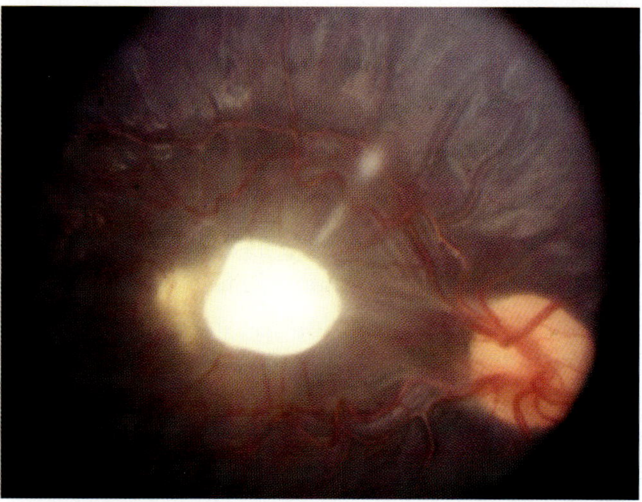

FIGURE 16.6: Toxocara: Posterior pole granuloma.

Posterior pole toxocariasis lesions are whitish or grayish-white in colour. They may be centered anywhere in the posterior pole including juxtapapillary and subfoveal location. The size of the lesion varies from less than one disk diameter to involvement of the entire macular region (Figure 16.6). Vitritis may range from minimal to severe and may mimic endophthalmitis.[14] Early lesions may be poorly visualized because of intense vitreous haze. Long-standing masses may have substantial secondary atrophy and hyperplasia of the retinal pigment epithelium. Dead larvae are sometimes seen as dark gray area within the whitish mass at the posterior pole. Choroidal neovascularization[15] and a subretinal toxocara granuloma has to be ruled out.[16]

Diagnosis and Differential Diagnosis

The diagnosis of ocular toxocariasis is based on clinical findings and the serological correlations. ELISA with *Toxocara* excretory-secretory antigen (TES-Ag) has been shown to be highly specific for toxocara infection. An increase of anti–TES-Ag IgE level indicates acute infection or progressive inflammation caused by toxocariasis. An increase in the immunoglobulin G (IgG) level confirms a past or present infection with minimum inflammation. ELISA with aqueous fluid is therefore useful when ocular toxocariasis is suspected. In addition to the above, ultrasound and to some extent CT findings may also aid in confirming the diagnosis. Calcification can occur in toxocariasis and can sometimes lead to a misdiagnosis of retinoblastoma. In children the differential diagnosis include endophthalmitis (exogenous/endogenous), intraocular neoplasm, severe inflammation such as pars planitis syndrome or juvenile rheumatoid arthritis associated uveitis, Coats' disease, persistent hyperplastic primary vitreous, late stages of retinopathy of prematurity or retinoblastoma.

Treatment

Medical treatment is directed toward the inflammatory response that produces structural damage and decreased vision. This includes initial treatment with local or systemic steroids. Since the disease process is usually seen in children, care should be taken to monitor the side effects such as growth retardation. No large case control trial as yet has compared antihelminthic therapy for ocular toxocariasis against observation alone. Most authors feel that although antihelminthic therapy may result in clinical improvement and a decrease in the antibody levels, the observed changes may simply represent the natural course of the disease.

Surgical treatment such as pars plana vitrectomy, cryopexy, laser photocoagulation has been used to treat patients with ocular toxocariasis. Vitrectomy may be beneficial for patients with endophthalmitis, unrelieved vitreoretinal traction and a tractional retinal detachment thereof.[1]

OCULAR TUBERCULOSIS (CHOROIDAL GRANULOMA AND SUBRETINAL ABSCESS)

Tuberculosis is an airborne communicable disease caused by *Mycobacterium tuberculosis* or by one of the three other closely related mycobacterial species (*M. bovis, M. africanum* and *M. microti*). The term tuberculosis implies active disease.[1]

Ocular tuberculosis includes primary, where the eye is the initial port of entry; and secondary tuberculosis, where the organisms spread to the eye hematogenously; this type includes tuberculous uveitis. Eye disease with active systemic tuberculosis was uncommon. A study from our centre noted that only 1.39% patients with systemic tuberculosis had tubercular uveitis.[17]

Clinical Features

The most common presentation of tuberculous uveitis is of disseminated choroiditis. Choroidal tubercles may be one of the earliest signs of disseminated disease.[18] The lesions may vary from few numbers to several hundred.[1] The lesions range from 0.5 to 3.0 mm in diameter and may vary in size and elevation within the same eye. They are deep, in the choroid; appear yellow; white or gray; and are fairly well circumscribed. In the vast majority of cases, the lesions present in the posterior pole.

The next most common presentation is a single tubercle, also termed focal choroiditis[19] (Figures 16.7A and B) which can occur at the posterior pole. A single

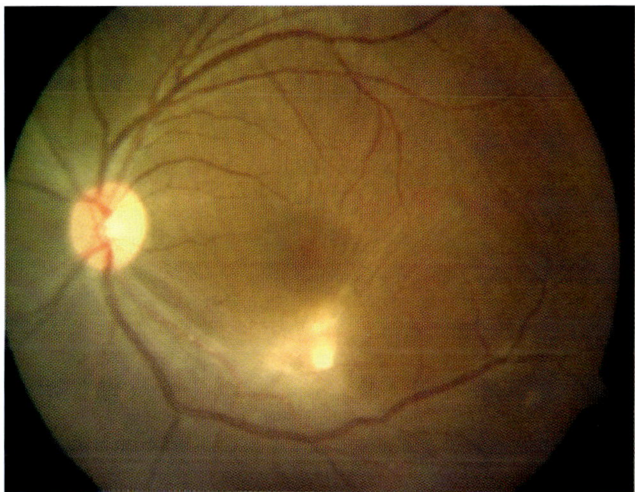

FIGURE 16.7A: Active tuberculoma of the choroid.

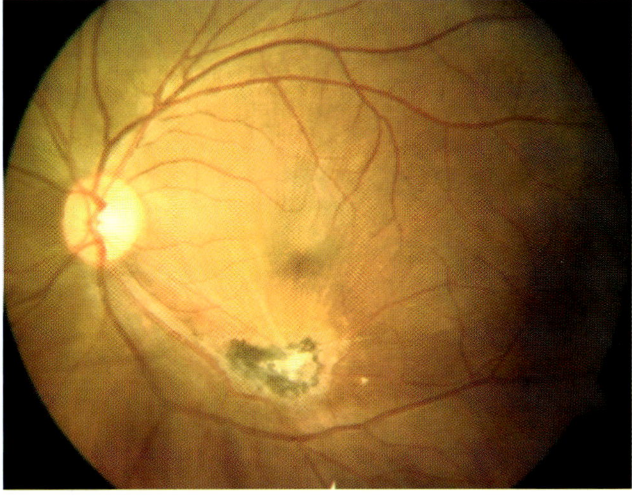

FIGURE 16.7B: Healed tuberculoma of the choroid.

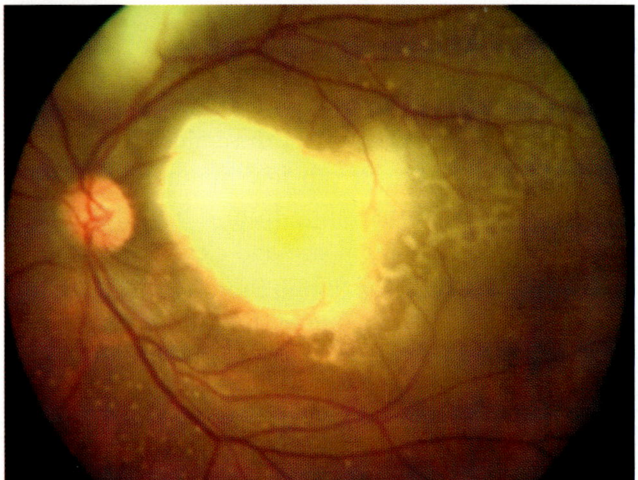

FIGURE 16.8A: Tuberculous subretinal abscess.

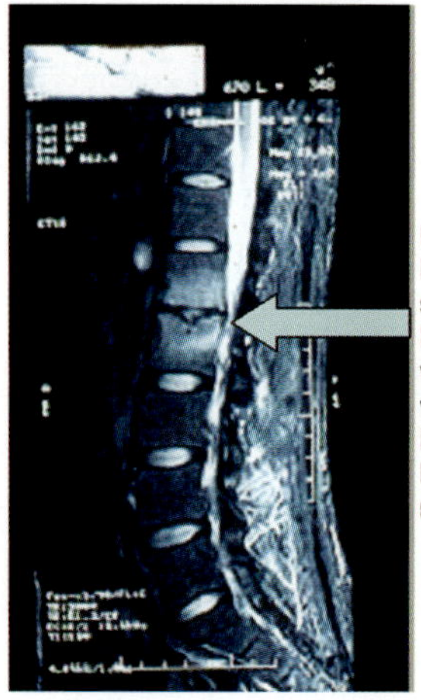

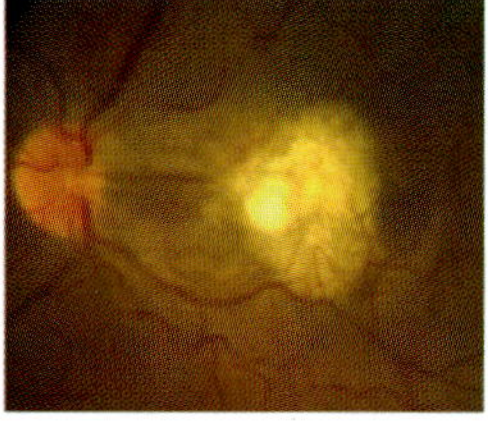

FIGURE 16.9A and B: Choroidal granuloma in a case of spinal tuberculosis.

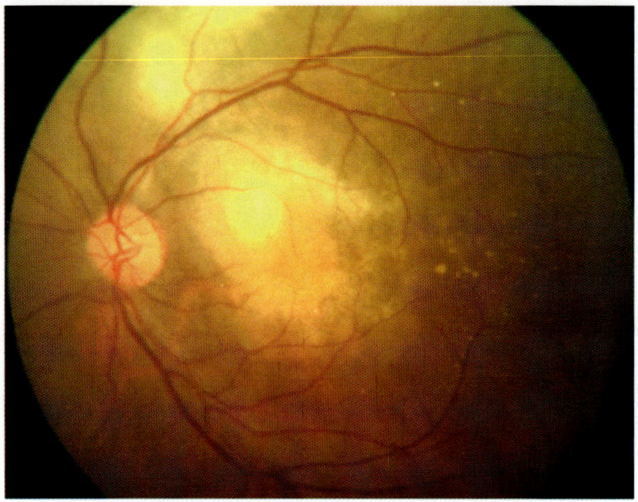

FIGURE 16.8B: Resolved tuberculous subretinal abscess .

choroidal mass is the characteristic feature on presentation, although multiple choroidal tubercles can be seen in cases of miliary tubercles and in immunosuppressed individuals. A large tubercle may measure up to 4.0 mm in diameter; however choroidal masses up to 14 mm in diameter have been reported.[20,21]

The mass is typically elevated, and may be accompanied by an overlying serous retinal detachment.[22, 23] A macular star may develop.[22] Subretinal abscess is formed progressively from a choroidal tubercle, which can be single or multiple (Figures 16.8A and B). Diagnosis is based on clinical features, suggestive systemic findings (Figure 16.9) and supportive investigations. Intraocular tuberculosis confirmed by histopathological and/or microbiological confirmation of mycobacterium infection especially by polymerase chain reaction has been reported.[24,25] However, a high index of suspicion is required in areas of low prevalence[26] as it is an important vision losing morbidity.[27] There have been reports of solitary tubercular choroidal granuloma misdiagnosed as choroidal melanoma.[28] The multiplicity of clinical findings is responsible for the delay of diagnosis.

Treatment

Primary treatment is with antituberculous therapy in collaboration with an internist, along with systemic steroids for control of the inflammatory process. Surgery should be the last resort done mostly for the complications. In case of doubt, microbiological studies of the vitreous biopsy or fine needle aspiration cytology material from the abscess can help to clinch the diagnosis. Recently, Gupta and associates[29] have reported the successful management of tubercular subretinal granulomas and have concluded that once the diagnosis of presumed or confirmed tuberculosis is established, surgical intervention should be avoided and responds well if treated promptly.[29]

Complications like choroidal neovascular membranes[30] have been reported in tubercular uveitis.

HERPETIC RETINITIS

Herpetic eye disease is among the most common causes for infectious uveitis. It may affect healthy as well as immunocompromised hosts, although its clinical presentation varies accordingly. Posterior uveitis caused by herpes viruses may appear as part of herpetic disease elsewhere (skin, brain, anterior segment of the eye) or as an isolated finding. Most forms of herpetic posterior uveitis are acute and fulminant, often resulting in serious complications such as retinal detachment and proliferative vitreoretinopathy.

Common presentation is of an acute retinal necrosis with the classical clinical triad of moderate to severe vitritis, arteritis and periphlebitis and confluent peripheral retinal necrosis. Although the posterior pole is not typically affected early in the disease process, it can also be involved primarily in necrotizing herpetic retinopathies. Polymerase chain reaction for viruses from the intraocular fluid specimen helps clinch the diagnosis in such cases with diagnostic dilemma. Treatment is long-term systemic antiviral drugs such as acyclovir. Necrotizing retinopathy due to *Toxoplasma* closely mimics this condition. Cytomegalovirus retinitis can also involve the posterior pole initially and can we found cotton-wool spots at the posterior pole in cases of HIV retinopathy (Figures 16.10A and B).

NON-NECROTIZING HERPETIC POSTERIOR UVEITIS

Several uncommon forms of non-necrotizing posterior uveitis may occur with herpetic infections. These include acute retinitis/choroiditis seen in children with varicella infection,[31-33] as well as chronic choroiditis or non-necrotizing retinal vasculitis in adults. Choroiditis may present as a solitary choroidal granuloma or as multifocal choroiditis with yellowish, punched out choroidal lesions.[34-40]

This condition is essentially a variant of acute herpetic retinitis occurring in profoundly immunosuppressed individuals, either from acquired immune deficiency syndrome (AIDS) [39] or from other disorders such as lymphoma or organ transplant. Progressive outer retinal necrosis (PORN) is most commonly caused by varicella-zoster virus but may be caused by herpes simplex virus (HSV) as well.[40] It differs from acute retinal necrosis (ARN) in some of its clinical characteristics. Although ARN

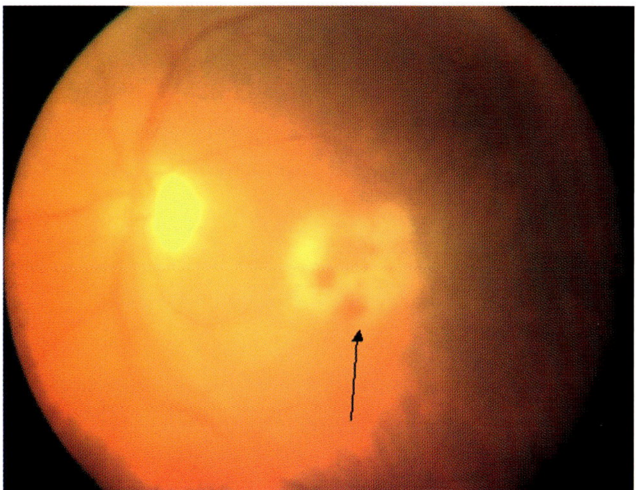

FIGURE 16.10A: Active herpetic necrotizing retinitis.

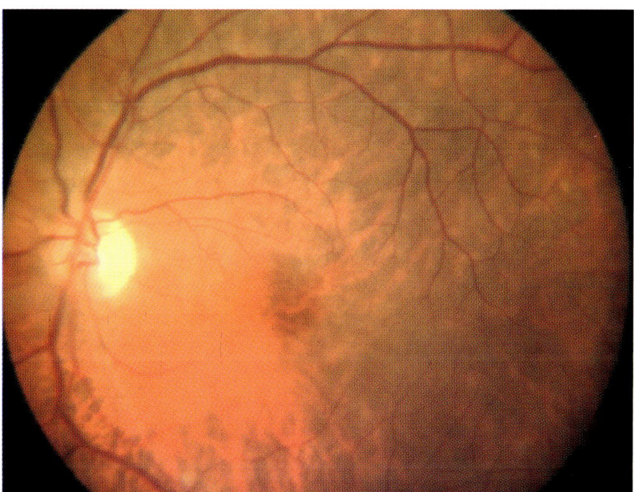

FIGURE 16.10B: Healed herpetic retinopathy: Post-treatment.

involves significant uveitis, PORN is characterized by necrotizing retinitis with a quiet vitreous and minimal or no signs of uveitis. The typical fundus picture consists of confluent areas of outer retinal whitening, involving the posterior pole early on, in contrast to ARN, which tends to spare it. Similar to ARN, it starts as patchy outer retinal areas that rapidly coalesce. Although early on the inner retina and vessels are spared, they do become involved later.[39]Although ARN and PORN are considered by some to be two different entities, they are essentially different manifestations of the same disease, with variations occurring due to different host immune response.[41] Progressive outer retinal necrosis is frequently bilateral and is associated with rapid development of rhegmatogenous retinal detachment. The principles of workup and treatment are similar to those of other viral retinitides. It is often resistant to treatment with acyclovir and requires a combination of systemic and intraocular antiviral therapy with foscarnet and ganciclovir.[42-46]

NON-INFECTIVE CAUSES

ACUTE POSTERIOR MULTIFOCAL PLACOID PIGMENT EPITHELIOPATHY

Acute Posterior Multifocal Placoid Pigment Epitheliopathy (APMPPE) was first described by Gass[47] in 1968. It is an inflammatory retinal/choroidal disease characterized by sudden loss of vision caused by the sudden appearance of multiple yellow-white, flat inflammatory lesions lying deep within the sensory retina, most notably at the level of the retinal pigment epithelium and the choriocapillaries.[1] The etiopathogenesis of this disorder remains obscure[47] till date. It is a self limiting ocular disorder with favorable visual outcome.[1, 48] Acute posterior multifocal placoid pigment epitheliopathy occurs predominantly in young adults, with the age distribution of 20 to 50 years with the mean age of 26.5 years.[1, 48] The true incidence and prevalence are not known.

Clinical Features

Patients present with acute, painless blurring of vision with associated photopsias, central and paracentral scotomas. Although usually bilateral in onset, the disorder may be asymmetric, with the involvement of other eye delayed by few days to several weeks. In approximately one-third of patients, symptoms of fever, myalgia, headache, and malaise are noted prior to the onset of ocular symptoms.[49] Anterior segment is usually quiet. Fundus examination reveals mild vitritis and characteristic multifocal, flat gray-white placoid lesions primarily in the posterior pole at the level of retinal pigment epithelium, ranging in size from 0.5 to several disk diameters (Figure 16.11). Depending on the localization of these lesions, patients may develop central or paracentral loss of vision. The overlying retina usually appears normal. After several days to weeks, the lesions begin to disappear and these areas are replaced by scattered areas of depigmentation and fine to coarse clumping of the pigment epithelium. The spontaneous healing of these lesions leaves behind varying degrees of retinal pigment epithelium atrophy and hyperpigmentation. During this time, a rapid improvement in the visual acuity may occur. Most patients completely recover; however, in a small percentage of patients, atrophy and scarring of the retinal pigment epithelium results in poor visual acuity. New lesions may be observed in the peripheral fundus for upto 3 weeks after the onset and these lesions tend to be more linear. Additional findings may include optic disk edema, keratic precipitates, retinal vasculitis, neurosensory detachments, and venous occlusions.[1]

Associated Findings

Acute posterior multifocal placoid pigment epitheliopathy has been associated with erythema nodosum, a vasculitic

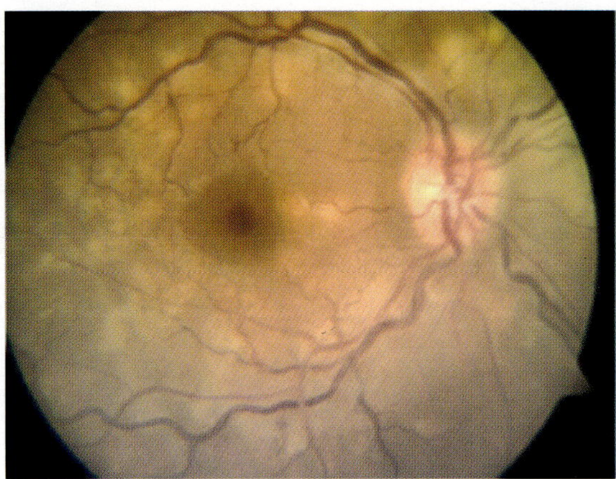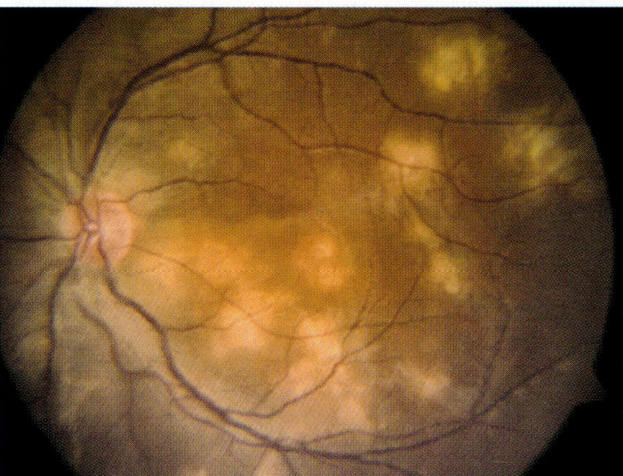

FIGURE 16.11: Acute stage of acute posterior multifocal placoid pigment epitheliopathy showing multiple flat gray placoid lesions.

condition that consists of painful subcutaneous nodules in the axilla and lower extremities. Acute posterior multifocal placoid pigment epitheliopathy with concomitant cerebral vasculitis also has been described.

Diagnosis

Fluorescein angiography in the acute, active stage shows hypofluorescence in the early phase and late hyperfluorescence of the active lesions with fluorescence persisting up to 30 minutes (Figures 16.12A and B). Inactive lesions may show window defects as a result of retinal pigment

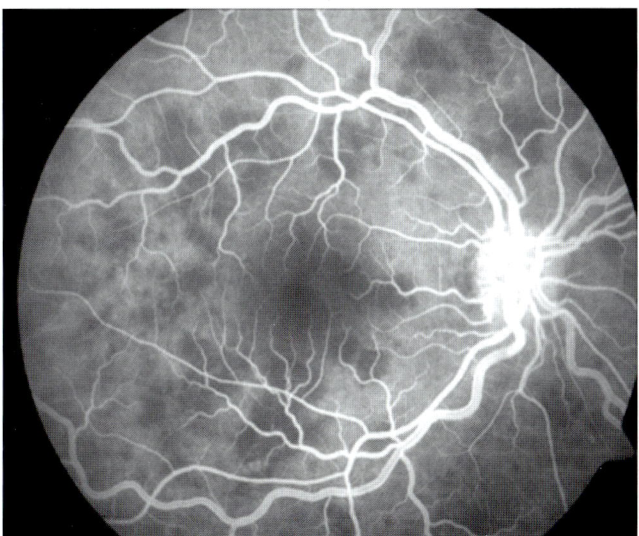

FIGURE 16.12A: Fluorescein angiography in the acute phase showing early hypofluorescence.

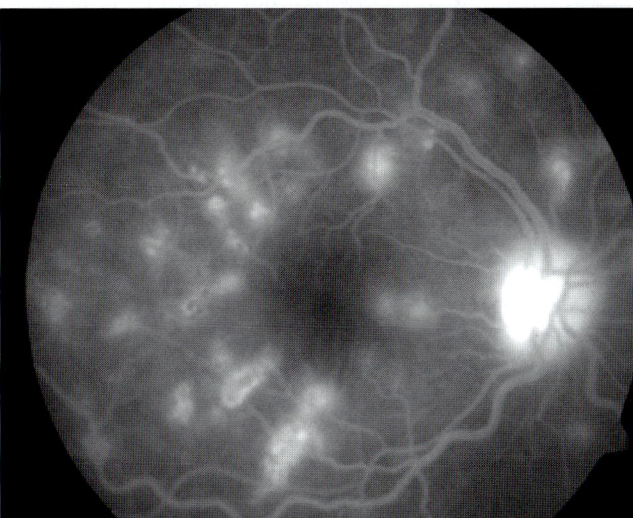

FIGURE 16.12B: Fluorescein angiography in the acute phase showing hyperfluorescence in the late phase.

epithelium atrophy and depigmentation. Indocyanine green angiography, with its ability to visualize the choroidal vascular structure, also has been used to diagnosis APMPPE. Acute lesions in APMPPE show marked choroidal hypofluorescence in both early and late phases of the indocyanine green angiogram. In the early phase, in addition, large choroidal vessels can be seen. In healed stage, choroidal hypofluorescence is seen.[48] OCT findings in conjunction with fluorescein angiography and microperimetry have been reported.[50] No consistent findings have been noted in electro-physiological testing.

Pathogenesis

The pathogenesis of APMPPE is still unknown. Occasionally, a viral prodrome occurs, and speculation exists that APMPPE may have an infectious etiology. In fact, adenovirus 5 has been isolated in one patient with a concurrent viral infection.[51] Acute posterior multifocal placoid pigment epitheliopathy also has been associated with human leukocyte antigen DR2 (HLA-DR2) and human leukocyte antigen B7 (HLA-B7), suggesting a genetic predisposition to the disease.[1] Delayed type of hypersensitivity or type IV hypersensitivity has been implicated in the pathogenesis.[52]

Differential Diagnosis

It has to be differentiated from other clinical conditions presenting with white dots in the posterior pole including non inflammatory conditions like multifocal chorio-capillaries infarcts due to hypertension, toxemia of pregnancy and disseminated intravascular coagulation.[48]

Management

Acute posterior multifocal placoid pigment epitheliopathy has a self-limited clinical course with spontaneous recovery of vision in most cases. Of those eyes that are affected, 90% of them typically achieve a visual acuity of more than 20/25 even.[53] In rare cases, recurrences may occur within 6 months of the initial episode, thereby giving a less favorable prognosis. In cases of macular involvement, corticosteroids may be considered, although their efficacy has not been proven in a controlled study.

Corticosteroids and cytotoxic drugs may be required in cases of associated cerebral vasculitis.[54] Choroidal neovascularization is a rare complication of APMPPE.

MULTIPLE EVANASCENT WHITE DOT SYNDROME

Multiple evanescent white dot syndrome is a rare disorder of unknown etiology characterized by the presence of white lesions deep in the outer retina or at the level of the retinal pigment epithelium.

The term multiple evanescent white dot syndrome was first used by Jampol and associates [55] in 1984 to describe a series of 11 young adults with transient loss of vision accompanied by white dots in the fundus. Multiple evanescent white dot syndrome occurs predominantly in young to middle-aged females in the 17 to 38 year age group,[48, 56] with a mean age of onset of 26.8 years. There have been reports of occurrence of multiple evanescent white dot syndrome more commonly in myopes especially in Japanese population.[57] In most cases, it is a unilateral disease, although bilateral involvement has been reported. A viral prodrome is known in 50 percent of the patients, and the multifocal nature of the disease, a viral prodrome is thought by many. Patients also present with acute, painless, unilateral loss of vision. In addition, patients may notice photopsias and scotomata, particularly in the temporal visual field.

Clinical Features

Examination of the fundus reveals multiple small (100 to 200 microns), round, slightly indistinct, white to yellow-white spots distributed over the posterior fundus, especially at the perifoveal and peripapillary regions. Each "dot" is composed of aggregates of many smaller dots found deep in the retina or at the level of the retinal pigment epithelium. These lesions are best appreciated by slit lamp biomicroscopy.[1] The lesions can be subtle in appearance, and careful examination is essential for accurate diagnosis. A characteristic finding of multiple evanescent white dot syndrome is foveal granularity. Additional findings that may be present include optic disk edema, mild vitritis (usually posterior vitreous cells), and a relative afferent pupillary defect. In a recent case series

of 5 patients, patients exhibited the newly recognized angiographic features termed dots and spots, which varied in size and location in the fundus. Small dots were in the inner retina or at the level of the retinal pigment epithelium, and larger spots were more external in the subpigment epithelial area.[56] There have been reports of atypical presentation with panuveitis, diffuse choroidal thickening.[58]

Diagnosis

It can be distinguished from other white dot syndromes by its distinct morphology, associated macular granularity, transient nature, characteristic angiographic appearance, unilaterality, self-limiting course, lack of significant sequelea, absence of associated systemic involvement, rapid recovery and excellent visual outcome.[1] Fluorescein angiography demonstrates early patchy or punctate hyperfluorescence with late deep staining of the retinal pigment epithelium and peripapillary area. These lesions are mostly located in the posterior pole. Occasionally leakage from the optic disk and retinal capillaries may be observed. Retinal pigment epithelium window defects may also be noted in severe cases. On closer examination, the early fluorescence of the lesions appears in a wreath-like pattern. The choroidal background fluorescence between lesions is usually normal.

Indocyanine green angiography demonstrates multiple hypofluorescent spots in the posterior pole and hypo-fluorescence around the optic nerve head, particularly in patients with enlarged blind spots. The hypofluorescent spots persist until the patient recovers.

Visual field testing usually shows considerable enlargement of the blind spot. The actual defect does not correlate with the distribution of white dots in the fundus, since the presence of white dots around the nerve are rare and the visual field defect persists even after the disappearance of the lesions.[48]

Electroretinographic studies during the acute stage demonstrates markedly reduced α-wave and early receptor potential amplitudes suggesting a primary involvement of the retinal pigment epithelium.[48] These abnormalities resolve with resolution of the disease. Multifocal ERG may be helpful in characterizing this and other blind spot enlarging conditions.[59,60]

Pathogenesis

The pathogenesis of multiple evanescent white dot syndrome is still unknown. The frequent viral prodrome may indicate an infectious etiology. Since the disease has a strong female predominance, hormonal status as a possible contributing factor is being investigated.

Management

Multiple evanescent white dot syndrome is a self-limited disease with almost all patients regaining good visual acuity within 3 to 9 weeks. Consequently, no treatment is recommended for patients with multiple evanescent white dot syndrome. The lesions disappear without scarring, and photopsias and scotomata gradually resolve. Occasionally, patients with multiple evanescent white dot syndrome may have persistent blind spot enlargement. Although uncommon, recurrences can occur. However, the prognosis is fairly good for these patients. A rare complication of multiple evanescent white dot syndrome is choroidal neovascularization that may require laser photocoagulation.[61]

MACULAR GEOGRAPHIC HELICOID PERIPAPILLARY CHOROIDOPATHY

Serpiginous choroiditis, also known as geographic helicoid peripapillary choroidopathy (GHPC), is a rare condition that typically affects middle-aged males. It was first described in 1932 by Junius.[1] It is a rare, chronic, progressive, and recurrent bilateral inflammatory disease involving the retinal pigment epithelium, the choriocapillaries and the choroid.[1] The cause is unknown. It is characterized acutely by irregular, gray-white or cream yellow subretinal infiltrates at the level of the choriocapillaries and the retinal pigment epithelium. Based on clinical presentation,[62, 63] it can be classified into:

1. Peripapillary,
2. Macular, and
3. Ampiginous types.

The clinical course, regardless of the presentation, is progressive with multiple recurrences leading to potentially significant visual loss.

Clinical Features

Patients present with unilateral or bilateral visual loss when the macula is involved, and they also may notice photopsias and scotomata. Anterior segment usually appears quiet, although a non granulomatous anterior uveitis has been described. Gray-white lesions are noted at the level of the retinal pigment epithelium. Active lesions usually are found at the border of inactive lesions (Figure 16.13A) and appear in an interlocking polygonal pattern that spreads out toward the periphery from the optic nerve. Macular involvement is common. Mild vitreous and anterior chamber inflammation is observed in one third of cases. Branch vein occlusions, although not common, have been reported.

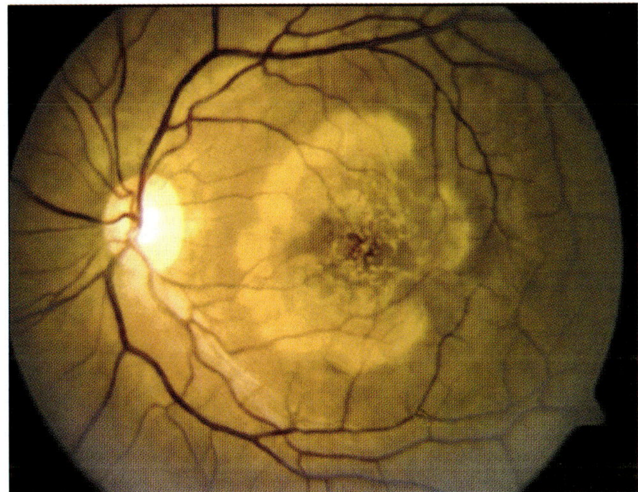

FIGURE 16.13A: Active macular geographic helicoid peripapillary choroidopathy.

Hardy and Schatz and many other workers have described a series of cases of serpiginous choroiditis in which the disease appeared initially in the macular area.[64-67] They termed the condition macular serpiginous choroiditis. This form of the disease can be unilateral or bilateral. Patients with the macular form present early in the course of the disease with an acute onset of central visual loss. Subretinal neovascularization, resulting in further visual loss, is relatively common in this type of serpiginous choroiditis.[1,68] In our case series (unpublished) 13 out of 107 eyes presented with macular involvement alone. There was no spread to the periphery in these patients even after a follow-up of almost 2 years.

Diagnosis

On fluorescein angiography, hypofluorescence is present in the center of the lesions (Figure 16.13B), and hyperfluorescence is present at the rim of the lesions in the early phase. Active lesions are hyperfluorescent in the late phase (Figure 16.13C). In addition, the choroidal vessels are easily seen on fluorescein angiography. Indocyanine green angiography does not contribute significantly toward the diagnosis. It is important to rule out other uveitic entities which involve the posterior pole.[69]

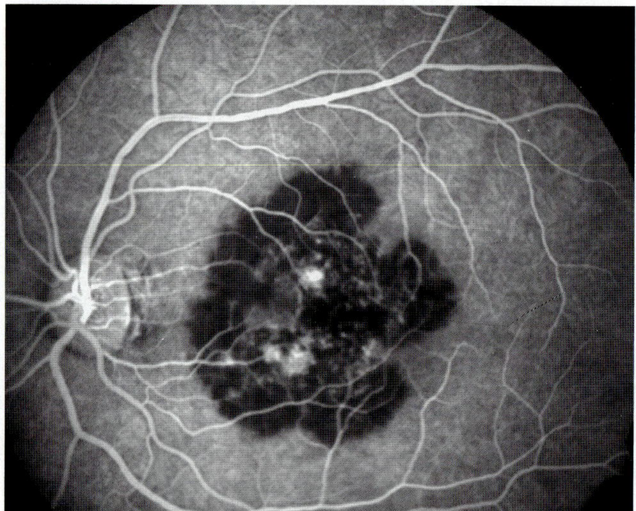

FIGURE 16.13B: Fundus fluorescein angiogram showing early hypofluorescence.

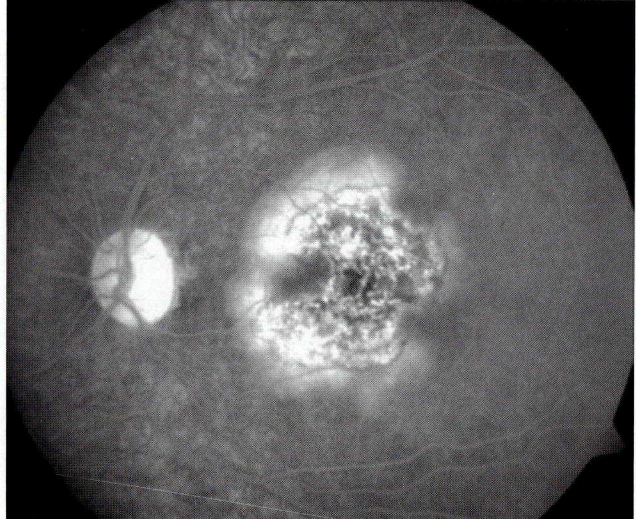

FIGURE 16.13C: Fundus fluorescein angiogram showing late hyperfluorescence.

Pathogenesis

The etiology of serpiginous choroiditis is unknown. The pathology of serpiginous choroiditis reveals lymphocytic infiltration in the affected choroid and the presence of fibroglial tissue surrounding the Bruch's membrane.

Management

It is a chronic, recurrent and progressive disease that is particularly resistant to treatment.[1] Macular GHPC is treated with an initial course of pulse therapy with IV methyl prednisolone[70] followed by systemic steroids and immunosuppressives.[71] Within a few weeks, the active lesions convert into inactive lesions with eventual retinal pigment epithelial atrophy (Figure 16.14). Inactive lesions are hypofluorescent in the early phase and staining of the sclera is visible in the late phase. If foveal involvement is absent, the visual prognosis is good. There have been successful reports with usage of intravitreal triamcinolone therapy for vision threatening serpiginous choroiditis.[72] Recurrences are common in serpiginous choroiditis. A serious complication of serpiginous choroiditis is choroidal neovascularization which can be treated appropriately.[73] However, it is of limited benefit, likely due to the abnormalities of the Bruch's membrane and the presence of lymphocytic infiltration.

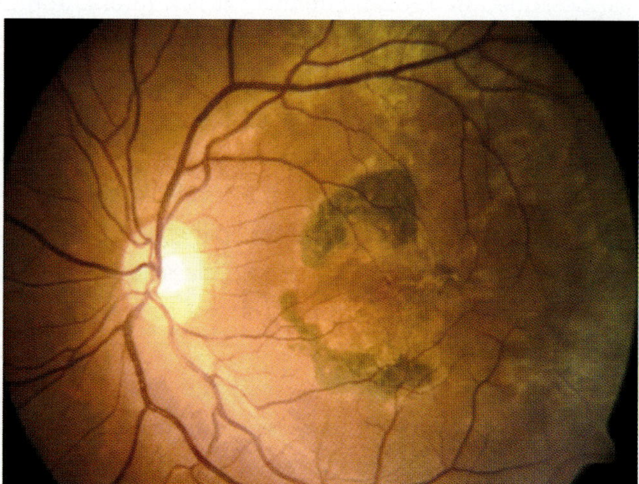

FIGURE 16.14: Fundus picture of healed geographic helicoid peripapillary choroidopathy.

MULTIFOCAL CHOROIDITIS

Multifocal choroiditis is a posterior chorioretinal inflammatory disease of unknown etiology with prominent elements of vitritis and anterior segment uveitis.[1] It occurs predominantly in myopic females between the second and sixth decades of life, [74] with a mean age of onset of 33 years. Patients usually present with an acute onset of blurred vision, photopsias, and scotomata. Bilateral involvement is present in approximately 66 to 79% of patients as reported by various studies.[75]

Ocular Findings

Examination of the fundus reveals multiple yellow or gray lesions at the level of the choroid and retinal pigment epithelium. These active lesions can range in size from 50 to 1000 μm and can be numerous (as many as several hundred at a time) (Figure 16.15A). The lesions usually are concentrated in the midperiphery. The active lesions can progress into chronic lesions, which are punched-out atrophic scars that develop pigmentation over time. The optic disk is usually normal, although, in some cases, it may be edematous. Peripapillary scarring and prominent linear chorioretinal streaks also may be present. Choroidal neovascularization can be present, in addition to peripapillary fibrosis. Almost all patients have vitreous inflammation, and many have anterior chamber inflammation. The patient also may present with cystoid macular edema.[1]

Diagnosis

The diagnosis is based on clinical examination and can be confirmed by angiographic studies. Fluorescein angiography demonstrates that active lesions show early hypofluorescence and late hyperfluorescence (Figures 16.15B and C). However, if patients present at a later stage, the active lesions usually have scarred or are in the process of scarring, thereby giving early

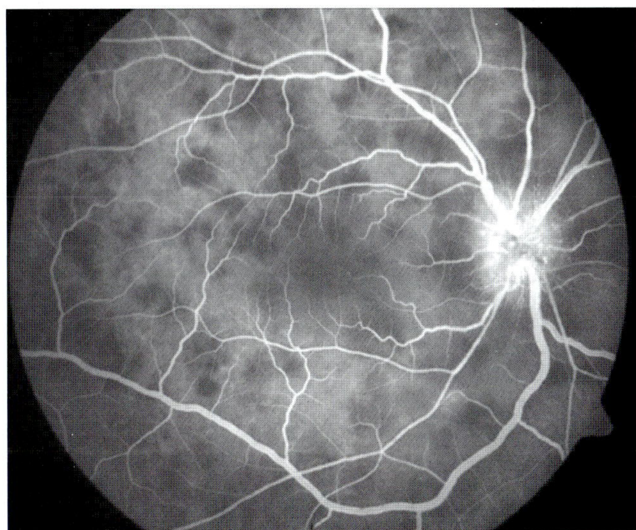

FIGURE 16.15B: Fluorescein angiography of active multifocal choroiditis showing early hypofluorescence.

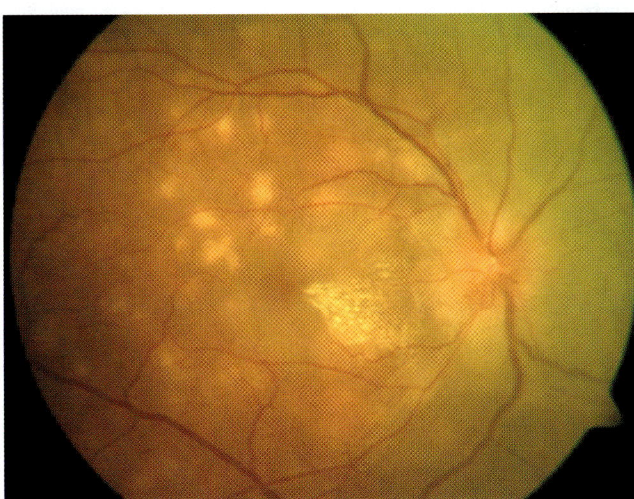

FIGURE 16.15A: Active multifocal choroiditis with hard exudates at the macula.

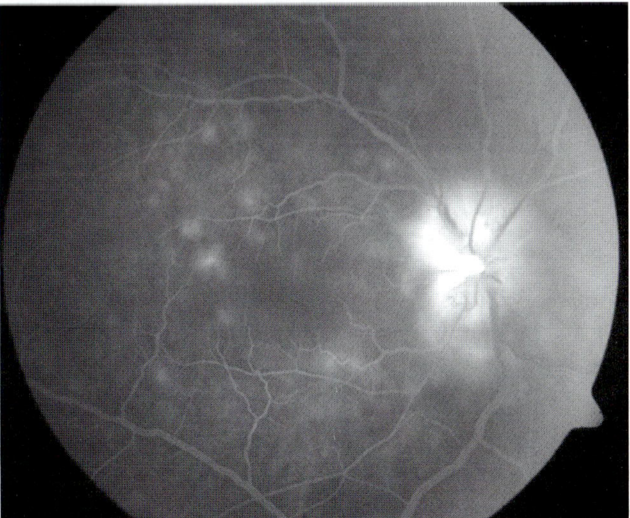

FIGURE 16.15C: Fluorescein angiography of active multifocal choroiditis showing late hyperfluorescence.

hyperfluorescence and late staining. If choroidal neovascularization is present, it usually is observed as early hyperfluorescence with a lacy appearance and a late leakage of dye. Indocyanine green angiography shows both active and chronic lesions as hypofluorescent. Indocyanine green angiography of choroidal neovascularization reveals hyperfluorescence.

Differential Diagnosis

The major disease to consider in the differential diagnosis is presumed ocular histoplasmosis syndrome.[76] The lesions in presumed ocular histoplasmosis syndrome are less numerous and smaller. However, the key distinguishing feature is that presumed ocular histoplasmosis syndrome does not present with anterior segment and vitreous inflammation. Other diseases to consider in the differential diagnosis of multifocal choroiditis with panuveitis include sarcoidosis and birdshot retinochoroidopathy.

Pathogenesis

The pathogenesis of multifocal choroiditis is unknown. Currently, controversy exists regarding the significance of a statistical association of the disease with the Epstein-Barr virus.[77]

Management

Patients with multifocal choroiditis have a chronic condition with recurrent bouts of active lesions and vitreous inflammation. These patients require long-term follow-up care. Overall, visual prognosis is variable, with final visual acuity of 20/40 or better in 66% of eyes. With each bout of inflammation, patients with multifocal choroiditis develop more active lesions, which later become atrophic with significant scarring (Figure 16.15D). Visual loss usually results from inflammatory scars in the fovea, cystoid macular edema, choroidal neovascularization, and iatrogenic induced by long-term corticosteroid use. The treatment of patients with multifocal choroiditis consists of corticosteroids. Oral steroids are helpful in patients with active posterior segment inflammation or with cystoid macular edema. Cantrill and Folk[78] noted that in their series of patients with multifocal choroiditis associated with progressive sub retinal fibrosis, the acute

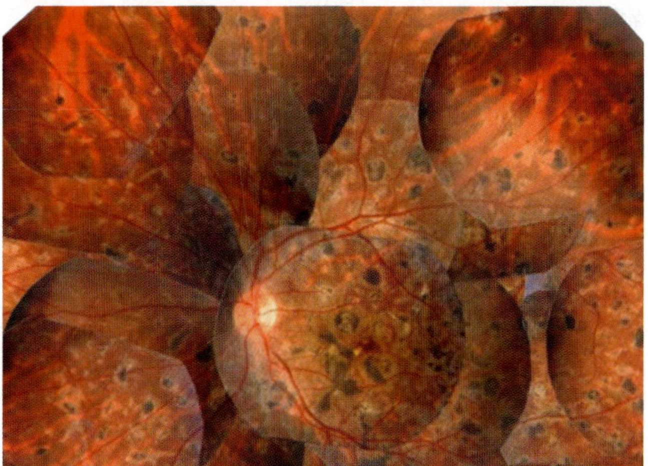

FIGURE 16.15D: Healed multifocal choroiditis.

lesions responded to systemic steroids initially in approximately 40% of cases whereas some progressed to the fibrotic stage despite treatment. Topical corticosteroids are helpful if there is severe anterior segment inflammation. However, cases in which corticosteroids have not improved the inflammation also have been described.

The most common complication of multifocal choroiditis is choroidal neovascularization (Figure 16.15E), which develops in 30% of patients. Photodynamic therapy may be indicated in these patients. Gerth and associates [79] have reported that photodynamic therapy in subfoveal or juxtafoveal classic choroidal neovascular membrane

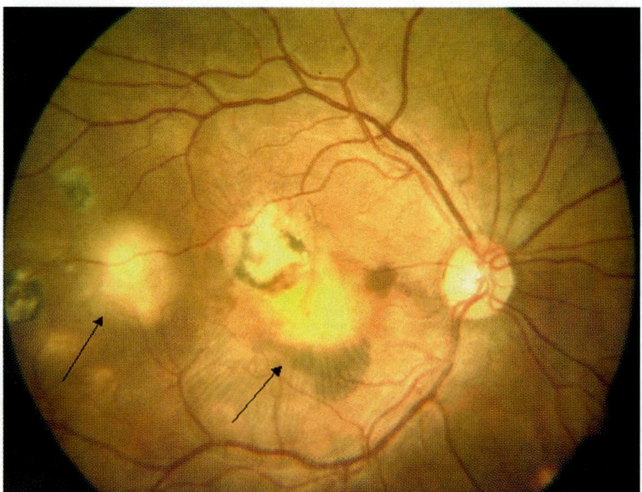

FIGURE 16.15E: Choroidal neovascularization in a case of multifocal choroiditis.

secondary to multifocal choroiditis and panuveitis stabilized or improved visual acuity in the majority of patients over a longer follow-up period. No risk factor for failed visual acuity rehabilitation could be defined. Oral steroids also may be used for choroidal neovascularization since they have been shown to decrease the neurosensory retinal detachments associated with choroidal neovascular membranes.

AMPIGENOUS CHOROIDITIS

Ampigenous choroiditis is a condition that resembles both the placoid lesions of APMPPE but some of these lesions

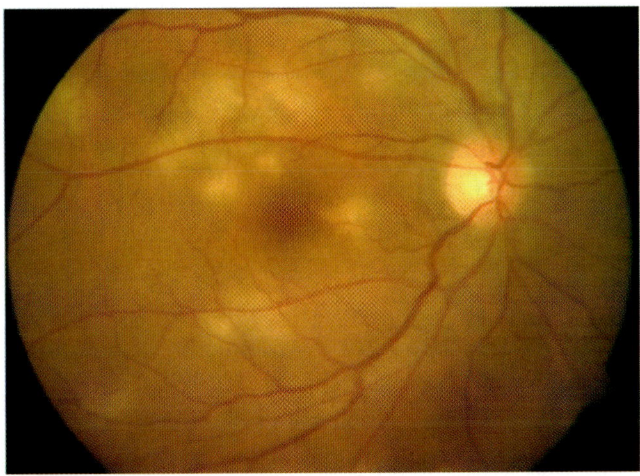

FIGURE 16.16A: Choroidal lesions resembling both placoid lesions of acute posterior multifocal placoid pigment epitheliopathy and active choroiditis patches.

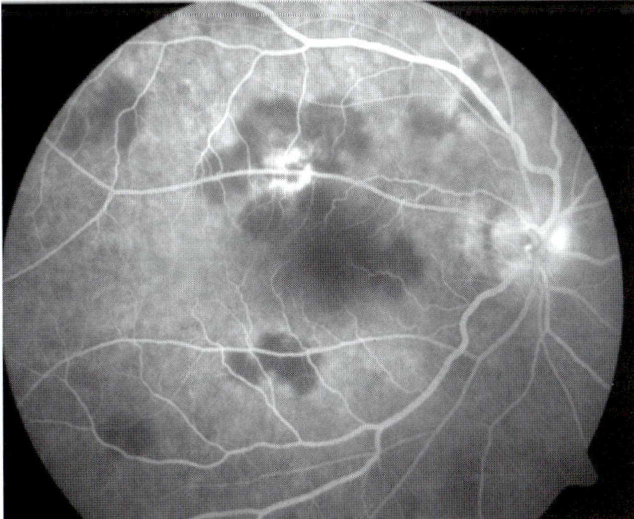

FIGURE 16.16B: Fluorescein angiography showing early hypofluorescence.

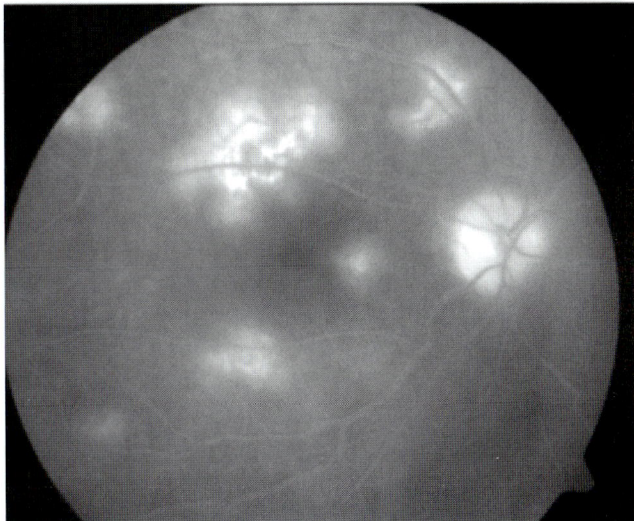

FIGURE 16.16C: Fluorescein angiography showing late hyperfluorescence.

coalesce as is seen in patients with GHPC (Figures 16.16A to C). The treatment is on similar lines as of GHPC.

PUNCTATE INNER CHOROIDOPATHY

Punctate inner choroidopathy is an inflammatory multifocal chorioretinopathy of unknown etiology. In 1984, Watzke and associates[80] described this condition in 10 myopic women.

Clinical Features

It presents with an acute bilateral loss of vision, photopsias and scotomata.[81,82] The anterior segment is quiet. The vitreous is clear without inflammatory cells. The lack of vitreous inflammation is a hallmark of punctate inner choroidopathy and the presence of vitritis should suggest a different diagnosis.[1] Fundus examination shows lesions which are multiple, discrete, flat, yellow, round lesion (50 to 300 microns) at the level of retinal pigment epithelium and the inner choroid. The numbers can vary[1] from 12 to 25 (Figures 16.17A to C). They are concentrated at the posterior pole which is different compared to multifocal choroiditis with panuveitis and sub retinal fibrosis with uveitis, where mid-peripheral lesions are more apparent. Fluorescein angiography and indocyanine green angiography[83] may assist in diagnosis.

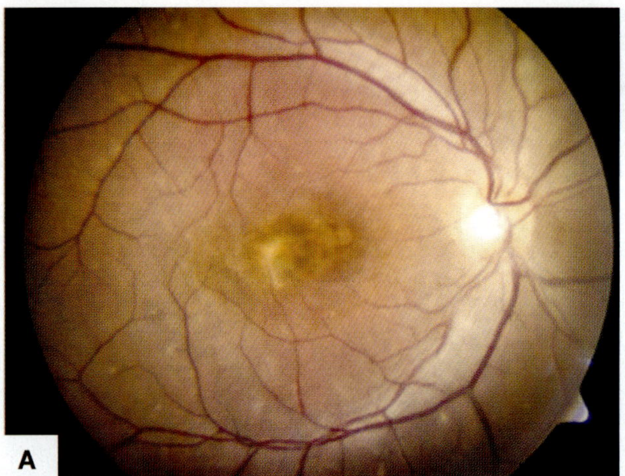

A

FIGURE 16.17A: Fundus photograph of a patient with punctate inner choroidopathy.

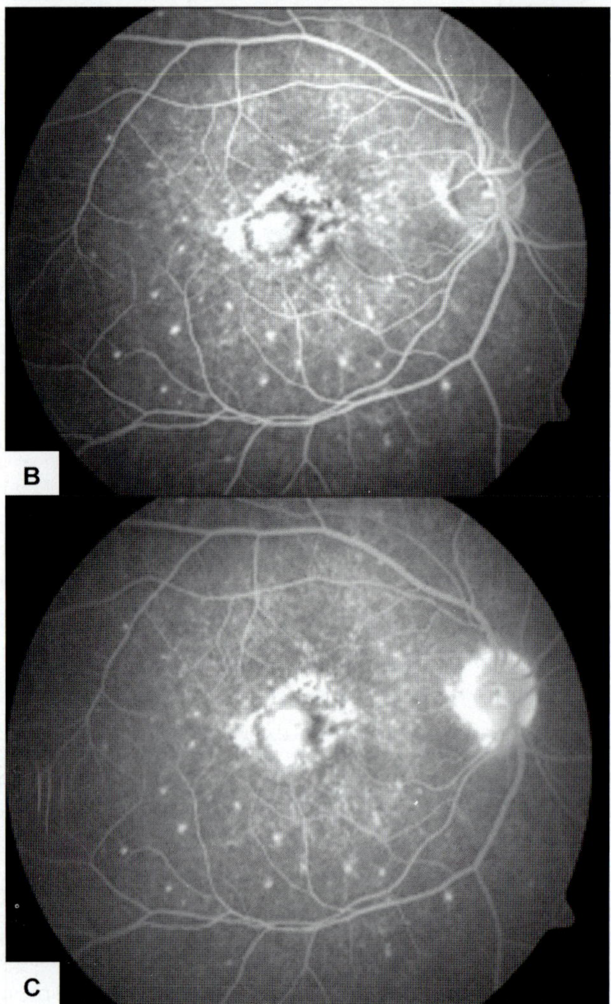

B

C

FIGURES 16.17B and C: Fluorescein angiography pictures of a patient with punctate inner choroidopathy showing punctate hyperfluorescent lesions.

Treatment

No treatment is advised for the majority of patients without evidence of choroidal neovascular membrane, as patients without choroidal neovascular membrane have excellent visual outcomes.[1] However, corticosteroids may be considered in some patients who present with poor initial visual acuity with an abundance of acute punctate inner choroidopathy lesions (with or without associated serous detachments) concentrated in the fovea.[1,84] Patients with punctate inner choroidopathy rarely have recurrences of the lesions. The initial lesions become atrophic and scarred; no new lesions erupt. In one third of patients, choroidal neovascularization develops at the site of the scar; thus, visual prognosis is causing visual loss.

SUBRETINAL FIBROSIS AND UVEITIS

The subretinal fibrosis and uveitis syndrome is a rare clinical entity that presents with a distinctive posterior uveitis and progresses to subretinal fibrosis. It belongs to the group of inflammatory conditions characterized by the presence of multifocal lesions of the retinal pigment epithelium and choroid and includes such entities as punctate inner choroidopathy and recurrent multifocal choroiditis. Although steroids in some cases have proved beneficial, the syndrome leads to progressive fibrotic sub retinal lesions with severe and permanent visual loss.[1,85] The fibrosis is predominantly at the area of previous inflammatory lesions, and a turbid, subretinal fluid that overlies the lesions also is present. Subretinal fibrosis has been reported in other inflammatory conditions, such as the late stage of serpiginous choroiditis, systemic lupus erythematosus associated central serous retinopathy and onchocerciasis.[1] This rare condition with poor visual prognosis has also been reported in other non uveitic conditions.[86]

BIRDSHOT RETINOCHOROIDOPATHY

Birdshot retinochoroidopathy is a clinically distinct, uncommon form of chronic intraocular inflammation characterized by vitritis and multiple, bilateral, hypopigmented, post equatorial inflammatory lesions in the fundus. The term birdshot retinochoroidopathy was coined by Ryan and Maumenee in 1980.[87] Also known as vitiliginous choroiditis, birdshot retinochoroidopathy typically affects females in the fourth to fifth decade of life.[88] Patients present with a painless gradual blurring of vision, floaters, and loss of color vision.[89] More than 90% of patients with birdshot chorioretinopathy are HLA-A29 positive.[90, 91] Research criteria for its diagnosis have been formulated by an international consensus conference recently.[92]

Clinical Features

The onset of visual symptoms may initially involve only one eye, but over time the fellow eye is almost always affected, although asymmetrically.[1] Examination reveals a quiet anterior chamber with rare non granulomatous uveitis in about 25% cases.[93] Ocular findings include multiple depigmented yellow-white patches scattered throughout the fundus. These lesions radiate from the optic nerve and follow the larger choroidal vessels. The term "birdshot" is given because the pattern of the lesions in the fundus is similar to the shotgun scatter of a birdshot[88] (Figure 16.18A). Vitritis, optic disk edema, and cystoid macular edema also may be present. A recent longitudinal cohort study has described the baseline clinical characteristics and has concluded that lesion pigmentation may be a marker of decreased visual function that is not reflected in central visual acuity.[94]

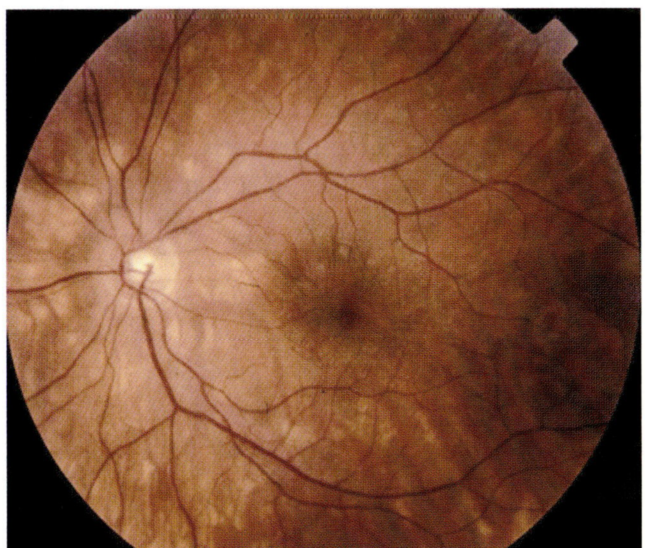

FIGURE 16.18A: Fundus photograph of birdshot choroidopathy.

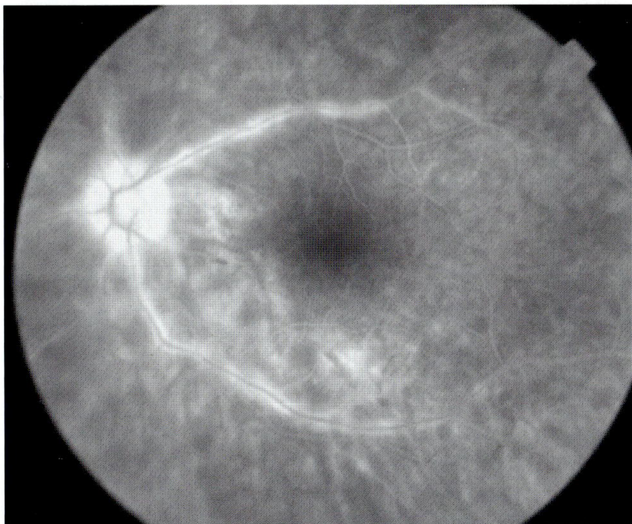

FIGURE 16.18B: Fluorescein angiography showing early hypofluorescence.

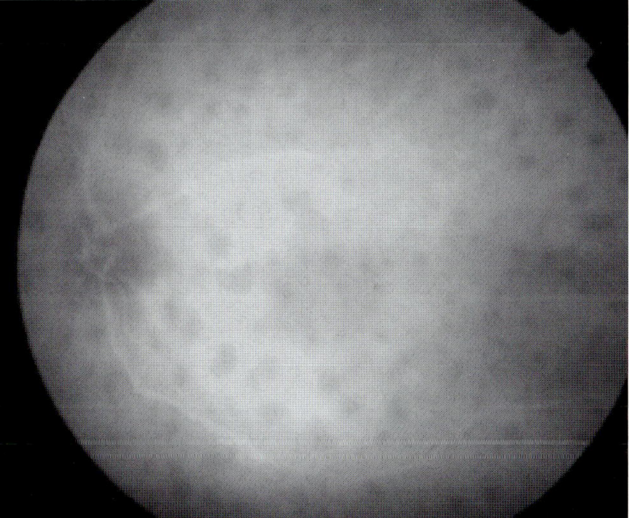

FIGURE 16.18C: Fluorescein angiography showing staining in the late phase.

Diagnosis is by clinical examination, fluorescein angiography, and HLA-A29 status. Fluorescein angiography demonstrates mild hyperfluorescence and staining in the late phase (Figures 16.18B and C).

The most common cause of a unilateral negative ERG is central retinal artery occlusion or birdshot chorioretinopathy.[95] The pathogenesis is unknown at this time; however, speculation exists regarding an autoimmune etiology. Systemic corticosteroids or immunosuppressive agents are generally the treatment of choice. Birdshot retinochoroidopathy is a chronic disease with multiple recurrences, and, consequently, the long-term visual prognosis generally is guarded.

PRESUMED OCULAR HISTOPLASMOSIS SYNDROME

Presumed ocular histoplasmosis syndrome usually occurs in endemic areas of *Histoplasma capsulatum,* which includes the Ohio and Mississippi River Valley,[1] though there are reports of its occurrence in non endemic areas.[96] Typically, adults in the fourth decade of life are affected. No sexual predilection exists. Associations of human leukocyte antigen DR2 (HLA-DR2)[97] and HLA-B7 with presumed ocular histoplasmosis syndrome has been described. Patients may be asymptomatic or may present with visual decline and a central scotoma.

On ocular examination, the vitreous is clear with no evidence of inflammation. Typically, peripapillary atrophy, atrophic chorioretinal lesions, and choroidal neovascularization are present. The lesions, which are yellow in color and resemble punched-out lesions, also may be present in the macula. Linear streaks in the midperiphery are found in a minority of the patients.[96]

The pathogenesis is presumed to be due to *H. capsulatum;* however, the organism has never been isolated from the choroid. Fluorescein angiography shows the typical features of choroidal neovascularization, i.e. early lacy hyperfluorescence with late leakage. Management of this condition includes argon laser photocoagulation for extrafoveal choroidal neovascularization, while krypton laser photocoagulation is beneficial for juxtafoveal choroidal neovascularization. Choroidal neovascularization has also been reported after LASIK procedure.[98] Dabil and associates [97] reported significant association between the HLA-DR15/HLA-DQ6 haplotype and development of choroidal neovascular lesions in presumed ocular histoplasmosis syndrome.

VOGT-KOYANAGI-HARADA SYNDROME

Vogt-Koyanagi-Harada (VKH) syndrome, formerly known as uveomeningitic syndrome, is a rare systemic disease involving various melanocyte-containing organs. Severe bilateral panuveitis associated with cutaneous, neurologic, and auditory abnormalities characterizes this syndrome. As first described by Vogt in 1906 and Koyanagi in 1929, predominantly anterior uveitis associated with poliosis, vitiligo, and auditory disturbances characterizes Vogt-Koyanagi syndrome. In 1926, Einosuke Harada reported a patient with idiopathic uveitis affecting the posterior segment with retinal detachment and meningeal irritation. At present, these 2 disorders are considered variations of a single entity referred to as Vogt-Koyanagi-Harada syndrome or uveoencephalitis[1]. It is seen predominantly in Asians, Hispanics, and Native Americans. Women are affected more commonly than men and most patients are in the 3rd to 5th decades of life at the onset of disease. The etiologic and pathogenic factors in VKH syndrome remain unclear. The clinical course of VKH syndrome with influenza like episode suggests a viral or post infectious origin. The major histopathologic feature of VKH is a diffuse granulomatous inflammation of the uveal tract with a preponderance of lymphocytes and epitheloid cells. The choriocapillaris is usually but not always involved.[1] In late stage, there is disappearance of choroidal melanocytes, chorioretinal scarring and occasionally, choroidal neovascularization.

Clinical Features

The classic course of VKH syndrome consists of the following 3 phases:

1. *Meningoencephalitis or the prodromal phase*—mimics a systemic viral infection. Symptoms include headache, fever, nausea, vertigo, orbital pain, generalized muscle weakness, hemiparesis, hemiplegia, dysarthria, and aphasia have been reported. Mental changes ranging from mild confusion to psychosis may occur. Tinnitus is a characteristic clinical symptom. It lasts for a few days.

2. *Acute uveitic phase*—most patients present to ophthalmologist at this phase. Patients with Harada's disease present with bilateral uveitis commonly. In 30% there may be asymmetric onset and presentation[99]

   a. Thickening of posterior choroid, manifested as an elevation of the peripapillary retinochoroidal layer and disk hyperemia are early findings (Figure 16.19A).

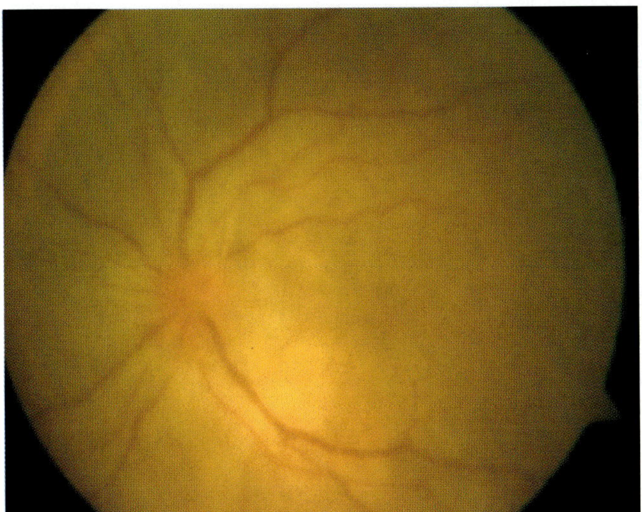

FIGURE 16.19A: Fundus picture showing disk edema with multiple pockets of fluid.

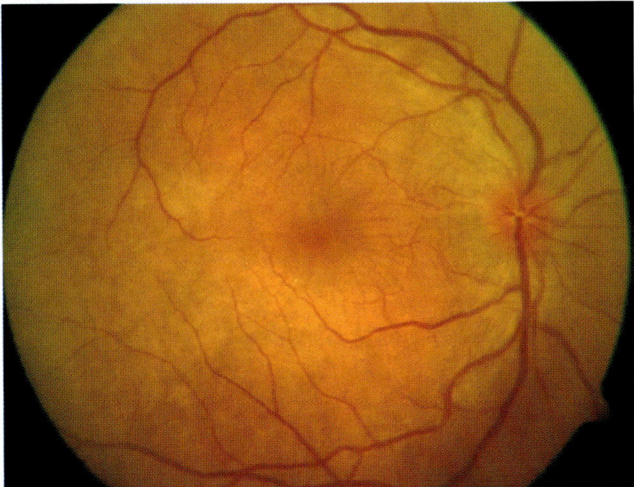

FIGURE 16.19B: Disk edema with retinochoroidal striae.

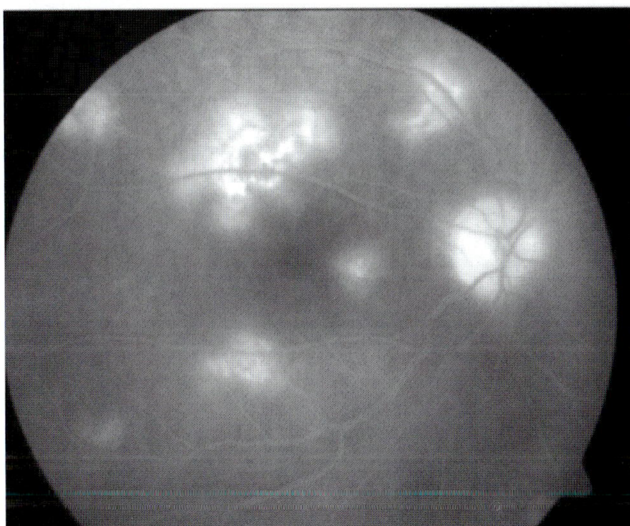

FIGURE 16.19C: Fundus picture showing multiple pockets of fluid –.

b. Retinal pigment epithelium barrier breakdown cause subretinal fluid accumulation and multiple serous retinal detachments.

c. Optic nerve head swelling is seen in 87% cases usually accompanying severe inflammation.

d. CSF pleocytosis.

e. Absence of extraocular manifestations

Early in the course of the disease, exudative retinal detachment may appear as retinal striae secondary to choroidal folds (Figure 16.19B). In addition exudative maculopathy may vary from loculated to multifocal (Figure 16.19C) to frank bullous exudative retinal detachment. The pathophysiology is choroidal inflammation leading to retinal pigment epithelium derangement and subsequent exudative retinal detachment.

Eventually the inflammation extends to the anterior segment and consists of mutton fat keratic precipitates and iris nodules. Dysacusis (usually bilateral) and tinnitus develop in 50% of patients.

Fluorescein angiography in the acute stage of VKH typically demonstrates multiple punctate hyperfluorescent dots at the level of the retinal pigment epithelium which gradually enlarge and pool in the subretinal fluid underlying areas of exudative retinal detachment (Figures 16.19D and E).

Ultrasound examination may reveal diffuse thickening of the posterior choroid, serous retinal detachment, or posterior thickening of sclera or episclera (Figure 16.20).

Optical coherence tomography is a valuable tool in picking up subtle retinal detachments and in follow up after treatment.[100]

3. *Convalescent phase*—characterized by cutaneous signs developing after uveitis begins to subside, usually within 3 months from the onset of the disease. Cutaneous signs typically occur several weeks to months after the onset of ocular inflammation.

a. Most patients have perilimbal vitiligo (Sugiura sign). Pigmentary changes tend to be permanent.

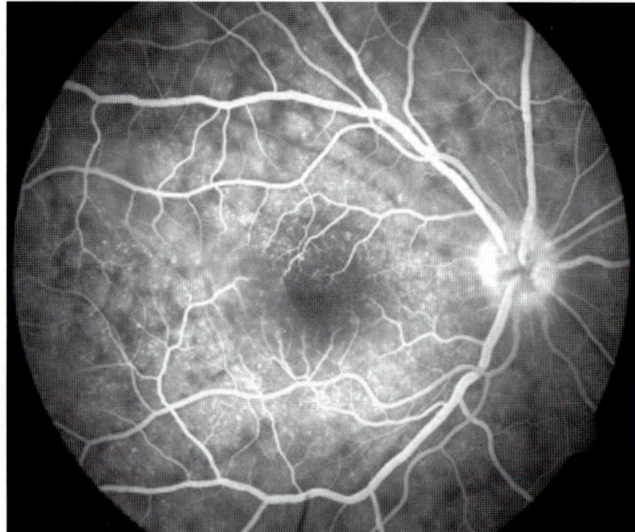

FIGURE 16.19D: Fluorescein angiography showing multiple pin point hyperfluorescence at the mid phase.

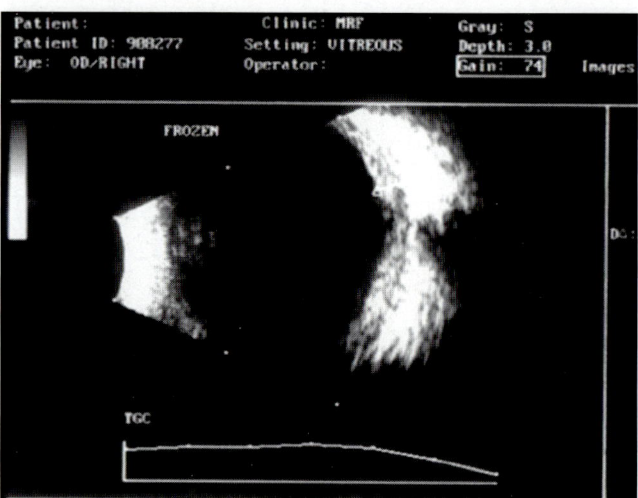

FIGURE 16.20: B scan showing increased choroidal thickness during acute phase.

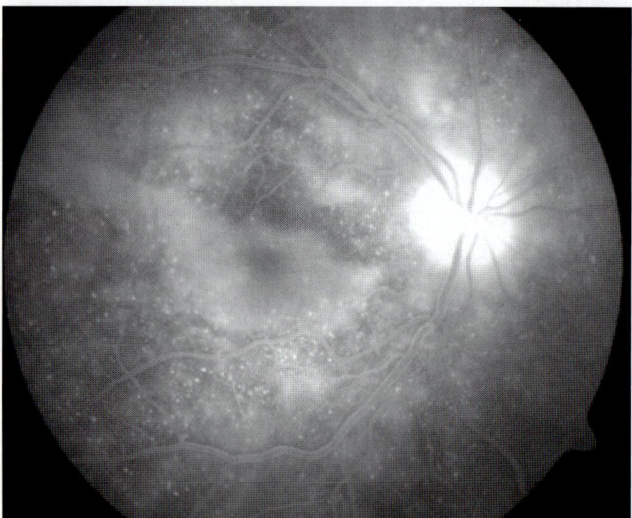

FIGURE 16.19E: Fluorescein angiography showing pooling of dye in the late phase.

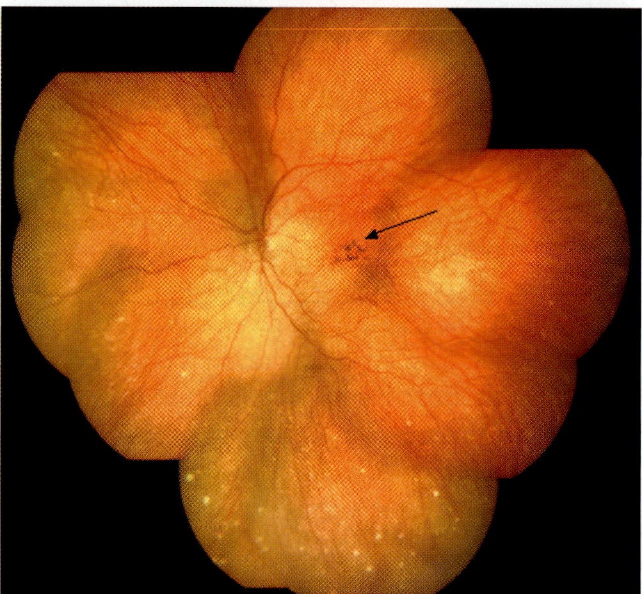

FIGURE 16.21: Typical sunset glow appearance with foveal stippling in the convalescent phase.

b. Depigmentation of the choroid causes a sunset glow fundus more commonly seen in the Asian patients (Figure 16.21).

c. Yellow white circumscribed lesions similar to Dalen Fuchs nodules are common usually in the mid periphery.

d. Poliosis, which occurs in 50% of patients, involves the eyebrows and eyelashes and, occasionally, the scalp and body hair. It usually appears after the onset of alopecia, which may be patchy or diffuse

e. Vitiligo manifests in 63% of patients and is often symmetric.

4. *Chronic recurrent phase—*

a. Complications like neovascularization of the disk or neovascularization occur.

b. Choroidal neovascularization.

Diagnosis

American Uveitis Society has recommended that, in addition to an absence of prior trauma or surgery, at least

3 of the following 4 criteria be met to confirm the diagnosis of VKH syndrome:

1. Bilateral iridocyclitis.
2. Posterior uveitis, which may include exudative retinal detachment, optic nerve swelling, or atrophy of the retinal pigment epithelium.
3. CSF pleocytosis or evidence of tinnitus, dysacusis, headache or meningismus, or cranial nerve involvement.
4. Cutaneous findings of vitiligo, alopecia, or poliosis. Read and associates[101] classified VKH based on 5 criteria into:

- Complete VKH
- Incomplete VKH
- Probable VKH (isolated ocular disease).

There have been reports of application of these for different populations and efforts for new diagnostic criterion of VKH.[102, 103]

Complete Vogt-Koyanagi-Harada Disease (Criteria 1 to 5 must be present):

1. No history of penetratring ocular trauma or surgery preceding the initial onsent of uveitis.
2. No clinical or laboratory evidence suggestive of other ocular disease entities.
3. Bilateral ocular involvement (a or b must be met, depending on the stage of disease when the patient is examined).
   a. Early manifestations of disease:
   i. There must be evidence of a diffuse choroiditis (with or without anterior uveitis, vitreous inflammatory reaction, or optic disk hyperemia), which may manifest as one of the following:
   a. Focal areas of subretinal fluid, or
   b. Bullous serous retinal detachments.
   ii. With equivocal fundus findings; both of the following must be present as well: (a) Focal areas of delay in choroidal perfusion, multifocal areas of pinpoint leakage, large placoid areas of hyperfluoresence, poling within subretinal fluid, and optic nerve staining (listed in order of sequential appearance) by fluoresceing

angiography and (b) Diffuse choroidal thickening, withtout evidenc of posterior scleritis by ultrasonography.
   b. Late manifestations of diseases. (i) History suggestive of perior presence of findings from 3a, and either both (ii) and (iii) below or multiple signs from (iii): (ii) Ocular depigmentation (either of the following manifestations is sufficient): (a) Sunset glow fundus, or (b) Sugiura sign.
   iii. Other ocular signs: (a) Nummular chorioretinal depigmented scars, or (b) Retinal pigment epithelium clumping and/or migration, or (c) Recurrent or chronic anteior uveitis.
4. Neurological/auditory findings (may have resolved by time of examination).
   a. Meningismus (malaise, fever, headache, nausea, abdominal pain, stiffness of the neck and back, or a combination of these factors: headache alone is not sufficient to meet definition of meningismus, howeve), or
   b. Tinnitus, or
   c. Cerebrospinal fluid pleocytosis.
5. Integumentary finding (not preceding onset of central nervous system or ocular disease):
   a. Alopecia, or
   b. Poliosis, or
   c. Vitiligo,

Incomplete Vogt-Koyanagi-Harada disease (criteria 1 to 3 and either 4 or 5 must be present):

1. No history of penetrating ocular trauma or surgery preceding the initial onset of uveitis, and
2. No clinical or laboratory evidence suggestie of other ocular disease entities and
3. Bilateral ocular involvement
4. Neurologic/auditory findings; as defined for complete Vogt-Koyanagi-Harada disease above, or
5. Integumentary findings; as defined for complete Vogt-Koyanagi-Harada disease above.

Probable Vogt-Koyanagi-Harada disease (isolated ocular disease; criteria i to iii must be prsent):

   i. No history of penetrating ocular trauma or surgery preceding the initial onset of uveitis.

ii. No clinical or laboratoy evidence suggestive of other ocular disease entities.

iii. Bilateral ocular involvement as defined for complete Vogt-Koyanagi-Harada disease above.

Differential diagnosis includes sympathetic ophthalmia, primary ocular B cell lymphoma, sarcoidosis, APMPPE, multiple evanescent white dot syndrome, uveal effusion syndrome, and other systemic disorders causing exudative retinal detachment such as toxemia of pregnancy and renal disease.

Patients who have evidence of neurologic involvement (headaches or meningism) may be considered for lumbar puncture which may reveal evidence of CSF pleocytosis (usually > 3 mononuclear cells/cu mm), supportive of the diagnosis.

Management

Treatment includes initial pulse corticosteroid therapy of IV methyl prednisolone 1 G daily for 3 consecutive days followed by oral steroids and immunosuppressive agents. Immunosuppressive agents[104] that can be used are cyclosporine or antimetabolites (eg, azathioprine, cyclophosphamide, methotrexate) may be required. Topical and periocular corticosteroids are also used. Cycloplegic-mydriatic eye drops are used for symptomatic relief.

Three major complications of VKH for which therapy or surgical intervention may be required are cataract, glaucoma, and choroidal neovascular membrane. Successful treatment with intravitreal triamcinolone has been reported.

The overall prognosis is fair, with the substantial number of patients achieving visual acuity of 20/50 or better with early and aggressive treatment. Ultimate visual potential may be limited by the development of cataract, glaucoma, and choroidal neovascular membrane which usually develop during the chronic recurrent phase of the disease.

SYMPATHETIC OPHTHALMIA

Sympathetic ophthalmia has been known since ancient times; however the first complete description of the disease dates back to the nineteenth century.[105] In 1865,

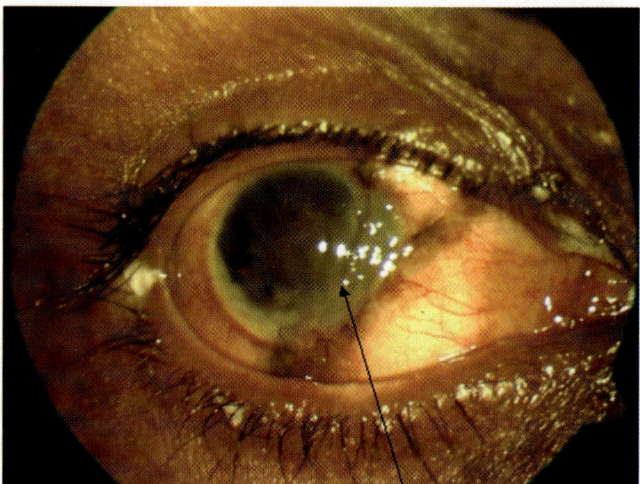

FIGURE 16.22: Slit lamp picture of the traumatized eye.

William Mackenzie described six patients, all of whom eventually became blind, who developed sympathetic ophthalmia following penetrating eye injury.

It is classically defined as a bilateral granulomatous panuveitis that occurs after either surgery or penetrating trauma to one eye. Traumatized eye is called the exciting eye (Figure 16.22) and the non-injured eye is called the sympathizing eye.[106]

The time from ocular injury to onset of sympathetic ophthalmia varies greatly, ranging from a few days to decades, with 80% of the cases occurring within 3 months after injury to the exciting eye and 90% within 1 year. Eye penetration is not essential for the development of sympathetic ophthalmia. Non-perforating procedures, such as laser cyclotherapies,[107] cyclocryotherapy[108] and proton beam irradiation for choroidal melanoma have also been associated with the disease.

In the past, trauma was the most common precipitating event; however, ocular surgery is now considered the major risk factor, particularly vitreoretinal surgery.[109,110,111]

There have also been few rare reports of sympathetic ophthalmia occurring following evisceration[112] or after surgical resection of an iridociliary melanoma.[113]

Rathinam and Rao[114] have studied the occurrence of sympathetic ophthalmia following postoperative bacterial endophthalmitis and have concluded that bacterial endophthalmitis cannot prevent the development of sympathetic ophthalmia. Early diagnosis of coexistent mixed infectious and inflammatory processes, and initiation of antimicrobial treatment directed at the infection followed by immunomodulatory agents to address the autoimmune component may improve the prognosis in such cases.

Etiology

The present theories are genetic predisposition, HLA association, ?infectious agent, retinal S antigen, primary immune dysregulation. Patients with sympathetic ophthalmia are more likely to express HLA-A11, HLA-DR4, and closely related HLADQw3 and HLA-DRw53 HLA-DRB1*04, DQA1*03, and DRB1*04 associated with sympathetic ophthalmia among Japanese, British, and Irish patients.[105]

An aberrant immune response to ocular self-antigens leads to specific ocular antigens and HLA-DR4 interaction. This triggers an inflammatory response directed at the choroid. Wu and associates[115] have postulated that retinal pigment epithelium may play a crucial role in the disease mechanism. The retinal pigment epithelium produces factors that provide a relative protection for the choriocapillaris, the retinal pigment epithelium, and the retina. Because retinal pigment epithelium has also been shown to produce cytokines that promote inflammation, it may be the unique balance of these factors in sympathetic ophthalmia that results in its manifestations.

Clinical Features

Patients with sympathetic ophthalmia may present with symptoms ranging from mild visual disturbance to significant visual loss. Near vision may be compromised, owing to change in accommodation. Patients typically present with bilateral acute anterior uveitis associated with mutton-fat keratic precipitates (Figure 16.23). In the posterior segment, the extent of inflammation can vary. Patients may have vitritis, retinal vasculitis, choroiditis and papillitis. The extent of inflammation may sometimes be represented by serous retinal detachment and optic nerve swelling in affected patients (Figure 16.24). White-yellowish lesions can be seen at the level of the choroid in the peripheral fundus of patients with sympathetic

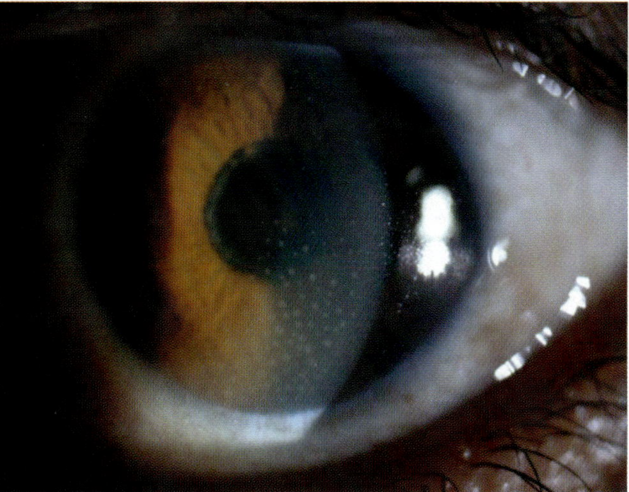

FIGURE 16.23: Slit lamp photograph showing granulomatous uveitis.

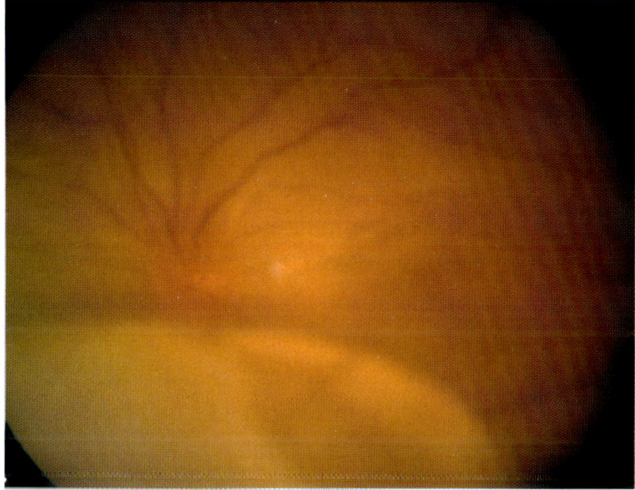

FIGURE 16.24: Disk edema with retinal detachment.

ophthalmia[106] (Figure 16.25). The clinical presentation of sympathetic ophthalmia covers a wide spectrum depending on the severity of the disease.[105]

Histopathology

Dalen-Fuchs nodules are found in approximately one-third of enucleated eyes thought to have sympathetic ophthalmia.[116] These nodules are clumps of lymphocytes and epithelioid cells usually located immediately anterior to Bruch's membrane, which may disclose breaks under visualization with electron microscopy.[117] The retinal pigment epithelium generally remains normal-appearing, but it may or may not be intact anteriorly to these nodules.

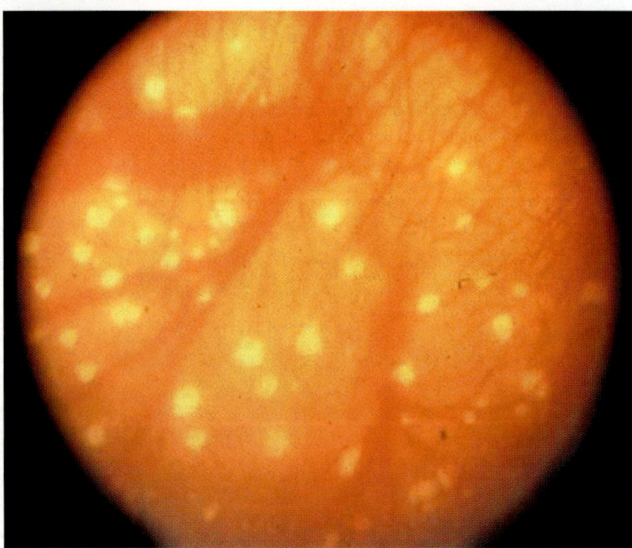

FIGURE 16.25: Dalen Fuchs nodules.

On the basis of these observations, Dalen-Fuchs nodules are postulated to be an extension of the choroidal inflammatory process in eyes affected by sympathetic ophthalmia.

Complications of sympathetic ophthalmia include secondary glaucoma, cataract, and chronic maculopathy. Choroidal neovascularization, chorioretinal and optic atrophy, and phthisis bulbi are rare and are usually related to a delayed diagnosis and inappropriate treatment.[1]

Clinical presentation of sympathetic ophthalmia and VKH are strikingly similar. Clinical differentiation is sometimes difficult[105]. Importantly, patients with VKH do not report a prior history of ocular injury. Also VKH patients usually present with systemic signs and symptoms: hearing dysfunction, skin changes, CSF pleocytosis and, meningeal signs (not classically associated with sympathetic ophthalmia) though sympathetic ophthalmia may present with extraocular findings similar to those observed with VKH disease. These findings reinforce the notion that sympathetic ophthalmia is a systemic disease requiring systemic therapy.

It is also important not to misdiagnose sympathetic ophthalmia as central serous retinopathy[118] especially in patients who have had penetrating trauma or surgical intervention in the other eye (Figures 16.26A to D). Fundus fluorescein angiography findings are similar to that seen in patients with VKH in the acute phase such as multiple pinpoint hyperflourescence in the early/mid phase and late pooling of dye due to subretinal fluid accumulation. OCT is an important tool in picking up subtle neurosensory detachments and is very useful during the follow up period (Figures 16.27A and B).

Treatment

Intra venous methyl prednisolone 1 G daily for 3 consecutive days, followed by high dose oral steroids and immunosuppressive agents in tapering doses with close monitoring of ocular and systemic status is common mode of therapy.

Triple agent immunosuppression in sympathetic ophthalmia have been found to be useful in patients with peripapillary atrophy.[119]

Cataract surgery in sympathetic ophthalmia has been found to be safe and successful if performed with vigilant preoperative and postoperative control of inflammation, careful surgical planning, and meticulous surgical technique. The final visual outcome, however, depended on the posterior segment complications of the disease.[120]

There have reports of favorable augmented response following treatment with intravitreal steroids along with systemic drugs.[121]

High degree of suspicion with early diagnosis and appropriate aggressive treatment can lead to a good prognosis in this condition.

SARCOIDOSIS

Sarcoidosis is a multisystem granulomatous disease that was first described by Jonathan Hutchinson in 1878. In 1899, Cesar Boeck demonstrated that non-caseating granulomatous inflammation was the pathologic hallmark of sarcoidosis.[1]

The clinical manifestations of sarcoidosis are variable and its course can be unpredictable. The organs affected more often are the lungs, skin and eyes. Definitive diagnosis is made by the demonstration of non-caseating granuloma by tissue biopsy. Noninvasive investigations like serum angiotensin converting enzyme and lysozyme, radiograph and CT scan of the chest, gallium scintillography, pulmonary function tests, bronchoalveolar lavage and measurement of serum and urinary calcium are helpful.[1]

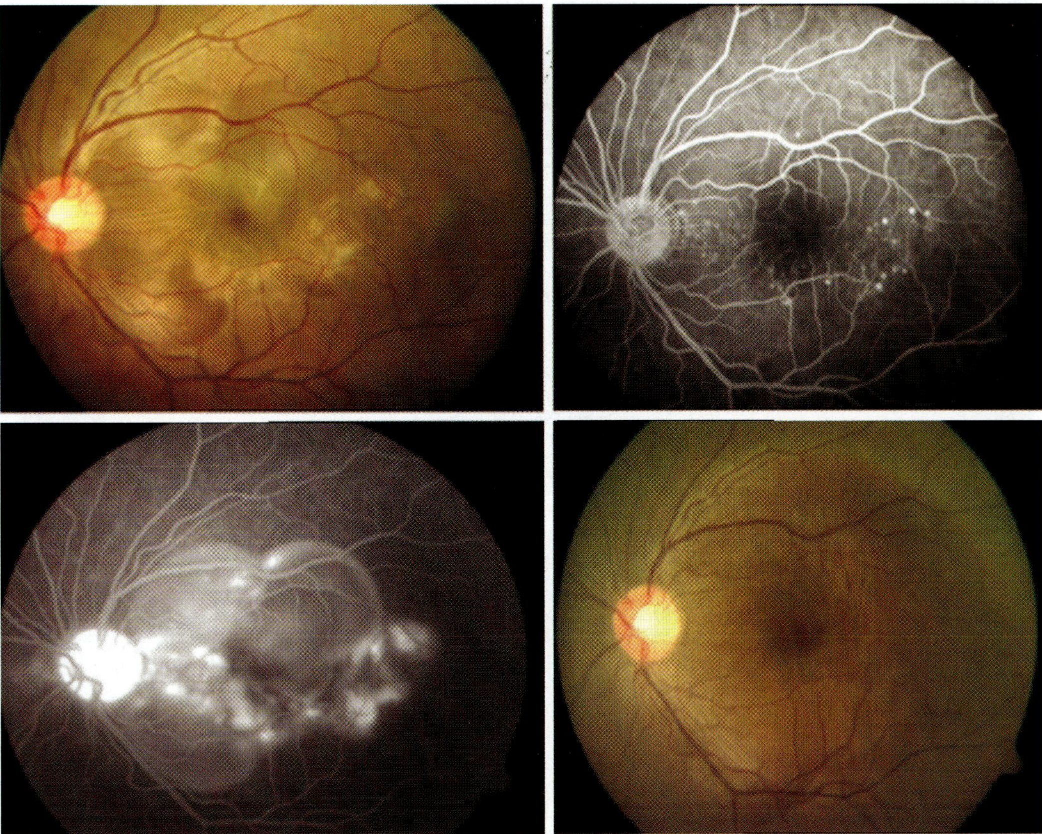

FIGURES 16.26A to D: (A) Status post-vitreoretinal surgery, misdiagnosed as central serous retinopathy. Fundus picture showing multiple pockets of fluid at the posterior pole. (B) Fluorescein angiography showing multiple pinhead leaks at the mid phase. (C) Fluorescein angiography showing pooling of the dye at the late phase. (D) Post-treatment fundus picture showing resolved lesions.

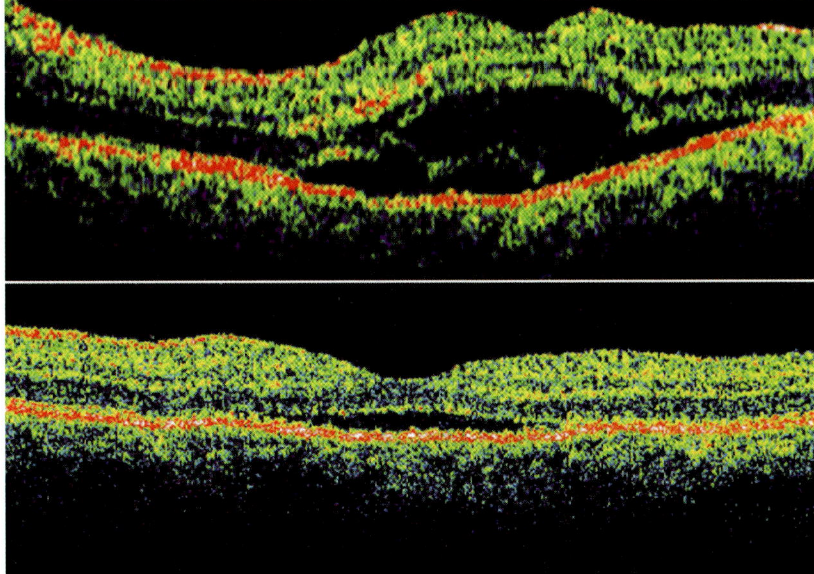

FIGURES 16.27A and B: (A) OCT scans showing neurosensory detachment in a case of sympathetic ophthalmia. (B) OCT scan showing almost complete resolution of neurosensory detachment 6 weeks after treatment.

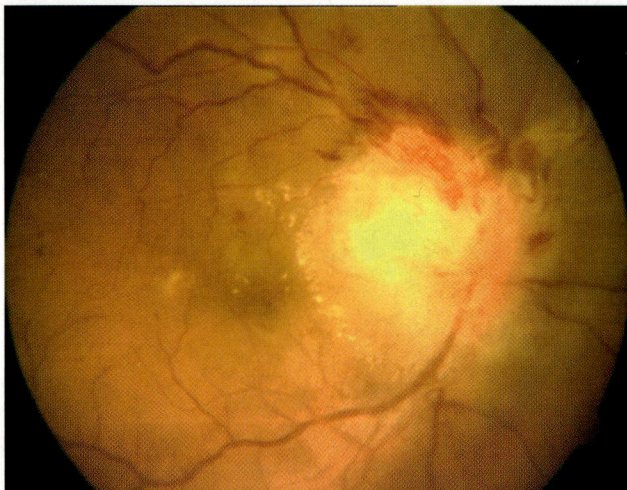

FIGURE 16.28: Sarcoid granuloma.

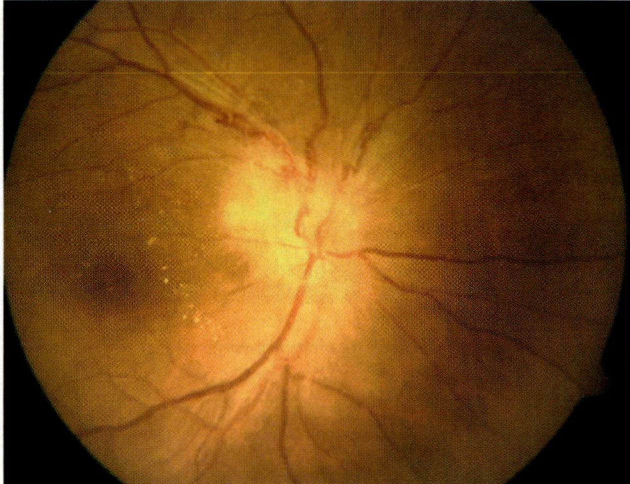

FIGURE 16.29A: Optic nerve head granuloma due to sarcoidosis: pre- treatment.

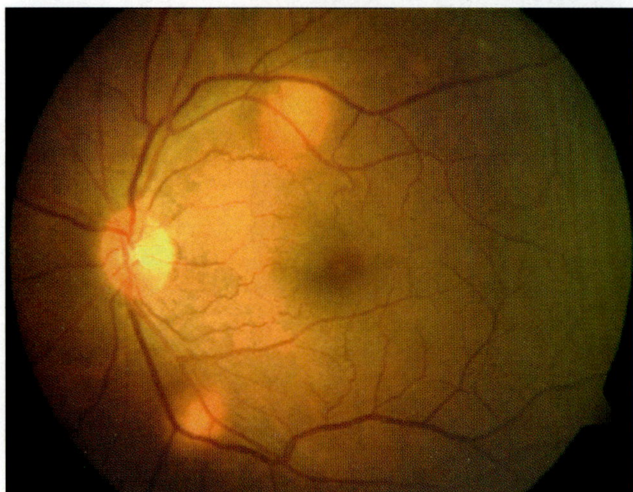

FIGURE 16.29B: Resolving optic nerve head granuloma due to sarcoid with treatment.

Ocular Features

Involvement of posterior segment is seen in 25% of the patients with ocular sarcoidosis and it can be the sole manifestation in 5 % of the patients. Posterior uveitis occurs in 12 % cases.[1] Sarcoid associated posterior uveitis has been known to be chronic with late onset of the disease. Sarcoid at the posterior pole can present with optic neuritis or neuroretinitis and as part of neurosarcoidosis. They can present as granuloma on the disk (Figure 16.28 and 16.29A and B) or at the macula. Choroidal granulomas are usually seen in about 12-15% cases.[122] Cystoid macular edema may be noted as part of posterior or panuveitis. Large inflammatory choroidal granuloma which can involve the macula have been noted (Figures 16.30A and B).

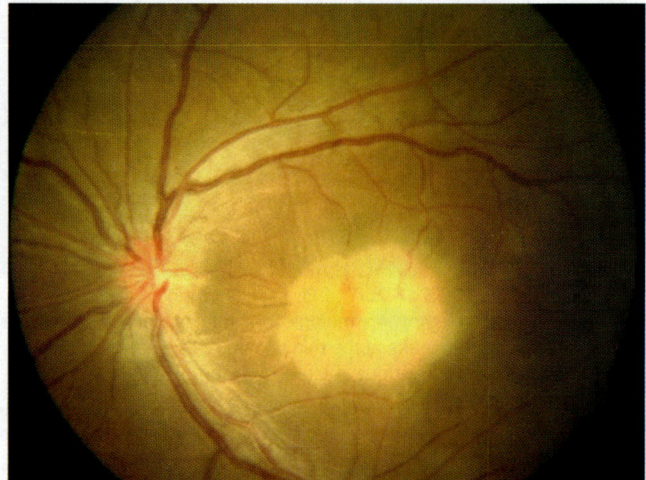

FIGURE 16.30A: Large inflammatory choroidal granuloma.

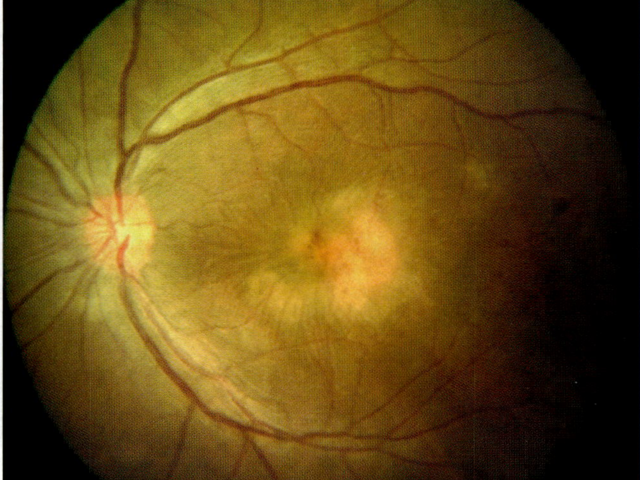

FIGURE 16.30B: Healed posterior pole choroidal granuloma.

Treatment

Once a clinical diagnosis of sarcoid uveitis has been made, the patient has to be subjected to systemic review. Sarcoid uveitis responds well to systemic steroids and immunosuppressive therapy. Dev and associates [123] have found methotrexate to be very effective in sarcoid posterior uveitis. There have been reports of good visual recovery of choroidal granuloma with intravitreal triamcinolone therapy.[124]

ACUTE RETINAL PIGMENT EPITHELITIS (KRILL'S DISEASE)

Acute retinal pigment epithelitis was first reported by Krill and Deutman.[125] They described a group of relatively young patients with subtle alterations in the retinal pigment epithelium.

It is a distinct clinical entity characterized by acute inflammation of the retinal pigment epithelium and manifested by the transient and relatively subtle alterations at the level of the retinal pigment epithelium. These are seen ophthalmoscopically as discrete clusters of small, dark-gray spots at the macular area, which clinically cause blurring of vision. Each of these spots appears to be surrounded by a yellow, halo-like zone.

Due to the acute nature of the disease the condition is often thought to be of viral origin[1].

Patients with acute retinal pigment epithelitis are typically young, healthy adults in the second to fourth decade of life. This condition has been reported to affect individuals from 16 to 75 years of age (median age of onset is about 45 years).[1]

Acute onset of unilateral blurred vision and metamorphopsia are common presenting symptoms.[48] There is usually no preceding history of illness or flu like symptoms in the otherwise healthy patient.[1]

Fundoscopy early in the disease shows the typical round macular lesions that are the hallmark of the disease. These are discrete clusters of small, hyperpigmented, dark gray spots at the level of the retinal pigment epithelium surrounded by a yellowish white halo or area of depigmentation. Each cluster typically contains one to four spots. As the condition resolves, the dark, grayish spots may further darken, displaying a pattern of pigment migration or they may fade and become difficult to detect clinically. The halo noted around these spots also becomes less distinct as the disease resolves. The lesions are generally confined to the macular region. However, extramacular lesions may also be observed, although rarely. Other structures such as optic nerve, retina and retinal vasculature are normal with absence of subretinal fluid, retinal edema or perivasculitis. Rarely vitritis may be present. The lesions resemble central serous retinopathy and fluorescein angiography is diagnostic. Fluorescein angiography shows an area of hypofluorescence surrounded by an area of hyperfluorescence.[48] In the late phase of the disease one may see lacy hyperflourescence. Visual evoked potential and ERG are usually normal, while EOG may be abnormal.[48]

Differential Diagnosis

It has to be differentiated from acute macular neuroretinopathy and APMPPE.

As the disease is known to resolve spontaneously, no treatment is needed.

SUMMARY

A host of infective and noninfective uveitic entities can involve the macula. The most common of them is toxoplasmosis. It is very important to have early diagnosis and appropriate treatment of these disorders. There can be significant loss of central vision if the treatment is delayed. Indirect ophthalmoscopy or examination with +78D or +90D lens examination of dilated fundus often provides the diagnosis. In addition, judicial usage of ancillary tests like fundus fluorescein or indocyanine green angiography, ultrasound and optical coherence tomography can be complementary to fundus examination to establish the diagnosis. While anti-infective agents are needed for infective uveitic entities like toxoplasmic retinochoroiditis, systemic steroids or immunosuppressive agents are needed for non infective (immunological) uveitic entities.

REFERENCES

1. Foster CS and Vittale AT (Eds). Diagnosis and Treatment of uveitis. Philadelphia, WB Saunders Company, 2002; pp. 264-72, 315-32, 710-25, 731-812.

2. Bonfioli and Orefice. Toxoplasmosis. Semin Ophthalmol 2005; 20:129-41.

3. Palanisamy M, Madhavan B, Balasundaram MB, et al. Outbreak of ocular toxoplasmosis in Coimbatore, India. Ind J Ophthalmol 2006; 54:129-31.

4. Kraushar MF, Gluck SB, Pass S. Toxoplasmic retino-choroiditis presenting as serous detachment of the macula. Ann Ophthalmol 1979; 11: 1513-4.

5. Eckert GU, Melamed J, Menegaz B. Optic nerve changes in ocular toxoplasmosis. Eye 2006; Published online 31 March, 2006

6. Mahalakshmi B, Therese KL, Madhavan HN, Biswas J. Diagnostic value of specific local antibody production and nucleic acid amplification technique-nested polymerase chain reaction (nPCR) in clinically suspected ocular toxoplasmosis. Ocul Immunol Inflamm 2006; 14:105-12.

7. De Groot-Mijnes JD, et al. Polymerase chain reaction and Goldmann-Witmer coefficient analysis are complimentary for the diagnosis of infectious uveitis. Am J Ophthalmol 2006; 141:313-8.

8. Balansard B, et al. Necrotising retinopathies simulating acute retinal necrosis syndrome.Br J Ophthalmol 2005; 89:96-101.

9. Atmaca LS, et al. Fluorescein and indocyanine green angiography in ocular toxoplasmosis. Graefes Arch Clin Exp Ophthalmol 2006 Published online on 4 May, 2006

10. Koo L, Young LH. Management of ocular toxoplasmosis. Int Ophthalmol Clin 2006 Spring; 46:183-93.

11. Baatz H, Mirshahi A, Puchta J, et al. Reactivation of *Toxoplasma* retinochoroiditis under atovaquone therapy in an immunocompetent patient. Ocul Immunol Inflamm 2006;14:185-7.

12. Benzina Z, Chaabouni S, Hentati N, et al. Recurrent toxoplasmic retinochoroiditis after clindamycin treatment J Fr Ophthalmol 2005; 28:958-64.

13. Wirthlin R, Song A, Song J, et al. Verteporfin photodynamic therapy of choroidal neovascularization secondary to ocular toxoplasmosis. Arch Ophthalmol 2006;124:741-3.

14. Stewart JM, Cubillan LD, Cunningham ET Jr. Prevalence, clinical features, and causes of vision loss among patients with ocular toxocariasis. Retina 2005; 25:1005-13.

15. Lampariello DA, Primo SA. Ocular toxocariasis: a rare presentation of a posterior pole granuloma with an associated choroidal neovascular membrane J Am Optom Assoc 1999; 70:245-52.

16. Higashide T. Optical coherence tomographic and angiographic findings of a case with subretinal toxocara granuloma. Am J Ophthalmol 2003;136:188-90

17. Biswas J, Badrinath SS. Ocular morbidity in patients with active systemic tuberculosis. Int Ophthalmol 1996;19: 293-8.

18. Thompson MJ, Albert DM. Ocular tuberculosis. Arch Ophthalmol 2005; 123:844-9.

19. Cangemi FE, Freidman AH, Josephberg R. Tuberculoma of the choroid. Ophthalmology 1980;87:252-8

20. Karim A, Laghmari M, Boutimzine N, et al. Choroidal granuloma revealing tuberculosis. A case report. J Fr Ophtalmol 2003; 26:614-7.

21. Lyon CE, Grimson BS, Pfeiffer RLL, et al. Clinicopatho-logical correlation of a solitary choroidal tuberculoma. Ophthalmol 1985;92:845-50.

22. Bernstein DM, Gentile RC, McCormick SA, Walsh JB. Primary choroidal tuberculoma. Arch Ophthalmol 1997;115: 430-1.

23. Chung YM, Yeh TS, Sheu SJ, Liu JH. Macular subretinal neovascularization in choroidal tuberculosis. Ann Ophthalmol 1989; 21:225-9.

24. Biswas J, Narain S, Das D, Ganesh SK. Pattern of Uveitis in a referral uveitis clinic in India. Int Ophthalmol 1996;20: 223-8.

25. Biswas J, Madhavan HN, Gopal L, Badrinath SS. Intraocular tuberculosis. Clinicopathologic study of five cases. Retina. 1995;15:461-8.

26. Varma D, Anand S, Reddy AR, et al. Tuberculosis: an under-diagnosed aetiological agent in uveitis with an effective treatment. Eye. 2005; Published online 7 October 2006;

27. Almeida SR, Finamor LP, Muccioli C. Ocular manifestation in patients with tuberculosis. Arq Bras Oftalmol 2006; 69:177-9.

28. Levecq LJ, De Potter P; Solitary choroidal tuberculoma in an immunocompetent patient. Arch Ophthalmol 2005; 123:864-6.

29. Gupta V, Gupta A, Sachdeva N, et al. Successful management of tubercular subretinal granulomas. Ocul Immunol Inflamm 2006; 14:35-40.

30. Chung YM, Yeh TS, Sheu SJ, Liu JH. Macular subretinal neovascularization in choroidal tuberculosis. Ann Ophthalmol 1989; 21:225-9.

31. MacKinnon JR, Lim Joon T, Elder JE. Chickenpox neuroretinitis in a 9 year old child. Br J Ophthalmol 2002; 86:475-6.

32. Kuo YH, Yip Y, Chen SN. Retinal vasculitis associated with chickenpox. Am J Ophthalmol 2001; 132:584-5.

33. Moinfar N, Wagner DG, Chrousos GA, et al. Paediatric varicella choroiditis. Br J Ophthalmol 1998; 82:1092-1093.

34. Roberts TV, Francis IC, Kappagoda MB, et al. Herpes zoster chorioretinopathy. Eye 1995; 9:594-8.

35. Chiquet C, Germain P, Burillon C, et al. Multifocal choroiditis associated with herpes zoster ophthalmicus. Apropos of a case. J Fr Ophtalmol 1996; 19:712-5.

36. Deegan WF; Unifocal choroiditis in primary varicella zoster (chickenpox). Arch Ophthalmol 1994; 112:735-6.

37. Frau E, Dussaix E, Offret H, et al. The possible role of herpes viruses in multifocal choroiditis and panuveitis. Int Ophthalmol 1990; 14:365-9.

38. Bloom SM, Snady-McCoy L. Multifocal choroiditis uveitis occurring after herpes zoster ophthalmicus. Am J Ophthalmol 1989; 108:733-5.

39. Forster DJ, Dugel PU, Frangieh GT, et al. Rapidly progressive outer retinal necrosis in the acquired immunodeficiency syndrome. Am J Ophthalmol 1990; 110:341-8.

40. Cunningham ET Jr, Short GA, Irvine AR, et al. Acquired immunodeficiency syndrome-associated herpes simplex virus retinitis. Clinical description and use of a polymerase chain reaction-based assay as a diagnostic tool. Arch Ophthalmol 1996; 114:834-40.

41. Gariano RF, Berreen JP, Cooney EL. Progressive outer retinal necrosis and acute retinal necrosis in fellow eyes of a patient with acquired immunodeficiency syndrome. Am J Ophthalmol 2001; 132:421-3.

42. Moorthy RS, Weinberg DV, Teich SA, et al. Management of varicella zoster virus retinitis in AIDS. Br J Ophthalmol 1997; 81:189-94.

43. Meffert SA, Kertes PJ, Lim PL, et al. Successful treatment of progressive outer retinal necrosis using high-dose intravitreal ganciclovir. Retina 1997; 17:560-2.

44. Perez-Blazquez E, Traspas R, Mendez Marin I, et al. Intravitreal ganciclovir treatment in progressive outer retinal necrosis. Am J Ophthalmol 1997; 124:418-21.

45. Ciulla TA, Rutledge BK, Morley MG, et al. The progressive outer retinal necrosis syndrome: successful treatment with combination antiviral therapy. Ophthalmic Surg Lasers 1998; 29:198-206.

46. Scott IU, Luu KM, Davis JL. Intravitreal antivirals in the management of patients with acquired immunodeficiency syndrome with progressive outer retinal necrosis. Arch Ophthalmol 2002; 120:1219-22.

47. Gass JDM. Acute posterior multifocal placoid pigment epitheliopathy. Arch Ophthalmol 1968; 80:177-85.

48. Biswas J, Dodds E. White dot syndrome. In Nema HV, Nema N (Eds): Recent Advances in Ophthalmology. New Delhi: Jaypee Brothers, 2000.

49. Jones NP. Acute posterior multifocal placoid pigment epitheliopathy. Br J Ophthalmol 1995; 79:381-9.

50. Souka AA, Hillenkamp J, Gora F, et al. Correlation between optical coherence tomography and autofluorescence in acute posterior multifocal placoid pigment epitheliopathy. Graefes Arch Clin Exp Ophthalmol 2006; Published online April 26, 2006.

51. Azar P Jr, Gohd RS, Waltman D, Gitter KA. Acute posterior multifocal placoid pigment epitheliopathy associated with adenovirus type 5 infection. Am J Ophthalmol 1975; 80:1003-5.

52. Park D, Schatz H, McDonald HR, et al: Acute multifocal posterior placoid pigment epitheliopathy: A theory of pathogenesis. Retina 1995; 15: 351-2.

53. Wolf MD, Alward WLM, Folk JC. Long-term visual function in acute posterior multifocal placoid pigment epitheliopathy. Arch Ophthalmol 1991; 109:800-3.

54. Sinan C, Thierry V, Jeffrey SR, Neil AB. Neurological manifestations of acute posterior multifocal placoid pigment epitheliopathy. Stroke. 1996; 27:996-1001.

55. Jampol LM, Sieving PA, Pugh D, et al. Multiple evanescent white dot syndrome. I Clinical findings. Arch Ophthalmol 1984; 102:671-4.

56. Gross NE, Yannuzzi LA, Freund KB, et al. Multiple evanescent white dot syndrome. Arch Ophthalmol 2006; 124:493-500.

57. Asano T, Kondo M, Kondo N, et al. High prevalence of myopia in Japanese patients with multiple evanescent white dot syndrome. Jpn J Ophthalmol 2004; 48:486-9.

58. Khurana RN, Albini T, Dea MK, et al. Atypical presentation of multiple evanescent white dot syndrome involving granular lesions of varying size. Am J Ophthalmol 2005; 139:935-7.

59. Feigl B, Haas A, El-Shabrawi Y. Multifocal ERG in multiple evanescent white dot syndrome. Graefes Arch Clin Exp Ophthalmol 2002; 240:615-21.

60. Chen D, Martidis A, Baumal CR. Transient multifocal electroretinogram dysfunction in multiple evanescent white dot syndrome. Ophthalmic Surg Lasers. 2002; 33:246-9.

61. Low U, Palmowski AM, Weich CM, Ruprecht KW. Choroidal neovascularization followed in a patient with "Multiple Evanescent White Dot Syndrome" (MEWDS) - a case report. Klin Monatsbl Augenheilkd. 2004; 221:1051-3.

62. Bock CJ, Jampol LM. Serpiginous choroiditis. In: Albert DM, Jakobiec FA (Eds): Principles and Practice of Ophthalmology. Vol. 1. Philadelphia: WB Saunders Co; 1994: 517-23.

63. Lim WK, Buggage RR, Nussenblatt RB. Serpiginous choroiditis. Surv Ophthalmol 2005; 50:231-44.

64. Mansour AM, Jampol LM, Packo KH, Hrisomalos NF: Macular serpiginous choroiditis. Retina 1988; 8:125-31.

65. Hardy RA, Schatz H: Macular geographic helicoid choroidopathy. Arch Ophthalmol 1987; 105:1237-42.

66. Laatikainen L, Erkkila H. Serpiginous choroiditis. Br J Ophthalmol 1974; 58:777-83.

67. Sahu DK, Rawoof A, Sujatha B. Macular serpiginous choroiditis. Ind J Ophthalmol 2002; 50:189-96.

68. Lee DK, Suhler EB, Augustin W, Buggage RR. Serpiginous choroidopathy presenting as choroidal neovascularization. Br J Ophthalmol 2003; 87:1184-5.

69. Sonika, Narang S, Kochhar S, et al. Posterior scleritis mimicking macular serpiginous choroiditis. Ind J Ophthalmol 2003; 51:351-3.

70. Markomichelakis NN, Halkiadakis I, Papaeythymiou-Orchan S, et al. Intravenous pulse methylprednisolone therapy for acute treatment of serpiginous choroiditis. Ocul Immunol Inflamm. 2006; 14:29-33.

71. Vianna RN, Ozdal PC, Deschenes J, Burnier MN Jr. Combination of azathioprine and corticosteroids in the treatment of serpiginous choroiditis. Can J Ophthalmol 2006; 41:183-9.

72. Karacorlu S, Ozdemir H, Karacorlu M. Intravitreal triamcinolone acetonide in serpiginous choroiditis. Jpn J Ophthalmol 2006; 50:290-1.

73. Lim JI, Flaxel CJ, LaBree L. Photodynamic therapy for choroidal neovascularization secondary to inflammatory chorioretinal disease. Ann Acad Med Singapore 2006; 35:198-202.

74. Joondeph BC, Tessler HH. Multifocal choroiditis. Int Ophthalmol Clin 1990; 30:286-90.

75. Dreyer RF, Gass JDM. Multifocal choroiditis and panuveitis. Arch Ophthalmol 1984; 102:1776-84.

76. Dreyer RF, Gass JDM. Multifocal choroiditis and panuveitis. A syndrome that mimics ocular histoplasmosis. Arch Ophthalmol 1984; 102:1776-84.

77. Tiedemann JS. Epstein Barr virus antibodies in multifocal choroiditis and panuveitis. Am J Ophthalmol 1987; 103:659-63.

78. Cantrill HL, Folk JC. Multifocal choroiditis associated with progressive subretinal fibrosis. Am J Ophthalmol 1986; 101:170-80.

79. Gerth C, Spital G, Lommatzsch A, et al. Photodynamic therapy for choroidal neovascularization in patients with multifocal choroiditis and panuveitis. Eur J Ophthalmol 2006; 16:111-8.

80. Watzke RC, et al. Punctate inner choroidopathy. Am J Ophthalmol 1984;98:572-84.

81. Brown J Jr, Folk JC, Reddy CV, Kimura AE. Visual prognosis of multifocal choroiditis, punctate inner choroidopathy and the diffuse subretinal fibrosis syndrome. Ophthalmology 1996; 103:1100-5.

82. Reddy CVV, Brown J Jr, Folk JC, et al. Enlarged blind spots in chorioretinal inflammatory disorders. Ophthalmology. 1996; 103:606-17.

83. Tiffin PAC, Maini R, Roxburgh STD, Ellingford A. Indocyanine green angiography in a case of punctate inner choroidopathy. Br J Ophthalmol 1995;90-1.

84. Levy J, Shneck M, Klemperer I, Lifshitz T. Punctate inner choroidopathy: resolution after oral steroid treatment and review of the literature. Can J Ophthalmol 2005; 40:605-8.

85. Palestine AG, Nussenblatt RB, Parver LM, et al. Progressive subretinal fibrosis and uveitis. Br J Ophthalmol 1984; 68:667.

86. Parodi MB. Progressive subretinal fibrosis in fundus flavimaculatus. Acta Ophthalmol 1994;72:260.

87. Ryan SJ, Maumenee AE. Birdshot retinochoroidopathy. Am J Ophthalmol 1980; 89:31-45.

88. Gasch AT, Smith JA, Whitcup SM. Birdshot retinochoroidopathy. Br J Ophthalmol 1999; 83: 241-9.

89. Priem HA, Oosterhuis JA. Birdshot chorioretinopathy: clinical characteristics and evolution. Br J Ophthalmol 1988; 72:646-59.

90. Priem HA, Kijlstra A, Noens L, et al. HLA typing in birdshot chorioretinopathy. Am J Ophthalmol 1988; 105:182-5.

91. Shah KH, Levinson RD, Yu F, et al. Birdshot chorioretinopathy. Surv Ophthalmol 2005; 50:519-41.

92. Levinson RD, Brezin A, Rothova A, et al. Research criteria for the diagnosis of birdshot chorioretinopathy: results of an international consensus conference. Am J Ophthalmol 2006; 141:185-7.

93. Opremcak EM. Birdshot retinochoroiditis. In Albert CM, Jakobiec FA (Eds): Principles and Practice of Ophthalmology, vol 1. Philadelphia: WB Saunders, 1994; p. 475

94. Monnet D, Brezin AP, Holland GN, et al. Longitudinal cohort study of patients with birdshot chorioretinopathy. I. Baseline clinical characteristics. Am J Ophthalmol 2006; 141:135-42.

95. Robson AG, Richardson EC, Koh AH, et al. Unilateral electronegative ERG of non-vascular aetiology. Br J Ophthalmol 2005; 89:1620-6.

96. Chryssafis C, Neubauer A, Haritoglou C, Gandorfer A. Presumed ocular histoplasmosis syndrome (POHS) in a non-endemic area. Klin Monatsbl Augenheilkd. 2004; 221:128-30.

97. Dabil H, Kaplan HJ, Duffy BF, Phelan DL, Mohanakumar T, Jaramillo A. Association of the HLA-DR15/HLA-DQ6 haplotype with development of choroidal neovascular lesions in presumed ocular histoplasmosis syndrome. Hum Immunol 2003; 64:960-4.

98. Fedorovich I, Mehr DS, Oz O, Akduman L. Choroidal neovascularization after laser in situ keratomileusis in a patient with presumed ocular histoplasmosis syndrome. Eur J Ophthalmol 2004; 14:261-3.

99. Damico FM, Kiss S, Young LH. Vogt-Koyanagi-Harada disease. Semin Ophthalmol 2005; 20:183-90.

100. Maruyama Y, Kishi S. Tomographic features of serous retinal detachment in Vogt-Koyanagi-Harada syndrome. Ophthalmic Surg Lasers Imaging. 2004;35:239-42.

101. Read RW, Holland GN, Rao NA, et al. Revised diagnostic criteria for Vogt-Koyanagi-Harada disease: report of an international committee on nomenclature. Am J Ophthalmol 2001; 131:647-52.

102. Kitamura M, Takami K, Kitachi N, et al. Comparative study of two sets of criteria for the diagnosis of Vogt-Koyanagi-Harada's disease. Am J Ophthalmol 2005; 139:1080-5.

103. Yamaki K, Hara K, Sakuragi S. Application of revised diagnostic criteria for Vogt-Koyanagi-Harada disease in Japanese patients. Jpn J Ophthalmol 2005; 49:143-8.

104. Paredes I, Ahmed M, Foster CS. Immunomodulatory therapy for Vogt-Koyanagi-Harada patients as first-line therapy. Ocul Immunol Inflamm 2006; 14:87-90.

105. Damico FM, Szil´ard K, Young LH. Sympathetic ophthalmia. Semin Ophthalmol 2005; 20:191-7.

106. Chu DS, Foster CS. Sympathetic ophthalmia. Int Ophthalmol Clin Vol 42, Summer 2002; pp 179-85.

107. Kumar N, Chang A, Beaumont P. Sympathetic ophthalmia following ciliary body laser cyclophotocoagulation for rubeotic glaucoma. Clin Experiment Ophthalmol 2004, 32: 196-8.

108. Biswas J, Fogla R. Sympathetic ophthalmia following cyclocryotherapy with histopathologic correlation. Ophthalmic Surg Lasers 1996; 27:1035-8.

109. Pollack AL, McDonald HR, Ai E, Green WR. Sympathetic ophthalmia following pars plana vitrectomy without antecedent penetrating trauma. Retina 2001; 21:146-54.

110. Vote BJ, Hall A, Cairns J, Buttery R. Changing trends in sympathetic ophthalmia. Clin Experiment Ophthalmol 2004; 32:542-5.

111. Su DH, Chee SP. Sympathetic ophthalmia in Singapore: new trends in an old disease. Graefes Arch Clin Exp Ophthalmol 2006; 244:243-7.

112. Griepentrog GJ, Lucarelli MJ, Albert DM, Nork TM. Sympathetic ophthalmia following evisceration. A rare case. Ophthal Plast Reconstr Surg 2005; 21:316-8.

113. Garcia-Arumi J et al. Sympathetic ophthalmia following surgical resection of iridociliary melanoma. A case report. Graefe Arch Clin Exp Ophthalmol 2006; published online on 8 March, 2006.

114. Rathinam SR, Rao NA. Sympathetic ophthalmia following post operative bacterial endophthalmitis: a case series. Am J Ophthalmol 2006; 141: 498-507.

115. Wu GS, Swiderek KM, Rao NA. A novel retinal pigment epithelial protein suppresses neutrophil superoxide generation: II. Purification and microsequencing analysis. Exp Eye Res 1996; 63:727-37.

116. Rao NA, Robin J, Hartmann D, et al. The role of the penetrating wound in the development of sympathetic ophthalmia experimental observations. Arch Ophthalmol 1983;101:102-4.

117. Chan CC, Benezra D, Rodrigues MM, et al. Immuno-histochemistry and electron microscopy of choroidal infiltrates and Dalen-Fuchs nodules in sympathetic ophthalmia. Ophthalmology 1985; 92:580-90.

118. Gomez V, Alcarcel M, et al. Central serous chorioretinopathy versus sympathetic ophthalmia. Case report. Arch Soc EsP Oftalmol 2004 Oct; 79: 507-10.

119. Ganesh SK, Narayana KM, Biswas J. Peripapillary choroidal atrophy in sympathetic ophthalmia and management with triple agent immunosuppression. Ocular Immunol Inflamm 2003; 11:61-6.

120. Ganesh SK, Sundaram PM, Biswas J, Babu K. Cataract surgery in sympathetic ophthalmia. J Cataract Refract Surg 2004; 30:2371-6.

121. Chan RV, Seiff BD, Lincoff HA, Coleman DJ. Rapid recovery of sympathetic ophthalmia with treatment augmented by intravitreal steroids. Retina 2006; 26:243-7.

122. Kirsch O, Frau E, Nodarian M, et al. Clinical course of ocular sarcoidosis in patients with histologically proven systemic sarcoidosis. J Fr Ophthalmol 2001; 24:623-7.

123. Dev S, McCallum RM, Jaffe GJ. Methotrexate treatment for sarcoid-associated panuveitis. Ophthalmology 1999; 106: 111-8.

124. Chan WM, Lim E, Liu DT, Law RW, Lam DS. Intravitreal triamcinolone acetonide for choroidal granuloma in sarcoidosis. Am J Ophthalmol 2005;139:1116-8.

125. Krill AE. Deutman AF. Acute retinal pigment epitheliopathy. Am J Ophthalmol 1972; 74:193-205.

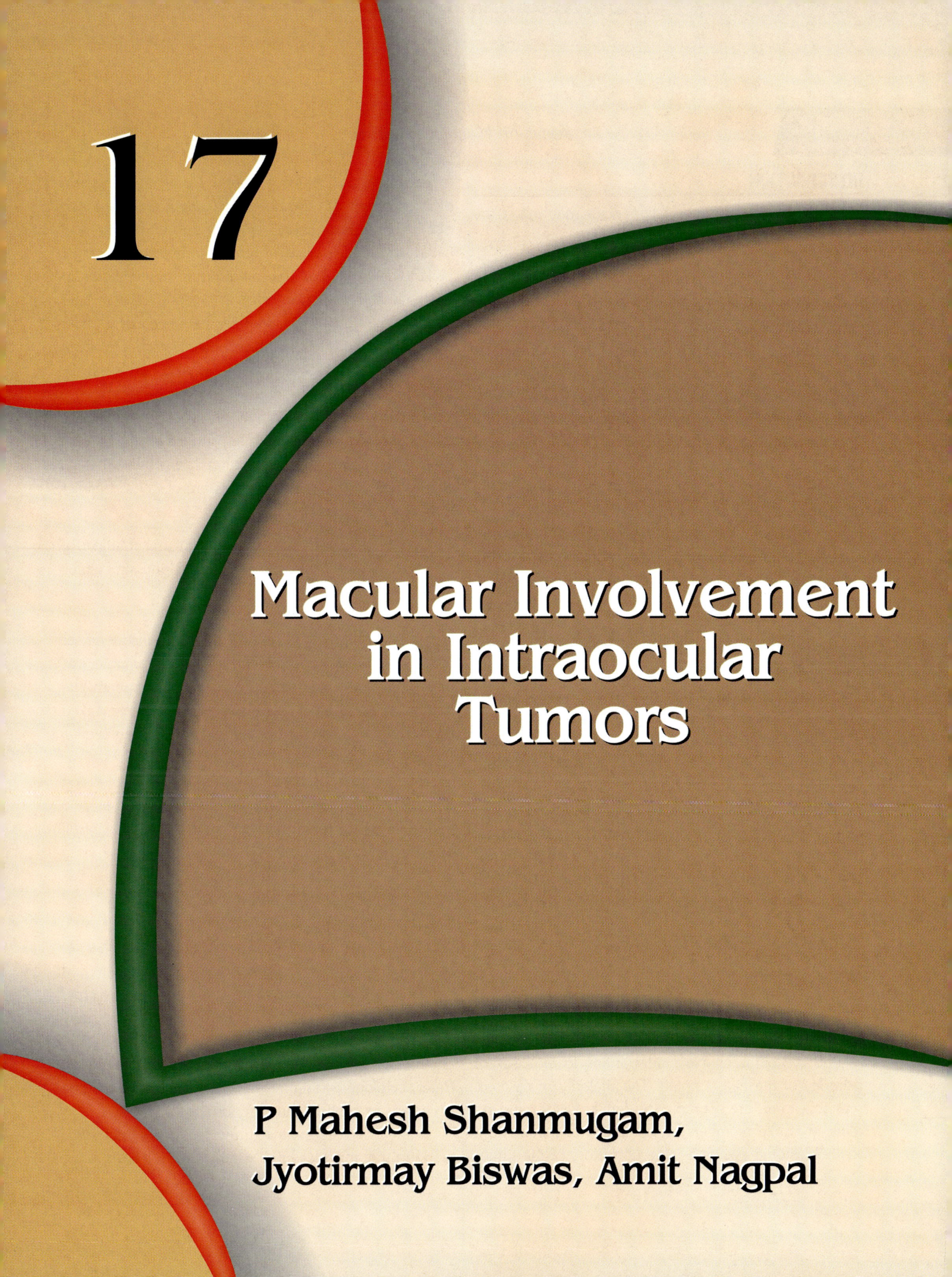

Macular Involvement in Intraocular Tumors

P Mahesh Shanmugam,
Jyotirmay Biswas, Amit Nagpal

INTRODUCTION

Intraocular and systemic malignancies may affect the macula:

- Directly by virtue of their macular location
- Indirectly by causing secondary effects on the macula
- Treatment of intraocular and systemic malignancies may adversely affect the macula.

In addition, the macular location of the tumor dictates selection of an appropriate treatment that will destroy the tumor but also cause minimal or no damage to the macula, thereby vision. Proximity to the macula and the optic disk is often a poor prognostic factor in many intraocular tumors.

Optical coherence tomography (OCT) is useful in early detection of secondary retinal changes caused by the tumors. It is not useful as a diagnostic tool in intraocular tumors. Optical coherence tomography may help the clinician evaluate the visual prognosis based on the severity of the macular changes caused by the tumor and also helps assess the resolution of the macular changes in response to treatment. Presence of subretinal fluid and intact photoreceptor layer as imaged by the OCT indicates recent activity of the tumor and possibly better visual prognosis; presence of intraretinal edema, retinoschisis, retinal pigment epithelium layer attenuation or thickening, photoreceptor loss indicates chronic macular changes and relatively poor visual prognosis. Optical coherence tomography can be performed in co-operative children as well thereby adding additional information in pediatric intraocular tumors such as retinoblastoma, angiomatosis retinae, astrocytic hamartoma and simulating conditions such as Coats' disease and toxocara granuloma.[1-7]

INTRAOCULAR TUMORS AND MACULA

RETINAL TUMORS

Retinoblastoma

Retinoblastoma occurs in approximately 1 in 14,000 to 34,000 live births.[8-10] No predisposition to race, sex or laterality of the eye is noted. The majority of cases of retinoblastoma are sporadic (no family history and no affected family members on ophthalmic examination). Retinoblastoma occurs as a result of loss of the tumor suppressor gene located on band 14, on the long arm of chromosome 13 (13q14).[11,12] In genetically transmitted disease, the abnormality results in the development of usually bilateral, multifocal tumors in relatively younger patients. This deletion also predisposes these children to other non-ocular tumors such as osteosarcoma in later stages of life. In contrast, sporadic tumors occur in older children and tends to be unifocal and unilateral. However, 10 to 20% of unilateral disease can also be genetically transmitted.

The average age at diagnosis of retinoblastoma in American children is 18 months, and evidence indicates that Asian children present later than their western counterparts.[8, 13-15] Bilateral cases are diagnosed earlier than unilateral cases.[8,16]

Clinical features: The most common presentation of retinoblastoma is leukocoria (61-70%) and strabismus (22-48%).[8,17,18]

On fundus examination retinoblastoma appears as a slightly white, flat, translucent lesion in the sensory retina. Moderately advanced lesions may present as unilateral or bilateral leukocoria. Based on the growth pattern, the tumor can be classified into endophytic, exophytic, mixed (both endophytic and exophytic) and diffusely infiltrative tumors.

Macular retinoblastoma results in early loss of vision due to loss of retinal function and anisometropic amblyopia and strabismus. Posterior location of the tumor may result in an early appreciation of the white reflex. The close proximity of macular retinoblastoma to the optic disk increases the risk of optic nerve spread; foveal and papillomacular bundle involvement impact visual prognosis. Local spread to the orbit, distant metastasis to brain, spinal cord, skull bones, distant bones, viscera and lymph nodes may occur in advanced retinoblastoma.

Ocular ultrasonography, computerized tomography and magnetic resonance imaging of the eye and orbit aid in diagnosis and evaluate local spread of the disease. Rarely cytology by fine needle aspiration biopsy may be necessary to confirm the diagnosis.

In advanced cases with extraocular disease, metastatic work-up that includes lumbar puncture, CT scan, bone marrow biopsy and routine blood investigations will be necessary.[19]

Management options in retinoblastoma include enucleation, in an eye without visual potential, if more than half the globe is involved by the tumor, or in the presence of glaucoma and anterior chamber involvement. Eyes with visual potential (unilateral/bilateral cases) are managed conservatively with modalities that include cryotherapy, laser photocoagulation, transpupillary thermotherapy (TTT), thermochemotherapy, chemoreduction, plaque brachytherapy and external beam radiotherapy.[8, 20]

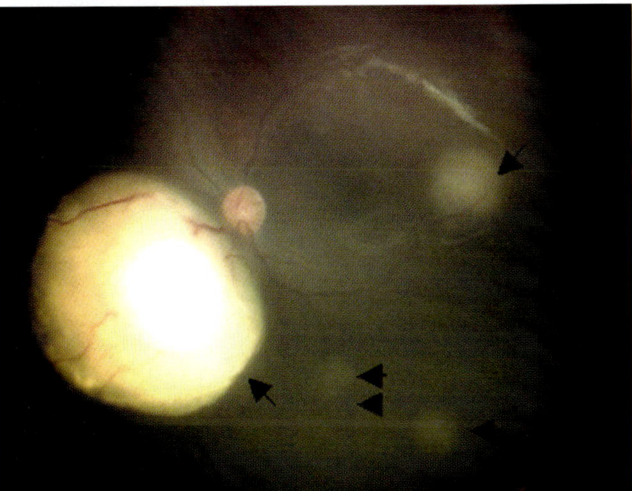

FIGURE 17.1A: Fundus Retcam photograph showing multiple retinoblastomas.

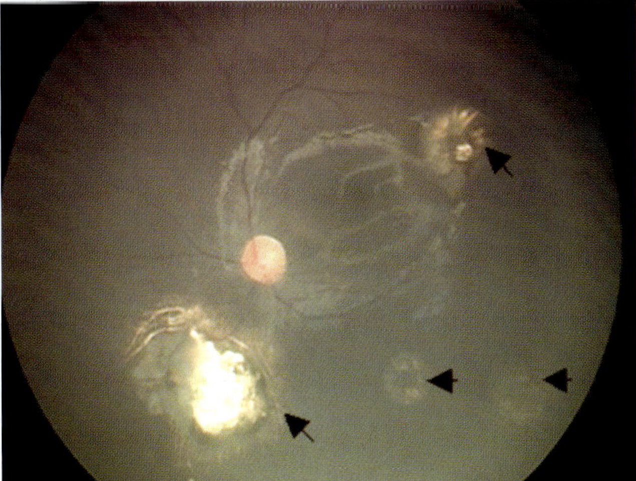

FIGURE 17.1B: Fundus Retcam photograph showing regressing retinoblastoma lesions after combined treatment with chemotherapy and focal consolidation.

Treatment: Studies have shown that macular retinoblastoma, particularly large tumors treated with various local treatment modalities or external beam radiation may be associated with a poor visual prognosis.[21,22] Migdal and Hall have reported 32% and 33% of eyes respectively with macular retinoblastoma had 20/40 or better vision after radiation. [23,24] Part of the visual loss may be related to the treatment itself; hence it is important to select a treatment that will control the tumor with least damage to the macula (Figures 17.1A and B).

Plaque radiotherapy has the benefit of limiting radiation exposure to the macula and also avoiding systemic toxicity associated with chemoreduction; but this technique was associated with radiation maculopathy in 25% of treated patients by 5 years when used to treat retinoblastoma in any fundus location.[25] The incidence of radiation maculopathy is likely to be higher if plaque therapy is used to treat macular tumors. Laser photocoagulation and cryotherapy are used less frequently to treat macular tumors as both can impart direct damage to the adjacent normal retina with profound treatment-related visual loss. Due to these limitations, triple drug chemoreduction using etoposide, vincristine and carboplatin with or without adjuvant treatment is preferred to treat macular retino-blastoma.

A study of 54 eyes treated with chemoreduction and local treatment, found only 24% of eyes with a macular tumor had a final visual acuity of 20/40 in contrast to 90% of eyes with extramacular tumor. This study showed tumors that were 3 mm away from the disk and macula and without subretinal fluid had a better visual prognosis.[26] Another study comparing the results of 6 cycles of chemoreduction alone vs. chemoreduction with fovea sparing thermotherapy in macular retinoblastoma found that combined treatment group had better tumor control at 4 years (83% vs. 65% tumor control combined group vs. only chemoreduction).[27] However, Gombos and associates [28] were able achieve tumors complete control in 84% of treated eyes with 6 to 8 cycles of chemoreduction alone. Both groups noted that tumors <2 mm had an increased risk of recurrence.

These studies indicate that chemoreduction alone may achieve adequate tumor control in at least 2/3rds of eyes with macular retinoblastoma; however adjuvant thermotherapy gives better results. However at present it is not known if visual results may be compromised by the adjuvant thermotherapy. In addition thermotherapy scars may extend a mean 0.72 mm 6-12 months after treatment and this has to be taken in to consideration when employing thermotherapy close to the fovea.[29]

Other factors such as status of vision in the other eye, age of the patient, size of the tumor, presence of vitreous / subretinal seeds, may also influence the selection of the treatment modality. In the presence of a normal macula in the other eye, addition of fovea-sparing thermotherapy to chemoreduction despite its potential for compromising vision may be acceptable, while in a patient with bilateral macular tumors or if the other macula is already compromised, only chemoreduction may be employed, with a close watch for tumor recurrence.

Treatment of amblyopia is also an important consideration in children with retinoblastoma; good results with occlusion can be obtained even in the presence of macular involvement and should be actively pursued.[26,30]

Enucleation may be considered in large macular retinoblastoma that is associated with extensive subretinal fluid, subretinal or vitreous seeds, particularly in unilateral disease.

Retinal Astrocytoma

Retinal astrocytomas are glial tumors arising from the optic nerve head or the retina. Though these tumors have a predilection to the posterior pole they may occur any where on the retina. The tumor may manifest in two clinical forms: as a glistening, white-yellow calcified tumor which has well defined borders and multiple small excrescences (mulberry or fish egg lesions) (Figures 17.2A and B) or as a flat, gray-white tumor that is round or oval and has a smooth surface.

Involvement of the macula or the optic disk by the astrocytic hamartoma or macular exudation may result in vision loss.[31,32] Rarely vitreous hemorrhage may occur.

Ultrasonography of calcified large astrocytoma show well demarcated, oval mass with a sharp anterior border, acoustic solidity and lack of choroidal excavation. There

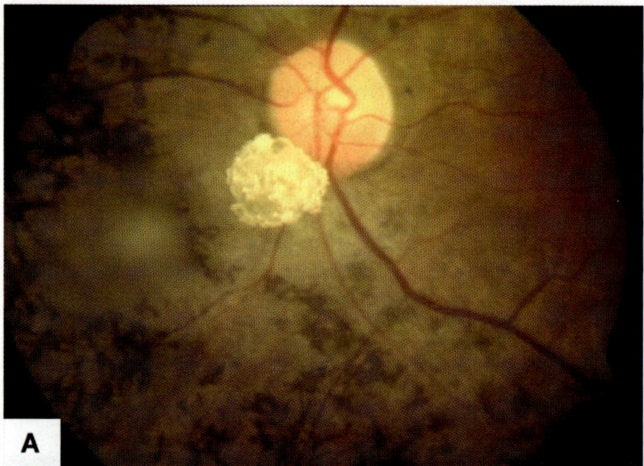

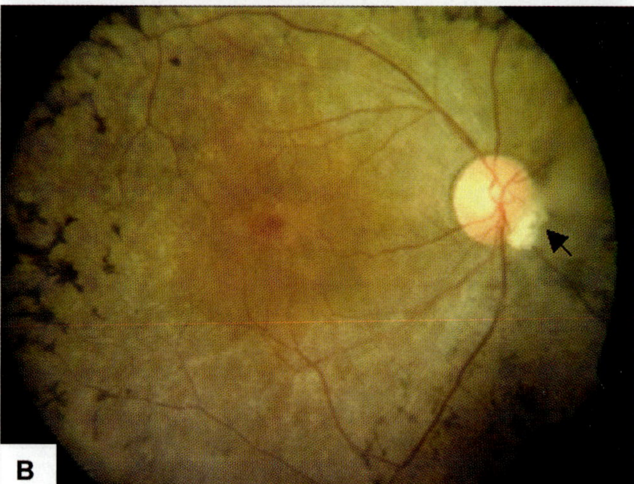

FIGURES 17.2A and B: Astrocytoma with retinitis pigmentosa.

may be orbital shadowing. The calcified astrocytoma may demonstrate autofluorescence in pre injection photographs of fluorescein angiography. There is diffuse hyperfluorescence in the late phases due to leakage from the tumor vessels.

Astrocytomas are relatively stable and rarely affect visual acuity; hence routine treatment is unnecessary. Direct light photocoagulation may aid in resorption of macular exudates if there is no spontaneous resolution of the detachment.[33,34]

Systemic associations: Approximately 50% of patients with tuberous sclerosis have retinal astrocytomas. They may also occur less commonly in patients with neurofibromatosis and retinitis pigmentosa.[35,36]

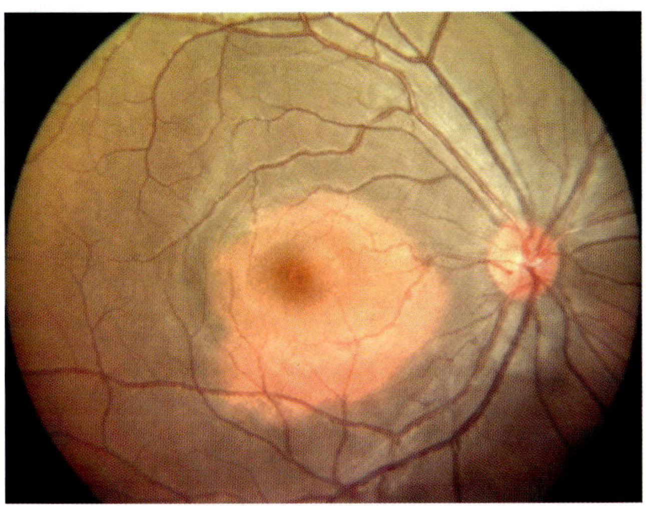

FIGURE 17.3: Capillary hemangioma.

VASCULAR TUMORS OF THE RETINA

Capillary Hemangioma of the Retina

Capillary hemangioma of the retina may occur as an isolated lesion within the retina (Figure 17.3) or as a part of phakomatosis with central nervous system and systemic tumors when it is called von Hippel-Lindau syndrome. It is genetically transmitted in an autosomal dominant mode with incomplete penetrance and variable expressivity. Von Hippel-Lindau syndrome is linked to a defect in short arm of chromosome 3 (3p 25-26).

The ocular lesions are usually diagnosed between 10 and 30 years of age. The early angioma appears as a yellow spot between a feeding arteriole and a draining

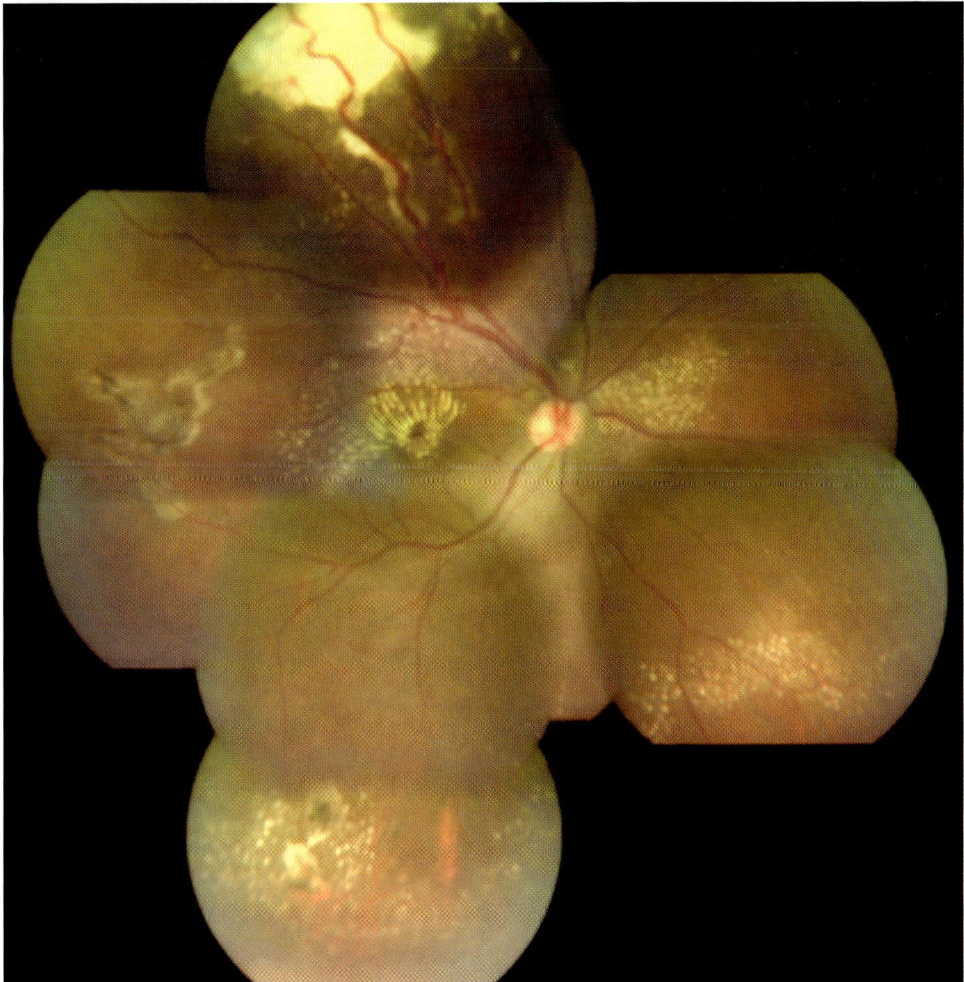

FIGURE 17.4: Appearance of capillary hemangioma superotemporally in a 23-year-old male. Note the chorioretinal atrophy of the previously treated healed lesions temporally and inferiorly. The other eye was blind due to extensive hemangiomas and exudation.

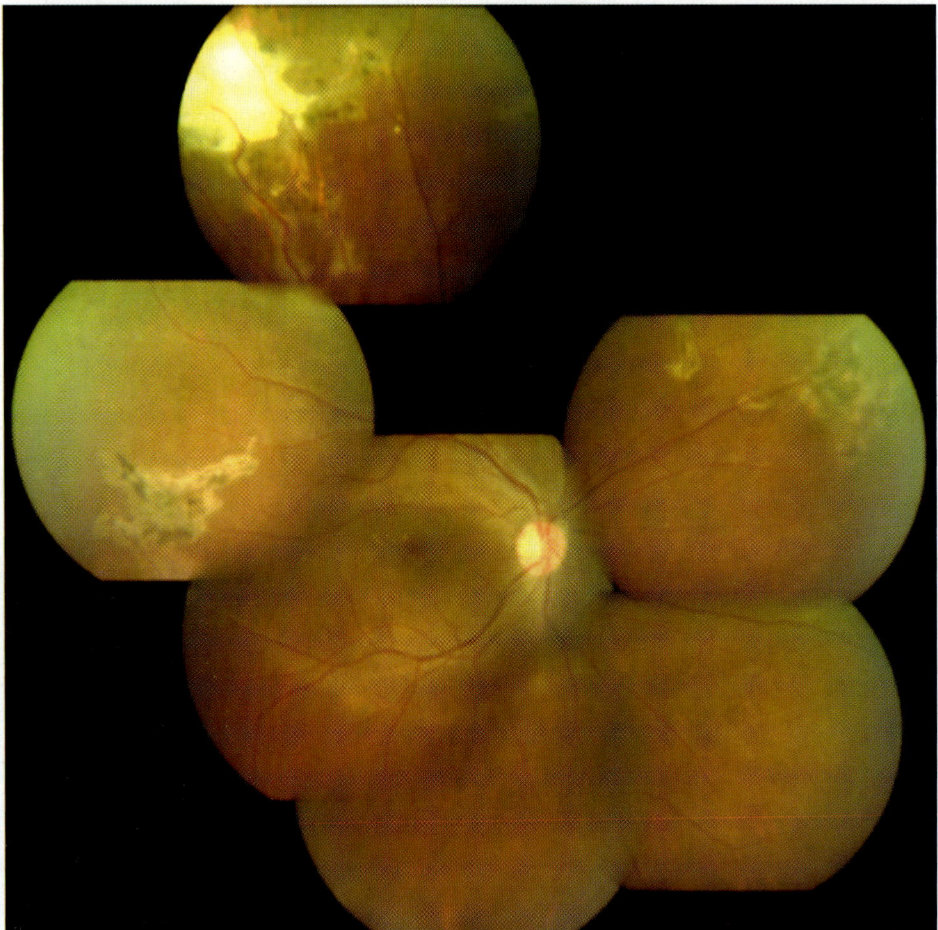

FIGURE 17.5: Regressed capillary hemangioma along the superotemporal arcade in the same patient following laser photocoagulation to the feeder vessels and the angioma along with transconjunctival cryopexy. Note the regressing exudation along the superotemporal arcade.

venule. As the angioma increases in size, the supplying vessels increase in diameter and become tortuous. Macular exudation or exudative macular detachment causes loss of vision (Figure 17.4). Epimacular proliferation, macular traction detachment, vitreous hemorrhage and combined traction rhegmatogenous retinal detachment can also lead to visual loss. Appearance of dilated pair of vessels in the posterior pole with macular exudates should prompt one to examine the periphery for a capillary angioma. Multiple or bilateral angiomas indicate the presence of von Hippel-Lindau tumor and screening for central nervous system or systemic disease should be performed. Without treatment, most eyes progress to total retinal detachment, neovascular glaucoma and a painful blind eye.

Angioma of the optic nerve head can simulate papilledema, wherein a defined feeder arteriole or a draining venule may not be seen. The orange red lesion is ill defined, involves an eccentric part of the optic disk with exudation that often involves the macula.

The diagnosis can be made most often on indirect ophthalmoscopy with the classic picture of an orange tumor with a feeding arteriole, draining venule associated with macular exudates. A fundus fluorescein angiogram will delineate early lesions that are not visible on clinical examination. Angiomas fill rapidly in the early phases of the angiogram and leak profusely in the late phases. The paired vessels are well delineated as well.

Treatment of retinal and papillary angioma: Patients with von Hippel-Lindau syndrome should undergo periodic neurological and systemic evaluation. A yearly urinary vanillyl mandelic acid estimation, ultrasonography of the abdomen and magnetic resonance imaging of the brain once in 3 years is essential screening for the systemic manifestations of von Hippel-Lindau syndrome.

Early treatment of retinal capillary angiomas leads to better visual results. Smaller tumors (<2 mm) can be treated with direct laser photocoagulation and larger tumors (2-5 mm) can be treated using the feeder vessel technique. Peripheral tumors or larger tumors can be treated with cryotherapy (Figures 17.4 and 17.5). In tumors associated with a bullous retinal detachment, drainage of the subretinal fluid, cryotherapy and scleral buckling may be necessary.

Transpupillary thermotherapy, plaque brachytherapy, proton beam irradiation and external beam radiation therapy have been employed in the management of retinal and disk angiomas.[37]

Transpupillary thermotherapy has been used to treat peripapillary and paramacular angiomas with regression of the tumor in 82% and improvement in vision in 55% of the treated cases over 18 months.[38] Transpupillary thermotherapy with indocyanine green has been used to treat peripheral angiomas with good results and minimal laser-induced effects in the vicinity of the tumor.[39]

Photodynamic therapy (PDT) has been used to treat large retinal angiomas with standard and modified PDT techniques where infusion times were shortened and longer light exposure was used. Multiple treatments were necessary, resulting in regression of the angiomas and improvement in vision. Some cases may additionally need vitrectomy to repair tractional retinal detachment or epiretinal membrane removal after successful regression of the angioma.[40]

Photodynamic therapy for peripapillary angioma is effective in causing regression of the tumor and resolve macular detachment. However, PDT treatment of peripapillary angioma appears to be associated with risk of iatrogenic retinal vascular occlusion and optic disk ischemia.[41-43]

Vitrectomy with epiretinal membrane removal and to repair of tractional or rhegmatogenous retinal detachment may be necessary in advanced vitreoretinal form of the disease. Rarely resection of the hemangioma, ligation of the feeder vessel has also been attempted.[44-46]

Intravenous vascular endothelial growth factor inhibitor infusion led to resolution of cystoid macular edema associated with multiple angiomas in one patient as long as the patient was on treatment.[47] Further studies may discern the role of antivascular endothelial growth factor agents in the management of neoplastic diseases of the eye.

Systemic associations: Cerebellar or spinal cord hemangioblastomas are the classic central nervous system lesions of von Hippel-Lindau syndrome. Cerebellar hemangioblastomas usually cause cerebellar symptoms in the 4th decade of life and can be imaged on a CT scan. The central nervous system tumors are managed by surgical resection if possible. Unilateral or bilateral pheochromocytomas, cysts of the kidney, pancreas, epididymis and renal cell carcinomas may occur in these patients.[48]

Cavernous Hemangioma of the Retina

Cavernous hemangioma of the retina is also recognized as a phakomatosis with involvement of the retina, skin and the central nervous system. It appears to have an autosomal dominant mode of inheritance.

Cavernous hemangioma may affect the macular region or peripheral retina. Macular location of the tumor or complications such as intraretinal hemorrhage at the macula, macular distortion due to epiretinal membrane proliferation, vitreous hemorrhage and amblyopia in children may cause loss of vision.[49,50] Exudation, however, is not a common feature of cavernous hemangioma of the retina. One patient with a superonasal cavernous angioma has been noted to have associated cone dysfunction.[51]

Cavernous hemangioma appears as a cluster of dark red saccules with associated fibroglial proliferation. No feeder arteriole or draining venule is usually seen though some authors have noted twin vessels to be associated with this tumor.[52] The lesion is non-progressive or may enlarge minimally over time.

The diagnosis is evident on fundus examination and fundus fluorescein angiogram is quite characteristic.

Cavernous hemangioma has a sluggish circulation which leads to the separation of the plasma from the blood cells, which settle down inferiorly within the saccule. Fluorescein enters the saccule slowly and fills the supernatant plasma, enhancing the fluid level, creating a "fluorescein cap".

Cavernous hemangioma of the retina does not require treatment and is usually observed. If vitreous hemorrhage were to occur, cryotherapy, photocoagulation, low energy plaque and vitrectomy to clear vitreous hemorrhage may be employed.[53]

Systemic associations: Cavernous hemangioma involving the central nervous system may lead to seizures and other neurological symptoms. Hepatic cavernous angiomas may also occur.[54] Cutaneous angiomas may involve the back or the neck.

Racemose Hemangioma

Racemose hemangioma is more of a vascular malformation than a tumor and if associated with systemic disease, is called the Wyburn Mason syndrome (Figure 17.6). No definite hereditary pattern has been noted.

Arteriovenous communications in Wyburn Mason syndrome have been classified in to 3 types.[55] In the first type, an abnormal capillary plexus is interposed between the arteriole and the venule. These lesions do not cause symptoms and are not usually associated with cerebral involvement. In type 2 no capillary bed is found and direct arteriovenous communication exists; patients experience few visual symptoms. Associated cerebral vascular malformation may be found. Group 3 patients have more complex and extensive arteriovenous malformation with visual loss and increased risk of cerebral disease. One or more dilated arterioles emanate from the disk, travel for a variable distance in the retina, form arteriovenous communication and return to the disk. Exudation or retinal detachment usually does not occur. Visual loss may occur due to vaso-occlusion, nerve fiber loss caused by pressure on the optic nerve or the anterior visual pathway by the tumor, intraretinal and vitreous hemorrhage and rarely macular exudation.[56-58]

The clinical appearance of racemose hemangioma is characteristic and a fluorescein angiogram may show

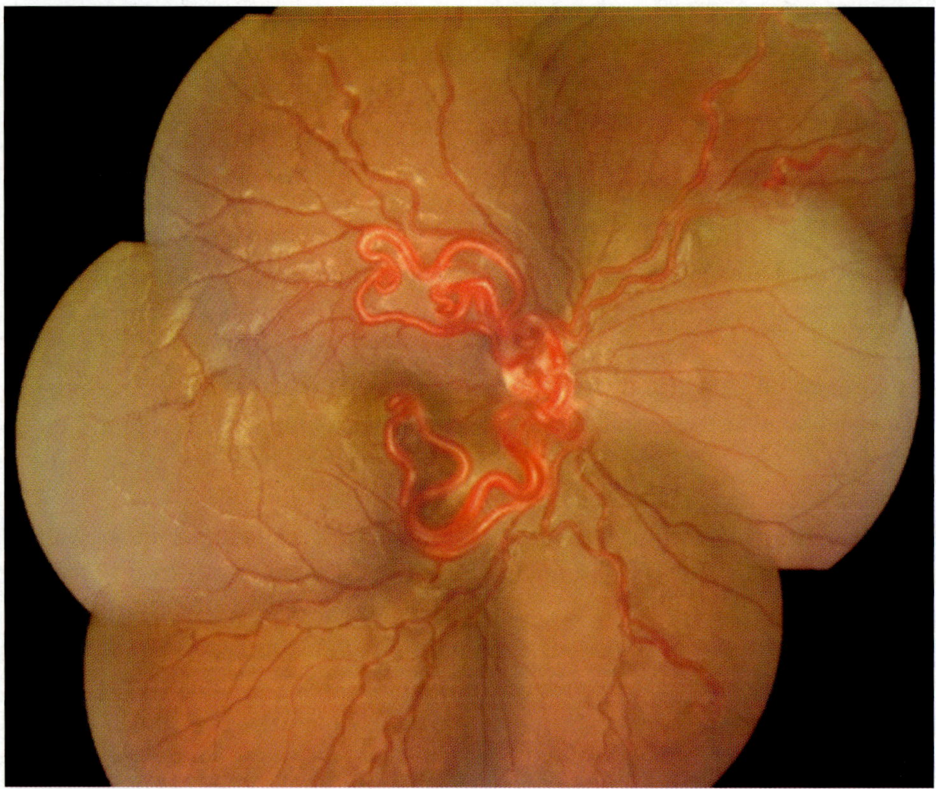

FIGURE 17.6: Fundus montage photograph of a case of racemose hemangioma.

rapid filling of the arteriovenous communication without dye leakage.

Most racemose hemangioma are stationary and do not need treatment. However, the visual prognosis is poor.

Systemic associations: Intracranial hemangiomas may be associated in 30% to 81% of patients with retinal angioma.[59-60] Spontaneous cerebral or subarachnoid hemorrhages may lead to neurological symptoms (hemiplegia, hemiparesis, cerebellar dysfunction, Parinaud's syndrome, mental changes affecting intelligence and memory, seizures. Ptosis or partial ophthalmoplegia due to III nerve involvement by intracranial tumor may occur. Facial (50% of patients, ipsilateral to the side of racemose hemangioma) and orbital hemangiomas, rarely hemangiomas involving the lung, spinal cord may co-exist.[61] Orbital vascular malformations may cause pulsating proptosis. Hemangiomas involving the bones of the skull, maxilla, and mandible may lead to massive bleeding during dental extraction. Intraocular racemose hemangioma communicating with intramuscular facial hemangioma has been reported.[62]

VASOPROLIFERATIVE TUMOR OF THE RETINA

Vasoproliferative tumors of the retina are solitary tumors that commonly involve the inferotemporal of inferior quadrants of the retina and may mimic a retinal angioma. The tumor is usually found in the 40 to 60 years age group. Vasoproliferative tumors may occur without any antecedent cause, but may be associated with prior uveitis, retinitis pigmentosa, Coats' disease and familial exudative vitreoretinopathy, sickle cell retinopathy, retinopathy of prematurity, long standing retinal detachment and toxoplasma scars.[63,64]

Vasoproliferative tumor appears as a solitary yellow or pink mass lesion with minimally dilated feeder vessels. Premacular fibrosis, cystoid macular edema, macular edema, intraretinal and subretinal exudation and hemorrhage, secondary retinal detachment, tractional retinal detachment, retinal pigment epithelium hyperplasia and vitreous hemorrhage may be associated and impair vision. Some patients may have multiple, bilateral or diffuse tumors. The pathogenesis of these lesions is unclear. Stellate macular exudates and gross dilated feeders seen in retinal angiomatosis are not found.

Fluorescein angiography shows early filling and late leakage and minimally or not dilated feeder vessels. Ultrasonography shows a mass lesion with low, medium or high internal reflectivity. If progressive exudation causes loss of vision, cryotherapy, photocoagulation, plaque brachytherapy may be necessary. Epiretinal proliferation may need vitreous surgery. Rarely PDT has been used to treat vasoproliferative tumor.[65]

CHOROIDAL TUMORS

Choroidal Hemangioma

Choroidal hemangioma is a benign vascular tumor that usually causes visual symptoms by early adulthood. Choroidal hemangioma may occur as a circumscribed, solitary lesion usually without systemic association or as a diffuse hemangioma associated with Sturge-Weber syndrome.

Circumscribed choroidal hemangioma presents as an orange-red mass. On ultrasonography, the mass shows a dome shape, medium to high internal reflectivity and no choroidal excavation or orbital shadowing. Fibrous or osseous metaplasia on the surface may however produce higher reflectivity and orbital shadowing. Fluorescein angiography shows filling of the lesion in the pre-arterial phase, coarse intratumor vessels and late leakage. On indocyanine green angiography the choroidal hemangioma exhibits extreme hyperfluorescence in the early frame by about 1 minute followed by moderate hyperfluorescence in the middle and late frames (8 and 20 minutes). This early hyperfluorescence followed by relative hypofluorescence is called washout and is characteristic of circumscribed choroidal hemangioma.

Circumscribed choroidal hemangioma is relatively hyperintense with respect to the vitreous in T1 weighted images and isointense to the vitreous in T2 weighted images.

Choroidal hemangioma may cause amblyopia by virtue of its location at the macula, vision loss by causing secondary macular changes such as exudative retinal detachment, cystoid macular edema, subretinal fibrosis and rarely neovascular glaucoma.

Diffuse choroidal hemangioma is usually diagnosed at a young age, either because of the visual impairment or the facial hemangioma that calls for attention. The pupil shows a brilliant red reflex (tomato catsup fundus) in the involved eye in contrast to the normal reflex in the opposite pupil. The lens and vitreous cavity are usually clear.

Diffuse choroidal hemangioma on ophthalmoscopy appears as a diffuse red-orange thickening of the posterior choroid most often involving the macula and often extending anterior to equator (Figure 17.7). The macular location of a unilateral tumor may result in anisometropic amblyopia. Exudative detachment of the macula, cystoid degeneration of the retina overlying the tumor surface and disruption of the retinal pigment epithelium over the tumor may result in visual loss. The overlying retinal vessels may appear tortuous. The diffuse choroidal hemangioma can produce a total secondary retinal detachment, cataract and an ipsilateral congenital glaucoma can develop, particularly when the upper lid is involved by the nevus flammeus. Ultrasonography demonstrates a markedly thickened choroid with medium to high internal reflectivity with an overlying retinal detachment. Fundus fluorescein angiography reveals diffuse leakage similar to circumscribed choroidal hemangioma but with more widespread involvement. Magnetic resonance imaging features are similar to circumscribed choroidal hemangioma.

Treatment: Refractive correction to avoid amblyopia is essential in young patients with submacular tumors, particularly those associated with diffuse hemangioma. Antiglaucoma surgery may also be necessary in these eyes.

Presence of visual symptoms, particularly due to exudative retinal detachment is an indication for treatment of choroidal hemangioma. Tumors with minimal overlying retinal detachment can be treated with laser photocoagulation, photodynamic therapy and transpupillary thermotherapy. Multiple sessions may be necessary to achieve resolution of the exudative retinal detachment, particularly with laser photocoagulation.

Photodynamic therapy with its potential for selective destruction of this vascular tumor is the preferred treatment of macular circumscribed choroidal hemangiomas.

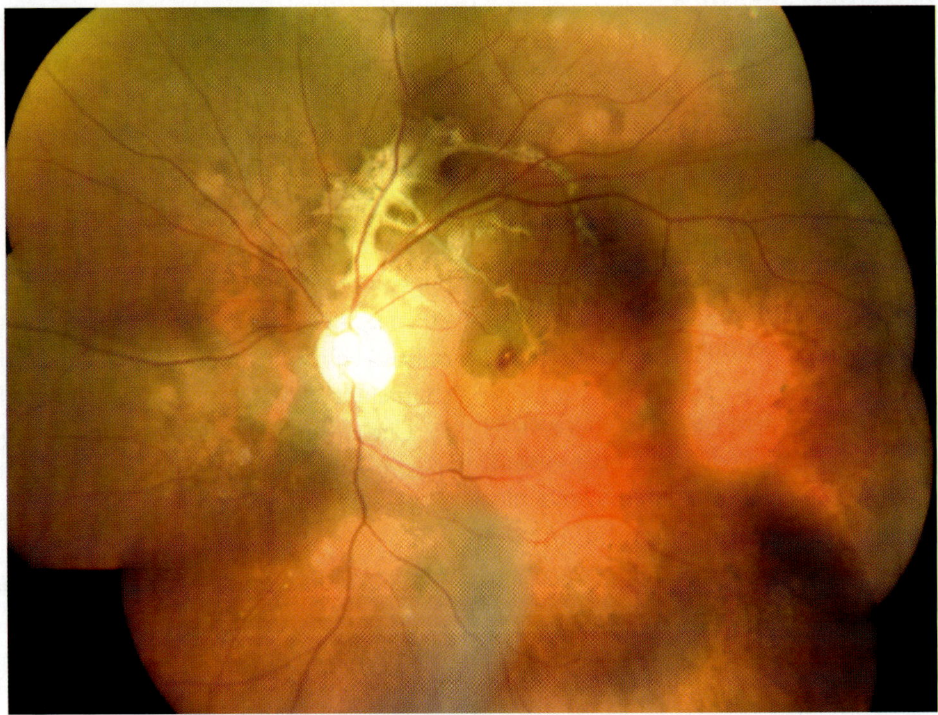

FIGURE 17.7: Fundus montage photograph of choroidal hemangioma.

Regression of the tumor, exudative retinal detachment and cystoid macular edema occurs after photodynamic therapy. Photodynamic therapy with 689 / 692 nm light using the macular degeneration protocol of using laser energy at 50 J/cm^2 15 minutes after infusion of 6 mg/m^2 dose verteporfin or modified techniques using 75 or 100 J/cm^2 laser energy, treatment duration of 75 or 186 (for tumors >2 mm thick) seconds, repeat PDT at 6 weeks intervals have been used to treat choroidal haemangioma.[66-68] Tumors up to 6.2 mm thick have been treated with PDT and long-term complete tumor regression with resolution of retinal detachment and visual improvement have been reported.[69-73] Multiple spot PDT with macular degeneration protocol has recently been used to treat diffuse choroidal hemangioma.[74] Photodynamic therapy has been found to be safe in treating choroidal hemangioma, though multiple treatments can cause minimal retinal pigment epithelium alterations.

Transpupillary thermotherapy can be used to treat circumscribed choroidal hemangiomas. Tumors <4 mm in thickness and <10 mm in basal diameter can be treated with transpupillary thermotherapy.[75] Indocyanine green enhancement may also be used, though many authors have achieved good results without the same. Transpupillary thermotherapy is applied using a spot size of 2 to 3 mm and a power of 200 to 300 mW with the end-point being mild whitening. Whole of the tumor is treated with overlapping burns. Forty-two percent of the treated tumors regressed completely while 53% regressed partially after treatment. Visual improvement of 2 or more lines has been documented in 77% of the treated eyes. Transpupillary thermotherapy leads to early resolution of subretinal fluid and tumor regression continuing for many months after treatment.[76-83] Cystoid macular edema, pre-retinal fibrosis, retinal vein occlusion and focal iris atrophy may occur as complications.

Circumscribed or diffuse choroidal hemangioma with extensive retinal detachment that precludes visualization of the tumor to deliver laser, can be treated with radiation utilizing external beam radiation, proton beam therapy or brachytherapy with Iodine-125 or Ruthenium-106 plaques. Resolution of the retinal detachment has been noted in 64 to 100% of treated cases though visual improvement may not always occur.[84-88] Visual recovery would depend on the duration of the retinal detachment, absence of atrophic changes in the retina and retinal pigment epithelium and absence of amblyopia. Recent onset of visual symptoms indicates a better visual prognosis. Stereo tactic radiotherapy delivering 20 Gy using a linear accelerator resulted in resolution of exudative retinal detachment and regression of the tumor in a small group of patients with peripapillary/macular circumscribed choroidal hemangioma.[89]

Systemic features: Diffuse choroidal hemangioma may be associated with glaucoma, facial hemangioma and ipsilateral leptomeningeal angioma (associated with abnormalities of the underlying cerebral cortex with intracranial calcification) forming the Sturge-Weber syndrome. The diffuse choroidal hemangioma is generally unilateral and ipsilateral to the facial hemangioma but may be bilateral if facial nevus flammeus is bilateral or of associated with variants of Klippel-Trenaunay-Weber syndrome.

Choroidal Osteoma

Choroidal osteoma is a rare, benign, ossifying tumor occurring in young adult women (Figure 17.8). It can be unilateral (70-80%) or bilateral and very rarely familial.[90-93]

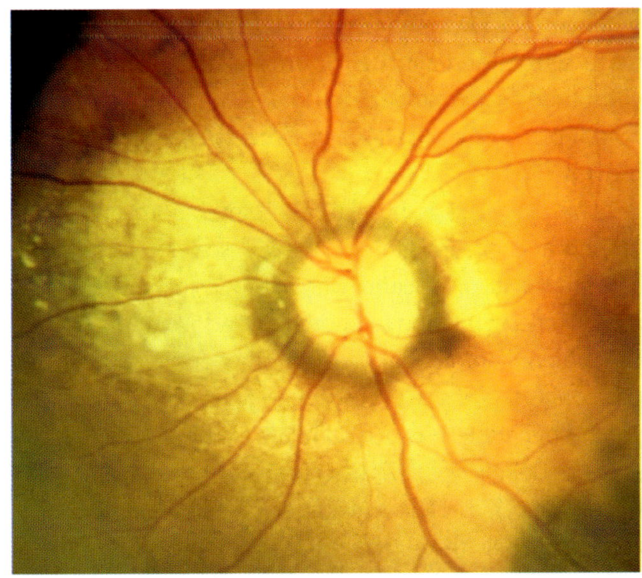

FIGURE 17.8: Choroidal osteoma.

Choroidal osteoma may be discovered on routine clinical examination or may cause gradual decrease in vision. Sudden loss of vision with metamorphopsia may rarely occur. Early osteoma begins in the peripapillary or macular region as an orange red lesion. With increasing calcification, the lesion assumes a yellow color and has well-defined borders with pseudopod like extensions. Osteoma may extend beneath the papillomacular bundle and the fovea. Capillary tufts simulating Haversian canal of bone, may be seen within the lesion. Morphology of the lesion may change over time with the lesion extending in one area and decalcifying in other. Degeneration of the overlying retinal pigment epithelium and retina, subretinal fluid or development of a choroidal neovascular membrane may lead to visual loss. Sudden unexplained loss of vision may rarely occur.

A recent study of 74 eyes with choroidal osteoma found that 22% of the tumors showed growth at 5 years and 51% at 10 years. Tumor decalcification occurred in 28% and 46% of eyes, choroidal neovascularization in 31% and 31% of eyes, visual acuity loss in 26% and 45% of eyes, and poor visual acuity in 45% and 56% of eyes at 5 and 10 years respectively, indicating that half of the eyes with choroidal osteoma may lose vision over time. Decalcification is associated with retinal pigment epithelium and choriocapillaris atrophy resulting in poor visual outcome and decalcified tumors have a decreased potential for growth. As can be expected, subfoveal tumors were associated with a poorer visual prognosis as compared to extrafoveal tumors. Absence of overlying retinal pigment epithelial alterations was associated with growth.[94]

The diagnosis is by clinical examination, ultrasonography and in rare situations, a CT scan or X-ray skull. The presence of calcium within the lesion gives rise to a high reflective lesion with orbital shadowing on B-scan. Curvilinear choroidal plaque of bone density can be seen on axial CT orbits. Fluorescein angiography shows early patchy hyperfluorescence with late staining of the lesion. A choroidal neovascular membrane, if present, will show up as early hyperfluorescence with late leakage that is more intense than that of the surrounding tumor. Indocyanine green angiography shows early tumor hypofluorescence (more in the orange region of the tumor as compared to the yellow-white part); intralesional blood vessels appear hyperfluorescent and late diffuse hyperfluorescence of the mass may be seen.[95,96]

Choroidal osteomas are observed periodically. Choroidal osteoma may cause loss of vision by virtue of its position beneath the macula, growth of a choroidal neovascular membrane, retinal pigment epithelium and choriocapillaris atrophy resulting in photoreceptor damage or by unknown mechanisms (Figure 17.9). Choroidal neovascular membrane may be treated with laser photocoagulation if extrafoveal or transpupillary thermotherapy and single or multiple sessions of photodynamic therapy using AMD protocol, can achieve stabilization of vision [97-102] Rarely, surgical excision of the choroidal neovascular membrane has also been attempted.[103]

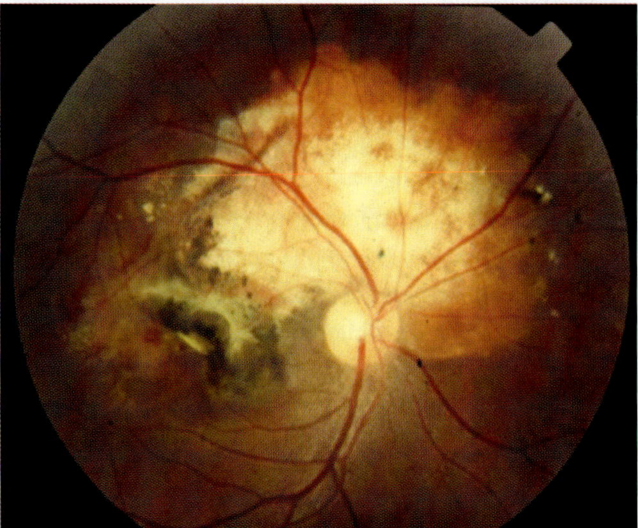

FIGURE 17.9: Choroidal osteoma with choroidal neovascular membrane, retinal pigment epithelium and choriocapillaris atrophy.

Choroidal Melanoma

Choroidal melanoma is a malignant neoplasm arising from neuroectodermal melanocytes within the choroid. The average age of detection of melanoma of the choroid and ciliary body is in the 5th and 6th decades.[104] Uveal melanoma (includes melanoma of the iris, ciliary body and choroid) has an incidence rate of 1.7 to 8.3 per million in the Caucasian population and is seen less frequently in pigmented population.[105] Uveal melanomas are rare in Indian population and appear at a relatively younger age (mean age 45.7+/–14.2 years, range 14-82 years).[106]

Predisposing factors for the development of uveal melanoma include:

1. Light colored skin, eyes.
2. Oculodermal melanocytosis.
3. Dysplastic nevus syndrome.
4. Uveal nevus.
5. Xeroderma pigmentosum.
6. Family history of melanoma.
7. Neurofibromatosis.
8. Exposure to intense artificial ultraviolet light.

Patients with choroidal melanomas may present with blurred vision due to a subfoveal tumor, cystoid macular edema, retinal detachment, vitreous hemorrhage, cataract, and if the tumor blocks the visual axis. They may also present with floaters due to vitreous hemorrhage, pain and field loss. A necrotic tumor may also induce an inflammatory reaction. Few patients may present with a blind, painful eye without prior diagnosis of uveal melanoma underlining the need for an ultrasound examination in blind eyes wherein the fundus could not be seen. Rarely, the tumor may remain asymptomatic and be discovered on routine fundus examination.

The typical choroidal melanoma appears as a dark brown, dome shaped, solid tumor (Figure 17.10). It can break through the overlying Bruch's membrane and form a dumb-bell or collar-button shaped nodular mass under

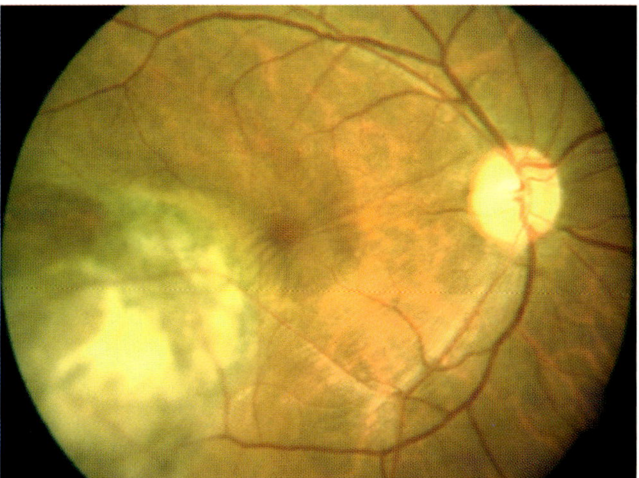

FIGURE 17.10: Choroidal melanoma.

the retina. Diffuse melanoma (height <15% of the base; also defined as <5mm thick and covering >25% of the uveal tract) may present as an ill-defined thickening of the choroid. Diffuse melanomas carry the risk of early extrascleral extension, greater number of malignant cytologic features and worse systemic prognosis.[107]

The tumor may lack pigment and appear amelanotic or more commonly show dense pigmentation and rarely the tumor may be multicentric or bilateral. Overlying retinal pigment epithelium and photoreceptor atrophy, drusen formation, retinal pigment epithelium detachment, cystoid degeneration of the retina, cystoid macular edema, and choroidal neovascularization may occur as secondary effects. Secondary retinal detachment usually occurs. Severe ocular pain may occur when the tumor impinges on the posterior ciliary nerves. Melanomas may exhibit orange colored lipofuschin pigment over their surface. Diffuse pigment indicates an active tumor while a localized pigment and drusen indicate a slow growing or a dormant tumor.

The tumor may grow anteriorly to involve the ciliary body causing cataract, trabecular meshwork causing glaucoma, erode blood vessels leading on to vitreous or anterior chamber hemorrhage. The tumor may also cause neovascular glaucoma secondary to rubeosis iridis and uveitis when undergoing necrosis. Subretinal hemorrhage and proptosis due to posterior extrascleral extension may occur.

Pathophysiology and prognosis: Uveal melanoma arises from melanocytes in the uveal tract. Although uveal melanomas may grow *de novo*, most develop from preexisting melanocytic nevi. Three distinct cell types, spindle A, spindle B, and epithelioid cell type are found. Modified Callender classification divides uveal melanocytic tumors into spindle cell A and B melanomas, mixed cell and epithelioid cell melanomas. Presence of the latter two types is associated with more aggressive behavior and carries a poorer prognosis for the patient's survival.

Tumor features such as larger size, anterior location, transcleral extension, proximity to the foveal avascular zone, advanced age of the patient, growth through

Bruch's membrane, optic nerve extension, lack of pigmentation, and histologic characteristics such as mitotic activity and cell type have been found to correlate with increased mortality.

Vascular networks, closed loops, parallel with cross linking microcirculation patterns noted on histopathological evaluation and chromosomal abnormalities appear to predict tumors that are likely to metastasize.

Uveal melanomas tend to metastasize to the liver, lung, central nervous system, bone and skin. Less frequently, transcleral growth of the tumor through emissary channels can result in orbital and conjunctival metastasis. An overall mortality rate of approximately 30 to 50% occurs from uveal melanoma within 10 years from diagnosis and treatment. The collaborative ocular melanoma study (COMS) found a 5-year mortality rate of 6% for small (1-3 mm height/at least 5 mm diameter), 18% for medium sized tumors (3.1 mm – 8 mm height and <16 mm in diameter) and 30% for large (>8 mm height and or >16 mm diameter) tumors.[108-110]

Management: Choroidal melanoma appear as a solid mass with a biconvex or mushroom shape on B scan ultrasonography and high surface spike with low amplitude internal reflectivity, with a decremental reduction of spike height from the surface to the depth of the mass on A scan. Acoustic hollowing and choroidal excavation are also seen.

Choroidal melanomas are predominantly hypofluorescent with pinpoint areas of hyperfluorescence due to retinal pigment epithelium loss in early frames and may show prominent intratumor blood vessels (double circulation). Leakage from the tumor and staining of the entire tumor with leakage into the subretinal fluid is seen in late phase of the angiogram.

Malignant melanomas block choroidal filling on indocyanine green angiography; late phase pictures may demonstrate intratumor vessels and minimal late dye leakage. Confocal indocyanine green angiograms may show complex microcirculation patterns that may indicate growth potential of the melanoma.[111]

CT scan can image most choroidal melanoma and a majority of them show enhancement on contrast CT. Choroidal melanoma appear bright (hyperintense) with respect to vitreous on T1 weighted images and dark (hypointense) with respect to vitreous in T2 weighted images on MRI scan.

Rarely, if the diagnosis cannot be made with reasonable certainty with non-invasive methods a fine needle aspiration biopsy may be necessary to obtain tissue specimen.

Pre-management evaluation of uveal melanoma includes, complete physical examination with particular attention to the liver, abdomen, skin and subcutaneous tissues, which are frequent sites of metastatic spread. Hepatic function tests (serum levels of gamma-glutamyl transpeptidase, lactic dehydrogenase, and glutamic-oxaloacetic transaminase), ultrasound/CT scan examination of the abdomen are essential to rule out hepatic metastasis. However, the imaging studies do not exclude micrometastasis. X-ray chest is also indicated to rule out lung metastasis, though it is often negative. These investigations are to be repeated 6 monthly after treatment, for early diagnosis of metastatic disease. However, most patients do not have detectable metastasis at the time of presentation.

Dormant, small and medium sized tumors, slow growing small and medium tumors in sick and one eyed patients may generally be observed periodically after proper documentation with color fundus photograph and ultrasonography.

Small nasal and temporal peripheral melanoma located away from macula and outside the arcade can be treated with laser photocoagulation. The tumors <3 mm in height and <9 mm to 10 mm in basal diameter without secondary retinal detachment and at least 1 disk diameter from the disk. Less than 5% of melanomas meet the criteria laid down for use of photocoagulation. Multiple treatment sessions may be necessary before satisfactory regression of the tumor. Cystoid macular edema, branch retinal vein occlusion, macular involvement with laser may occur as complications of laser treatment.[112]

Transpupillary thermotherapy has found wide use in treating small melanomas (<3 mm in thickness) that are away from the disk and macula. With proper selection of tumors 91 to 94% of treated small choroidal melanomas showed regression.[113-115] In a series of 256 consecutive melanomas (mean 2.7 mm in height) treated only with mean 3 sessions of TTT, 91% of the tumors remained regressed at 3 years. More than 3 TTT sessions and tumor overhanging the optic disk were risk factors for recurrence. Risk factors for visual acuity < 20/200 were documented tumor growth before treatment, mushroom tumor configuration, initial symptom of blurred vision, poor initial visual acuity, superior quadrant tumor location, underlying diabetes mellitus, and tumor overhanging the optic disk. Treating tumors larger than 3 mm in thickness increases the risk of recurrence.[115]

Though TTT results in good short-term regression of the tumor, persistence of choroidal vessels beneath the tumor after TTT indicates that there may be a higher risk of tumor recurrence after TTT.[116,117] Transpupillary thermotherapy is preferred in the treatment of small melanomas so that radiation induced complications can be avoided; however a study comparing the visual results with TTT and brachytherapy found no difference in the visual outcome. There was an increased risk of recurrence of the tumor with TTT alone; suggesting that TTT is better used as an adjuvant treatment rather than a primary treatment.[118] Dense scotomas due to nerve fiber defects, epiretinal gliosis and macular abnormalities may also limit visual recovery after TTT (Figures 17.11A and B).[119]

Indocyanine green enhanced TTT is also effective in treating small and medium melanomas, particularly amelanotic tumors (100 mg indocyanine green dye in 10 min, 2 minutes after starting TTT).[120,121]

Photodynamic therapy has used as a primary treatment or as an adjunct to treat tumor close to the posterior pole to avoid radiation related complications. A bolus dose of verteporfin and treatment at 1 minute with double the light dose for 166 seconds and multiple sessions have been employed. Photodynamic therapy may be particularly suitable to treat amelanotic melanomas that do not respond well to TTT.[122-124]

Conventional external beam radiotherapy is not used in the management of choroidal melanoma as the large radiation dose involved will invariably cause radiation related complications leading to blindness. The COMS study failed to show any benefit of pre enucleation radiation in decreasing mortality. Post-enucleation irradiation may be useful in cases where extrascleral extension has been transected intra operatively.[125]

Uveal melanomas up to 24 mm in diameter and 14 mm in height have been treated with charged particle irradiation. Tumors involving the fovea, optic nerve head, those with small extrascleral extension are also treatable with proton beam radiation. The five-year survival rate following proton beam radiation has been to be comparable with of plaque therapy. The disadvantage of the current charged particle radiation systems is that they are expensive to install and maintain and hence are available in few centers in the world. Risk of radiation maculopathy is high after proton beam radiation of paramacular melanomas. A study or 218 eyes with paramacular melanoma treated with proton beam radiation, 89% developed some degree of radiation

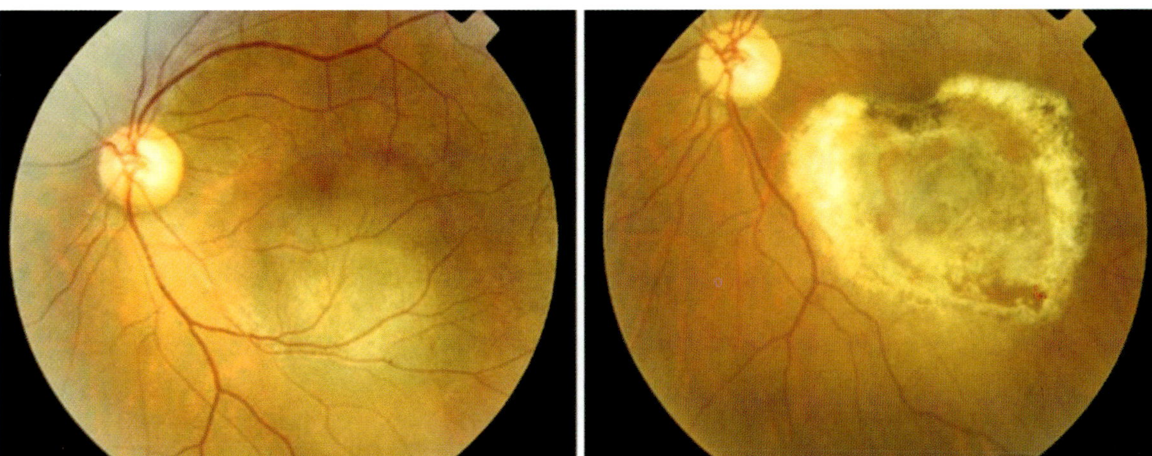

FIGURES 17.11A and B: Choroidal melanoma: Pre- and post-transpupillary thermotherapy.

maculopathy and 67% had <20/200 vision 3 years after treatment.[126]

Brachytherapy: The current relative indications of plaque therapy are:

1. Selected small melanomas that are documented to be growing or that show clear-cut signs of activity on the first visit.
2. Most medium sized and some large choroidal and ciliary body melanomas in an eye with potential salvageable vision.
3. Almost all actively growing melanomas that occur in the patients' only useful eye.

Radiation induced complications can result in poor vision after brachytherapy. Forty-nine percent of the eyes with medium melanoma in COMS had lost >6 lines of vision 3 years after treatment. Patients with a history of diabetes and patients whose eyes had thicker tumors, tumors close to or beneath the foveal avascular zone, tumor-associated retinal detachment, or tumors that were not dome shaped were those most likely to have a poor visual acuity.[127]

Posterior tumors need higher dose of radiation to the macular region which may adversely affect visual acuity; older patients and tumors close to the optic disk are also adverse risk factors for poor visual outcome after brachytherapy.[128-130] In a study of 630 macular melanoma treated with brachytherapy, though 91% local tumor control could be achieved, visually significant maculopathy developed in 40% of the patients, papillopathy in 13% and vision decrease by >3 Snellen lines was found in 40% of the patients.[131] A study comparing the incidence of retinopathy between anterior posterior uveal melanoma of comparable size treated with similar dose of brachytherapy found that radiation maculopathy occurred in 52% of the posterior tumor eyes as compared to 4% of anterior tumor eyes, indicating that treatment of posterior tumors increases the risk of radiation retinopathy.[132]

Larger melanomas are associated with increased chances of visual morbidity and local recurrence of tumor with radiation therapy.[133] A study of brachytherapy for large melanomas found that 91% of the treated eyes had lost > 6 lines of vision 3 years after treatment. Tumor height and location posterior to ora serrata were associated with poor visual results.[134]

Combined plaque radiotherapy and laser photocoagulation or thermotherapy increase the likelihood of complete local tumor destruction particularly in patients with tumor adjacent to the optic disk.[135,136] Macular location of the tumor epicenter, diffuse tumor configuration, and tumor margin extending underneath the foveola may however limit visual recovery.[135] Epiretinal gliosis and macular edema may also result in poor vision after combined therapy.[136]

Ciliary body tumors, not extending more than 4 clock hours of pars plicata, choroidal melanoma not greater than 15 mm in diameter, anterior to the equator can be considered for iridocyclectomy or partial lamellar sclerouvectomy respectively if the retina is spared, and penetrating sclerochorioretinovitrectomy if the retina and sclera are involved.[137-139] The concerns are of residual tumor and recurrence, other than tumor dissemination during surgery. The current concept of combining brachytherapy prior to or following resection ensures eradication of the tumor more completely. Internal resection of melanoma after delimiting preoperative photocoagulation around the tumor followed by vitrectomy and internal removal of the tumor piece-meal has been attempted for posterior melanoma that are not amenable to lamellar sclerouvectomy and also have an increased risk of radiation maculopathy.[140,141] Short-term results do not report increased metastatic or recurrence risk.. Combining brachytherapy with resection and pre-enucleation radiation is said to reduce the risk of tumor recurrence and metastasis.

Eyes with melanoma >8 mm in height or >16 mm in diameter are usually enucleated. Small or medium sized tumors with optic nerve invasion, posterior uveal melanomas with total retinal detachment or severe glaucoma however are also managed by enucleation. Pre-enucleation radiation does not alter the mortality rate and hence not advised.[142] A "no touch technique" has been advocated to prevent hematogenous dissemination of the tumor.[143,144]

Choroidal Nevus

Choroidal nevi are slate grey or brown pigmented lesions that are less than 2 mm in thickness and may be associated with drusen, orange pigment, overlying retinal pigment epithelium alteration and rarely retinal detachment and choroidal neovascularization. Visual symptoms, greater tumor thickness and diameter, presence of orange pigment, absence of drusen, absence of retinal pigment epithelial changes adjacent to the tumor, posterior tumor margin adjacent to the disk, and subretinal fluid and growth are considered risk factors for malignant transformation.[145-147] The annual rate of malignant transformation of a choroidal nevus was estimated to be 1 in 8,845 in a recent study.[148]

Macular detachment associated with choroidal nevi may resolve spontaneously or by employing steroid therapy, gas injection, TTT or photocoagulation.[149,150] Choroidal neovascularization associated with choroidal nevi can be treated successfully with PDT.[151-154]

INTRAOCULAR METASTASIS

Intraocular metastasis is thought to be the commonest form of intraocular malignancy. However, due to the advanced nature of the malignant disease, these patients are most often not seen by the ophthalmologist. Approximately 50 to 70% of patients with metastatic ocular disease are women and 70 to 80% of intraocular metastasis in women is from the breast.[155]

Metastatic tumors may affect any part of the eye but most commonly affect the vascular, posterior choroid. Ninety percent of metastatic tumors affect the posterior choroid, 10% involve the iris and or ciliary body.[156-159] Metastatic tumors to the retina, optic nerve, and vitreous are uncommon.

Carcinomas are most often seen as metastatic tumors in the eye as compared to the sarcomas and melanomas, which are less common as primary malignancies. Breast in women and the lung in men are the common sites of origin of uveal metastasis. Tumors of the thyroid, prostate, alimentary tract, pancreas, kidney and other organs may rarely metastasize to the eye. Twenty five percent of patients present with uveal metastasis without history of a primary malignancy and 10% may not have a detectable primary despite evaluation.

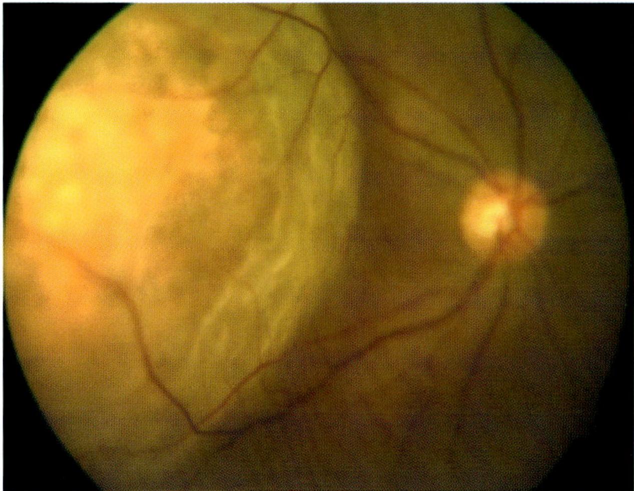

FIGURE 17.12: Fundus photograph of choroidal metastasis with exudative retinal detachment.

Patients with choroidal metastasis frequently present with loss of vision and may also report photopsias, floaters or metamorphopsia or may be asymptomatic. Choroidal metastasis may be multiple, bilateral, yellow or cream colored, associated with disproportionate secondary retinal detachment and are usually not highly elevated (Figure 17.12). However, metastatic lesions may be solitary, and of orange (carcinoid, thyroid, renal cancer) or gray/black color (cutaneous melanoma). Retinal pigment epithelial hyperplasia overlying the metastatic tumor (leopard skin pigmentation), choroidal detachment and rarely a mushroom shape may also occur with choroidal metastasis.

Retinal metastasis may seed the vitreous and may simulate an occlusive vasculitis. Optic disk metastasis will appear as a unilateral disk swelling or as a mass lesion.[160] Disk edema and posterior vitritis may also develop.

Diagnosis of metastatic tumors is essentially by the clinical features and the history of a primary malignancy. A metastatic lesion shows moderate to high internal reflectivity on A-scan and a dome shaped mass without orbital shadowing or choroidal excavation on B-scan ultrasonography. Fundus fluorescein angiography shows early hypofluorescence and hyperfluorescence in the late venous phase with late leakage. In cases of diagnostic uncertainty or an unknown primary a fine needle aspiration biopsy may be required to establish the diagnosis and identify the site of the primary tumor. If the site of primary is unknown, a systemic evaluation consisting of mammography, chest radiography and liver function tests is indicated. Other tests such as prostate-specific antigen (elevated in prostate cancer), human chorionic gonadotropin (elevated in seminoma) and 5-hydroxyindoleacetic acid (carcinoid tumor) may also assist in locating the primary malignancy.

Treatment

Small asymptomatic choroidal metastasis or those improving systemic chemotherapy may be observed.

Small breast cancer and carcinoid metastasis has been treated with laser photocoagulation resulting in regression of the tumor, resorption of subretinal fluid and improvement in vision. Secondary macular detachment caused by small peripheral thyroid metastasis has been treated with cryotherapy.[161-163]

If the primary tumor is responsive to chemotherapy, choroidal metastasis can also be treated using the same protocol used for systemic disease.

Large, growing tumors or those associated with secondary retinal detachment and unresponsive to systemic chemotherapy are treated with radiation. Solitary metastasis can be treated with brachytherapy.

Transpupillary thermotherapy has been used to treat select, solitary, small metastatic tumors.[164]

Photodynamic therapy has been employed to treat solitary carcinoid choroidal metastasis at the macula that was resistant to chemotherapy and radiation. Multiple spots of PDT using AMD protocol resulted in regression of the exudative retinal detachment and some regression of the mass.[165]

Rarely, solitary metastatic tumors from tumors with favorable systemic prognosis have been resected.[166]

Painful, blind eyes resulting from secondary glaucoma may be enucleated to make the patient comfortable or to help diagnosis in patients with an unknown primary.

Systemic prognosis of patients with intraocular metastasis depends on the systemic malignancy; patients with carcinoid, breast and thyroid cancer metastasis have the longest survival while those with metastasis from kidney, pancreas, gastrointestinal tract and cutaneous melanoma tumors have a poor prognosis.

OPTIC DISK TUMORS

Melanocytoma

Melanocytoma is a specific variant of nevus, located on the optic disk or elsewhere in the uveal tract, characterized clinically by a dark brown to black color. Histopathological examination shows deeply pigmented, round to oval cells with small, round, uniform nuclei. Melanocytomas occur more commonly in blacks.

Melanocytomas may rarely involve the iris, ciliary body or elsewhere in the choroid. Optic disk melanocytoma is a benign tumor of the optic nerve head.[167] It may probably be present at birth, but the usual age at diagnosis is 50 years (range: 14-79 years). There is no sex and eye predilection. Bilaterality is extremely rare.

Most patients with optic nerve head melanocytomas are usually asymptomatic, but if the tumor is fairly large, may experience slight blurring of vision to severe loss of vision. Some patients may have afferent pupillary defect even if visual acuity is excellent.

The tumor appears as a flat to slightly elevated dark black mass located eccentrically over the edge of optic disk commonly occupying inferior temporal quadrant. Some tumors may completely obscure the disk and retinal vessels. The tumor has a fibrillary edge as it extends in to the nerve fiber layer (Figures 17.13A and B). A choroidal nevus contiguous with the disk portion of the melanocytoma is present in about 50% of cases. Choroidal and or retinal component may be found in continuation to the optic disk tumor. Uninvolved portion of the optic nerve can appear clinically normal or may have edematous appearance. Sheathing of overlying retinal vessels is quite common. Rarely melanocytomas may undergo malignant transformation.[168-169] Signs of malignant transformation are increase in the size of the tumor associated with or without vitreous seeding.

No specific treatment is indicated for optic disk melanocytoma and periodic observation with baseline color fundus photograph and ultrasound measurement of the tumor will aid in the follow-up of these patients. Necrosis within the tumor or growth of the tumor may result in complications such as neuroretinitis [170,171] central retinal vein occlusion [172,173] obstruction of adjacent blood vessels or optic neuritis, subretinal fluid [174] may have affect

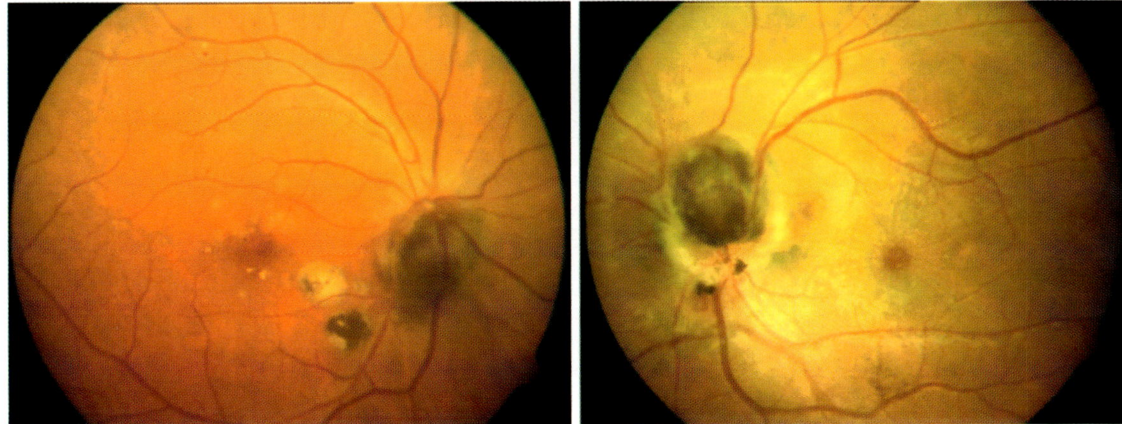

FIGURES 17.13A and B: Melanocytoma of the optic nerve head.

the macula and vision. Spontaneous visual recovery with resolution of neuroretinitis and optic neuritis has been reported. Enlarged blind spot, altitudinal defects, arcuate scotoma and paracentral field defects may also occur.

RETINAL PIGMENT EPITHELIAL TUMORS

Combined Hamartoma of the Retina and Retinal Pigment Epithelium

A hamartoma is a benign overgrowth of cells that are normally present at the involved site, and combined hamartomas of the retina and retinal pigment epithelium characteristically contain pigment epithelium, vascular, and glial components.[175]

Most patients with combined hamartoma of the retina and retinal pigment epithelium present with painless visual loss, due to macular distortion, caused by retinal striae and epiretinal membrane. Patients may present with strabismus, floaters, leukocoria and ocular pain. Direct involvement of optic nerve and papillomacular bundle may also reduce visual acuity.

Combined hamartoma of the retina and retinal pigment epithelium appear as a slightly elevated black or charcoal gray mass involving the retinal pigment epithelium, retina and overlying vitreous. Most lesions are peripapillary some macular and rarely peripheral in location (Figure 17.14).[176] Base of each lesion is composed of a relatively flat sheet of highly pigmented tissue and the outer more pigmented portion of tumor is covered centrally by gray-white retinal and preretinal tissue. Contraction of inner surface of the lesion is associated with distortion and displacement of neighboring retina and retinal blood vessels toward the center of the lesion. In early-phase fluorescein angiography, hyperpigmentation of the tumor results in hypofluorescence. Tractional distortion of the retina leads to marked vascular tortuosity and telangiectasia. Vascular anomalies are more evident in the mid phase and late hyperfluorescence due to leakage from the tortuous vessels. Indocyanine green may show patchy hyperfluorescence corresponding to the location of the tumor in late phases.

Combined hamartoma of the retina and retinal pigment epithelium is usually not associated with retinal detachment, hemorrhage, exudation, and vitreous inflammatory cells; although superficial hemorrhages can rarely occur with these lesions. However, retinal capillary non-perfusion with preretinal neovascularization resulting in vitreous hemorrhage may occur.[177-179] Other complications such as choroidal neovascularization and macular hole formation may also result in visual loss.[180-182]

Combined hamartoma of the retina and retinal pigment epithelium may be associated with neurofibromatoses 1 and 2, facial hemangiomas, incontinentia pigmentii and tuberous sclerosis.[183]

There is no established treatment for the combined hamartoma. In those cases that produce visual loss because of retinal traction in the fovea, vitrectomy and membrane peeling can be attempted to improve visual acuity.[184-186] A functional component of amblyopia may be superimposed on visual loss caused by structural abnormalities, and in some cases this can be treated.[187] Subfoveal choroidal neovascular membrane associated with combined hamartoma of the retina and retinal pigment epithelium has been surgically excised with good visual recovery in one patient.[188]

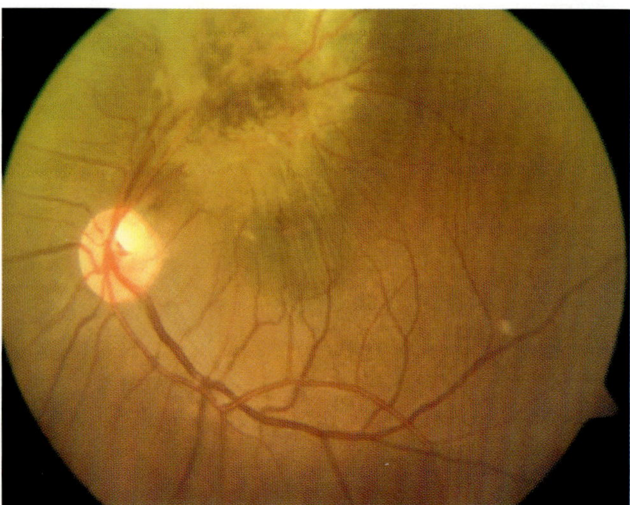

FIGURE 17.14: Combined hamartoma of the retina and retinal pigment epithelium.

Miscellaneous Tumors of the Retinal Pigment Epithelium

Rare tumors such as adenocarcinoma of the retinal pigment epithelium (arising from a focus of congenital hypertrophy of retinal pigment epithelium), multiple myeloma, adenoma of the non-pigmented ciliary epithelium may affect the macula leading to cystoid macular edema, exudative retinal detachment and surface wrinkling maculopathy, resulting in vision loss.[189-191]

PRIMARY INTRAOCULAR LYMPHOMA

Primary Intraocular lymphoma is a subtype of lymphoma, which was formerly called reticulum cell sarcoma. It is a non-Hodgkin's large cell lymphoma. Patients usually belong to the age group of 60 to 70 years and commonly present with diminished vision and floaters. Retinovitreal involvement is associated with central nervous system lymphoma, most of which are diffuse large B-cell lymphoma; this form is more common than the choroidal form which is associated with systemic lymphoma. Fifteen to 25% of patients with primary CNS lymphoma have

intraocular lymphoma at diagnosis; 25% of those without intraocular lymphoma at diagnosis of CNS lymphoma will develop the same over time. Sixty to 80% with intraocular lymphoma will develop CNS lymphoma over time.

Patients present with floaters, blurred vision or a red painful eye as in uveitis. Two-thirds of those with CNS disease may present with behavioral and cognitive impairments. Ocular examination reveals a uveitis like picture. There may be signs of anterior uveitis with cells and keratic precipitates with diffuse cellular infiltration of the vitreous. These cell clumps differ from vitreous cells associated with vitritis in that they are larger and are clumped together. There may be accumulation of lymphoma cells in the sub retinal pigment epithelial space. These appear yellowish white, geographic choroidal elevations, with pigmentation due to clumping of retinal pigment epithelium at the borders (Leopard skin appearance). Small satellite lesions can occur at the vicinity of larger lesions. Macula may be affected by the associated exudative retinal detachment, macular edema and subfoveal tumor. Retinal involvement appears as punctuate lesions with retinal pigment epithelium atrophy. Viral retinitis like presentation with large yellow creamy infiltrates, retinal hemorrhages, vasculitis, retinal detachment and necrosis may occur.

Fundus fluorescein angiogram shows hypofluorescence of the punctuate lesions and retinal infiltrates and late hyperfluorescence and late staining. Extensive retinal pigment epithelial changes demonstrated by fluorescein combined with the absence of perivascular staining or leakage and macular edema may be noted. In eyes that have undergone prior surgery, cystoid macular edema and venous staining may also be noted. Ultrasonography may reveal choroidal thickening in the choroidal form of the disease. The diagnosis requires a strong index of suspicion, particularly in elderly patients presenting with signs of chronic uveitis not responding to steroids. If suspected, a CNS evaluation consisting of MRI of the brain, lumbar puncture must be carried out. Periventricular lesions that show diffuse and homogenous enhancement with contrast are seen. In HIV patients, lesions with ring enhancement are seen which may be confused with toxoplasmosis infection. If a systemic lymphoma is suspected evaluation of the chest, abdomen, pelvis and bone marrow biopsy would be necessary. Diagnostic vitreous biopsy may demonstrate malignant lymphoid cells with cytological features of large lymphoid cells in an undiluted, unfixed vitreous specimen. Immuno-histochemistry with B cell markers, flow cytometry, polymerase chain reaction for gene rearrangements in immunoglobulin heavy (rearrangement at the comple-mentary determining region III (CDR3) is the most common) and light chains, bcl-2, or T-cell receptor gamma gene, cytokine levels in the eye (IL-10 to IL-6 ratio of >1 is suggestive) are also useful for diagnosis.[192,193] Rarely a fine needle aspiration biopsy may be necessary to prove the diagnosis.

Treatment

Primary intraocular lymphoma responds to low dose ocular radiation and chemotherapy and whole brain irradiation was recommended for patients with central nervous system lymphoma. However due to delayed neurological sequelae whole brain radiation for CNS lymphoma is not recommended now and hi-dose methotrexate (0.8–1.5 g/m^2) is recommended. To avoid late complications of radiation to the eye, hi-dose chemo-therapy with autologous bone marrow transplantation is recommended. Repeated injections of intravitreal methotrexate 400 μg/0.1 ml has been used primarily or in the treatment of recurrent intravitreal lymphoma.[193-195]

INTRAOCULAR LEUKEMIA

The leukemias are malignant transformations of the blood forming cells of the body. They include lymphocytic and myelogenous groups. Intraocular deposits of leukemic cells have been noted in 31% of patients post mortem. Clinical signs of intraocular leukemia may be subtle but are said to occur in ~40% of all patients with newly diagnosed disease.[196] Eye changes indicate advanced disease and suggest an unfavorable prognosis. Intraocular leukemia can occur even if the peripheral blood smear and the bone marrow biopsy suggest disease remission.[197]

The ocular manifestations of leukemia may be because of the blood dyscrasias caused by leukemia or because of leukemic infiltrates. Leukemic infiltrates may involve the cornea, sclera, iris, vitreous, retina, choroid and optic nerve. Pseudohypopyon, iris nodules, secondary glaucoma and rubeosis are other anterior segment mani-festations. Anemia, hyperviscosity and thrombocytopenia can result in cotton-wool spots, intraretinal hemorrhages, vitreous hemorrhage, vascular occlusions, microaneur-ysms and leukemic infiltrates can result in Roth's spots (white centered retinal hemorrhages), periphlebitis, optic disk swelling.[198] Anticardiolipin antibodies causing bilateral central retinal vein occlusion has been described in one case.[199] Macular changes may be secondary to the vascular effects of blood dyscrasias or primary macular infiltration. Bilateral serous macular detachment, cystoid macular edema may occur which can also result in visual symptoms.[200-202] Overlying retinal pigment epithelial disturbance with resultant degeneration and clumping (leopard spot pattern) may be seen. Opportunistic fungal and viral infections have to be differentiated from leukemic infiltrates.

A history of treated leukemia is important in suspecting the diagnosis. In patients with pseudohypopyon or vitritis, cytological analysis of the aqueous tap or vitreous aspirate/biopsy may be necessary. Treatment is as that of the primary disease which includes systemic or intrathecal chemotherapy and ocular radiation.[107]

SYSTEMIC MALIGNANCIES AND MACULA

Systemic tumors, other than causing ocular metastatic disease, may affect the macula by causing paraneoplastic syndromes or other secondary effects. Treatment of systemic malignancy with chemotherapy and bone marrow transplantation, radiation to structures close to the eye may adversely affect the macula.

PARANEOPLASTIC SYNDROMES

Cancer Associated Retinopathy

Cancer-associated retinopathy syndrome (CAR) is a paraneoplastic disorder in which autoantibodies against tumor antigen cross react with retinal proteins resulting in cone and rod dysfunction.[203]

Small cell carcinoma of the lung is the most common systemic malignancy associated with CAR; ovarian, uterine, cervical, endometrial, prostate, colon and breast cancers, have been associated with CAR.

Patients may present with symptoms similar to retinitis pigmentosa due to rod dysfunction—nyctalopia, reduced peripheral fields, prolonged dark adaptation. Cone dysfunction may cause photosensitivity, reduced color vision, central scotomas and decreased vision. Fundus may be normal in early stages; progressive disease results in arteriolar attenuation, disk pallor, generalized retinal pigment epithelium alteration. Electroretinogram shows reduced rod and cone amplitudes.

Etiology

At least 15 antigens expressed by rods, cones and ganglion cells have been identified to act as potential autoantigens in CAR. The most common antigen is the 23 kD recoverin, a calcium-binding protein that regulates phosphorylation of the visual pigment rhodopsin during visual transduction. Circulating autoantibodies against the tumor cross react with recoverin in CAR resulting in closure of ion channels, depolarization of cells and photoreceptor cell death.[204] Photoreceptor death due to apoptosis may also occur in CAR.[205] Increased levels of anti-recoverin antibodies may be demonstrated in the patient's serum. It is not clear how the retinal antigens are expressed outside the eye; it is postulated that the genetic sequences coding for the retinal proteins may be closely associated with other cancer-related foci and a mutation in such a focus may result in expression of the retinal protein outside the eye along with the occurrence of the malignancy.[206] An ectopic expression of a autoantigen alone is probably not enough to cause tumor induced retinal degeneration; additional stress events and possibly a genetic predisposition to autoimmunity play a role.[207]

Treatment

There are anecdotal reports of steroid therapy resulting in visual improvement. However, treatment of the underlying malignancy, steroid therapy, and plasmapheresis has led to disappointing results. Intravenous immunoglobulin has restored vision in one of three patients treated; visual recovery may be possible if treated before significant loss of photoreceptors occurs.[208]

MELANOMA-ASSOCIATED RETINOPATHY

Melanoma-associated retinopathy (MAR) is associated with an established diagnosis of cutaneous melanoma and affects males predominantly.[209] Patients may notice shimmering, photopsia, mildly progressive visual loss, mild peripheral field constriction, and acute onset of night blindness. Electroretinogram (ERG) shows markedly decreased B-wave amplitude indicating bipolar cell dysfunction. "A" wave is normal. Blue cone ERG may be severely reduced as blue cones are affected in MAR.[210,211] Acute anterior or posterior uveitis and patchy choroidal depigmentation may be seen.[212]

Bipolar cells appear to be the primary site of paraneoplastic damage in MAR. However, no specific antigen has been identified as etiologic in MAR. An atypical presentation involving antibody activity with transducin and interphotoreceptor retinoid-binding protein has however been reported recently.[213,214] Steroid or plasmapheresis has not resulted in visual improvement in MAR.

LYMPHOMA-ASSOCIATED RETINOPATHY

Lymphoma-associated retinopathy with night blindness, slight constriction of visual fields, reduced mixed rod cone responses on ERG in a patient with Hodgkin's lymphoma has been reported. A previously unrecognized antigen of approximately 65 kD molecular weight was suspected to be responsible. Steroid therapy was not useful in arresting the progression of this condition, which appeared to stabilize after a few years.[215]

SECONDARY EFFECTS OF SYSTEMIC TUMORS ON THE EYE

Hyperviscosity syndrome associated with systemic tumor such as multiple myeloma may result in venous occlusions that may result in macular edema.[216,217]

BILATERAL DIFFUSE UVEAL MELANOCYTIC PROLIFERATION

In contrast to uveal metastasis, bilateral diffuse uveal melanocytic proliferation (BDUMP) is non-metastasizing uveal tumors that occur as a hamartomatous response to systemic malignancies such as adenocarcinoma of the gall bladder, ovarian cancer, carcinoma of the colon and lung.[218]

Patients may present with focal pigmented or non-pigmented iris tumors, cataracts, exudative retinal detachment and flat or elevated pigmented lesions of the choroid, simulating metastatic cutaneous melanoma. Macula may be affected by the exudative retinal detachment or photoreceptor damage. Fluorescein angiography may show blocked fluorescence corresponding to the uveal tumors surrounded by hyperfluorescence. Ultrasonography shows choroidal thickening.

The melanocytic proliferation is probably a response to a trophic hormone produced by the systemic tumor.[219] Retinal pigment epithelium and retinal receptor damage in this disorder is postulated to be secondary to toxic and immune factors and not because of the melanocytic proliferation.[220] No treatment has proved effective in curtailing the progression of BDUMP.[218]

CONGENITAL HYPERTROPHY OF RETINAL PIGMENT EPITHELIUM (CHRPE)

Multifocal haphazardly arranged small (<0.1 disk diameter), round, flat darkly pigmented retinal pigment epithelium lesions with irregular borders, simulating bear-tracks may occur as an indicator to Gardner's syndrome. Four or more such pigmented fundus lesions in each eye (Figure 17.15) is a reliable indication that the patient may eventually develop colorectal cancer. These lesions are hamartomas of retinal pigment epithelium composed of tall, columnar densely pigmented retinal pigment

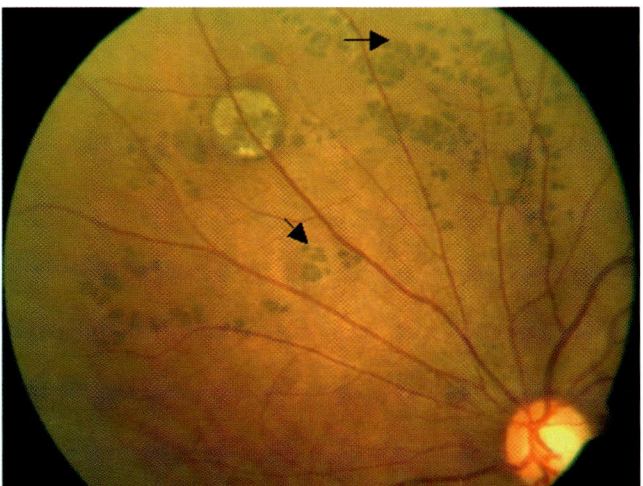

FIGURE 17.15: Congenital hypertrophy of retinal pigment epithelium.

epithelium surrounded by halo of depigmented retinal pigment epithelium cells.[218]

EFFECTS OF TREATMENT OF SYSTEMIC MALIGNANCY ON THE MACULA

Interferon Retinopathy

Patients with systemic malignancies such as cutaneous melanoma, lymphoma, and leukemia undergoing treatment with hi-dose interferon may develop ischemic retinopathy (cotton wool spots and retinal hemorrhages, capillary non perfusion, arteriolar occlusion), macular edema and optic neuropathy that may compromise vision.[221-223]

Retinal Complications of Chemotherapeutic Agents for Systemic Malignancies

Chemotherapeutic agents for systemic malignancies may have side effects on nasolacrimal duct, cornea, conjunctiva, lens vitreous, retina and optic nerve. Some of the chemotherapeutic agents may have to be administered for very long periods resulting in cumulative toxicity. Others may be given in extremely high doses causing ocular problems due to peak concentrations. Intra-arterial or intracerebral administration may lead to more serious side effects than intravenously administered drugs. Combination therapies may enhance the toxicity of certain compounds and renal and hepatic insufficiency may also increase the risk of toxicity due to impaired excretion of chemotherapeutic agents. Chemotherapeutic agents may cause direct changes on the macula such as pigmentary changes, retinal crystals and macular edema or indirectly by causing vascular occlusion, ischemia and vasculitis.

Alkylating agent cisplatin somewhat commonly and carboplatin rarely can cause macular pigmentary changes. Carboplatin and antibiotic anthracycline doxorubicin and estrogen antagonist tamoxifen have been rarely associated with maculopathy. Antimetabolite pyrimidine analog cytosine arabinoside, antimetabolite folic acid analog methotrexate and estrogen antagonist tamoxifen have rarely been associated with macular edema. Cisplatin and methotrexate can cause retinal pigment epithelium mottling rarely. Cisplatin, mitotic inhibitor (topoisomerase inhibitor) etoposide and alkylating agent nitrosurea carmustine are associated with central retinal artery occlusion. Alkylating agent nitrogen mustard derivate chlorambucil, nitrosurea carmustine, estrogen antagonist tamoxifen are associated with retinal hemorrhages and carmustine has been associated with arterial narrowing, retinopathy with exudates and cotton wool spots. Antimetabolite pyrimidine analog cytosine arabinoside can also cause cotton-wool patches and neovascularization. Carmustine has also been associated with retinal periarteritis and periphlebitis.[224] Tamoxifen and toremifene used in breast cancer patients is associated with macular crystals, drusen and yellow-white spots in the retina.[225] Imatinib used to treat leukemia and gastrointestinal tumors may cause retinal edema and visual disturbance.[226,227]

Effects of Bone Marrow Transplantation on the Retina

Bone marrow transplantation may be necessary in the treatment of hematogenous malignancies. To facilitate colonization of the bone marrow with the transplanted cells, cytoreductive chemotherapy with or without whole body radiation is used to destroy all malignant and host marrow to decrease host immune response. Bone marrow and solid organ transplantation may result in significant ophthalmic complications because of the underlying disease process, conditioning regimen, and long-term immunosuppression.

Bone marrow transplant (BMT) retinopathy usually occurs 6 months after transplantation. Retinal findings are bilateral and symmetric. Clinical features include multiple cotton wool spots, telangiectasia, micro-aneurysms, macular edema, hard exudates, and retinal hemorrhages. Fluorescein angiography reveals capillary nonperfusion and dropout, intraretinal microvascular abnormalities, microaneurysms, and fluorescein leakage around the fovea consistent with macular edema. Neovascularization, vitreous hemorrhage and neovascular glaucoma have also been reported.

Pre-transplant radiation is a contributing factor to BMT retinopathy and high dose and short time interval between radiation and BMT are associated with an increased risk of BMT retinopathy. Conditioning chemotherapy chemotherapeutic agents may be one of the factors that lead to BMT retinopathy.

Though the clinical picture is similar to radiation retinopathy, in contrast to radiation retinopathy, BMT retinopathy may be reversible and occurs within 6 months of BMT. In addition, radiation retinopathy is often refractory to treatment. Bone marrow transplantation retinopathy resolves 2 to 4 months after stopping or lowering the dose of cyclosporine with or without the use of systemic prednisolone.

Cytomegalovirus and herpes virus infections, aspergillus, candida, fusarium fungal infections, toxoplasmic retinochoroiditis infections may occur after BMT. Anemia, thrombocytopenia, hyperviscosity that may occur after BMT and chemotherapy can result in retinal hemorrhages, vascular occlusion and vitreous hemorrhage, complications that may adversely affect the macula.[228]

Central serous retinopathy may occur after bone marrow transplantation and graft vs. host disease. The pathogenesis of central serous chorioretinopathy after bone marrow transplantation is believed to be due to combined effects of high doses of corticosteroids, emotional stress, systemic hypertension and cyclosporine. Retinal pigment epithelium changes caused by choriocapillaris ischemia have also been postulated to be the cause of the serous retinal detachment.[229] The visual prognosis of central serous chorioretinopathy in these patients is generally good, and treatment with photocoagulation may be needed only in refractory cases.[230,231]

Radiation Retinopathy

Radiation retinopathy can occur following radiation to the *eye*, orbit, intracranial lesions, and nasal and paranasal tumors or following total body irradiation in bone marrow transplant patients. Radiation retinopathy usually does not occur within 6 months or after 3 years of radiation.[232-234]

Radiation retinopathy is rare if the radiation dose is less than 4500 cGy at 180 to 200 cGy per fraction. Higher the total dose and higher dose per fraction (recommended 180 to 200 cGy/ fraction) more is the risk of radiation retinopathy. Doses of 4500 to 5500 cGy range delivered to half or more of the retina is likely to produce radiation retinopathy. More than 6500 to 7000 cGy dose entails a risk of 85 to 100% of developing radiation retinopathy.[235,236] Mean duration to developing retinopathy after radiation appears to be 12.6 to 18.7 months depending on the dose delivered and delivery method. Brachytherapy appears to be safer than external beam radiation in that, much higher doses of local therapy must be delivered to produce vascular damage than with external beam radiation.[237,238] External beam radiation also produces a more diffuse retinopathy that is more evident in the posterior pole than local therapy. Cumulative 5-year rates for radiation maculopathy, radiation papillopathy, and vision loss were 64%, 35%, and 68%, respectively in a study of 558 patients treated with proton irradiation for small to medium choroidal melanoma located within 4 disk diameters of the macula or optic nerve. Radiation exposure to the macula and optic disk were risk factors for development of radiation complications. History of diabetes was a significant risk factor for maculopathy and optic neuropathy.[239]

Diabetes mellitus, hypertension, collagen vascular diseases increase the risk of radiation retinopathy; pre-existing diabetic retinopathy increases the risk further.[140,237] Administration of adjunctive chemotherapy, and bone marrow transplantation soon after radiation increases the risk of radiation retinopathy.[237,241-243]

Patients may present with metamorphopsia, blurred vision, central scotoma or sudden complete loss of vision. Clinical findings include microaneurysms, retinal telangiectasia, dot and blot intraretinal hemorrhages, cotton-wool spots, macular exudates, macular edema, perivascular sheathing and intraretinal microvascular abnormalities, vascular occlusions (Figures 17.16A and B). Progression of retinopathy results in neovascular proliferation of the disk, retina and iris. Vitreous hemorrhage, neovascular glaucoma and tractional retinal detachment may occur as complications. Subretinal neovascular membranes may occur. Pigmentary changes including retinal pigment epithelium atrophy and a salt and pepper pattern may appear.

The most common macular change is macular edema, followed by telangiectasia and microaneurysms and intraretinal hemorrhages, hard exudates, nerve fiber layer infarcts and capillary non-perfusion, vascular

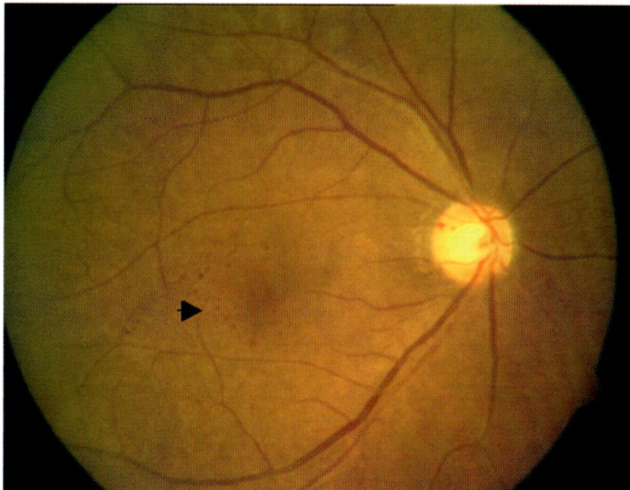

FIGURE 17.16A: Radiation retinopathy.

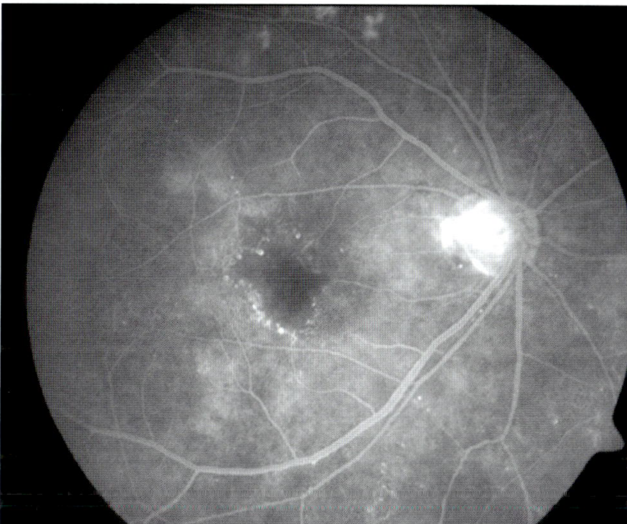

FIGURE 17.16B: Fundus fluorescein angiogram of radiation retinopathy showing multiple perifoveal microaneurysms and distorted foveal avascular zone due to ischemia.

sheathing follow later.[126] Hard exudates seem to appear earlier following brachytherapy and neovascularization more common with teletherapy (due to large area of retina irradiated).[237] Radiation optic neuropathy may occur with retinopathy or may occur without concurrent retinal changes. Radiation dosage more than 5500 cGy and fractions of more than 250 cGy/fraction seem to increase the risk of radiation optic neuropathy.[244]

Fluorescein angiogram shows areas of capillary non-perfusion, retinal vascular abnormalities, neovascularization, window defects due to retinal pigment epithelium loss.

Spontaneous regression of radiation retinopathy may occur rarely; usually there is progression of the disease over 3 to 6 months with neovascularization, tractional retinal detachment and neovascular glaucoma. Nerve fiber infarcts may disappear but macular edema, microaneurysms and capillary non-perfusion and telangiectasia usually persist.

Pathogenesis

Low doses of radiation result in tight junctions of the endothelium to lose their integrity causing increased vascular permeability, retinal edema and exudation. Increase in radiation dose results in death of the endothelium resulting in vascular occlusion resulting in capillary occlusion and cotton-wool spots. Telangiectasia (may cause subretinal neovascular membrane) and retinal hemorrhages also occur. In animal experiments rod photoreceptor damage was noted with single dose of 200 cGy of radiation and single dose of 1000 cGy or more results in photoreceptor death. Cone photoreceptors are more resistant to radiation damage. Damage to ganglion cells and nerve fiber thinning has also been documented. Retinal pigment epithelium damage is seen with single dose of 500 cGy radiation, though cell death does not occur until single dose of 2000 cGy dose is reached.[245] Preferential inner retinal damage due to its dependence on retinal circulation is seen.

Treatment

Treatment of radiation retinopathy is similar to that of diabetic retinopathy. Laser techniques used in the management of diabetic retinopathy are to be followed to treat radiation retinopathy as well. Background retinopathy without macular edema or exudates is not treated but the patient is followed periodically. Focal macular edema or exudates are treated with macular photocoagulation directed at leaking areas identified on fluorescein angiogram; gross macular ischemia does not benefit with photocoagulation and is not treated. Diffuse macular edema is treated with grid laser photocoagulation. Patients are followed up monthly after treatment. Focal laser therapy resulted in resolution of macular edema in 26% and >1 Snellen line vision improvement in 42% of treated patients at 6 months in a study; however there was no difference between treated and untreated eyes at 2 years.[246] Another study found 2 line improvement in vision in 60% of patients after grid photocoagulation over 3 to 22 months follow-up.[247] A recent study on photocoagulation for radiation retinopathy (includes cases with only retinopathy/maculopathy and both) after plaque therapy for posterior uveal melanoma, found that 64.4% regressed after laser photocoagulation. There was evidence to suggest that prophylactic laser photocoagulation before the onset of retinopathy may yield better visual results. However, this has to be confirmed by further studies.[248]

Intravitreal injection of triamcinolone results in temporary resolution of macular edema and visual improvement in eyes with radiation maculopathy.[249,250] Proliferative retinopathy is treated with panretinal photocoagulation.[247,251]

Photodynamic therapy has been performed in 4 patients with macular edema due to radiation maculopathy, resulting in regression of hard exudates in all eyes and visual improvement in one eye.[252]

Vitreous hemorrhage, tractional retinal detachment and fibrovascular proliferation will need vitreous surgery.

Various intraocular tumors may affect the macula directly or by causing secondary effects. Less destructive treatments such as photodynamic therapy, transpupillary thermotherapy and chemotherapy may allow the clinician to destroy the tumor and also limit iatrogenic visual loss. Systemic malignancies may cause an auto-immune reaction affecting the macula. Various modalities used to treat systemic malignancy, such as chemotherapy and radiation may also affect the macula causing vision loss.

REFERENCES

1. Shields CL, Materin MA, Shields JA. Review of optical coherence tomography for intraocular tumors. Curr Opin Ophthalmology 2005; 16:141-54
2. Shields CL, Mashayekhi A, Luo CK, et al. Optical coherence tomography in children: analysis of 44 eyes with intraocular tumors and simulating conditions. J Pediatr Ophthalmol Strabismus. 2004; 4:338-44.
3. Espinoza G, Rosenblatt B, Harbour JW. Optical coherence tomography in the evaluation of retinal changes associated with suspicious choroidal melanocytic tumors. Am J Ophthalmol 2004; 137:90-5.

4. Ide T, Ohguro N, Hayashi A, et al. Optical coherence tomography patterns of choroidal osteoma. Am J Ophthalmol 2000; 130:131-4.
5. Fukasawa A, Iijima H. Optical coherence tomography of choroidal osteoma. Am J Ophthalmol 2002; 133:419-21.
6. Stallman JB. Visual improvement after pars plana vitrectomy and membrane peeling for vitreoretinal traction associated with combined hamartoma of the retina and retinal pigment epithelium. Retina 2002; 22:101-4.
7. Mashayekhi A, Shields CL, Eagle RC Jr, Shields JA. Cavitary changes in retinoblastoma: relationship to chemoresistance. Ophthalmology. 2005; 112:1145-50.
8. Shields JA, Shields CL. Retinoblastoma. Clinical and pathologic features. In Intraocular tumours: A Text and Atlas. WB Saunders, Philadelphia, 1992, pp 305-31.
9. Senft S, al-Kaff A, Bergqvist G, et al. Retinoblastoma. The Saudi Arabian experience. Ophthalmic Paediatr Genet 1988; 9:115-9.
10. Kock E, Naeser P. Retinoblastoma in Sweden 1958—1971. A clinical and histopathological study. Acta Ophthalmol 1979:57:344-50.
11. Francke U. Retinoblastoma and chromosome 13. Cytogenet Cell Genet 1976; 16:131-4.
12. Yunis JJ, Ramsay N. Retinoblastoma and subband deletion of chromosome 13. Am J Dis Child 1978; 132:161-3.
13. Shanmugam MP, Biswas J, Gopal L, et al. The clinical spectrum and treatment outcome of retinoblastoma in Indian children. J Pediatr Ophthalmol Strabismus. 2005; 42:75-81.
14. Vemuganti G, Honavar S, John R. Clinicopathological profile of retinoblastoma in Asian Indians. Inv Ophthalmol Vis Sci 2000; 41(S790):4.
15. Sahu S, Banavali SD, Pai SK, et al. Retinoblastoma: problems and perspectives from India. Pediatr Hematol Oncol 1998; 15:501-8.
16. Rubenfeld M, Abramson DH, Ellsworth RM, et al. Unilateral vs. bilateral retinoblastoma. Correlations between age at diagnosis and stage of ocular disease. Ophthalmology 1986; 93:1016-9.
17. Kayembe L. Retinoblastoma: 21-year review. J Fr Ophthalmol 1986; 9:561-5.
18. Mathew L, Miale TD, Rao S, et al. Retrospective analysis of 58 children with retinoblastoma. Ophthalmic Paediatr Genet 1984; 4:67-74.
19. Mohney BG, Robertson DM. Ancillary testing for metastasis in patients with newly diagnosed retinoblastoma. Am J Ophthalmol 1994; 118:707-11.
20. Epstein J, Shields CL, Shields JA. Trends in the management of retinoblastoma: evaluation of 1,196 consecutive eyes during 1974–2001. J Pediatr Ophthalmol Strabismus 2003; 40:196-203.
21. Desjardins L, Charif Chefchaouni M, Lumbroso L, et al. Functional results of retinoblastoma treatment with local treatment used in isolation or associated with chemotherapy. J Fr Ophthalmol 2005; 28:725-31.
22. Weiss AH, Karr DJ, Kalina RE, et al. Visual outcomes of macular retinoblastoma after external beam radiation therapy. Ophthalmology 1994; 101:1244-9.
23. Migdal C. Bilateral retinoblastoma: the prognosis for vision. Br J Ophthalmol 1983; 67:592–5.
24. Hall LS, Ceisler E, Abramson DH. Visual outcomes in children with bilateral retinoblastoma. J AAPOS 1999; 3:138-42.
25. Shields CL, Shields JA, Cater J, et al. Plaque radiotherapy for retinoblastoma: long term tumor control and treatment complications in 208 tumors. Ophthalmology 2001; 108:2116-21.
26. Demirci H, Shields CL, Meadows AT, Shields JA. Long-term visual outcome following chemoreduction for retinoblastoma. Arch Ophthalmol 2005; 123:1525-30.
27. Shields CL, Mashayekhi A, Cater J, et al. Macular retinoblastoma managed with chemoreduction: analysis of tumor control with or without adjuvant thermotherapy in 68 tumors. Arch Ophthalmol 2005; 123:765-73.
28. Gombos DS, Kelly A, Coen PG, et al. Retinoblastoma treated with primary chemotherapy alone: the significance of tumor size, location and age. Br J Ophthalmol 2002; 86:80-83.
29. Lee TC, Lee SW, Dinkin MJ, et al. Chorioretinal scar growth after 810-nanometer laser treatment for retinoblastoma. Ophthalmology 2004; 111:992-6.
30. Watts P, Westall C, Colpa L, et al. Visual results in children treated for macular retinoblastoma. Eye 2002; 16:75-80.
31. Brown CG, Shields JA. Tumors of the optic nerve head. Surv Ophthalmol 1985; 29:239-64.
32. Atkinson A, Sanders MD, Wong V. Vitreous haemorrhage in tuberous sclerosis. Br J Ophthalmol 1973; 57:773-9.
33. Vrabec TR, Augsburger JJ. Exudative retinal detachment due to small noncalcified retinal astrocytic hamartoma. Am J Ophthalmol 2003; 136:952-4.
34. Bloom SM, Mahl CF. Photocoagulation for serous detachment of the macula secondary to retinal astrocytoma. Retina 1991; 11:416-22.
35. Lagos JC, Gomez MR. Tuberous sclerosis, Reappraisal of a clinical entity. Mayo Clin Proc 1967; 42:26-49.
36. Reeser FH, Aaberg TM, Van Horn D. Astrocytic hamartoma of the retina not associated with tuberous sclerosis. Am J Ophthalmol 1978; 86:688-98.
37. Garcia-Arumi J, Sararols LH, Cavero L, et al. Therapeutic options for capillary papillary hemangiomas. Ophthalmology 2000; 107:48-54.
38. Gill HS, Simpson R. Transpupillary thermotherapy in the management of juxtapapillary and parafoveal circumscribed choroidal hemangioma. Can J Ophthalmol 2005; 40:729-33.
39. Costa RA, Meirelles RL, Cardillo JA, et al. Retinal capillary hemangioma treatment by indocyanine green-mediated photothrombosis. Am J Ophthalmol 2003; 135:395-8.
40. Aaberg TM Jr, Aaberg TM Sr, Martin DF, et al. Three cases of large retinal capillary hemangiomas treated with verteporfin and photodynamic therapy. Arch Ophthalmol 2005; 123:328-32.

41. Obana A, Goto Y, Ikoma M. A case of von Hippel-Lindau disease with papillary capillary hemangioma treated by photodynamic therapy. Nippon Ganka Gakkai Zasshi 2004; 108:226-32.

42. Schmidt-Erfurth UM, Kusserow C, Barbazetto IA, Laqua H. Benefits and complications of photodynamic therapy of papillary capillary hemangiomas. Ophthalmology 2002; 109:1256-66.

43. Atebara NH. Retinal capillary hemangioma treated with verteporfin photodynamic therapy. Am J Ophthalmol 2002; 134:788-90.

44. McDonald HR, Schatz H, Johnson RN, et al. Vitrectomy in eyes with peripheral retinal angioma associated with traction macular detachment. Ophthalmology 1996; 103:329-35.

45. Farah ME, Uno F, Hofling-Lima AL, et al. Transretinal feeder vessel ligature in von Hippel-Lindau disease. Eur J Ophthalmol 2001; 11:386-8.

46. Peyman GA, Rednam KR, Mottow-Lippa L, Flood T. Treatment of large von Hippel tumors by eye wall resection. Ophthalmology 1983; 90:840-7.

47. Girmens JF, Erginay A, Massin P, et al. Treatment of von Hippel-Lindau retinal hemangioblastoma by the vascular endothelial growth factor receptor inhibitor SU5416 is more effective for associated macular edema than for hemangioblastomas. Am J Ophthalmol 2003; 136:194-6.

48. Kreusel KM, Bornfeld N, Bender BU, et al. Retinal capillary angioma. Clinical and molecular genetic studies. Ophthalmologe 1999; 96:71-6.

49. Naftchi S, la Cour M. A case of central visual loss in a child due to macular cavernous haemangioma of the retina. Acta Ophthalmol Scand 2002; 80:550-2.

50. Yamaguchi K, Yamaguchi K, Tamai M Cavernous hemangioma of the retina in a pediatric patient. Ophthalmologica 1988; 197:127-9.

51. Gunduz K, Ozbayrak N, Okka M, et al. Cavernous hemangioma with cone dysfunction. Ophthalmologica 1996; 210:367-71.

52. Bottoni F, Canevini MP, Canger R, Orzalesi N. Twin vessels in familial retinal cavernous hemangioma. Am J Ophthalmol 1990; 15:285-9.

53. Haller JA, Knox DL. Vitrectomy for persistent vitreous hemorrhage from a cavernous hemangioma of the optic disk. Am J Ophthalmol 1993; 15:116:106-7.

54. Drigo P, Mammi I, Battistella PA, et al. Familial cerebral, hepatic, and retinal cavernous angiomas: a new syndrome. Childs Nerv Syst 1994; 10:205-9.

55. Archer DB, Deutman A, Ernest JT, et al. Arteriovenous communications of the retina. Am J Ophthalmol 1973; 75:224-41.

56. Bernth-Petersen P. Racemose haemangioma of the retina. Report of three cases with long term follow-up. Acta Ophthalmol (Copenh) 1979; 57:669-78.

57. Mansour AM, Wells AM, Jampol LM, et al. Ocular complications of arteriovenous communications of the retina. Arch Ophthalmol 1989; 107:232-6.

58. Schatz H, Chang LF, Ober RR, et al. Central retinal vein occlusion associated with retinal arteriovenous malformation. Ophthalmology 1993; 100:24-30.

59. Wyburn-Mason R. Arteriovenous aneurysm of mid-brain and retina, facial nevi and mental changes. Brain 1943; 66:163-203.

60. Theron J, Newton TH, Hoyt WF. Unilateral retinocephalic vascular malformations. Neuroradiology 1974; 7:186-96.

61. Albert DM, Jakobiec FA, (eds.). Phakomatoses. In: Principles and practice of ophthalmology, 2nd ed. Philadelphia: WB Saunders, 2000:3779.

62. Goh D, Malik NN, Gilvarry A. Retinal racemose haemangioma directly communicating with a intramuscular facial cavernous haemangioma. Br J Ophthalmol 2004; 88:840-2.

63. Shields CL, Shields JA, Barrett J, De Potter P. Vasoproliferative tumors of the ocular fundus. Classification and clinical manifestations in 103 patients. Arch Ophthalmol 1995; 113:615-23.

64. Heimann H, Bornfeld N, Vij O, et al. Vasoproliferative tumours of the retina. Br J Ophthalmol 2000; 84:1162-9.

65. Barbezetto IA, Smith RT. Vasoproliferative tumor of the retina treated with PDT. Retina 2003; 23:565-7.

66. Madrepala SA. Choroidal hemangioma treated with photodynamic therapy using verteporfin. Arch Ophthalmol 2001; 119:1606-10.

67. Robertson DM. Photodynamic therapy for choroidal hemangioma associated with serous retinal detachment. Arch Ophthalmol 2002; 120:1155-61.

68. Sheidow TG, Harbour JW. Photodynamic therapy for circumscribed choroidal hemangioma. Can J Ophthalmol 2002; 37:314-7.

69. Barbazetto I, Schmidt-Erfurth U. Photodynamic therapy of choroidal hemangioma: two case reports. Graefes Arch Clin Exp Ophthalmol 2000; 238:214-21.

70. Schmidt-Erfurth UM, Michels S, Kusserow C, et al. Photodynamic therapy for symptomatic choroidal hemangioma. Visual and anatomic results. Ophthalmology 2002; 109:2284-94.

71. Michels S, Michels R, Beckendorf A, Schmidt-Erfurth U. Photodynamic therapy for choroidal hemangioma. Long-term results. Ophthalmologe 2004; 101:569-75.

72. Porrini G, Giovannini A, Amato G, et al. Photodynamic therapy of circumscribed choroidal hemangioma. Ophthalmology 2003; 110:674-80.

73. Landau IM, Steen B, Seregard S. Photodynamic therapy for circumscribed choroidal haemangioma. Acta Ophthalmol Scand 2002; 80:531-6.

74. Huiskamp EA, Muskens RP, Ballast A, Hooymans JM. Diffuse choroidal haemangioma in Sturge-Weber syndrome treated with photodynamic therapy under general anaesthesia. Graefes Arch Clin Exp Ophthalmol 2005;243:727-30.

75. Gunduz K. Transpupillary thermotherapy in the management of circumscribed choroidal hemangioma. Surv Ophthalmol 2004; 49:316-27.

76. Shields JA, Shields CL, Materin MA, et al. Changing concepts in management of circumscribed choroidal hemangioma: the 2003 J. Howard Stokes Lecture, Part 1. Ophthalmic Surg Lasers Imaging 2004; 35:383-94.

77. Garcia-Arumi J, Ramsay LS, Guraya BC. Transpupillary thermotherapy for circumscribed choroidal hemangiomas. Ophthalmology 2000; 107:351-6.

78. Kamal A, Watts AR, Rennie IG. Indocyanine green enhanced transpupillary thermotherapy of circumscribed choroidal haemangioma. Eye 2000; 14:701-5.

79. Othmane IS, Shields CL, Shields JA, et al. Circumscribed choroidal hemangioma managed by transpupillary thermotherapy. Arch Ophthalmol 1999; 117:136-7.

80. Rapizzi E, Grizzard WS, Capone A Jr. Transpupillary thermotherapy in the management of circumscribed choroidal hemangioma. Am J Ophthalmol 1999; 127:481-2.

81. Mosci C, Polizzi A, Zingirian M. Transpupillary thermotherapy for circumscribed choroidal hemangiomas: first choice in therapy. Eur J Ophthalmol 2001; 11:316-8.

82. Fuchs AV, Mueller AJ, Grueterich M, Ulbig MW. Transpupillary thermotherapy (TTT) in circumscribed choroidal hemangioma. Graefes Arch Clin Exp Ophthalmol 2002; 240:7-11.

83. Vianna RN, Fernandes L, Muralha A, et al. Transpupillary thermotherapy in the treatment of circumscribed choroidal hemangiomas. Int Ophthalmol 2004; 25:117-21.

84. Zografas L, Bercher L, Chamot L, et al. Cobalt-60 treatment of choroidal hemangiomas. Am J Ophthalmol 1996; 121:190-9.

85. Madreperla SA, Hungerford JL, Plowman PN, et al. Choroidal hemangiomas: visual and anatomic results of treatment by photocoagulation or radiation therapy. Ophthalmology 1997; 104:1773-9.

86. Ritland JS, Eide N, Tausjo J. External beam irradiation therapy for choroidal hemangiomas. Visual and anatomic results after a dose of 20-25Gy. Acta Ophthalmol Scand 2001; 79:184-6.

87. Schilling H, Sauerwein W, Lommatzsch A, et al. Long term results after low dose ocular irradiation for choroidal hemangiomas. Br J Ophthalmol 1997; 81:267-73.

88. Shanmugam MP, Sharma T. External beam irradiation in the management of choroidal haemangioma. Ind J Ophthalmol 1997; 45:45-8.

89. Kivela T, Tenhunen M, Joensuu T, Tommila P, Joensuu H, Kouri M. Stereotactic radiotherapy of symptomatic circumscribed choroidal hemangiomas. Ophthalmology 2003; 110:1977-82.

90. Gass JDM, Guerry RK, Jack RL, et al. Choroidal Osteoma. Arch Ophthalmol 1978; 96:428-35.

91. Shields JA, Shields CL. Intraocular tumors. A text and atlas. Philadelphia: WB Saunders, 1992, pp 261-71.

92. Cunha SL. Osseous choristoma of the choroid. A familial disease. Arch Ophthalmol 1984; 102:1052-4.

93. Noble KG. Bilateral choroidal osteoma in three siblings. Am J Ophthalmol 1990; 109:656-60.

94. Shields CL, Sun H, Demirci H, Shields JA. Factors predictive of tumor growth, tumor decalcification, choroidal neovascularization, and visual outcome in 74 eyes with choroidal osteoma. Arch Ophthalmol. 2005; 123:1658-66.

95. Yuzawa M, Kawamura A, Haruyama M, Matsui M. Indocyanine green video-angiographic findings in choroidal osteoma. Eur J Ophthalmol 1994; 4:191-8.

96. Lafaut BA, Mestdaugh C, Kohno T, et al. Indocyanine green angiography in choroidal osteoma. Graefes Arch of Clin Exp Ophthalmol 1997; 235:330-7.

97. Grand MG, Burgess DB, Singermann LJ, Ramsey J. Choroidal osteoma. Treatment of associated subretinal neovascular membranes. Retina 1984; 4:84-90.

98. Morrison DL, Magargal LE, Ehrlich DR, et al. Review of choroidal osteoma: successful krypton red laser photocoagulation of an associated subretinal neovascular membrane involving the fovea. Ophthalmic Surg 1987; 18:299-03.

99. Shanmugam MP, Sharma S, Bhargava S. Transpupillary thermotherapy for choroidal neovascularization in choroidal osteoma. Ind J Ophthalmol 2004;52:329-30.

100. Battaglia PM, da Pozzo S, Toto L, et al. Photodynamic therapy for choroidal neovascularization associated with choroidal osteoma. Retina 2001;21:660-61.

101. Shukla D, Tanawade RG, Ramasamy K. Transpupillary thermotherapy for subfoveal choroidal neovascular membrane in choroidal osteoma. Eye 2005 Oct 21; [Epub ahead of print]

102. Singh AD, Talbot JF, Rundle PA, Rennie IG. Choroidal neovascularization secondary to choroidal osteoma: successful treatment with photodynamic therapy. Eye 2005; 19:482-4.

103. Foster BS, Fernandez-Suntay JP, Dryja TP, et al. Clinicopathologic reports, case reports, and small case series: surgical removal and histopathologic findings of a subfoveal neovascular membrane associated with choroidal osteoma. Arch Ophthalmol 2003; 121:273-6.

104. Egon, KM, Seddon JM, Glynn RJ, et al. Epidemiologic aspects of uveal melanoma. Survey of ophthalmology 1998; 32:239-51.

105. Iscovich J, Abdulrazik M, Pe'Er J. Posterior uveal malignant melanoma: temporal stability and ethnic variation in rates in Israel. Anticancer Res 2001; 21:1449-54.

106. Biswas J, Kabra S, Krishnakumar S, Shanmugam MP. Clinical and histopathological characteristics of uveal melanoma in Asian Indians. A study of 103 patients. Ind J Ophthalmol 2004; 52:41-4.

107. Ou JI, Wheeler SM, O'Brien JM. Posterior pole tumor update. Ophthalmol Clin North Am 2002; 15:489-501.

108. The Collaborative Ocular Melanoma Study Group. Mortality in patients with small choroidal melanoma. COMS report no. 4. Arch Ophthalmol 1997; 115:886-93.

109. The Collaborative Ocular Melanoma Study Group. The collaborative ocular melanoma study randomized trial of

iodine 125 brachytherapy for choroidal melanoma, III: initial mortality findings. COMS report no. 18. Arch Ophthalmol 2001; 119:969-82.

110. The Collaborative Ocular Melanoma Study Group. The collaborative ocular melanoma study randomized trial of pre-enucleation radiation of large choroidal melanoma II: initial mortality findings. COMS report no. 10. Am J Ophthalmol 1998; 125:865-7.

111. Mueller AJ, Freeman WR, Schaller UC, Kampik A, Folberg R and Munic/San Diego/Iowa city collaboration. Complex microcirculation patterns detected by confocal indocyanine green angiography predict time to growth of small choroidal melanocytic tumors. MuSIC report II. Ophthalmology 2002; 109:2207-14.

112. Qiang Z, Cairns JD. Laser photocoagulation treatment of choroidal melanoma. Aust N Z J Ophthalmol 1993; 21:87-92.

113. Oosterhuis JA, Journee-de Korver HG, Kakebeeke-Kemme HM, et al. Transpupillary thermotherapy in choroidal melanomas. Arch Ophthalmol 1995; 113:315-21.

114. Shields CL, Shields JA. Transpupillary thermotherapy for choroidal melanoma. Curr Opin Ophthalmol 1999; 10:197-203.

115. Shields CL, Shields JA, Perez N, et al. Primary transpupillary thermotherapy for small choroidal melanoma in 256 consecutive cases: outcomes and limitations. Ophthalmology 2002; 109:225-34.

116. Stoffelns BM. Primary transpupillary thermotherapy (TTT) for malignant choroidal melanoma. Acta Ophthalmol Scand 2002; 80:25-31.

117. Stoffelns BM. Tumor regression and visual outcome after transpupillary thermotherapy (TTT) for malignant choroidal melanoma Klin Monatsbl Augenheilkd 2006;223:74-80.

118. Robertson DM, Buettner H, Bennett SR. Transpupillary thermotherapy as primary treatment for small choroidal melanomas. Trans Am Ophthalmol Soc 1999; 97:407-27.

119. Harbour JW, Meredith TA, Thompson PA, Gordon ME. Transpupillary thermotherapy versus plaque radiotherapy for suspected choroidals melanomas. Ophthalmology 2003; 110:2207-14.

120. Liggett PE, Lavaque AJ, Chaudhry NA, et al. Preliminary results of combined simultaneous transpupillary thermotherapy and ICG-based photodynamic therapy for choroidal melanoma. Ophthalmic Surg Lasers Imaging 2005; 36:463-70.

121. Stoffelns BM. Kinetics of indocyanine green (ICG) and clinical use for enhancement of transpupillary thermotherapy (TTT) in hypopigmented small choroidal melanomas Klin Monatsbl Augenheilkd 2004; 221:374-8.

122. Kim RY, Hu LK, Foster BS, et al. Photodynamic therapy of pigmented choroidal melanomas of greater than 3-mm thickness. Ophthalmology 1996; 103: 2029-36.

123. Barbazetto IA, Lee TC, Rollins IS, et al. Treatment of choroidal melanoma using photodynamic therapy. Am J Ophthalmol 2003; 135: 898-9.

124. Donaldson MJ, Lim L, Harper CA, et al. Primary treatment of choroidal amelanotic melanoma with photodynamic therapy. Clin Experiment Ophthalmol 2005; 33:548-9.

125. Robertson DM. Changing concepts in the management of choroidal melanoma. Am J Ophthalmol 2003; 136:161-70.

126. Guyer DR, Mukai S, Egan KM, et al. Radiation maculopathy after proton beam irradiation for choroidal melanoma. Ophthalmology 1992; 99:1278-85.

127. Melia BM, Abramson DH, Albert DM, et al; Collaborative Ocular Melanoma Study Group. Collaborative ocular melanoma study (COMS) randomized trial of I-125 brachytherapy for medium choroidal melanoma. I. Visual acuity after 3 years COMS report no. 16. Ophthalmology 2001; 108:348-66.

128. Jones R, Gore E, Mieler W, et al. Post treatment visual acuity in patients treated with episcleral plaque therapy for choroidal melanomas: dose and dose rate effects. Int J Radiat Oncol Biol Phys 2002; 52:989-95.

129. Char DH, Kroll S, Quivey JM, Castro J. Long term visual outcome of radiated uveal melanomas in eyes eligible for randomization to enucleation versus brachytherapy.Br J Ophthalmol 1996; 80:117-24.

130. Seddon JM, Gragoudas ES, Polivogianis L, et al. Visual outcome after proton beam irradiation of uveal melanoma. Ophthalmology 1986; 93:666-74.

131. Gunduz K, Shields CL, Shields JA, et al. Radiation complications and tumor control after plaque radiotherapy of choroidals melanoma with macular involvement. Am J Ophthalmol 1999; 127:579-89.

132. Finger PT. Tumour location affects the incidence of cataract and retinopathy after ophthalmic plaque radiation therapy. Br J Ophthalmol 2000; 84:1068-70.

133. Jampol LM, Moy CS, Murray TG, et al. The collaborative ocular melanoma study randomized trial of I-125 brachytherapy for choroidal melanoma. IV. Local treatment failure and enucleation in the first five years after brachytherapy. COMS Report No.19. Ophthalmology 2002; 109:2197-06.

134. Puusaari I, Heikkonen J, Summanen P, et al. Iodine brachytherapy as an alternative to enucleation for large uveal melanomas. Ophthalmology 2003; 110:2223-34.

135. Shields CL, Cater J, Shields JA, et al. Combined plaque radiotherapy and transpupillary thermotherapy for choroidals melanoma: tumor control and treatment complications in 270 consecutive patients. Arch Ophthalmol 2002; 120:933-40.

136. Stoffelns BM, Kutzner J, Schopfer K, Frising M. Prospective nonrandomized analysis of "Sandwich Therapy" for malignant melanoma of the choroid] Klin Monatsbl Augenheilkd 2002; 219:211-5.

137. Damato BE, Foulds WS. Surgical resection of choroidal melanoma. In: Ryan SJ. (ed.). Retina St. Louis, CV Mosby, 2001, pp 762-72.

138. Shields JA, Shields CL. Surgical approach to lamellar sclerouvectomy for posterior uveal melanomas: The Schoenberg lecture. Ophthalmic Surg 1988; 19:774-80.

139. Peyman GA, Juarez CP, Diamond JG, Raichand M. Ten years experience with eye wall resection of uveal melanomas. Ophthalmology 1984; 91:1720-24.

140. Peyman GA, Charles H. Internal eyewall resection in the management of uveal melanoma. Can J Ophthalmol 1988; 23:219-23.

141. Garcia-Arumi J, Sararols L, Martinez V, Corcostegui BF. Vitreoretinal surgery and endoresection in high posterior choroidal melanomas Retina 2001; 21:445-2.

142. The Collaborative Ocular Melanoma Study Group. The collaborative ocular melanoma study randomized trial of pre-enucleation radiation of large choroidal melanoma II: initial mortality findings. COMS report no. 10. Am J Ophthalmol 1998; 125:865-7.

143. Fraunfelder FT, Boozman FW, Wilson RS, et al. No touch technique for intraocular malignant tumors. Arch Ophthalmol 1977; 95:1616-20.

144. Midgal C. Effect of the method of enucleation on the prognosis of choroidal melanoma. Br J Ophthalmol 1983; 67:385-8.

145. Shields CL, Shields JA, Kiratli H, et al. Risk factors for growth and metastasis of small choroidal melanocytic lesions. Ophthalmology 1995; 102:1351-61.

146. Collaborative Ocular Melanoma Study Group. Factors predictive of growth and treatment of small choroidal melanoma: COMS report No. 5. Arch Ophthalmol 1997; 115:1537-44.

147. Shields CL, Cater JC, Shields JA, et al. Combination of clinical factors predictive of growth of small choroidal melanocytic tumors. Arch Ophthalmol 2000; 118:360-64.

148. Singh AD, Kalyani P, Topham A. Estimating the risk of malignant transformation of a choroidal nevus. Ophthalmology 2005; 112:1784-9.

149. Duquesne N, Hajji Z, Jean-Louis B, Grange JD. Choroidal nevi associated with serous macular detachment. Fr Ophtalmol 2002; 25:393-8.

150. Muscat S, Srinivasan S, Sampat V, et al. Optical coherence tomography in the diagnosis of subclinical serous detachment of the macula secondary to a choroidal nevus. Ophthalmic Surg Lasers 2001; 32:474-6.

151. Levy J, Shneck M, Klemperer I, Lifshitz T. Treatment of subfoveal choroidal neovascularization secondary to choroidal nevus using photodynamic therapy. Ophthalmic Surg Lasers Imaging 2005; 36:343-5.

152. Parodi MB, Boscia F, Piermarocchi S, et al. Variable outcome of photodynamic therapy for choroidal neovascularization associated with choroidal nevus. Retina 2005; 25:438-42.

153. Zografos L, Mantel I, Schalenbourg A. Subretinal choroidal neovascularization associated with choroidal nevus. Eur J Ophthalmol 2004; 14:123-31.

154. Stanescu D, Wattenberg S, Cohen SY. Photodynamic therapy for choroidal neovascularization secondary to choroidal nevus. Am J Ophthalmol 2003; 136:575-6.

155. Freedman MI, Folk JC. Metastatic tumors to the eye and orbit: a clinicopathologic study of 227 cases. Arch Ophthalmol 1987; 105:1215-9.

156. Ferry AP, Font RL. Carcinoma metastatic to the eye and orbit. I. Clinicopathologic study of 227 cases. Arch Ophthalmol 1975; 92:276-86.

157. Shields JA, Shields CL. Intraocular tumors. A text and atlas. Philadelphia, WB Saunders, 1992, pp 207-38.

158. Shields CL, Shields JA, Gross N, et al. Survey of 520 uveal metastases. Ophthalmology 1997; 104:1265-76.

159. Shields JA, Shields CL, Kiratli H, De Potter P. Metastatic tumors to the iris in 40 patients. Am J Ophthalmol 1995; 119:422-30.

160. Gallie BL, Graham JE, Hunter WS. Optic nerve head metastasis. Arch Ophthalmol 1975; 19:983-7.

161. Levinger S, Merin S, Seigal R, Pe'er J. Laser therapy in the management of choroidal breast tumor metastases. Ophthalmic Surg Lasers 2001; 32:294-9.

162. Harbour JW, De Potter P, Shields CL, Shields JA. Uveal metastasis from carcinoid tumor. Clinical observations in nine cases. Ophthalmology 1994; 101:1084-90.

163. Gysin P, Gloor B. Cryo- and photocoagulation for choroidal metastases of a thyroid carcinoma (author's transl)] Klin Monatsbl Augenheilkd 1979; 174:978-81.

164. Vianna RN, Pena R, Muralha A, et al. Transpupillary thermotherapy in the treatment of choroidal metastasis from breast carcinoma. Int Ophthalmol 2004; 25:23-26.

165. Harbour JW. Photodynamic therapy for choroidal metastasis from carcinoid tumor. Am J Ophthalmol 2004; 137:1143-5.

166. Eagle RC Jr, Ehya H, Shields JA, Shields CL. Choroidal metastasis as the initial manifestation of a pigmented neuroendocrine tumor. Arch Ophthalmol 2000; 118:841-5.

167. Zimmerman LE, Garon LK. Melanocytoma of the optic disc. Int Ophthalmol Clinics 1962; 2:431-40.

168. Lauritzen K, Augsburger JJ, Timmes J. Vitreous seeding associated with melanocytoma of the optic disc. Retina 1990; 10:60-62.

169. Meyer D, Jayne GE, Blinder KJ, et al. Malignant transformation of an optic disc melanocytoma. Am J Ophthalmol 1999; 127:710-14.

170. Garcia-Arumi J, Salvador F, Corcostegui BF. Neuroretinitis associated with melanocytoma of the optic disc. Retina 1994; 14:173-6.

171. Shanmugam MP, Khetan V, Sinha P. Optic disc melanocytoma with neuroretinitis. Retina 2004; 24:317-8.

172. Shields JA, Shields CA, Eagle RC, et al. Central retinal vascular obstruction secondary to melanocytoma of the optic disc. Arch Ophthalmol 2001; 119:129-33.

173. Agarwal S, Shanmugam MP, Gopal L, et al. Necrotic melanocytoma of the optic disk with central retinal vascular obstruction. Retina 2005; 25:364-7.

174. Shields JA, Demirci H, Mashayekhi A, Shields CL. Melanocytoma of optic disc in 115 cases: the 2004 Samuel Johnson Memorial Lecture, part 1. Ophthalmology 2004; 111:1739-46.

175. Ryan SJ. Combined hamartoma of the retina and retinal pigment epithelium In: Retina St. Louis, Missouri, Mosby, Inc., 2001, pp 640-46.

176. Font RL, Moura RA, Shetlar DJ, et al.. Combined hamartoma of sensory retina and retinal pigment epithelium. Retina 1989; 9:302-11.

177. Helbig H, Niederberger H. Presumed combined hamartoma of the retina and retinal pigment epithelium with preretinal neovascularization. Am J Ophthalmol 2003; 136:1157-9.

178. Moschos M, Ladas ID, Zafirakis PK, et al. Recurrent vitreous hemorrhages due to combined pigment epithelial and retinal hamartoma: natural course and indocyanine green angiographic findings. Ophthalmologica 2001; 215:66-9.

179. Kahn D, Goldberg MF, Jednock N. Combined retinal-retina pigment epithelial hamartoma presenting as a vitreous hemorrhage. Retina 1984; 4:40-43.

180. Schachat AP, Shields JA, Fine SL, et al. Combined hamartomas of the retina and retinal pigment epithelium. Ophthalmology 1984; 91:1609-15.

181. Mason JO, Kleiner R. Combined hamartoma of the retina and retinal pigment epithelium associated with epiretinal membrane and macular hole. Retina 1997; 17:160-62.

182. Verma L, Venkatesh P, Lakshmaiah CN, Tewari HK. Combined hamartoma of the retina and retinal pigment epithelium with full thickness retinal hole and without retinoschisis. Ophthalmic Surg Lasers 2000; 31:423-6.

183. Vianna RN, Pacheco DF, Vasconcelos MM, de Laey JJ.Combined hamartoma of the retina and retinal pigment epithelium associated with neurofibromatosis type-1. Int Ophthalmol 2001; 24:63-6.

184. McDonald HR, Abrams GW, Burke JM, Neuwirth J. Clinicopathologic results of vitreous surgery for epiretinal membranes in patients with combined retinal and retinal pigment epithelial hamartomas. Am J Ophthalmol 1985; 100:806-13.

185. Sappenfield DL, Gitter KA. Surgical intervention for combined retinal-retinal pigment epithelial hamartoma. Retina 1990; 10:119-24.

186. Stallman JB. Visual improvement after pars plana vitrectomy and membrane peeling for vitreoretinal traction associated with combined hamartoma of the retina and retinal pigment epithelium. Retina 2002; 22:101-4.

187. Kushner BJ. Functional amblyopia associated with organic ocular disease. Am J Ophthalmol 1981; 91:39-45.

188. Inoue M, Noda K, Ishida S, et al. Successful treatment of subfoveal choroidal neovascularization associated with combined hamartoma of the retina and retinal pigment epithelium. Am J Ophthalmol 2004; 138:155-6.

189. Shields JA, Shields CL, Eagle RC Jr, Singh AD. Adenocarcinoma arising from congenital hypertrophy of retinal pigment epithelium. Arch Ophthalmol 2001; 119:597-02.

190. Brody JM, Butrus SI, Ashraf MF, et al. Multiple myeloma presenting with bilateral exudative macular detachments. Acta Ophthalmol Scand 1995;73:81-82.

191. Suzuki J, Goto H, Usui M. Adenoma arising from nonpigmented ciliary epithelium concomitant with neovascularization of the optic disk and cystoid macular edema. Am J Ophthalmol 2005; 139:188-90.

192. Chan CC, Buggage RR, Nussenblatt RB. Intraocular lymphoma. Curr Opin Ophthalmol 2002; 13:411-8.

193. Coupland SE, Heimann H. Primary intraocular lymphoma. Ophthalmologe 2004; 101:87-98.

194. Helbig H, Cerny T, de Smet MD. Intravitreal chemotherapy for intraocular lymphoma. Ophthalmologe 2003; 100:145-9.

195. Batchelor TT, Kolak G, Ciordia R, et al. High-dose methotrexate for intraocular lymphoma. Clin Cancer Res 2003; 9:711-5.

196. Kincaid MC, Green WR, Ocular and orbital involvement in leukemia. Surv Ophthalmol 1983; 27:211-32.

197. Leonardy N J, Dent G, Rupani M, Klintworth GK. Analysis of 135 autopsy eyes for ocular involvement in leukemia. Am J Ophthalmol 1990; 109:436-44.

198. Rosenthal AR. Ocular manifestations of leukemia. Ophthalmology 1983; 90:899-05.

199. Al-Abdulla NA, Thompson JT, LaBorwit SE. Simultaneous bilateral central retinal vein occlusion associated with anticardiolipin antibodies in leukemia. Am J Ophthalmol 2001; 132:266-8.

200. Malik R, Shah A, Greaney MJ, Dick AD. Bilateral serous macular detachment as a presenting feature of acute lymphoblastic leukemia. Eur J Ophthalmol 2005; 15:284-6.

201. Horgan SE, Fraser SG, Ferrante PF, et al. Macular serous detachment revealing acute lymphoblastic leukemia. J Fr Ophtalmol 2005; 28:39-44.

202. Abdallah E, Hajji Z, Mellal Z, et al. Cystoid macular oedema in chronic myeloid leukemia: treatment with acetazolamide and response to bone marrow transplantation. Eye 1996; 10 (Pt 3):394-6.

203. Solomon SD, Smith JH, O'Brien J. Ocular manifestations of systemic malignancies. Curr Opin Ophthalmol 1999; 10:447-51.

204. Keltner JL, Thirkill CE. Cancer-associated retinopathy vs. recoverin-associated retinopathy (editorial) Am J Ophthalmol 1988; 126:296-02.

205. Adamus G, Machniki M, Elerding H, et al. Antibodies to recoverin induce apoptosis of photoreceptors and bipolar cells in vivo. J Autoimmun 1998; 11:523-33.

206. McGinnis JF, Austin B, Kisak I, et al. Chromosomal assignment of the human gene for the cancer-associated retinopathy protein (recoverin) to chromosome 17p13.1. J Neurosci Res 1995; 40:165-8.

207. Thirkill CE. Cancer induced immune-mediated ocular degenerations. Ocul Immunol and Inflamm 2005; 13:119-31.

208. Guy J, Aptsiauri N. Treatment of paraneoplastic visual loss with intravenous immunoglobulin. Arch Ophthalmol 1999; 117:471-7.

209. Boeck K, Hofmann S, Klopfer M, et al. Melanoma-associated paraneoplastic retinopathy: case report and review of literature. Br J Dermatol 1997; 137:457-60.

210. Gittinger JW, Smith TW. Cutaneous melanoma-associated paraneoplastic retinopathy: histopathologic observations. Am J Ophthalmol 1999; 127:612-4.

211. Kellner U, Bornfeld N, Foerster MH. Severe course of cutaneous melanoma associated paraneoplastic retinopathy. Br J Ophthalmol 1995; 79:746-52.

212. Gass JDM. Neoplastic diseases of the retinal and optic disc. In Stereoscopic Atlas of Macular Diseases: Diagnosis and

Treatment, edn 4. Edited by Craven L. St. Louis: Mosby; 1997:894-6.

213. Potter MJ, Adamus G, Szabo SM, et al. Autoantibodies to transducin in a patient with melanoma-associated retinopathy. Am J Ophthalmol 2002; 134:128-30.

214. Thirkill CE, Keltner JL, Yip P, et al. Atypical antigen/antibody reaction in amelanoma-associated retinopathy (MAR). Ocul Immunol Inflamm 2001; 9:277-8.

215. To KW, Thirkill CE, Jakobiec FA, et al. Lymphoma-associated retinopathy. Ophthalmology 2002; 109:2149-53.

216. Hayasaka S, Ugomori S, Kodama T, et al. Central retinal vein occlusion in two patients with immunoglobulin G multiple myeloma associated with blood hyperviscosity. Ann Ophthalmol 1993; 25:191-4.

217. Aggio FB, Cariello AJ, Almeida MS, et al. Bilateral central retinal vein occlusion associated with multiple myeloma. Ophthalmologica 2004; 218:283-7.

218. Amin AR, Jakobiec FA, Dreyer EB. Ocular syndromes associated with systemic malignancy. Int Ophthalmol Clin 1997; 37:281-02.

219. Margo CE, Lowery RL, Kerschmann RL. Lack of p53 protein immunoreactivity in bilateral diffuse uveal melanocytic proliferation. Retina 1997; 17:434-6.

220. Gass JDM, Gieser RG, Wilkinson CP, et al. Bilateral diffuse uveal melanocytic proliferation in patients with occult carcinoma. Arch Ophthalmol 1990; 108:527-33.

221. Guyer DR, J. Tiedeman J, Yannuzzi LA, et al. Interferon-associated retinopathy. Arch Ophthalmol 1993; 111:350-6.

222. Lohmann CP, Kroher G, Bogenrieder T, et al., Severe loss of vision during adjuvant interferon alfa-2b treatment for malignant melanoma [letter]. Lancet 1999; 353:1326.

223. Shimura M, Saito T, Yasuda K, Tamai M. Clinical course of macular edema in two cases of interferon-associated retinopathy observed by optical coherence tomography. Jpn J Ophthalmol 2005; 49:231-4.

224. Schmid KE, Kornek GV, Scheithauer W, Binder S. Update on ocular complications of systemic cancer chemotherapy. Surv Ophthalmol 2006; 51:19-40.

225. Parkkari M, Paakkala AM, Salminen L, Holli K; Finnish Breast Cancer Group. Ocular side-effects in breast cancer patients treated with tamoxifen and toremifene: a randomized follow-up study. Acta Ophthalmol Scand 2003; 81:495-9.

226. Kusumi E, Arakawa A, Kami M, et al. Visual disturbance due to retinal edema as a complication of imatinib. Leukemia 2004; 18:1138-9.

227. Masood I, Negi A, Dua HS. Imatinib as a cause of cystoid macular edema following uneventful phacoemulsification surgery. J Cataract Refract Surg 2005; 31:2427-8.

228. Moon SJ, Mieler WF. Retinal complications of bone marrow and solid organ transplantation. Curr Opin Ophthalmol 2003; 14:433-42.

229. Stewart MW, Gitter KA, Cohen G. Acute leukemia presenting as a unilateral exudate retinal detachment. Retina 1989; 9:110-14.

230. Ebner R, DaCol E, Bullorsky E. True, true and related? Surv Ophthalmol 2001; 45:489-92.

231. Fawzi AA, Cunningham ET Jr. Central serous chorioretinopathy after bone marrow transplantation. Am J Ophthalmol 2001; 131:804-5.

232. Kaiser PK, Gragoudas ES. Radiation retinopathy In Guyer DR, Yannuzzi LA, Chang S, Shields JA, Green WR (eds):Retina-Vitreus-Macula, 1st edition. Philadelphia, WB Saunders Co, 1999, pp 477-87.

233. Bagan SM, Hollenhorst RW. Radiation retinopathy after irradiation of intracranial lesions. Am J Ophthalmol 1979; 88:694-7.

234. Augsburger JJ. Radiation retinopathy. In: Tasman WS (ed.). Clinical Decision in Medical Retinal Diseases. Philadelphia, Mosby, 1994, pp 216-75.

235. Parsons JT, Bova FJ, Fitzgerald CR, Mendenhall WM, Million RR. Radiation retinopathy after external-beam irradiation: analysis of time-dose factors. Int J Radiat Oncol Biol Phys 1994; 30:765-73.

236. Merriam GR, Szechter A, Focht EF. The effects of ionizing radiations on the eye. Front Radiat Ther Oncol 1972; 6:346-85.

237. Brown GC, Shields JA, Sanborn G, et al. Radiation retinopathy. Ophthalmology 1982; 89:1494-1501.

238. MacFaul PA, Bedfore MA, Ocular complications after therapeutic irradiation. Br J Ophthalmol 1970; 54:237-47.

239. Gragoudas ES, Li W, Lane AM, et al. Risk factors for radiation maculopathy and papillopathy after intraocular irradiation. Ophthalmology 1999; 106:1571-77.

240. Viebahn M, Barricks ME, Osterloh MD. Synergism between diabetic and radiation retinopathy: case report and review. Br J Ophthalmol 1991; 75:629-32.

241. Wara WM, Irvine AR, Neger RE, et al. Radiation retinopathy. Int J Radiat Oncol Biol Phys 1979; 5:81-83.

242. Lopez PF, Sternberg P Jr, Dabbs CK, et al. Bone marrow transplant retinopathy. Am J Ophthalmol 1991; 112:635-46.

243. Chan RC, Shukovshy LJ, Effects of irradiation on the eye. Radiology 1976; 120:673-5.

244. Harris JR, Levene MB. Visual complications following irradiation for pituitary adenomas and craniopharyngiomas. Radiology 1976; 120:167-71.

245. Amoaku WM, Frew L, Mahon GJ, et al. Early ultrastructural changes after low-dose X-irradiation in the retina of the rat. Eye 1989; 3 (Pt 5):638-46.

246. Hykin PG, Shields CL, Shields JA, Arevalo JF. The efficacy of focal laser therapy in radiation-induced macular edema. Ophthalmology 1998; 105:1425-9.

247. Kinyoun JL, Chittum ME, Wells CG. Photocoagulation treatment of radiation retinopathy. Am J Ophthalmol 1988; 105:470-78.

248. Finger PT, Kurli M. Laser photocoagulation for radiation retinopathy after ophthalmic plaque radiation therapy. Br J Ophthalmol 2005; 89:730-38.

249. Sutter FK, Gillies MC. Intravitreal triamcinolone for radiation-induced macular edema.) Arch Ophthalmol 2003; 121:1491-3.

250. Shields CL, Demirci H, Dai V, et al. Intravitreal triamcinolone acetonide for radiation maculopathy after plaque radiotherapy for choroidal melanoma. Retina 2005; 25:868-74.

251. Chaudhuri PR, Austin DJ, Rosenthal AR. Treatment of radiation retinopathy. Br J Ophthalmol 1968; 65:623-5.

252. Bakri SJ, Beer PM. Photodynamic therapy for maculopathy due to radiation retinopathy. Eye 2005; 19:795-9.

18

Oxidative Stress in Macular Diseases

Vinay K Khanna, Aditya B Pant,
Prachi Srivastava, Asheesh Mehrotra,
Sandeep Saxena

INTRODUCTION

Eyes are one of the most invaluable organs of human body which receive inputs from the external source and feed the brain accordingly. Macular diseases if not treated properly may lead to blindness. Preventable blindness has been identified as a global public health problem since long.[1,2] It has been estimated that about 28 million people are blind worldwide and out of these, 2/3rd live in developing countries.[3]

Although the list of ocular disorders is long, the prevalence differs from developing to developed nations. The incidences of disorders are more in the developing countries due to obvious reasons. Most common of these disorders are cataract, uveitis, macular degeneration, diabetic retinopathy, Eales' disease, etc. Studies carried out on clinical cases and experimental models have provided important clues in understanding the etiopathogenesis of these ocular disorders; however, the mechanisms of these disorders is not clearly understood.

Free radical mediated oxidative stress has been implicated in the pathogenesis of a variety of human diseases including ageing, degenerative disease and age-related ocular disorders.[4-8] An imbalance in the ratio of pro-oxidants (free radicals)/anti-oxidants, where the concentration of pro-oxidants is relatively high leads to the state of oxidative stress. In aerobic organisms, reactive oxygen species (ROS) in body tissues are generated by various mechanisms both under pathological and physiological conditions by enzymatic and non-enzymatic pathways. The ROS formed with in the cells may oxidize biomolecules like DNA, proteins, lipids, carbohydrates and lead to tissue injury. The superoxide anion is produced by addition of one electron to molecular oxygen which joins with the other anion to form hydrogen peroxide. The addition of an electron to it forms the highly reactive hydroxyl radical.[9] The free radicals can act both as oxidants and reducing agents and induce chain reactions. These primary radicals may generate secondary radicals and produce biological effects. Interestingly, when two molecules combine, a stable molecule is formed. The ROS formed in most of the aerobic cells are reported to be involved in chemotaxis and regulate lymphocyte functions. Besides, platelet aggregation and prostaglandin synthesis are also modulated by free radical species.[10-12]

FREE RADICALS

It is known since long that life and free radicals have gone together in the journey of evolution.[13] The ionizing solar radiation initiated free radical reaction and led to the formation of basic chemicals of life. The defense mechanism against these ubiquitous and omnipresent free radicals also developed as per requirement. Any species that contains one or more unpaired electrons and is capable of independent existence is known as free radical.[14] An unpaired electron remains alone in the orbital of such molecules (Figure 18.1).

FORMATION OF FREE RADICALS

Free radical species can either be positively or negatively charged. These reactive species can also be electrically neutral and are formed by three different reactions:[14,15]

i. Homolytic cleavage of a covalent bond of a normal molecule with each fragment retaining one of the paired electrons and radicals are electrically neutral,
$$X : Y \longrightarrow X\bullet + Y\bullet$$
ii. Loss of an electron from a normal molecule leading to produce positively charged radicals, and
$$X - e^- \longrightarrow X^+\bullet$$
iii. Addition of a single electron to a normal molecule resulting to a negatively charged radical.
$$X + e^- \longrightarrow X^-\bullet$$

In the biological system, formation of free radical by electron transfer, i.e. either by loss or addition is more common than the homolytic fission since it requires high energy input through high temperature, UV light or ionizing radiation. In case of heterolytic cleavage, electrons of the covalent bond are retained by only one of the fragments of the parent molecule. Therefore, it will not form a free radical but produce ions which have charge on it.
$$X : Y \longrightarrow X :^- + Y^+$$

SOURCES OF FREE RADICALS IN BIOLOGICAL SYSTEM

Production of free radicals in animal cell can be either under physiological processes of the body or accidental.

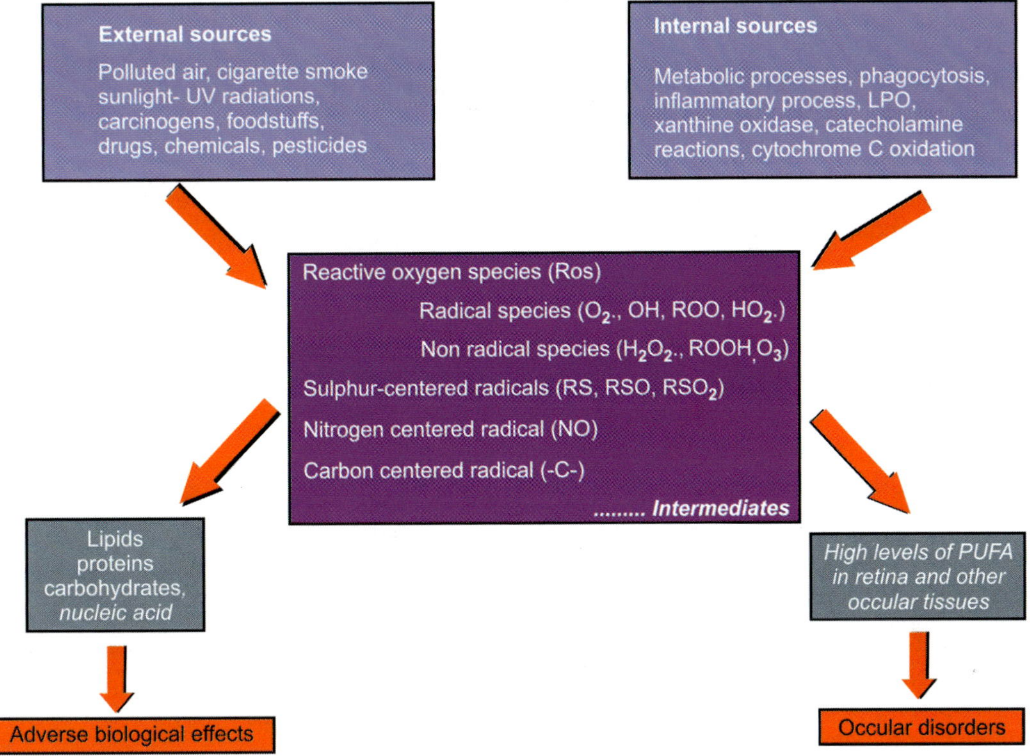

FIGURE 18.1: Free radicals in the biological system

These are highly reactive and short-lived species [15] and are produced both through the external and internal sources.

A variety of sources in the environment have been reported to produce free radical species. Polluted air, cigarette smoke, foodstuffs, carcinogens, sunlight, ionizing radiation are the potent external source for free radical generation. Besides, a number of drugs, chemicals and pesticides have been reported to produce these reactive species. [16-18]

Endogenously, cellular metabolism, phagocytosis, lipid peroxidation are the primary sources of free radical generation. Reactive species are also produced by xanthine, oxidase, catecholamines and mitochondrial cytochrome-C oxidase by various reactions. Inflammatory conditions and enzymatic reactions also generate free radicals in the cell. [19-24] The mechanisms by which free radicals are formed in the cell and their potential sources have been reviewed from time to time. [20]

GROUPS OF FREE RADICALS

Free radicals have been classified broadly into four groups in the biological system:

i. Oxygen derived free radical
ii. Sulphur-centered free radicals
iii. Carbon-centered free radicals, and
iv. Nitrogen-centered free radicals.

Amongst these, oxygen derived free radicals, viz. superoxide anion, singlet oxygen, hydroxyl radical and lipid peroxyl radical are quite common and omnipresent.[18, 25] Hydrogen peroxide does not contain unpaired electron but generates a free radical through the Fenton reaction in the biological system. Thiyl radicals (RS·) are formed during oxidation of glutathione and have been reported to be active and produce detrimental effects in the biological system.

Attack of an oxidizing radical, like OH· on a biological molecule (RH) like lipid, nucleic acid, carbohydrates, or proteins produce the carbon-centered free radicals. These radicals rapidly react with oxygen to form corresponding peroxyl radical (ROO·). These peroxyl radicals participate in other biological reactions and generate alkoxyl radicals (RO·). Metabolic activation of CCl_4 is a classical example of carbon centered radical formation in aerobes. The damaging effects Of CCl_4 On the liver have been suggested due to metabolic conversion Of CCl_4 to the primary free radical intermediate CCl_3.

Among the nitrogen centered free radicals, nitric oxide (NO·) is an important physiologically active species. It is produced by vascular endothelium as relaxing factor and also by phagocytes.[26] Although NO· has considerable physiological significance, excess production of NO· is reported to be toxic.[27] Under certain circumstances, NO· combines with O_2 and generate more active species.

Inspite of the fact that the *eye* is small and anatomically distinct; it readily captures photons which exposes them to harmful effects of light induced changes. Several regions in the *eye* are highly enriched with polyunsaturated fatty acids which readily and extensively utilize oxygen and lead to peroxidation and therefore cause oxidative stress. The fact that oxygen consumption by the retina is much greater than any other tissue also enhances the risk of oxidation from free radicals produced by sunlight, cigarette smoke and environmental pollutants. The outer segment membrane of photoreceptors and other regions in the *eye* are rich in polyunsaturated fatty acids that is readily oxidized.

A number of enzymatic and non-enzymatic antioxidants exist in the cells to protect them from potentially harmful attack of the reactive oxygen species. The antioxidants, based on their properties, are classified into four types.[28] Preventive antioxidants provide the first line of defense and suppress the formation of free radicals. The chain initiation and/or breaking chain propagation reactions are controlled by the radical scavenging antioxidants which are of the second type. Repair and *de novo* antioxidants are the third class of antioxidants. The fourth class of antioxidant provides adaptation where the signal for the production and reaction of free radicals induces formation and transport of the appropriate antioxidant to the target site.

To counteract the effect of free radicals, the body is equipped with several antioxidant enzymes which have selective functions of maintaining the homeostasis. The enzyme superoxide dismutase (SOD), catalyzes the dismutation of superoxide radical (O_2^-) to yield hydrogen peroxide (H_2O_2) which is decomposed to water and oxygen either by catalase or glutathione peroxidase. These enzymes are preventive antioxidants as they remove the species involved in the initiation of free radial chain reaction. Vitamin E, a non-enzymatic lipid soluble antioxidant is present in high quantities in body tissue including eyes and maintains cellular integrity by inhibiting lipid peroxidation and prevents intracellular peroxidation of free radicals. Other non-enzymatic antioxidants, viz. beta-carotene, vitamin A, ascorbate (vitamin C) and sulfhydryl group are also present in eyes. Ascorbate and tocopherol function together to protect membrane lipid damage and quench residual free radicals. Besides vitamins, micronutrients like zinc, copper, selenium and manganese are also reported to serve as potent antioxidants.[29,30] These antioxidants are able to inactivate the oxidizing radicals directly.

Preventive role of antioxidants in many diseases including ocular disorders is well documented.[31-33] The eyes possess considerably high amount of anti-oxidant enzymes and other anti-oxidants.[34] Epidemiological studies on anti-oxidant levels and risk of cataract and macular degeneration have found a close association between the anti-oxidant status and these diseases. The risk to develop cataract and macular degeneration decreases if the plasma anti-oxidant level goes up.[35-37]

Retina is the primary target both in age-related macular degeneration (AMD) and diabetic retinopathy while in uveitis, the uvea is affected selectively. Studies on ocular tissues and fluids have provided useful information on the basic understanding of the mechanism and management of the disease. These studies have also been found to be useful in developing suitable therapeutic targets and strategies. Such studies are however, limited due to ethical considerations. Realizing these difficulties, peripheral fluids including blood and its components (plasma, serum, lymphocytes, neutrophils, etc.) have been widely utilized to understand the mechanisms in diabetic retinopathy, uveitis, cataract, Eales' disease, etc. Although several studies have been carried out, precise mechanisms involved at cellular and molecular level are yet to be understood. In the present chapter, role of oxidative stress in the etiopathogenesis of selected ocular disorders has been reviewed based on the clinical and experimental studies.

AGE-RELATED MACULAR DEGENERATION

Age-related macular degeneration is a leading cause of blindness in Caucacians (54.4%) as compared to blacks (4.4%) and Hispanics (14.3%) [38] permanent visual loss in the elderly. Among two types of AMD, dry AMD is more common and occurs due to slow degeneration of the macula while wet AMD is caused by an abnormal growth of blood vessels behind the retina. A decrease in the central visual activity due to accumulation of cellular waste products called drusen is a characteristic feature of AMD. Drusen, pale yellowish spots are often seen in the retina of elderly persons over 50 years. Some individuals however may develop more severe form of the disease due to eventual loss of the retinal pigment epithelium and photoreceptors. Decreased contrast and color sensitivity, increased glare sensitivity, metamorphosia and central scotomas which inhibit the ability to read or identify faces are other symptoms of this disease.

Evolutionary theory of aging suggests a close association between oxidative stress and aging and age related disorders. [39] Enhanced oxidative stress due to generation of reactive oxygen intermediates has been suggested both in aging and age related disorders. [39] The theory is quite convincing as it helps explain the complex relationship between longevity and metabolic rate, enhanced degenerative diseases at advance stage of life, enhanced life span due to caloric restriction, etc. [40] An increase in oxidative load with age has been reported that may cause oxidative damage in collagen elastin and DNA and enhance the lipofuscin, a degradative product formed following lipid peroxidation. [41-44] The antioxidant defenses are also impaired with the age. [5-47]

Like other organs, eye is also affected with the age. Further risk of blindness, health problems and mortality significantly increases with age. [48] In a population based study on AMD, Klein[49] found consistent and significant association of age with AMD irrespective of ethnic and racial background.

Role of oxidative stress in the etiology of age related macular degeneration has been suggested. [39] Keeping in view of the fact that oxidative stress and aging are intimately involved, a number of studies have suggested that oxidative stress contributes to AMD. [39,50,51] Disturbance in the antioxidant and oxidant balance has been found to be associated with the development of ocular disorders including AMD. [52]

A number of pro-oxidants have been suggested to be associated with the development of AMD. High dietary intake of polyunsaturated fatty acids has been linked with early AMD. [53, 54] However, Sanders and associates [55] in a case control study did not find significant change in plasma cholesterol levels between the cases of age related maculopathy and controls.

Enhanced thiobarbituric acid reactive substances (TBARS) in plasma were found in elderly rhesus macaques. [56] It was observed that circulating plasma TBARS levels were higher in monkeys with >10 drusen. [56] Hammes and associates[57] found that N(epsilon) (carboxymethyl)-lysin (CML), an oxidative product of lipoprotein or sequential glycation and oxidation and the AGE receptor RAGE colocalize in the subfoveal age related neovascular membranes. As CML was not identified in the healthy retina of a donor eye, it was correlated with the development of AMD. Ishibashi [58] found that CML is present in soft drusen and adjacent retinal pigment epithelium well before the development of choroidal neovascularization and not in control eyes. Feeney-Burns [59] found a good correlation between age and lipofuscin in retinal epithelium cells. Higher amount of lipofuscin, an oxidative product were found in retinal epithelium cells with atrophic AMD. [60] It was suggested that N-retinylidene-N-retinylethonolamine, present in high amount in retinal epithelial cells may cause cell membrane blebbing and cytoplasm extrusion in to Bruch's membrane leading to drusen formation. [61-64] It may be closely linked to the development of AMD. [65]

Age-related macular degeneration is considered to be a multifactorial disease. Although gene-environment interaction has been suggested in the etiology of the disease, not much is known about the interplay.[51] A number of twin studies have supported the genetic association of the disease;[66] however, the genetic etiology is quite complex and difficult to correlate with the disease.[51] Risk of AMD has been linked with the cumulative life time exposure to sun light.[67-71] The hypothesis is of concern since high exposure to blue or visible light and AMD are interrelated.[67,70]

Smokers are at an increased risk of AMD.[72,73] It was suggested that smoking may deplete the antioxidant capacity and therefore the macula lutea may be an easy target of free radicals.[74] Incidence of the disease are also associated with the family history. Light-colored eyes are thought to be more susceptible to AMD. In a case control study on Australian population Darzins[68] reported that excessive exposure to the sun is a risk factor to develop AMD. Angiogenesis and inflammatory process also play an important role in AMD.[75]

There is currently no effective treatment for AMD. A significant interest has arisen among the health scientists about the dietary factors, particularly antioxidants since these have been reported to prevent or impede the progress of macular degeneration. Several mechanisms for such an effect have been suggested. One such reason is that the retina, rich in polyunsaturated fatty acids, may be altered by free radical production and oxidation and, conversely, may be protected by nutrients that block this oxidative damage. Antioxidant status, particularly of carotenoid intake appears to play an important role, since formation of drusen in the retina has been shown to occur faster in those deprived of carotenoids. Population studies show that people who eat more carotenoid-rich vegetables, particularly those containing lutein and zeaxanthin such as spinach and kale, have a significantly lower risk of developing AMD.[54] Supplementation with these carotenoids has been reported to exhibit an inverse relationship between macular density and lens density and therefore retard the age related increase in the lens density.[76,77] Khachik and Bernstein[78] suggested that both lutein and zeaxanthin may act as antioxidants and protect the macula against short wave length visible light. The study also suggested that oxidative and reductive pathways for lutein and zeaxanthin in human retina may

play a key role in the prevention of age related macular degeneration. Supplementation with vitamin-mineral antioxidants (a mixture of vitamins E and C, selenium and beta-carotene) was reported to be effective clinically as compared to placebo in the treatment of AMD.[79] Antioxidants have also been reported to maintain the integrity of the choroidal blood vessels that supply the macular region of the retina and therefore could be of prophylactic/therapeutic use.

There are reports that a high intake of lutein and zeaxanthin either through food or other sources increases the pigment's density. In addition to the macula lutea, yellow is also a characteristic color of the lens, which gradually yellows with age. An important function of macular carotenoids is to filter blue light which is important at a young age when the lens is clear.[80]

DIABETIC RETINOPATHY

Diabetic retinopathy is a retinal vascular disorder and has been identified a major cause of blindness throughout the world. The prevalence of the disease is quite high and it affects individuals between the ages 20 and 65 years.[81] Approximately 8 percent of legally blind individuals are reported to have diabetes and approximately 1.2 percent of new blindness is due to diabetic retinopathy.[82] Approximately 25% of all diabetics have some form of retinopathy. The disease occurs both in the cases with insulin dependent diabetes mellitus (IDDM, type I) and non-insulin-dependent diabetes mellitus (NIDDM, type II), however, cases of IDDM are at a greater risk to develop diabetic retinopathy.

It is widely accepted that diabetics have a 50- to 80-fold greater risk of becoming blind than non-diabetics. The diabetics develop some degree of retinopathy. In the United States diabetics account for 10% or more of all cases of blindness and 20% of new cases in patients over the age of 45 years.[83] The main determinants in incidence of diabetic retinopathy are duration of disease, age of patient and type of diabetes viz, Type I or Type II. In IDDM diabetics no clinically discernible retinopathy usually occurs for 4 to 5 years after the original diagnosis of the disease.[84] By 10 to 15 years after diagnosis 25% to 50% of patients show signs of retinopathy which are found in 75 to 95% of the population and the proportion approaches 100% after 30 years. Proliferative diabetic retinopathy reported in 14 to 17% of the population at after 13 to 14 years of diabetes.[85]

Duration of diabetes and poor metabolic control are important risk factors of diabetic retinopathy. In patients diagnosed with diabetes before the age of 30 years, the incidence of diabetic retinopathy was found to be 50% after 10 years of diabetes. There was a significant increase in percent cases with diabetic retinopathy after 30 years of diabetes. However, diabetic retinopathy is rarely seen with in 5 years of the onset of diabetes and before puberty. Good metabolic control of diabetes delays the development of diabetic retinopathy by few years but may not prevent the disease. In view of this, there is a continuous stress to keep the blood glucose normalized in diabetics. The miscellaneous factors related with diabetic retinopathy are pregnancy, hypertension, and renal disease.[86]

Diabetic retinopathy is a microangiopathy which affects the retinal precapillary arterioles, capillaries and venules. However, larger vessels may also be involved. Retinopathy has features of both microvascular occlusion and leakage.

Besides, the duration and type of diabetes, numerous other factors have been suggested to be involved in the development and progression of the diabetic retinopathy. It was suggested that onset of puberty is linked with diabetic retinopathy.[87-89] Rapid development of proliferative retinopathy was observed in patients with Mauriae's syndrome.[90] It was suggested that individuals with type I diabetes and proliferative diabetic retinopathy had much higher level of insulin-like growth factor I (IGF-1, previously known as somatomedin-C) which may enhance the proliferative capacity of several types of cells including vascular endothelium. It was also found that elevated levels of IGFs may enhance the development of proliferative diabetic retinopathy.[87] Both background and proliferative diabetic retinopathy is directly related to levels of systemic systolic and diastolic blood pressure.[91] Rand and associates[92] observed the effect of myopia on the prevalence of diabetic retinopathy.

Role of free radical in pathogenesis of diabetic retinopathy has been well accepted. Generation of reactive oxygen species (oxidative stress) has played an important role in the etiology of diabetic complications including diabetic retinopathy. This hypothesis is supported by evidence that many biochemical pathways strictly associated with hyperglycemia (Glucose auto-oxidation, polyol pathway, prostanoid synthesis, protein glycation) can increase production of free radical. Jenning and associates[93] reported that homeostatic abnormalities possibly generated excess free radicals and reduced antioxidant scavenger mechanisms. Losada and Alio[94] during their study in plasma described that oxidative stress may be a causative factor in case of diabetic retinopathy Wolf[95] suggested that free radical mechanisms may be associated with the development of diabetic microangiopathy. Lunec and associates[96] stated that lipid hydroperoxides (LHP) are produced from a variety of long chain polyunsaturated fatty acid precursors via free radical, reactions and themselves have been implicated in vascular endothelial damage and are also intimately involved in prostaglandin biosynthesis and both of these (i.e. vascular endothelial damage and altered prostanoid metabolism) factors are evident in microangiopathy. Lipid hydroperoxides may be formed due to accumulation of retinal hard exudates which are results of lipoprotein leaking from retinal capillaries into extracellular space of retina.

Observations of Rema and associates[97] further supported involvement of oxidative stress in diabetic retinopathy. They found low levels of both vitamins E and C (which are key substance for maintaining the levels of SOD in body) in patients of diabetic retinopathy. There are reports that, high doses of vitamin C and nicomartine (A lipid lowering compound) regimens are associated with reversal of early signs of retinopathy and normalization of capillary strengths in diabetes mellitus, confirming the role of antioxidants against the development of the pathology in blood vessels.[98] Hammes and associates[99] and Grattaglianio[100] carried out their experiment in subretinal fluid of patients suffering from diabetic retinopathy and compared with patients of diabetes only and again with healthy controls. Results suggested that involvement of free radical damage was highest in case of diabetic retinopathy than the diabetics and controls. All these studies implicate that involvement of free radical may be one of the etiological factor in the pathogenesis underlying the development of diabetic retinopathy.

UVEITIS

Uveitis is a major cause of blindness, mainly due to the inflammation of the uveal tract.[101] However, other ocular structure viz. retina, optic nerves and intraocular cavities may also be affected during the disease process. The disease has been reported to be more common in cases with immunological abnormalities like sarcoidosis, Behcet's disease, etc.[102-105] Involvement of T cell mediated responses has been well recognized both in clinical uveitis and experimental autoimmune uveitis (EAU).[104-106]

Several studies have been carried out on clinical cases and experimental models to unravel and understand the mechanism of the uveitis. It has been suggested that the loss of vision is due to damage caused by inflammatory cell infiltration following release of various cytokines or other mediators like oxygen metabolites.[107] Lymphocytes phagocyte cells such as macrophages which device from circulating monocytes are the major inflammatory cells involved in chronic uveitis, although the other tissue cellular components may also participate and may enhance or reduce the inflammation. Interestingly, in the retina, the cellular components involved in the inflammatory process are microgilla, astrocytes, muller cells, photoreceptors and retinal pigment epithelium while in the uvea these cellular components are vascular endothelia and melanocytes. [108-110]

Recently, role of reactive oxygen species has been suggested to be foremost in the etiology of uveitis. [107,111] Experimental studies indicate that phagocyte-generated oxidants and nitric oxide (NO) related species play an important role in the initiation of peroxidation of cellular lipid components, which may further amplify inflammatory mechanism.[107, 112, 113] Oxygen metabolites such as O_2^-, H_2O_2, hypochlorus acid, OH and peroxynitrite (ONOO) have been reported to be involved in the initiation of photoreceptor cell disintegration and the amplification of inflammatory processes in uveitis. [107,112,114-115] Studies on experimental model of uveitis demonstrated that the generation of oxygen metabolites (O_2^-, H_2O_2 and OH)

was 20 times higher at the peak severity of uveitis. It was also reported that activated phagocytes easily infiltrate the uvea and retina and are the major source of O_2^- products.[107,112]

Excessive generation of NO^- at the site of inflammation has also been reported by various investigators in experimental uveitis.[112, 116-118] In an interesting study, Rao and Wu[111] reported that retinal proteins and the oxidized lipid products of the outer retina may enhance generation of oxidants, superoxide and NO^- and therefore the retina is more vulnerable to oxidative stress. The NO generated during the process readily interacts with O_2^- and forms $ONOO^-$ which is a potent oxidant capable of oxidizing and nitrating a variety of cellular macromolecules. The generation of O_2^- and H_2O_2 may enhance the production of OH, which reacts with various cellular macromolecules including lipids, proteins and DNA and enhance the process of peroxidation. Since photoreceptors are enriched with PUFA these are an easy target for oxidants and reactive radicals and lead to lipid peroxidation. [119] Amplification of pathological retinal degeneration in uveitis has been reported due to enhanced lipid peroxidation. The activity of antioxidant enzymes and antioxidants are other important factors which regulate the level of oxidants and free radicals in the eye.

Studies on the protective role of antioxidants in experimental uveitis have also been carried out. Treatment with hydroxyl radical scavangers and antioxidants was reported to decrease the retinal lipid peroxidation in experimental uveitis.[120-122] In another study, treatment with an iron chelator, deferoxamine could reduce inflammation. [123] Extensive experimental studies using antioxidants and free radical scavengers have been carried out to investigate their preventive/therapeutic effect in uveitis. Animals treated with SOD, catalase and glutathione peroxidase enzymes or hydroxyl radical scavengers were found to have low levels of lipid peroxidation products and a reduced severity of the disease.[114, 121-125]

The available literature suggests that excessive free radical generation may be associated with a variety of ocular disorders and that an impaired antioxidant defense capacity is the contributory factor for increased incidences of such disorders. However, detailed clinical studies are required to establish a precise link and develop suitable therapeutic antidotes through pharmacological interventions.

REFERENCES

1. WHO The prevention of blindness: Report of a WHO study group. WHO Tech Rep Ser 1973; 518: 5-17.
2. WHO The prevention of blindness: Report of a WHO study group. WHO Chron 1976; 30:391-7.
3. WHO Programme Advisory Group on the Prevention of Blindness. Data on blindness throughout the world. WHO Chron 1979; 33:275-83.
4. Bohr V, Anson RM, Majur S, Dianov G. Oxidative DNA damage processing and changes with aging. Toxicology Letters 1998; 102:47-52.
5. Zhang Y, Dawson VL, Dawson TM. Oxidative stress of genetics in the pathogenesis of Parkinson's disease. Neurobiol Dis 2000; 7:240-50.
6. Butterfield DA, Lauderback CM. Lipid peroxidation and protein oxidation in Alzheimer's disease, brain potential causes and consequences involving amyloid beta-peptide associated free radical. Free Rad Bio Med 2002; 32:1050-60.
7. Kubo E. Cataract formation through the polyolpathways is associated with free radical production. Exp Eye Res 1999; 68:457-67.
8. Frank RN, Amin RH, Puklin JE. Antioxidant enzymes in the macular retinal pigment epithelium of eyes with neovascular age related macular degeneration. Am J Ophthalmology 1999; 127:694-709.
9. Thomas PAD, Jayshree P. Free radicals, antioxidants in human disease. EMSI Newslett 1999: 23:1.
10. Martin W, Loschen G, Gunzler WA, Flone L. Superoxide dismutase inhibits LTB2-induced leukotaxis. Agents Actions 1985: 16;48-49.
11. Freed BM, Patterson DA, Repoport R, et al. Inhibition of human T cell response by hydrogen peroxide. Pharmacol Ther 1988; 39:267-8.
12. Del Princie D, Menichilli A, Dematteis W, et al. Hydrogen peroxide has a role in the aggregation of human platelets. FEBS Lett 1985; 185:142-6.
13. Harman D. The aging process. Proc Natl Acad Sci USA 1981;78:4712-28.
14. Halliwell B, Hoult IRS, Blake DR. Oxidants, inflammation and the anti inflammatory drugs. FASEB J 1989; 2:2867-73.
15. Cheeseman KH. Mechanisms and effects of lipid peroxidation. Mol Aspects Med 1993; 14:191-7.
16. Niwa Y, Hanseen M. Protection far life. Jhorsone Publishers Ltd. Wellingbrough. England, 1989; pp 9-11.
17. Pryor WA. Oxy radicals and related species: then formation life times and reaction. Ann Rev Physiol 1984; 48: 657-67.
18. Halliwell B, Gutteridge JMC. Lipid peroxidation, oxygen radicals, cell damage and antioxidant therapy. Lancet 1984;1: 1396-8.
19. Grisham MB. Oxidants and free radicals in inflammatory bowel disease. Lancet 1994; 344: 859-61.
20. Simon RI., Maxwell I. Prospects for the use of antioxidant therapies. Drugs. 1995; 49: 345-61.
21. Grisham MB, Rursell WJ, Roy R.S, Mc Cord, JM. In: Rotilloi G (ed). Superoxide and superoxide dismutase in chemistry Biology and Medicine. 1986; p 571.
22. Augustine AJ, Spitznas M, Sekundo W, et al. Effects of allopurinol and steroid on inflammation and oxidative tissue in experimental lens induced uveitis: A biochemical and morphological study. Br J Ophthalmol 1976; 80:451-7.
23. Freeman BA, Crapo JD. Free radical and tissue injury. Lab Invest. 1982; 47:412-26.
24. Esterbauer H, Zollner H, Schaur RI. Aldehydes formed by lipid peroxidation mechanism of formation, occurrence and termination. In: Vigo-Pelfrey C (Ed): Membrane Lipid Oxidation. Bqco. Raton. Rc. 1990; pp 239-83.
25. Fridovich I. The biology of oxygen radicals: The superoxide radical is an agent of oxygen toxicity. Superoxide dismutase provides an important defense. Science 1978; 201:875-80.
26. Moncadd S, Higgs A. The L-arginine nitric oxide pathway. M Eng J Med 1993; 329: 2002-12.
27. Beckman JS, Chen J, Ischiroprocilos H, Crow JP. Oxidative chemistry of peroxy nitrite. Methods in Enzymology 1994; 233: 229-40.
28. Noguchi N, Watanabe A. Diverse function of antioxidants. Free Rad Res 2000; 33:809-17.
29. Zaman Z, Roche S, Fielden P, et al. Plasma concentration of vitamin A and E and carotenoids in Alzheimer's disease. Age and Aging 1992; 21:91-4.
30. Chandra RK. Effect of vitamin and trace element supplementation on immune responses of infection in elderly subjects. Lancet 1992; 340:1124-7.
31. Perrig WJ, Perrig P, Stahelin HB. The relation between antioxidants and memory performance in old and very old. J. Am Geriatr Soc 1997; 45:718-24.
32. Smith W, Mitchell P, Web K, Leeder SR. Dietary antioxidants and age related maculopathy—the blue mountain eye study. Ophthalmology 1999; 106:761-7.
33. Serdar A, Yesilbursa D, Serder Z, et al. Relation of functional capacity with the oxidative stress and antioxidants in chronic heart failure. Congest Heart Fail 2002; 7:309-11.
34. Halliwell and Gutteridge Ed. 1985. Free radicals in biology and medicine. Claredon Press, Oxford, USA.
35. Leska MC, Chylack LT, He Q, et al. Longitudinal study of cataract group antioxidant vitamins and nuclear opacities. Ophthalmology 1998; 105:831-6.
36. Lyle BJ, Mares Perlman JA, Klein BEK, et al. Serum carotenoids and tocopherols and incidence of age related nuclear cataract. Am J Clin Nutr 1999; 69:272-7.

37. Teikari JM, Laatikainin L, Virtamo J, et al. Six year supplementation with alpha-tocopherol and beta carotene and age related maculopathy. Acta Opthalmol Scand 1998; 76:224-9.

38. Friedman DS, O'Colman G, Munoz B, et al. The eye diseases prevalence research group. Prevalence of age related macular degeneration in the United States. Arch Ophthalmol 2004; 122:564-72.

39. Beatty S, Koh HH, Henson D, Boulton M. The role of oxidative stress in the pathogenesis of age related macular degeneration. Surv Ophthalmol 2000; 45: 115-34.

40. Harman D. The aging process. Proc Natl Acad Sci USA 1981; 78: 7124-8.

41. Cortopassi GA, Shibata D, Soong NW, et al. A pattern of accumulation of a somatic deletion of mitochondrial DNA in aging human tissues. Proc Natl Acad Sci USA 1992; 89:7370-4.

42. La Bella FS, Vivian S, Thornhill DP. Amino acid composition of human aortic elastin as influenced by age. J Gerontol 1966; 21:550-5.

43. Matsumura G, Herp A, Pigman W. Depolymerization of hyalouronic acid by autoxidants and radiations. Radiat Res 1966; 28:735-52.

44. Tas S, Tam CF, Walford RL. Disulfide bonds and the structure of the chromatin complex in relation to aging. Mech Ageing Dev 1980; 12:65-80.

45. Kritchevsky SB, Muldoon MF. Oxidative stress and aging: still a hypothesis [editorial; comment]. Jam Geriatr Soc 1996; 44:873-5.

46. Paolisso G, Tagliamonte MR, Rizzo MR, et al. Oxidative stress and advancing age: results in healthy centenarians. Jam Geriatr Soc 1998; 46:833-8.

47. Rondanelli M, Melzi dEril GV, Anesi A, Ferrari E. Altered oxidative stress in healthy old subjects. Aging Clin Exp Res 1997; 9:221-3.

48. Weale R. The eye within the framework of human senescence: biological decline and morbidity. Ophthalmic Res 1998; 30:59-73.

49. Klein R, Klein BE, Linton KL. Prevalence of age related maculopathy: The beaver dam eye study. Ophthalmology 1992; 99:933-43.

50. Blodi BA. Nutritional supplements in the prevention of age related macular degeneration. INSIGHT 2004; 24:15-16.

51. McConnell V, Silvestri G. Age related macular degeneration. Ulster Med J 2005; 74: 82-92.

52. Webb M: Toxicological significance of metallothionein. Experientia Suppl 1987; et al 52:109-34.

53. Mares-Perlman JA, Brady WE, Klein R, et al. Dietary fat and age-related maculopathy. Arch Ophthalmol 1995; 113:743-8.

54. Seddon J, Ajani V, Sperduto R. Dietary fat intake and age-related macular degeneration (abstract). Invest Ophthalmol Vis Sci 1994; 35(Suppl):2003.

55. Sanders TAB, Hanes AP, Wormald R, et al. Essential fatty acids, plasma cholesterol and fat soluble vitamins in subjects with age related maculopathy and matched control subjects. J Clin Nutr 1993; 57:428-34.

56. Olin KL, Morse LS, Murphy C, et al. Trace element status and free radical defense in elderly rhesus macaques (Macaca mulatta) with macular drusen. Proc Soc Exp Biol 1995; 208: 370-7.

57. Hammes HP, Hoerauf H, Alt A, et al. N (epsilon) (carboxymethyl) lysin and the AGE receptor RAGE colocalize in age-related macular degeneration. Invest Ophthalmol Vis Sci 1999; 40:1855-9.

58. Ishibashi T, Murata T, Hangai M, et al. Advanced glycation end products in age-related macular degeneration. Arch Ophthalmol. 1998; 116:1629-1632.

59. Feeney-Burns L, Eldred GE. The fate *of* the phagosome: conversion to age pigment and impact in human retinal pigment epithelium. Trans Ophthalmol Soc UK 1983; 103:416-21.

60. Sarks JP, Sarks SH, Killingsworth MC. Evolution of geographic atrophy of the retinal pigment epithelium. Eye 1988; 2:552-77.

61. Eldred GE, Lasky MR. Retinal age pigments generated *by* self-assembling lysosomotropic detergents. Nature 1993; 361:724-6.

62. Ishibashi T, Patterson R, Ohnishi Y, et al. Formation of drusen in the human eye. Am J Ophthalmol 1986; 101:342-53.

63. Ishibashi T, Sorgente N, Patterson R, et al. Pathogenesis of drusen in the primate. Invest Ophthalmol Vis Sci 1986; 27:184-93.

64. Weiter JJ, Delori FC, Wing GL, et al. Retinal pigment epithelial lipofuscin and melanin and choroidal melanin in human eyes. Invest Ophthalmol Vis Sci 1986; 27:145-52.

65. Feeney-Burns L, Gao CL, Tidwell M. Lysosomal enzyme cytochemistry *of* human RPE, Bruchs membrane and drusen. Invest Ophthalmol Vis Sci 1987; 28:1138-47.

66. Hammond CJ, Webster AR, Snieder H, et al. Genetic influence on early age related maculopathy: a twin study. Ophthalmology. 2002; 109:730-6.

67. Cruickshanks KJ, Klein R, Klein BE. Sunlight and age-related macular degeneration. The Beaver Dam *Eye* Study. Arch Ophthalmol. 1993; 111:514-8.

68. Darzins P, Mitchell P, Heller RF. Sun exposure and age-related macular degeneration. An Australian case-control study. Ophthalmology. 1997; 104:770-6.

69. Hyman LG, Lilienfeld AM, Ferris FL 3d, et al. Senile macular degeneration: a case control study. Am J Epidemiol 1993; 118:213-27.

70. Taylor HR, West S, Munoz B, et al. The long-term effects of visible light on the eye [see comments]. Arch Ophthalmol 1992; 110:99-104.

71. Taylor HR, Munoz B, West S, et al. Visible light and risk of age related macular degeneration. Trans Am Ophthalmol Soc 1989; 88:163-73.

72. Age related eye disease study research group. Risk factors associated with age related macular degeneration: A case control study in the age related eye disease study: Age related eye disease study report number 3. Ophthalmology 2000; 107: 2224-32.

73. Smith W, Assink J, Klein R, et al. Risk factors for age related macular degeneration: Pooled findings from three continents. Ophthalmology 2001; 108: 697-704.

74. Christen WG, et al. A prospective study of cigarette smoking and risk of age-related macular degeneration in men. JAMA 1996; 276:1147-51.

75. Penfold P, Provis JM, Billson FA. Age related macular degeneration: Ultrastructural studies of the relationship of leucocytes to angiogenesis. Graefes Arch Clin Exp Ophthalmol. 1987; 225:70-76.

76. Hammond BR, et al. Dietary modification of human macular pigment density. Invest Ophthalmol Visual Sci 1997; 38:1795-1801.

77. Hammond BR, et al. Density of the human crystalline lens is related to the macular pigment carotenoids, lutein and zeaxanthin. Optomet Vis Sci 1997; 74: 499-504.

78. Khachik BF, et al. Identification of lutein and zeaxanthin oxidation products in human and monkey retinas. Invest Ophthalmol Vis Sci 1997; 38:1802-11.

79. Seddon JM, et al. A prospective study of cigarette smoking and risk of age-related macular degeneration in women. JAMA 1996; 276:1141-6.

80. Schalch W, et al. Carotenoids in the retina - a review of their possible role in preventing or limiting damage caused by light and oxygen. Free radical and ageing. 1992; 7:280-98.

81. Dutta LC. Ophthalmology Principle and Practice. New Delhi: Jaypee. 1995; pp 106-40.

82. Klein R, Klein BEK. Epidemiology of eye diseases in diabetes. In: Flynn HW Jr, Smiddy WE (eds.). Diabetes and ocular diseases. San Francisco: American Academy of Ophthalmology 2000;19-67.

83. Kahn HA, Hillu R. Blindness caused by diabetic retinopathy. Am J Ophthalmol 1974; 78:58-67.

84. Klein R, Klein BEK, Moss SE, et al. The Wisconsin epidemiological study of diabetic retinopathy II. Prevalence and risk of diabetic retinopathy when age at diagnosis is less than 30 years. Arch Ophthalmol 1984; 102:520-6.

85. Chatterjee BM. Text Book of Ophthalmology. CBS Publishers, 1993; 210-20.

86. Kanski JJ. Clinical Ophthalmology. Butterworth Heinemann Publishers, USA, 2000; pp 463-508.

87. Knowler WC Jr., Guest GM, Lampe J, et al. The course of juvenile diabetics treated with unmeasured diet. Diabetes 1965; 14:239-73.

88. Klein R, Klein BEK, Moss SE, Davis MD, Dermets DL. Retinopathy in young onset diabetic patients. Diabetic Care 1985; 8:311-5.

89. Nanda M., Murphy RP, Plotnick L, et al. The effects of puberty on the prevalence of diabetic retinopathy. Invest Ophthalmol Vis Sci. 1986; 27(Suppl):5.

90. Daneman D, Drash AL, Lobes LA, et al. Progressive retinopathy with improved control in diabetic dwarfism (Mauriac's syndrome). Diabetes Care. 1981; 4:360-5.

91. Knowler WC, Beunett PH, Ballintne EJ. Increased incidence of retinopathy in diabetic with elevated blood pressure: a six year follow up study in Pima Indians IV. Eng J Med 1980; 302:645-50.

92. Rand JI, Krolewski AS, Aiello LM, et al. Multiple factors in the prediction of risk of proliferative diabetic retinopathy. New Eng J Med 1985; 313:1433.

93. Jenning PE, Mc Laren M, Scott NA, et al. The relationship of oxidative stress to the thrombotic tendency in type 1 diabetic patients with diabetic retinopathy. Diabet Med 1991; 8:860-5.

94. Losada M, Alio JL. Malondialdehyde serum concentration in type I diabetic with and without retinopathy. Doc Opthalmol 1997; 93:223-9.

95. Wolf SP. The potential role of oxidative stress in diabetes and its complications: Novel implications for theory and therapy. In: Crabbe MJC (ed.) Diabetic Complications: Scientific and Clinical Aspects Churchill Livingston, London. 1987; pp167-221.

96. Lunec CJ, Malloran SP, White AC, Dormand TL. Free radical oxidation (peroxidation) in serum and synovial fluid in rheumatoid arthritis. J Rhematol 1981; 8:233-45.

97. Rema M., Mohan V, Bhaskar A, Shanmugasumdaram KR. Does oxidant stress play a role in diabetic retinopathy? Indian J Ophthalmol 1995; 43:17-21.

98. Cox BD, Butterfield WJH. Vitamin C supplementation and diabetic cutaneous capillary fragility. Br Med J. 1971; 3:205-9.

99. Hammes HP, Barmann A, Engel L, Welforth P. Antioxidant treatment of experimental diabetic retinopathy in rats with macanartine. Diabetologica 1997; 40:629-34.

100. Grattagliono I, Vendemiale G, Boscia F, et al. Oxidative retinal products and ocular damages in diabetic patients. Free Rad Biol Med 1998; 25:369-72.

101. Yato H, Matsumoto Y. CD56+T cells in the peripheral blood of uveitis patients. Br J Ophthalmol 1999; 83:1386-1388.

102. Khan MA. HLA-B27 and its subtypes in world population. Curr Opin heumatol. 1995; 7: 263-9.

103. Linssen A, Rothava A, Valkenberg HA, et al. The life time cumulative incidence of acute anterior uveitis in a normal population and its relation to ankylosing spondylitis and histocompatibility antigen HLA-B27. Invest Ophthalmol Vis Sci 1991; 32:2568-78.

104. Ohta K, Norose K, Wang X, et al. Abnormal native and memory T-lymphocyte subsets in the peripheral blood of patients with uveitis. Curr Eye Res 1997; 16:650-5.

105. Mochizuki M, Lwase K, Numaga J, et al. Behcet's disease in Japan. In: Belfort RJ, Petrilli AM, Nussenblatt RB (Eds): Proceedings of the First World Uveitis Symposium. Sao Paulo: Roca, 1988: p401.

106. Lightman S, Chan CC. Immunopathology of ocular inflammatory disorders. Lightman S. (ed.) Immunology of eye diseases. London: Kluwer Academic, 1988; pp 87-99.

107. Rao NA. Role of Oxygen free radical in retinal damage associated with experimental uveitis. Trans Am Ophthalmol Soc 1990; 88: 797-850.

108. Planck SR, Dang TT, Ansel JC, et al. Expression of granulocyte macrophage colony stimulating factor (GM-CSF) and interleukin-1 by retinal pigment epithelial (RPE) cells. Invest Ophthalmol Vis Sci 1991; 32 (Suppl). 1056.

109. Planck SR, Dang TT, Graves D, et al. Retinal pigment epithelial cells secret interleukin-6 in response to interleukin-1 Invest Ophthalmol Vis Sci 1992; 33:78-82.

110. Forrester JV, Liversidge J, Dua HS. Regulation of the local immune response by retinal cells. Curr Eye Res 1990; 9(Suppl):193-9.

111. Rao NA, Wu GS. Free radical mediated photoreceptor damage in uveitis. Prog Ret Eye Res 2000; 19:41-68.

112. Wu GS, Zhang J, Rao NA. Peroxynitrite and oxidative damage in experimental autoimmune uveitis. Invest Ophthalmol Vis Sci 1997; 38:1333-9.

113. Goto H, Wu, GS, Gritz DC, et al. Chemotactic activity of the peroxidized retinal membrane lipid in experimental autoimmune uveitis. Curr Eye Res 1991; 10:1009-14.

114. Rao NA, Romero JL, Fernandez MAS, et al. Role of free radicals in uveitis. Surv Ophthalmol 1987; 32:209-13.

115. Wu GS, Sevanian A, Rao NA. Detection of retinal lipid hydroperoxides in experimental uveitis. Free Rad Biol Med 1992; 12:19-27.

116. Zhang J, Wu GS, Rao NA. Role of nitric oxide (NO) in experimental autoimmune uveitis (EAU). ARVO Abstract Invest Ophthalmol Vis Sci 1993:34.

117. Hoey A, Grabowski PS, Ralston SH, et al. Nitric oxide accelerates the onset and increase the severity of experimental autoimmune uveoretinitis through an IFN-y dependent mechanism. J Immunol 1997; 159:5132-42.

118. Jacquemin E, De Kozak Y, Thillaye B, et al. Expression on inducible nitric oxide synthase in the eye from endotoxin-induced uveitis rats. Invest. Ophthalmology Vis Sci 1996; 37:1187-96.

119. Goto H, Wu GS, Chen F, et al. Lipid peroxidation in experimental uveitis sequential studies. Curr Eye Res 1992; 11: 489-99.

120. Marak, GE Jr., Rao NA, Scott JM, et al. Antioxidant modulation of phacoanaphylactic endopthalmitis. Ophthalmic Res 1985; 17:297-301.

121. Rao NA, Calandra AJ, Sevanian A, et al. Modulation of lens induced uveitis by superoxide dismutase. Ophthalmic Res 1986; 18:41-6.

122. Rao NA, Fernandez MA, Sevanian A, et al. Antiphologistic effect of catalase on experimental phacoanaphylactic endophthalmitis. Ophthalmic Res 1986; 18:185-91.

123. Rao NA, Romero JL, Fernandez MA, et al. Effect of iron chelation on severity of ocular inflammation in an animal model. Arch Ophthalmol 1986; 104:1369-71.

124. Rao NA, Bowe BE, Sevanian A, et al. Modulation of lens-induced uveitis by dimethyl sulfoxide. Ophthalmic Res 1986; 18:193-8.

125. Rao NA, Thaete MD, Delmage JM, Sevanian A. Superoxide dismutase in ocular structures. Invest Ophthalmol Vis Sci 1985; 26:1778-81.